Cooney's EMS Medicine

Cooney's EMS Medicine

Editor

Derek R. Cooney, M.D., FF/NREMT-P, FACEP
Associate Professor of Emergency Medicine
Program Director, EMS Medicine Fellowship
State University of New York Upstate Medical University
Syracuse, New York

Assistant Editor

John W. Lyng, M.D., NREMT-P, FACEP
Medical Director, Office of the Medical Directors
North Memorial Ambulance & Air Care
North Memorial Medical Center
Minneapolis, Minnesota

Art Advisor

Jeremy Joslin, M.D., FAWM, FACEP
Assistant Professor of Emergency Medicine
Program Director, Wilderness and Expedition Medicine Fellowship
State University of New York, Upstate Medical University
Syracuse, New York

Mc
Graw
Hill
Education

New York   Chicago   San Francisco   Athens   London   Madrid   Mexico City
New Delhi   San Juan   Singapore   Sydney   Toronto

Cooney's EMS Medicine

1 2 3 4 5 6 7 8 9 0   CTP/CTP   19 18 17 16 15

ISBN 978-0-07-177564-9
MHID 0-07-177564-1

This book was set in Minion Pro 9/10.5 by MPS Limited.
The editors were Brian Belval and Regina Brown.
The production supervisor was Catherine Saggese.
Project management was provided by Asheesh Ratra, MPS Limited.
Cover photo courtesy of Upstate Medical University
China Translation & Printing Services, Ltd. was printer and binder.

Library of Congress Cataloging-in-Publication Data

EMS medicine / [edited by] Derek Cooney.—First edition.
    p. ; cm.
Emergency medical services medicine
Includes bibliographical references and index.
ISBN 978-0-07-177564-9 (hardcover : alk. paper)—ISBN 0-07-177564-1 (hardcover : alk. paper)
I. Cooney, Derek, editor.   II. Title: Emergency medical services medicine.
[DNLM: 1. Emergency Medical Services—methods.   2. Emergencies.   3. Emergency Responders—education.   WX 215]
RA975.5.E5
362.18—dc23
                                                                                                    2015030069

To the dedicated and courageous men and women who answer the call for help from their fellow man, and to the physicians who have dedicated their careers, and their lives, to guiding and supporting them in their mission.

To my wife, Norma, whose love and intellectual support has made this project possible.

In memoriam:
Donald Robert Cooney, MD
February 7, 1943-June 21, 2008
Celebrated professor, dutiful physician, learned scholar, loyal mentor, healer of sick and injured children, and beloved father. His absence from the world leaves a great sense of loss which is only outweighed by the grand legacy of his good acts and inspiring teaching.

Contents

Contributors

Roy Ary, MD, FACEP
Assistant Clinical Professor
Section of Emergency Medicine
Department of Internal Medicine
Louisiana State University Health Sciences Center
New Orleans, Louisiana

Jean B. Bail Ed.D, RN, MSN, CEN, EMT-P
Program Director
Disaster Medicine and Management Program
Philadelphia University
Philadelphia, Pennsylvania

Edward A. Bartkus, EMT-P, MD, FACEP
EMS Medical Director
Indiana University Health Methodist Hospital
Indianapolis, Indiana

Charles I. Beaudette, MD, MS
Department of Emergency Medicine
SUNY Upstate Medical University
Syracuse, New York

Oliver M. Berrett, MD
Emergency Medicine/EMS Physician
Einstein Medical Center
Philadelphia, Pennsylvania

Anthony J. Billittier IV, MD, FACEP
Clinical Associate Professor of Emergency Medicine
State University of New York at Buffalo, School of Medicine and
    Biomedical Sciences
Assistant Professor
Department of Social and Preventive Medicine
State University of New York at Buffalo, School of Public Health and
    Health Professions
Chief Medical Officer
Millennium Collaborative Care
Performing Provider System
New York State Delivery System Reform Incentive Payment (DSRIP)
    Program
Buffalo, New York

Tanner S. Boyd, MD
Attending Physician of Emergency Medicine
Williamson Medical Center
Franklin, Tennessee

Adin J. Bradley
Division General Manager
Rural/Metro Medical Services of Western NY
Buffalo, New York

Darren Braude, MD, MPH, FACEP, EMT-P
Associate Professor of Emergency Medicine and Anesthesia
University of New Mexico School of Medicine
Albuquerque, New Mexico

Clifford J. Buckley II, MD, MBA
Assistant Professor
Department of Emergency Medicine
Scott & White Healthcare
Temple, Texas

Donna Burns, BSN, EMT
Prehospital Coordinator
University of Virginia
Charlottesville, Virginia

Ella K. Cameron MD, MPH, MSc
Staff Physician- Pediatric Emergency Department
Mary Bridge Children's Hospital
Tacoma, Washington

Richard M. Cantor, MD, FAAP/FACEP
Professor of Emergency Medicine and Pediatrics
Upstate Medical University
Syracuse, New york

Hugh H. Chapin, MD, MS
Project Manager
Mount Sinai Health System
New York, New York

Brian Clemency, DO, MBA, FACEP
Assistant Clinical Professor & EMS Medical Director
Department of Emergency Medicine
University at Buffalo
Buffalo, New York

Craig Cooley, MD, MPH, EMT-P, FACEP
EMS Fellowship Program Director
    Assistant Clinical Professor
Department of Emergency Medicine
University of Texas School of Medicine
Associate EMS Medical Director
San Antonio Fire Department
San Antonio, Texas

Norma L. Cooney, MD, FACEP
Assistant Professor of Emergency Medicine
Emergency Department
Upstate University Hospital
Syracuse, New York

Jimmy L. Cooper, MD
Major, Medical Corps, US Army
Chief, Clinical Operations
Department of Combat Medic Training
Army Medical Department Centre and School
Fort Sam Houston, Texas

Jeremy T. Cushman, MD, MS, EMT-P, FACEP

Assistant Professor of Emergency Medicine
Division of Prehospital Medicine and Department of Emergency
   Medicine
University of Rochester School of Medicine and Dentistry
Monroe-Livingston Regional EMS Medical Director
City of Rochester and County of Monroe, New York

Peter J. Cuenca, MD

Major (Promotable), Medical Corps, US Army
Chief, Academics
Department of Combat Medic Training
Army Medical Department Centre and School
Fort Sam Houston, Texas

Garreth C. Debiegun, MD

Staff Physician
Maine Medical Center
Department of Emergency Medicine
Portland, Maine

Theodore R. Delbridge, MD, MPH

Department of Emergency Medicine
East Carolina University
Greenville, North Carolina

Gerard DeMers, DO, DHSc, MPH

Naval Medical Center San Diego
Department of Emergency Medicine
San Diego, California

Robert Donnarumma, MD

Attending Emergency Physician
Saratoga Hospital
Saratoga Springs, New York

Rebecca Dreher, MD

Attending Physician, Emergency Department
Mercy Hospital
Portland, Maine

Jerome Emmons, MD, AEMT-P

Medical Director
Oswego Hospital Emergency Department
Oswego County Ambulance Service
Greater Baldwinsville Ambulance Corps
Donald McFee Memorial Ambulance
Baldwinsville, New York

Tracy Fricano Chalmers, MS

Program Manager, Public Health Emergency Preparedness
Erie County Department of Health
Buffalo, New York

Christopher J. Fullagar, MD, EMT-P, FACEP

Department of Emergency Medicine
SUNY Upstate Medical University
Syracuse, New York

Molly A. Furin, MD, MS

Fellowship Co-Director - EMS
Attending Physician, Department of Emergency Medicine, Einstein
   Medical Center Philadelphia & Elkins Park
Albert Einstein Medical Center
Philadelphia, Pennsylvania

Deb Funk, MD, FACEP

Medical Director
Albany MedFlight
Albany, New York

Jeffrey M. Goodloe, MD, NREMT-P, FACEP

Professor and Director of the EMS Division
Department of Emergency Medicine
The University of Oklahoma School of Community Medicine
Tulsa, Oklahoma

Dario Gonzalez, MD, FACEP

Assistant Professor, Emergency Medicine
Albert Einstein College of Medicine
Medical Director, NYC FDNY EMS
Medical Director, NYC Office of Emergency Management
New York

Prasanthi Govindarajan, MBBS, MAS

Associate Professor of Surgery
Division of Emergency Medicine
Stanford University Medical Center
Stanford, California

Robert D. Greenberg, MD, FACEP

Regional Medical Director of Emergency Services
Director, Division of Prehospital Medicine
Department of Emergency Medicine
Baylor Scott & White Health Central Texas Division
Associate Professor, Texas A & M Health Science Center College of
   Medicine
Temple, Texas

Sean Hardy, MD

Assistant Professor
Louisiana State University Health Sciences Center
Department of Internal Medicine, EMS Section
New Orleans, Louisiana

Andrew J. Harrell, IV, MD

Emergency Medicine
University Of New Mexico Hospital
Albuquerque, New Mexico

Lori L. Harrington, MD, MPH

Assistant Professor
Department of Emergency Medicine
Boston University School of Medicine
Boston, Massachusetts

Jesse L. Hatfield, MD, MS

Department of Emergency Medicine
University of Oklahoma School of Community Medicine
OU Schusterman Center
Tulsa, Oklahoma

Teresita M. Hogan, MD, FACEP
Director Geriatric Emergency Medicine
University of Chicago
Chicago, Illinois

William Hughes, MD, FACS
University of Massachusetts Medical School
Department of Emergency Medicine
Worcester, Massachusetts

Doug Isaacs, MD
Medical Director FDNY EMS
FDNY- EMS Fellowship Director
Assistant Professor of Emergency Medicine
Albert Einstein College of Medicine
New York

Rebecca Janes, NREMT-P
Assistant Professor
University of Maryland, School of Medicine
Department of Emergency Medicine
Baltimore, Maryland

Jeffrey L. Jarvis, MD, MS, EMT-P, FACEP
EMS Medical Director
Williamson County EMS
Georgetown, Texas
Emergency Medicine Physician
Baylor Scott & White Healthcare
Temple, Texas

Jeremy Joslin, MD
Assistant Professor of Emergency Medicine
Program Director, Wilderness and Expedition Medicine Fellowship
State University of New York
Upstate Medical University
Syracuse, New York

Bradley Kaufman, MD, MPH, FACEP
Assistant Professor, Emergency Medicine
Albert Einstein College of Medicine
Medical Director, NYC FDNY EMS
Medical Director, NYC Office of Emergency Management
New York

Marie King, MD, PhD
University of Massachusetts Medical School
Department of Emergency Medicine
Worcester, Massachusetts

Anne Klimke, MD, MS, EMT-HP
Attending Physician
Department of Emergency Medicine
Einstein Medical Center
Philadelphia, Pennsylvania

Christian C. Knutsen, MD, MPH, FACEP
Assistant Professor
SUNY Upstate Medical University
Department of Emergency Medicine
Syracuse, New York

Melissa Kohn, MD, MS, FACEP
Emergency Medicine/EMS Physician
Einstein Medical Center
Philadelphia, Pennsylvania

Michael Kowalski, DO
Attending Physician
Department of Emergency Medicine
Einstein Medical Center
Philadelphia, Pennsylvania

Ricky C. Kue, MD, MPH, EMT-T, FACEP
Assistant Professor of Emergency Medicine
Boston University School of Medicine
Associate Medical Director
Boston EMS, Police and Fire Departments
Boston, Massachusetts

Pam Lai, MD
Instructor
Medicine
Columbia University College of Physicians and Surgeons
New York City, New York

David M. Landsberg, MD, FACP, FCCP
Chief of Medicine Crouse Hospital
Associate Professor of Medicine
Clinical Associate Professor, Emergency Medicine, Upstate Medical
    University
Syracuse, New York

Jeff Larson
Paramedic
Vehicle Operations Safety/Education Coordinator
North Memorial Ambulance Service
Brooklyn Center, Minnesota

Debra Lee, MD, FACEP
Assistant Professor
University of Maryland, School of Medicine
Department of Emergency Medicine
Baltimore, Maryland

Tracy Leigh LeGros, MD, PhD, UHM, FACEP, FAAEM
Fellowship Program Director
Undersea and Hyperbaric Medicine
Associate Professor
Department Of Medicine (Emergency Medicine Section)
Assistant Professor
Department Of Surgery, Tulane Medical Center
Medical Director
Nunez Community Paramedic College
Attending Hyperbaric Medicine Physician
West Jefferson Medical Center
New Orleans, Louisiana

Erryn Leinbaugh, MD
University of Massachusetts Medical School
Department of Emergency Medicine
Worcester, Massachusetts

Ryan Lewis, MD, FACEP

TEMS Physician, LEMT-P (ret)
Lubbock, Texas

Joshua J. Lynch, DO

Vice President - Medical Operations
Medical Director, & Flight Physician
Partner & Emergency Physician
FDR Medical Services
Emergency Physician/Medical Director of Stroke Services
United Memorial Medical Center
New York

John W. Lyng, MD, NREMT-P, FACEP

Medical Director, Office of the Medical Directors
North Memorial Ambulance & Air Care
North Memorial Medical Center
Minneapolis, Minnesota

Russell D. MacDonald, MD, MPH, FCFP, FRCPC

Medical Director, Ornge Transport Medicine
Mississauga, Ontario, Canada
Associate Professor and Co-Director, Fellowship Programs
Division of Emergency Medicine, Faculty of Medicine
University of Toronto
Toronto, Ontario, Canada

Darryl J. Macias, MD

Professor, Department of Emergency Medicine
Medical Director, Wilderness Medicine & International Health
Assistant Chief of Clinical Operations
University of New Mexico
Albuquerque, New Mexico

James Mangano, DO

Assistant Professor of Emergency Medicine
State University of New York
Upstate Medical University
Syracuse, New York

Stephen McConnell, MD

Emergency Physician
Scott & White Healthcare
Waco, Texas

Kevin R. McGee, DO

Assistant Clinical Professor of Emergency Medicine
School of Medicine and Biomedical Sciences
University at Buffalo
Buffalo, New York

Joshua M. Mularella, DO

Emergency Medicine Physician
Cambridge Health Alliance
Cambridge, Massachusetts

Kevin G. Munjal, MD, MPH

Assistant Professor, Emergency Medicine
Assistant Professor, Health Evidence & Policy
Associate Medical Director of Prehospital Care
Icahn School of Medicine at Mount Sinai
New York, New York

Marc-David Munk, MD

VP Accountable Care
Iora Health
Cambridge, Massachusetts

Jared Novack, MD

Clinical Assistant Professor
NorthShore University Health System
Chicago, Illinois

Shannon D. O'Keefe, MD

Clinical Instructor of Emergency Medicine
University of Washington
Seattle, Washington

Steven J. Parrillo, DO, FACOEP-D, FACEP

Division Director, EMS and Disaster Medicine
Einstein Healthcare Network
Medical Director, Disaster Medicine and Management Master's
    Program
Philadelphia University
Philadelphia, Pennsylvania

Douglas Patton, MD, MSEd

Emergency Professional Services, Inc
Phoenix, Arizona

Debra G. Perina, MD

Division Director, Prehospital care
University of Virginia
Charlottesville, Virginia

Bradley M. Pinsky, JD, MHA

Attorney and Owner
Pinsky Law Group, PLLC
Syracuse, New York

Andrew R. Poreda, MD

Department of Emergency Medicine
SUNY Upstate
Syracuse, New York

Mark Quale, MD

University of Massachusetts Medical School
Department of Emergency Medicine
Worcester, Massachusetts

Taylor Ratcliff, M.D. FF/EMT-LP

Assistant Professor of Emergency Medicine
Texas A&M Health Science Center College of Medicine
Emergency Physician
Scott & White Healthcare
Temple, Texas

Michael A. Redlener, MD

Medical Director for Prehospital Care/Emergency Department
    Physician
St. Luke's Roosevelt Hospital Center
New York City, New York

Susan M. Schreffler, MD, EMT-P
Medical Director
Durham County Emergency Medical Services
Medical Director of Prehospital Medicine and Emergency Physician
Duke University Hospital
Durham, North Carolina

Naveen B. Seth, MD, MBA
Emergency Physician
Department of Emergency Medicine
Crouse Hospital
Syracuse, New York

Deepali Sharma, MD
Emergency Medicine
Upstate Emergency Medicine
Syracuse, New York

J. Matthew Sholl, MD, FACEP
Director, Emergency Medical Services
Maine Medical Center
Portland, Maine

Karl A. Sporer, MD, FACEP, FACP
EMS Medical Director
Alameda County EMS Agency
San Leandro, California

Danniel J. Stites, MD
Physician
John C Lincoln Deer Valley Hospital
Phoenix, Arizona

Margaret Strecker-McGraw, MD, FACEP
Assistant Professor of Emergency Medicine
Texas A&M Health Science Center College of Medicine
Emergency Physician
Scott & White Healthcare
Temple, Texas

David K. Tan, MD, FAAEM, EMT-T
Washington University School of Medicine
Division of Emergency Medicine, EMS Section
St. Louis, Missouri

Joseph Tennyson, MD, FACEP
Assistant Professor, Emergency Medicine
University of Massachusetts Medical School
Department of Emergency Medicine
Worcester, Massachusetts

Stephen H. Thomas, MD MPH
Department of Emergency Medicine
University of Oklahoma School of Community Medicine
OU Schusterman Center
Tulsa, Oklahoma

David P. Thomson, MS, MD, MPA, FACEP, CMTE
Clinical Professor of Emergency Medicine
Medical Director, EastCare
East Carolina University
Greenville, North Carolina

Peter Tilney, DO, EMT-P
Emergency Physician
Albany Medical Center
Albany, New York

Gary M. Vilke, MD
University of California, San Diego School of Medicine
Department of Emergency Medicine
San Diego, California

Noel Wagner, MD, NREMT
Synergy Medical Education Alliance
Department of Emergency Medicine/Division of EMS
Saginaw, Michigan

Harry Wallus, DO, MPH
EMS Medical Director
Portsmouth Regional Hospital
Medical Director
Seacoast Emergency Response Team
Portsmouth, New Hampshire

Alvin Wang, DO, FAAEM
Division of Emergency Medical Services
Department of Emergency Medicine
Temple University School of Medicine
Philadelphia, Pennsylvania

Stacy N. Weisberg, MD, MPH, FACEP
Associate Professor, Emergency Medicine
University of Massachusetts Medical School
Department of Emergency Medicine
Worcester, Massachusetts

Abigail R. Williams, RN, JD, MPH, MS
Lead Trial Counsel
Abigail Williams & Associates, LLC
Worcester, Massachusetts

Kenneth A. Williams, MD, FACEP
Director, Division of EMS & EMS Fellowship
Medical Director, LifePACT Critical Care Transport Associate
    Professor of Emergency Medicine
Rhode Island Hospital
The Alpert Medical School of Brown University
Providence, Rhode Island

Michael P. Wilson, MD, PhD
University of California, San Diego School of Medicine
Department of Emergency Medicine
San Diego, California

Gerald Wydro, MD, FAAEM
Division of Emergency Medical Services
Department of Emergency Medicine
Temple University School of Medicine
Philadelphia, Pennsylvania

Ernest Yeh, MD, FAAEM
Division of Emergency Medical Services
Department of Emergency Medicine
Temple University School of Medicine
Philadelphia, Pennsylvania

Andrew Young, MD
Physician
Emergency Medicine
Emergency Services Northwest
UW Medicine
Northwest Hospital and Medical Center
Seattle, Washington

Preface

The practice of EMS Medicine continues to evolve, bringing greater expectations of the physicians who provide field care and medical oversight. Physicians are integral components in the medical direction of ambulance agencies, fire departments, rescue squads, law enforcement organizations, and emergency management agencies. Physician field response is becoming a more regular component of modern EMS systems and EMS physicians are becoming more defined in their scope of practice. The breadth of knowledge and skills required to serve as a competent EMS physician is unique and rapidly expanding. The advent of board-certification, start of ACGME-accreditation of fellowship programs, and the continuous broadening of the clinical practice of EMS Medicine has made the formal study of the art and practice even more essential than ever before.

There have been many milestones along the road of the development of the specialty. In 1966 when the white paper entitled *Accidental Death and Disability: The Neglected Disease of Modern Society* was released there was little attention paid to the practice of emergency care in the prehospital arena or even within the hospital setting. Dr Zoll had performed the first successful defibrillation and Drs Elam and Safar had introduced cardiopulmonary resuscitation (CPR) almost a decade earlier and yet EMS had not yet even begun its "Renaissance." Even after the passage of the *Highway Safety Act* in 1966 and the *EMS Systems Act* in 1973 the medical component of EMS systems was slow to develop. EMS physicians of today have many of their predecessors to thank for the development of the modern EMS system. Pioneers like Drs Frank Pantridge, Leonard Cobb, Eugene Nagal, William Grace, and J. Michael Criley laid the foundation. Organizations like the National Associate of EMS Physicians (NAEMSP), Society for Academic Emergency Medicine (SAEM), American College of Emergency Physicians (ACEP), American College of Surgeons (ACS), and the National Association of Emergency Medical Technicians (NAEMT) pushed for the development of the science, education, and medical practices that formed the basis for our understanding of EMS Medicine well into the 1990s. In the early 1990s, EMS physicians made their first attempt at gaining official recognition as a subspecialty. Meeting fierce opposition, and lacking clear evidence of their unique area of practice, the movement suffered a significant defeat in 1995 with the disbanding of the American Board of Emergency Medicine's (ABEM) task force.

As we moved forward out of the 20th century, the practice of evidence-based medicine and the advancement of prehospital clinical research began to strip away the dogma of the past and gave rise to the early beginnings of the "Renaissance" of EMS Medicine. In 2003, the Institute of Medicine again exposed some glaring inadequacies of our EMS systems and at the same time made a very clear statement about the need for EMS Medicine physician specialists stating: "*Delivery of clinical care in the field is quite different from delivering care in the hospital or other medical facility, and the oversight of EMS is complex.*" Armed with enhanced data and medical literature, along with new-found recognition and political support, EMS physicians were able to successfully petition the American Board of Medical Specialties (ABMS) and in September 2010 ABMS unanimously voted in favor of creating the subspecialty.

EMS Medicine has taken its place in the House of Medicine. Now it is our duty to ensure we show our worth and never-ending commitment to improving patient care across the entire scope of our practice as EMS physicians. Now is the time of our "Renaissance" and it is our most sincere hope that this text serves you well on your journey, wherever the practice of EMS Medicine may take you.

On behalf of the authors of this textbook,

Derek R. Cooney, MD, FF/NREMT-P, FACEP (Editor)

PART I

Medical Oversight, Research and Quality Improvement

EMS Medicine as a Subspecialty

Theodore R. Delbridge

INTRODUCTION

This book is dedicated to the premise that emergency medical services (EMS) represent a bona fide field of physician subspecialty, that certain knowledge and skills are required, and that there is broad interest in learning about these matters. This chapter describes the subspecialty and begins the process of providing clarity to the roles of an EMS physician and the practice of EMS.

OBJECTIVES

- Define the scope of EMS medicine.
- Contrast EMS medicine to the practice of emergency medicine.
- Define EMS physician.
- Describe the necessary skill sets of an EMS physician.

THE BASIS FOR A SUBSPECIALTY

Indeed, since the earliest developments of EMS there have been physicians who applied their expertise to the nuances of providing care to the ill and injured in the field. They came from diverse clinical backgrounds, but they shared perspectives that optimal care provided as soon as a life-threatening condition could be recognized provided opportunities for improved outcomes. Though they may not have thought of themselves as such, they were the pioneer EMS subspecialists.

The next chapter will provide a historical overview of EMS. Among the various milestones of EMS development, there was generally a physician using his clinical knowledge, understanding of pathophysiology, and patients' needs to prompt innovation and advances of all sorts. Some might be considered logistical, such as when Jean Dominique Larry, Napoleon's chief military physician, built "ambulance volantes" to evacuate wounded soldiers from the battlefield.[1] Others might be considered clinical advances, such as the development of cardiopulmonary resuscitation (CPR) or Dr Frank Pantrindge's delivery of life-saving defibrillatory shocks to patients not yet at a hospital.[2,3] Still, others advanced the concept of medical oversight, as were the lessons of Drs Cobb and Copass in Seattle. Collectively, these examples help reveal the breadth of knowledge and skill required among EMS subspecialists.

Nevertheless, for some time there was a considerable struggle to define the nature of the EMS subspecialty and designate it as such. Among the challenges was the necessary distillation of a multifaceted and blended discipline to reveal and capture its clinical essence, upon which various administrative and health care management roles may be layered. That culminated on September 23, 2010, when the American Board of Medical Specialties (ABMS) officially recognized EMS as a physician subspecialty as requested by the American Board of Emergency Medicine (ABEM).

The journey to that point is revealing, and in some respects is not unlike the path to recognition of emergency medicine as a specialty with its own unique fund of knowledge and purview.

The often-cited 1966 paper *Accidental Death and Disability: The Neglected Disease of Modern Society* pointed out a number of shortcomings in the American health care system related to trauma and emergency care.[4] John M Howard, MD, was an army surgeon during the Korean Conflict and one of the paper's authors. He has recalled that the impetus for the study and a report of its findings was the observation by him and similar physicians that the lessons learned in Korea had not translated to home in the United States.[5] The American health care system remained woefully ill prepared to deal with what was described as an injury epidemic.[4] At the time, although new patterns of staffing hospital emergency departments were evolving, many hospitals required all medical personnel, regardless of specialty, to share emergency department responsibility. The 1966 paper proclaimed that no longer can emergency department responsibility be assigned to the least experienced member of the medical staff or solely to specialists who, by the nature of their training and experience, cannot provide adequate care without the support of other staff members.[4] Indeed, emergency department care represented early intervention in the continuum of care required by seriously ill or injured people. It demanded special expertise and both breadth and depth of clinical skills and knowledge. Subsequently, the Emergency Medical Services Act of 1971, among other things, made "seed money" available to help develop new emergency medicine residency programs.[6] Emergency medicine became recognized as a primary board by ABMS in 1979.

Part of the rationale for emergency medicine to be a distinct specialty rested in its interface with EMS systems and personnel. While care in an emergency department was undoubtedly early in the continuum, care in the field was earlier and it required active oversight by physicians with attentive interest and appropriate insights. At the time, EMS often represented the notion of taking the emergency department to the patient. Thus, by natural extension emergency physicians became the most active physician participants within EMS systems, offering a distinction from the rest of medicine.

EMS, as we know, has evolved. The need for specific expertise has intensified. It is no longer acceptable to uniformly bring the emergency department to every patient. Whether or not a specific intervention or pharmaceutical agent ought to be translated from the emergency department to out-of-hospital scenes requires careful analyses of risks and benefits and cost-effectiveness in the context of local circumstances. Decisions regarding use of thrombolytics, neuromuscular blocking agents, and even steroids are all examples. These sorts of analyses are done on a patient-by-patient basis numerous times a day by physicians of all genres. However, the knowledge and perspectives required by these specific questions and those like them have demanded special expertise and understanding the needs of EMS patients and the intricacies of often complex EMS care delivery systems.

As defined by the Institute of Medicine of the National Academies, EMS comprises the crucial early phases of the continuum of emergency medical care for acutely ill and injured persons. It encompasses prehospital and out-of-hospital emergency care, including 9-1-1 access and dispatch, field triage and initial stabilization, and treatment and transport in specially equipped ambulances or helicopters to hospitals or between medical facilities.[7]

EMS PHYSICIANS

EMS physicians provide emergency medical care for patients in out-of-hospital settings and medical oversight of EMS systems. According to ABEM, the unique clinical elements that characterize EMS medical practice stem from its position early in the continuum of patient care, its physical location outside of fixed medical facilities, and the relatively higher acuity of its patient population compared to emergency medicine. The treatments developed by EMS physicians, and either delivered or overseen by them, affect patients' ultimate outcomes as patient safety and proper treatment are ensured.[8] It is the EMS physician who brings medical decision making to the patient's side at the site of accident or injury, ensuring appropriate care until arrival at a hospital or other advancement further in the continuum of care. According to ABEM, the purpose of subspecialty certification in EMS is to standardize physician training and qualifications for EMS practice, to improve patient safety and enhance the quality of emergency medical care provided to patients in the prehospital environment, and to facilitate integration of prehospital patient treatment into the continuum of patient care.[8]

In 2011, ABEM published *The Core Content of EMS Medicine*. It incorporates four principal topic categories (**Table 1-1**) that include more than 400 total elements.[9] Each element relates to one or more core competencies as described by the Accreditation Council for Graduate Medical Education and ABMS, including patient care, medical knowledge, practice-based learning, professionalism, interpersonal skills, and system-based practice.[10]

In developing the core content, the ABEM EMS Examination Task Force surveyed clinically active EMS physicians to determine the frequency and importance of each element. The core content subsequently represents what those physicians perceive as relevant to their professional practice.[10] Thus, it provides an excellent overview of the nature of knowledge and skills required of an EMS physician.

Another practical way of evaluating EMS physician skill sets is by considering them as related to clinical, medical oversight, or administrative issues. While there is typically substantial overlap among them, it can be helpful to think about them this way.

TABLE 1-1   The Core Content of EMS Medicine Major Topics[9]

1.0 Clinical Aspects of EMS Medicine
   1.1 Time/life critical conditions
   1.2 Injury
   1.3 Medical emergencies
   1.4 Special clinical considerations
2.0 Medical Oversight of EMS
   2.1 Medical oversight
   2.2 EMS systems
   2.3 EMS personnel
   2.4 System management
3.0 Quality Management and Research
   3.1 Quality improvement principles and programs
   3.2 Research
4.0 Special Operations
   4.1 Mass casualty management
   4.2 Chemical/biological/radiological/nuclear/explosive (CBRNE)
   4.3 Mass gathering
   4.4 Disaster management
   4.5 EMS special operations

Adapted from American Board of Emergency Medicine. The core content of emergency medical services medicine. East Lansing, MI 2011. https://www.abem.org/public/subspecialty-certification/emergency-medical-services/the-core-content-of-ems-medicine.

CLINICAL SKILLS

Among clinical knowledge and skills, there are several features of practice that distinguish EMS medicine from the general practice of emergency medicine or any other specialty for that matter. As already noted, the focus is at the earliest points in a patient's continuum of care after recognition of acute illness or injury. Thus, the culprit illness or injury is the least differentiated and earlier in its dynamic process of evolution. Further, the tools available to refine the differential are limited to what can be cost-effectively taken to the patient's side no matter where that might be. The environment of care has considerable influence, including such factors as ambient lighting, uncontrollable noise, temperature, and humidity. Each of these may present specific challenges to patient evaluation, treatment, and evacuation. For example, the noise and vibration of an EMS helicopter mandate a greater degree of technology-driven patient monitoring. Auscultation of blood pressure and lung sounds is not possible. Bright ambient light may affect the ability to perform laryngoscopy and adaptive or alternate tactics must be readily available.

In the final analysis, EMS physicians are responsible for understanding the appropriate prehospital or out-of-hospital care for the full spectrum of potential illness and injury among the entire extent of the population in their communities. As noted in the core content, some conditions are undoubtedly time or life critical, such as cardiac arrest, airway compromise, respiratory failure, hypotension, and shock. Others include the broadest range of trauma, respiratory, cardiac, and other medical illnesses; obstetrical and gynecologic emergencies; poisoning and toxicological emergencies with special attention to containment and decontamination; and communicable diseases.

The nature of some patients' illnesses or injuries mandate that EMS physicians are technically competent to perform or facilitate a number of procedures that, depending on local circumstance, may be required to sustain patients to definitive care and improve outcomes. These are outlined in **Table 1-2**.

MEDICAL OVERSIGHT

Medical oversight of EMS systems demands an understanding of applicable state laws, rules, and regulations and, in some cases, local ordinance. While there are several well-accepted tools or approaches, there is anything but a standard method of ensuring appropriate medical oversight for any given system. Instead, it is akin to any other form of management or leadership, where the leader adapts the style he or she is most comfortable with and pulls out the necessary tools when the time or situation is right.

EMS physicians must be skilled at providing direct medical oversight. This occurs via direct communication with EMS providers caring for a particular patient. In some cases, the physician may be present at the scene. The merits of medical director response to the field have been well described.[11] The advantages include contemporaneous direction of EMS personnel, observing the system and its personnel in action at the tip of the spear, so to speak (eg, what works well and not so well), delivering real-time education, and, when appropriate, participating in patient care. Most often, however, direct medical oversight occurs via radio, telephone, or audio/video communication with EMS providers caring for a patient. While this may often be in the purview of general emergency physicians, EMS physicians should provide expertise and guidance regarding both best ways to extract information from EMS providers and to provide the best possible direction. Asking questions or giving orders that are difficult to understand or not applicable to the field situation is not helpful. For example, an inquiry to get precise information might be to ask how many boxes wide a QRS complex is as opposed to asking whether or not a wide-complex rhythm is present or how many milliseconds wide it is. Giving an order to transport a patient who the EMS providers, by their report, are already transporting is redundant or inconsequential and could be construed as out of touch or insulting. Advising EMS providers to solicit law enforcement help to restrain a

TABLE 1-2 EMS Physician Clinical Procedures

Airway Management
- Manual airway-opening techniques
- Bag-valve-mask ventilation
- Glottic airways
- Supraglottic airways
- Direct laryngoscopy
- Use of intubation adjuncts
- Rapid sequence intubation; neuromuscular blockade
- Medically facilitated intubation without paralysis
- Cricothyroidotomy
- Nasal intubation
- Control of airway bleeding including posttonsillectomy hemorrhage

Respiratory Management
- Prehospital continuous positive airway pressure
- Portable ventilator management

Cardiovascular Management
- Peripheral intravenous access
- Central intravenous access
- Intraosseous access
- Pericardiocentesis
- Intra-aortic balloon pump management
- Prehospital administration of thrombolytic agents

Trauma Management
- Needle and tube thoracostomy
- Hemorrhage control
- Controlled hyperventilation
- Selective spinal immobilization
- Application of splints and traction devices
- Limb amputation

Obstetrics Management
- Routine childbirth
- Management of abnormal fetal presentations
- Postpartum hemorrhage control
- Peri/Postmortem cesarean section

Ultrasonography
- Focused assessment with sonography for trauma
- Intravenous access

patient to enable transport is likely to be unhelpful unless there is precedent for such in the community.

Indirect medical oversight is about everything that happens off-line to affect the scope and quality of care provided by the EMS system. EMS physicians must be skilled at developing protocols and patient care procedures, overseeing quality improvement projects and programs, and assessing and improving the competency of the system and its people.

ADMINISTRATIVE SKILLS

The administrative skill set of EMS physicians is necessarily broad. It includes financial management and allocation of resources; working with administrative leaders, public officials, and elected representatives of the community; and human resources management.

Potentially, among the most necessary administrative skills of an EMS physician are those of political survival. Dr Norm Dinerman has described these as five political senses to be mastered over a career.[12] They are:

- *Mission*: knowing his or her mission, that of the specialty, and that of the agency and interfacing institutions
- *Tradition*: understanding the history of the community and service so that goals can be best integrated into the larger context of community and agency
- *Position*: understanding the position of the EMS physician within the agency structure and the agency relative to others in the community
- *Humor*: knowing when and how to bring an element of levity to a situation and not taking oneself too seriously
- *Sense of timing*: taking advantage of appropriate opportunities to advance new ideas, tactics, or strategies.

What differentiates EMS physicians from administrators elsewhere in the health care system is, again, the breadth of their necessary knowledge and influence in diverse environments, serving the most diverse of populations, and interfacing with an incredible array of other professionals and stakeholders. A hospital administrator may have incredible responsibility and authority. However, his or her primary focus is what is happening within or affects the physical plant he or she oversees. For an EMS physician, the realm of responsibility is as amorphous as the community he or she serves, with a constant state of flux, and personal interfaces that are potentially infinite. For a hospital administrator a discussion of safety probably conjures attempts to improve patient safety in the hospital. For an EMS physician, the topic could easily and immediately turn to issues of patient safety as well as personnel safety and the safety of the general public that is encountered as fellow motorists, bystanders, and future potential patients.

SUMMARY

EMS physicians are the clinical champions of the EMS system, possessing perspectives, expertise, and professional passion for prehospital care like no other member of the health care team. History has demonstrated the power of ideas to move certain care to the point soonest after recognition of an acute illness or injury and the value of physicians with clinical expertise, administrative skill, and attentiveness to medical oversight. Chapter 3 will lend further justification to the notion that EMS is a bona fide subspecialty with its own fund of knowledge and skill set focused on the earliest parts of the continuum of care for acute injury and illness as well as community health.

KEY POINTS

- The Core Content of EMS Medicine includes four categories: clinical aspects of EMS medicine, medical oversight of EMS, quality management and research, and special operations.
- Five political senses are needed by a successful EMS physician: mission, tradition, position, humor, and a sense of timing.

REFERENCES

1. Garrison FH. *An Introduction to the History of Medicine*. Philadelphia, PA: WB Saunders; 1929.
2. Kouwenhoven WB, Jude JR, Knickerbocker GB. Closed chest cardiac massage. *JAMA*. 1960;173:1064.
3. Pantridge JF, Geddes JS. A mobile intensive care unit in the management of myocardial infarction. *Lancet*. 1966;1:807.
4. Committee on Trauma and Shock, Division of Medical Sciences, National Academy of Sciences National Research Council. *Accidental Death and Disability: The Neglected Disease of Modern Society*. Washington, DC: National Academies Press; 1966.
5. Howard JM. MD: Personal Communication, May 1998.

6. EMS System Act of 1973, Public Law 93-154, Washington, DC; 1973.

7. Institute of Medicine, Committee on the Future of Emergency Care in the United States Health System, Board of Health Care Services. *Emergency Medical Services at the Crossroads*. Washington, DC: National Academies Press; 2006.

8. American Board of Emergency Medicine. Application for subspecialty certification. East Lansing, MI 2009.

9. American Board of Emergency Medicine. The core content of emergency medical services medicine. East Lansing, MI. 2011. https://www.abem.org/public/subspecialty-certification/emergency-medical-services/the-core-content-of-ems-medicine. Accessed on March 10, 2015.

10. Perina DG, Pons PT, Blackwell TH, et al. The core content of emergency medical services medicine. *Prehosp Emerg Care*. 2012;16:309.

11. Pepe PE, Stewart RD. Role of the physician in the prehospital setting. *Ann Emerg Med*. 1986;15:1480.

12. Dinerman N. Political realities for the medical director. In: Bass RR, Brice JH, Delbridge TR, Gunderson MR, eds. *Medical Oversight of EMS*; Cone DC, O'Connor RE, Fowler RL, eds., *Emergency Medical Services: Clinical Practice and Systems Oversight*. Olathe, KS: National Association of EMS Physicians; 2009:148.

Historical Aspects

Derek R. Cooney

INTRODUCTION

Emergency care of the sick and wounded in the field has deep historical roots as far back as the ancient times when Roman soldiers were carried off the field of battle on their own shields or by chariots and wooden carts. Homer describes medical care being provided in the field by surgeons for those who were too badly injured to be moved. The Brothers of the Benedictine Monastery of Saint Mary Latina began providing care in AD 1080, and later as the Knights Hospitaller[1] of the order of St John began rendering emergency medical care on the battlefield and evacuating the victims to a hospital for continued care. Historical references demonstrate stretcher movements of nonambulatory injured or sick persons in Native American North America, India, Egypt, and Europe throughout early history and into the more modern times.[2] In the 15th century, King Ferdinand and Queen Isabella of Spain established deployable field hospitals called *ambulancia*. George Washington's Continental Army possessed mobile field hospitals with organized systems for retrieving the wounded and delivering them to the field hospital for care. However, Napoleon's surgeon, Dominique-Jean Larrey, is credited with creating one of the first most recognizable EMS systems, centered on his *ambulance volante* (or flying ambulance) that had been inspired by his observation that the injured waited long time periods without care and that the same basic cart design was a proven mode for rapidly moving artillery.

OBJECTIVES

- Discuss key historical points in the evolution of EMS.
- Name key leaders and their contributions.
- Name key organizations and their contributions.
- Discuss the evolution and changing role of the EMS physician.
- Describe historical milestones for EMS physicians.

AMERICAN HISTORY OF EMS

The American Civil War offered more experience with triage, field care, and movement to field hospitals for damage control medicine before movement to a hospital. Due to the success of this concept the US Congress passed "an act to establish a uniform system of ambulances in the United States" (also known as the Ambulance Corps Act) in 1864. During this time American hospitals began to develop their own ambulance services. World War I saw the use of motorized ambulances as a regular part of military operations. Despite the existence of ambulance services, and even rescue squads (like the Roanoke Life Saving Crew, Roanoke, VA, est. 1928), modern EMS in the United States did not take form until the late 1960s and early1970s. This chapter will focus on key events and developments in the evolution of modern EMS in the United States.

THE LATE 1800s

In 1864, President Abraham Lincoln signed into law "an act to establish a uniform system of ambulances in the United States." Around the same time in Europe (1863) the Red Cross of Europe was founded. The 1860s would also see the first hospital-based ambulance services. The first civilian hospital-based ambulance service in the United States was founded at the Commercial Hospital (now Cincinnati General) in Cincinnati, Ohio, in 1865. Four years later, Bellevue Hospital began ambulance service in 1869 under the direction of Dr Dalton. These services provided

transportation of patients to the hospital, however, little care was provided until they arrived. Although paramedics would not exist until the 1970s, the first civilian prehospital care system staffed by nonphysicians (who provided care) began operation in 1872 in England under the direction of a surgeon by the name of Major Peter Shepard. In 1877, this service became St Johns Ambulance Association. Boston City Hospital began operation of its own ambulance service in 1892 and the first automobile ambulance began operation out of Michael Reese Hospital in Chicago in 1899.

THE EARLY 1900s

The 1900s saw the birth of air medical transport with one of the first air medical flights in1910 which took off from Fort Barrancas and unfortunately crashed after takeoff after about 500 yards of travel.[3] In 1917, an injured English soldier was airlifted successfully in Turkey, and in 1918 two American officers successfully demonstrated the use of a modified Curtis JN-4 biplane for air medical evacuation.[3] The US Army Air Corps designed and placed into service three air medical transport planes in 1929. These aircraft were designed to carry two patients and an attendant. Helicopters were placed in use in the Korean War for medical evacuation in 1951 and the value of this concept became apparent in both the military and civilian realms.

On the ground things had also been developing. During World War I (1914-1918), the US Army had assembled a fleet of motorized ambulances and in the civilian world, the first Rescue Squad known to have been formed in the United States was founded in Roanoke, Virginia. The Roanoke Life Saving Crew was formed in 1928. By 1939, the American Red Cross had nearly 5000 units and incorporated mobile aid units and training posts. These were typically manned by trained volunteers and had the ability to call upon local medical assets such as physicians and ambulances. By 1948 around 40,000 citizens were trained in First Aid by the American Red Cross.

In 1952, Dr Paul Zoll performed the first successful external electrical defibrillation at Beth Israel Hospital in Boston. This raised interest in the potential for improved responses to cardiac emergencies. In 1956, Drs Elan and Peter Zafar develop mouth-to-mouth resuscitation which further contributed to the interest in advancing emergency care. In 1959, Johns Hopkins developed the first portable defibrillator on record. These were some of the prerequisite elements needed to drive forward the early concept of prehospital medical care.

THE 1960s

In 1960, Dr Zoll further developed the use of defibrillation when he demonstrated external electrical countershock and showed it could successfully terminate supraventricular tachycardia (SVT) and ventricular tachycardia (VTach). In that same year (1960), Drs Kouwenhoven, Knickerbocker, and Jude published their report on the use of cardiopulmonary resuscitation (CPR). Los Angeles County Fire Department, in an effort to advance care in the prehospital setting, equipped every fire engine, ladder truck, and rescue truck with a resuscitator in 1960, signifying a significant commitment to the idea of prehospital emergency care. The year 1965 marked a dubious epidemiological point in American history when it was found that more people died in automobile accidents (50,000) than in 8 years of armed conflict during the Vietnam War. In response to this fact, and due to growing concern for public safety, President Lyndon Johnson signed into law the National Highway Safety Act of 1965. In an interesting turn of events, just 5 years later (1970) President Johnson was, himself, a patient of a newly formed rescue squad while visiting his son-in-law in Charlottesville, Virginia. The Charlottesville-Albemarle Rescue Squad, under the medical direction of Dr Richard Crampton, was the first volunteer paramedic agency in the county. The now famous white paper on trauma and motor vehicle related deaths entitled "Accidental Death & Disability—The Neglected Disease of Modern Society" was published by the National Research

Council in 1966 and sparked continued interest and political efforts to address the need for improved emergency care in the United States. The following government acts, including the EMS Systems Act of 1973, were intended to create research, funding, and regulatory structure for EMS systems in America and in many ways have helped shape the development of modern EMS since the 1970s.

■ DEVELOPMENT OF ADVANCED PREHOSPITAL CARE

In 1966, Dr Pantridge developed coronary care ambulances and showed improved survival in out-of-hospital cardiac arrest in Belfast, Ireland. He had developed a portable defibrillator and much of his published work focused on the acute management of cardiac injury and arrest (**Figure 2-1**). One paper in 1977 describing the energy needed to successfully defibrillate patients in ventricular fibrillation reported data including shocks delivered by a Pantridge portable defibrillator.

In 1967, the American Ambulance Association published an article that claimed that around 25,000 Americans had been left permanently disabled due to the improper care that they had received from undertrained prehospital providers. That same year the City of Miami (Miami, Florida) Fire Department began training paramedics in what would be the first of such programs in the United States. Dr Eugene Nagal championed the development of prehospital cardiac care advocating for CPR and developing first radio ECG telemetry program with the help of a colleague, Dr Jim Hirschmann. These transmitted ECGs demonstrated the presence of cardiac rhythms in the victims likely responsible for their death, further illustrating the need to bring defibrillation to the prehospital arena.

In 1968, just 2 years after Dr Pantridge introduced a similar concept, Dr Grace of St Vincent's Hospital in New York City launched the United States' first mobile coronary care units. The program was originally designed with ambulances staffed by physicians. The year 1968 also saw three other important events in the development of American EMS. The same year as St Vincent's Hospital launched its new program, the American Telephone & Telegram Company (AT&T) began an initiative to systematically reserve the telephone digits 9-1-1 for planned use as a universal emergency number. At the same time, the state of Virginia

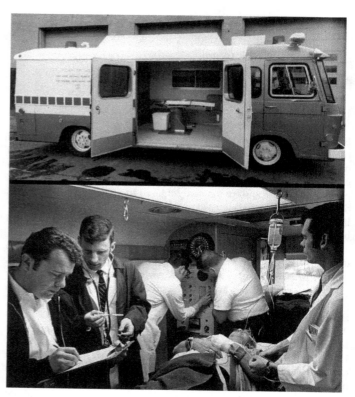

FIGURE 2-2. The Heartmobile. (Reprinted with permission from Central Ohio Fire Museum.)

made an important distinction recognizing ambulances and their unique role by establishing legislation regulating ambulances, required training, and providing permits for their use. And possibly what would prove to be the most significant pro-EMS event of 1968 and one that would help aid in the professional development of prehospital medicine was the establishment of the American College of Emergency Physicians.

In 1969, several other notable events related to the development of prehospital cardiac care were recorded. Dr Leonard Cobb from Harbor View Hospital in Seattle, Washington, formed a relationship with the Seattle Fire Department and together they developed the "Medic 1" program. They utilized firefighters with special training in a converted recreational vehicle that was equipped and dispatched from the hospital in response to calls for cardiac events. In Toronto, Canada, a program known as "Cardiac One" was established to provide advanced cardiac life support measures utilizing a hospital physician and a portable cardiac monitor. That same year, the Ohio State University Medical Center (Columbus, Ohio) placed a unit in service, staffed by three firemen and one physician, designed to respond to prehospital coronary events. The program was dubbed "The Heartmobile" and was later absorbed by the Columbus Division of Fire, then removing the physician from the standard crew (**Figure 2-2**). The Miami Fire Department (Miami, Florida) documented the first successful prehospital cardiac defibrillation in June 1969, resulting in the patient experiencing full recovery with normal neurological outcome at the time of hospital discharge. Notably, the Florida legislature passed 10-D-66 that same year, making the provision of prehospital emergency care legal under the laws of the State of Florida.

PARAMEDICINE IN THE MEDIA

In 1972, the American public began to have some additional exposure to the concept of advanced prehospital care and the relationship with emergency "room" physicians through the popularization of the concept by the television program "Emergency!" featuring two Los Angeles County Fire Department paramedics and their prehospital exploits. The characters of Johnny Gage (Randolph Mantooth) and Roy DeSoto

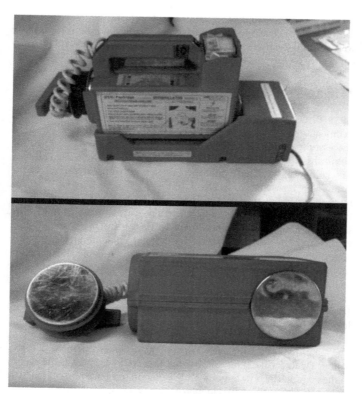

FIGURE 2-1. Pantridge defibrillator. (Reprinted with permission from National EMS Museum.)

(Kevin Tighe), and their now famous Squad 51, graced the screens of American televisions from January 1972 until 1979 with 5 years of regular broadcasts and six 2-hour specials and introduced the "paramedic" to most Americans who had never heard the term. The show introduced some basic concepts surrounding the relatively new concept of paramedicine, including emergency medical dispatching, advanced life support, and on-line medical control as well as introducing some to the concepts of CPR and first aid, that many Americans had never seen much less had received training. At the start of broadcast there were only six paramedic-level units in the country and by the end of production there was one in every state.[4]

AIR MEDICAL SERVICES

The first air medical evacuation in recorded history is that of a Serbian officer that was airlifted by the French Air Service during World War I. The French noted a reduction in battlefield mortality from 60% down to 10% using their fixed wing medical evacuation strategy. In 1917, a British soldier with a gunshot wound on his ankle made the trip to hospital in 45 minutes, when by ground the trip would have taken 3 days. In the 1920s, the French and English continued to experiment with military air medical evacuation. The French documented over 7000 air evacuations.[5] The concept spread and became more widely adopted into the 1930s and World War II saw the first use of helicopters for the purpose, with the evacuation of three wounded British pilots by a US Army Sikorsky in Burma. The US Army continued use of helicopters in the Korean War and the French did as well in the First Indochina War. By the time the United States entered into the Vietnam War, medical corpsmen were incorporated into the air medical evacuation operation. This practice sparked the concept of civilian helicopter air medical programs and is a vital component of the military medical operation to this day.

Although civilian air medical evacuation had existed around the world since the 1920s, the United States did not see civilian air medical service until 1947. J Walter Schaefer started the program as an additional component of the Schaefer Ambulance Service in Los Angeles, California, and was the first FAA-certified air ambulance program. Prior to the point, air medical evacuation was typically based out of wilderness and remote locations and was done out of pure necessity. In the late 1960s, in response to the increasing interest in helicopter-based medical

evacuation born of the military experience, the federal government funded two research programs to access the concept of civilian air medical helicopter programs.[6] *Project CARESOM* was based in Mississippi in three separate communities (**Figure 2-3**). The project was found to be a success; however, only one of the sites chose to continue operation after completion of the project. In doing so, Hattiesburg, Mississippi, became the site of the first civilian medical helicopter program in the country.[5] In 1969, the second demonstration project, based out of Fort Sam Houston in San Antonio, began operation by utilizing military aircraft to augment the civilian EMS system. The *Military Assistance to Safety and Traffic* (MAST) program was deemed a successful project and local governments recognized the value of employing helicopters in their EMS systems based on these results.

Flight for Life Colorado was the first hospital-based air medical helicopter program in the United States, beginning operation in 1972 out of St Anthony Central Hospital in Denver, Colorado. In 1977, the Ontario Ministry of Health began operation of a helicopter service in Toronto with a predominantly paramedic-based staffing and has grown to a service of over 30 aircraft.[5] Air medical programs are now a standard, yet many times debated, component of EMS systems in the United States.

LEGISLATING THE MODERN EMS SYSTEM

In 1960, John F. Kennedy stated that: "Traffic accidents constitute one of the greatest, perhaps the greatest, of the nation's public health problems."[2] This was one of the first public acknowledgments by the government for the need for improved organization, regulation, and funding of EMS from the federal government. In 1965, when Medicare was created by the Congress, funding for EMS as part of the reimbursement model was included. This was a key feature in the development of the system. In 1966, following the final report of the *President's Commission of Highway Safety*, President Lyndon Johnson's administration supported passage of what would become the *National Highway Safety Act* (Public Law 89-564) outlining the standards for the development of the EMS System in each state. Previously created by the *National Traffic and Motor Vehicle Safety Act* (Public Law 89-563), the *National Traffic Safety Agency* was merged with the *National Highway Safety Advisory Committee* (from Public Law 89-564) to form one body that was then moved under the newly formed *Department of Transportation* and was now overseen by Dr William J. Haddon, Jr.

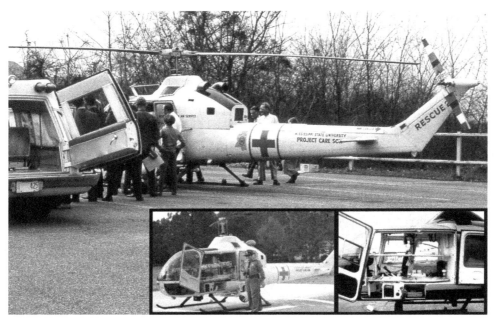

FIGURE 2-3. Mississippi State University CARE-SOM FH1100 helicopter. (Reprinted with permission from FH1100 Manufacturing Corp.)

President Richard Nixon's administration also contributed to the early development when in 1972 the *Department of Health, Education and Welfare's* (DHEW) *EMS Division* was focused on a more health care–oriented approach to the issues. Under the direction of Dr David R. Boyd, the Division of EMS provided funding to more than 300 demonstration projects across the United States.[2] These programs and structure were the result of the *EMS Systems Act of 1973* (Public Law 93-154) and were enacted under President Gerald Ford, who appointed Dr Boyd to his position.

PHYSICIANS IN RECENT EMS HISTORY

Throughout the recent history of EMS there are many important individuals who have contributed greatly to the development of this field. Many of these individuals are not noted here; however, this listing is meant to provide some prospective on the importance of the contributions of individual physicians. These individuals are listed in alphabetical order.

BRYAN BLEDSOE, DO, EMT-P

Dr Bledsoe was born in 1955 and became an EMT in 1974 and a paramedic in 1976. As an EMS physician he has contributed much to the literature and to provider education. He is the principal author of *Paramedic Care: Principles & Practice, Essentials of Paramedic Care, Intermediate Emergency Care: Principles & Practice, Critical Care Paramedic, Anatomy & Physiology for Emergency Care, Prehospital Emergency Pharmacology*, and *Pocket Reference for ALS Providers*. Dr Bledsoe stands out because of his place in modern EMS education, as well as his ability to communicate important EMS medicine concepts to physicians, EMS providers, other health care providers, and to lay people. He is an internationally recognized and cited EMS physician.[7]

DAVID R. BOYD, MD

Dr Boyd began his career as a resident in surgery at Cook County where he and his colleagues sought to improve the management of gunshot wounds and automobile trauma. He became the Illinois State EMS Medical Director and oversaw the development of a comprehensive trauma system that coordinated prehospital and hospital assets from 1970 to 1974. Under his leadership the program realized successful improvements in communication and utilization of more advanced staffing on ground and air ambulances. In 1974, Boyd was appointed to oversee the Department of Health Education and Welfare EMS Division by President Ford. Under his direction a "wall-to-wall" nation-wide EMS system began to take shape. In addition, Dr Boyd successfully advocated for EMS to President Ford, resulting in the White House conferences on EMS and the declaration of EMS Week. He served in the office until 1981 when the position was dissolved in favor of state-administered block grant programs.

NANCY CAROLINE, MD (1944-2002)

Dr Caroline started her career in EMS during her training in critical care medicine under Dr Peter Safar at the University of Pittsburg. Safar had begun work on the Freedom House Ambulance Service and much of the responsibility of organization and training of participants to become paramedics was delegated to Dr Caroline. She excelled at paramedic education and authored a textbook to suite the unique curriculum and scope of practice entitled *Emergency Care in the Streets*. She was a courageous field provider and innovator. In addition to her work in the United States, she had also been a bush doctor in Africa and after leaving in the States in 1976 became one of the most influential individuals in the development of EMS in Israel. She worked with prehospital programs, developed terrorism medical response tactics, and served as the medical director of Magen David Adom. Her textbook for paramedics was the only dedicated educational text on the topic for a decade and is still one of the most well known to this day.[8]

LEONARD COBB, MD

In many ways Seattle is considered one of the epicenters of EMS advancement in the United States. One of the key figures in the development of that reputation is Dr Leonard Cobb. In 1967, Dr Cobb was practicing cardiology in Seattle when he learned of the work of Dr Frank Pantridge at the Royal Victoria Hospital in Belfast, Ireland. In an effort to bring this new prehospital cardiac intensive care concept to Seattle, he worked with colleagues to bring about a paramedic training program based on the fire service that could provide similar advance cardiac care in the field. The resulting program developed by the University of Washington, Harborview Medical Center, and the Seattle Fire Department began serving King County under the name *Medic One*.[9]

DAVID CONE, MD

Physicians practicing (and holding board certification in) EMS medicine have a number of key people to thank for the academic and political development of the subspecialty. One of the key concerns during the development of the subspecialty of EMS medicine was a lack of organized scientific productivity. In addition to his publications in peer-reviewed journals on EMS specific topics he also served to guide others in academic productivity in the field. Some of his notable positions from which he effectively served in this role have been as the editor-in-chief of the NAEMSP textbook, project leader for the development of the NAEMSP proposal that was used to petition the American Board of Emergency Medicine (ABEM) to pursue subspecialty board recognition, and also as the editor-in-chief of Academic Emergency Medicine. Dr Cone has provided significant mentorship to young EMS physicians in training and also served as the president of NAEMSP during a critical time in the development of the subspecialty. Dr Cone was the first chair of the Council of EMS Fellowship Directors.[10]

RICHARD CRAMPTON, MD

Dr Richard Crampton had worked with Dr William Grace who had founded the mobile coronary care unit at St Vincent's Hospital in Manhattan and he had taken the time to visit Dr Pentridge personally in order to better understand program developed there in Belfast, Ireland. He successfully implemented these concepts in Charlottesville, Virginia, and in doing so by 1971 the Charlottesville Rescue Squad was trained and certified in CPR and became the nation's second all-volunteer mobile coronary care unit. They operated in a rural environment. Dr Crampton's program did require a physician to respond in order to utilize the advanced coronary care concept.[11]

J MICHAEL CRILEY, MD

Dr Criley is credited with founding the Los Angeles County Paramedic Program in 1969 at the time he served as the Chief of the Division of Cardiology at Harbor—UCLA medical center. One of his chief accomplishments was convincing medical and public safety stakeholders as well as politicians that a well-designed prehospital coronary care program could be performed by paramedics. Recognizing legislative shortfalls he successfully petitioned state government, including the then governor Ronald Reagan, to approve legislation making it legal for paramedic personnel to provide advanced level coronary care in the prehospital environment.[12]

RALPH FLEICHER, MD

Dr Fletcher, along with Dr Ernie Goodwin, is credited with forming the nation's very first paramedic-level volunteer rescue squad. The Haywood County volunteer rescue squad became a paramedic-level service offering advanced coronary care and the prehospital setting in 1969.[13,14]

RAYMOND FOWLER, MD

In addition to participating in the formation of the National Association of EMS physicians he also served as one of the early presidents of the organization. He has contributed as an author and as an editor for a number of textbooks. He has worked diligently to develop multidisciplinary training programs for providers and educators at all levels in the fields of EMS, disaster medicine, tactical medicine, and emergency medicine.[15,16]

WILLIAM GRACE, MD (-1974)

Dr William Grace is credited with founding the nation's first mobile coronary unit based on the program started in Belfast, Ireland, by Dr Pantridge. The program was based out of St Vincent's Hospital and Medical Center in New York. Dr Grace and his associate Dr John Chadbourn recognized the potential for improve survival if cardiac patients could be reached with advanced care in a more immediate fashion. In 1968, St Vincent's first mobile coronary care unit went into service in a van with a driver and attended, an attending physician, a resident physician, an emergency room nurse, an ECG technician, and a student nurse observer. The vehicle carried a portable battery power to defibrillator/ monitor, electrocardiograph, intravenous kit with drugs, and a resuscitation/oxygen kit. It was noted that it could take up to 25 to 30 minutes to reach the patient; however, the effect of the program's prehospital cardiac care was published with a reported reduction in mortality from 21% down to 8%.[2] Many consider this first American version of the mobile coronary care unit concept to have directly inspired the development of such programs around the country.[17,18]

RICHARD LEWIS, MD

Dr Lewis is credited with participating in the development of the Heartmobile along with Dr James Warren. The City of Columbus Fire Services along with the Ohio State University Medical Center developed the Heartmobile paramedic program in 1969.[13]

NORMAN MCSWAIN, MD

Dr Mc Swain is best known for his work as a trauma surgeon. However, while on faculty at the University of Kansas he helped develop paramedic education and push for the development of the EMS system. At the time of his move to Tulane in New Orleans, he was credited with helping bring about the evolution of the Kansas EMS system to a point where 90% of citizens were covered by paramedic response in less than 10 minutes. While working with stakeholders in New Orleans he was selected to develop a comprehensive emergency medical services system for the city. This led to the introduction of BLS and ALS prehospital provider education and the development of a citywide EMS system. During his work with the American College of Surgeons Committee on Trauma (ACS-COT) he noted gaps in the education of prehospital providers as part of the trauma care team care team and was enlisted to help develop the Pre-Hospital Trauma Life-Support (PHTLS) program, a joint venture between the ACS-COT and the National Association of Emergency Medical Technicians (NAEMT).[19]

EUGENE NAGEL, MD

Dr Nagel is credited as being one of the first physicians to recognize that there was a potential impracticality to basing out of hospital coronary care on response of the physician to the field. Working with Miami-Dade fire officials and a cardiologist colleague, Dr Hirschman, to develop a system by which paramedics could transmit an ECG to the hospital and receive voice medical control by a physician. They enlisted the help of a little known company in developing their telemetry package with a defibrillator into a unit known as the Physio-Control LifePak 33. Although the LifePak device required redesign to allow for the rugged field environment, coupling this concept together with fire rescue personnel taught to defibrillate, provide intravenous medications, and advanced airway techniques proved to be a workable combination. At that time, however, there was no legal authority for them to implement their new paramedic skill set. It has been reported that Dr Nagel actually went to the city manager's office and allowed his newly trained paramedics to intubate him in the office to prove their skill set. Ultimately Dr Nagel was able to spearhead the creation of a law (10-D-66) in the state of Florida that made it illegal for paramedics perform the skills and is considered the cornerstone for EMS law in that state. Dr Nagel was also successful in advocacy at the national level and was one of the key individuals who petitioned successfully for the passage of the EMS Systems Act.[20,21]

FRANK PANTRIDGE, MD (1916-2004)

In one very important way it could be said that Dr Pantridge is in fact the father of prehospital advanced coronary care. Dr Pantridge was a cardiologist working at Royal Victoria Hospital in Belfast, Ireland, when he determined that it would be most appropriate to deliver electrical therapy and advanced coronary care in the prehospital setting rather than delaying care until arrival at the hospital. In order to accomplish this, he developed a portable mobile defibrillator 1965. This was integrated into a prehospital care team which Pantridge then studied and published in the *Lancet* in 1967. The first prehospital advanced coronary care units in the United States were based on Pantridge's program.[22]

PAUL PEPE, MD

Dr Pepe is an outspoken and prolific academic and lecturer in EMS medicine. He has held numerous prestigious positions, but is well known for his work to develop and popularize many of the clinical concepts focal to our understanding of modern prehospital care. Dr Pepe has been cited as authoring over 400 published papers and abstracts and has provided high-level medical direction in multiple major systems. He coordinates the Eagles Consortium, comprised of medical directors for the nation's major metropolitan areas. He has provided mentorship and leadership to numerous EMS and emergency medicine physicians and is considered by many to be the chief expert on EMS physician interaction with the media.[23]

DEBRA PERINA, MD

Dr Perina is a notable EMS physician and educator who has served since 1999 as the EMS fellowship director at the University of Virginia. She has contributed greatly to the development of the subspecialty through her work at NAEMSP and as the president of the American Board of Emergency Medicine (ABEM). Her leadership was critical during the development of the application to the American Board of Medical Specialties (ABMS) to create the new subspecialty. Her mentorship and guidance (along with other key members of the EMS physician community) in the development of the subspecialty and training program certification process has led to the realization of ACGME-accredited fellowship training programs and board certification.[24]

PETER SAFAR, MD (1923-2003)

Dr Safar is credited with popularizing the important concepts of CPR and developing the "ABCs" of resuscitation. In 1956, he and Dr James Elan invented mouth-to-mouth resuscitation after demonstrating the effectiveness of mouth-to-mouth rescue breathing through a series of experiments on human volunteers who had been paralyzed. He also advocated for and effectively showed that laypeople could serve as the initial prehospital rescuers for CPR. He partnered with Asmund Laerdal, who at the time was a doll maker, in the development of the initial (and now internationally recognized) prehospital cardiac training tool, Resusci Anne. Dr Safar is also credited with the successful development of one of the first modern ambulances, which he identified as a required replacement for the hearses and station wagons that were being used at the time. While working in the Baltimore system he trained fire department rescuers to add intubation skills to their CPR technique. He developed standards for emergency medical technician education and initiated the Freedom House Enterprise Ambulance Service in Pittsburgh in 1967. In 1976, he cofounded the World Association for Disaster and Emergency Medicine and in 1979 founded the International Resuscitation Research Center. He was nominated three times the Nobel Prize in Medicine.[25]

RONALD STEWART, MD

Dr Stewart, although a now famous contributor to the development of emergency medicine and EMS medicine, began his career as a general practitioner in Neil's Harbour, Nova Scotia. After completing his training in emergency medicine he became the founding medical director of the Los Angeles County paramedic program and served that community until accepting a position in Pittsburgh, Pennsylvania, where he was the founding director of the Center for Emergency Medicine and the medical director of the Department of Public Safety of the City of Pittsburg. This program soon became one of the preeminent centers for the development of EMS medicine in the country. He eventually returned to Canada and continued to develop his role in the political landscape of health care after taking up a post at Dalhousie University. In 1993, Dr Stuart became a member of the Nova Scotia legislature and was eventually appointed as the Minister of Health and Registrar General for the province until 1996. Dr Stewart's influence on the development of EMS medicine is evidenced by many publications and the productivity of his former students and colleagues in various areas of emergency medicine and EMS.[26,27]

ROBERT SWOR, DO

Like many of the former presidents of the National Association of EMS Physicians, Dr Swor has provided significant academic contributions to the field. He has been politically active in his advocacy for the development of EMS medicine and serves as an advisor to multiple key stakeholder organizations, including the National Highway Traffic Safety Administration and the American Heart Association.[28] His book on quality improvement was one of the first publications to address this area of medical direction in an organized and detailed fashion. He remains one of the most prominent EMS educators in the country.

JAMES WARREN, MD

Dr Warren of Columbus Ohio participated in the early development of advanced out-of-hospital coronary care through collaboration with the Ohio State University and the Columbus Division of Fire. In 1969, the *Heartmobile* program was initiated. The program included three firefighters and the physician responding in the Heartmobile from the hospital.[29] In 1971, it was apparently clear to Dr Warren that the firefighters could be trained to operate the Heartmobile without the on-scene presence of the physician. On July 1, 1971, the Columbus vision division of fire took over Heartmobile operations.

PAUL M. ZOLL, MD (1911-1999)

In 1952, Dr Zoll published his work on the use of "external electrical stimulation" (transcutaneous pacing). In 1956, he and his colleagues published the paper detailing the successful termination of ventricular fibrillation with "electric countershock" (transcutaneous defibrillation) and in the same year developed an oscilloscope-based cardiac monitor with built-in audible alerts. Dr Zoll is also credited with advancing the concept of using countershock (electrocardioversion) as a viable alternative to antidysrhythmic medications in the termination of dysrhythmias.

KEY PROFESSIONAL ORGANIZATIONS

A number of organizations have contributed to the evolution of modern emergency medical services in the United States and beyond. The *International Association of Fire Chiefs* (IAFC) was founded in 1873 as the National Association of Fire Engineers. The IAFC has a long history of advocacy and the development of standards and guidelines for fire and EMS operations and has supported the development of a number of other EMS organizations throughout the development of EMS systems and the evolution of the practice of prehospital emergency care. The *National Registry of EMTs* (NREMT) was formed in 1970 in response to President Lyndon Johnson's Committee on Highway Traffic Safety recommended the creation of a national certification agency. The NREMT focuses on the development and proliferation of national standards for education of EMS providers. The *American Ambulance Association* (AAA) was founded in 1979 and has contributed much to the early studies and more to ongoing political advocacy and the creation of industry guidelines. The *American College of Emergency Physicians* (ACEP), founded in 1968, was the primary voice of the new specialty of emergency medicine and spearheaded to creation of the specialty in 1979. Much of the unique nature of emergency medicine was tied directly to the developing prehospital emergency care in the nation.[30] The *National Association*

of Emergency Medical Technicians (NAEMT) was founded in 1975 and served to provide significant educational programs to prehospital providers, including Pre-Hospital Trauma Life Support (PHTLS) and Advanced Medical Life Support (AMLS).[31] NAEMT has a strong advocacy mission and supports political and scientific advancement in the field. The *National Association of State EMS Officials* (NASEMSO) was formed in 1980 and focuses on formation and development of policy and standards relating to oversight of EMS systems across the country. The *Society for Academic Emergency Medicine* (SAEM) was formed from University Association for Emergency Medicine (UAEM) and the Society of Teachers of Emergency Medicine (STEM) in 1989 and was instrumental in development of EMS Medicine fellowship curricula and funding of EMS research.[32] *National Association of EMS Physicians* (NAEMSP) was founded in 1984 to represent a peer group of EMS physicians and to devise key resources to serve the EMS community. This organization has developed research, education, and advocacy programs that have had major influence in the evolution of EMS in North America and beyond. NAEMSP was a lead organization in the development of the proposals that ultimately led to the EMS Medicine board certification under ABMS and the advent of ACGME accreditation for EMS Medicine fellowship programs. The *National Association of EMS Educators* (NAEMSE) was founded in 1995 and is dedicated to the development of resources and advocacy directed at support EMS educators.[33]

KEY POINTS

- In 1864, President Abraham Lincoln signed into law "an act to establish a uniform system of ambulances in the United States."
- In 1966, Dr Pantridge developed coronary care ambulances and showed improved survival in out-of-hospital cardiac arrest in Belfast, Ireland.
- In 1968, Dr Grace of St Vincent's Hospital in New York City launched the United States' first mobile coronary care units.
- In 1965, funding for EMS as part of the reimbursement model was included in Medicare.
- In 1966, following the final report of the President's Commission of Highway Safety, President Lyndon Johnson's administration supported passage of what would become the National Highway Safety Act (Public Law 89-564).
- The American College of Emergency Physicians (ACEP) was founded in 1968.
- In 1973, the EMS Systems Act (Public Law 93-154) was enacted under President Gerald Ford.
- National Association of EMS Physicians (NAEMSP) was founded in 1984.

REFERENCES

1. Wikipedia. The Knights Hospitaller. http://en.wikipedia.org/wiki/Knights_Hospitaller. Accessed September 10, 2013.
2. Robbins VD. A history of emergency medicine services & medical transportation systems in America. March 2005. https://www.monoc.org/bod/docs/History%20American%20EMS-MTS.pdf. Accessed August 11, 2013.
3. The history of the air ambulance. www.airambulanceservice.com/history.html. Accessed December 18, 2013.
4. Wikipedia. Paramedics in the United States. http://en.wikipedia.org/wiki/Paramedics_in_the_United_States. Accessed December 18, 2013.
5. Wikipedia. Air medical services. http://en.wikipedia.org/wiki/Air_medical_services. Accessed December 18, 2013.
6. Our history: Forrest General Hospital. www.forrestgeneral.com. Accessed December 4, 2010.

7. Wikipedia. Bryan E. Bledsoe. http://en.wikipedia.org/wiki/Bryan_E._Bledsoe. Accessed December 18, 2013.

8. National EMS Museum. Nancy Caroline, MD. http://www.emsmuseum.org/virtual-museum/publications/articles/398276-1976-Nancy-Caroline-MD; http://old.post-gazette.com/obituaries/20021221caroline2.asp. Accessed January 12, 2014.

9. National EMS Museum. Leonard Cobb, MD. http://www.emsmuseum.org/virtual-museum/biographies/articles/398250-1967-Leonard-Cobb-MD. Accessed January 12, 2014.

10. Yale School of Medicine. David C Cone MD: biographical information. http://medicine.yale.edu/emergencymed/people/david_cone-2.profile. Accessed January 12, 2014.

11. National EMS Museum. Richard Crampton, MD. http://www.emsmuseum.org/virtual-museum/By_Era/articles/398163-1968-Richard-Crampon-MD. Accessed January 12, 2014.

12. National EMS Museum. J. Michael Criley, MD. http://www.emsmuseum.org/virtual-museum/history/articles/399756-J-Michael-Criley-MD. Accessed January 12, 2014.

13. Wikipedia. Paramedic. http://en.wikipedia.org/wiki/Paramedic. Accessed October 12, 2013.

14. Haywood County Resuce Squad. HCRS history. http://www.haywoodrescue.org/history-2/history. Accessed January 16, 2014.

15. UT Southwestern Medical Center. Raymond Fowler, M.D.: biography. http://profiles.utsouthwestern.edu/profile/51235/raymond-fowler.html. Accessed January 12, 2014.

16. Raymond L. Fowler, M.D., FACEP. http://www.csi.edu/emsconference/documents/Fowler_Resume.pdf. Accessed January 12, 2014.

17. Grace WJ, Chadbourn JA. The mobile coronary care unit. *Dis Chest.* June 1969;55(6):452-455.

18. National EMS Museum. William Grace, MD. http://www.emsmuseum.org/virtual-museum/history/articles/398198-1968-William-Grace-MD. Accessed January 8, 2014.

19. Tulane Universtiy School of Medicine. Norman E. McSwain, Jr., MD, FACS. http://tulane.edu/som/departments/surgery/faculty-staff/upload/bio-080608-short-1.pdf. Accessed January 12, 2014.

20. National EMS Museum. Eugene Nagal, MD. http://www.emsmuseum.org/virtual-museum/history/articles/398203-1964-Eugene-Nagel-MD-First-Telemetry-Radio. Accessed October 12, 2013.

21. City of Miami, Department of Fire-Rescue. About us. http://www.miamigov.com/Fire/pages/AboutUs/OurHistory.asp. Accessed October 12, 2013.

22. EMS World. Remembering Dr. Frank Pantridge, 1916-2004. http://www.emsworld.com/article/10324106/remembering-dr-frank-pantridge-1916-2004. Accessed April 1, 2015.

23. UT Southwestern Medical Center. Paul Pepe, M.D. http://profiles.utsouthwestern.edu/profile/43741/paul-pepe.html. Accessed January 12, 2014.

24. National Library of Medicine. MEET LOCAL LEGEND: Debra G. Perina, M.D. http://www.nlm.nih.gov/locallegends/Biographies/Perina_Debra.html. Accessed October 12, 2013.

25. Wikipedia. Peter Safar. http://en.wikipedia.org/wiki/Peter_Safar. Accessed October 12, 2013.

26. Ronald Stewart, M.D. EMS revisited: down the rabbit hole and through the looking glass. http://www.emsworld.com/article/10319905/ems-revisited-down-the-rabbit-hole-and-through-the-looking-glass. Accessed October 12, 2013.

27. Cape Breton University. Ronald Daniel Stewart. http://www.cbu.ca/honorees/ronald-stewart. Accessed October 12, 2013.

28. National Registry of EMTs. Board bios: Robert Swor, D.O., FACEP. http://www.nremt.org/nremt/about/board_bios.asp?member=Swor. Accessed January 12, 2014.

29. The Ohio State University College of Medicine, Department of Emergency Medicine. OSU EMS history—The "Heartmobile" 1969. http://www.osuem.com/about/ems-history.shtml. Accessed December 18, 2013.

30. American College of Emergency Physicians. History of ACEP. http://www.acep.org/Content.aspx?id=22594. Accessed January 5, 2014.

31. The National Association of EMTs. History of NAEMT. http://www.naemt.org/about_us/history/history_home.aspx. Accessed January 5, 2014.

32. Society for Academic Emergency Medicine. About SAEM. http://www.saem.org/about-saem. Accessed January 5, 2014.

33. The College Network. National Association of EMS Educators. http://www.collegenetwork.com/corporate/CorporatePartners/NAEMSE.aspx. Accessed February 20, 2014.

Training and Board Certification

Debra G. Perina

INTRODUCTION

In the United States, over 15.9 million patients per year are transported to emergency departments (ED) by emergency medical services (EMS), and 40% of all hospital inpatient admissions arrive by ambulance.[1] Physicians have dedicated a significant portion of their practice to EMS since the late 1960s. EMS physicians acquired their expertise primarily by direct experience and together built the subspecialty through professional association, collaborative research, and standards development. EMS medicine has many roots, with growth spurts largely coming out of casualty care during warfare. Modern EMS started in Great Britain and Los Angeles in the early 1960s, driven by cardiologists who wanted a way to resuscitate cardiac arrest patients in the field.[2] In the late 1960s with Death and Disabilities white paper, EMS saw exponential growth at the hands of surgeons who wanted a rapid way to evacuate and treat trauma victims on the nation's highways similar to the care and resuscitation of trauma victims during the Vietnam War.[3] The majority of these surgeons also worked and staffed the "accident units," precoursers of today's ED. When emergency medicine became an organized specialty in the late 1970s, it was a natural transition for these "new kids on the block" to take an active role in EMS since the interface was far more than that for physicians from other specialties. The growth of EMS medicine actually parallels the growth of emergency medicine to a large degree.

OBJECTIVES

- Discuss education and training backgrounds of practicing EMS physicians.
- Describe available EMS medical director training courses.
- Describe formal EMS physician fellowship training.
- Describe the current state of EMS board certification and qualifications for examination.
- Describe scientific and educational conferences that provide EMS physicians with state-of-the-art EMS research and clinical practice CME.
- Discuss additional areas of training useful to EMS physicians fulfilling specific operational roles.

EMS PHYSICIANS

In 2003, the Institute of Medicine (IOM) convened the Committee on the Future of Emergency Care in the United States Health System "to examine the emergency care system in the U.S., to create a vision for the future of the system, and to make recommendations for helping the nation achieve that vision." One volume of this IOM report focused exclusively on EMS.[1] The IOM noted that: *Delivery of clinical care in the field is quite different from delivering care in the hospital or other medical facility, and the oversight of EMS is complex.* Furthermore, the IOM acknowledged that EMS physician involvement improves the quality of care delivered by EMS systems.

As defined by the IOM, EMS comprises the crucial, early phases of the continuum of emergency medical care for acutely ill and injured persons including (a) 9-1-1 access and dispatch, (b) field triage and initial stabilization, and (c) treatment and transport in specially equipped ambulances or helicopters to hospitals or between medical facilities.

The term *EMS system* describes the organizational structure that integrates all of the essential components of EMS care. In their practice, EMS physicians provide direct emergency medical care for patients and

medical oversight of EMS systems. They practice in every state, in a variety of different venues including industry, academia, private, municipal, fire-based and hospital-based systems. All states have regulations governing the role and responsibility of EMS physicians. Many states require specific medical director training which is often based on the national medical director curriculum developed by the National Highway Traffic Safety Administration (NHTSA).[4]

EMS medical practice is unique due to its position early in the continuum of patient care, physical location outside of fixed medical facilities, and relatively higher acuity of the patient population compared to emergency medicine. The majority of the most severely ill and injured patients presenting to ED arrive via EMS. EMS physicians provide direct patient care and medical oversight in unique settings such as mass gatherings, firefighting operations, disaster scenes, hazardous materials incidents, tactical law enforcement missions, and air medical and critical care inter-facility transports. As part of their clinical practice, EMS physicians are responsible for medical oversight of the EMS team. This includes daily direct medical decision making, control of care provided by EMS personnel, developing treatment guidelines, and ensuring procedural competency training of EMS personnel. EMS physicians also lead quality management activities relating to medical care delivered by the entire EMS system.

EMS physicians have developed treatments and techniques in the EMS environment that allow for patient safety and ensure proper treatment affecting the patient's final outcome.[5-9] Extensive peer-reviewed articles address the roles of EMS physicians in the science and practice of EMS.[10-18] EMS physicians are uniquely trained and positioned to provide the clinical care and leadership to mold prehospital- and hospital-based care into regionalized systems of care. The unique expertise gained from EMS physician field practice and system oversight improves patient safety and clinical outcomes.[5]

For over four decades, steadily increasing numbers of physicians have defined their professional practice as caring for patients in the EMS environment. Emergency medicine physicians comprise the principal physician group that has driven the growth of EMS practice since 1984. Current estimates are roughly 75% of EMS physicians are emergency medicine trained, 23% Family Medicine trained, with the remaining 2% being pediatricians, surgeons, and obstetrics and gynecology physicians. EMS physicians are often leaders in their communities concerned with meeting the needs of the public and provision of quality EMS care. Most academic emergency medicine departments employ an EMS physician who supervises the exposure of residents to EMS and engages in research activities to expand the scientific body of knowledge of this practice. EMS physicians hold key positions in several federal government agencies involved in EMS issues. Complex and sophisticated medical procedures previously only performed in hospitals, or completely unavailable a few decades ago, are now routinely integrated in EMS due to EMS physicians.[19-22]

EMS physicians play many pivotal roles. They serve as providers, expert consultants, and educators. Many EMS physicians plan prevention efforts implemented through the EMS system, with goals directed at reducing the societal costs of injury and illness. They facilitate optimal care through education and continual oversight of providers. EMS physicians reduce variability in care, limit interventions that are of no benefit, and facilitate delivery of care that enhances patient safety and improves outcomes.[23-27] As the EMS subspecialty matures, patient outcomes will be further improved with continued advancement of scientific knowledge and treatments adding further sophistication to this area of practice.

EMS MEDICAL DIRECTOR TRAINING COURSES

EMS medical director training courses exist that are designed to allow physicians to acquire basic knowledge of EMS practice. These are primarily 1- to 3-day courses, and are offered by individual states or professional associations. These courses provide a basic introduction to EMS practice, EMS system quality improvement, and medical oversight. However, the

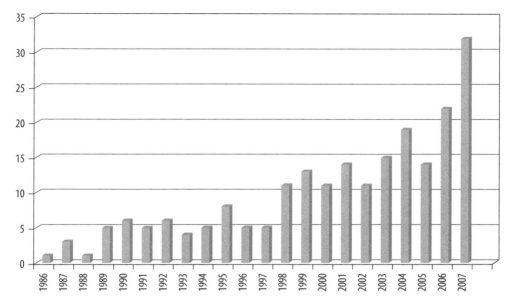

FIGURE 3-1. The number of EMS fellowship graduates (1986-2007). (Data from American Board of Emergency Medicine (ABEM). https://www.abem.org/public/.)

content does not delve deeply into the clinical practice of EMS or its scientific basis due to intrinsic time constraints. Some are online, while others are delivered in classroom format. Many states require such training by regulation for physicians who wish to be EMS medical directors. These mandated courses are provided through each state and are frequently based on the National Highway Safety and Traffic Association (NHTSA) National Standard Medical Directors Curriculum. Both the National Association of EMS Physicians (NAEMSP) and the American College of Emergency Medicine (ACEP) have courses devoted to physician medical direction. NAEMSP offers the 2-day basic EMS medical director course and the 1-day advanced EMS medical directors course in conjunction with its annual scientific meeting. ACEP offers a preconference (Eagles conference) concentrating issues related to large EMS system management.

EMS PHYSICIAN FELLOWSHIP TRAINING

Presently at least 268 fellowship-trained EMS physicians are practicing in 41 states as well as several foreign countries. The first known EMS fellowship program was at Adam R Crowley Shock Trauma Institute, graduating one fellow in 1983. Three EMS fellowships sponsored by emergency medicine programs began in 1985, with the first of these fellows graduating from Wright State University in 1987. The number of graduates has steadily increased since that time (**Figure 3-1**). It is believed that there may be more graduates than represented by the graph as some original training programs are no longer in existence and no graduation records are accessible. EMS fellowships are located in most states across the country. **Figure 3-2** depicts the location of all EMS fellowships, accredited and unaccredited. Most fellowship programs offer

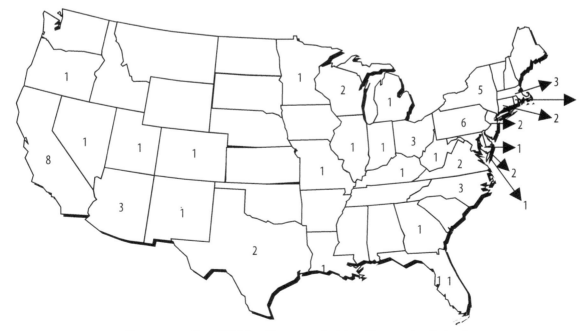

There are currently no EMS fellowship programs in states with no number displayed

FIGURE 3-2. Accredited and unaccredited EMS fellowship programs depicted by state (October 2013). (Data from Accreditation Council for Graduate Medical Education (ACGME). https://www.acgme.org/acgmeweb/.)

TABLE 3-1	Original ACGME-Accredited EMS Medicine Fellowships (2012-2013 Academic Year)	
Program	**Director**	**Phone/Fax/E-mail**
Los Angeles County-Harbor- UCLA Torrance, California	Marianne Gausche-Hill, MD	Ph: (310) 222-3503 Fax: (310) 222-6101
Orlando Health Orlando, Florida	George A Ralls, MD	Ph: (407) 836-7611 Fax: (407) 836-7634
Indiana University School of Medicine Program Indianapolis, Indiana	Daniel O'Donnell, MD	Ph: (317) 695-2042 Ph: (317) 962-3003
HealthPartners Institute for Education and Research Saint Paul, Minnesota	Ralph J Frascone, MD	Ph: (651) 264-7781 Fax: (651) 778-3778
Washington University/B-JH/SLCH Consortium St Louis, Missouri	William S Gilmore, MD	Ph: (314) 362-9279 Fax: (314) 362-0478
University of New Mexico School of Medicine Albuquerque, New Mexico	Darren Braude, MD	Ph: (505) 220-7422 Fax: (505) 272-6503
SUNY Upstate Medical University Program Syracuse, New York	Derek R Cooney, MD, FF/NREMTP, FACEP	Ph: (315) 464-4851 Fax: (315) 464-4854
North Shore-Long Island Jewish Health Brooklyn, New York	Douglas Isaacs, MD	Ph: (718) 999-2790 Fax: (718) 999-0119
University at Buffalo School of Medicine Buffalo, New York	Brian Clemency, DO, MBA	Ph: (716) 898-3600
University of Texas School of Medicine at San Antonio San Antonio, Texas	Craig Cooley, MD, MPH, FACEP	Ph: (210) 567-4297 Fax: (210) 567-0757
University of Virginia Medical Center Charlottesville, Virginia	Debra Perina, MD	Ph: (434) 243-6720 Fax: (242) 924-2877

Original accredited fellowships by state: CA = 1, FL = 1, IN = 1, MN = 1, NM = 1, NY = 3, TX = 1, VA = 1 (Total = 11)

Data from Accreditation Council for Graduate Medical Education (ACGME). https://www.acgme.org/acgmeweb/.

one to two positions per year. EMS fellowships are generally 1 year in length. Some programs offer an optional second year leading to an advanced degree (eg, MPH, MHA, MBA, MEd). A small minority of programs are 2-year training programs. ACGME-accredited programs (the first-round approvals were for the 2012-2013 academic year) were required to comply with a 12-month curriculum. The original round of accredited programs included 11 EMS medicine fellowships (3-1). As of a report generated from the ACGME Web site on October 15, 2014, there are now 40 accredited programs.

The EMS Medicine Core Content, first published in 1985 and revised several times since, describes the domain of EMS medicine and is the basis for fellowship training curricular development.[28] Fellowship curricula have become relatively standardized as a result of the work of the Society of Academic Emergency Medicine (SAEM) and NAEMSP.[29] The curriculum is designed to provide specific training in general and specific core competencies for EMS physicians, including medical knowledge, clinical expertise, operations, education, research, and administration. It contains all topic areas in the EMS Medicine Core Content covered through a combination of didactics, self-study, case review, and direct clinical experience. This was culminated in the official documents defining the core content and curriculum which now dictate content for ACGME-accredited programs. EMS fellows provide direct patient care in the prehospital setting, educate other physicians and allied health personnel, perform quality improvement activities of EMS systems, and create treatment guidelines for EMS systems. Participation in local and state EMS systems and specialty societies is required. The fellowships are designed to allow fellows to develop proficiency in managing the breadth of clinical conditions encountered by EMS systems in nontraditional health care settings with limited resources in uncontrolled circumstances. Specific procedural skills, such as patient extrication, airway management in water, use of alternative airway devices such as the King airway, spinal immobilization with long board and KED, application of Hare traction splint, and field triage are integrated into the training. Specific funding for EMS research fellowships is available. NAEMSP sponsors a resuscitation fellowship to prepare and train individuals for a career in prehospital resuscitation research, as well as a fellowship designed to encourage the development of high-quality medical director leaders. SAEM also sponsors and provides grant funding for an EMS research fellowship.

As of Spring 2013, there are 29 accredited EMS medicine fellowships, with 62 total in existence (**Table 3-1**). The Accreditation Council for Graduate Medical Education (ACGME), parent body of the Residency Review Committee for Emergency Medicine (RRC-EM), recognized EMS as a subspecialty area in June 2010 and opened the application process for fellowship programs in December 2012. The number of accredited programs will likely increase over the next several years. This will lead to greater standardization in training and promotion of consistent knowledge with the defined curriculum in fellowship graduates.

EMS MEDICINE BOARD CERTIFICATION

EMS medicine subspecialty certification recognizes the unique body of knowledge and clinical practice of EMS physicians and their important contributions to the safety and clinical outcomes of patients. Physician specialty and subspecialty certification is achieved through recognition by the American Board of Medical Specialties (ABMS) by request of a member Board who makes a case of need for the subspecialty. The journey to creation of the EMS subspecialty began in 1992 when the American Board of Emergency Medicine (ABEM) created the first subspecialty task force exploring the possibility of creating an ABMS application for recognition. EMS medicine was in its infancy at that time. There were few fellowship programs. The first EMS fellowship curriculum was not published until 1994.[29] The ABEM task force disbanded in 1995 concluding that EMS medicine needed more growth in scientific underpinnings of the specialty, number of fellowships, dedicated physicians in practice, and standardization of training. Between 1995 and 2001, dedicated EMS physicians furthered a research base, created fellowships, and attempted to standardize fellowship training. In 2001, it was felt that perhaps EMS had matured to the point that another attempt was possible. In 2001, joint collaboration between NAEMSP and the ACEP EMS Committee focused on addressing issues necessary to complete an EMS subspecialty application to forward to ABEM.

In 2003, the IOM report noted a lack of standardization in the training and qualifications of EMS physicians currently limited their impact in many parts of the country. For this reason, the IOM formally recommended that "… *ABEM create a subspecialty certification in EMS. The certification would be analogous to those available in toxicology, sports medicine, and pediatric emergency medicine. Creating this type of designation would acknowledge the unique challenges and complexities introduced by the out-of-hospital environment. The certification would ensure that physicians providing medical direction are trained specifically in Prehospital EMS and are prepared to meet the challenges it consistently presents.*"[1] This provided renewed interest and impetus for efforts to achieve board certification and subspecialty recognition for EMS physicians. Various committees and meetings contributed to this effort, with a completed EMS subspecialty application submitted to ABEM in 2008. This application went through several revisions before being finally accepted by ABEM in 2009 and forwarded to ABMS for subspecialty recognition.

Physician subspecialty certification is achieved through recognition by ABMS of a unique body of knowledge, scientific underpinnings for the specialty, sufficient training programs, and dedicated physicians to have a positive impact on patients and society. Every ABMS specialty board is concerned with setting and promoting the standards for quality patient care and practice in their field. As such, member boards are concerned that new specialties enhance quality in patient care, and where there is overlap with their specialty there is the ability of their diplomates to access training and certification should they wish to do so. Representatives from all other specialty boards must vote approval to create a new subspecialty such as EMS medicine. During the application process, the biggest hurdle faced was helping other boards understand what EMS medicine was and how it impacted their diplomates. ABMS unanimously voted to create the subspecialty of EMS medicine in September 2010.

The parent board for EMS medicine is ABEM. As such, ABEM is responsible for creating and administering the certification examination, the blueprint for the exam, and periodic revisions to the core content. As is customary for any new specialty, candidates will initially qualify through training in unaccredited EMS fellowship programs or by virtue of meeting practice hour requirements (practice track). Further information can be found on the ABEM Web site under subspecialty certification.[30] Eventually as the subspecialty matures, the only route to achieve board certification will be through completion of an ACGME-accredited EMS medicine fellowship. To become board certified, the candidate must successfully pass a secure proctored multiple-choice-question examination based on the core content. The first exam was conducted in October 2013.

The birth of the subspecialty will have many consequences. The ability to achieve board certification has already increased interest among residents in pursuing careers in EMS medicine. As we have seen in the growth of other specialties, over time board certified specialists will be sought for positions. State regulators and hospital credentialing committees will produce language requiring appropriate training and certification to practice in the specialty. Regulators will promote EMS specialists for medical direction positions on a state level, and over time EMS agencies and the public will seek the same. Greater coordination and communication between EMS physicians, EM physicians, and other specialties will enhance patient care and ultimately improve patient outcomes.

SCIENTIFIC MEETINGS AND CONTINUING EDUCATION

There are several EMS-related scientific meetings and continuing education opportunities available. The National Association of EMS Physicians (NAEMSP) was founded in 1984 to address the professional needs of career EMS physicians, provide leadership, and foster excellence in prehospital patient care.[31] Since its inception, NAEMSP membership has grown from a handful of dedicated founders to include 827 physician members located in all 50 states, Puerto Rico, Guam, and Washington, DC. NAEMSP has secured multiple state and federal EMS-related grants, including EMS medical direction core content development, EMS medical directors' national standard training curriculum, and EMS research agenda that have shaped EMS system design and set national EMS patient care guidelines. It publishes *Prehospital Emergency Care*, the premier journal on EMS medicine. It also sponsors and runs the National EMS Medical Directors Course & Practicum in conjunction with its annual scientific meeting.

The Air Medical Physician Association (AMPA) is a physician organization dedicated to EMS medical practice involving air medical and critical care ground transports. AMPA has 342 members representing extensive expertise in these areas.[32] AMPA offers opportunities for education and research promoting patient safety and quality patient care during transports. AMPA publishes the *Air Medical Journal* and sponsors the Air Medical Transport Conference and the Critical Care Transport Medicine conferences held annually. It also sponsors the two-part Air Medical Directors Core Curriculum course.

Other emergency medicine organizations have EMS committees or membership sections, and a portion of their annual scientific meeting content covers EMS related topics. These include the American College of Emergency Physicians (ACEP), Society for Academic Emergency Medicine (SAEM), and American Academy of Emergency Medicine (AAEM). ACEP EMS activities also include several committees (EMS and Disaster and Emergency Preparedness) and special-interest sections (EMS, Trauma Care and Injury Prevention, Air Medical and Tactical Medicine) which seek to address EMS issues and promote relationships with outside organizations. SAEM has EMS and disaster medicine interest groups. AAEM has an EMS committee that provides education to its membership on EMS-related topics and communicates prehospital medical issues to the general membership.

Almost all states have an EMS related statewide meeting that includes educational offerings for physicians. Team-based training is prevalent at these meetings, as well as operational specialized EMS training in which the physician may elect to participate (see the next section). Attendance at these meetings can not only be educational, but can afford networking opportunities as well as participation in statewide EMS meetings.

OPERATIONAL EMS TRAINING

There are several specialized areas in EMS where specific 1- to 2-day courses exist designed to provide in-depth operational understanding to the participant. Some of these courses lead to certificates of completion, and can be very helpful to EMS medical directors in gaining understanding of specific types of responses.

The Counter Narcotics and Terrorism Operational Medical Support (CONTOMS) course provides specialized medical training for civilian providers to support tactical law enforcement operations. It was first developed in the late1980s by the Casualty Care Research Center (CCRC) in the Department of Military and Emergency Medicine at the Uniformed Services University (USU). It is focused on the broad range of knowledge and skills required for crisis management medical response including care under fire; weapons of mass destruction (WMD); medical counterterrorism; counternarcotics; protective operations; hostage rescue; explosive ordnance disposal; maritime operations; civil disorder; and major national security events. The CONTOMS Program has become one of the academic and scientific anchors for tactical emergency medicine. To meet evolving aspects of the tactical medicine field, the CCRC has built on the CONTOMS Program to develop other evidence-based educational and applied science courses including EMT-Tactical: the Advanced School, the Public Safety Commanders course, the Medical Directors course, and the Tactical Medicine Instructor Development School.

Emergency Medical Dispatch (EMD) courses are designed to train dispatchers how to appropriately question callers and provide prearrival instructions to bystanders to render aid prior to EMS arrival. There are two basic sponsors of these courses: APCO Institute and Medical Priority. These courses are typically 4 to 6 days and include didactic and Web-based components leading to certification. Both programs require medical direction of dispatch centers to ensure proper oversight and quality management.

HAZMAT courses are designed for the student to understand OHSA requirements in the workplace as related to chemical, radiological, and biologicals, with emphasis on learning decontamination, proper storage and handling, and recognition of exposures. The Advanced HAZMAT Life Support (AHLS) course was developed and is cosponsored by the American Academy of Clinical Toxicology and the University of Arizona research center. It is designed to provide the critical skills needed to treat victims exposed to toxic substances.

Search and Rescue (SAR) courses are usually 2 to 3 days in length but may be up to a week. Most have both urban and wilderness components. Content can also include swift water rescue and structural collapse. Basic courses offer training in map and compass reading and basic search theory. Intermediate courses address search design, team leading, and practice searches.

Wilderness medicine has many educational course offerings per year often in wilderness locations. Educational objectives include acquiring an understanding of common wilderness injuries and illnesses with hands-on practical instruction for improvised treatments. There is also a certification course, Advanced Wilderness Life Support, developed by the University of Utah.

Confined space rescue is a subset of technical rescue operations that involves the rescue and recovery of victims trapped in a confined space. Classes typically cover the OSHA regulations along with all the typical equipment used in an entry. Rescue operations are explained and demonstrated, with students expected to have hands-on participation in scenarios practiced in simulators.

KEY POINTS

- Approximately 270 fellowship-trained EMS physicians in 41 states as of 2010.
- The first EMS fellowship at the Adam R. Crowley Shock Trauma Institute graduated its first fellow in 1983.
- ABMS recognized EMS as a subspecialty in 2010.
- EMS physicians have a wide background of primary medical specialty training including emergency medicine, family medicine, pediatrics, surgery, and obstetrics and gynecology.
- Newly accredited EMS fellowship programs are 1 year long.
- EMS medicine became a subspecialty of emergency medicine in 2010.
- EMS physicians are regulated by states and initial and recurrent training is frequently required.
- Multiple specialized training courses exist to help EMS physicians acquire additional knowledge concerning special responses (ie, confined space, HAZMAT, tactical).
- Accreditation of EMS fellowship programs began in 2012 and around 40 programs are now accredited.
- Certification examination for EMS medicine began through the American Board of Emergency Medicine in 2013.

REFERENCES

1. Institute of Medicine, Committee on the Future of Emergency Care in the United States Health System, Board of Health Care Services. *Emergency Medical Services at the Crossroads*. Washington, DC: National Academies Press; 2006.
2. Ambulances and the injured. *Br Med J*. March 19, 1966;1(5489):691-692.
3. Resuscitation and survival in motor vehicle accidents (editorial). *J Trauma*. 1969;9(4):356.
4. National Highway Traffic Safety Administration, Department of Transportation, and the Maternal and Child Health Bureau, Health Resources Services Administration, Department of Health and Human Services. EMS agenda for the future. 2001. http://www.nhtsa.gov/people/injury/ems/ems-agenda/EMSResearchAgenda.pdf. Accessed April 5, 2015.
5. Pepe PE, Mattox KL, Duke JH, Fisher PB, Prentice FD. Effect of full-time, specialized physician supervision on the success of a large, urban emergency medical services system. *Crit Care Med*. 1993;21(9):1279-1286.
6. Benitez FL, Pepe, PE. Role of the physician in prehospital management of trauma: North American perspective. *Curr Opin Crit Care*. 2002;8(6);551-558.
7. Falk JL. Medical direction of emergency medical service systems: a full-time commitment whose time has come. *Crit Care Med*. 1993;21(9):1259-1260.
8. Alonso-Serra H, Blanton D, O'Connor RE. Physician medical direction in EMS. *Prehosp Emerg Care*. 1998;2(2):153-157.
9. Klein KR, Spillane LL, Chiumento S, Schneider SM. Effects of on-line medical control in the prehospital treatment of atraumatic illness. *Prehosp Emerg Care*. 1997;1(2):80-84.
10. Matera P. Medical direction of prehospital care. *Ann Emerg Med*. 1994;24(6):1200.
11. Callaham M. Quantifying the scanty science of EMS [comment]. *Ann Emerg Med*. 1997;30(6):785-790.
12. Brazier H, Murphy AW, Lynch C, Bury G. Searching for the evidence in prehospital care: a review of randomized controlled trials. On behalf of the Ambulance Response Time Sub-Group of the National Ambulance Advisory Committee. *J Accid Emerg Med*. 1999;16(1):18-23.
13. Brice JH, Garrison HG, Evans AT. Study design and outcomes in out-of-hospital emergency medicine research: a ten-year analysis. *Prehosp Emerg Care*. 2000;4(2):144-150.
14. Singer AJ, Homan CS, Stark MJ, Werblud MC, Thode HC, Jr., Hollander JE. Comparison of types of research articles published in emergency medicine and non-emergency medicine journals. *Acad Emerg Med*. 1997;4(12):1153-1158.
15. Seidel JS, Henderson D, Tittle S, et al. Priorities for research in emergency medical services for children: results of a consensus conference. *Ann Emerg Med*. 1999;33:206-210.
16. Maio RF, Garrison HG, Spaite DW, et al. Emergency Medical Services Outcomes Project I (EMSOP I): prioritizing conditions for outcomes research. *Ann Emerg Med*. 1999;33:423-432.
17. National Highway Traffic and Safety Administration, DOT and Maternal and Child Health Bureau, National EMS Research Agenda for the Future. December 2001. www.researchagenda.org.
18. Sayre MR, White LJ, Brown LH, McHenry SD; National EMS Research Strategic Plan Writing Team. The national EMS research strategic plan. *Prehosp Emerg Care*. 2005;9:255-266.
19. Gaxmuri RJ, Nadkarni VM, Nolan JP, et al. Scientific knowledge gaps and clinical research priorities for cardiopulmonary resuscitation and emergency cardiovascular care identified during the 2005 International Consensus Conference on E and CPR science with treatment recommendations: a consensus statement from the International Liaison Committee on Resuscitation. *Circulation*. 2007;116:2501-2512.
20. Gausche M, Lewis RJ, Stratton SJ, et al. Effect of out-of-hospital pediatric endotracheal intubation on survival and neurological outcome: a controlled clinical trial [see comments] [published erratum appears in JAMA 2000Jun 28;283(24):3204]. *JAMA*. 2000;283(6):783-790.
21. Kaye K, Frascone RJ, Held T. Prehospital rapid-sequence intubation: a pilot training program. *Prehosp Emerg Care*. 2003;7(2):235-240.
22. Aufderheide TP, Kereiakes DJ, Weaver WD, Gibler WB, Simoons ML. Planning, implementation, and process monitoring for prehospital 12-lead ECG diagnostic programs. *Prehosp Disast Med*. 1996; 11(3):162-171.
23. Hobgood C, Bowen JB, Brice JH, Overby B, Tamayo-Sarver JH. Do EMS personnel identify, report, and disclose medical errors? *Prehosp Emerg Care*. 2006;10(1):21-27.
24. Holroyd BR, Knopp R, Kallsen G. Medical control. quality assurance in prehospital care. *JAMA*. 1986;256(8):1027-1031.
25. Hoyt BT, Norton RL. Online medical control and initial refusal of care: does it help to talk with the patient? *Acad Emerg Med*. 2001;8(7):725-730.
26. Davis EA, Billitier AJ 4th. The utilization of quality assurance methods in emergency medical services. *Prehosp Disast Med*. 1993;8(2): 127-132.
27. American College of Emergency Physicians, Position Statement. Medical direction of emergency medical services. *Ann Emerg Med*. 1998;31(1):152.
28. Krohmer J, Swor R, Benson N, Meador S, Davidson S. A prototype core content for a fellowship in emergency medicine services. *Ann Emerg Med*. 1994;23:109-114.
29. Krohmer J, Swor R, Benson N, Meador S, Davidson S. A prototype curriculum for a fellowship in emergency medicine services. *Prehosp Dis Med*. 1994;9(1):93-97.
30. American Board of Emergency Medicine. www.abem.org.
31. National Association of EMS Physicians. www.NAEMSP.org.
32. Advancing Air & Ground Critical Care Transport Medicine. www.AMPA.org. Accessed April 5, 2015.

CHAPTER
4

Medical Control, Direction, and Oversight

Kenneth A. Williams

INTRODUCTION

EMS in the United States is a hierarchical care delivery system, with physician leaders working in partnership with EMT/paramedic providers to rescue, care for, and transport patients. Alternative system structures are possible, and work well in other countries and settings. These include both systems with more physician involvement (physicians routinely staffing ambulances), and systems where EMS providers organize and manage their system with little or no physician input. The US model includes a robust prehospital emergency care network in which care is directly provided by predominantly nonphysician prehospital providers. The physician role in this type of system is heavily weighted toward oversight and direction of the system and through direct contact with providers in the field when called for medical control. This chapter will provide an overview of these topics and following chapters will provide greater detail on each of the elements discussed.

OBJECTIVES

1. Define the terms *medical control*, *medical direction*, and *medical oversight*.

2. Describe online (telecommunications and in person) and off-line medical direction.

3. Discuss qualifications for providing medical direction.

4. Describe proper base-station training for EM and EMS physicians.

5. List the components of medical oversight.

PHYSICIAN ROLES IN THE EMS SYSTEM

Although not explicitly stated in some of the original governmental documents describing the EMS system in the United States, medical direction and physician oversight have always been key components to the development and operation of prehospital emergency care services. Although it has been surmised that physician involvement was always assumed, later documents specifically call for medical oversight. This function has evolved over time and can be described in terms of four general types of physician involvement.

ONLINE MEDICAL CONTROL

Online medical control, also known as *direct medical control*, refers to consultation between EMS providers and a physician, typically by radio or telephone, to guide care for an individual patient or EMS incident. These physicians are usually required to take a base-station course and maintain up-to-date knowledge of the EMS treatment protocols. The majority of the physicians providing this type of medical control are not EMS physicians or EMS agency medical directors. Typically, they are the emergency physicians on duty in receiving emergency departments (**Figure 4-1**). However, in some cases they may also be assigned

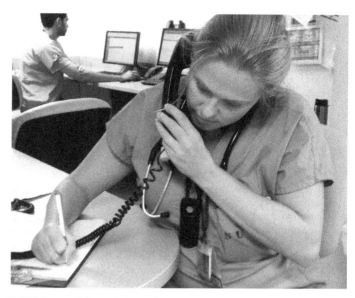

FIGURE 4-1. Online medical control. A physician answers the radio-phone. (Reproduced with permission from Dr. Susan Schreffler.)

this duty exclusively when working a medical control shift in a larger system. Another form of online medical control is *on-scene medical control*. This refers to the presence of the physician at the patient's side during EMS care, working directly with EMS providers to deliver care (**Figure 4-2**). These physicians may be referred to as EMS physicians or flight physicians. When the on-scene EMS physician is also the medical director, this allows for four components: (1) provision of orders and direction of care, (2) evaluation of provider performance, (3) provision of postincident education, and (4) evaluation of system design and operational parameters. Physicians responding to the field should have proper training, awareness, and equipment. Minimum requirements include operational proficiency in operation of an emergency vehicle,

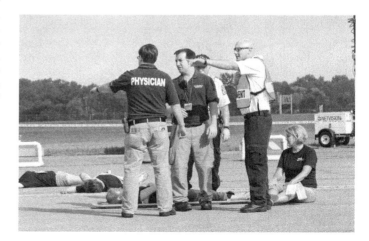

FIGURE 4-2. On-scene medical control. MCI drill with EMS physicians providing on-scene medical control. (Photo by Bob Mescavage/Upstate Medical University.)

radio communications, scene size-up and safety, proper attire and personal protective equipment, use of EMS equipment, and regional procedures for utilization of prehospital resources and response plan(s) for mass casualty incidents and disasters.

OFF-LINE MEDICAL CONTROL

Off-line medical control, *also known as indirect medical control*, typically refers to physician duties performed at an ambulance service or local level. The physician reviews care reports and other data to provide feedback on care delivered to improve quality and other aspects of care. The medical director will oversee continuous quality improvement (CQI) programs, primary and continuing education programs, verification of skills and competencies, criteria for determining overall fitness for duty, and the controlled substance handling and antidiversion program. Off-line medical control also includes development of medical care policies, protocols, and procedures. This type of medical control also includes the authorization of licensed prehospital providers to participate in care as a member of an agency or system. It may also include the authorization of ambulances and other response vehicle for use in patient care and to care medical equipment and medications.

MEDICAL DIRECTION

Medical direction is sometimes considered the same as off-line medical control. Although it does include this activity, it is a higher level of involvement at the agency level. This refers to advising agency administrators on minimum standards for providers, setting educational standards, reviewing policies and procedures, and advising on medication and equipment choices. Despite some administrative functions, the medical director is not the EMS system administrator in the vast majority of cases. Administrative directors (CEO, COO, director of operations, etc), as opposed to medical directors, typically focus on finance, human resources, staffing, contracts, political relations, and protection of corporate interest.

MEDICAL OVERSIGHT

Medical oversight is typically performed by a medical director(s) at the local, regional, and state levels, in collaboration with regulatory authorities, regional/county medical directors, and advisory committees in many jurisdictions.[1] In addition to the duties described under off-line medical control and medical direction, medical oversight involves interaction with local, regional, and state authorities and stakeholders. Medical oversight requires a broad understanding of the emergency medical system as a whole and ensuring proper policies and procedures exist to ensure safe transitions of care and the utilization of appropriate resources in the field.

MEDICAL CONTROL, DIRECTION, AND OVERSIGHT

The four EMS physician roles (online medical control, off-line medical control, medical direction, and system oversight) may overlap, have multiple and ambiguous titles, or receive variable focus depending on individual system parameters, but they should be understandable as a progression from direct patient care through consultation regarding that care, review of care, and system design/oversight to optimize care.

Medical control, both on-scene (EMS physician) and online (direct), implies a concurrent process with patient care. In other words, the physician input occurs during the care of a specific patient or patients (in a multiple casualty incident where simultaneous consultation occurs regarding a group of patients). The on-scene EMS physician may be an integral part of the ambulance or helicopter crew, serve in a responding supervisory role for a region or system, be a service medical director who supports the service through scene presence, or may be a member of a major incident, search and rescue, or disaster response team. These physicians should be integrated and accepted members of the EMS scene presence, and their role (which may vary significantly) should be clearly

understood by the EMS providers, the EMS physician, local emergency departments/hospitals, and the system oversight authority. Otherwise, conflict may occur between the on-scene EMS physician and the system's physician substituted judgment as reflected in guidelines and protocols. Online (direct) medical control also occurs concurrent with patient care, typically during a telephone, radio, or computer communication between EMS providers and an emergency physician at the intended receiving hospital, "resource" hospital, or designated medical control base station (or telemetry station). The online medical control physician must be rapidly available, have sufficient understanding of the communications technology employed and the EMS system to interact in a helpful manner, and be able to promptly provide concise guidance to EMS providers based on current protocols and available drugs and equipment.

Medical direction typically includes both off-line (indirect) medical control and other functions of a service or system medical director, such as training, quality assurance, pharmaceutical, and other responsibilities. However, in many jurisdictions, off-line medical control is provided by a physician or committee at a designated hospital or governmental entity. In these situations, quality assurance review of EMS charts is augmented by (HIPAA-appropriate) access to emergency department and hospital records. Ideally, the service medical director collaborates with the off-line medical control process to institute quality improvements when the two functions are performed by different people or institutions.

EMS *system oversight* is a collaborative process that includes physician consultation with a regulatory/licensing authority (often at the state department of health, public safety, or department of transportation) and cooperation with various committees and boards comprised of physicians, EMS providers, and other stakeholders (hospital staff, specialty clinicians, representatives of various interest groups, etc). Physicians involved in system oversight must have an understanding of public health, financial and political influences on the system, human resources issues, and other administrative aspects of EMS. In some states, a physician medical director holds strong authority over system design, scope of practice, and other aspects of EMS practice. In other cases, the state-level authority functions in an empowering and coordinating role, and most aspects of EMS practice are controlled at a regional, county, or even individual service level.

PHYSICIAN KNOWLEDGE AND INVOLVEMENT IN EMS

In order to prevent substandard medical control, direction, and oversight, systems should require formal standardized training for physicians providing these important functions.

ONLINE MEDICAL CONTROL

The most basic qualifications for physician involvement in EMS apply to online medical control physicians. These physicians are in communication with EMS providers during patient care. Therefore, they must understand the local EMS system, including provider levels and scope of practice, use of guidelines and/or protocols, and communications technology. There may be additional knowledge required depending on the use of special EMS resources (tactical teams, urban search and rescue teams, wildfire or wilderness EMS providers, mass or sports event EMS, etc) in the area. In almost all cases, they should be emergency physicians or pediatric emergency physicians as indicated by patient age. Prompt availability for consultation implies either presence in an emergency department or a system where the online medical control physician is designated to provide this service and equipped with the necessary communications tools. Training for these physicians, assuming that they are residency trained in emergency medicine and have immediate access to relevant documents (guidelines, protocols, patient destination plans, etc) can be brief, likely fewer than 5 hours, and may be significantly amenable to online or other distance learning techniques. While many of these topics are covered in the emergency medicine residency curriculum, local system variation mandates additional training/orientation. After

TABLE 4-1 Education for Online Medical Control Physicians

EMS system overview	Overview of EMS providers, system design, and scope of practice
Regional system structure	Regional structure including legal authority, regulatory oversight, guidelines, disaster response plans
Local system	Local practices and protocols
EMS response practices	Refusals, specialty centers, alternative destinations, air medical, physician response teams
Role of physicians	Online, on-scene, off-line, medical oversight
Providers	Provider types and scope of practice
Vehicles	Ground, air, special rescue
Documentation and review	PCRs, signing physician orders, chart review process
Communications	Radio system, physician operation, radio etiquette
Medical control practical	Hands-on practice with equipment in scenarios with providers

TABLE 4-2 Additional Training for On-Scene Medical Direction

Scene safety	Driving, parking, vehicle operations, hazards of extrication and rescue, use of police or special teams (HAZMAT, USAR) to secure scenes
Scene operations	Physician roles in directing care, integration with incident command and EMS providers, providing care, particularly if there are hazards from extrication, etc
Special operations	Role in extrication, tactical situations, psychiatric emergencies, technical rescue, etc
Communications	Hierarchy of operation, operation of equipment, and maintenance of communications equipment
Care and transport	Practices involving physician transport, vehicle operations, altitude physiology, report to receiving facilities, patient handoff, documentation and readiness for future responses
Quality assurance	Integration with the off-line medical control system, including documentation, flagging of issues, concerns, or examples of excellence, review process, etc

confirming initial competence, recurrent training and verification are necessary when there are system changes (protocol updates, new treatments, changes in destination plans, etc). Specific topics that should be covered in training include a number of important introductory concepts (**Table 4-1**).

ON-SCENE MEDICAL CONTROL

More extensive training is necessary for physicians who provide on-scene medical control. In addition to the knowledge necessary to provide online medical control, physicians who respond to the scene must be familiar with EMS equipment and practices, scene safety, local incident management hierarchy, and system-specific practices related to physicians at EMS scenes. If driving emergency vehicles or responding to incident scenes, these physicians should have experience or training in emergency driving techniques, safe scene parking practices, and use of warning lights and sirens. To effectively integrate into the EMS system, these physicians should be familiar with, and be accepted by, the leadership and EMS providers they work with, and with staff at local emergency departments. Training requirements for these physicians will vary depending on their background and system parameters. Those who worked as EMS providers prior to becoming physicians may require shorter training and should achieve competency more rapidly. Systems where the physician is more hands-on with extrication, rescue and other technical aspects of EMS will need more training time, whereas systems using on-scene medical control in a more hands-off advisory role may achieve competence (including training the physician regarding safety around technical EMS efforts) in a shorter period of time. Systems where the physician provides transport care (by ground ambulance, helicopter, or other vehicle) will need to include training for those aspects of care, perhaps including vehicle operations, inventory, altitude physiology, etc.[2] Topics that should be covered in training in addition to those for online medical control are listed in **Table 4-2**.

OFF-LINE MEDICAL CONTROL

Physicians providing off-line medical control should have a thorough understanding of the EMS system beyond that required for online medical control, and a basic understanding of the system's use of on-scene medical control, if any. In addition, these physicians should be comfortable with topics such as CQI, risk management, HIPAA requirements, liability protection, and understand their responsibilities and authorities as system managers (**Table 4-3**).

A key component of the provision of off-line medical control is the review of documentation. For the physician to be effective in this role, they must possess a detailed understanding of the mechanics of charting (Which EMTs complete the record? Is it electronic, paper, or both? Do all members of the care team sign the record? What about EMTs

who did not accompany the patient during transport? What path does the record follow through the QA process and beyond?). Maintaining regulatory compliance and ensuring high-quality care require the physician to understand the role of quality assurance/improvement systems in improving care, reducing risk, identifying both excellence and concerns in care variations, aggregating data, protecting data, and transmitting results of review to providers, services, regulators, and others.

Processes vary from agency to agency and the medical director must know the mechanics of review for their agency (Does the review occur by computer, on paper, or both? Is there a committee or an individual reviewer involved? How are the results recorded? Are they peer protected, and what is the mechanism for ensuring this protection throughout the process? How are the review results transmitted to providers and others? Supervised practice reviews are recommended). In order to protect themselves, the providers, patients, and the agency from unnecessary distraction from the prehospital care mission, the medical director must be aware of certain legal issues (How is liability protection provided for the reviewer? How is due process protected for the EMS provider? How is patient confidentiality protected during the review process? Are meetings or hearings open, or closed? May services or providers present evidence, witnesses, or be represented by union officials or legal counsel at such meetings? How is peer review protection (if claimed) protected throughout the process?).

TABLE 4-3 Key Areas of EMS Medical Director Expertise

Guidelines, policies, protocols, and procedures	Development of documents designed to allow for prehospital providers to provide high-quality care
EMS personnel	Utilization of different types of providers (EMT, paramedic, flight nurse) for maximum benefit of the system, patients, and providers
Continuous quality improvement	Development and maintenance of a culture of quality and safety
Provider education	Development of a successful educational program (primary and CME)
Controlled substance program	Development of safe, secure, practices with accountability
EMS system design	Ensure best practices for resource management and delivery of high-value prehospital medical care
Communications and dispatching	Provide oversight for 9-1-1 and dispatch centers to ensure best practices in medical dispatch and prearrival instruction
Community relations and public health	Participate in public education and support advancement of public health and integration of the health care network
EMS research	Ensure availability of meaningful data for advancement of care and the utilization of evidence-based medicine in protocol design

▨ AGENCY MEDICAL DIRECTORS

Agency medical directors responsible for local or regional EMS systems will need additional training depending on their role. They should have a good understanding of the medical control topics discussed above, particularly if they serve in those roles for their service(s). Medical directors develop, review, and revise medical policies, protocols, and procedures. They authorize levels of practice of providers. They establish policies relative to difficult medicolegal issues such as refusal of care/transport, end-of-life issues, and termination of resuscitation. Medical directors must be up-to-date with pertinent medical literature and research interpretation and design. While systems vary, ideally the service medical director should have final authority over all aspects of the service that involve health and medical care, and be responsible for all relevant aspects of the service. In some situations, medical directors have limited arrangements with ambulance services, and therefore additional topics that may be relevant include:

- *EMS provider safety*: EMS is a dangerous profession, with a significant risk of injury from vehicle operations, infection or injury from patient care interaction, psychological stress, physical stress during operations, and fitness issues. The service medical director should be aware of these issues, be involved in service decisions that affect EMS provider safety, and be an advocate for safety within the EMS system.

- *Guidelines and/or protocols*: some service medical directors practice in systems where they author individual service guidelines or protocols, and the EMS providers practice under the physician's license by following these guidelines/protocols. In these systems, understanding the authority and authorship of guidelines/protocols is important.

- *Human resources*: Essential if the medical director is involved in interviewing, hire/fire/discipline decisions, setting workplace parameters and accommodations for employees, etc. In most cases, it is more appropriate for the medical director to understand, but not to participate in this component. Rather, they should strictly restrict their activities to authorization to practice and fitness for duty.

- *Billing and reimbursement*: Important if the medical director is involved in verification of billing levels, attests to levels of care required, helps decide destination facilities, vehicle or crew choices, or treatment options that influence billing, etc.

- *System integration*: How does the service obtain mutual aid, assist with disaster operations, fit into regional plans for care, interact with regulatory authorities, etc?

- *Vehicle and equipment options*: How does the service choose and maintain vehicles and equipment? Do they provide for safe EMS operations and meet the standard of care for patient treatment? Is provider training sufficient to provide safe and optimal care? The physician medical director, as final arbiter of all aspects of the service affecting patient care and the health and safety of employees, must be involved in these decisions and may be held responsible for the service's choices.

- *Service management*: Does the service's management structure, scheduling, reimbursement, benefit package, and other aspects of business operations respect EMS providers as professionals with their own health and safety needs? If the service is staffed by volunteers, how are they provided with equipment, a safe schedule, adequate training, personal protective equipment, etc?

Different agency types and structures can incorporate their medical director in various ways. Knowing the organizational chart for the agency receiving medical direction will help the physician understand their role and chain of command in the eyes of the agency leadership (**Figure 4-3**).[3]

▨ MEDICAL OVERSIGHT

In order to provide medical oversight as a regional, county, or state medical director, the emergency physician should be generally knowledgeable about the above topics and have a detailed and specific knowledge of a number of relevant areas. Understanding the interplay between *public health and EMS* and how the state EMS system integrates into general public health efforts is key. Being able to evaluate the metrics that justify (or could help support improvement in) the state's EMS system and knowing how the state is working to advance EMS, for providers, services, and patients, can guide physician efforts and program initiative development. Taking part in the state addressing challenges facing EMS, such as financial constraints, EMS provider workforce issues, patient obesity, infection risks, major incident/terrorism threats, integration of air and ground EMS services, matching available level of care to patient need, and other basic controversies can lead to greater integration and help focus efforts on patient outcome across the system.

Mastery of the *state-specific EMS system structure* leads the physician to answers to important questions—How are licensing, regulation, discipline, quality assurance, scope of practice, and other issues decided and managed at the state level? What committees and boards are involved? What is the authority and expectation of each? What are the state's special interests or challenges (geography, climate, disease prevalence, etc)? What laws and regulations control EMS in the state, and do they need modification? Without specific operational knowledge of these components, it is impossible to actively develop relationships and programs aimed at process improvement and increase in health care quality and value.

Knowing the occupational and legal expectations and protections afforded to a physician providing system medical oversight is essential in order to avoid experiencing incapacitating shortfalls and surprises. The physician must understand what liability protection is extended and how much time is needed to perform the job properly. Key occupational components such as required travel, compensation, and employment (or contractor) status are essential parts of any medical oversight agreement. Ultimately the physician must also know what the physician's authority is within the system, who they may answer to (politically or otherwise), and how conflicts of interest are managed.

Finally, there must be recognition of the way in which the system is meant to integrate into the larger EMS System. Important questions need to be asked in every system—How does the system obtain mutual aid from neighboring states? How does it handle response across borders? Does the state follow national standards for training, patient care, EMS provider safety, and physician involvement? Are the state's EMS physicians active in relevant organizations at a state and national level? How are the state's EMS physicians participating in EMS research and education to advance the field?

PERSPECTIVES ON EMS PHYSICIAN ROLES

The above discussion assumes a patient-centered role for the physician involved in an EMS system. However, there are other ways that physician involvement in EMS can be organized. For example:

- *Patient care*: Primarily as described above, but most of the focus above is on "9-1-1 emergencies," and not on critical care transport, or transport of special needs patients, for example.

- *EMS research*: Some physicians participate in the EMS system primarily or solely through their research efforts to improve EMS care.

- Product development – some physicians are involved in EMS product development, pharmaceutical applications in EMS, etc.

- *Special response/incident teams (mass events/sports, HAZMAT, tactical, wilderness, marine, dive rescue, search, cave rescue, disaster, urban/structure, fire (particularly wildland fires), ski patrol*: All of these response types present special challenges and opportunities for the interested physician, and require specific training.

- *Training and education*: Physician educators can integrate with the EMS system through various educational efforts, including injury prevention efforts provided for the public, EMS provider training, and training of

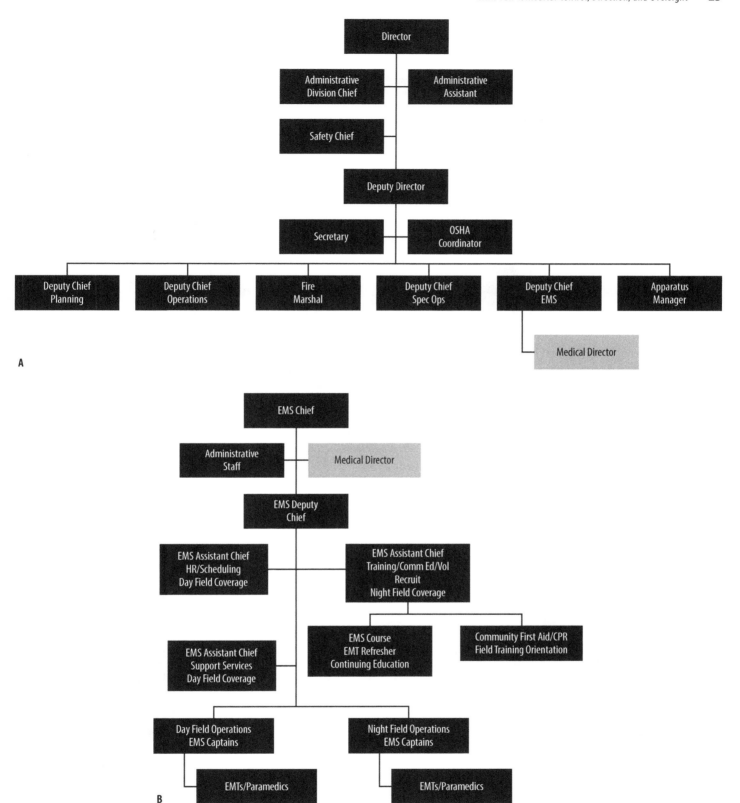

FIGURE 4-3. Examples of agency organizational charts. A: Fire department (Memphis, Tennessee, Fire Department). B: Third service model (Town of Colonie, New York, Department of Emergency Medical Services). C: Fire department (Prince William County, Virginia, Department of Fire and Rescue). D: Private for-profit (LifeCare Medical Transports, Virginia). (Modified from International Association of Fire Chiefs. Emergency Medical Services Section; Department of Homeland Security. Office of Health Affairs. *Handbook for EMS Medical Directors*. Emmitsburg, MD : Department of Homeland Security. Federal Emergency Management Agency. United States Fire Administration; March 2012.)

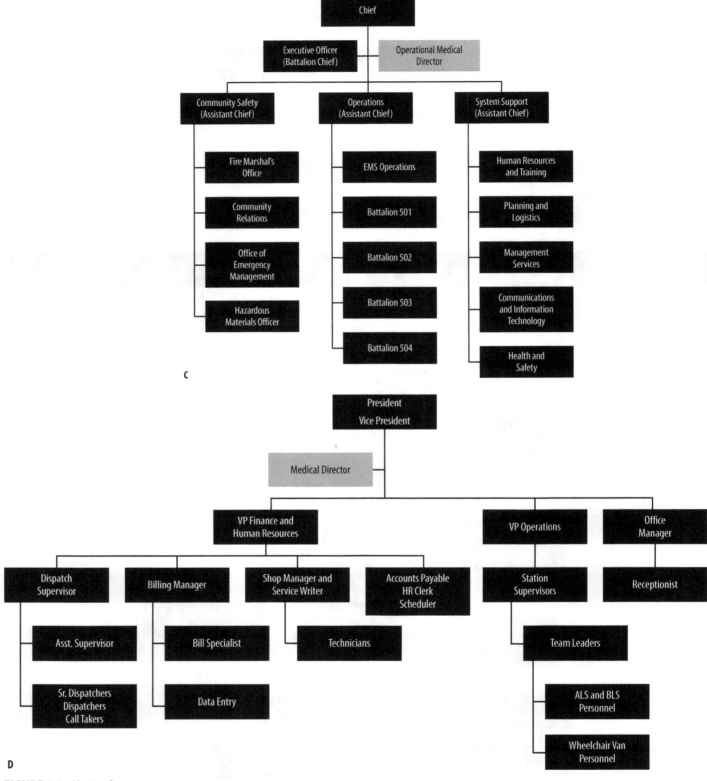

C

D

FIGURE 4-3. (*Continued*)

EMS physicians. Use of distance learning, adult learning techniques, just-in-time training, high-fidelity simulation, and other techniques make this an exciting and challenging aspect of EMS, particularly since manual skill is just as important as book knowledge. With the advent of EMS as a recognized subspecialty of emergency medicine, physicians will be more involved in EMS as both teachers and learners.

- *Documentation and billing*: Physicians have developed billing companies, software to document care, integrated EMS dispatch/tracking/ documentation/billing suites, and other technologies to assist with EMS documentation, quality assurance, and reimbursement.

- *Policy*: EMS is an evolving field, and therefore subject to policy scrutiny. Recent efforts by NHTSA to develop research and education (provider levels and scope of practice) agendas[4] are evidence that physician input is essential in this area.

- *Organizations/associations*: Many physicians are active in EMS at a national or international organization level, usually as an adjunct to other EMS activities. The National Association of EMS Physicians (NAEMSP), the Air Medical Physician Association (AMPA), and the National Association of EMS Officials (NASEMSO) are three major EMS-focused associations. There are also active EMS sections within ACEP, SAEM, and other physician organizations.

REGULATION OF EMS PHYSICIANS

Individual ambulance services may, through job description, contract, or typical practice, impose limits and expectations on EMS physicians they interact with—typically with a service medical director, but also with hospital-based providers of online (direct) medical control and other physicians. Local, regional, or state EMS authorities may similarly have expectations for the EMS physicians practicing in (or visiting) their area, including those providing on-scene care, medical direction, and system oversight. This regulation may take the form of minimum qualifications, required training, certification, contractual requirements, authorization to participate in the system, limits on authority, etc. Similarly, EMS physicians should have expectations of the EMS system, services, and providers they interact with. This may include reassurance regarding liability protection, access to technology, compensation, authority to direct care and other practices in accordance with standards of care and their wishes, input into budget, equipment, and personnel decisions, and other important areas of practice.

Some states have formalized EMS physician interaction with their system at a statewide, regional, or service level. This involvement can be centralized, or distributed among regions, counties, or even individual ambulance services. For example, in Maine EMS authority is centralized by a law which requires appointment of a state EMS medical director and regional medical directors. Together with a representative from the Maine Chapter of the American College of Emergency Physicians, these EMS physicians develop statewide EMS protocols and perform other duties.[5] Maryland has a more distributed system, with the physician authority empowered by regulation, including state, regional, and local "operational program" (service level) medical directors all regulated by a board of stakeholders appointed by the governor.[6] In Massachusetts and Rhode Island, the actual authority is held by the state EMS office, and the physician EMS medical director and various boards and councils have advisory input.[7,8] In Ohio, a more distributed system, a state board with physician input sets maximum limits on scope of practice, but individual service physician medical directors control the actual practice protocols for each service.[9]

Various professional organizations provide guidance on EMS physician practice, and offer education, position statements, research forums, and other support. To a large extent, these efforts provide a forum for and repository of EMS physician practice and training guidelines in the United States. Several offer position papers on training and qualifications of EMS physicians in various roles, and provide training for physicians seeking to meet those qualifications.

NAEMSP

The National Association of EMS Physicians, founded in 1984, is a US association focused entirely on EMS physician practice. It publishes a journal, hosts conferences, publishes texts, and coordinates efforts such as a Council of EMS Fellowship Directors and a curriculum for EMS fellowships (www.naemsp.org).

AMPA

The Air Medical Physician Association, founded in 1992, is a US-based international association focused on physician involvement in ground and air critical care transport aspects of EMS. It publishes a textbook, collaborates in publication of a journal and organization of several annual conferences, has position papers, and supports EMS research (www.ampa.org).

SAEM

The Society for Academic Emergency Medicine also has an EMS interest group and offers an EMS fellowship scholarship (www.saem.org).

ACEP

The American College of Emergency Physicians has a standing EMS committee and interest sections including EMS and Air Medical Transport (www.acep.org).

Both ACEP and NAEMSP have provocative position statements concerning the medical direction of EMS services and are relevant to EMS physician studies. The ACEP position statement covers components and medical director qualifications for off-line medical control, online medical control, local EMS medical directors, regional/state medical directors, and medical directors for air medical, nonemergency, wilderness EMS, tactical EMS, interfacility transport programs. The ACEP site reviews the ideal qualifications, responsibilities, and authority for each type of medical direction and discusses how the system should support these activities.[10]

EMS PHYSICIAN TRAINING

Many physicians involved in EMS are former, or current, EMS providers, having begun their medical careers as EMTs or other first responders. Emergency medicine residency training, according to the ACGME Residency Review Committee, must include "Residents must have experience in emergency medical services (EMS), emergency preparedness, and disaster management.

1. EMS experiences must include ground unit runs and should include direct medical command.
2. This should include participation in multi-casualty incident drills.
3. If programs require residents to ride in air ambulance units, the residents must be notified of this requirement and associated liabilities during the resident recruitment process.

Residents should have experience teaching out-of-hospital Emergency Medicine emergency personnel.[11] While no specific time parameters are included in these requirements, many residencies fulfill them in the equivalent of 2- or 4-week rotations during 3 or 4 years of residency training. For those emergency physicians seeking deeper understanding of EMS, and a career focused on EMS, fellowship training is available. On September 23, 2010, the American Board of Medical Specialties unanimously voted to make EMS a medical subspecialty, under the auspices of the American Board of Emergency Medicine (ABEM),[12] but exact training and certification requirements were not clear until the ACGME accreditation process began in 2013. The advent of this subspecialty certification begins a process where EMS fellowship training, and subspecialty certification are likely to become highly recommended or required for physicians focusing their career on EMS. More detail on this area is contained in Chapter 3.

KEY POINTS

- The American Board of Medical Specialties (ABMS) approved EMS as a subspecialty under the American Board of Emergency Medicine (ABEM) on September 23, 2010.
- There are four major roles for physician involvement in EMS: on-scene medical control, online medical control, off-line medical control, and EMS system oversight.
- Other physician roles also include research, education, product development, disaster response, mass event/sports coverage, and integration of EMS with the rest of the health care system.
- All physician EMS roles require training, integration with the EMS system, and continuous efforts to improve quality, safety, and patient care.

REFERENCES

1. Summary of EMS Boards Survey by NASEMSO Medical Director's Council, communication from Carol Cunningham (Council Chair), September 7, 2011.
2. Thomas SH, Williams KA, for the 2002-2003 Air Medical Services Task Force of the National Association of EMS Physicians. Flight physician training program—Core content*. http://www.naemsp.org/Documents/Position%20Papers/POSITION%20Flight%20Physician%20Training%20Program.pdf. Accessed April 9, 2015.
3. International Association of Fire Chiefs. Emergency Medical Services Section; Department of Homeland Security. Office of Health Affairs. *Handbook for EMS Medical Directors*. Emmitsburg, MD: Department of Homeland Security. Federal Emergency Management Agency. United States Fire Administration; March 2012. http://www.usfa.fema.gov/downloads/pdf/publications/handbook_for_ems_medical_directors.pdf. Accessed April 9, 2015.
4. Emergency Medical Services. http://www.ems.gov/. Accessed September 8, 2011.
5. Maine Revised Statutes. http://www.mainelegislature.org/legis/statutes/32/title32sec83.html. Accessed September 12, 2011.
6. Title 30 Maryland Institute For Emergency Medical Services Systems (MIEMSS) http://www.dsd.state.md.us/comar/subtitle_chapters/30_Chapters.aspx. Accessed September 12, 2011.
7. http://www.mass.gov/eohhs/gov/departments/dph/programs/hcq/oems/public-health-regulations-emergency-services.html. Accessed April 9, 2015.
8. http://www.health.ri.gov/regulations/?parm=Emergency%20Medical%20Services. Accessed April 9, 2015.
9. 4765.02 State board of emergency medical, fire, and transportation services. http://codes.ohio.gov/orc/4765.02. Accessed September 12, 2011.
10. American College of Emergency Physicians. Clinical & practice management. Medical direction of emergency medical services PREP. http://www.acep.org/Clinical---Practice-Management/Medical-Direction-of-Emergency-Medical-Services-PREP/. Accessed October 1, 2013.
11. http://www.acgme.org/acgmeweb/Portals/0/PFAssets/2013-PR-FAQ-PIF/110_emergency_medicine_07012013.pdf. Accessed April 9, 2015.
12. http://www.abms.org/member-boards/contact-an-abms-member-board/american-board-of-emergency-medicine/. Accessed April 9, 2015.

CHAPTER 5

Protocols, Policies, and Guidelines

Kenneth A. Williams
Derek R. Cooney

INTRODUCTION

Prehospital emergency medical care by EMS providers can be defined as physician-directed medical care in the prehospital setting with or without ambulance transport. A wealth of details clarifies this definition within specific jurisdictions and for particular circumstances. The care provided by prehospital providers as a part of the EMS system is a practice of medicine with standards of care established by the training and experience of practitioners and system leaders. Therefore, a key component of the EMS system is physician oversight and medical direction. A well-developed and well-designed EMS system usually incorporates four opportunities for physician input:

- System design
- Operational policies and guidelines
- Patient care protocols
- Medical direction

In an excellent EMS system, all four opportunities are coordinated by EMS physicians collaborating with EMS professionals to produce excellent and efficient care for patients while improving all aspects of the system and the providers working within it. System design, at a national and state level, provides guidance regarding curriculum, scope of practice, regulatory & licensing structure, and other overall aspects of the EMS system. Medical direction, provided at the time of care (online) and all other activities of the medical director (off-line), is discussed in chapter 4. This chapter focuses on the development of protocols, policies, procedures, and guidelines and defining important concepts relative to these activities.

OBJECTIVES

- Define the terms *guidelines*, *policies*, *procedures*, *protocols*.
- Define the terms *scope of practice* and *standard of care*.
- Discuss how the above concepts relate to the medical care provided in the field.
- Describe the processes involved in development of guidelines, policies, procedures, and protocols.

In order to fully appreciate the importance of clear and definitive documents defining prehospital medical operations, it is essential to know the purpose of the different document types and understand how they serve to define the parameters by which prehospital care is delivered. If the medical director confuses these components, and their purpose, there is potential for inappropriate development of these documents that could lead to operational, regulatory, legal, and medical complications.

KEY TERMS AND DEFINITIONS

Guidelines: provide broad parameters for management of a particular problem. They should be the result of expert consensus, based on evidence, and typically apply at a national or international level. An example would be recommending early 12-lead ECG acquisition for EMS patients with possible cardiac ischemia as a method to triage STEMI patients to the best treatment option.

Scope of practice: is the range of care expected and allowed for a particular type of care provider, such as an EMT or paramedic, but the term applies to all types of providers. It typically is described in laws, regulations, and protocols and includes allowed procedures, medications, and requirements for each type of provider in a system. Scope-of-practice documents define the bounds of practice expectation and procedural limits for providers. An example would be describing the level of provider and training required to acquire and interpret a 12-lead ECG. In many cases performing and intervention outside a provider's scope of practice could have legal implications, even if they were given an order by a physician to performing an intervention.

Standard of care: is the minimum acceptable quality of practice expected of a provider of similar level or type facing a particular situation. The standard of care for any particular instance is usually derived from review of medical literature, position papers from expert panels, and by examining local practices. It is typically limited by the scope of practice and defined during legal proceedings through review of these materials and the expert opinion of providers with the same or similar training as the provider being evaluated, and should be applied to the same or similar clinical circumstances. *Acceptable practice* is performed above the standard of care; practice below the standard of care is *negligent practice*. While some aspects of the standard-of-care apply without regard to geography, variability in EMS scope of practice, guidelines and protocols may create local and regional variations in the standard of care. An example would be the expectation that trained and equipped providers would obtain a 12-lead ECG early in the care of a 48-year-old patient with acute onset of atraumatic chest pain. Breaches in the standard of care can be ground for the allegations of malpractice in cases where harm and causality can be established.

Policies: set forth the general operational parameters for a system or service. They encompass all aspects of operation (eg, human resources, equipment maintenance, and response for patient care, etc). They may reflect these elements of a national organization, a state agency, or an individual ambulance agency. Examples would be the ACEP Policy on Leadership in Emergency Medical Services,[1] or an ambulance agency policy that sets out a clinical goal to provide the best possible patient care.

Protocols: specify care, often including the chronological order of care, for a specific situation or patient complaint. They are often service or system specific. They implement guidelines and policies. An example would be a protocol that sets forth the steps expected by the EMS system in the care of a 48-year-old patient with chest pain.

Procedures: are delineated methods to perform tasks or implement policies and protocols. They are typically detailed, ordered, and specific to the service, piece of equipment, or task. An example would be the exact steps necessary to acquire a 12-lead ECG using the particular brand and model of monitor available at a particular ambulance service.

OTHER DEFINITIONS

Physician directed: means that properly committed, knowledgeable, and collaborative physicians provide oversight for the EMS system. EMS is a developing subspecialty, and board-certified EMS physicians will eventually become the logical choice to serve in this role, supported by consultation with other medical specialties as indicated. Currently, many physicians with varied training and backgrounds provide EMS system oversight. This physician oversight may take many forms, and does not require that a physician be present at every EMS incident, communicate with EMS providers during every patient transport, review every document, or teach every EMS course, although these circumstances may be indicated at times. Instead, what we mean is that physician oversight is reflected throughout the EMS system wherever patient care is involved. This oversight may, for example, take the form of EMS provider scope of practice and curriculum guidance, direct and indirect education, research, efforts to seek and secure system funding, provider standards and supervision, development and interpretation of guidelines, policies, protocols and procedures, and other measures that implement physician judgment throughout the EMS system. The degree and mechanism of physician direction will vary from system to system, as designated by the laws, regulations, and other guidance of the jurisdiction.

Ambulance: refers to any vehicle or conveyance used to transport patients or personnel and equipment used to treat patients, including all associated equipment, supplies, and medications. These vehicles may or may not be dedicated to sole use as ambulances, may or may not be motorized, and may be designed for a variety of travel environments (ie, air, on and off road, water, snow, mud, wilderness, urban structures, etc). Ambulances and their associated equipment may be specified by, inspected by, and their operation and use controlled by the EMS system. The degree and mechanism of ambulance control and regulation will vary from system to system, as designated by the laws, regulations, and other guidance of the jurisdiction.

Transport: means the potential that a patient or patients may be best served by physical relocation from their current location to another for medical care, safety, or other associated purpose. This may include evaluation and care to determine if such transport is indicated, the actual movement of patients within or between entities or facilities, and any associated vehicles, mechanisms, and personnel. It also includes search for and rescue of patients from entrapment or other hazardous circumstances, evacuation of persons during a time of hazard, care at gatherings and mass events, and transportation to, from, or between temporary, emergency, or alternate health care entities.

Patient: any person to whom the EMS system owes, or may owe, a duty of care. Patients may include those who have gathered at a mass event and are potentially in need of medical care, persons living in or located in a particular area or circumstance (such as a flood zone or epidemic area), persons in routine or emergency need of medical evaluation, care, and/or transportation, and any other person within the jurisdiction of the EMS system who may be affected by the design, operation, regulation, or other aspects of the EMS system and its personnel and equipment.

Care: is that medical evaluation and treatment provided to a patient by an EMS provider. It may include physical relocation to a place of greater safety, remote evaluation of patient circumstances or risk, efforts to identify a patient, obtaining a medical history from the patient or others, hands-on physical examination, testing (including laboratory testing, imaging, and other evaluation), and treatment with medications, devices, equipment, and transport. Care includes ensuring the safety of patients, providers, and others through the use of accepted means to immobilize, restrain, protect, splint, isolate, and otherwise provide measures that protect patients, providers, and others from harm.

GUIDELINES, POLICIES, PROCEDURES, AND PROTOCOLS AS TOOLS FOR DEFINING EMS SYSTEM STRUCTURE

Organization of EMS systems is, ideally, logical and transparent. When asked, "Why do we do it that way?" it is helpful to have both evidence and structure supporting the answer. Proper development of (or reference to) relevant guidelines when defining scope of practice, creating protocols, and drafting policies and procedures provides the foundation for good quality EMS practice. The tools then available to system leaders (protocols, procedures, etc) are used to ensure that best practices are provided throughout the system. Of course, a thorough quality improvement system is necessary to close the loop.

■ GUIDELINES

Guidelines paint, in broad strokes, current best practice information (or the lack thereof—such as the lack of a single recommended outcome measure for cardiac arrest studies[2]). They are a means to promulgate current best practice information throughout the EMS system. They should be developed using an objective, transparent, and commonly accepted approach to evaluating the evidence, and should answer important clinical questions. However, guidelines require interpretation and review before application during patient care.

The development of guidelines probably does not occur at a local level. As a statement of expert consensus after review of the best available evidence, guidelines are typically beyond the scope of a local EMS

system. However, to be applied locally they need to be examined and interpreted to ensure that their local use matches needs, operational capabilities, and realities, and can be measured through a quality assurance process to assess both positive and negative influences on the local EMS system. A number of national professional organizations maintain guidelines (sometimes referred to as positions) relevant to EMS systems (eg, National Association of EMS Physicians, American College of Emergency Physicians, American Heart Association, American College of Surgeons). A process should be described for the evaluation of the evidence used in development of these guidelines, including scoring of the evidence considered[3] and conflict of interest management during involvement of the experts involved in the guideline development process.[4]

■ POLICIES

Policies generally flow from the overall system mission and operational goals. They should have a standard format that transparently identifies the author or authors, the authority for the policy, date of origination and any revisions, and a system to catalog revisions as they occur. Policies reflect the personality of the agency and set out goals for operations and practices, but do not provide details about how those goals are carried out. Flowing from administration and vetted through an established process, policies must also be checked to be certain they comply with applicable laws, regulations, and accreditation standards. If review by state or regional regulatory organizations (or officials) is necessary, an inherent delay must be anticipated in the implementation of these policies. Policies should be clear, concise, and as brief as possible.

■ PROCEDURES

Procedures are used to itemize the exact process by which policies and protocols are implemented. Procedures are very specific to a particular brand of equipment, for example, or to local circumstances. While a policy may call for adherence to state protocols for management of patients with various emergencies, a procedure will tell the EMS provider how to operate the patient monitoring equipment, where the medications are kept in the ambulance, and how to complete the agency's documentation.

■ PROTOCOLS

Protocols specify patient care. By the nature of being a protocol, they imply a protocol-based approach to medical care. Typically this means giving specific directions to be used in response to identified problems, symptoms, findings, and situations. This may vary in implementation from a loose structure to a strict algorithm. **Box 5-1** illustrates the function of the above types of documents in an EMS system.

PROTOCOL DEVELOPMENT

Medical director input on the development of policies and procedures is important to the overall ability of the EMS physician to provide oversight to areas pertaining to medical operations (eg, controlled substances, dispatching, infection control, etc); however, protocol development is arguably the most important off-line component of medical direction. The protocol by which prehospital care is provided is an extremely important document around which the majority of the medical directors' other off-line duties revolve (ie, CQI and education).

■ DESIGN TEAM

The medical director should consider the system for which the protocol is intended and seek to involve key members of the system in the design process. A protocol being designed for a single agency in a defined geographic location may need a team of stakeholders that simply includes the medical director and several senior prehospital providers or supervisors who can help fact check and provide feedback on the usability and applicability of the protocol. These individuals will also provide the medical director with essential information about the perception and interpretation of

---

Box 5-1

Guidelines, Policies, Procedures, and Protocols

As an example:

Guidelines for resuscitation from sudden atraumatic death are promulgated by the American Heart Association. A typical ambulance agency, "Example EMS", seeks to implement this guideline.

When making this determination, the Example EMS leadership should review their policies, procedures, and current practices, which should include a description of the system's operational parameters and personnel, goals, mission, and vision.

Example EMS has a *policy* stating that one goal of the agency is improved survival from sudden death within their service area. Example EMS leadership would then discuss the resuscitation guideline recommendations with key personnel, including EMS physicians, and consider improvements to their practices. Once potential options are considered, they should be discussed with and considered by key involved parties, including EMS providers, affiliated services, and the regional

hospitals. New *protocols* on cardiac arrest derived by the EMS system after reviewing the guidelines would outline the expectations for mutual aid response for timely ALS support, transport destinations and priority, and notification and telemetry to the receiving hospital.

Procedures are then developed to state exactly how Example EMS dispatchers will arrange mutual aid, what numbers they call and frequencies they use to coordinate the response, how these efforts are documented, which hospitals would be primary receiving hospitals for these patients, which patient transports would be done using lights and sirens, what information would be relayed and how, and how to transmit telemetry, including 12-lead ECGs in cases where there was return of spontaneous circulation.

In this example, international guidelines were interpreted and implemented at the local level. This process involved review and interpretation of the guidelines, as well as review of and modification to policies and procedures. It may also have included modification to or the development of protocols for patient treatment. See **Figure 5-1** *for a flowchart example of the process.*

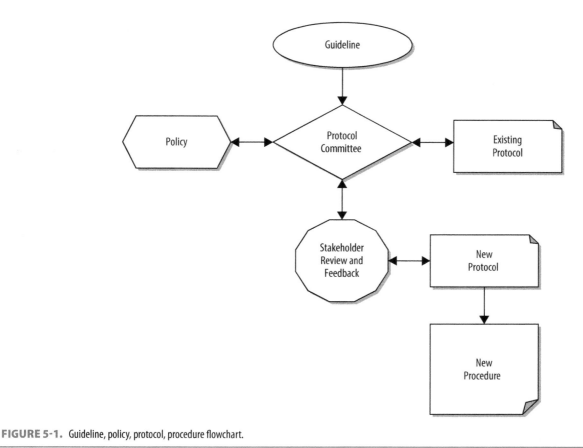

FIGURE 5-1. Guideline, policy, protocol, procedure flowchart.

---

the language and flow of the document. At times, these individuals may also note errors in design relative to scope of practice issues and help point out areas of significant educational deficits that will need to be addressed at the time of protocol rollout education. In cases of larger systems (ie, regional or state), there may be multiple medical directors and specialty physicians involved in development. Stakeholders from various type of agencies (ie, fire based, commercial, municipal third service, volunteer) from various geographical areas (ie, urban, suburban, rural, super rural) should be consulted and/or actively involved in the development of the protocols to ensure that the document represents a deliverable level of care that serves the needs of the agencies and patients it is designed to serve.

▉ DESIGN STRUCTURE

Protocol design includes decisions about how to reflect the system's structure, goals, capabilities and limitations, and philosophy. Graphic layout and structure is an important feature of design. The quality of the

flow and usability of the protocol by all levels of provider is an important area of focus and a number of questions should be asked (**Box 5-2**).

Specific physical features of the protocols may be, in part, determined by the size and environment in which they are used. Most systems favor a

---

Box 5-2

Questions That Determine Design

- Are there size constraints? (pocket guide, smart phone, kept in a binder)
- Are they to be primarily visual (flowchart), textual, or both?
- Are the protocols strictly ordinal? (sequential steps to be followed in order)
- What is the depth of information to be conveyed?
- What is the system's approach regarding protocol use?

protocol book than can be carried in a pocket in some format. This allows the provider to efficiently reference the protocol in times of question or if there is a need for clarification. This limits the content and design somewhat in that a lengthy and verbose text would not logically provide for this requirement. Due to the desire to have a convenient reference for providers, many protocols have taken on a somewhat graphic appearance. In some cases this means they are color coded or in the form of a flow diagram. This may allow conveyance of more information with less text. If the steps of the protocol are to be followed exactly in order, they may actually be numbered or represented in a vertical fashion (**Figure 5-2**) instead of being designed as a branching algorithm (**Figure 5-3**) or flow chart. The depth of the information presented in the protocol can vary and some have

a large amount of reference detail added to each page in order to provide some educational component and allow providers to "study" the protocol and look up referenced material during downtime. Other reference material, such as guidelines, standards, call centers, and online databases may also be included in protocols that are designed in this fashion. Another approach is to streamline the protocol to show only the core steps in care and to provide separate reference documents and protocol education. The advantages of this style might be size and easy of reading.

IMPACT OF INTENDED IMPLEMENTATION ON DESIGN

Although the definition of a protocol is fairly specific, there is a significant amount of variability in the way in which they are employed in the

---

ROUTINE MEDICAL CARE

INTERMEDIATE

The following procedures will be performed on medical emergencies requiring Advanced Life Support:

- Assure scene safety
- Bring ALS equipment to the patient and utilize as indicated:
  - AED, Pulse oximetry, Oxygen, Suction
  - Advanced airway equipment, Continuous waveform capnography
  - IV access, Glucometer (Agencies with Regional approval)
  - Capability for field to hospital communications
- Initial patient assessment and vital signs; blood pressure, pulse, and respirations every 5–15 minutes and after every treatment (first BP manually)
- Reassurance and proper positioning
- Medical Control notification as soon as reasonable
- ● INTERMEDIATE STOP

CRITICAL CARE

- Bring ALS equipment to the patient and utilize as indicated:
  - Monitor/defibrillator
  - Medications
  - Obtain 12 Lead ECG if appropriate
- ● CRITICAL CARE STOP

PARAMEDIC
- ● PARAMEDIC STOP

MEDICAL CONTROL ORDER

Key Points/Considerations

- Multiple Patient Procedures:
  If a potential MCI exists, contact 9-1-1 center and medical control ASAP. The medical control physician may authorize standing orders during the MCI. Document incident commander's name and affiliated agency.
- Upon completion of patient assessment and identification of need for ALS, ILS transporting units need to request and then rendezvous with ALS units or transport to hospital, whichever is closer.

A

Drowning, Submersion and Diving Injuries
ESSENTIALS OF PATIENT CARE

- Remove from water (if trained and safe to do so).
- Initiate rescue breathing as soon as patient's airway can be opened (if safe to do so).
- Airway management and supplemental oxygen via non-rebreather as soon as possible.
- Pulse oximetry.
- Spinal motion restriction as indicated.
- Remove wet clothing.
- Provide and maintain patient warmth.
- Suction the airway as needed; do not attempt abdominal thrusts to remove water from the airway.

ADULT	**PEDIATRIC**
BLS CARE	**BLS CARE**
Bronchospasm secondary to water immersion • Nebulized albuterol 2.5 mg repeated as needed. • Ipratropium bromide 0.5 mg be added to albuterol.	*Bronchospasm secondary to water immersion* • Nebulized albuterol 2.5 mg repeated as needed. • Ipratropium bromide 0.5 mg be added to albuterol.
ALS CARE	**ALS CARE**
• Monitor cardiac rhythm and obtain a 12-lead ECG, and capnography (if available), if time and patient condition permits. • Consider intubation for persistent hypoxia or airway compromise.	• Monitor cardiac rhythm and obtain a 12-lead ECG, and capnography (if available), if time and patient condition permits. • Consider intubation for persistent hypoxia or airway compromise.
Evidence of hypoperfusion or hypovolemia IV Normal Saline 1 liter bolus. Repeat as needed to maintain a SBP > 90 or unitl two (2) liters.	*Evidence of age related hypotension or hypovolemia* IV or IO Normal Saline 20 ml/kg bolus. Repeat as needed.
Evidence of pulmonary edema • Do not administer Nitrates • Consider CPAP • If intubated, initiate PEEP. Begin at 5 cm H_2O and increase in increments of 5, as needed, up to 15 cm H_2O.	*Evidence of pulmonary edema* • Do not administer Nitrates • Consider CPAP • If intubated, initiate PEEP. Begin at 5 cm H_2O and increase in increments of 5, as needed, up to 15 cm H_2O.
Hypotension unresponsive to fluid therapy • Dopamine 5–20 mcg/kg/min IV infusion to maintain a SBP of >90.	*Age related hypotension unresponsive to fluid therapy* • Dopamine 5–20 mcg/kg/min IV/IO infusion to improve perfusion.
ADVANCED AUTHORIZATION	**ADVANCED AUTHORIZATION**
• Consider RSII	• Consider RSII

ON-LINE MEDICAL CONTROL

- Notify for all patients with altered mental status, hypotension or intubation.

Standing Orders and Patient Care Guidelines

B

FIGURE 5-2. Two examples of vertical flow protocols. (A: Reproduced with permission from *Collaborative Protocol Handbook*, 2013, Central New York EMS, Midstate EMS, North Country EMS. New York. B: Reproduced with permission from *EMS Protocols: Standing Orders and Patient Care Guidelines*, 2009, Harker Heights Fire and Rescue, Harker Heights, Texas.)

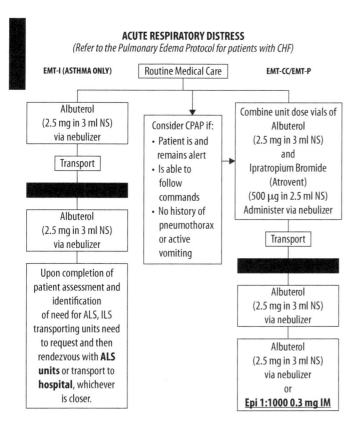

ACUTE RESPIRATORY DISTRESS
(Refer to the Pulmonary Edema Protocol for patients with CHF)

★ Contact On-line Medical Control if CPAP is utilized.

★ Aerosol therapy may be administered prior to establishing IV access.

★ Entire protocol is standing order for **Paramedics**. Epinephrine is standing order option only for patients < 50 years old.

FIGURE 5-3. Example of algorithm protocol. (Reproduced from *Protocol Handbook*, 2009 ed., Central New York EMS. Central New York Region, New York.)

provision of care by prehospital providers. Based on variability in scope of practice, regulatory limitations, and local standards of care, the medical director may need to adjust the protocol design to fit with the needs of the system. In some cases, protocols may appear almost like guidelines with open-ended points that seem to represent recommendations and reminders, whereas others may be so detailed and ordinal that they appear to represent an algorithmic recipe with little to no room for interpretation or judgment. The protocol development team must consider this variability and choose a style and structure that best suits the needs of the system. When considering a protocol they should ask a number of questions (**Box 5-3**).

Approach to Protocol Application Clinical features of a particular patient encounter can change during the prehospital phase of care. This is true in time of discovery of new information when caring for a patient who is found to be a poor historian, during reevaluation, or in response to therapy. These changes in clinical state and presentation may change the prehospital treatment goals for the patient at that time. If the intent of the protocol is that the prehospital provider will choose a protocol and "stick" to it through the rest of the care, it may be necessary to ensure that more extensive, and at times redundant, steps are contained in every one of the protocols. Alternatively, if the provider is allowed to move from protocol to protocol in response to new and changing clinical information each one could be more concise and potentially contain prompts referencing other protocols.

Protocols also typically contain prompts that usually include criteria for contacting online medical control. Typically this is when unusual circumstances are encountered, notification is needed in order to activate specialty services at the receiving facility (eg, trauma team,

Box 5-3

Questions to Ask When Evaluation a Protocol

What is the system's approach regarding application of the protocol?

• *Must EMS providers "pick-and-stick" to a protocol?*

• *Can EMS providers combine protocols to individualize for a patient?*

• *When do EMS providers need to consult medical direction?*

• *What level(s) of EMS providers are included in the protocols?*

    How does the protocol set reflect the system's philosophy?

• *Do the protocols reflect strict control over many aspects of EMS care?*

    Is there a logical structure to the protocols?

    What documentation do the protocols require? *(ECG, handoff reports, capnography waveforms)*

    Do the protocols specify destinations for particular patient problems? *(stroke, trauma, STEMI)*

    Do the protocols include instructions on use of prearrival information and instruction from dispatch, patient data, hospital records, or other sources?

catheterization lab, stroke team) or in the field (eg, helicopter, EMS physician field response), when local regulatory or scope-of-practice constraints are met, or when a perceived high-risk action is to be taken (eg, termination of resuscitation, high-risk refusal). The basis for the need to contact online medical control must be based on the specific needs of the particular system. In some systems, this may be required for the administration of controlled substances and the signing off of a patient refusal, whereas other systems may require almost no online medical control unless the provider deems it necessary or when a deviation from protocol is requested.

Provider Discretion In some systems, protocols are designed to provide the prehospital provider with options to allow for clinical judgment and provider discretion. The protocols are written in such a way as to allow for some choice in care paths or in medication utilization. In some instances, this represents a choice of whether or not to utilize a particular intervention (eg, may ask the provider to "consider" obtaining a 12-lead ECG) and in others it may be a choice of a range of dose or choice of medications to treat a particular condition (eg, β-blocker or calcium channel blocker, morphine or fentanyl, ketamine or versed).

Logical Structure Protocol design should include a consistent organizational structure to improve utility and access for providers. If the protocols are disorganized or difficult to follow, unintended delays and errors could occur when providers seek to reference them during patient care. A logical structure and organization of protocols also aids in protocol review and revision efforts.

Required Documentation There are a number of potential documentation requirements that can be considered during protocol development that should relate directly to key elements of patient care and CQI. Some elements that are sometimes required as parts of the patient care record (PCR) are depicted in **Table 5-1**. Documentation demands must consider a balance between provider workload and impact on patient care and input from providers and stakeholders may help delineate useful components from those that may incur less positive impact.

Defining Specialty Centers In some locations, there are recognized specialty centers that mat be considered for primary transport destination over other (sometimes closer) hospitals in cases where there is a perceived benefit due to a particular identified condition (eg, major trauma, stroke, STEMI). In addition to evaluating the documented evidence of patient benefit the medical director and protocol development team should consider local and state regulations, as well as political and financial impacts on the system. Some states have designated centers for trauma, stroke, STEMI, and others which may mandate inclusion into the protocol, or may simply offer additional information concerning the capability of specific centers. Designing bypass into the protocol could have negative impacts and

TABLE 5-1 Requiring Additional Documentation Components

Required Element	Potential Benefit
ECG, monitoring strips (rhythm and capnography)	Immediately available cardiac tracings and waveform capnography may provide important clinical information to the receiving hospital
Handoff report	Brief written report available at the time of transfer of care to the hospital staff may prevent errors due to a delay in receipt of complete information documented on the PCR
First responder report	Prevent loss of initial scene and patient presentation/intervention information
Signature of all providers (on the PCR)	Provides an opportunity for all providers to review the PCR for accuracy and completeness and potentially prevent errors in reporting

careful consideration of the criteria and provider education should occur. In addition, discussions with stakeholders should occur during the development, implementation, and redesign of this component of the protocols.

CATEGORIZATION

Categorization of protocols reflects the method used to organize the system's scope of practice and approach to various clinical challenges. While this issue appears trivial, it is an important reflection of system design, provider expectations, timing of physician involvement, and error reduction. One common categorization is general, medical, trauma, and procedural. Pediatric specific protocols are interspersed. However, another arrangement that may avoid limiting diagnostic considerations and premature closure (all chest pain becomes cardiac, all motor vehicle crashes become trauma, etc)[5] is to categorize conditions according to acuity and severity, attempting to avoid diagnostic categorization. A sample table of contents is shown in **Figure 5-4**.

INDEX

INTRODUCTION	PEDIATRIC PROTOCOLS continued
4 Medical Control Agreement	43 Altered Mental Status
5 Responsibilities of Providers	44 Asystole/PEA
ADULT PROTOCOLS	45 Facilitated Intubation
6 Routine Medical Care	46 Fluid Challenge
7 Routine Trauma Care	47 IV/IO Therapy
8 Acute Coronary Syndrome	48 Neonatal Resuscitation
9 12 Lead ECG	49 Neonatal Resuscitation - continued
10 Acute Resp. Distress Asthma/COPD	50 Pain Management
11 Airway Management	51 Percutaneous Airway
12 Airway Obstruction	52 Poisoning/Overdose
13 Allergic Reaction/Anaphylaxis	53 Seizures
14 Altered Mental Status	54 Symptomatic Bradycardia
15 Antiemesis	55 Tachycardia - Stable
16 Asystole/PEA	56 Tachycardia - Unstable
17 Burns	57 Tension Pneumothorax
18 Facilitated Intubation	58 V. Fib and Pulseless V. Tach
19 Fluid Challenge	SPECIAL PROTOCOLS
20 Hypoperfusion/Cardiogenic Shock	59 Air Medical Protocol
21 IV/IO Therapy	60 Continuous Positive Airway Pressure
22 OB Complications/Emer. Childbirth	61 Do Not Resuscitate/MOLST
23 Pain Management	62 Interfacility Transfers
24 Patient Restraint	63 Left Ventricular Assist Device (LVAD)
25 Percutaneous Airway	64 Left Ventricular Assist Device - continued
26 Poisoning/Overdose	65 Physician On Scene
27 Post Cardiac Arrest Induced Hypothermia	66 Physician On Scene Card
28 Pulmonary Edema	67 Radio Failure
29 Rapid Sequence Intubation (RSI)	68 Patient Refusals Against Medical Advice
30 Seizures	69 Termination of Resuscitation
31 Stroke	70 Transfer of Care
32 Symptomatic Bradycardia	71 Trauma Triage Criteria
33 Tachycardia - Stable	CHARTS
34 Tachycardia - Unstable	72 Adult Protocol Drug Chart
35 Tension Pneumothorax	73 Adult Protocol Drug Chart - continued
36 V.Fib and Pulseless V.Tach	74 Adult IV Drip and Pediatric Drug Charts
PEDIATRIC PROTOCOLS	75 APGAR and Abnormal Pediatric Vital Signs
37 Routine Medical Care	76 Glasgow Coma and Cincinnati Stroke
38 Routine Trauma Care	77 Cranial Nerve Exam and Visual Pain Scale
39 Acute Resp. Distress	78 Rule of Nines Chart
40 Airway Management	79 Hospital Telephone and Fax Numbers
41 Airway Obstruction	80 Hospital Telephone and Fax Numbers
42 Allergic Reaction/Anaphylaxis	81 Notes

FIGURE 5-4. Sample table of contents. (Reproduced with permission from *Collaborative Protocol Handbook,* 2013, Central New York EMS, Midstate EMS, North Country EMS. New York.)

Box 5-4

Implementation of the Protocol Design Process

1. Determine the *need* for a new protocol, or a revision.
   a. Is there new knowledge (guideline or otherwise)?
   b. What is the source for this knowledge?
   c. Should this new knowledge be applied to the EMS system?
   d. Is this knowledge an educational issue, or does it require protocol intervention?
   e. Can an existing protocol be revised, or is a new protocol needed?
2. Assemble a protocol *development* team/committee.
   a. Key members of the EMS community including EMS physician representation.
   b. Should include affected stakeholders and interest groups.
3. *Draft* the new/revised protocol.
   a. Circulate drafts to stakeholders and interest group representatives.
   b. Edit and redraft until the protocol is acceptable and medically optimal.
4. Determine the *effects* of the new/revised protocol on the system and propose a plan for managing these effects.
   a. What education will be needed?
   b. What new errors or challenges must be managed through quality assurance?
   c. Will there be expense for education, supplies, equipment, or medications?
   d. How long will it take to safely manage these effects?
5. *Introduce* the draft protocol through a transparent process.
   a. A wider audience, including emergency departments, professional groups, medical society, various state agencies, may be included.
   b. Revise, if necessary.
6. *Publish* the protocol, with effective date.
   a. Ensure that outdated versions are marked as such, or removed from circulation.
   b. Accept suggestions to correct errors, spelling mistakes, etc.

team. This can also cause confusion among providers as to when this change would take effect and how and when they are required to obtain new training to meet this change in guideline, which is now codified as protocol due to their referencing in the protocols themselves. While reviewing protocols from other systems can be very beneficial during protocol development, medical directors should be cautious when considering adoption of another system's protocols. Even when systems are geographically nearby or under a similar set of regulatory requirements, other local factors may make this practice unsound (ie, difference in hospital capabilities, provider demographics, patient demographics, associated emergency services). Medical directors and EMS systems administrators should not underestimate the need to review drafts and gain ongoing input from field providers, supervisors, and participating hospitals during the development process. Failure to involve key stakeholders and end users in the process can lead to catastrophic failure of implementation in some cases.

KEY POINTS

- Guidelines set forth best practices as described after expert review of available evidence. They require interpretation for local implementation.
- Policies set goals and expectations. They reflect standards set by law, regulation, and accreditation requirements.
- Protocols describe methods for providing care. They should be carefully designed, categorized, and implemented. Protocols are one means to define the scope of practice and standards of care for EMS providers and agencies.
- Procedures delineate procedural detail for performance of a task. They are specific to the referenced equipment, agency, or task, and should be clear, concise, and simple.
- Scope of practice defines the range of care expected from and allowed for by a specific type of care provider.
- Standard of care is defined as the minimum acceptable quality of practice expected of a provider facing a particular situation.

IMPLEMENTATION OF THE DESIGN PROCESS

Implementation of the principles discussed in this chapter results in an organized and well structured process that takes into account the key features of a system in order to ensure development of a viable protocol with high likelihood of successful implementation. The process is summarized in **Box 5-4** noting the key components: need, development, draft, introduce, publish.

In some systems, protocols are revised on a regular schedule (annually, etc) while in others they are revised or introduced based on need, administrative resources, etc. There are benefits to both approaches; the scheduled system facilitates a standardized process with expectations for development, education, expense, and implementation, while the episodic system is more agile and avoids "change for change's sake."

POTENTIAL PITFALLS

Consider avoiding the use of referencing outside guidelines in the protocol (eg, "start ACLS algorithm"). Although in most cases it is unlikely that a medical director would strongly object to an updated algorithm from a respected nation or international professional organization (eg, American Heart Association/International Liaison Committee on Resuscitation) this applies a variable to the protocols that are outside the control of the medical director and the protocol development

REFERENCES

1. American College of Emergency Physicians. Clinical & practice management. Leadership in emergency medical services. http://www.acep.org/Content.aspx?id=29540. Accessed November 29, 2011.
2. Becker LB, Aufderheide TP, Geocadin RG, et al. Primary outcomes for resuscitation science studies: a consensus statement from the American Heart Association. *Circulation.* November 8, 2011;124(19):2158-2177.
3. Morley PT, Atkins DL, Billi JE, et al. Part 3: Evidence evaluation process: 2010 International Consensus on Cardiopulmonary Resuscitation and Emergency Cardiovascular Care Science With Treatment Recommendations. *Circulation.* October 19, 2010;122(16 suppl 2):S283-S290.
4. Billi JE, Shuster M, Bossaert L, et al. Part 4: Conflict of interest management before, during, and after the 2010 International Consensus Conference on Cardiopulmonary Resuscitation and Emergency Cardiovascular Care Science With Treatment Recommendations. *Circulation.* October 19, 2010;122(16 suppl 2):S291-S297.
5. Croskerry P. Achieving quality in clinical decision making: cognitive strategies and detection of bias. *Acad Emerg Med.* November 2002;9(11):1184-1204.

CHAPTER 6

Patient Safety and Continuous Quality Improvement

Rebecca Janes

Brian Clemency

Derek R. Cooney

INTRODUCTION

Emergency medical services providers, like other health care workers, are dedicated to improving the lives of their patients. Unfortunately, even with the best of intentions, there are times where the care provided may be suboptimal. This may be the result of an error by an individual provider or a larger system issue. Providers and organizations should embrace quality improvement efforts as a means of reducing errors and improving clinical care to benefit the overall health of the patients they serve.

OBJECTIVES

- Describe the components of an EMS agency CQI program.
- Describe the components of an EMS system CQI program (local, regional, state).
- Discuss how the CQI process interfaces with protocol design (Chapter 5) and provider education (Chapter 7).
- Discuss surveillance of high-risk call types and procedures.
- Define retrospective and prospective CQI, and give examples of their use.
- Determine how patient care can be evaluated through analysis of tasks and outcomes.
- Describe how the Plan-Do-Check-Act model can be used to evaluate system changes.
- Understand the legal protections that may, or may not, be afforded to the CQI process.
- Discuss what it means to develop a culture of quality and safety.
- Discuss the importance of utilizing a Just Culture approach.

Oversight and active involvement in continuous quality improvement (CQI) is a key component of any medical director's duties to an EMS agency. CQI has been defined as a "structured organizational process for involving personnel in planning and executing a continuous flow of improvements to provide quality health care that meets or exceeds expectations."[1] When considering CQI in the EMS system it is logical to consider the components of a quality improvement program (**Box 6-1**).[1] In examining a provider, agency, or system, quality measures (now better known as performance indicators [PI]) must be examined and applied to programs and initiative designed to improve quality and patient safety.

HISTORY OF QUALITY MANAGEMENT

The basics of modern day quality improvement can be traced back to manufacturing principles from the Industrial Age. As mass production spread, it was necessary to ensure products looked similar, worked the same, and had minimal flaws or defects. Initially, these principles were limited to manufacturing and other "product"-based industries. Manufacturing is often seen as a linear process where an idea is developed and ultimately sold. The actual making of the product is typically straightforward, with high repetition and limited variability. In manufacturing, quality is often considered "conformance to requirements."[2] Historically, health care was not thought of as a product, but instead a

---

Components of a CQI Program

1. A link to key elements of the organization's strategic plan
2. A quality committee made up of representative leadership
3. Training programs for personnel
4. Mechanisms for selecting improvement opportunities
5. Formation of process improvement teams/initiatives
6. Staff support for process analysis and redesign
7. Policies that motivate and support participation in process improvement
8. Application of the scientific method and statistical process control

Modified for EMS agencies from Sollecito, WA, Johnson, JK. The global evolution of continuous quality improvement: from Japanese Manufacturing to Global Health Services. *McLaughlin and Kaluzny's Continuous Quality Improvement in Health Care*. 4th ed. Burlington, MA: Jones & Bartlett Learning; 2011. www.jblearning.com. Reprinted with permission.

---

process to maintain and improve an individual's state of health. In health care, the focus is typically on health outcomes and not defects in a product. The process is individualized to the patient and situation. As a result, provider input and variability is never completely standardized.[2] Over time, however, efforts have been made to bring TQM principles to light in health care and are the basis for the development of CQI. When examined more generally, some of the characteristics of manufacturing TQM can again be seen in the evaluation of the delivery of modern health care. In EMS, the call taking and dispatch processes are similar to an assembly line (**Figure 6-1**). When quality is redefined as customer satisfaction and improved outcomes, the so-called "product" of patient care and transport is more easily assessed. While the focus on improving efficiencies can apply in the EMS setting, the main focus is on reducing errors and improving patient outcomes.

KEY POINTS IN THE DEVELOPMENT OF MEDICAL QUALITY

Two very important publications lead to a significant cultural impact on physicians and the health care system that helped drive the system toward evidence-based medical practice and quality assessment. The *Flexner Report* (published by Abraham Flexner in 1910) exposed the serious failings of the American medical education system and detailed some of the major deficits in the practice patterns of American physicians. The resulting pressure from the American public strengthened the mission of the newly founded Council on Medical Education and a large number of medical schools were closed and the number of schools was less than half in just 25 years after the report. Around the same time *Dr Ernest Amory Codman* was pushing for hospital reform and advancing his idea of the "end-result system." He was possibly the first doctor to champion an organized system for evaluation of the outcome of medical practice on patients and advocated not only for the use of this information to guide medical practice, but also believed the information should be made public so that patients could choose their doctors and hospitals based on their outcome performance. *Sir William Osler* is credited with many accomplishments that advanced medical education and patient care, including moving medical student education the bedside, creation of residency training, and emphasizing the importance of the patient interview. Dr Olser has also been credited with introducing morbidity and mortality discussions to standard medical education for students and practicing physicians. In 1952, the *Joint Commission on Accreditation of Hospitals* (JCAH) was formed and began its work based on evaluation of hospital-based medical care and the policies and procedures that guided patient safety, leading to an "accreditation" that now has significant financial implications based on eligibility for reimbursement for care provided. Standardization and benchmarking of modern hospital patient safety efforts have been credited to this organization and their accreditation process. Most EMS medical directors know this organization as the Joint Commission on Accreditation

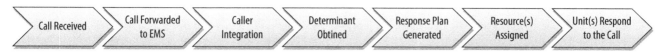

FIGURE 6-1. Process diagram for call dispatching.

of Healthcare Organizations (JCAHO); however, they have changed the name again, and it is now known as The Joint Commission (TJC). *Dr Avedis Donabedian*'s work in the 1950s to 1960s to develop an organized study and approach to health care quality is also a key component of the development of the modern CQI process. His 1966 paper entitled "Evaluating the Quality of Medical Care" is still considered an important work for study.

MODERN QUALITY MANAGEMENT STRATEGIES

In many ways the worlds of corporate business and medical practice are now intertwined, and as the recognition of medical care as an industry has matured they have increasingly been recognized as sharing many quality management goals. The pioneers of the modern quality management movement included W. Edwards Deming, Walter Shewhart, Joseph Juran, Philip Crosby.[2,4] Deming and Shewart developed the Plan-Do-Check-Act (PDCA) model (described later); Juran was among the first to directly link the quality improvement processes of manufacturing to the health care setting.[4] Juran also broke the process down into three steps: *quality planning* or ensuring the process will meet standards; *quality control* or checking to make sure the product is correct; and *quality improvement*, focusing on making the process and product better.[3] These strategies were building blocks of the modern concept of total quality management (TQM) described in 2001 by Cua, McKone, and Schroeder that went beyond these principles and pulled in concepts relevant to customers and supply as well; however, this is not always easily translated into a program focused on patient outcomes.[5] There are also several other well-known names associated with the principles of quality improvement, including ISO 9001:2000, Six Sigma, and Baldridge. Both Six Sigma and Baldridge have been studied and applied extensively to hospital settings, with degrees of success in improved efficiencies and processes.[6,7] The Lean methodology, commonly combined with Six Sigma, relates to streamlining processes and is not necessarily germane to the focus of patient safety and CQI in EMS, however, may be employed by administrators managing the operational components of an agency or system. These concepts can be compared by their component areas of focus (**Box 6-2**).

Box 6-2

Comparison of Quality Improvement Concepts

ISO 9001:2000	Baldridge	Six Sigma	Lean (Eight Areas of Waste)
1. Define system	1. Leadership	1. Define	1. Waiting
Processes	2. Strategic planning	2. Measure	2. Transportation of parts/materials/tooling
Controls	3. Customer/market focus	3. Analyze	
2. Management of system		4. Improve	3. Nonvalue-added processing
	4. Measurement, analysis and knowledge management	5. Control	4. Excess inventory
Set objectives			5. Overproduction
Review performance	5. Human resource focus		6. Defects
3. Measure, analyze, improve			7. Excess motion
	6. Process management		8. Underutilized people
	7. Business results		

EMS CQI AT MULTIPLE LEVELS

It is important for the EMS physician and medical director to recognize that key personnel and leadership at multiple levels of the EMS system must be actively engaged in CQI. Each level of organization has slightly different ideal roles in the overall system and participants at these levels must be careful to maintain their focus on important task relative to the particular level of CQI being performed. Although the highest level or system administration could attempt to perform, or be directly involved at all levels, this would prove impractical and very inefficient.

AGENCY CQI

At the agency level the CQI committee and other key personnel should consider focusing on surveillance and improvement of specific provider PI and the overall performance of the agency. Individual providers should be compared to their peers using statistics (usually evaluating for a deviation from the mean) that can allow CQI committee members and the medical director to identify individual providers that may need additional education of remediation in the identified areas. In addition, agency level CQI should include review of the agency means for PI and consider comparison to other agencies in the system or to national benchmarks. Derivation from these means could signify a need for agency-wide education and/or process improvement. CQI done at this level allows for understanding of procedural detail that may be causing some poor performance and members may be able to derive specific initiatives or process/procedure changes in an effort to improve outcomes.

SYSTEM (COUNTY/REGIONAL) CQI

At the system level, the focus should shift to evaluation of patient outcomes and the review of policies, procedures, and protocols that affect overall delivery of patient care. In some cases, a county or regional level agency may have a regulatory duty/authority over individual provider CQI when certain types of errors are made or other criteria are met. This may also be a function of state-level CQI and may result in the suspension of privileges or revocation of licensure. CQI at this level should also focus on the sharing of PI findings among agencies in the system. Errors should be reviewed in an effort to alert other agencies to the possibility of similar problems, and for the purpose of sharing quality improvement initiatives. This level of CQI should also be used to demonstrate examples of exceptional care, and to share this information with other agencies for their benefit by modeling examples of successful practice.

STATE CQI

Some functions of the state-level CQI may be somewhat similar to the system-level program; however, the state usually has regulatory authority concerns that guide the particular goals of CQI. Protocol review, narcotic diversion issues, scope-of-practice determinations, licensure concerns, and grant funding programs aimed at supporting quality improvement and best practices may all be the focus of CQI at this level.

NATIONAL CQI

Establishing national standards and setting benchmarks for PI are among the CQI goals at the national level. In some cases, nation-wide CQI efforts may guide the legislative process, set criteria for receipt of grant funding, and alter the parameters for reimbursement from Medicare and Medicaid. The National EMS Information System (NEMSIS) database serves as a platform for data collection for research into trends and could be used to assess value. Value in health care is usually defined as the impact of an intervention, or a PI, divided by the cost of the intervention or service. This concept could also be developed into a methodology by which EMS agencies reimbursement could be transitioned to a pay-for-performance model.

QUALITY ASSURANCE VERSUS IMPROVEMENT

Quality assurance is defined as, "retrospective review or inspection of services or processes that is intended to identify problems."[3] In this process, the review begins after an event has occurred, and the focus is often on the actions of individual providers measured against some standard or threshold. Providers receiving feedback may consider it punitive or subjective. Some quality can be achieved with quality assurance, but the effect is often to settle for "good enough" if a subjective standard is met.[8]

CQI focuses on the improvement of processes, systems, or organizations as a whole.[3] Individual providers may be the focus of education and training, but most focus is on the systemic problems with a process. The improvement process is data driven, and the focus is in education and improvement, not discipline.[8]

In medicine, CQI principles are seen prominently in clinical practice guidelines.[9] Guidelines are developed using best practices to improve the processes of patient care. These guidelines help decrease the types of variations in clinical practice that can lead to poor outcomes. In EMS, providers practice understanding orders or protocols supplemented by online medical control orders. Protocols can be considered similar to clinical practice guidelines, though it is important to ensure protocols are based on up-to-date information.

MAKING QUALITY A PRIORITY

With limited budgets in EMS, the focus tends to be drawn toward reacting to the present crisis. Thinking of quality in general is a proactive process. This makes planning, budgeting, and prioritizing quality improvement activities difficult. Quality assurance, at minimum, is often a requirement at the state level for ambulance service licensing/certification.[10] Many states require evidence of or participation in activities such as patient care report reviews, data collection, continuing education. Organizations may choose to go no further than the required quality assurance activities, but this will not result in improvement. Quality improvement starts with the deliberate decision by an organization to be proactive in improving the patient care it provides.

Since the 2006 Institute of Medicine report "Emergency Medical Services at the Crossroads" a greater emphasis has been placed on developing system-wide (and nation-wide) quality improvement initiatives with established benchmarks for PI. In addition to agencies' and providers' interest in ensuring high-quality patient care, and the desire to maintain regulatory compliance, there is also a possible direct financial consideration that can justify an increased focus on CQI. Based on the "pay-for-performance" reimbursement model that continues to become an ever-greater influence on health care finance, these PI are likely to become the basis for reimbursement in the future.

EVALUATING TASKS

One way to evaluate care is by task performance. EMS protocols lend themselves well to this type of evaluation by providing benchmarks. A reviewer can turn to the appropriate protocol for a chief complaint and compare the protocol to the actual care performed. A similar task-based evaluation is common in practical skills testing. While this method is useful, the binary "did" or "did not" approach to procedures may lead to an oversimplification. It may also fail to recognize how well the procedure was performed, or whether it was done at the appropriate time during the encounter.

When a case is reviewed retrospectively, some tasks are easy to point out when they are done versus when they are not done. Spinal immobilization is one task that traditionally has been easy to review retrospectively when not performed. The lack of immobilization in the setting of

a significant mechanism raises a red flag, which is easy for a reviewer to find. Conversely, it may be difficult for a reviewer to identify a case where spinal immobilization was performed though not indicated. Spinal immobilization will continue to be an important topic of conversation as the EMS community continues to focus on the iatrogenic effects of immobilization and has moved away from reflexive immobilization of all trauma patients.[11]

Administering dopamine to a hypertensive patient is a clear error of commission. However, evaluating a patient with a mild allergic reaction who receives epinephrine inappropriately may be more difficult to evaluate. The patient may have been adequately treated with diphenhydramine, but the reviewer may be unable to determine this retrospectively from a case review.

Medication errors have been well studied in the hospital setting and are estimated to account for one of the largest portions of preventable medical errors.[12] While usually only one patient is being cared for in the EMS setting, the other medication "rights" still apply and errors can occur with these. A medication could be given in the wrong site, such as IV access obtained in the same arm as a fistula; the wrong concentration, such as epinephrine 1:1000 versus 1:10,000; the wrong route, such as IV versus IM administration; or the wrong medication, such as with two similarly shaped or colored vials. Evaluating the tasks associated with medication administration ensures that potential errors are recognized, and processes can be improved if needed.[13]

When evaluating the events that make up an error, a *root cause analysis* (RCA) style approach can be considered. The nature, magnitude, and the timing of the error are all potentially important to determining the root cause(s). RCAs usually require a team approach and it may be helpful to construct a patient care timeline from available data and documentation. In some cases, multiple root causes may be identified. As in RCA for production and business, the CQI RCA should result in identification of causes that can then be addressed by remediation, education, and institution of preventative measures. The goal is to reach proactive solutions, rather than simply deriving reactive ones.

MEASURING OUTCOMES

Outcome-based reviews are important for all health care professionals. Outcome measures are especially difficulty for prehospital providers who have a single, brief interaction with their patient. There are some changes that can be measured in transport: return of spontaneous circulation (or loss of pulse), improvement in vital signs, and reduction in pain are all potential short-term outcome measures that can be identified within a single EMS patient encounter. However, these may not always reflect the patient's long-term outcome.

Many EMS providers have traditionally held the myopic view that any patient who is "alive when we get to the hospital" is a success. In truth, a patient dying during transport because of an error, though critically important, is probably fairly infrequent. These events must be reviewed extensively when they do occur. Morbidity or mortality later on as a result of prehospital care is more likely. Improper oxygenation of a head injury patient, leading to a poor neurologic recovery, is one such example. Obtaining feedback from the hospital allows agencies to better understand the bigger picture and their role in the overall care of the patient.

Hospital feedback is especially important in missed diagnosis/missed identification of conditions. For example, an agency may believe it is treating ST-elevation myocardial infarction (STEMI) patients correctly if a review of their records shows that 100% of patients with a provider impression of STEMI are taken to a PCI-capable center. Unfortunately, such a review is limited to cases where the provider had correctly identified the patient condition. This type of review would overestimate compliance by only reviewing cases where a diagnosis was made. Without hospital feedback, the agency may miss cases of STEMI that were not identified in the first place and as a result taken to an inappropriate destination.

CHOOSING WHAT CASES TO REVIEW

What cases are reviewed is key issue for any QA program. While some programs strive for 100% case review, resource constraints often hamper the ability to perform a meaningful review on all calls. A random sampling of calls is a good way to begin any review. By creating a sampling protocol that provides a mixture of call types and providers, the sample will reflect the overall composition of patient encounters. In addition, certain high-risk conditions, high-risk procedures and high frequency events may warrant increased scrutiny. A breakdown of procedures by risk and frequency can be useful in analyzing where a CQI program's attention should be focused. A set list of triggers for 100% case review should be created by the CQI staff in conjunction with the medical director. An example of such a list is seen in **Box 6-3**; please note that a single case may fall under multiple triggers.

■ EXAMPLE: INTUBATION

Intubation is a high-risk, low-frequency skill that should be scrutinized in all EMS quality assurance programs. The desire to provide patients with a definitive airway is balanced by the alarming rates of procedural failure. Tracking the intubation success rate is one important step. Intubations success rates should be monitored on an individual call, provider and agency level (and perhaps a system level). Quality in intubation, like most complex skills, goes beyond a simple "success/failure." The number of attempts required, time spent on each attempt, as well as the resulting trauma to the airway, hypoxia, and the time opportunity cost of not performing other tasks (such as CPR) are all adverse events associated with intubation attempts.[14] In addition to chart review prospective CQI, including use of scenarios and simulation, should always be a component of the review process as chart review alone is inadequate for revealing potential deficits in provider proficiency in these types of high-risk, low-incident procedures.

REVIEWING COMPLAINTS

Complaint-driven reviews may originate from patients, families, hospitals, first responders, crewmembers, or the providers themselves. Though patients and families may not understand the intricacies of patient care, their concerns are no less valid. Often their complaints stem from a non-medical concern such as crew demeanor or rough patient handling. It is reasonable to review all such cases from a medical perspective. A review of seemingly nonmedical complaints may reveal clinical errors. Hospitals and other first responders are other important sources of feedback. Complaints that originate from fellow crewmembers are often the most concerning. Partner complaints must be investigated extensively, and whenever possible, with sensitivity for the confidentiality of the reporter.

SELF-REPORTING

A culture that encourages self-disclosure of errors is important part of a CQI program. Due to concerns of embarrassment, liability, or job action, a provider may choose to hide or at least not disclose an error. From an individual perspective, the provider may lose an opportunity to grow as a professional. From an agency perspective, it may mask a larger systemic issue within the organization. Few agencies have 100% call review, and even those that do will not pick up every error. Policies that protect individuals who self-report their errors from discipline or termination assuage some of the concerns surrounding self-reporting. Such policies should protect providers who make good faith efforts, with possible exceptions for intentional or fraudulent acts. In jurisdictions where there exists local, regional, and/or state oversight of quality there are typically criteria for what types of errors require reporting to these regulatory authorities. When an agency has discovered it has committed an error or regulatory violation, self-reporting incidents that require regulatory review is usually advantageous and shows initiative and a willingness to comply with review and remediation. In the case of provider errors that must be reported, agencies should strongly advocate for their providers to self-report to the agencies and should make it a point to include this fact when forwarding to regulatory organizations (eg, New York State Department of Health Bureau of Emergency Medical Services).

NONCLINICAL EVENTS

Response times are historically the most scrutinized metric, yet paradoxically, they are the least related to direct patient care and have not been shown to represent quality in patient outcomes. Response times have been embraced because of their ease of monitoring despite this fact and are commonly a component of a municipal contractual obligation. Systems use fixed (although varied) starting point for this interval which ends when a unit radios it is on the scene. There is little room for interpretation as this is a discrete value. The response time can then be measured against a predetermined standard to determine compliance. Response times are internally monitored because they are closely scrutinized externally by municipalities, contracting agencies, the media, and others. This should not be a benchmark for the CQI process, but may be tracked due to monetary contractual concerns of the agency administration.

Stretcher Drops and Ambulance Response Collisions are important causes for harm for patients, responders, and the community.[14,15] These are generally seen as operational issues, and not under the direct review of the medical director or the CQI committee. If an agency chooses to review these events outside of their CQI system, they must still ensure these cases are treated with appropriate attention and scrutiny.

PLAN-DO-CHECK-ACT MODEL

CQI can be used to evaluate system change in a circular manner.

The classic model developed by Shewhart and Deming and used in CQI is Plan-Do-Check-Act, or PDCA.[16] In this model, each step flows into the next and is a continuous cycle (**Figure 6-2**).

Using a defined model helps prevent the improvement process from being arbitrary. When time, money, and effort are being expended, an organization should strive to develop the most efficient and well-designed program, process, or improvement. A model helps guide our process and thinking so we can focus on the steps necessary to affect change. This also prevents an all too common occurrence: the "great idea" model of improvement that is not data driven or fact based.

Box 6-3
Example of Triggers for CQI Case Review
Clinical Triggers for CQI Reviews
1. Cardiac arrest
2. Intubation attempt
3. Interosseuous access attempt
4. STEMI
5. New provider for the first 30 cases
6. New procedure for the first 30 cases
7. Patient sign offs (50% of cases reviewed)
8. Random case review (20% of cases reviewed)
Nonclinical Triggers for CQI Review
1. Patient drop/injury
2. External complaint
3. Internal complaint
4. Provider self-reported event
5. State reportable event

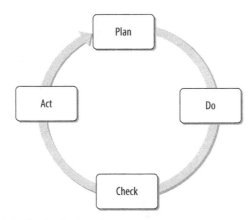

FIGURE 6-2. Plan-Do-Check-Act diagram.

The PDCA model is especially helpful when planning a new improvement project or work process. It should also be utilized whenever implementing a change, defining a repetitive work process, and planning data collection and analysis. Anytime there is change or improvement involved, the PDCA model can be applied.

PLAN

The basic steps of the PDCA cycle follow the names given to them. The first step is to recognize that an opportunity for improvement exists and begin planning the improvement process. The foundation of planning is the process of assessment, including needs assessment or situational assessment. During the planning phase, multiple different techniques may be employed in an effort to derive potential solutions. Creative development techniques such as brainstorming, the Delphi method, value engineering, morphological analysis, and others should be employed during this phase to ensure a breath of ideas have been considered and explored.

DO

The second step is beginning implementation of the plans. This is also the step to begin testing and reevaluating the plan set forth based on your assessment. Note that incremental changes are more easily accommodated and tested. "Pilot" programs or projects are useful to work out the kinks identified in the planning stage.

CHECK

It is important to step back and evaluate the successes and weaknesses of the plans you have implemented. The check is essential to the improvement process—without looking at the lessons learned from a pilot program or testing of implementation, we cannot improve in the next iteration.

ACT

Using what has been learned or discovered from the previous three steps, we must take action and begin the planning phase again. Have we met a "best practice" standard? What else could be done to improve? Be prepared to go through this process repeatedly and continuously—incremental changes and improvements are more easily attained than a complete overhaul.

PROTECTION FOR CQI DOCUMENTS

While protection for quality assurance and improvement proceedings are clearly enumerated for physicians and the hospital setting, these protections are less defined in the prehospital setting.[17] Major concerns include whether CQI processes are discoverable, the extent of protection provided to those performing CQI functions, and how CQI documents may be used in disciplinary action against individual providers. CQI documents may include data gathered, such as the patient care reports or statistics on providers; written records of audits, improvement plans, and investigations; and written or oral deliberations, disclosures, and statements.

Confidentiality of CQI records, both from legal proceedings as well as for individual providers, should be addressed specifically in setting up a CQI program. Some states may address the issue of confidentiality for documents produced or related to CQI in the EMS setting, and additional research into the state of practice laws is essential. The EMS agency type—for example, a municipal service that falls under "freedom of information" disclosure rules, a hospital-based system using an existing review board, or a private entity that may function independently—may also determine what protections apply.

With a hospital-based system, prehospital CQI activities fall under umbrella of the hospital's existing peer review mechanism, which may alleviate some concerns over the discoverability of CQI documents. State statutes may exist that allow confidential review by a centralized party, while others may allow for confidential review by the individual EMS agency.

To help strengthen the case for confidentiality of documents produced by CQI activities, the CQI program should specify how documents are produced, stored, distributed, and protected. Policies and procedures should be written specifying the private and confidential nature of CQI documents and information, including the use of a watermark or other means to mark documents used for CQI if possible. The program staff should be defined, and responsibility for data collection and analysis determined. Finally, documents should be securely stored and protected against unauthorized distribution.

The Health Insurance Portability and Accountability Act of 1996 specifically allows for the sharing and use of patient information without individual authorization for health care operations including "quality assessment and improvement activities, including case management and care coordination."[18] This includes the sharing of hospital data with an EMS agency for the purpose of EMS quality assurance.

LIMITATIONS OF CHART REVIEWS

A common method of retrospective quality assurance and improvement is review of the patient care record, or PCR. A PCR may be handwritten on paper forms or electronic. With the advent of electronic medical records and "ePCR," data mining and reporting is even more accessible and useful. Regardless of the method of documentation, PCRs are the foundation for gathering data from the field. Limitations to PCR reviews do exist and must be acknowledged to prevent misuse of the possible data.

The PCR is a record of what happened and what actions the provider may have taken on a call. Documentation is often completed after the patient care has ended—hopefully immediately after leaving a patient's side but could be potentially hours to days later. The record is only as accurate as the information gathered and inputted. If a provider purposely or accidentally fails to include details such as assessment findings or treatment provided, these data are not captured and cannot be analyzed. Unfortunately, it is not uncommon for providers to omit an unsuccessful IV attempt from the PCR, for example, thus skewing the data for reporting. When using paper forms, documentation can be inconsistent, incomplete, and illegible. Even if accidental, missing data elements may prevent accurate reporting and statistics. Similar to the possible lag in documentation, review of the PCR is usually not in real time. Typically, days or even weeks may pass before a call is reviewed by CQI. Potential quality issues may not be uncovered in time to prevent another incident.

While reviewing a PCR, it is important to remember that the intricacies of patient care may not have been precisely described. A provider who struggles with documentation may be unable to relate what happened effectively. Additional information can be obtained through the audit process or interviews. Poor documentation does not always mean poor care was provided, and conversely, poor care can be provided even with excellent documentation.

PROSPECTIVE CQI

Prospective CQI refers to the active review of provider skills, policies, protocols, and procedures. Evaluation and CQI relative to policies, protocols, and procedures should be a component of the protocol development process; however, CQI committee members should forward any findings relative to system errors and negative impacts that can be tied to these documents. Regular evaluative activities including, but not limited to, oral exam scenarios, high-fidelity and low-fidelity patient encounter simulations, and skills check-offs are examples of potentially high-yield prospective CQI. Conducting surveillance of the agency providers and identifying the agencies' potential deviations from regional, state, or national benchmarks can lead to increased continuous medical education efforts in identified areas. This increased educational component should also be accompanied by evaluative tools to ensure efficacy.

IDENTIFICATION OF ERRORS

When an error is discovered, by any process, it is important to define the error in terms of the general type of the error. This is usually considered a two-component system: (1) provider error and (2) system error.

PROVIDER ERROR

Provider errors are those directly related to a failure of the individual to perform the correct actions and could represent an error of omission or commission. The causes of this type of error can be of a number of types, including educational deficit, skill incompetence, impairment (substance abuse, emotional distress, fatigue), negligence, reckless conduct, malicious intent. These errors can be further characterized as *diagnostic* (error in diagnosis/field impression, failure to perform diagnostic intervention, or failure to act on results of monitoring or testing) or *therapeutic* (error in the performance of a procedure, error in administering a treatment, error in the dose or administration of a drug, or providing a therapy that is not indicated). Evaluation of underlying features (or root causes) and choosing the appropriate response to the error is discussed further in the section *Just Culture* in this chapter on *Just Culture*.

SYSTEM ERROR

System errors are those that stem primarily from process failures that allow for otherwise preventable occurrences. In some cases, processes and/or policies themselves create confusion or develop into new risk for error occurrence. When an error is identified that should have been prevented by a better process, policy, or protocol, this is referred to as a system error. The distinction is important, in that remediating one provider based on a patient care error that was primarily a system error, not only does not aid in enhancing the provider's ability to care for future patients, but it also fails to prevent another provider from encountering the same situation and potentially committing the same preventable error. It is crucial when reviewing cases of medical error that the determination be made concerning the presence of provider error and/or system error. If both types are present, then both must be addressed. An example would be a case in which a medication shortage led to the stocking of the same medication in a different (higher) concentration. The provider draws the same volume and mistakenly injects twice the dose due to the high concentration. It is then easy to see that the provider failed to check the concentration and ensure administration of the correct does; however, there was a lack of system safety policy to alert the provider to double-check the dose due to the replacement stocking. The system failed to provide for patient safety, when simply marking the vials with sticker or packing them in such a way as to identify them as being different than the usual concentration. Other system errors include failure of communication and equipment failure.

REMEDIATION

Remediation is not a disciplinary action, but rather a customized educational program aimed at enhancing provider knowledge and/or skill in a determined area of deficiency. This concept is covered in Chapters 7 and 27. Remediation should be carried out by the training director, medical director, or other appropriate designee, but should ideally not be the duty of any member of the CQI committee that was or will be party to CQI review of the same provider, or by the individual who is known to be responsible for instituting disciplinary action.

LIABILITY

Liability is an important concern for those performing CQI functions, as well as EMS agencies in general. The goal of any case review should be to have a candid discussion with the providers. Many barriers may exist to having an open, candid discussion. Fear of discipline, termination, legal liability, and professional embarrassment are all potential concerns for individual providers. CQI should be used to improve patient care, not for disciplinary reasons, and any data gathered or improvement plans required should be shared only with those necessary. In instances where discipline or termination results from CQI review, confidentiality and adherence to proper human resources procedures may be helpful. If implemented incorrectly, it is possible for the medical director to suffer from legal action related to claims on the part of the provider of a lack of appropriate *due process* or even *defamation of character*. Because the CQI process can lead to reduction in (or removal of) authorization to practice, it is possible to claim that the medical director has interfered with the providers' property (license) or their ability to conduct business. Therefore due process must be followed and CQI procedures must be clear and clearly followed. In order to avoid suit brought under Federal Civil Rights Statute 42 USC 1983, the medical director must ensure due process—*(1) notice, (2) hearing, (3) opportunity to challenge, (4) fair and nondiscriminatory process.* If the CQI process is not properly protected or not kept confidential, a provider could claim that the medical director is to blame for loss of fame (reputation and respect) that could impact their state of mind and ability to earn an income and could then bring suit against the medical director and agency for defamation of character.

ELECTRONIC MEDICAL RECORDS

Electronic medical records streamlined quality assurance programs.[19] What used to take hours of meticulous hand searching through patient records can now be done automatically via computerized reports. Once a report is written, it can be applied to various time periods, allowing a similar search to be done quickly at a future date. Electronic patient care records typically have a mixture of free text sections and defined fields. Although some free text can be searched by individual word or by hand, encouraging or mandating crews to use defined fields improves the ability to review specific interventions. Predefined subfields allow further review of particular interventions. This allows review of overall success rates of procedures for an agency or a particular provider. Tracking intubation success rates is one frequently measured procedure. Finally, the use of closed call rules can ensure all preselected fields are entered before the electronic PCR is completed.

As electronic patient care records become more popular, the NEMSIS will allow us to begin looking at data from prehospital encounters all over the country. NEMSIS is a data repository designed to collect patient data from every state to allow for reporting on a state and national level. This national data set will permit research into evidence-based prehospital interventions and benchmarking of PI. Most prehospital electronic records systems are designed around the required NEMSIS data points, though not every state and agency is able to submit data at this time.[20]

SETTING UP YOUR CQI TEAM

How a specific EMS organization sets up the CQI team may depend on local, state, and company guidelines, but there are two general paradigms—a CQI committee or a CQI person.

A committee draws upon the experiences and background of multiple stakeholders to help guide a service in its improvement activities. Ideally, the committee should consist of the service's medical director, several members of the management, and several field providers at all levels of practice. Additionally, stakeholders in the surrounding medical community, such as hospital staff or other public safety personnel, may be included. Decisions and activities are guided by the committee, though single members may be responsible for tasks such as PCR reviews. The committee must meet regularly to be effective, thus potentially being a significant time commitment to its members.

If a committee is not possible, a single provider may be assigned to perform CQI duties independently. This should be an experienced provider who is able to build and maintain relationships with providers, management, and local hospitals. This person would be responsible to guide the organization toward quality improvement, as well as tasks such as PCR reviews, data collection and reporting, and investigations. The use of a single person may be more cost-effective but prevents buy-in from providers and other stakeholders.

A blend of the two paradigms is possible, with a "CQI coordinator" becoming the leader of a guidance committee. The CQI coordinator would regularly meet with stakeholders, but would be responsible to lead the organization and CQI department. Organization size and workload may necessitate additional members of the CQI team to assist, but the coordinator acts as the champion to put everything together.

QUALITY ASSURANCE PITFALLS

Quality assurance and similar medical direction activities are often outside of collective bargaining between an organization and its employees. Similarly, quality assurance activities also provide a level of protection for disclosure, which operational activities do not enjoy. As a result, an organization may be tempted to move activities unrelated to CQI under the CQI umbrella. In doing so, the medical director may be drawn into issues that are outside of his or her purview. Establishing clear expectations for an agency's medical director and CQI program will prevent issues of under- or overreach later on.

CULTURE OF QUALITY AND SAFETY

One of the most important components of a successful CQI program is to work toward development of a culture of quality and safety. Focusing on group delivery of initiatives and ensuring education and encouragement are included in every change to the system. Group consensus building can lead to improved communication and employing such techniques as affinity grouping and utilizing surveys, town meetings, and small group discussions ensures an appreciation for the need to establish communication at all levels. The Agency for Healthcare Research and Quality (AHRQ) states that five basic features must be present for this type of environment to exist (**Box 6-4**).[21] The development of this culture also requires a support of another concept known as *Just Culture*.[22]

JUST CULTURE

The recognition of four different behavioral causes of individual provider error leads to a more "just," and arguably more effective, response to each error event. The recognition and participation of members of the agency lead to increased trust in the CQI process and the eventual increase in self-reporting and the recognition and reporting of near-misses and process failures. The CQI personnel must first consider these behaviors: human error, negligence, reckless conduct, and intentional rule violations. (**Box 6-5**)

Box 6-4

Features of a Culture of Quality and Safety

1. *Acknowledgment* of the high-risk nature of an organization's activities
2. *Determination* to achieve consistently safe operations.
3. *Blame-free environment* where individuals are able to report errors or near misses without fear of reprimand or punishment.
4. *Collaboration* across ranks and disciplines to seek solutions to patient safety problems.
5. *Commitment* of resources to address safety concerns.

Modified from Agency for Healthcare Research and Quality. Safety Culture. U.S. Department of Health and Human Services. http://psnet.ahrq.gov/primer.aspx?primerID=5. Accessed October 1, 2013.

■ ERROR-PRODUCING BEHAVIOR

This section describes the four types of behavior that contribute to commission of an error. It is important to note that a medical error may be related to the presence of one or more of these behavior types. *Human error* is when an individual is recognized as having done something other than the desired course of action, which then resulted (or could have resulted) in an undesirable outcome. Despite the outcome, these events need to be considered carefully, as they may be due to fatigue or knowledge gaps that could otherwise have been avoided, or can be avoided in the future. This type of error implies that the provider could not have detected the error prior to performing it and should result in a review and remediation to allow for improvements in the provider's performance. If the provider is found to have been impaired by substance abuse and/or emotional disturbance, they should be referred for appropriate medical and psychological care and counseling. Provider impairment is also discussed in Chapter 8. *Negligence* is the concept that the human error was performed by an individual that should have recognized the risk inherent to the action and is therefore culpable for the outcome. *Reckless conduct* is when the provider chose to disregard the risk, even when it was apparent to them, and is also known as *gross negligence*. *Intentional rule violation* is the act of knowingly and willfully acting in a way that is contrary to the rules, policies, or procedures. When a provider does this, they display their disregard for the authority of those who have established the rule and for those the rule is meant to protect. There are three ways to respond to these behaviors: *outcome-based*, *rule-based*, and *risk-based* decision making.

Box 6-5

Just Culture Behavior Types—Simplified Response Strategy

Behavior	Character	Response
Human error	Mistake—took wrong action (low culpability)	Remediation (and evaluate for signs of impairment)
Negligence	Failure to recognize a risk that should have been recognized (high culpability)	Remediation (and possible discipline)
Reckless conduct (gross negligence)	Conscious disregard of a significant visible risk (high culpability)	Discipline (and remediation)
Intentional rule violations	Knowingly and willfully broke the rule(s) (high culpability if associated with risk)	Discipline if based on unnecessary risk

The above represents a simplification based on the risk-based decision-making model.

Multiple error types can occur as components of the same wrong act (commission or omission).

*Impaired providers require assistance and should be referred for care and then remediated (especially if self-reported).

DECISION MAKING

In *outcome-based* decision making, a provider would receive remediation and/or disability action based on the outcome of the error. Because of the tremendous potential for the provider to only be corrected when their errors result in harm, and the potential for a minor error to result in a major outcome issue, this is probably the least "just" and least prospectively effective method. For example, if an individual were to knowingly give an IV β-blocker multiple times during a transport and ignore the protocol requirement for cardiac monitoring and repeat blood pressures and the patient had no significant detected harm from the *intentional rule violation* and *reckless conduct* of the provider, then there could be determined little to no need to provide remediation of discipline and the providers would have no incentive to correct their behavior, potentially leading to future harm or death of a patient.

In *rule-based* decision making, a provider who breaks a rule is found to require remediation and/or discipline based on the infraction alone. This may have the desired outcome for the example provider above whose rule violation was risky and potentially life-threatening to his or her patient. However, if the breaking of the rule is judged on its own, then infractions of rules in an effort to comply with operational norms or patient needs may also result in remediation and/or discipline that does not suit the circumstances. For example, if a provider fails to fully restock the ambulance after a call with nonessential items in order to respond from the hospital to a high-priority call for which there is no other available unit, that provider has knowingly committed an *intentional rule violation*. However, this behavior is more beneficial to the patient and the system than strict adherence to that particular rule.

In *risk-based* decision making, the inherent risk of the behavior is the major factor in assigning the need for remediation and/or discipline, in that it focuses on the intent of a provider with regard to an undesirable outcome. Where a provider commits a human error there is no presumed level of inherent risk to their behavior and therefore was not an obviously preventable act. In a case where a provider commits gross negligence through *reckless conduct* they have committed an error with a high level of risk and would then be subject to remediation and discipline, possibly with the emphasis on the disciplinary action due to the grave nature of the knowing acceptance of risk toward the patient and the need for the agency to maintain standards among its providers. In the case of straight *negligence* it may be significantly unclear how much remediation verses discipline is warranted and there may be a need for both depending on the particular reason that the provider was unaware of the perceivable, yet unperceived, risk. The *risk-based* approach supports Just Culture as the preferred method on which to base these decisions.

MASTERING JUST CULTURE

The volume of work in this area is staggering and is beyond the scope of this chapter. However, those EMS physicians seeking to involve themselves in CQI at the system level and/or are involved in the active development of health policy should spend considerable effort toward achieving greater mastery of this area. Reviewing and understanding the work of Reason (Reason culpability Decision Tree, Reason Foresight test) and Hudson (Just Culture diagram) may enhance this process.[23-25] College and graduate level classes, as well as webinars and seminars, are available on these topics.

PERFORMANCE INDICATORS

One of the important features of prospective CQI is the ability to look for trends or areas of improvement without the alert of a particular incident or even recognizable poor outcome. In order to perform meaningful system surveillance, PI must be developed in order to gather and analyze data leading to discovery of trends and the establishment of baselines and benchmarks.

NFPA 1710

As expected, this standard was developed for fire services, but does contain standards for EMS activities. The standard recommends a 4-minute response time for first responders and an 8-minute response for ALS.

In addition to this arbitrary designation, the standard also calls for no less than two paramedics and two EMTs for every ALS activation. The standard also requires the existence of a quality review process and a medical director to oversee this process. Conflicting studies exist on the effect of response times and therefore utilizing the only PI in NFPA 1710 for routine CQI would seem less than advantageous.

NHTSA MEDICAL SERVICE PERFORMANCE MEASURES

In response to the lack of meaningful PI and the need to express a uniform set of quality measures to the medical community, administrators, payers, and policy makers, the National Association of State EMS Officials (NASEMSO) and the National Association of EMS Physicians (NAEMSP) partnered with the National Highway and Safety Administration (NHTSA) to develop a system for standardized PI development. The document "Emergency Medical Services Performance Measures: Recommended Attributes and Indicators for System and Service Performance" was published in 2009 and broke down PI into areas of focus: system design and structure, human resources, clinical care and outcome, response, finance/funding, quality management, community demographics. The 30 PI that were developed for data collection and review were derived through expert opinion and review of the literature (**Box 6-6**).

Box 6-6

NHTSA Medical Service Performance Measures

1. Annual turnover rate
2. Average defibrillation time
3. 90th percentile defibrillation time
4. Average initial rhythm analysis time
5. 90th percentile initial rhythm analysis time
6. Major trauma triage to trauma center rate
7. Pain relief rate
8. Pain worsened rate
9. Pain unchanged rate
10. PARKED pain intervention rate
11. 12-Lead performance rate
12. Aspirin administration for chest pain/discomfort rate
13. ST-elevation myocardial infarction (STEMI) triage to specialty center rate
14. Mean emergency patient response interval
15. 90th percentile emergency response interval
16. Mean emergency scene interval
17. 90th percentile emergency scene interval
18. Mean emergency transport interval
19. 90th percentile emergency transport interval
20. PARKED per capita agency operating expense
21. PARKED patient care satisfaction rate
22. Patient care satisfaction survey rate
23. Rate of appropriate oxygen use
24. Undetected esophageal intubation rate
25. Delay-causing crash rate per 1000 EMS responses
26. EMS crash rate per 100,000 fleet miles
27. EMS crash injury rate per 100,000 fleet miles
28. EMS crash death rate per 100,000 fleet miles
29. EMS cardiac arrest survival rate to ED discharge
30. EMS cardiac arrest survival rate to hospital discharge

CALIFORNIA EMS SYSTEM CORE QUALITY MEASURES

The Emergency Medical Services Authority of the California Health and Human Services Agency has developed a set of "core quality measures" relating to 10 different areas in which they sought to measure as PI: trauma, acute coronary syndrome/heart attack, cardiac arrest, stroke, respiratory, pain intervention, pediatric, skill performance by EMS providers, EMS, response and transport, public education bystander CPR. The project was designed to test and develop data gathering and analysis from across the state and to compare California to the national data through submission to the NEMSIS. The design of the investigation included data gathering from April 2012 to April 2013 and included specific PI values (**Box 6-7**).

Box 6-7

California EMS System Core Quality Measures

Scene time for severely injured trauma patients

Direct transport to trauma center for severely injured trauma patients

Aspirin administration for chest pain/discomfort

12-Lead ECG performance

Scene time for suspected heart attack patients

Advance hospital notification for ACS

Direct transport to PCI center for suspected ACS

AED prior to EMS arrival

Out-of-hospital cardiac arrests ROSC

Out-of-hospital cardiac arrests survival to ED discharge

Out-of-hospital cardiac arrests survival to hospital discharge

Identification of stroke in the field

Glucose testing for suspected stroke patients

Scene time for suspected stroke patients

Advance hospital notification for suspected stroke

Direct transport to stroke center for suspected stroke patients

CPAP given for patients with respiratory distress

β_2-Agonist administration for respiratory distress

Pediatric asthma patients receiving bronchodilators

Transport to pediatric trauma center when criteria met

Pain intervention

Results of pain intervention

Endotracheal intubation success rate

End-tidal CO_2 performed on any endotracheal intubation

Ambulance response time (emergency)

Ambulance response time (nonemergency)

Transport of patients to hospital

Out-of-hospital cardiac arrests receiving bystander CPR

FUTURE OF PERFORMANCE INDICATORS IN EMS

Hospitals are being reimbursed based on PI in more situations than ever before. No such measures currently exist for EMS operations that link reimbursement to quality of care provided. Federal and commercial payers, such as the Centers for Medicare and Medicaid Services, may begin to apply the same type of focus on quality prehospital as in hospital patient care. Measures may include out-of-hospital cardiac arrest survival rates, response times, patient satisfaction, and transportation to the appropriate facility.[26]

EMS is also in a position to assist hospitals in meeting their PI. Strengthening EMS protocols for STEMIs will help reduce door-to-balloon times, for example. In addition, the growing field of community paramedicine has potential to reduce emergency department visits and hospital readmissions. A randomized controlled trial in the United Kingdom showed that adequately prepared paramedic practitioners were able to safely provide basic care and follow-up for elderly patients without the need for transport or hospital admission.[27] CQI in EMS can help foster relationships with hospital partners while improving the care we provide to every patient we encounter.

SUMMARY

Quality management originated in manufacturing and has slowly moved into the health care field. Many hospitals have adopted CQI principles and EMS has begun to move in the same direction. QA/CQI programs are often required by regulation, but are also important to assess and ensure that quality patient care is being provided. The focus of any CQI program should be on improvement of processes and practices, not disciplinary action against individual providers. The Plan-Do-Check-Act model is a continuous process used to evaluate system change. Anytime there is change or improvement involved, the PDCA model can be applied. Although CQI documents may be protected under state regulations, it is important to address the protection and confidentiality of all CQI activities in the planning process. In some states there is only limited protection for these materials. The most common type of retrospective quality assurance, chart reviews, can be hindered by poor data collection and missing information. Electronic medical records may help this process, as well as provide methods of data mining and reporting. Currently, no standard EMS specific guidelines for reimbursement tied to PI exist on a national level, though EMS can assist hospital partners in achieving their PI. Future directions may include collecting EMS quality data, for example, on out-of-hospital cardiac arrests and response times.

KEY POINTS

- Medication errors are estimated to account for one of the largest portions of preventable medical errors.
- Quality assurance and continuous quality improvement practices are a necessary component of a functional EMS agency or system.
- QA/CQI focus should be on improvement of processes and practices, not on disciplinary action against an individual provider.
- Confidential discussions and documents generated by the CQI process are usually protected as "nondiscoverable" with regard to court proceedings.
- EMS-specific guidelines for reimbursement tied to performance indicators do not currently exist on a national level.
- The Plan-Do-Check-Act (PDCA) model is a well-defined process guide for continuous quality improvement.
- Always utilize Just Culture in all CQI activities.

REFERENCES

1. Sollecito WA, Johnson JK. The global evolution of continuous quality improvement: from Japanese manufacturing to global health services. *McLaughlin and Kaluzny's Continuous Quality Improvement in Health Care.* 4th ed. Burlington, MA: Jones & Bartlett Learning; 2013.
2. McLaughlin CP, Kaluzny AD. *Continuous Quality Improvement in Health Care: Theory, Implementation, and Applications.* Sudbury, MA: Jones & Bartlett Learning; 2004:31.
3. National Highway Traffic Safety Administration. *A leadership guide to quality improvement in emergency medical services systems.* Washington, DC. 1998. http://icsw.nhtsa.gov/people/injury/ems/leaderguide/.
4. Manos A, Sattler M, Alukal G. Make healthcare lean. *Qual Prog.* 2006;39(7):24-30.
5. Cua KO, McKone KE, Schroeder RG. Relationships between implementation of TQM, JIT, and TPM and manufacturing performance. *J Oper Manag.* 2001;19(6):675-694.
6. Sehwail L, DeYong C. Six Sigma in health care. *Leadersh Health Serv.* 2003;16(4):1-5.
7. Mazzocato P, Savage C, Brommels M, Aronsson H, Thor J. Lean thinking in healthcare: a realist review of the literature. *Qual Saf Health Care.* 2010;19(5):376-382.
8. Goldstone J. The role of quality assurance versus continuous quality improvement. *J Vasc Surg.* 1998;28(2):378-380.
9. Carnett WG. Clinical practice guidelines: a tool to improve care. *J Nurs Care Qual.* 2002;16(3):60-70.
10. Michigan Public Health Code (Excerpt), 333.20919. 1978.
11. Hauswald M, Braude D. Spinal immobilization in trauma patients: is it really necessary? *Curr Opin Crit Care.* 2002;8(6):566-570.
12. Kohn LT, Corrigan JM, Donaldson MS. *To Err Is Human: Building a Safer Health System.* Washington, DC: National Academy Press; 2000.
13. Allard J, Carthey J, Cope J, et al. Medication errors: causes, prevention and reduction. *Br J Haematol.* 2002;116(2):255-265.
14. Goodloe JM, Crowder CJ, Arthur AO, Thomas SH. EMS stretcher "misadventures" in a large, urban EMS system: A descriptive analysis of contributing factors and resultant injuries. *Emerg Med Int.* 2012; 2012:745706.
15. Slattery DE, Silver A. The hazards of providing care in emergency vehicles: an opportunity for reform. *Prehosp Emerg Care.* 2009; 13(3):388-397.
16. Tague NR. *The Quality Toolbox.* 2nd ed. Milwaukee, WI: ASQ Quality Press; 2005: 390-392.
17. Health Care Quality Improvement Act, 1986.
18. Health Insurance Portability and Accountability Act, 1996.
19. Landman AB, Lee CH, Sasson C, et al. Prehospital electronic patient care report systems: Early experiences from emergency medical services agency leaders. *PLoS ONE.* 2012;7(3):e32692.
20. Dawson DE. National Emergency Medical Services Information System (NEMSIS). *Prehosp Emerg Care.* 2006;10(3):314-316.
21. Agency for Healthcare Research and Quality. Safety culture. U.S. Department of Health and Human Services. http://psnet.ahrq.gov/primer.aspx?primerID=5. Accessed October 1, 2013.
22. Marx D. Patient safety and the "just culture": a primer for health care executives. April 17, 2001. Prepared for Columbia University under a grant provided by the National Heart, Lung, and Blood Institute. www.mers-tm.net/support/marx_primer.pdf. Accessed October 1, 2013.
23. Reason J. *Managing the Risks of Organisational Accidents.* Hants, England: Ashgate Publishing Ltd; 1997.
24. Safety culture. In: Reason J, Hobbs A, eds. *Managing Maintenance Errors: A Practical Guide.* Aldershot, Hampshire, England: Ashgate; 2003:chap 11.
25. Hudson P. Presentation: Aviation Safety Culture, Safe skies Conference, Canberra, Australia. 2001.
26. El Sayed MJ. Measuring quality in emergency medical services: a review of clinical performance indicators. *Emerg Med Int.* 2012; 2012:161630.
27. Mason S, Knowles E, Colwell B, et al. Effectiveness of paramedic practitioners in attending 999 calls from elderly people in the community: cluster randomised controlled trial. *BMJ.* 2007;335:7626.

CHAPTER 7

Provider Education

Jeffrey L. Jarvis
Douglas Patton

INTRODUCTION

All US states and territories require that providers staffing EMS vehicles have successfully completed a program of initial training and passed an examination process. These providers are also required to complete continuing education in order to continue practice. EMS medical directors are responsible for the oversight of these education programs. Additionally, they should continually evaluate the actual clinical performance of their providers and, through their quality improvement process, implement an ongoing education program designed to continually improve provider practice. EMS education in the United States, although guided and supported by national guidelines and curricula, is regulated at the state level. As a result, the specific provider levels of training and the corresponding educational requirements vary from state to state. Fortunately, there are generalizations about provider education that can be made about the overall education and training processes and requirements.

OBJECTIVES

- Describe the national basis for the education of prehospital providers.
- Describe the levels of prehospital providers and typical training requirements at each level.
- Describe the types of educational organizations providing EMS education and the role of accreditation in preparing candidates for national EMS certification.
- Detail the use of high-fidelity simulation.
- Discuss the use of distance learning, including advanced self-study and Web-based education.
- Detail the development of a field preceptor program and criteria for clearing a provider for independent practice.
- Define remediation and discuss its use in educational programs and for providers identified during CQI as having additional education needs.
- Contrast National Registry certification to state-specific EMS provider certification.
- Discuss continuing education requirements and recertification pathways.

The most common levels of training include emergency medical technician (EMT) basic, EMT-intermediate, and paramedic. Many states also include some type of formal first responder training level. This training is provided by a wide variety of institutions ranging from formal degree programs in traditional educational institutions such as colleges and universities to system-based training programs. In all states, this training is, at least loosely, based on national standards, as is the standardized examinations administered either at the state level or by a national organization (new national standard levels: EMR, EMT, AEMT, paramedic).

Many EMS systems have advanced evaluation tools that medical directors can use to measure actual clinical performance. These tools are typically used by field training officers (FTOs)/preceptors to determine and institute "stretcher-side" training aimed at continuous teaching. Additionally, EMS educators and medical directors utilize a variety of mechanisms, including simulations and distance learning methodologies, to carry out their educational goals.

As with all of EMS, the medical director bears ultimate responsibility for ensuring that the education provided at both the initial and continuing levels is clinically and scientifically appropriate and up to date.

BASIS FOR THE EMS EDUCATIONAL SYSTEM

Authority for defining and regulating EMS provider education, certification, and licensure in the United States is held by each individual state. While the federal government has a role in providing technical support, it is the states that ultimately define the education required to become an EMS provider. As a result, there has historically been a large disparity between provider levels among the states, a situation that has made providing for interstate reciprocity a difficult task. Partly in recognition of this, and in response to the education vision outlined in the 1996 EMS Agenda for the Future document, the National Highway Traffic Safety Administration published the EMS Education Agenda for the Future in 2000. This document is becoming the foundation for the state's regulation of EMS education. It describes a national EMS education system comprising five related components as depicted in **Figure 7-1**.

The National EMS Core Content is analogous to the Model of the Clinical Practice of Emergency Medicine (formerly the "Core Content") upon which emergency medicine residency and board certification is based. Because the Core Content defines the medical knowledge required for the profession, physician organizations such as the National Association of EMS Physicians (NAEMSP) will be primarily responsible for maintenance and revision of this document. The EMS Core Content defines the knowledge and skills required of EMS providers but does not dictate the differences between levels of providers. The distinction of what is required of each level of provider, that is, the definitions of provider levels, is described in the National EMS Scope of Practice Model. The knowledge and skills, thus divided up among provider levels, is broken down into learning objectives in the National EMS Education Standards. These Education Standards are meant to replace the prior National Standard Curriculum for each provider level. The standards are what EMS education programs and publishers will use to create lesson plans and textbooks.

Additionally, the standards will be used as the basis for what will be on the standardized examinations used for National EMS Testing. Finally, the EMS Education Agenda recommends that, as a requirement to sit for the national examination, a candidate must have completed an education program that has been accredited by a national accrediting organization.

Currently, the organization that is developing and offering national examinations is the National Registry of EMTs (NREMT). Likewise, the Committee on Accreditation of Educational Programs for the EMS Professions (CoAEMSP) is the organization that ensures an accredited education program has demonstrated that their curriculum adequately covers the material described in the EMS standards.

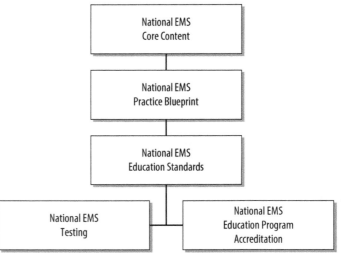

FIGURE 7-1. Five components of a national EMS education system. (From diagram 1 found in the National EMS Core Content. National Traffic Safety Administration. http://www. nhtsa.gov/people/injury/ems/FinalEducationAgenda.pdf.)

EDUCATION, CERTIFICATION, LICENSING, AND CREDENTIALING: WHAT IS IN A NAME?

Few things in EMS have given rise to more angst than the terms certification and licensing. Unfortunately, these terms are frequently used imprecisely, interchangeably, or incorrectly. It is important to review these terms in order to avoid this angst and understand how these different components overlap. While there may be some States that have specifically defined these terms in different ways, we will describe them here in the context used by national documents and organizations to illustrate the concepts involved. The Venn diagram in **Figure 7-2** helps define the relationship between these domains.

Education refers to the knowledge and skills gained by the provider during his or her initial preparation for practice as well as his or her continuing education. Certification is provided by a national testing organization, currently the NREMT, attesting that the provider has demonstrated competence, through written and skills testing, as a "minimally competent" provider at a given level, that is, paramedic. Licensure is granted by each state to those individuals who have been certified by the testing agency. Finally, and most importantly at a system level, a licensed provider may only practice if credentialed by the local EMS medical director. In some systems, credentialing may also be referred to as authorization to practice.

PROVIDER LEVELS

The National EMS Scope of Practice document describes the four levels of EMS provider: emergency medical responder, EMT, advanced emergency medical technician (AEMT), and paramedic. Emergency medical responders have been called first responders in the past as have AEMTs been referred to with names such as EMT-intermediate and EMT-special skills. Training at each level includes didactic instruction (traditional classroom lectures), procedure labs where psychomotor skills are taught and practiced, hospital-based clinical rotations, and field-based clinical rotations. Some programs will also require a field preceptorship that is roughly analogous to a physician's internship. It is done after the student has completed all other program requirements and is focused on integration of the knowledge and skills. It is typically completed with the same field preceptor over the course of multiple shifts and, optimally, should be based on well-defined objectives with progressive clinical responsibilities ending with completely managing all aspects of the call as though they are no longer a student. **Table 7-1** lists typical requirements for each provider level. While some states may require specific hours but

TABLE 7-1 Typical Clock Hours, Including Hospital and Field Rotations			
EMR	EMT	AEMT	EMT-P
48-60 (*No clinical/field rotations*)	150-190	300-440	1000-1300

Compiled from the CoAEMSP Interpretations of the Standards & Guidelines. http://coaemsp.org/Documents/Standards_Interpretations_CoAEMSP-8-2-2014.pdf. Accessed April 12, 2015.

the recommendations of the CoAEMSP is that requirements be based on achievement of specific objectives and demonstration of defined competencies rather than specific hours.

EDUCATIONAL PROGRAMS AND ACCREDITATION

EMS education is provided in very diverse fashion throughout the country with sponsoring organizations ranging from local EMS systems/fire departments and private training programs to 4-year universities and medical schools. This diversity is probably most noticeable at the basic levels (EMR and EMT) and less so at the paramedic level where there has been some coalescence behind academic affiliations. Much of the nation's paramedic education programs, and the vast majority of accredited programs, are now offered through community colleges and universities. The requirements for approval of a training program vary by level and from state to state. The specificity of these requirements also increases with provider level with the requirements at the paramedic level being more detailed than at the lower levels.

Accreditation is a widely accepted mechanism for ensuring that an educational program meets recognized standards in their educational processes. The agency recognized by the National Association of EMS State Officials (NAEMSO) to provide accreditation services is the Commission on Accreditation of Allied Health Education Programs (CAAHEP). CAAHEP is composed of multiple committees that specialize in the various allied health professions. CoAEMSP is the CAAHEP committee dedicated to EMS accreditation. NAEMSO, composed of state regulators, voted in 2010 to require CAAHEP accreditation in order to sit for the NREMT's national EMS paramedic certification examination beginning January 1, 2013.[1] CoAEMSP only accredits paramedic level programs, although these programs frequently offer options to "test out" at lower levels such as EMT.

The process of becoming accredited involves the program completing a rigorous self-study that describes how it complies with the accreditation criteria or standards. These standards are based on accepted educational processes and supported by the EMS Education Standards as published by NHTSA. The program then develops a report based on this self-study and submits it to CoAEMSP, which then assigns a trained site visit team to come review the program in person. This team then prepares a report detailing, in objective terms, the program's compliance with the standards. The CoAEMSP board will then review the site visit team's report and make a recommendation to the full CAAHEP regarding accreditation. Ultimately, it is CAAHEP that issues the accreditation. The program must then submit ongoing progress reports to CoAEMSP and undergo periodic reaccreditation similar to the initial process.

FIELD TRAINING AND EVALUATION

While the initial education, certification, and licensing of a medic are clearly very important, it is but the beginning of a continuing process of evaluation, training, and reevaluation. The medical director is responsible for this process but will likely need the assistance of FTOs. While it would be ideal for the medical director himself to perform these evaluations, it often is not feasible in all systems. These FTOs are valued employees who have demonstrated superior clinical, teaching, and interpersonal communication skills and are specifically trained to evaluate medics using objective performance criteria. The FTO process is the most accurate means of evaluating a medic's *actual* performance in a real-world environment. The criteria used should have several features: they

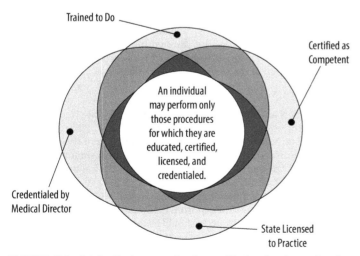

FIGURE 7-2. Relationship between education, certification, licensing, and credentialing. (From Figure 1 found in the National EMS Scope of Practice. National Traffic Safety Administration. http://www.ems.gov/education/EMSScope.pdf.)

should be specific, measurable, attainable, and tied to desired job-related competencies.

The evaluation process should be a one-on-one relationship between an assigned employee and a single FTO to promote continuity of the evaluation. It should begin with the FTO reviewing the criteria with the medic and ensuring that they understand what is required for successful completion. Any time-related requirements should also be reviewed, that is, "you have 2 months to achieve these objectives." The FTO should then teach the employee the desired knowledge/skills in a didactic fashion reinforced with manikin/simulation practice. Once this has been accomplished, the FTO should demonstrate the objective and then observe the medic demonstrate the objective, after which they should provide appropriate feedback. Next, the medic should demonstrate the objective independently with the FTO providing no feedback. Finally, the medic should demonstrate the objective to an FTO not involved in his training. This process should be completed for each objective deemed critical for successful practice by the medical director. Obviously, multiple objectives may be demonstrated concurrently rather than in series. The FTO should utilize a formal tracking system for the completion of these objectives.

When providing feedback, it is useful to utilize a standard format. One such format involves the following steps, in order: (1) ask the medic how they feel about their performance, (2) tell them what they did right, (3) tell them what they did wrong citing specific objectives and examples, (4) reiterate how the objective should have been performed and, finally, (5) briefly summarize the performance and reinforce what they did well.[2]

This process of evaluation is most detailed when the FTO is "clearing" new employees for practice as part of the process by which the medical director credentials the medic. A modified version may also be used when rolling out new skills, medications, or clinical approaches.

HIGH-FIDELITY SIMULATION

■ A BRIEF HISTORY OF SIMULATION

For centuries, professors of medicine have been challenged with a dilemma: how can a student practice and gain the skills necessary to care for critically ill patients, while still giving patients safe and competent care? A wide variety of patient simulation devices have been employed to address this problem, including the use of cadavers, animal labs, static models of wood (and later, plastic) in an attempt to give students the feel of performing life-saving techniques without risking the lives of actual patients (**Figure 7-3**). It was not until the introduction of SimOne in 1968, followed by the Harvey cardiology trainer that same year, that the potential of mechanical patient simulators became widely acknowledged.[3] Today, there are dozens of models designed to train professionals in a variety of procedures ranging from airway management to colonoscopy. Many of these models now feature important physical examination findings, such as pupils that react to light, pulses that bound and ebb, and heart and lung sounds that can suggest complex physiological changes. As these models evolve to better approximate critical illness and trauma, influential reports such as *To Err is Human: A Call to a Safer Health System* have increasingly called to incorporate simulation into all levels of medical training.[4]

The immediate safety of a trainee's patient is not the only benefit of a properly conceived and implemented simulation training program. Studies show improved knowledge and medical skills for the participants, high levels of satisfaction to both learners and instructors, and effective transfer of these skills into field practice. For example, students who learn basic CPR skills using HFS manikins are significantly more proficient at delivering appropriate chest compressions and ventilation than students who train using traditional manikins such as Resusci Anne.[5] Nonetheless, great care must be taken in designing a simulation program if its full benefits are to be realized.

■ IMPLEMENTING A SUCCESSFUL HFS PROGRAM

Naturally, the first element of any HFS program involves access to a simulation laboratory. The details of creating and staffing such a lab are beyond the scope of this chapter; however, as noted above, most EMS

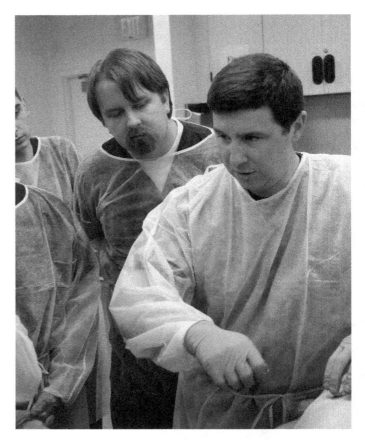

FIGURE 7-3. Cadaver lab for paramedic students. An EMS physician teaching anatomy and procedures to paramedic students in a cadaver lab. (Reproduced with permission from Doug Sandbrook, NRP, SUNY Upstate Medical University.)

training programs are associated with a community college or local university with an existing simulation laboratory; therefore, the specifics will vary depending upon the host institution.

Components of HFS Design One popular course framework (proposed by Jeffries) identifies five major components that contribute to a successful HFS program. Competent and supportive teachers, motivated and well-prepared students, and a well-defined set of demonstrable, objective criteria form three of the five components. In addition, a program should be designed using educational practices that create an active, collaborative learning environment characterized by high expectations on the part of the faculty, directed toward achievable and measurable objectives.[6] In the section below we address the most complex component: design of the simulation experience.

■ SIMULATION DESIGN

The first critical action in implementing an HFS program is to develop a list of learning objectives. These should be measurable skills that the student should be able to demonstrate upon completion of the simulation exercises. Because simulator time is typically limited, simulation objectives should focus on the psychomotor skills and clinical problem-solving exercises that best exploit its use.

While simulation attempts to be lifelike (**Figure 7-4**), the experience is not usually natural to the student from the start. After measurable objectives are communicated, students should be introduced to each feature of the simulator, as well as the role of each piece of equipment in the room that they will be expected to use. Early simulation encounters should be simple, typically involving just one clinical problem or derangement. From the first encounter, all simulations should be made to be as "real" as possible, following a typical clinical course, in an environment

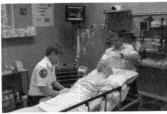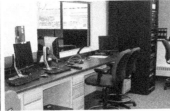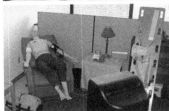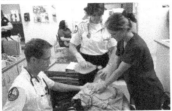

FIGURE 7-4. High-fidelity simulation lab. (Photos provided by Temple College and SUNY Upstate Medical University. All photos reproduced with permission.)

that mimics a real-life scenario as closely as practical. As learners gain experience, the level of scenario complexity can be increased to include multiple medical problems, equipment challenges, and irrelevant or distracting data, to more closely approximate situations that providers encounter in the field. Lastly, all simulations should be followed by a debriefing session, where the student reviews her perceptions of the simulation, identifies performance strengths and weaknesses, and receives constructive feedback to be applied to future scenarios. This debriefing session should focus on developing the student's critical thinking skills, rather than fumbles or "misses," with an aim to improve self-confidence and readiness to tackle field work.[7]

Finally, as departmental goals develop and change, so should simulation exercises. New techniques and equipment constantly pose new training challenges, even for veteran providers. Thus, students should come to see the simulation lab as a lifelong method of improving old skills and obtaining new ones, as a part of the EMS provider's relentless quest to deliver the finest possible care for living patients.

DISTANCE LEARNING

Throughout this chapter, we have paid attention to the considerable psychomotor skills that EMS providers must acquire, as well as the vast content area of practical knowledge that must be mastered in order to become a credentialed medic. Traditionally, this education has taken the form of classroom teaching in lecture format, using assignments to ensure appropriate progress and written tests to confirm mastery of key concepts. This is usually referred to as "traditional learning." Alternatively, long-distance communication has been successfully used for many years as an adjunct to, and occasionally as a replacement for, traditional learning. In distance learning (DL), course materials are typically mailed (or, more recently, e-mailed) to the student, regular assignments are given, examinations are administered, and grades or certificates distributed, sometimes without the student and teacher ever physically meeting. With the advent of ubiquitous computers and the World Wide Web, the practice of instructing students over great distances has become an accepted and valuable mode of education in nearly all fields of study. EMS students may learn as well in DL as they do in traditional learning[8]; however, the medical director who wishes to incorporate DL into a department's educational plan should be aware that there are significant pitfalls to be avoided.

ADVANTAGES OF DISTANCE LEARNING

Students report that they are attracted to, and value, the enormous flexibility that DL offers. The ability to learn, study, and take examinations at virtually any time of day can be of critical importance to working trainees. Many students also find that they can pursue their studies at a pace that suits that individual's learning style. This greater freedom necessitates greater responsibility, and many students appreciate the opportunity to take charge of their own learning plan and gain valuable confidence from their own self-directed success.

DISADVANTAGES OF DISTANCE LEARNING

Unfortunately, the very factors that attract students to this learning format, such as a difficult working schedule or significant family demands, can impair the success of the program as well. A student can significantly underestimate the amount of time required for his or her assignments and fail to plan ahead for large projects and examinations. Another may overestimate his or her own self-discipline and fail to make steady progress without daily classroom structure. Certain students, despite the best of intentions, may require classroom interaction in order to make sure that appropriate learning takes place.

In addition, certain content does not adapt well to an electronic-only format. In particular, procedural knowledge (such as CPR, venous cannulation and intubation skill) is best taught one-on-one, under direct supervision with immediate feedback and correction. For these reasons, most EMS training programs are not suited to a DL-only format.

HYBRID MODEL

A hybrid model of DL uses a combination of traditional learning format with elements of DL, in order to capitalize on the most effective qualities of each model. Student groups form and interact more effectively in person than online, while at the same time the smaller number of physical meetings to attend allows students greater freedom to incorporate coursework into a busy work and family schedule. Nonetheless, great care must be taken to preserve these advantages when designing a hybrid course, in order to avoid some of the pitfalls noted above. Since procedural knowledge is key to EMS training, most EMS DL programs will, by necessity, be hybrid programs.

IMPLEMENTING A SUCCESSFUL DL PROGRAM

Technological Requirements The vast majority of contemporary DL programs take place using a World Wide Web–based platform; therefore, most DL requires that both the student and the instructor have reliable access to relatively modern computers at convenient times of day with up-to-date Web browsers installed and reliable access to the Internet. Most students meet these requirements at home; however, local libraries, community colleges, and Internet cafés can provide acceptable alternatives. In these cases, it must be stressed to the students that they are responsible for making sure that their access is reliable before undertaking the course.

Many commercial platforms are available for the instructor to organize and deliver both content and testing materials. Ideally, selection of a particular platform will depend upon the content to be delivered, types and frequency of assignments, and the desired method of evaluation. Alternatively, an ambitious instructor could design a course using nothing but a basic word-processing program and standard e-mail; however, between tallying assignments and maintaining testing rigor, administration tasks could quickly become onerous. Practical instructors usually opt for the platform currently in use at the department's affiliated community college. In this case, refer to that college's information systems department for specific computer and Internet requirements before undertaking a DL program.

SETTING STUDENT EXPECTATIONS

One underappreciated aspect of course implementation is the communication of expectations to students. Instructors should be explicit: readings should be finished on time, assignments will be marked down (or not accepted) after their due date, and all efforts are to be the original work of the student and no one else. Students should also be told the approximate number of hours per day (or week) that the course requires, including meetings, readings, assignments, and testing. Early and appropriate action should reinforce these standards if any expectation is not met.

▨ EVALUATING LEARNING GOALS

The appropriate assessment of learning in the student is a complex and sometimes contentious topic; however, a few brief guidelines should be kept in mind. Assignments should probe for depth of knowledge in particular topics, while testing should assess breadth of knowledge across content areas. When designing a test, every test item or procedure should relate to a previously presented learning objective, and all important learning objectives should be represented at some point in testing. Test items should be clear, unambiguous questions regarding physiological knowledge, or clinical presentation. If a question seems "too easy," move into more difficult content rather than rewriting the question to obscure its base content. Multiple choice questions better discriminate knowledge when there are at least four alternatives to choose from, and when all alternatives could be plausible to a novice. A good question can be recognized when a top student can answer it without looking at the alternatives. Finally, if more than half of the students cannot answer a test item, consider replacing it.

▨ DISTANCE LEARNING AND CONTINUING EDUCATION

Distance learning can provide an effective method for established, motivated learners to maintain and broaden the skills and knowledge they need in order to continually improve the level of care they provide for patients. As in certification education, only those aspects that are easily taught and assessed on paper or the computer screen should be attempted via DL. Also, a medical director may find that once the goal of credentialing has been reached, students may not be as motivated to keep up with their educational commitments. Regular progress reports and coursework deadlines can help keep students on track when undertaking continuing education, and modest incentives may serve to help keep students abreast of new technology and training techniques.

CONTINUOUS QUALITY IMPROVEMENT

Lasting excellence in a training program is not simply a goal to be achieved and maintained, but rather an ongoing process of inquiry, adjustment, data collection, and revision. These four actions form the core process of "total quality management," a business philosophy first developed in the 1950s by W. Edwards Deming, who went on to develop an influential set of management principles. These principles have been successfully adapted (as "continuous quality improvement") to diverse industries, and have improved the performance of many EMS departments to date using the following key aspects[9]:

- Everyone is responsible for quality improvement. Each employee from the medical director to each responder should feel empowered to identify and address areas where training can be improved or made more efficient. Medical directors must exemplify this commitment by taking interest in any detail that can lead to better training.

- Impediments to quality are due solely to errors in the system, not the people. EMS providers are attracted to the field because they naturally want to learn how to help, and it should be the attitude of the departmental leadership that failures to meet training goals are not personal failures, but instead represent opportunities to uncover and correct systemic flaws. This philosophy shifts the approach from an adversarial relationship to a professional collaboration with the common goal of improving education and job performance.

- Sound data are essential to improvement. Appropriate tests and performance data should be collected with the intent of using that data to recognize and reinforce good performance as well as to identify potential areas of systemic improvement.

Many strategies can be employed in the pursuit of training excellence; however, an improvement plan should always include the following elements:

1. The development of a descriptive and inspirational vision statement.
2. Identification of key driving factors (sometimes called "critical indicators").
3. The adoption of measurable, achievable objectives for the department.
4. Meticulous collection and analysis of relevant data.

Other strategies may include the use of trainee focus groups, which can help identify obstacles and provide leadership feedback, comparison to statewide benchmarks to ensure that goals are realistic and achievable, and trainee well-being programs to make sure that trainees remain connected to the core reasons that motivated them to become providers.[10]

In instituting all of the above, the core process of inquiry, adjustment, data collection, and revision (sometimes called PDCA, for "plan, do, check, act") should organize continuous improvement. Through feedback from instructors and trainees as well as data analysis, leadership *plans* a change that is projected to have a measurable impact on a specific key driver, members of the department *do* their part to make the change, followed by *checking* of data to ensure that measurable change has occurred. If not, swift *action* is taken to correct whatever flaws in the process persist. Care must be taken not to allow the department to become solely "number driven," however. Only when the focus remains upon delivering high-quality training can the process be relied upon to lead to new cycles of improvement and better performance.

REMEDIATION

It should be the goal of training and remediation to give every opportunity to the motivated student to reach his or her goals within the department. Thus, when a student fails to pass qualifying examinations, or when an FTO determines that a trainee has not mastered the skills necessary to deliver independent care, the student should be entered into a formal process to identify deficient areas and to help the student achieve mastery of the necessary knowledge or skills. This process is called "remediation," and it should never be approached as a personal failure, but as an opportunity to strengthen the training program so that it can better serve its trainees.

▨ IDENTIFYING REMEDIATION CANDIDATES

Most students who are candidates for remediation are aware that they are not achieving their learning goals long before their instructors realize that there is a problem, so it is important to create an atmosphere where students can feel free to come forward and ask for help. Many students will not feel comfortable admitting that their education plan is not working, however; therefore, each department should set and communicate benchmarks that students should pass in order to be maintained in the standard education plan. If these benchmarks are not met—usually minimum test scores or passing assessments on practical skills—then remediation begins.

▨ GOALS OF REMEDIATION

Remediation should be seen as a collaborative effort to remove learning obstacles for the student so that educational goals can be met. In the end, the goal of remediation is to return the student to a strengthened and more robust training program with new tools and confidence.

▨ IMPLEMENTING A SUCCESSFUL REMEDIATION PROGRAM

Setting Expectations As with any educational endeavor, the expectations of the student and department must be clearly communicated at the start of remediation. The student must be open to making changes and committed to giving his best effort to the course. The instructor must be willing to put extra time and resources into ensuring success for the student. The approach to remediation must always stress the "win-win" nature of training, with the ultimate goal of ensuring that all providers deliver outstanding patient care. The department must communicate faith that this can be achieved, and the student must believe that he or she can and will succeed, in order for remediation to work.

Remediation Strategies First, the instructor should inquire into the conditions of the student's learning environment, including the amount of time and conditions under which the student studies, materials used, attitudes toward the content material, and so on. Often, this discussion will reveal key obstacles of which the instructor was unaware, and many times simple adjustments can be prescribed to the student's schedule or study habits that can have a profound impact on performance.

There are as many remediation strategies as there are students; however, no program can be considered complete unless the student has access to the following:

- *Private tutoring*: This can come in the form of extra time with an instructor, help from a former graduate, or simply pairing the student with a successful classmate. Whatever the method, one-on-one tutoring has the highest chance of improving test and procedural performance over any other remediation strategy.
- *Alternative materials*: No single textbook works well for all students, and often a student can improve dramatically through presenting the material in a different way. Instructors should always have alternative materials on hand, and be willing to try new materials when a student does not seem to be responding to the standard text.
- *Formative examinations*: Giving remediation students examinations that do not count toward their personal benchmarks allows greater feedback in areas of concern and also reinforces which areas of knowledge are of most concern to the program.[11]

MONITORING PROGRESS AND TERMINATING REMEDIATION

Of course, students in remediation require close monitoring; however, the instructor should not project an attitude of "how are you doing?," but rather "how are we helping you?" There is always another book to try, or a different tutor who might help. Some students will only be made more uncomfortable with these offers, however, and the tactful medical director will know when to make more materials available and when to leave students to find their own path. In some cases, multiple adjustments must be made before an effective combination of strategies can be found.

Ultimately, an EMS department is responsible to its patients, and students must show that they have mastered the knowledge and skills necessary to appropriately care for those patients in order to proceed. Thus, remediation ends when a student has either reached appropriate benchmarks or exhausted all of the above strategies for improvement and cannot identify any further ones. Most students will recognize at this point that they will be unable to serve the department as they would like, at which point the student's future role in the department will have to be discussed.

CONCLUSION

In addition to the myriad clinical oversight and practice responsibilities, the EMS medical director is essential in all phases of EMS education. This involvement begins with the planning and development of the initial education program, its operations and ongoing evaluation, as well as the specific evaluation of students both in the classroom, lab and in the field. A solid understanding of the education and regulatory foundation for this education is essential. Additionally, as the technology of simulations and DL continues to advance, so too will the opportunities for the medical director to leverage these tools to meet their responsibilities of ensuring a well-educated, well-trained, and appropriately credentialed EMS provider.

- All levels of prehospital provider education should be based on the National EMS Core Content as described in the National EMS Education Standards, peer-developed, and reviewed documents published by the National Highway Traffic Safety Administration (NHTSA).
- Educational programs each develop their own curricula and may seek accreditation sponsored by the Committee on Accreditation of Educational Programs for the EMS Professions (CoAEMSP).
- Prior to practice, providers must achieve *certification* by successfully completing the national examination developed and administered by the National Registry of EMTs (NREMT), and/or apply to be *licensed* by their state EMS office and finally successfully complete the local process defined by their EMS medical director in order to be *credentialed* to practice.
- The most common levels of EMS provider, being standardized nationally, are the emergency medical responder (EMR), emergency medical technician (EMT), advanced emergency medical technician (AEMT), and paramedic.
- Providers receive their initial education through a variety of institutions including EMS and fire departments, educational consortiums, and, most commonly, community colleges and universities.
- The NREMT will require candidates for paramedic certification to have graduated from a nationally accredited paramedic program beginning January 1, 2013.
- The field training officer (FTO) is responsible, under the supervision of the EMS medical director, for providing education and evaluation of providers during initial and ongoing training using written objectives that are specific, measurable, attainable, and tied to desired job-related competencies.
- Simulation training must be based on well communicated and measurable objectives in as realistic a setting as possible and should be followed by debriefing session in which specific, objective, and actionable feedback is provided immediately to the learner.
- Distance learning technologies are advancing rapidly, however, may require greater self-discipline from the learner and greater preparation time for the instructor.
- A remediation program should be available at all levels of provider education, be flexible and based on the individual learner's needs, and may include private tutoring, peer assistance, alternative source materials, and formative or "practice" examinations.

REFERENCES

1. NAEMSO Resolution 2010-04. National EMS Certification and Program Accreditation. http://www.nasemso.org/documents/Resolution2010-04NationalCertificationandProgramAccreditation20101013.pdf. Accessed August 30, 2011.
2. From training materials for the FTO, developed by David Phillips, BS, LP.
3. Cooper J, Taqueti V. A brief history of the development of mannequin simulators for clinical education and training. *Postgrad Med J.* 2008;84:563-570.
4. Kohn L, Corrigan J, Donaldson M. *To Err is Human: Building a Safer Health System*. Washington, DC: National Academy Press; 1999.
5. Oermann MH, Kardong-Edgren S, Odom-Maryon T, et al. HeartCode BLS with voice assisted manikin for teaching nursing students: preliminary results. *Nurs Educ Perspect*. September-October 2010;31(5):303-308.

6. Jeffries P. A framework for designing, implementing and evaluating simulations used as teaching strategies in nursing. *Nurs Educ Perspect*. 26(2):77-81.

7. Issenberg SB, McGaghie WC, Petrusa ER, Lee Gordon D, Scalese RJ. Features and uses of high-fidelity medical simulations that lead to effective learning: a BEME systematic review. *Med Teach*. 2005;27(1):10-28.

8. Hobbs GD, Moshinskie JF, Roden SK, Jarvis JL. A comparison of classroom and distance learning techniques for rural EMT-I instruction. *Prehosp Emerg Care*. July-September 1998;2(3):189-191.

9. Eastham JN, Champion HR, Bass RR, et al. A leadership guide to quality improvement for Emergency Medical Services (EMS) Systems. July 1997. http://www.nhtsa.gov/people/injury/ems/leaderguide/. Accessed September 10, 2011.

10. Repar PA, Patton D. Stress reduction for nurses through Arts-in-Medicine at the University of New Mexico Hospitals. *Holist Nurs Pract*. July-August 2007;21(4):182-186.

11. Doty C, Lucchesi M. The value of a Web-based testing system to identify residents who need early remediation: what were we waiting for? *Acad Emer Med*. March 2004;11(3):324.

CHAPTER 8

Controlled Substance Programs

Debra G. Perina

Donna Burns

INTRODUCTION

An emergency medical services (EMS) agency medical director usually focuses primarily on the oversight of the care provided directly to patients and their families. One of the medical director's other main concerns is that of the health and safety of the EMS providers. These concerns overlap in a number of ways. This chapter specifically deals with diversion issues and identifying and managing potentially impaired providers. The more an EMS physician knows about diversion of narcotics and other substances, the more likely they are to be able to properly oversee the EMS agency–controlled substance program and to help safeguard the health and safety of patients and EMS providers alike.

OBJECTIVES

- Describe the components of an EMS agency narcotics control program.
- Describe the process by which EMS agencies obtain, stock, and utilize controlled substances.
- Discuss DEA regulations and the differences between using a personal DEA registration versus an agency DEA registration.
- Discuss state narcotics laws and regulations that affect EMS agencies.
- Describe proper storage and handling of controlled substances.
- Discuss wasting and accountability for controlled substances.
- Discuss diversion of controlled substances by providers, how surveillance may prevent and/or identify a problem, and what to do when a diversion issue has been identified.
- Discuss risk factors and warning signals associated with a provider who is impaired by drugs and/or alcohol use/abuse.

EMS AGENCY NARCOTICS CONTROL PROGRAM

Diversion means different things to different people. In its strictest sense, diversion means to move attention away from themselves through finger pointing, nit picking, manipulation, sleight of hand, or misdirection. For law enforcement purposes, diversion means the misappropriation of DEA scheduled medications from approved and/or legitimate patient usage, through doctor shopping, prescription forgery, theft, or substitution. Those who divert drugs often utilize skills mentioned in the above definition. EMS providers are not immune to diversion and agencies and medical directors need to be vigilant to ensure that such is not occurring in their systems. Drug addiction is an occupational hazard among EMS professionals, who have easy access to controlled substances such as Fentanyl, Morphine, Demerol, Versed, and other highly addicted drugs. Tampering is the diversion of medications done in such a way that it looks like drugs were never stolen. The tampered medication is then left in the system, to be used by an unsuspecting health care professional. EMS provider reports of patients not experiencing pain relief after the administration of pain medication may be a red flag indicating drug tampering.

Structured programs should be in place to account for and stocking, use, and restocking of controlled medications. EMS professionals cannot consistently divert drugs if the system has adequate physical security and an effective record-keeping system with a comprehensive audit trail. Most EMS health care professionals are unaware of the magnitude

of the legal hazard associated with failing to provide adequate security and maintaining complete and accurate controlled substance records. EMS agencies should have a narcotics control program and written policies covering the acquisition, storage, and use of controlled substances. Elements of this program should include ordering and stocking of drugs, controlled access storage, crew shift counts and checklists, quality improvement programs that monitor use of drugs on specific patients, and medical director sign off on drug counts. **Box 8-1** further describes elements that should be incorporated into an agency-controlled substance program.

Agencies should also have wellness programs, which are a systematic approach for professionals to get assistance in overcoming alcohol or drug addiction. When identified, these individuals enter into a contract where they maintain sobriety to maintain their employment. Model systems use medical models and inpatient services (when needed) for the initial stages followed by regular counseling and continual drug and alcohol screening.

DEA REGULATIONS AND AUTHORITY

The Federal Drug Enforcement Agency (DEA) regulations cover narcotic dispensing and use. All physicians prescribing narcotics are required to maintain a separate license for dispensing narcotics that must be periodically renewed. Historically, many medical directors have used their own DEA license, either directly or through hospital pharmacies, to order controlled substances for their EMS agencies. Presently, this practice is discouraged and has all but disappeared in some areas due to lack of accountability, diversion issues, and increased DEA scrutiny. Obtaining separate physician DEA licenses for each EMS agency for which a physician is providing medical direction is being recommended and even required in some states. The DEA requires absolute accountability by an EMS agency that uses controlled substances during patient care. Areas of accountability are specified clearly in DEA regulations (**Box 8-2**).[1]

Box 8-1

Elements of an Agency-Controlled Substance Program

- Each vial has unique tracking number.
- Providers assigned specific numbered narcotic pouches.
- Providers required to fill out narcotic resupply forms when using narcotics.
- Resupply occurs only after patient care reports and narcotic resupply forms match.
- Weekly reports are made of providers' controlled substance administrations.
- Medical director sign off at least weekly on reports.
- Scheduled and random controlled substance audits are conducted.
- Random provider drug testing conducted as well as ability to conduct testing "for cause" if concerns arise.

Box 8-2

DEA-Required Areas of Drug Accountability

- Ordering and receipt of medications in a manner compliant with DEA regulations
- Proper completion and signature on the third copy of the DEA-222 forms
- Controlled, proper distribution of medications within the agency
- Documentation of all usage and wastage
- Resupply based only on documented usage
- Auditing procedures that use both routine and random inspections
- Investigative procedures in place in the event of incorrect audits

The EMS agency must keep records compliant with all DEA requirements. The DEA has the authority to schedule inspections and audits at any time of controlled substance usage by any "entity" that maintains inventory of these substances, including EMS. EMS agencies should educate all employees that each has a responsibility to report drug diversion according to the Code of Federal Regulations, Section 1301.91. The DEA's stance is an employee who has knowledge of drug diversion by a fellow employee is obligated to report such information to a responsible official of the agency. The agency should treat this information as confidential and take all reasonable steps to protect the confidentiality of the information and identity of the employee furnishing it. The DEA considers failure by an employee to report diversion to directly impact the ability of continuing to allow that employee to work in a drug secured area. Furthermore, the DEA believes employers have a responsibility to inform their employees accordingly of the requirements of the code. All agencies should ensure the above has occurred. Individuals found tampering with or diverting narcotics is charged under the Federal Anti-tampering Act which carries maximum penalties of $25,000 and 10 years in prison. If a death results from these actions the maximum penalty is $100,000 and life imprisonment.

Many of the narcotics, depressants, and stimulants manufactured for legitimate medical use are subject to abuse and have, therefore, been brought under legal control. Under federal law, all businesses that import, export, manufacture, or distribute controlled substances; all health professionals licensed to dispense, administer, or prescribe them; and all pharmacies authorized to fill prescriptions must register with the DEA. Registrants must comply with regulatory requirements relating to drug security and record keeping. The DEA is also obligated under international treaties to monitor the movement of controlled substances across US borders and to issue import and export permits for such.

Title 21 is the portion of the Code of Federal Regulations that governs food and drugs (21 CFR). Individuals having knowledge of drug diversion are obliged to report such knowledge to law enforcement and the DEA through 21 CFR. Specific items that must be reported to the DEA as specified in 21 CFR are noted in **Box 8-3**. The Office of Diversion Control is the component of the DEA which investigates and ensures that the regulations are followed. Diversion investigations can involve physicians who sell prescriptions to drug dealers or abusers; pharmacists who falsify records and sell drugs; employees who steal from inventory or falsify records to cover illicit diversion; prescription forgers; and individuals who commit armed robbery of pharmacies. The DEA considers the theft of controlled substances from a registrant to be a criminal act, and a source of controlled substances diversion requiring notification of DEA (FR Doc 03-17127). The DEA registrant is required to notify the area DEA field office immediately upon discovery of any theft of controlled substances. If the circumstances are known, online DEA form 106 should be filed. When an investigation is needed to determine circumstances, initial notice to the DEA may be done by faxed statement and form 106 submitted after the investigation is completed. Local law enforcement should also be notified, and this may be mandatory in some states. If the medical director is the DEA registrant, this responsibility falls to them. However, if the DEA license belongs to the EMS agency it becomes their responsibility to ensure that law enforcement is properly notified and DEA forms filed.

Box 8-3

Reports Required by 21 CFR*

- Destruction of controlled substances
- Import/export declarations (chemical reports)
- Import/export permit applications and declarations (controlled substances)
- Quota applications and year-end reports
- Theft or loss of controlled substances

* These reports are available online from the DEA.

STATE LAWS AND REGULATIONS

All states have EMS and pharmacy regulations governing the dispensing of narcotic and controlled substances. Compliance with these is overseen by state departments of EMS and pharmacy boards. Pharmacy boards license pharmacists, pharmacies and oversee the distribution of drugs within the state. There are also national organizations dedicated to drug monitoring. The National Association of State Controlled Substance Authorities (www.nascsa.org) is a 501(C)³ nonprofit educational organization whose primary purpose is to provide a mechanism through which state and federal agencies and others can work to increase effectiveness and efficiency of state and national efforts to prevent and control drug diversion and abuse. NASCSA works cooperatively with the DEA, US Food and Drug Administration, Substance Abuse and Mental Health Services Administration, National Institute on Drug Abuse, National Alliance for Model State Drug Laws, state professional licensing boards, pharmaceutical companies, and other national associations. NASCA also sponsors another organization, Alliance of States With Prescription Monitoring Programs (http://www.nascsa.org/rxMonitoring.htm), to facilitate exchange of information across states with prescription monitoring programs. Both the state pharmacy and EMS agencies will conduct monitoring programs for compliance with regulations. These often include periodic on-site inspections of drug storage and records.

State regulations contain explicit instructions as to agency responsibilities in monitoring and dispensing of controlled substances as well as actions to take when loss or diversion is suspected. Failure to comply may lead to loss of licensure or certification of the pharmacy or agency involved. Medical directors should be knowledgeable of the regulations governing controlled substance storage and usage in their states. Administration of drugs by EMS personnel is limited to their scope of practice, as determined by the state office of EMS, the individual's certification level, and the protocols established by the medical director. State regulations also allow drug administration when the EMS provider is acting within their certification level under a direct prescriber's orders received over an active communication link (ie, online medical command).

HANDLING OF CONTROLLED SUBSTANCES

EMS agencies obtain controlled substances either through direct ordering or a hospital exchange program. Many hospitals have a program whereby EMS can do a one-to-one exchange of medications either in the emergency department or pharmacy itself. This often takes the form of obtaining medications through a pyxis device, limiting access to approved personnel. If hospital exchange programs are utilized there generally is also an administrative cost, particularly if the EMS agency bills for service, as federal anti-kickback laws come into play if the hospital provides this service for free.

If EMS agencies choose to pack their own drug boxes rather than hospital exchange of boxes, there are increased responsibilities. EMS agencies must comply with federal and state regulations concerning storage of controlled substances. General security requirements are listed in the Code of Federal Regulations—Title 21 CFR Sections 1301.72-1301.76. Key components of these requirements for schedule II drugs (narcotics) are they must be stored in a safe, steel cabinet or secured room/vault that must be locked at all times when not in use. The safe or cabinet must meet specifications that include 10 man-minutes against forced entry and 20 man-hours against lock manipulation. If the safe or cabinet weighs less than 750 pounds it must be bolted or cemented to the floor. Secure room/vault specifications are also listed. Depending on the quantities and types of controlled substances stored an alarm system may be required. Entry into the safe, cabinet, or secured room/vault should be limited to a limited number of supervising staff. Ideally the secured area should keep a log of who enters at all times. Inventories should be done at least daily, and ideally at each change of shift. Inventory and administration records of controlled substances should be maintained separately from all other records and kept in chronological order. Records of receipt of drugs must also be kept including date of receipt, name and address of person who received, and kind and quantity of drug.

Regardless of how the drugs are obtained, overall supervision and control of these drugs are the responsibility of EMS organization personnel who hold appropriate certification to access the drugs for which they are responsible. All drugs must be secured in a tamper-evident setting with access limited to EMS personnel based on their certification status. All licensed entities that can possess controlled substances are mandated to provide effective controls and procedures to deter and detect theft and drug diversion.

PROPER STORAGE

EMS agencies should have written accountability practices. Controlled substances should be inventoried and recorded at the change of each shift. Both the off-going and on-coming staff members should sign the inventory records, which should be kept for a minimum of 2 years. Discrepancies are most often caused by someone forgetting to sign out a drug for restocking, and should be swiftly corrected when discovered. All shift paperwork must be reviewed until the missing controlled substance documentation is found. It is also helpful to have shift supervisors review inventory sheets frequently and at least on a weekly basis to ensure that compliance is occurring. As stated previously, the DEA registrant is ultimately held responsible for the security and proper use of the controlled substance. As such, the medical director has ultimate responsibility and should periodically review these logs for compliance also. It is suggested that at a minimum this should be done weekly. In some states, physician signature on these logs is actually required by the pharmacy board.

Individual stocked drug boxes should be kept in secured locked compartments within ambulances. If the agency restocks its own drug boxes, those kept at agency headquarters should also be locked in a special area as noted previously at all times. This area should be restricted to only a few personnel who are responsible for dispensing new boxes and inventory of the returned used drug boxes. Best practices would dictate that when a box is returned, both the provider exchanging the box and the supervisor dispensing a new box sign the log and verify the returned drug box contents. Drug inventories should be performed by each EMS agency on a routine basis, tracking drug box expiration dates and ensuring that they are exchanged or used before expiration dates. A rotational system should be developed to place older boxes in service before they expire and replace stock with newly exchanged boxes. Medications and drug boxes should be kept in locked ambulances at all times or removed from vehicles and stored in a properly maintained and locked secure environment if that is not possible.

Drug boxes are to be sealed at all times. EMS agencies should have policies and procedures detailing what providers should do if this is compromised. If accidentally broken or opened and not used, the drug box should be immediately returned for restocking. If a provider finds a box with a broken seal, the contents should be inspected and if missing drugs are found or appear to have been tampered with, the provider should avoid handling the box and notify law enforcement. The box should be returned to the pharmacy where box was packed, or if stocked by the agency, returned to a supervisor so it can be secured until further processing can occur. A drug diversion form should be completed according to state regulations. Many states have regulations requiring EMS agencies to notify the state office of EMS for any suspected diversion, loss, theft, or tampering of controlled substances, medication delivery devices, or other regulated materials from an agency, facility, or vehicle. It behooves the medical director to familiarize themselves with their agencies' policies and to ensure compliance with regulations.

Sealed drug boxes, either from the pharmacy or the agency itself if it does its own restocking, can also be a source of discrepancies. Occasionally, a field provider may open a drug box and find certain medications or supplies missing from the box. There should be a drug box incident reporting form available (preferably placed in each sealed box) for the provider to document what was missing upon opening the

box so that an investigation can ensue to determine what occurred. EMS providers should be instructed to check for the presence of all controlled substances every time they open a drug box. If there are missing controlled substances discovered upon opening the box it is most likely a restocking error. This should be easily detected retrospectively with a review of the records. If the missing controlled substances are not discovered until the box is returned to for exchange, there are more possibilities to consider including diversion which likely will result in increased scrutiny and stress for the provider. The medical director should be cognizant of these occurrences to ensure a pattern does not arise with specific providers. This can be done by asking the agency to provide a copy of any incident report generated as a result of missing controlled substances during restocking, or working collaboratively with the pharmacy involved to alert you of occurrences.

WASTING AND ACCOUNTABILITY

Success of any accountability system is based on the full understanding and support by EMS providers, hospital pharmacies, medical directors, and emergency department physicians. It is common for EMS providers to have small amounts of unused portions of controlled substances left at the end of a call. The most common practice is for the unused portion to be drawn up out of the vial/ampoule and wasted in the presence of a witness. Partially used controlled medications should not be administered to any other patient other than the individual the medication was opened for. The remainder should be disposed of immediately following completion of the transport, and disposal witnessed by an EMS crew member, registered nurse, or pharmacist. Some systems specify who the witness should be, such as an ED nurse. The EMS provider and witness document the waste on the run sheet along with their signatures. Both the amount in milligrams given to the patient and the amount wasted should both be documented on the same record (eg, morphine 6 mg given, 4 mg wasted). Unused portions of controlled substances should never be passed on to other agencies (such as flight programs the agency might have turned the patient over to) or returned to an open drug box. Instead unused portions should be wasted by the provider who opened the vial.

Some systems use reverse distribution where all narcotic containers are returned to headquarters for wasting instead of wasting any unused medication immediately after use. This return allows for random analysis of the medications to ensure that diversion and replacement with substances other than the appropriate narcotic have occurred. When this system is used, all parts of the narcotic container should be returned, especially the lids from vials and the wrappers that held the Carpujects. Benefits to this type of system are that any evidence is retained, rather than discarded, and personnel know that all returned stock or a fraction thereof will be analyzed. This accountability system is quite effective. Fear of getting caught causes addicts to tamper with narcotics rather than outright steal them. Fear of having returned narcotics through reverse distribution programs coming back as saline after analysis has prevented any further cases of diversion in systems that had such difficulties in the past.

The type of controlled substance storage system will depend on the narcotic exchange program used by the EMS agency. Some systems use drug boxes packed in hospital pharmacies. These boxes are generally sealed with a numbered plastic lock by a pharmacist and have a unique identifying number written on the box. The drug boxes are then stored in locked compartments on EMS vehicles. The storage compartment should be temperature controlled. After use, the EMS provider returns the opened drug box with documentation of what was administered and wasted to the pharmacy exchanging it for another sealed box. The pharmacy staff verifies that all controlled substances have been accounted for. Records are kept by the pharmacy of the identifying number on the box, the seal number, agency name, and name of the provider exchanging the box. A similar system should be in place at EMS agency headquarters, if the agency stores and stocks its own drug boxes. Disposal of large amounts of outdated controlled substances must be done in accordance with CFR. The code states that a controlled substance can be returned to a manufacturer who accepts returns, the registrant (DEA license holder) can dispose of the controlled substance under the procedures outlined in 21 CFR 1307.21, or the controlled substance can be turned over to the registered reverse distributor.[2]

DIVERSION OF CONTROLLED SUBSTANCES

The Code of Federal Drug Regulation in Section 1301.91 delineates employee responsibility to report drug diversion. Reports of drug diversion by fellow employees are not only a necessary part of an overall employee security program but also serve the public interest at large. Therefore, it is the position of DEA that an employee, who has knowledge of drug diversion by a fellow employee, has an obligation to report such information to the designated official of the employer. The employer shall treat such information as confidential and take all reasonable steps to protect the confidentiality of the information and identity of the employee furnishing the information. Failure to report information or knowledge of drug diversion can result in the employee not being allowed to work in a drug-secure area. The employer (EMS agency) should inform all employees of this code and policy.

Diversion of controlled substances can occur in many creative ways limited only by the creativity of the involved individuals. There are numerous and probably still to be discovered ways for providers to divert controlled substances. The most common involves replacing the controlled substance with another fluid, hopefully sterile saline. Of all the types of narcotic diversion, tampering with or substituting saline for the narcotic is nearly the most insidious, while also inhumane and selfish as the tampered container is left in the system to be used by an unsuspecting paramedic on an unsuspecting patient. Seemingly tamper proof packaging has proven not to be, as providers develop creative ways of altering packaging. (**Figure 8-1**). Another common ruse is "lost" or "broken" vials. As a certain amount of this occurs in normal operations, it takes vigilance to determine diversion utilizing this method. An anti-theft design by some manufacturers is to use plastic caps that spin before the seal is broken and the cap removed. If a vial cap is removed and glued back on, the cap will not spin, making tampering more noticeable. To circumvent this anti-theft design providers use very small gauge needles to puncture through the plastic cap and rubber stopper and remove the controlled substance. These minute punctures are very difficult to detect, and can only been viewed with a magnifying glass.[3]

Controlled substances can be stolen out of drug boxes. Some drug boxes are similar to fishing tackle boxes with front and side latches. The pharmacy or agency will place plastic seals on the front latch area, but this can be circumvented by removing the top part of the front latch, allowing the front flap to be opened without disturbing the plastic seal. To prevent this, the plastic seal can be placed through drilled holes in the front flap and top cover of the drug box. In addition, plastic seals can be numbered by the pharmacy or agency when dispensed to ensure that a seal is not discarded and replaced with another before returning the box for restocking. It is extremely rare for a provider to need to waste more than one or an entire vial or ampoule of a controlled substance. If

this occurs, extra vigilance is appropriate. Provider explanations of these occurrences include that the medication was drawn up and not given it to the patient or the vial/ampoule was broken or missing when the drug box was opened. Providers who are noted to be wasting or missing multiple units of controlled substances should be counseled, and their controlled substance documentation audited.

Narcotic diversion is insidious, and it is difficult to recognize providers at risk for diversion. There are few common denominators and all levels of providers are involved. The one common denominator is access. Those that divert narcotics often have nearly unconstrained access to the drugs or know how to get access. Effective narcotic control and accountability systems are built to prevent field personnel from having direct physical access to narcotics except for times needed to treat a patient. Otherwise, they are stored inside a tamper-evident lock box. One must remember that access is still available to a supervisor, who is also not immune or above involvement in diversion. Multiple checks and balances should be built into the system to ensure that multiple eyes are on the box count should diversion occur. Narcotics restock programs where medications are stored in a locked area where a single person can access them at any time is a system asking for trouble. A far more secure and better approach would be to have narcotic cabinets utilize two keys: one key for the supervisor or administration and another key for field personnel. An electronic lock that requires two separate combinations, codes, or electronic key card can also be a deterrent and can track those who enter. No supervisor or single person, for their own sake, should ever have unrestricted access to narcotics stock. While the vast majority of EMS personnel are ethical people, unfortunately some are susceptible to temptation.

EFFECTIVE SURVEILLANCE PROGRAMS

An effective surveillance program can help prevent or identify drug diversions if they occur. Radio-frequency identification (RFID) tags can be placed on controlled substances which track location of vials and deter theft, but this can be cost prohibitive. Some form of nonremovable ID tags placed on every container can be helpful and less costly. A commercial shrink wrap machine can be used to secure items. The entire drug box can be closed with tamper evident tape with unique serial numbers. Some systems have used shrink wrap to enclose narcotics vials after placing a metal slug over the cap to prevent needles from being used to withdraw content illicitly. Pharmacy sealed containers can provide accountability if one-to-one exchange of medications occur directly after use, and the exchange is accompanied by a patient report sheet detailing the use of the drugs being restocked.

Some containers are more tamper proof than others. Certain glass ampoules are tamper proof, but have been known to cause provider injury and necessitate the use of filter needles. Agencies who self-stock should develop special secured drug lockers to secure medications before deployment to individual provider units as mentioned previously. It is recommended that the area be key secured and that only two providers have access. These providers would preferably be at the supervisor level. Two are preferred over single access as each can serve as a check on the other. Daily inventories should be conducted and a signed log kept to identify problems should they occur.

An effective quality improvement program is necessary for proper surveillance and heightened awareness to prevent diversion. Audits of run sheets benched against narcotic use should be routine part of the quality improvement program. EMS agencies should educate providers to verify that the medication they give works. If the patient states they are not getting relief from the narcotic, they should question why. Quite often, the first things that come to mind are that the patient is a drug seeker, has low tolerance for pain, or that not all people get relief from narcotics. Sadly we do not tend to keep track of these occurrences as well as we track our resuscitative efforts. If we tracked relief or improvement of pain in those patients whom we administer narcotics, it may trigger problems and the narcotics need to be analyzed for efficacy, environmental damage, and tampering if there is a pattern of no or little relief

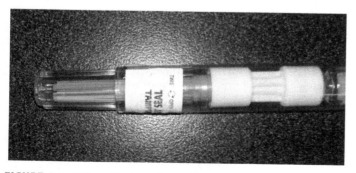

FIGURE 8-1. With a quick glance this morphine carpuject appears unopened, but on closer inspection one can see tampering with the seal. (Reproduced with permission of Heidi M. Hooker, Executive Director, Old Dominion EMS Alliance (ODEMSA), Richmond, Virginia.)

with pain medication administration. These occurrences should also be tracked for patterns relative to specific providers.

IMPAIRED PROVIDERS

As previously stated health care workers are as likely as anyone else to abuse drugs and are unfortunately involved in controlled substances diversion. With easy access to controlled substance medications available, some will divert and abuse these drugs for relief from stress, self-medication, or to improve work performance and alertness. Drug abusers often exhibit similar behaviors, and certain signs may indicate a drug addiction problem in a health care professional (**Box 8-4**).[4,5]

There is a natural reluctance to approach a coworker suspected of drug addiction. Many tend to assume they are overreacting and misinterpreting behaviors. There are fears that speaking out might anger the coworker, result in retribution, or result in termination of the suspected individual. Many employers or coworkers simply end up being "enablers" of health care practitioners as a result. Drug impaired coworkers are frequently protected from the consequences of their behavior. Addicted colleagues are often given lighter work schedules, switched among partners, or excuses made for their poor job performance. Excessive absences from the work site are often overlooked in long time employees who had previously demonstrated good work ethic. Unfortunately, this allows them to continue to rationalize their addictive behavior or continue denial that a problem exists. In addition, there are mandated federal laws regarding reporting that should be followed (see "DEA Regulations and Authority" section earlier in the chapter) with real consequences to the agency and individual if not followed.

If signs or symptoms of impairment are recognized in a provider, it is time to demonstrate concern. Drug abuse and drug dealing are serious problems that should be handled by qualified professionals. If it is suspected that an addiction problem exists or diversion is occurring, employees should be encouraged to *not* intervene on their own and report concerns to their supervisors. As noted in CFR 21, all efforts must be made to protect the identity of the information source if at all possible. Some states have mandatory reporting laws when a health care worker is found to be impaired secondary to drug use. However, most allow for return to work after successful completion of a remediation program with ongoing checks after return to work.

Confrontation techniques for those suspected of impairment start with an expression of concern. This should ideally come from an individual the suspected party respects and is likely to listen to. The denial that often comes with impairment may limit the effectiveness of this approach. Resistance can lead to the next step which is an intervention. This is a

---

Box 8-4

Warning Signs of Impaired Providers

- Chronic tardiness or work absenteeism without notice
- Degradation of performance due to poor decisions, inattention, or bad judgment
- Increasing personal and professional isolation
- Deterioration or lack of personal hygiene
- Increased irritability, mood swings
- Personality changes, anxiety, or depression
- Relationship breakup
- Heavy "wastage" of drugs
- Insistence on personal administration of injected narcotics to patients
- Excessive amounts of time near drug supply
- Volunteer for overtime and are at work when not schedule to be there
- Wearing long sleeves when not appropriate
- Frequent disappearances or long unexplained absences at work, trips to bathroom or stockroom
- Poor record keeping, suspect ledger entries and drug shortages

---

Box 8-5

Recommendations for Successful Interventions

- The intervention should be conducted by a team, not an individual.
- The team leader should be experienced in interventions.
- Team members should be educated about interventions and treatment possibilities.
- It is important to collect and evaluate as much data as possible prior to the intervention.
- Presentations during the intervention process should be focused on facts.
- The team should include only members whose attitude is conducive to the objective tone of the intervention.

---

formal group process whereby the individual meets with a group of individuals who "confront" the individual in a supportive fashion while insisting that he get help. This step should not be undertaken lightly nor before resources are identified and available to help the provider. A member of this group should include a close friend who can offer support and act as an independent supportive voice for the individual. When confrontation occurs, the group should be ready to intervene immediately by getting the provider into a program to receive necessary help. Immediately after confrontation is the most dangerous time for an impaired provider, who may feel they have nothing to lose and possibly resort to self-harm. See **Box 8-5** for effective confrontation recommendations.[6] For some, the mere fact that a supervisor talks to them is enough to help them change. For others the problem may be more severe and require drastic measures such as the threat of termination. The threat of losing a job may have more influence on a drug abuser than a spouse's threat to leave or a friend's decision to end a relationship. Many drug abusers will seek help for their problem if they believe their job is at stake, even though they have ignored such pleas from other people important in their life.[7]

Prior to speaking with an employee suspected of impairment, one should consult with the human resources department regarding applicable policies and procedures. In some settings, immediate drug screening can be mandated for cause. In situations where the employee is a member of a union, there may be a policy that the member has the right to have a union advocate with him during any discussions. He may also have the right to refuse drug screening until such time as a hearing occurs. Violation of processes and policies on the part of a supervisor may leave the agency open to legal redress or personal charges of slander. Therefore, it behooves agency leadership to familiarize themselves with such policies and to contact human resources in every case before any action, including verbal discussions with the employee, is taken.

Drug addicts can recover with appropriate intervention and help. There are effective programs available. Treatment programs range from guided self-help to formal inhospital recovery programs. A number of state licensing boards, employee assistance programs, state diversion programs, and peer assistance organizations are available to individuals and their families for appropriate counseling and treatment services. These services maintain the confidentiality of those seeking assistance to the greatest extent possible. EMS services and medical directors should be familiar with services that exist in their state.[8]

- Title 21 of the Code of Federal Regulations governs food and drugs.
- Title 21 CFR Section 1309.91 defines employee responsibility to report diversion of controlled substances.
- Title 21 CFR Sections 1301.72-76 define general security measures with regard to controlled substances.
- Tampering with or diverting a controlled substance incurs a fine of $25,000 and/or 10 years in prison.
- A death resulting from tampering or diversion of a controlled substance incurs a life prison sentence and $100,000 fine.

REFERENCES

1. Office of Diversion Control. www.deadiversion.usdoj.gov/. Accessed December 12, 2011.
2. Coombs RH, Zeidonis. *Handbook of Drug Abuse Prevention: A Comprehensive Strategy to Prevent the Abuse of Alcohol and Other Drugs.* New York, NY: Oxford University Press; 1995.
3. Solis K. Ethical, legal, and professional challenges posed by "controlled medication seekers" to healthcare providers, Part 2. *Am J Clin Med.* Spring 2010;7(2):86-92.
4. Coombs RH. *Drug-Impaired Professionals.* Cambridge, MA: Harvard University Press; 1997.
5. Beeson J, Ayres C. EMS & the DEA. *JEMS.* January 2010; 35(1):S18-S20.
6. Karp D. Dealing with an impaired colleague. *Med Econ.* 2007;84(8):30.
7. Baldisseri MR. Impaired healthcare professional. *Crit Care Med.* 2007;35(2 suppl):S106-S116.
8. Angres D, Talbott G, Bettinardi-Angres K. *Healing the Healer: The Addicted Physician.* Madison, CT: Psychosocial Press, International University Press Inc; 1998.

CHAPTER 9
Community Relations and Public Health

Anthony J. Billittier IV
Tracy Fricano Chalmers
Robert Donnarumma

INTRODUCTION

Public health as defined by Charles-Edward A. Winslow is "the science and art of preventing disease, prolonging life, and promoting health through the organized efforts and informed choices of society, organizations, public and private, communities, and individuals."[1] The World Health Organization (WHO) defines the whole of public health as "a state of complete physical, mental, and social well-being and not merely the absence of disease or infirmity."[2] Public health's charge is to protect the health of the population, which can range in size from a small group of people to several continents. Overall, public health strives to *prevent* illness and injury by *protecting* individuals from things they cannot directly control (eg, drinking contaminated water, inhaling tuberculosis bacteria) and *promoting* healthy behaviors for things they can directly control (eg, eating healthily, exercising regularly, not smoking).

Public health utilizes the elements of epidemiology, surveillance, and prevention. Epidemiology is the study of the distribution and determinants of health-related states or events in specified populations, and the application of this study to control health problems.[3] Epidemiological investigations are conducted to determine the distribution and determinants of disease and to attempt to categorize disease by person, place, and time.

Surveillance is the ongoing process of collecting, analyzing, and interpreting health data, and disseminating the conclusions to relevant entities. There are several types of surveillance utilized in routine public health practice including passive, active, sentinel, and syndromic. Passive surveillance is frequently utilized at the local and state levels in the form of case reporting. Depending on the locale, there may be well over 50 communicable diseases that must be reported to public health officials when diagnosed or suspected by physicians, laboratories, hospitals, and others. This differs from active surveillance in which public health agencies attempt to proactively identify individuals meeting specific criteria. Finding sexual partners of an individual with HIV or another confirmed sexually transmitted disease would be an example.[4]

Primary prevention, one of the most common public health strategies, includes actions to stop disease from occurring. Examples of primary prevention are childhood immunizations, hand washing, and seat belt use. Secondary prevention involves screening asymptomatic individuals to detect disease in the early stage and thereby preventing clinical manifestations. Examples of secondary prevention include blood pressure screening to detect hypertension, mammography to detect breast cancer, colonoscopy to detect colon cancer, and urine screening in adolescent girls to detect occult sexually transmitted diseases like chlamydia. Tertiary prevention is treatment of clinically manifested disease to halt the progression and complications of the disease.

OBJECTIVES

- Display a general understanding of the history, principles, and core disciplines of public health.
- Discuss the differences between governmental public health departments and the public health system.
- Understand primary, secondary, and tertiary prevention and how they relate to public health and EMS.
- Understand many of the commonalities, synergies, and partnerships, as well as some of the differences between EMS and public health.
- Understand the benefits from partnerships between EMS and public health.

HISTORY OF PUBLIC HEALTH

Public health concepts are evident from ancient times and developed out of necessity as primitive civilizations began to establish cities. Municipal water supplies and sewage systems have been documented by archeologists from ancient cities in Africa, Asia, Europe, and South America. Ancient sanitary engineering peaked in Rome where aqueducts supplied the city with water as effectively as modern water systems do today.

The practice of isolation (separating those with a communicable disease from those without) was practiced in early medieval times. Special rules created separate housing to exclude lepers from communities.

The Renaissance marked the beginning of a period of cultural growth and was also the beginning of a series of epidemics that devastated Europe and the Near East. This included the Black Death (bubonic plague), which killed 25% of the European population in 4 years. These events led to three important contributions to public health: the organization of boards of health, the promulgation of a theory of contagion, and the introduction of vital statistics (contagious disease and mortality data).[5,6]

Concepts emerged during the Enlightenment (1750 through mid-19th century) that encouraged government programs designed to protect the population against disease and to promote health. Theories of Utilitarianism (greatest good for the greatest number) led to legislation regarding prison reform, birth control, establishment of a ministry of health, and sanitary measures. Implementation of these ideas was championed by Edwin Chadwick in his publication *General Report on the Sanitary Condition of the Labouring Population of Great Britain (1842)*. This report illustrated many population-based inequities and resulted in movement toward sewage systems, potable water supplies, refuse disposal, ventilation of housing and work locations, and supervision of public works by qualified individuals.

In 1854, a cholera outbreak in London resulted in a defining moment in epidemiology founded by physician John Snow. Snow was skeptical of the then current miasma theory, which postulated that diseases like cholera or plague were caused by breathing "bad air." Snow's study of the pattern of cholera in London led to the removal of the Broad Street pump based on his conclusion that ingestion of water contaminated with fecal matter resulted in illness. In the 1870s and 1880s tremendous advances were made by French scientist Louis Pasteur and German physician Robert Koch. Together these two scientists are known as the fathers of the germ theory and bacteriology. Pasteur is best known for his recognition that fermentation is caused by growth of microorganisms and spoiling of beverages like beer, wine, and milk. The process of heating liquids to kill harmful bacteria was later termed pasteurization. Pasteur also developed vaccinations for rabies and anthrax. Koch furthered the support of the germ theory with his development of the Koch postulates that outline the characteristics an organism must have to cause disease. He is also famous for isolating several organisms including *Bacillus anthracis*, tuberculosis bacillus, and *Vibrio cholerae*.[5,6]

MODERN PUBLIC HEALTH

The improvements in sanitary conditions and development of bacteriology in the early 20th century reduced mortality from enteric diseases and shifted the focus of public health interventions to other problems. Development of maternal and child health programs to reduce infant mortality, government regulation of the food processing industry, industrial hygiene and occupational health programs to address occupational injury and disease, and focus on mental health and nutrition were among the highlights of this period.

A developmental process known as *epidemiological transition* occurs as a country undergoes modernization from Third World to First World. Population rates sharply increase and then level off due to declining fertility rates. Infectious disease rates decrease because of immunization and communicable disease control, and public health initiatives shift to chronic diseases like heart disease and cancer.[6] In the second half of the 20th century, the role of public health expanded to address aging populations in industrialized nations, recognition of the importance of

---

Box 9-1

10 Essential Functions of Public Health

1. Monitor health status to identify and solve community health problems.

2. Diagnose and investigate health problems and health hazards in the community.

3. Inform, educate, and empower people about health issues.

4. Mobilize community partnerships and action to identify and solve health problems.

5. Develop policies and plans that support individual and community health efforts.

6. Enforce laws and regulations that protect health and ensure safety.

7. Link people to needed personal health services and ensure the provision of health care when otherwise unavailable.

8. Ensure competent public and personal health care workforce.

9. Evaluate effectiveness, accessibility, and quality of personal and population-based health services.

10. Research for new insights and innovative solutions to health problems.

From http://www.cdc.gov/nphpsp/essentialServices.html.

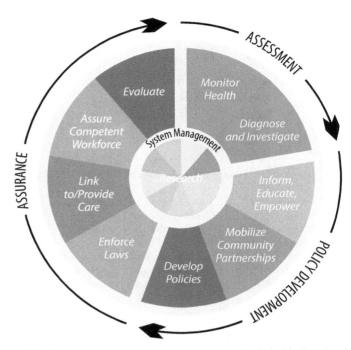

FIGURE 9-1. Core elements and 10 essential functions of public health. (From http://www.cdc.gov/nceh/ehs/EPHLI/core_ess.htm.)

behavioral risk factors (eg, diet, tobacco use, obesity, high-risk sexual practices), increasing social inequalities in health, and violence.[5]

As we move into the 21st century, public health faces challenges such as naturally emerging infections like severe acute respiratory syndrome (SARS) and the H1N1 pandemic; bioterrorism by the intentional release of anthrax and diseases previously eradicated such as smallpox; health inequities and lack of access to affordable health care; childhood obesity; and long-term effects of natural disasters including the Indian Ocean tsunami (2004), Hurricane Katrina (2005), and the Haiti earthquake (2010).

The 1988 Institute of Medicine (IOM) report *The Future of Public Health* describes three core functions of public health that are necessary to maintain and improve the health of the community. These include assessment, policy development, and assurance. Assessment involves the ongoing collection of community health data, and the analysis of these findings to identify trends in illness, injury, and death. Priorities determined from assessment are used to develop local, state, and federal health policies, which must consider community, political, and social infrastructures for successful implementation. Assurance is making sure that all members of the population have access to appropriate and cost-effective health services including those for prevention and health promotion along with evaluation of the effectiveness of these efforts.[7]

The 1994 Vision of Public Health in America "Healthy People in Healthy Communities" outlined the goals of public health to prevent epidemics and the spread of disease, protect against environmental hazards, promote and encourage healthy behaviors and injury prevention, respond to disasters and assist communities in recovery, and ensure the quality and accessibility of health services.[8] The 10 essential functions of public health (**Box 9-1**) are those public health services necessary to achieve these goals. Together, they provide a working definition of public health and a guiding framework for the responsibilities of public health systems. These essential services operationalize the core functions of public health. The relationship between the core functions and the essential services are illustrated in **Figure 9-1**.

TEN GREATEST PUBLIC HEALTH ACHIEVEMENTS

Although somewhat subjective, health scientists at the CDC nominated the most noteworthy public health achievements in the United States from 2001 to 2010. These include vaccine-preventable diseases, prevention and control of infectious diseases, tobacco control, maternal and infant health, motor vehicle safety, cardiovascular disease prevention, occupational safety, cancer prevention, childhood lead poisoning prevention, and public health preparedness and response. These advances in public

health led to significant contributions in the decrease in the age-adjusted death rate from the leading causes of death in the United States.[9]

ORGANIZATION OF PUBLIC HEALTH AGENCIES

Effective delivery of services by public health organizations at the federal, state, tribal, and local levels requires a capable and qualified workforce, up-to-date data and information systems, and public health agencies capable of assessing and responding to public health needs.[10] A strong public health infrastructure depends on effective coordination among all of these organizations.

INTERNATIONAL PUBLIC HEALTH

WHO is the directing and coordinating authority for health within the United Nations system. It is responsible for providing leadership on global health matters, shaping the health research agenda, setting norms and standards, articulating evidence-based policy options, providing technical support to countries, and monitoring and assessing health trends. WHO fulfills these objectives through its core functions that include providing leadership on matters critical to health and engaging in partnerships where joint action is needed; shaping the research agenda and stimulating the generation, translation, and dissemination of valuable knowledge; setting norms and standards and promoting and monitoring their implementation; articulating ethical and evidence-based policy options; providing technical support, catalyzing change, and building sustainable institutional capacity; and monitoring the health situation and assessing health trends.[11]

FEDERAL HEALTH AGENCIES

Most US governmental health agencies fall under the Department of Health and Human Services (HHS). HHS is the principal department responsible for protecting the health of all Americans along with providing essential human services especially for those who are least able to help themselves. HHS comprises the Office of the Secretary (18 staff divisions) and 11 operating divisions including the Centers for Disease

Control and Prevention (CDC), the Food and Drug Administration (FDA), the Health Resources Services Administration (HRSA), and the National Institutes of Health (NIH).

The CDC is considered the national authority on public health. It promotes health and quality of life by preventing and controlling disease, injury, and disability. The CDC is composed of the Office of the Director, the National Institute for Occupational Safety and Health, the Center for Global Health, and five offices including Public Health Preparedness and Response; State and Local Support; Surveillance, Epidemiology and Laboratory Services; Non-communicable Diseases, Injury, and Environmental Health; and Infectious Diseases.[12]

The FDA is responsible for protecting the public health by ensuring the safety, efficacy, and security of human and veterinary drugs, biological products, medical devices, cosmetics, products that emit radiation, and our nation's food supply. Ideally, this is accomplished while simultaneously helping speed innovations that make medicines and foods more effective, safer, and more affordable. In addition, the FDA ensures that the public receives accurate, science-based information on medicines and food to improve their health.[13]

The HRSA is the primary federal agency responsible for improving access to health care services especially for people who are uninsured, isolated, or medically vulnerable. The Indian Health Services (IHS) provides a comprehensive public health and health care delivery system for approximately 1.9 million American Indians and Alaska Natives who belong to 564 federally recognized tribes in 35 states.[14]

In addition to the agencies that fall under the HHS umbrella, there are several other agencies responsible for protecting specific aspects of the public's health. The Environmental Protection Agency (EPA) is tasked with protecting human health and the environment by writing and enforcing regulations based on laws passed by Congress. Since 1970, the EPA has been working for a cleaner, healthier environment for the American people. The Occupational Safety and Health Administration (OSHA) ensures the health and safety of America's workers by setting and enforcing standards; providing training, outreach, and education; establishing partnerships; and encouraging continual improvement in workplace health and safety. The mission of the National Highway Traffic Safety Administration or NHTSA is to save lives, prevent injuries, and reduce economic costs due to road traffic crashes through education, research, safety standards, and enforcement activity. It includes the office of EMS, which leads federal EMS efforts.

STATE HEALTH AGENCIES

The US Constitution delegates the main responsibility for protecting the public's health to the states that may, in turn, delegate authority to the local level. As a result, there are considerable differences in state approaches. At least half of the states report having a free-standing public health agency (state department of health), and the remainder include public health under a larger umbrella such as a department of human services.[15] Although there is some variability in the functioning of state health departments, most distribute funds to local health departments and other agencies; maintain datasets of vital statistics (birth and death certificates); collect and report information on reportable communicable diseases; credential health care professionals; and oversee public health laboratories, rural health, special needs children, and minority health.[16] In some states, the lead EMS agency is a division of the state health department.

LOCAL HEALTH DEPARTMENTS

As the level of authority moves to the local level, an even greater variability in governance, organizational structure, and roles and responsibilities exist. The National Association of City and County Health Officials (NACCHO) developed the National Profile of Local Health Departments (LHD) in 2008 to characterize the jurisdiction and governance of LHD.[12] Only a small percentage (5%) of the 2794 LHD in the United States

Rank	Activity or Service	Percentage of Jurisdictions
1	Adult immunizations provision	88%
2	Communicable/infectious disease surveillance	88%
3	Child immunizations provision	86%
4	Tuberculosis screening	81%
5	Food service establishment inspection	77%
6	Environmental health surveillance	75%
7	Food safety education	74%
8	Tuberculosis treatment	72%
9	Tobacco use prevention	70%
10	Schools/daycare center inspection	68%

TABLE 9-1 Percentage of LHD Jurisdictions With 10 Most Frequent Activities and Services Available Through LHDs Directly

serve populations larger than 500,000 persons, and the majority (64%) serve populations less than 50,000 persons. Most LHD (60%) are county based. An additional 11% serve combined city-county jurisdictions; 9% serve multicounties, districts, or regions; 7% serve cities; and 11% serve towns. The services provided at the local level depend on the roles and responsibilities performed by the state, and the size of the population served. The top 10 activities provided by LHD are presented in **Table 9-1**.

Emergency medical services (EMS) were provided by less than 5% of the LHD surveyed. The majority of EMS at the local level was provided by other governmental agencies or nongovernmental organizations (NGO).[17]

NONGOVERNMENTAL ORGANIZATIONS AND COMMUNITY-BASED ORGANIZATIONS

NGO and community-based organizations (CBO) including private, nonprofit agencies play an important role in the delivery of public health services. Many were created to target education, funding, advocacy, and legislation for specific public health issues. The American Cancer Society, National Safety Council, and American Lung Association are a few examples. In some localities NGO and CBO provide public health services either in partnership with the LHD or directly through contractual services.

THE PUBLIC HEALTH SYSTEM

The public health *system* comprises governmental public health departments and other local, state, and federal agencies together with all other entities that play a part in protecting the public's health. These other entities include, but are not limited to, NGO/CBO, public health laboratories, health care providers, hospitals, medical and health related schools, and EMS agencies. A high degree of collaboration and cooperation among these partners is challenging, yet extremely important to ensure a seamless, efficient, and effective system.

Given the diversity and complexity of modern threats to the health and wellness of the community, the public health system must ensure the delivery of a broad spectrum of services. Although there is often considerable overlap, specialization into various public health disciplines is necessary to ensure adequate expertise in each area of public health. Most consider chronic and communicable disease control, environmental health, social and behavioral health, maternal and child health, laboratory services, and, more recently, public health emergency preparedness and response (PHEP) to be core public health disciplines. Other public health disciplines may include school health, home health care, occupational health, forensic death investigation, and EMS.

Communicable diseases control is accomplished through prevention, investigation, and intervention including treatment. Hand washing, respiratory etiquette, and immunizations are important components of infectious disease prevention. Guidelines and schedules for immunizations are typically recommended at the federal level (Advisory Committee on Immunization Practices), mandated by public health law at the state level, and operationalized (immunization clinics) and enforced (exclusion from work or school) at the local level.

Local and state health agencies investigate outbreaks of infectious disease to determine and eliminate the source and to prevent further spread. Foodborne illness, various respiratory infections (pertussis, TB, *Legionella*), and sexually transmitted diseases occur routinely and often require case investigation, contact tracing, and information gathering through interviews. Somewhat extraordinary measures are sometimes employed to enhance disease control efforts. Directly observed therapy (DOT) to ensure medication compliance by tuberculosis patients has become a standard of care. Expedited partner therapy (EPT), which is the provision of additional prescriptions for sexual partner(s) of patients diagnosed with chlamydia infections, has also been utilized to improve eradication.

Environmental health encompasses the theory and practice of assessing and controlling factors in the environment that can potentially affect health.[18] WHO includes those external physical, biological, and chemical factors that affect human health, , and related behaviors. Environmental health services vary by jurisdiction but generally ensure the safety of food, water, air, soil, and the built environment.

Food safety and protection may include permitting and inspection of food establishments, training for food handlers, and investigation of foodborne disease outbreaks. Environmental health programs ensure the safety of public facilities frequented by members of the community such as day care centers, children's camps, swimming pools and spas, beaches, hotels and motels, migrant worker camps, body piercing and tattoo parlors, and hair salons and barber shops. Statutory and/or regulatory requirements often mandate lifeguards, adequate chlorination, safety plans, sterilization, and placement of automated external defibrillators (AED). Other threats addressed by environmental health include childhood lead poisoning; radon and indoor air quality; tobacco use in public places; public and private water systems; septic systems; land-use planning; rabies; and vectors such as mosquitoes, ticks, and rodents.

Human behavior is one of the important determinants of health. Social and behavioral health attempts to change individual behaviors using "the carrot" and/or "the stick" approach. Education may be used to encourage safe, healthy behaviors, and governmental regulation may be used to discourage unhealthy behaviors. Behavioral change is typically difficult and gradual. There are many examples of behavioral modification addressing sexual activity; drug, alcohol, and tobacco use; and injury prevention. The "Click it or Ticket" campaign has included both education and fines to successfully increase seatbelt use to 85%.[19] Recently, much attention has been focused on the use of social media to impact health-related behaviors.

Following the tragic events on September 11, 2001, the discipline of public health emergency preparedness and response has mushroomed within health departments nationwide. In large part, this is a result of the CDC's annual Public Health Emergency Preparedness Cooperative Agreements that infuse significant funds and provide guidance and technical assistance to states, territories, and LHD. This has led to a readiness to respond to a variety of emergencies and disasters ranging from severe weather events to incidents involving chemical, biological, radiological, nuclear, and explosive (CBRNE) agents. Successful mitigation hinges on an all-hazards approach and close working relationships with many local and state partners such as the American Red Cross, health care providers, schools and universities, businesses, and traditional first responders including law enforcement, fire, HAZMAT, emergency management, and EMS.

EMS AS PART OF THE PUBLIC HEALTH SYSTEM

By their very nature EMS systems are uniquely positioned in most communities since they typically fall into many camps. EMS has traditionally been closely aligned with the public safety and emergency services community. However, EMS delivers health care in the austere out-of-hospital environment and rightly should also be considered a component of the health care delivery system. In fact, EMS providers are often the true frontline of the health care system for some patients, interacting with them in their homes, workplaces, and communities. More recently, the concept that EMS is actually part of the public health system has emerged. These overlapping partnerships provide both EMS providers and EMS physicians with exciting bridging opportunities to greatly impact their communities through beneficial exploitation.

COMMONALITIES BETWEEN EMS AND PUBLIC HEALTH

A natural commonality among emergency departments, EMS systems, and public health is their service to communities at large. They provide access to all comers regardless of ability to pay. They often serve the disadvantaged. They care for citizens with all types of health needs, as well as many nonmedical needs. Perhaps most significantly, they all serve as safety nets for the population at large, and thereby support the public health initiative to reduce health disparities. EMS systems offer universal access (anyone can call for an ambulance at any time for any reason) and equitable resource availability (same equipment, same personnel every time).[20] Also common to public health, effective EMS must delve into many disciplines both within and peripheral to the health care. These include adult and pediatric medical and injury care, maternal and child health, mental health, lifestyle behaviors, environmental issues, community service, social service, public education, public advocacy, and even transportation service. Therefore, in addition to competent clinical knowledge and skills, EMS providers and EMS physicians should be well versed in those economic, social, cultural, psychological, environmental, and other community conditions that greatly impact their EMS systems and their patients.

A working group assembled by NHTSA, the National Association of EMS Physicians (NAEMSP), and the American Public Health Association (APHA) identified eight potential benefits in partnering EMS and Public Health efforts (**Table 9-2**).[21] Key components of this collaborative include surveillance, disaster response, screening, community education, neutralization of socioeconomic disparities, workforce development and safety, and allocation of resources. Both EMS and public health stand to gain from this symbiosis. More importantly though, leveraging this partnership will ultimately benefit the health and wellness of the populations they commonly serve.

TABLE 9-2	**Benefits of Collaboration Between EMS and Public Health**
Reduced health care costs	A greater range of resources and options for delivery of services, offering improvements in efficiency and reduced costs
Greater accountability	Reduce uncertainty about roles and improve accountability for community health
Education	A simplified delivery system and improved community outreach
Coverage	Combining the unique surveillance and access resources to improved reach into underserved areas and populations
Security and stability	Assess the relative value of health services and allocate health care funding to provide the greatest value to the community
Access	Extend the reach of EMS and the mobility of EMS to enhance the delivery of public health services
Adaptability	A combined EMS and public health system will be capable of quickly detecting and responding to community health needs
Improved health	Improved responsiveness, greater efficiency, and enhanced effectiveness will lead to improved health in the community

PARTNERSHIP BENEFITS PRIMARILY TO PUBLIC HEALTH

Originally developed to stem the tide of infectious disease, traditional surveillance efforts have broadened to include the scope of injuries, domestic violence, occupational hazards, chronic medical conditions, environmental hazards, and more. Data acquisition by public health is often challenging, and EMS can be a valuable source of information. EMS frequently interfaces with impoverished, underserved, and difficult to reach communities that are also typically the focus of public health actions. Thanks to modern technology, EMS data can be made available in near real time, which is important for some public health needs. Scene information to which only EMS providers might be privy can be particularly helpful to public health for developing injury prevention strategies. From a more social perspective, EMS data may be useful for identification of unsafe living conditions for at-risk populations who can then be guided to appropriate resources.

Public health access to EMS data for surveillance purposes will likely continue to expand with the ever-increasing promotion of electronic health information. As a unique example, the US Customs and Border Protection on the US-Mexico border has used EMS call logs to screen travelers for infectious disease and then enact isolation precautions when indicated.[22] In Seattle, Baer et al analyzed emergency department and EMS databases to detect an increase in carbon monoxide intoxications following a wind storm that was associated with power outages.[23] Inclusion of electronic prehospital care records by regional health information organizations or RHIOs will likely help continue to facilitate this information age transition.

EMS AGENCY ROLES IN DISEASE PREVENTION

Relevant findings from public health community health assessments may lead to primary or secondary prevention interventions. While the primary role of EMS in the community has traditionally been tertiary prevention, EMS resources can support public health–driven primary and secondary prevention programs. Prevention efforts during EMS downtime may be most cost-effective since the costs of EMS provider salaries are already fixed. However, these interventions should be flexible and brief given the unpredictable nature of the EMS schedule. Distribution of condoms along with brief sexually transmitted infection and teen pregnancy prevention information is one of numerous examples.

More involved prevention efforts can be undertaken by EMS during off-duty time. An example of the interplay between surveillance and health promotion was the creation of the Eliminating Preventable Injuries in Children (EPIC) Foundation in San Diego by local paramedics. After the tragic drowning of a young boy, EMS system data were used to create a community education and advocacy campaign to reduce childhood drowning.[24] Other successes include education on the use of public access AEDs[25]; helmet and child car seat distribution; and health-fair style hypertension, diabetes, and other chronic disease screenings that often include an educational component designed to change health behaviors.

When studied by Lerner et al,[26] a majority of EMS professionals thought that they should participate in disease and injury prevention programs, and about a third of them reported that they actually had already provided prevention services. There are, however, barriers and shortcomings to EMS-based health promotion activities especially in the clinical arena. Health behaviors are deeply seeded and may not be amenable to change because of any single interaction. Patients may not be receptive to EMS provider educational efforts for various reasons including distraction by the acuity of their illness, inadequate respect for EMS provider advice, or simply because of minimal contact time. EMS providers may be resistant to this additional responsibility for various reasons including time constraints of the emergency clinical interaction and reluctance to acquire necessary, new skills especially without increased compensation. Brownson et al. has listed 10 strategies for overcoming these difficulties with Brown and Devine adapting these strategies for EMS-based health promotion (**Table 9-3**).[27]

TABLE 9-3	Sample Approaches for Overcoming Barriers to Health Promotion
Start with environmental and policy interventions	Working to create healthy environments or healthy public policy avoids some of the difficulties associated with directly trying to change individual attitudes and behaviors or the structure of the EMS system, has less immediate impact on clinical caregiving, and may be less threatening than an initiative that requires explicit patient-oriented action by paramedics.
Think comprehensively and across multiple levels	Health problems are multifaceted, and there is rarely one single intervention that can solve a health problem. Develop health-promotion initiatives that attack a problem on more than one front. They probably will not all be successful, but they might not all fail, either.
Use economic evaluations	Demonstrating the economic benefits of improved health, or at least the continued costs of poor health, can facilitate change at the individual (patients and paramedics), institutional (EMS and health care system), and governmental levels.
Use existing tools	Adapt health-promotion initiatives and materials that have been successfully implemented in other areas and by other disciplines.
Understand local context	Determine the kinds of EMS-based health-promotion initiatives the community (individuals, organizations, business, government) will be most receptive to and start with those.
Understand politics	Identify key stakeholders in the community, and engage them in the efforts early. Be as inclusive as possible.
Build new and nontraditional partnerships	Pursue an intersectoral approach to every initiative and be creative.
Address health	Keep the focus on improving health and participate in health-promoting initiatives that arise from other sectors.
Learn from others	Keep abreast of what other EMS-based health-promotion programs are doing, the obstacles they are encountering, and the successes they are experiencing. Adopt things that have been shown to work elsewhere; do not waste resources on things that have already failed.
Participate in research	Conduct ongoing evaluations of health-promotion efforts, and revise programs appropriately. Initiate, or participate in, scientific analyses of the results of health-promotion programs. Data supporting the effectiveness of EMS-based health promotion will help generate support for expanded and new programs.

Reproduced with permission from Table II of Brown LH and Devine S. EMS & health promotion: a next step in the collaboration between EMS and public health. *EMS World*. Oct. 2008;37(10):113.

In addition to population-based surveillance data, EMS can actively and passively provide relevant individual patient information to public health. On a day-to-day basis this may take the form of screening and case reporting of various conditions and suspected diseases such as TB, meningitis, individuals living in squalor, and clusters of individuals with similar presentations that could have resulted from common ingestion of contaminated food, inhalation of carbon monoxide, etc. During events that are widespread and ongoing, EMS can assist public health efforts by targeted screening of individuals with radiological or chemical contamination and identification of individuals who may require isolation or quarantine because of exposure to a circulating infectious agent.

EMS SYSTEM RESPONSE TO PUBLIC HEALTH EMERGENCIES/DISASTERS

The roles EMS can play during disasters and other emergency events could also go well beyond basic information sharing. The shrinking public health workforce could be supplemented by EMS providers functioning within, as well as beyond their scope of practice. One of the marquee public health emergency preparedness functions is mass prophylaxis during epidemics and other communicable disease exposures such as might occur from a food handler with hepatitis A infection. EMS

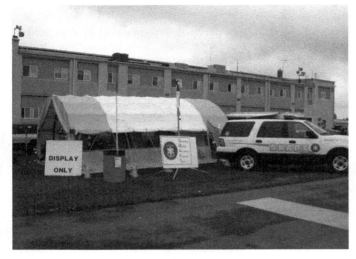

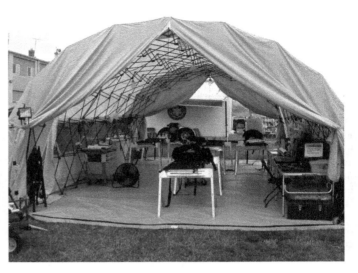

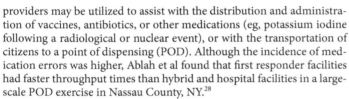

FIGURE 9-2. Medical Reserve Corps deployment.

providers may be utilized to assist with the distribution and administration of vaccines, antibiotics, or other medications (eg, potassium iodine following a radiological or nuclear event), or with the transportation of citizens to a point of dispensing (POD). Although the incidence of medication errors was higher, Ablah et al found that first responder facilities had faster throughput times than hybrid and hospital facilities in a large-scale POD exercise in Nassau County, NY.[28]

EMS providers and EMS physicians can play many other roles in support of public health. These include triage during mass casualty and epidemic events, medical screening in POD, recovery of remains from mass fatality sites such as a plane crash, decontamination of victims, provision of comfort care to moribund patients, medical support for public health workers and other responders, medical care in shelters and alternate care facilities, and assistance with infectious disease containment. This latter role could include support of voluntary and mandatory quarantine and isolation enforcement, as well as dissemination of respiratory masks, other supplies, and information to the populous to help prevent the spread of pathogens.

This concept has been formalized and operationalized in western New York. A partnership between the Erie County Department of Health (ECDOH) and the Department of Emergency Medicine at the University at Buffalo has created the Specialized Medical Assistance Response Team (SMART). Emergency medicine residents, EMS fellows, and EMS physicians remain available 24/7 to respond to events throughout the western New York region in fully equipped emergency response vehicles. Initially created in the 1990s as a way to train emergency medicine residents and EMS fellows, SMART has since grown through recruitment of other physician specialists, midlevel clinicians, nurses, EMS providers, pharmacists, respiratory therapists, mental health professionals, funeral directors, and other technical specialists who are deployed as a Medical Reserve Corps during prolonged public health events (**Figure 9-2**). However, along with local EMS, the EMS physician component of SMART continues to serve as the first response arm of the ECDOH to large and small public health events with any patient involvement. This partnership has led to better utilization and availability of limited resources throughout the eight county region of western New York,[29] and is a win-win for all parties.

PARTNERSHIP BENEFITS PRIMARILY TO EMS

EMS may benefit from guidance and other support provided by public health. Guidelines provided by public health regarding alternate standards of care and allocation of limited resources may be beneficial to EMS. These guidelines may allow EMS providers and EMS physicians to extricate themselves from ethically difficult (and perhaps impossible) rationing decisions and to redirect any criticism and legal challenges to public health.

■ PUBLIC HEALTH IMPACT ON EMS PROVIDER HEALTH AND WELLNESS

EMS providers themselves may be the direct beneficiaries of various public health programs including worksite wellness, immunization, and smoking cessation. Other protective actions by public health such as guidelines for personal protective equipment use, fit testing, and EMS provider isolation and quarantine measures may prove invaluable to EMS providers during communicable disease events. This became reality during the SARS outbreak that impacted Toronto EMS in 2003.[30] Following exposure to patients with SARS, isolation of symptomatic paramedics became necessary. In addition, a working quarantine program was developed to ensure an adequate EMS workforce remained available while minimizing the risk of further spread of the virus.

■ PUBLIC HEALTH SUPPORT OF EMERGENCY SERVICES

Shrinking budgets continuously threaten most public and private industries and subject them to ongoing close scrutiny. EMS is no different and may, in fact, face bigger challenges given its sizeable governmental funding. All the positive aspects of EMS may be tampered by ongoing debate regarding overuse and abuse of emergency care. As recently as this year, Governor Cuomo of New York created a Medicaid Redesign Team that quickly identified ambulance "frequent fliers" as a target to reduce costs and achieve savings.[31] It will be important for EMS physicians and other EMS leaders to advocate on behalf of EMS to ensure that a balance is struck between cost-effectiveness and the potential for missing a true emergency.

The success of EMS leaders to advocate on its behalf will hinge in part on the overall public perception of EMS and the stature it enjoys within the community. The approval of EMS as a subspecialty of emergency medicine by the American Board of Emergency Medicine (ABEM) in September, 2010, solidified the academic history and promise of the field. Weaving EMS fellowships, as well as resident and medical student rotations in EMS into the community fabric will help further ingrain the indispensability of EMS. Arguably, the more value-added services EMS provides, the stronger the voice it will have. Insertion of EMS into public health activities and other facets of the community such as EMT classes in high schools, community CPR and first-aid training, and safety demonstrations may also help solidify its future and prevent further degradation of this community safety net.

COMMUNITY PARAMEDICINE

An emerging practice model that joins EMS and public health in many ways is currently referred to *community paramedicine*. In many systems, it has long been apparent that the expansion of the practice of paramedicine into a more complete health care enterprise would be considered a method of meeting the increasing need for access to health care, especially in rural environments. Community paramedicine has been described as "an organized system of services, based on local need, provided by emergency medical technicians and paramedics, that is integrated into the local or regional health care system and overseen by emergency and primary care physicians."[32] In addition to addressing the needs of patients who frequently call 9-1-1 due to a lack of access to nonemergency primary care services, there appear to be very real possibilities of utilizing paramedics for home health assessments, physical therapy, and to enhance hospital-based admission avoidance (aversion) programs. Demonstration projects are underway in numerous communities around the county and professional organizations like the National Association of Emergency Medical Technicians (NAEMT), the American Academy of Family Physicians (AAFP), the American College of Emergency Physicians (ACEP), and the National Association of EMS Physicians (NAEMSP) are working to evaluate this new area of practice and to help guide the development of this new area of EMS medicine. The utilization of prehospital providers to immunize, treat, and provide preventative health services without transport will require continued development of an alternative funding methodology, including changes in the reimbursement of services by government and private insurance programs.

CONCLUSION

EMS providers and EMS physicians have a somewhat comprehensive and extraordinary perspective of the interface between the health care system and society at large. This affords them with an opportunity to contribute to, and potentially influence, public health policy decisions. Active EMS involvement in advocacy, research, and other public health endeavors can spark excitement and job satisfaction among both EMS providers and EMS physicians. Career ladders in EMS are often limited for EMS providers, and expansion into various public health programs could be another source of vocational fulfillment. EMS physicians can help plug many gaps in the limited clinical expertise in many governmental public health departments. Their support of public health is truly valuable, and could lead to other career opportunities, as well as funding, academic, research, and other partnering possibilities.

KEY POINTS

- Public health is the "the science and art of preventing disease, prolonging life, and promoting health through the organized efforts and informed choices of society, organizations, public and private, communities, and individuals."[1]
- Public health focuses on primary prevention (interventions to avert the onset of disease) and secondary prevention (screening for asymptomatic disease to avoid disease progression and onset of clinical symptoms). EMS focuses on tertiary prevention (treatment of symptomatic disease).
- The public health *system* includes governmental public health departments along with many other governmental and nongovernmental entities including EMS that have the common goal of protecting the public's health.
- The National Highway Traffic Safety Administration's Office of EMS leads federal EMS efforts.
- Partnerships between EMS and public health can be mutually beneficial and can increase vocational, advocacy, funding, academic, research, and other opportunities for EMS providers and EMS physicians.
- Three core functions of public health include assessment, policy development, and assurance.

- Public health focuses on primary prevention to avert onset of a disease or injury and secondary prevention to screen for asymptomatic disease, while EMS typically focuses on tertiary prevention which includes treatment of symptomatic disease or injury.
- Key components of EMS and public health collaboration include surveillance, disaster response, screening, community education, neutralization of socioeconomic disparities, workforce development and safety, and allocation of resources.

REFERENCES

1. Winslow CE. The untilled fields of public health. *Science*. 1920; 51:23.
2. Preamble to the Constitution of the World Health Organization as adopted by the International Health Conference, New York, 19-22 June, 1946; signed on 22 July 1946 by the representatives of 61 States (Official Records of the World Health Organization, no. 2, p. 100) and entered into force on April 7, 1948.
3. Last JM, ed. *A Dictionary of Epidemiology*. 4th ed. New York, NY: Oxford University Press; 2000.
4. Centers for Disease Control and Prevention. Summary of notifiable diseases-United States. *MMWR Morb Mortal Wkly Rep*. 2009;58(53);1-100.
5. Answers.com. History of public health. http://www.answers.com/topic/history-of-public-health. Accessed July 27, 2011.
6. Wikipedia.com. Public health history. http://en.wikipedia.org/wiki/Public_Health#History_of_public_health. Accessed June 21, 2011.
7. Institute of Medicine. *The Future of Public Health*. Washington, DC: National Academies Press; 1988.
8. Public Health Steering Committee, Office of Disease Prevention and Health Promotion. Public Health in America. Fall 1994. http://www.health.gov/phfunctions/public.htm. Accessed April 5, 2015.
9. Centers for Disease Control and Prevention. Ten great public health achievements-United States, 2001-2010. *MMWR Morb Mortal Wkly Rep*. 2011;60(19);619-623.
10. Healthy People 2020. Public health infrastructure. http://www.healthypeople.gov/2020/topicsobjectives2020/overview.aspx?topicid=35. Accessed July 27, 2011.
11. World Health Organization. http://www.who.int/en/. Accessed July 21, 2011.
12. Centers for Disease Control and Prevention. www.cdc.gov. Accessed July 25, 2011.
13. Food and Drug Administration. www.fda.gov. Accessed July 25, 2011.
14. Indian Health Services. www.ihs.gov. Accessed July 25, 2011.
15. Beitsch LM, Brooks RG, Grigg M, Menachemi N. Structure and functions of state public health agencies. *Am J Public Health*. 2006;96(1):167-172.
16. State and local health departments. In: *Encyclopedia of Public Health*. Lester Breslow, ed. Gale Cengage, 2002. eNotes.com. 2006. http://www.enotes.com/public-health-encyclopedia/state-local-health-departments. Accessed August 8, 2011.
17. National Association of County and City Health Officials. 2005 National profile of local health departments. Washington, DC. 2009. http://www.naccho.org/topics/infrastructure/profile/resources/2008report/upload/NACCHO_2008_ProfileReport_post-to-website-2.pdf. Accessed April 5, 2015.
18. World Health Organization. Environmental health. http://www.who.int/topics/environmental_health/en/. Accessed July 25, 2011.
19. National Highway Traffic and Safety Administration. National Seat Belt Enforcement Mobilization. May 21 - June 3, 2012. http://www.nhtsa.gov/CIOT. Accessed August 27, 2011.
20. Brown LH, Devine S. EMS & public health. http://www.emsworld.com/article/10320821/ems-health-promotion. Accessed April 5, 2015.

21. National Highway Traffic Safety Administration. *EMS & Public Health: Building a Partnership for Community Health Care [electronic version]*. Washington, DC: National Highway Traffic Safety Administration; 2000.

22. CDC. Public health surveillance using emergency medical service logs—U.S.-Mexico land border, El Paso, Texas, 2009. *MMWR.* June 4, 2010;59(21):649-653.

23. Baer A, Elbert Y, Burkom HS, Holtry R, Lombardo JS, Duchin JS. Usefulness of syndromic data sources for investigating morbidity resulting from a severe weather event. *Disaster Med Public Health Prep.* 2011 Mar;5(1):37-45.

24. Griffiths K. Best practices in injury prevention: National award highlights programs across the nation. *JEMS.* 2002;27(8):60-74.

25. Winkle RA. The effectiveness and cost effectiveness of public-access defibrillation. *Clin Cardiol.* July 2010;33(7):396-399.

26. Lerner EB, Fernandez AR, Shah MN. Do emergency service professionals think they should participate in disease prevention? *Prehosp Emerg Care.* January-March 2009;13(1):64-70.

27. Brown LH, Devine S. A next step in the collaboration between EMS and public health. *EMS World.* October 2008;37(10):113.

28. Ablah E, et al. A large-scale points-of-dispersing exercise for first responders and first receivers in Nassau County, New York. *Biosecr Bioterror.* March 2010;8(1):25-35.

29. Billittier AJ. Regional emergency preparedness efforts by local health departments in Western New York. *J Public Health Manag Pract.* 2003;9(5):394-400.

30. Verbeek PR, McClelland IW, Silverman AC, Burgess RJ. Loss of paramedic availability in an urban emergency medical services system during a severe acute respiratory syndrome outbreak. *Acad Emerg Med.* September 2004;11(9):973-978.

31. New York State. Department of Health. Redesigning New York's Medicaid Program. http://www.health.ny.gov/health_care/medicaid/redesign/. Accessed June 15, 2011.

32. DeLucia JA. Innovations: what is community paramedicine. *Urgent Matters E-Newsletter.* http://smhs.gwu.edu/urgentmatters/news/innovations-what-community-paramedicine. Accessed April 5, 2015.

CHAPTER 10

EMS Research

Derek R. Cooney
Tracy Leigh LeGros

INTRODUCTION

Clinical research is an essential feature of modern medical practice. Although most areas of medicine present challenges to conducting high-quality controlled studies, the prehospital and emergency care environments are particularly challenging due to numerous uncontrolled variables inherent in developing and implementing meaningful and ethical consent processes. Despite this, an ever-growing body of research in the area of EMS Medicine has helped solidify the subspecialty and moved prehospital care toward a more evidence-based practice. EMS physicians and medical directors must be able to interpret the literature and should aid in its advancement whenever possible.

OBJECTIVES

- Describe basic research concepts and definitions.
- Describe patient groups and study designs.
- Describe scientific levels of evidence and grades of recommendation.
- Standardized reporting of clinical trials.
- Describe the development of EMS research.
- National Research EMS Agenda.
- Describe the design of an EMS study, including development of the research question.
- Describe the usual IRB process and approach to clinical research.
- Describe the concept of emergency exception for informed consent.
- Describe community consultation and public disclosure.
- Define basic statistical terms.
- Describe some basic research pitfalls.
- List existing EMS research databases and discuss how to request access to the data.
- List sources of potential funding for EMS-related research.

RESEARCH

Scientific research is meant to draw investigators and readers of the scientific literature closer to "the truth." Study design and limitations of conducting research in the clinical environment can drastically affect the results of clinical research, potentially altering the truth being sought. In cases where meticulous design considerations have limited the presence of bias and error, it is possible to utilize study results to advance the practice of medicine. This is the basis for the concept of *evidence-based medicine*. Acknowledging that not all research study results lead to applicable medical practices, it is important to consider how to best interpret current EMS research results and design future studies.

BASIC SCIENTIFIC CONCEPTS AND TERMS

In order for EMS physicians to provide state-of-the-art medical direction and oversight of EMS systems, a basic grasp of the methodology behind clinical research is required. Research concepts and the definitions of common research terms are prerequisites for this understanding.

EFFICACY

Efficacy is a description of how well the treatment works in clinical trials ("explanatory").

EFFECTIVENESS

Effectiveness refers to how well the treatment works in the practice of medicine ("pragmatic").

VALIDITY

Validity in research is the degree to which a *tool measures* what it *claims to measure*. The validity of a study refers to determining the likelihood that the conclusions drawn from the study are correct or reasonable. A valid study asks the *appropriate questions*, uses the *correct sample* (in size and character), collects the *correct outcome measures*, and utilizes *correct statistical methods*. This is a very complex process that requires strict adherence and reassessments to produce a truly valid study.

Internal validity: Internal validity considers the direct effect of one variable (the independent variable) on another variable (the dependent variable). It is important in studies designed to show cause-and-effect relationships. At times, even properly designed studies may have confounding variables that interfere with internal validity.

Confounding variables: There are eight types of confounding variables that interfere with internal validity: (1) *history*—specific events occurring between measurements (in addition to any experimental variables); (2) *maturation*—participant changes over time (eg, becoming tired, growing older, etc); (3) *testing effect*—the effect that taking the first test has on taking any additional testing; (4) *instrumentation*— refers to changes in measurement tool calibration or the changes in observers that may change measurements; (5) *statistical regression*—when selected groups are selected based on their extreme score; (6) *selection bias*—results from the differential (nonrandom) selection of respondents for the comparison groups; (7) *experimental mortality*—the loss of participants from comparison groups; (8) *selection-maturation interaction*—occurs when participant variables (eg, hair or skin color) and time variables (eg, age, obesity) interact.[1]

External validity: Relates to the extent to which the results of a (internally valid) study *remain true* in other cases (ie, different populations, places, or times). *Can the study findings be generalized?* Are the research participants representative of the general population? Many studies are performed in a single geographic area, with smaller samples or patients, who also possess unique characteristics or are representative of a specific population only (ie, volunteers, military cadets, medical students). Studies that are not generalizable have low external validity. Other factors adversely affect external validity include (1) *testing effect*; (2) *selection bias*; (3) *experimental arrangements*—which are not generalizable to patients in a nonexperimental setting; and (4) *multiple-treatments interferences*—effects of previous treatments that interfere with present testing and are not erasable.

Internal versus external validity: It might appear as if internal and external validity contradicts each other. If a strict adherence to experimental designs control as many variables as possible, the study may have high internal validity. Yet, this highly artificial setting lowers the external validity. Alternatively, in performing observational research, it is difficult to control for interfering variables and lowers the low internal validity. However, the study of environmental or other measures in a natural setting results in higher external validity. Fortunately, these apparent contradictions are resolvable, as a great many studies primarily wish to deductively test a theory, in which the major consideration is the rigor (internal validity) of the study.

BLINDING

Blinding refers to procedures undertaken to ensure that neither the study participants nor any member of the study team know to which group the participant belongs (treatment or nontreatment). Some studies have been classified as single, double, or triple blinded, depending on whether it was the participants, care team, or outcome assessors that were blinded. It is currently accepted that investigators should refrain from this terminology and simply state the type of blinding within the test of the paper.[2]

Unblinded/open/open label: These are trials without blinding.

INCLUSION CRITERIA

Inclusion criteria are conditions that must be met for the appropriate recruitment of subjects into a clinical study.

EXCLUSION CRITERIA

Exclusion criteria are conditions that must be met for the appropriate rejection of subjects from a clinical study.

STUDY ANALYSES

There are different paradigms for performing analysis of data from clinical studies. When attempting to limit bias and evaluate the effect of introducing a clinical intervention on a particular population it is best to utilize a study design that incorporates intention-to-treat analysis. Other poststudy analysis and interim analysis may be appropriate in some circumstances, but the conclusions drawn from these may be less accurate.

Intention–to–treat (ITT) analysis: The objective is to analyze each group exactly as they existed upon randomization. A true ITT analysis is possible only when complete outcome data are available for all randomized subjects. This means to include all subjects, including those that drop out. ITT analyses decrease outcome bias.

Subgroup analysis: Analyzing groups within the groups being studied. Subgroup analyses are discouraged because multiple comparisons may lead to false-positive findings that cannot be confirmed.

Interim analysis: A pretrial strategy for stopping a trial early if the results show large outcome differences between groups. It allows for periodic assessments for beneficial or harmful effect of treatment compared to concurrent placebo or control group while a study is ongoing. It is used as a cost-saving measure and importantly the ethical obligation that only the minimum number of patients should be entered into a trial to achieve the study's primary objective and reduce the participants' exposure to the inferior treatment. This analysis may occur following the inclusion of a certain number of treatments or after a set period of time. However, the way in which the interim analysis is to be conducted must be expressly stated in the study protocol. Additionally, the results of the interim analysis should be evaluated by an independent data monitoring committee.[3] Other reasons to stop an interim analysis are that there are unacceptable side effects or toxicity, accumulation is so slow that the trial is no longer sufficient, outside information makes the trial unnecessary or unethical, poor execution compromises the studies' ability to meet its objectives, or disastrous fraud or misconduct.

SCIENTIFIC BIAS

Bias usually refers to any unintended influence that a particular facet of the study design may have that will alter or skew the results. Typically investigators seek to limit bias as much as possible; however, much of the medical literature is affected by bias in some form.

Selection bias: Usually results from an error in choosing the individuals or groups to participate in a study. It distorts the statistical analyses and may result in drawing incorrect conclusions regarding the study outcome(s). It weakens internal validity.

Sampling bias: A systematic error in a study that occurs because the participants do not represent a random sampling of the population. This occurs in some instances due to participant self-selection or prescreening of trial participants. The result is that some members of the population are less likely to be included than others. It weakens external validity.

Attrition bias: A kind of selection bias caused by the loss of participants. It includes patients that dropout or do not respond to a survey (nonresponders), or who withdraw or deviate from the study protocol. It results in biased results because a study intervention or nonintervention is unequal or underrepresented in the outcome.

Publication bias: A bias regarding what is most likely to be published, positive or negative findings. If negative findings are underreported, it leads to a misleading bias in the overall published literature. Studies suggest that positive studies are three times more likely to be published than negative studies. Trial registration is now required by many journals to ensure that unfavorable results are not withheld from publication.[4]

RANDOMIZATION

Participants are arbitrarily assigned to a treatment (intervention) or nontreatment (control) group. Randomization eliminates bias in group assignment, aids in blinding the investigator, participants, and other assessors from knowing the grouping of study participants, and allows the use of probability theory to express the likelihood that any outcome differences between groups merely indicate a chance finding.

Cluster randomization: A preexisting group of study participants (schools, poisoning victims, families) are randomly selected to receive (or not receive) an intervention. Cluster randomization is sometimes done due to factors related to study participants (ie, all family members are placed in the same treatment or nontreatment group)

Factorial randomization: Each participant is randomly assigned to a treatment (or nontreatment group) that receives a particular combination of interventions (or noninterventions).

Randomization procedure: Generation of an unpredictable sequence of allocations to be distributed to participants to treatment or control groups using an element of chance, following the patient's evaluation of eligibility and recruitment into the study.

Allocation concealment: Very strict protocols to ensure that patient group assignments are not revealed prior to their allocation to a group. *Sequentially numbered, opaque, sealed envelopes* (SNOSE) is a type of allocation concealment

TRIAL REGISTRATION

As of July 1, 2005, the International Committee of Medical Journal Editors (ICMJE) announced that all RCTs must be registered to be considered for publication in member journals. This registration may occur late.[5]

PATIENT GROUPS

During the design phase of a study, it is important to define groups. Based on the study type, there may be several different types of groups needed for a particular study.

Control group: A patient group that receives no treatment

Placebo control group: A patient group that receives no treatment, but will receive a "sham" or "placebo" treatment that will mimic what is being performed in the "test group" but without physiological or real effect.

Parallel group: Participants are randomly allocated to a group, and study participants either receive or do not receive an intervention.

Crossover group: Participants are randomly allocated to a group, and, over time, all study participants receive and do not receive an intervention in a random sequence.

EVALUATING THE SCIENTIFIC LITERATURE

Certain attributes of studies produce better evidence than others. It is important to consider the design of the study when determining how to interpret a study. Some studies may have seemingly ideal designs, whereas others do not. The constraints of design related to the clinical environment many times limit the investigators' ability to design a study with all of the ideal parameters. In general, the following attributes can be used to distinguish between stronger and weaker level of evidence.

- Randomized studies are superior to nonrandomized ones.
- Prospective studies are superior to retrospective studies.
- Blinded studies (in which patients, and clinicians and data analysts where possible, do not know which intervention is being used) are superior to unblinded studies.
- Controlled studies are superior to uncontrolled ones.
- Experimental study designs are superior to observational study designs.
- Contemporaneous (occurring at the same time) control groups are superior to historical control groups.
- Internal control groups (ie, managed within the study) are superior to studies with external control groups.
- Large studies (ie, involving enough patients to detect with acceptable confidence levels any true treatment effects) are superior to small studies (ie, properly powered studies are superior to underpowered studies).
- Studies that clearly define patient populations, interventions, and outcome measures are superior to those that do not clearly define these parameters.

TYPES OF CLINICAL TRIALS

RANDOMIZED CONTROLLED TRIAL

In a randomized controlled trial (RCT), subjects are assessed for eligibility and recruitment into the trial. Then, before the intervention or treatment begins, the patients are randomly allocated to receive one treatment or another of the treatments being studied. After the patients are randomized to one treatment arm or the other(s), they are followed in exactly the same way, with the only difference between the two groups being the randomly allocated treatment(s). RCTs are the gold standard for a clinical trial. They are often used to test the efficacy or effectiveness of various types of medical interventions within a patient population. An RCT must contain a control group or a previously tested treatment (a positive-control study). The advantage of an RCT is that they are so strictly controlled that they reduce study bias and the confounder of causality. The disadvantages of RCTs are that they are very expensive, time consuming, may have lower external validity, and perhaps unethical for certain orphan diseases (rare) or rapidly morbid or mortal conditions or injuries which do not lend themselves to RCT evaluation. The types of RCTs are listed below.

Superiority trials: Most RCTs are superiority trials, wherein one intervention is hypothesized to be significantly superior to another.

Noninferiority trials: These RCTs seek to determine whether a new treatment is no worse than an established treatment.

Equivalence trials: These RCTs seek to determine whether two interventions are indistinguishable from each other.

RANDOMIZED (UNCONTROLLED) CLINICAL/COMPARATIVE TRIAL

A randomized (uncontrolled) clinical/comparative trial is a trial that compares multiple treatment groups with each other in the absence of a control group.

NONRANDOMIZED TRIAL

These types of studies also called *quasi-experimental studies*. They do not have random assignments to either a control or treatment group. In these studies, the researcher controls the assignment to a grouping (ie, sicker patients receive the treatment) or circumstances dictate grouping (ie, patients presenting on nights and weekends are allocated to the control arm). These studies typically have lower internal validity because the two groups may not have comparable baselines.

OBSERVATIONAL STUDIES

Observational studies typically are designed to follow patients of a particular type, or whom have specific common features or risk factors.

Cohort studies: These studies are longitudinal studies, in that they look at an effect of an intervention on a patient population over time. It may assess risk factors in a group of patients who share common characteristics (ie, diabetes or heart disease risk factors) and it may or may not compare the effect of the study intervention to a comparison group (ie, a similar group of patients without the intervention) or to historical groupings previously studied. Several types of cohort studies are discussed below.

Prospective cohort studies: A study that sets out to evaluate patients that present forward from some set time. They usually seek to determine risk factors that affect the studied group over time. These are important studies in that it is unethical to perform such as study as an RCT and purposely expose patients to risk factors. Prospective studies are of a higher level of evidence than retrospective studies.

Retrospective cohort studies: These studies are also called historic (post hoc) cohort studies. They review the records of patients that have already been treated or an event that has already taken place. These studies are easier to complete than prospective studies, less expensive and may allow for the study of rare diseases. The disadvantages are that some important statistical measures cannot be made and significant biases (selection and informational) may confound the results. Moreover, these studies rely on precise record taking that has already taken place, which may have key data points, epidemiological, or treatment information missing or unavailable.

TIME SERIES STUDIES

Time series studies are studies run through a period of time, in order to test a hypothesis or make an observation.

Case-controlled study: This is an observational study in which two groups with different outcomes are identified and compared. These studies are often performed to identify contributing factors in patients with a particular condition with patients who do not have that particular condition. They are simpler to perform than other studies and less expensive. Additionally, they are usually used as preliminary studies for research questions related to topics that have limited known information. However, the conclusions drawn may be weaker than more rigorously performed studies.

Nested case-control study: This variation of a case-controlled study evaluates only a subset of controls from the cohort to the incident cases. This subset is selected to match risk sets with the incident cases. In a case-cohort study all incident cases are compared. These studies may be analyzed using methods that take missing covariates into consideration.

Cross-sectional studies: These studies are also called cross-sectional analyses, transversal studies, or prevalence studies. These are observational studies involving either all members of a population or a representative subset of that population, at a specific point in time.

Ecological study: This is an epidemiological study in which large populations, rather than individuals are evaluated. These studies are considered inferior to cohort and case-controlled studies because of the concept of ecological fallacy (a false interpretation of the data made because inferences are made regarding individuals based on inferences from the group to which those individuals belong).

SCIENTIFIC LEVELS OF EVIDENCE

This is a ranking system used in evidence-based medicine to assign a strength rating to a clinical trial or research study. There are five levels of evidence (I, II, III, IV, and V) with alphanumeric subsets (**Table 10-1**).

TABLE 10-1	Level of Evidence
I a	Systematic reviews (with homogeneity) of more than one RCT
I b	Evidence from at least one well-designed RCT with a narrow confidence interval
II a	Systematic review (with homogeneity) of at least one well-designed nonrandomized controlled trial or cohort study
II b	Evidence from at least one well-designed cohort study or a lower quality RCT (> 80% follow-up)
III a	Systematic review (with heterogeneity) of case-controlled studies
III b	Evidence from individual case-controlled studies
IV	Evidence from case series and lower quality cohort studies
V	Expert opinion based on physiology, bench research, or "first principles"

Modified from Oxford Centre for Evidence-Based Medicine (updated 2009).

TABLE 10-3	Examples of Endpoints by Type of Data
Continuous measurements	Blood pressures, weight, blood chemistry variables
Event times	Time to recurrence of CHF exacerbation, survival time, length of stay
Counts	Frequency of occurrence of migraine headaches, number of uses of rescue meds for asthma
Binary endpoints	Recurrence (yes or no), major cardiac event in 30 days (yes or no)
Ordered categories (scales)	Absent-mild-moderate-severe pain, NYHA class status
Unordered categories	Categories of adverse experiences: GI, cardiac, etc

Modified with permission from STAT 509 – Design and Analysis of Clinical Trials. Penn State. https://onlinecourses.science.psu.edu/stat509/node/32. Accessed November 1, 2013.

GRADES OF RECOMMENDATION

These are ranking of the strength of medical evidence. These "grades" are based on the level of scientific evidence on the subject matter and used in clinical practice guidelines to summarize work quality of the literature (**Table 10-2**).

STANDARDIZED REPORTING OF CLINICAL TRIALS

The interpretation of clinical trials measuring effects of interventions on clinical outcomes is made more complex by inherent variability in the way trials have been designed and their results reported. This is made even more clear when attempting to compare and contrast results of multiple trials on the same intervention. Meta-analysis studies can be made more complex (a potentially less meaningful) when the body of literature on a particular intervention is limited by nonstandard reporting of outcomes/results.

OUTCOMES

Outcome research was introduced by health care research leaders such as Codman (1910) and Donabedian (1966). Outcome measurement is clearly a defining component of medical research. The various types of outcome measures include physical/clinical (mortality), performance/function (self-care), economic (cost/benefit), and humanistic (quality of life).[6] When measuring outcomes it is common to utilize outcome measurement/indicator tools. These may be general health/generic measures, disease-specific measures, or functional status measurement tools. The tools may represent a direct measure of a desired outcome, or a tool designed to demonstrate an outcome that cannot be directly measured. These may be considered surrogate endpoints in some cases. Clinical endpoints may also be categorized as *primary* (one of more endpoints that have been powered for rejection of the null hypothesis), *secondary* (other prespecified endpoints that have been powered for hypothesis testing), and *tertiary* (exploratory). Endpoints can also be categorized by type of data as well (**Table 10-3**).[7]

In some cases, authors will combine endpoints after data analysis and may show statistic significance based on the combined outcome, despite the lack of significance when evaluating each independently. This may lead to some confusion and is not considered to be the preferred methodology.

TABLE 10-2	Grades of Recommendation
A	Consistent Level 1 Studies
B	Consistent Level 2 or 3 studies or Extrapolations from Level 1 studies
C	Level 4 studies or extrapolations from Level 2 or 3 studies
D	Level 5 evidence or troublingly inconsistent or inconclusive studies of any level

Reproduced with permission from Oxford Centre for Evidence-Based Medicine (updated 2009).

Consolidated Standards of Reporting Trials Consolidated standards of reporting trials (CONSORT) is a collection of initiatives developed by the CONSORT Group to help ameliorate problems that may arise from inadequate reporting of RCTs. The main objective of the CONSORT Group is the development of the CONSORT Statement.[8] This is a minimum set of recommendations for the reporting of RCTs that is standardized and promotes "transparent reporting," the reduction of bias, and aids readers in their appraisal and interpretation of the RCT. The most recent version contains a 25-item checklist for researchers as well as a flow diagram with descriptive text. There is an additional document called the CONSORT "Explanation and Elaboration" document that is advocated strongly for concomitant use with the CONSORT Statement.[9]

DEVELOPMENT OF EMS RESEARCH

CURRENT AREAS OF FOCUS

The current areas of focus in EMS research are in the prehospital clinical sciences, EMS systems, and the EMS education realms. The current *clinical* areas of focus are out-of-hospital cardiac arrest (OHCS), major trauma, stroke, shock, and spinal immobilization. *Systems*-based areas of focus include transport of specialty patients, STEMI coordinated care, stroke coordinated care, trauma coordinated care, and ED crowding/off-load times. Some *educational* areas of focus include evidence-based decision making in EMS, advanced-airway adjuncts, integration of advanced practice providers (ie, physician assistants, nurse practitioners), and community paramedicine.

COMPONENTS OF A SUCCESSFUL PROGRAM

Development of a successful research program can be a significant undertaking and may represent considerable investment in time and funds. In order to maximize return on the investment it is important to consider the components required for successful development.

Training: In an EMS system, researchers may come from a variety of different backgrounds. Basic and advanced training in study design, participant expectations, ethical principles, study development, and statistical analyses is advised. Many institutions provide modules on these topics, and the facility's Institutional Review Board (IRB) may be an invaluable resource.

Mentorship: In many studies, mentorship is essential. For those just beginning a research study, the mentorship of a seasoned investigator is very much advised. Many institutions, universities, and medical centers have such experienced mentors available.

Collaboration: Teaming up with like-minded researchers from related fields is advisable in many situations (**Figure 10-1**). For example, a study related to an advanced airway adjunct may benefit from collaborators from emergency medicine, surgery, and anesthesiology.

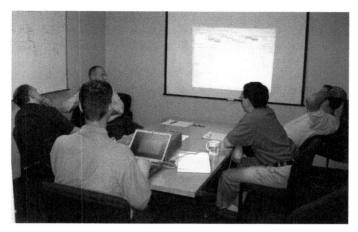

FIGURE 10-1. EMS research group meeting. Like-minded collaborators including a simulations expert, education program director, prehospital providers, and EMS physicians discuss their local research agenda.

Collaboration allows different viewpoints and experience to be shared among researchers, often leading to a more efficient and streamlined area of focus.

NATIONAL EMS RESEARCH AGENDA

The National EMS Research Agenda, published by the National Highway Transportation and Safety Administration in 2001, provides an assessment of the state of EMS research and recommendations for the continued advancement of this critical area.[10] This document outlines areas of weakness and specific challenges that limit the advancement of EMS research programs. It advocates for policy changes and enhanced funding for the development of researchers, research centers, and studies. Additionally, it proposes a greater organization of stakeholders to ensure research finders are utilized in the development of evidenced-based practice. The recommendations of the authors of the document are illustrated in **Table 10-4** (*paraphrased from the executive summary*).

TABLE 10-4	NHTSA National EMS Research Agenda
Recommendation 1	Large cadre of career EMS investigators should be developed and supported in the initial stages of their careers; training programs with content directed toward EMS research methodologies should be developed
Recommendation 2	Centers of excellence should be created; bring together experienced investigators, institutional expertise, and resources such as budgetary and information systems support
Recommendation 3	Federal research sponsoring agencies should acknowledge commitment to EMS research
Recommendation 4	States, corporations, and charitable foundations should be encouraged to support EMS research
Recommendation 5	Organize efforts of EMS professionals, delivery systems, academic centers, and public policy makers to support and apply results of research
Recommendation 6	EMS professionals of all levels should hold themselves to higher standards of requiring evidence before implementing new procedures, devices, or drugs
Recommendation 7	Standardized data collection methods at local, regional, state, and national levels; EMS provider agencies should adopt the uniform prehospital data elements for data collection
Recommendation 8	Food and Drug Administration (FDA) and Office for Human Research Protections (OHRP) should work with EMS research stakeholders to evaluate requirements for exception from informed consent in emergency situations and address serious impediments to conducting EMS research

STUDY DESIGN

FORMING A WORK GROUP

There is a new trend in scientific research termed *team science*. It involves the collaboration of researchers to enhance and further research goals. There are several types of research teams, including:

Independent research: Usually a single investigator working independently on a research question or with one or more collaborators.

Collaborative efforts: May range from independent research, to collaborative efforts among several investigators, to fully integrated research teams.[11]

FORMULATING THE RESEARCH QUESTION(S)

One of the most apparently simply but challenging steps in the research process is formulation of the "research question." It is the first, and possibly the most important step in the research design. It sets the basis from which the study is designed and is supposed to ensure that the study actually answers the proposed question. Prior to formulating the hypothesis and null hypothesis for any proposed study, the researcher(s) must carefully develop the research question(s).

PICO process: This process is used in evidenced-based medicine research to properly frame and answer a clinical question (**Box 10-1**).

FINER criteria: This is a set of criteria developed to promote the development of a good research question. (**Box 10-2**)[12]

REFINEMENT OF RESEARCH QUESTIONS, HYPOTHESES, AND RESEARCH OBJECTIVES

After the initial development of the research question is complete and stakeholders are satisfied with the basic principles surrounding the investigation, the question and hypotheses must be further elucidated and refined in order to define the specific research objectives. This can be accomplished by following a basic set of steps.

1. *Systematic literature review*: This is often the first step undertaken. It is performed to develop an understanding of previous work, the overall level of evidence of the subject matter, controversies in the literature, and knowledge gaps within the field study.

2. *Intensive review of scientific trends and technological advancements within the field of study*: This is important to assess the rigor with

Box 10-1
The PICO Process
Patient problem or population to be studied
Intervention to be evaluated
Comparison between group(s)
Outcome of Study

Box 10-2
The FINER Criteria
Feasible: Adequate numbers of subjects, appropriate technical expertise, affordable study in terms of time and funding, and with an a study that is manageable in its scope
Interesting: The project outcome is intriguing to researchers, peers, and the community
Novel: The study will confirm, refute, or extend previous work
Ethical: The study conforms to IRB specifications and moral principles
Relevant: The study outcome is pertinent to existing scientific knowledge, clinical and/or health care policy, and future research

which the proposed study must be performed in order to align with the current highest levels of investigation.

3. *Question refinement review(s)*: The question, once developed, must be shared with mentors, colleagues, and collaborators so that it can be refined and honed into the simplest yet most complete question that encompasses the proposed scope of the investigation.

4. *FINER criteria review*: Is then used to further test the appropriateness of the research question.

5. *PICO criteria*: Reapplied to ensure that appropriate aspects of the question are addressed.

6. Development of a research hypothesis: From the research question.

7. *Development of primary and/or secondary objectives*: This is done prior to commencement of the study and listed in the IRB and the formal study protocol.

Null Hypothesis This is the standard or "default" assumption/prediction made at the outset of scientific inquiry. It reasons that there will be no significant difference in outcomes between two groups treated in different ways. One can reject or disprove a null hypothesis. However, a null hypothesis cannot be accepted or proven.

Alternative Hypothesis This is the rival hypothesis to the null hypothesis. It states that there will be a significant difference in outcomes between two groups treated in different ways. If the null hypothesis is rejected, the alternative hypothesis is accepted.

BASIC STATISTICAL CONCEPTS

At times it may be appropriate to review study results and then apply a particular statistic methodology in order to satisfy a previously undefined research objective. However, in most cases the study design should include the statistical methodology by which results are to be sought prior to submission and implementation of the study design. It is important to understand the types of measures and the errors that can occur during this phase, and to choose appropriate statistical methodology.

MEASURES OF CENTRAL TENDENCY

Mean: This is probably the most often used descriptive statistic measured. It measures the "central tendency" of a variable and is usually reported with confidence intervals. It is usually calculated as the mathematical average of a set of values. For numbers 1, 3, 5, 7, 13, 25, 27, and 30, the mean is 15.85.

Median: The median is the value for which 50% of the observations will lie above that value and 50% will lie below that value (when all values are ranked). For numbers 1, 3, 7, 13, 25, 27, and 30, the median is 13.

Mode: The mode is the value that appears most often in a data set. It is the value most likely to be sampled. For numbers 1, 3, 7, 13, 13, 13, 25, and 27, the mode is 13.

Type I errors: or "false-positive" errors—an incorrect rejection of a *true* null hypothesis. It wrongly concludes that a treatment has a positive effect when it does not.

Type II errors: or "false-negative" errors—an incorrect acceptance of a *false* null hypothesis. It wrongly concludes that a treatment has a negative effect, when it actually is a positive study with regard to treatment significance.

P Value: A P value helps determine the significance of study results. It is a number between 0 and 1. The smaller the P value (≤ 0.05), the stronger the evidence against the null hypothesis (the null hypothesis is rejected). The larger the P value (> 0.05), the weaker the evidence against the null hypothesis and the null hypothesis is not rejected.

MEASURES OF DISPERSION

Standard deviation (SD): The SD determines how much variation from the average exists with a data set. A low SD indicates that the data are very close to the mean. A high SD indicates that the data are spread out over a large range of values. The SD is the square root of its variance. It is used to measure confidence in statistical conclusions.

Standard error of the mean (SEM): The SEM is the standard deviation (SD) of the different sample means. Approximately 68.3% of the sample means would be within one SEM and 95.4% would be within two SEMs and 99.7% would be within three SEMs.

Confidence intervals: A range of values around the mean where it is expected that the true mean is located. For example, if the mean = 23 ($p = 0.05$) and the lower and upper confidence intervals are 19 and 27, respectively, then there is a 95% probability that the population mean is > 19 and < 27. Smaller P values result in wider confidence intervals. The confidence interval depends on the sample size and the variation of data values. Confidence intervals are based on the assumption that the variable is normally distributed in the population being studied. Larger sample sizes have more reliable means. The larger the variation, the less reliable the mean.

DIAGNOSTIC TESTING

Sensitivity: Sensitivity is also called the true positive rate or the recall rate. It describes how well a test can detect a disease or condition in those that have the disease or condition. Sensitivity helps rule out disease when the result is negative (**Se**nsitivity Rule **Out** = "Snout"). Sensitivity = true positives/(true positives + false negatives).

Specificity: Specificity refers to the percentage of people who test negative for a specific disease among a group of people without the disease. A highly specific positive test, it is highly certain that the patient actually has the disease (**Sp**ecificity Rule **In** = "Spin"). A very specific test rules in a disease with a high degree of confidence. Specificity = true negatives/(true negatives + false positives).

Positive predictive value: This test asks the question: "If the test result is positive, what is the probability that the patient actually has the disease?" PPV = true positives/(true positives + false positives).

Negative predictive value: This test asks the question: "If the test result is negative, what is the probability that the patient does not have the disease?" NPV = true negatives/(true negatives + false negatives).

Likelihood ratios: A likelihood ratio is the ratio of two probabilities of the same event under different circumstances. It uses the sensitivity and specificity of a test to determine whether a test result usefully changes the probability that the condition exists. A positive likelihood ratio = sensitivity/1 – specificity. A negative likelihood ratio = 1 – sensitivity/specificity. A likelihood ratio > 1 indicates that the test result is associated with the disease. A likelihood ratio < 1 indicates that the result is associated with absence of the disease.

Odds ratios: The odds ratio measures the association between an exposure and an outcome. It represents the odds that an outcome will occur given a particular exposure, compared to the odds of the outcome occurring in the absence of that exposure. It is calculated by using a two-by-two frequency table.

STATISTICS TERMS

Sample size calculation: This is a very important part of a study design that is performed to determine the appropriate number of subjects in each group that will be needed to make a valid inference about the population from which the subjects are taken.

Variable: An object or event that is being measured or evaluated.

Independent variable: A variable that is not changed by other variables being measured or assessed (ie, age, gender, education). When assessing the relationship between variables, one is usually attempting to discern if the independent variable caused a change in the other variables (the dependent variables). Independent variables may cause a change in a dependent variable. However, dependent variables cannot cause a change in an independent variable.

Dependent variable: A variable that may change, depending on the effects of other variables (ie, a test score is dependent upon prior night's restfulness and/or the duration or quality of pretest preparation).

Correlation: A correlation is a measure of the relation between two or more variables.

Pearson correlation: The most widely used type of correlation coefficient. It is also known as the linear or product correlation. It is used to determine the extent to which values of two variables are proportional to each other.

Proportionality: The extent to which two or more variables are linearly related (approximated by a straight line sloping either upward or downward). The line is called a regression line (or least squares line) and is determined such that the sum of the squared distances of all of the data points from the line is the lowest possible.

Correlation coefficients: Can range between −1.00 and +1.00.

Negative correlation: The value of −1.00 represents a perfect negative correlation. With a negative correlation, the relationship between two variables is such that as the value of one variable increases, the value of the other variable decreases.

Positive correlation: The value of +1.00 represents a perfect positive correlation. With a positive correlation, the relationship between two variables is such that as the value of one variable increases, the value of the other variable also increases.

No correlation: The value of 0.00 represents a complete lack of correlation between two or more variables.

TRADITIONAL STATISTICAL METHODS

STUDENT *T* TEST

The Student *t* test is used to determine if two sets of data are significantly different from each other. It is usually used to assess if any significant difference occurs between groups in response to an intervention measured with the same statistical unit or whether the slope of a regression line differs significantly from zero.

ANALYSIS OF VARIANCE

Analysis of variance (ANOVA) is a collection of statistical models used to analyze differences between group means and their associated interventions. It is used for comparing three or more groups' means for statistical significance. It assesses the "variation" both among and between groups. It tests whether or not the "means" of groups are equal. It generalizes the *t* test to more than two groups. When three or more groups are being compared, it is better to use ANOVA rather than performing multiple two-sample *t* tests (which might increase the chance of a type I error).

REGRESSION ANALYSIS

This is a process for evaluating the relationships among measured variables. It focuses on the relationship between a dependent variable and one or more independent variables and aids in the understanding of how the value of the dependent variable changes when any one of the independent variables is varied (while the other independent variables remain fixed.).

THE USE OF HUMANS IN RESEARCH STUDIES

There have been a large number of experiments that have been performed on humans that were unethical, illegal, and immoral. These experiments include deliberately infecting people with debilitating or deadly diseases, exposing subjects to biological weapons, chemical weapons, radiation, torture, interrogation techniques, mind-altering substances, and other similar types of testing. Often these "studies" were performed on at-risk patient populations (pregnant women, children, racial minorities, the

mentally disabled, the sick, the elderly, the poor, and prisoners). These types of studies have been banned for 40 years and stringent regulations have been instituted to ensure human subjects are heavily protected from exploitation and dangerous clinical trials.

THE NUREMBERG CODE

The Nuremberg Code is a set of research ethics and principles for human experimentation that resulted from the Nuremberg trials at the end of World War II (1947). It was developed in response to the "Doctors Trial" involving 23 doctors that conducted human experiments in concentration camps on German citizens.

THE DECLARATION OF HELSINKI

The Declaration of Helsinki is a set of ethical principles on human experimentation developed in 1964 by the World Medical Association and is considered the "cornerstone" document of human research ethics.

POLICIES FOR THE PROTECTION OF HUMAN SUBJECTS

This document was created by the *National Institutes of Health* in 1966. It recommended the establishment of IRBs to oversee clinical studies involving human subjects.

THE NATIONAL RESEARCH ACT

This legislation was established by the *National Commission for the Protection of Human Subjects* in 1974 and mandated that the *Public Health Service* develop regulations to protect the rights of humans involved in research studies.

BELMONT REPORT

The Belmont Report was issued in 1979 by the National Commission for the Protection of Human Subjects of Biomedical and Behavioral Research. It outlines the ethical principles for research on humans. It was initiated at the Belmont Conference Center, which was once part of the Smithsonian Institution. The report was prompted by concerns related to the *Tuskegee Syphilis Study*. It outlines three fundamental ethical principles for any human subject research:

Respect for persons: Especially as it relates to the autonomy of all people and in treating them with courtesy and respect. It discusses informed consent and the duty that all researchers have to be truthful and without deception.

Beneficence: This is the philosophy of "do no harm" and in minimizing research subject risk while maximizing research benefits.

Justice: This doctrine ensures that reasonable, nonexploitive, and well thought-out procedures are administered fairly and equally.

The "Common Rule": The Federal Policy for the Protection of Human Subjects came into effect in 1981, following the 1975 revision to the Declaration of Helsinki. It was fully encapsulated and published in 1991. It contains five subparts.

Subpart A: Contains the "Common Rule" which outlines the basic provisions for IRBs, informed consent, and assurances of compliance.

Subpart B: Provides additional protections for pregnant women, fetuses, and neonates.

Subpart C: Provides additional protections for prisoners.

Subpart D: Provides additional protections for children.

Subpart E: Provides additional protections for the registration of IRBs.

INSTITUTIONAL REVIEW BOARDS

Institutional Review Boards (IRBs) are also called ethical review boards and have been instituted worldwide to formally approve, monitor, and review all biomedical and behavioral research involving human subjects. These tasks are accomplished through uniform procedures and reviews that involve a risk-benefit analysis of the proposed research.

DUTIES OF AN IRB

The primary focus of any IRB is to ensure that human subjects are protected from exposure to any potential harm.

EXEMPTIONS FROM IRB REVIEWS

IRB reviews are universally mandated in all but a few circumstances. Some of these exceptions include those involving the study of differing educational practices or testing, staffing instructional studies, curriculum studies, management methods, some surveys, observation studies (unless electronically recorded or those that contain identifiable information), and in some cases research involving the collection of existing data already in a system (deidentified data).

INFORMED CONSENT

A cornerstone of an IRB process is the obtainment of permission prior to performing an intervention. The subject must understand the risks, benefits, implications, and future consequences of either treatment or nontreatment. The patient must also have appropriate reasoning faculties and the capacity to understand the entire informed consent document. It is very important that the patient understand that in research trials, the patient may *not* be allocated to the treatment group. Studies have consistently shown that many RCT subjects believe that they are certain to be in the treatment group, not understanding the difference between research treatment (therapeutic misconception).[13]

EMERGENCY CONSENT

In the United States, between 1979 and 1993 emergency research involving critically ill patients who could not reasonably consent was often considered to be performed under a concept known as waived consent. However, in 1993 the branches of the Department of Health and Human Services (DHHS) charged with review and development of policy relative to clinical research found that there was no clear guidelines by which investigators could safely and ethically evoke waiver of consent for emergency research. This led to an ensuing debate and a 1993 *federal moratorium* on all research without prospective informed consent. Due to disagreement concerning the specific intent of components of the Common Rule, in 1995 the Final Rule was introduced and was intended as a mechanism investigator to establish enrollment parameters for emergency research and exception from informed consent in place of the previous waiver method.

EXCEPTION FROM INFORMED CONSENT

Final Rule, 61 Fed. Reg. 51498 (Oct. 2, 1996) 21 CFR 50.24 defined the new standard for this process. The new 1996 standard for emergency research involves the investigator(s), study sponsors, IRB, and also the general public.

In order to be considered for eligibility for granting of exception from informed consent (EFIC) by the IRB a specific set of eligibility criteria must be met.[14] The human subjects are in a life-threatening situation, available treatments are unproven or unsatisfactory, and the collection of valid scientific evidence is necessary to determine the safety and effectiveness of particular interventions.

1. Obtaining informed consent is not feasible because:
   a. The subjects will not be able to give their informed consent as a result of their medical condition
   b. The intervention under investigation must be administered before consent from the subjects' legally authorized representatives is feasible
   c. There is no reasonable way to identify prospectively the individuals likely to become eligible for participation in the clinical investigation
2. Participation in the research holds out the prospect of direct benefit to the subjects because:
   a. Subjects are facing a life-threatening situation that necessitates intervention

b. Appropriate animal and other preclinical studies have been conducted, and the information derived from those studies and related evidence support the potential for the intervention to provide a direct benefit to the individual subjects
   c. Risks associated with the investigation are reasonable in relation to what is known about the medical condition of the potential class of subjects, the risks and benefits of standard therapy, if any, and what is known about the risks and benefits of the proposed intervention or activity
3. The clinical investigation could not practicably be carried out without the waiver.
4. The proposed investigational plan defines the length of the potential therapeutic window based on scientific evidence, and the investigator has committed to attempting to contact a legally authorized representative for each subject within that window of time and, if feasible, to asking the legally authorized representative contacted for consent within that window rather than proceeding without consent.
5. The IRB has reviewed and approved informed consent procedures and an informed consent document consistent with 50.25.

The process requires five major components:

1. *Community consultation*: There must be consultation with the leaders of the community about the research design and plans.
2. *Public disclosure*: The investigators (and sponsor) must inform the community about the research.
3. *Multiple consent process*: Investigators must prepare and utilize informed consent: a standard informed consent for the participant, a form for the family or legally authorized representative (proxy informed consent), and a consent to continue in the research.
4. *Independent data monitoring*: The study data must be monitored independently to ensure ethical practices relative to early termination in cases of harm (or poor risk/benefit ratio) based on interval results.
5. *Community reporting*: Investigators are also required to inform the community of the study's results and the demographic characteristics of the participants.

SUMMARIZING DATA

TYPES OF SCIENTIFIC ABSTRACTS

There are two basic types of abstracts:

Informational abstracts: These are short abstracts that contain an introduction or purpose, methods, scope, results, conclusions, and recommendations.

Descriptive abstracts: These are also short abstracts, sometimes less than 100 words. They contain a purpose, methods, scope. They do not contain results, conclusions, or recommendations.

HIGH-QUALITY ABSTRACTS

High-quality abstracts are effective and succinct. It is helpful to reread your abstract several times, focusing on the main components, individually and as part of the whole document. Work to remove extraneous information and wordiness. Analyze the work for errors in grammar and mechanics. Have a scientific mentor review your work, correcting weaknesses in organization and coherence.

PRESENTATION OF RESULTS

Scientific abstracts can be presented in a number of ways. Typically preliminary results or the initial report of a study result will take the form of a poster presentation of an oral abstract presentation. Peer-reviewed manuscripts are the backbone of the scientific literature and require more stringent review and presentation of the study results and therefore take more preparation and work to submit.

Oral Presentation These are usually 15- to 30-minute presentations containing the background, methods, results, discussion, conclusions, and areas for future research. Afterward, time is allotted for questions and discussions with the audience. Important points to remember for an oral presentation are to have something important to say, in a meaningful and easy-to-understand manner. First impressions are important. The message is important. However, body language and vocal tone are the qualities your audience evaluates first. The best oral presenters appear earnest, competent, trustworthy, and do not seek to belittle or humiliate others. Allow the audience to interact with you in a friendly and congenial manner. Slides should be simple (5-7 lines per slide), of a readable sized font with bullets (not sentences). Stick to one key point per slide. Use color only to gain attention (avoid overuse of red).

Poster Presentation A poster is the visual representation of scientific work. It is usually 48 in wide × 36 in tall and attached to poster boards. The submitting presenter is expected to be alongside the poster to discuss its contents at specific times when the judges will be reviewing the submitted works. The top of the poster contains the title, authors and affiliations, and an institutional logo (ensure that it is approved for use). The title should be legible from across the room (4 cm high). The text should be in bullets and contain an introduction, material and methods, results, discussion, conclusions, references, and acknowledgments. The results are best represented in tables, charts, or graphs. These tables or graphs should have explanations and be able to standalone in the information they impart. Informative pictures are desired. Vivid contrasting colors may be beneficial in this setting (as opposed to their use in oral presentations). Poster handouts, typically an 8 in × 11 in copy of the presentation with contact information should be on hand. It is as important to practice poster presentations as it is to practice oral presentations. There is a tendency to under-review a poster presentation, as the information is readily available for reference. However, fluid flow and smooth delivery are important components of a well-presented poster, and cannot be extemporaneously produced.

Manuscript Submission Abstracts may also be submitted as part of scientific manuscript submission to a medical journal. Every journal has its own set of author instructions. However, some rules are fairly ubiquitous:

- *Journal's aim and scope*: Each journal has its own area of interest and expertise. They desire manuscripts that are technically sound and of interests to the specialists within their field. Additionally, the work must *not* have been published or submitted elsewhere.

- *Journal format/author's instructions*: This must be adhered to stringently. Most journals will have a typeset maximum for pages, usually double-spaced with guidelines for tables and graphs and a word count. The abstract will usually also have a word count. These limitations are to be strictly followed. The journal will also dictate the exact format for the presentation: abstract, introduction, background, material, methods, statistics, results, discussion, and references. Many journals limit the number of references and disallow footnotes.

- *Electronic submissions*: Some journals have electronic submissions that do not allow for fancy fonts, bold or italic lettering, and many have only online submission systems. Journals may also specify that the text be submitted only as .doc or .docx documents. Similarly, figures may only be accepted only in jpeg form. Ensure compliance with all instructions, check for typos numerous times, and submit before the deadline.

EMS SYSTEM DATA COLLECTION

UTSTEIN TEMPLATE

The Utstein-style template is a standardized data set and form of reporting that allows for the comparison of different studies and their results as they relate to cardiac arrest. The latest version was updated by the International Liaison Committee on Resuscitation (ILCOR) in 2004

and the reporting template (for use by study investigators) is shown in **Figure 10-2**.[15] It may be reasonable to expect EMS and event medicine (mass gathering) study investigators to also report cardiac arrest related data using this format.

(NHTSA) UNIFORM PREHOSPITAL EMS DATA SET

In 1993, the National Highway Traffic Safety Administration released their Uniform Prehospital EMS Data Set. The data set contains data elements that have been determined to be essential components of the patient care report that lead to database population in many states and at the national level. The purpose of the uniform (standardized) data set is to allow local, regional, state, and national EMS organizations and agencies to perform analysis on key system indicators and allows benchmark comparisons to be made across systems and throughout published EMS research studies. The current version of the data set is version 3.3.1 although many systems are still currently using a version 2 build. The data are expected to be collected and incorporated into electronic databases in all participating states. The states (and territories) then upload data to *NEMSIS*. NEMSIS is the National EMS Information system and currently 90% of states and territories are participating (http://www.nemsis.org). The goals of NEMSIS are to allow "reporting capabilities, allowing Federal, State and Local EMS stakeholders access to

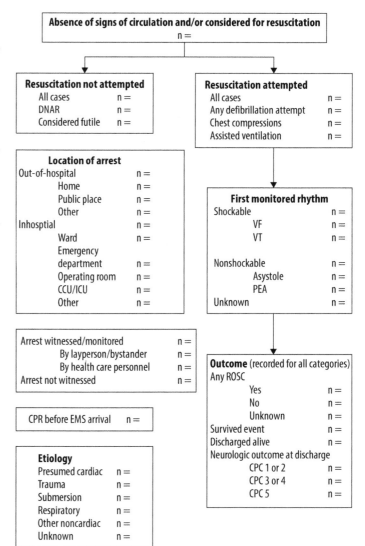

FIGURE 10-2. Utstein template for reporting cardiac arrest data. Utstein reporting template for core data elements. ED, emergency department; OR, operating room; CCU/ICU, critical care unit/intensive care unit; and PEA, pulseless electrical activity.

performance and benchmarking metrics." NEMSIS has obvious research value as well.

NATIONAL TRAUMA DATA BANK

The National Trauma Data Bank (NTDB) is associated with the American College of Surgeons and comprises a large network of participating hospitals that maintain a trauma database (usual designated trauma centers). The NTDB utilizes a standardized data dictionary and contains many data fields including some prehospital data and ultimately outcome data. This is another excellent source for EMS quality improvement and research investigation. Each participating hospital maintains the ability to perform studies with their own data set.

CRASH OUTCOME DATA EVALUATION SYSTEM

Each state has members of the nationwide database designed to bring further clarity to the causes and outcomes of motor vehicle crashes. Crash Outcome Data Evaluation System (CODES) is also an administrative and cost-benefit database including crash data with special attention to "type, severity and cost in relation to the characteristics of the crash, vehicles, and persons involved." Researchers with special focus and interest in injury prevention may find utilizing these type of data in conjunction with other data may lead to greater in-depth investigation and more meaningful conclusions concerning motor vehicle-related injuries and death.

OTHER SOURCES OF DATA

Other databases that may provide some data of interest to EMS researchers include the Hospital Available Beds for Emergencies and Disaster (HAvBED) system, the Emergency System for Advanced Registration of Volunteer Health Professionals (ESAR-VHP), and the Health Alert Network (HAN) maintained by the Centers for Disease Control.

CONCLUSION

Much advancement and evolution has occurred in the field of EMS medicine due to increasing development of research based in the prehospital arena. Failure to maintain vigilance in the design and implementation of prehospital EMS research investigations will lead to improper information on the effectiveness and appropriateness of current and future EMS practices. It is essential to utilize proper ethical procedures in compliance with established standards and to utilize standardized data systems when possible. Failure to implement these tools will lead to a failure to advance EMS medicine as an evidence-based field of medical practice. EMS physicians and medical directors should utilize available science to gauge and modify their practice when appropriate.

KEY POINTS

- EMS research design and interpretation require understanding of key components and statistics.
- Emergency research utilizing exception from informed consent (EFIC) requires adherence to specific qualifying attributes and adherence to specific procedural guidelines.
- EMS data should be recorded and reported using standardized/uniform formats to allow for research result comparisons and system benchmarking.
- Building a research team with incorporation of education, mentorship, and collaboration is a key component to successfully engaging in EMS research.

REFERENCES

1. Trochim WMK. Internal validity. Research Methods Knowledge Base. 2006. http://www.socialresearchmethods.net/kb/. Accessed October 1, 2013.
2. Moher D, Hopewell S, Schulz KF, et al. CONSORT 2010 explanation and elaboration: updated guidelines for reporting parallel group randomised trials". *Br Med J*. 2010;340:c869.
3. Buyse M. Interim analyses, stopping rules and data monitoring in clinical trials in Europe. *Stat Med*. March 1993;12(5-6):509-520.
4. Dickersin K, Chan S, Chalmers TC, et al. Publication bias and clinical trials. *Control Clin Trials*. 1987;8(4):343-353.
5. Edwards SJL, Lilford RJ, Hewison J. The ethics of randomised controlled trials from the perspectives of patients, the public, and healthcare professionals. *Br Med J*. 1998;317(7167):1209-1212.
6. Maloney K, Chaiken BP. An overview of outcomes research and measurement. *J Healthc Qual*. November-December 1999;21(6):4-9.
7. STAT 509 – Design and Analysis of Clinical Trials. PennState. 5.1– Endpoints. https://onlinecourses.science.psu.edu/stat509/node/32. Accessed November 1, 2013.
8. Schulz KF, Altman DG, Moher D; CONSORT Group. CONSORT 2010 statement: updated guidelines for reporting parallel group randomised trials. *BMJ*. 2010 Mar 23;340:c332.
9. Moher D, Hopewell S, Schulz KF, et al. CONSORT 2010 explanation and elaboration: updated guidelines for reporting parallel group randomised trials. *BMJ*. 2010;340:c869
10. Sayre MR, White LJ, Brown LH, McHenry SD; National EMS Agenda Writing Team. National EMS Research Agenda. *Prehosp Emerg Care*. July-September;6(3 suppl):S1-S43. Review.
11. Bennett LM, Gadlin H, Levine-Finley S. *Collaboration and Team Science: A Field Guide*. Bethesda, MD: National Institutes of Health. August 2010, NIH Publication, no. 10-7660.
12. Hulley S, Cummings S, Browner W, et al. *Designing clinical research*. 3rd ed. Philadelphia, PA): Lippincott Williams and Wilkins; 2007.
13. Appelbaum PS, Roth LH, Lidz C. The therapeutic misconception: informed consent in psychiatric research. *Int J Law Psychiatry*. 1982;5(3–4):319-329.
14. U.S. Department of Health and Human Services, Food and Drug Administration, Office of Good Clinical Practice, Center for Drug Evaluation and Research, Center for Biologics Evaluation and Research, Center for Devices and Radiological Health. Guidance for institutional review boards, clinical investigators, and sponsors exception from informed consent requirements for emergency research. March 2011. Updated April 2013. http://www.fda.gov/downloads/RegulatoryInformation/Guidances/UCM249673.pdf. Accessed November 1, 2013.
15. ILCOR Task Force on Cardiac Arrest and Cardiopulmonary Resuscitation Outcomes. Cardiac arrest and cardiopulmonary resuscitation outcome reports: update and simplification of the Utstein templates for resuscitation registries: a statement for healthcare professionals from a task force of the International Liaison Committee on Resuscitation. *Circulation*. November 23, 2004;110(21):3385-3397.

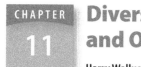

Diversion, Bypass, and Offload Delay

Harry Wallus
Derek R. Cooney

INTRODUCTION

Although the primary focus of an advanced EMS system is typically the patient care rendered in the field and during transport, the act of delivering the patient to the most appropriate facility, performing a safe transfer of care, and returning to service to await the next emergency call is an important and sometimes overlooked by EMS physicians as part of the "operational component." Diversion and bypass may increase transport distance and delays in offload of patients in crowded emergency departments can cause EMS crews to be out of service for longer periods, reducing system efficiency. Clearly this component has a direct impact on patient care, both current and for those who have not yet dialed 9-1-1. Defining and understanding the different components and facets of this part of the medical operation is critical to medical directors seeking to ensure patient high-quality care.

OBJECTIVES

- Define terms ambulance diversion, hospital bypass, patient demand, ambulance offload delay, alternative destination, and emergency department crowding.

- Discuss the historical and contemporary effects of ambulance diversion.

- Describe the practice of hospital bypass and specialty hospital designations (eg, trauma, ACS/PCI, stroke).

- Describe the NEDOCS scoring system and its potential use in EMS resource management.

- Discuss state regulations, as well as legal, financial, and ethical implications of patient demand.

- Discuss the use of alternative destinations, such as urgent care centers, psychiatric facilities, and doctors' offices.

- Discuss the concept of "treatment, no transport" as an alternative to transport to the emergency department.

Emergency departments and EMS personal serve as the country's so-called medical safety net. As such, both are expected to be able to handle any and all patients at all times. The population within the United States continues to increase and as such, so do its medical need and the demands it places on the EMS system. Emergency department crowding and extended wait times have both become the norm and the focus of the press, legislature, and public.[1,2] Several strategies have been implemented in an effort to decrease ED wait times and crowding. Prominent and controversial among these is ED diversion. Depending on the communities in which you serve, ED diversion may play a significant role in day-to-day EMS operations and present particular challenges to the prehospital provider.

Emergency medical personnel face many unique and challenging situations in the prehospital environment aside from that of direct patient care. Ideal patient management often requires careful consideration of the final destination for the patient and selection of a facility optimally equipped to deal with their particular emergency. For example, it may be appropriate to bypass the local community hospital in favor of the closest trauma center, focused pediatric emergency department, or high-risk labor and delivery hospital depending on the situation and the patient. Other decisions such as to potentially transport a patient by air as opposed to ground must also be considered and must factor in variables such as patient acuity, weather, and availability of aircrews.

Selection of the most appropriate facility for the patient is significantly influenced by real-time variables such as time of transport (traffic delays during peak travel periods, etc), distance of transport, and patient acuity, among others. As a general rule, getting the patient to the closest most appropriate facility is always the goal. This is not always as straightforward as it may sound. If there is a question as to the most appropriate disposition for the patient, it may be necessary to get medical control involved in the decision-making process. If there is significant concern about the stability of a patient, they should be transported to the closest emergency department for further stabilization, assessment, and subsequent transfer. A relatively newer facet of emergency care referred to as ED diversion is further complicating these already complex decisions as well as affecting prehospital providers in a number of other ways.

DEFINING THE TERMS

Ambulance diversion (AD) is the practice of redirecting or limiting destination of an ambulance carrying a patient to a hospital as its destination. Typically AD occurs as part of the EMS system, where it is an excepted practice for hospitals to signal the system that their ED is crowded and there is likely to be a significant delay, or lack of patient care services if additional patients were to arrive by ambulance during that time.

Hospital bypass (HB) is the practice of directing prehospital providers to transport patients needing specialty care to a specialty center instead of the nearest hospital. This sometimes means significant increases in travel time and is usually in cases where time to definitive care is believed to be the primary clinical factor affecting patient outcome (eg, major trauma, ST-elevation MI, acute stroke).

Patient demand (PD) refers to the right of the patient to choose their hospital destination, even when the prehospital provider advises a different destination, or in some systems, even when the chosen hospital is on diversion.

Ambulance offload delay (AOD) is the time between arrival of an ambulance, and the time that the patient is both (1) off the stretcher and (2) EMS report has been given. AOD is a relatively new quality measure in the United States, but has been evaluated in Canada for some time due to the fact that it represents a delay in patient care that is sometimes significant.

Transport to *alternative destinations* in response to 9-1-1 calls is not a new concept, but is not yet widely accepted. In many systems, ambulances on 9-1-1 calls may only transport patients to an emergency department. In some systems, prehospital providers are allowed to use clinical judgment and/or specific criteria to determine the appropriateness of transporting to an urgent care center, doctor's office, or psychiatric facility. In some cases, the providers may also be able to determine the appropriateness of treating the patient and leaving them at their home or initial call location. If the patient requires no emergency care and it is determined that the patient should seek primary care services (rather than emergency care) some systems allow providers to decline treatment and transport and provide the patient with a list of resources and clinics instead.

Emergency department crowding (EDC) is a significant problem in many systems across the country. Hospital throughput issues and limited primary care access are thought to be significant contributing factors. Expanding ED facility size has not been found to be a particularly successful solution to this problem.

AMBULANCE DIVERSION

It is important for the EMS physician to have a general understanding of the background basis for ED diversion as well as the evidence-based results of its implementation as it can significantly affect the field provider in real time as well as the administrator looking to optimize unit hour utilization (UHU). First described by Lagoe and Jastremski in 1990 as a novel approach to alleviating EDC in an urban environment, AD has swept across the nation and is increasingly utilized in one form or another by most busy medical systems.[3-6] While there are variations on its definition, essentially an ED which is placed on diversion is closed to all incoming ALS and BLS traffic. Exceptions to this rule can include PD and specialty services (trauma, burn, etc). Proposed benefits of incorporating some type of diversion system include a decrease in mortality and morbidity by avoiding crowded (overwhelmed) EDs, a decrease in waiting times and crowding, and increased efficiency in utilizing resources. Proposed detriments to the system include complex patients being transported to facilities both unfamiliar with their history and lacking the patient's primary physicians, increased turnaround times for EMS personal traveling outside of normal service areas, and public perception of an institution turning away individuals requiring emergency care. This public perception can also be transferred to the prehospital provider. While ideal in concept, actual implementation and experience with diversion status have yielded conflicting research and brought the practice into question. Not only is the process being scrutinized by many different researchers and medical systems, the growing problem of EDC has clearly been shown to be much more complex than simply numbers of patients presenting to the Emergency Department via ALS and BLS ambulance.[7,8]

EFFECTS OF AMBULANCE DIVERSION

A first glance at the research and data surrounding diversion yields seemingly conflicting results. A number of researchers have demonstrated some association between AD and increased patient mortality and morbidity.[9-11] However, a recent systematic review of the literature relating to AD has suggested no such association exists.[12] This same review also concluded that based on the summary of the literature AD is common and increasing in frequency, is associated with EDC, is reducible through redesign or addition of resources, is associated with a small increase in patient transport and treatment times, slightly decreases ambulance flow, and appears to be associated with estimated losses to hospital revenue. Based on initial studies and this review, one could conclude diversion either has no demonstrable effect on mortality and morbidity or may slightly increase it.

As stated above, a theoretical benefit of diversion is greater utilization of available resources, and this is where the role of the prehospital provider is introduced as they are one of the obvious key available resources. Somewhat surprisingly studies have shown diversion results in only slightly increased turnaround times or has no significant negative effect on EMS resources.[12,13] Carter and Grierson sought to determine how diversion impacts ambulance resources. They evaluated 1563 instances of response times during an hour of diversion and 30 minutes before and after for 2002. These were compared with 1403 calls in 2001 when hospitals were not on diversion. They concluded their findings did not support a significant negative effect on EMS resources when one hospital in their study city was on diversion. They additionally state no difference was noted in transport, hospital turnaround, or total out-of-service times. The review by Pham and colleagues identified six articles evaluating AD and transport and treatment times. These articles demonstrated a 1.7 to 5 minute delay in transport times associated with AD. Delays in treatment times have been associated with increased patient mortality and morbidity.[14,15]

REDUCTION OF DIVERSION TIME

Several studies have shown institution of protocols and plans to both EMS systems and hospitals to decrease diversion hours have been effective. Based on the aforementioned articles demonstrating either no delay or minimal delay in treatment of patients when hospitals are on diversion, it would seem evident a reduction or elimination of diversion hours would benefit patients. Early intervention has been shown to be an important predictor in patient outcomes.[16,17] Asamoah, Weiss, and colleagues implemented a novel diversion protocol among a county of 600,000 people and 10 hospitals over a period of 6 months.[18] The protocol utilized limited diversion hours to one out of every eight (a total of 90 hours/month). The protocol was successful in reducing diversion hours during the trial (305 hours/month pretrial to 54 hours/month posttrial). The authors do note, however, they did see a small but statistically significant increase

in turnaround times for EMS providers as they waited longer to off load patients in busy emergency departments.

Vilke et al also examined a community intervention to decrease diversion hours.[19] They looked at a community of 2.8 million people and implemented a policy where hospitals could be on diversion for 1 hour only, could not go back on diversion until they had received at least one ambulance patient, and lastly, while on diversion, the hospital would take patient requests unless a significant patient safety issue existed. The trial took place over a 3-month period during which 235,766 patients were transported to emergency departments in the county. During the study, AD was decreased by 73% and the number of patients who could not be transported to their hospital of choice was decreased by 75%. In a review of the literature, Pham et al identified nine studies where individuals sought to limit diversion time through similar methods as those listed above (putting limitations on diversion status only).[12] An additional seven studies looked at emergency department and hospital-wide interventions to decrease diversion time (mainly through increasing throughput and admissions). They concluded that diversion rates can be reduced by adding resources to decrease EDC or closely monitoring diversion. No definite conclusions could be drawn with regard to EDC or patient outcome simply based on changing or limiting diversion.

CONCLUSIONS CONCERNING IN AMBULANCE DIVERSION

After reviewing the relevant literature, it is difficult to endorse uniform use of AD. Diversion appears to have either no effect on mortality and morbidity or results in a slight increase. Therefore, based on mortality and morbidity data, the practice cannot be supported. The majority of studies indicate diversion can result in increased turnaround and therefore response times for EMS personal as they are unable to access the closest appropriate hospital during times of diversion. This must also take into account the complex issues the prehospital provider is faced with when attempting to deliver optimal patient care as stated at the beginning of the chapter. Practices to decrease diversion times have proven to be successful and have allowed patients' greater access to primary hospitals where their medical records and primary providers are located. Some important references on AD are listed in **Table 11-1**.

HOSPITAL BYPASS

Some attention has been paid to the concept of bypassing local hospitals to provide primary transport to specialty centers for specific conditions. In a 2009 study comparing bypass for primary transport to a percutaneous intervention (PCI) center versus transport to a community hospital to receive thrombolytics, there was a somewhat less than impressive result in the expected benefit of bypass.[20] Wang et al noted that patients receiving "best-case" thrombolytics and "best-case" PCI have the same overall outcomes (relative risk of 1.000). Survival at 30 days for all cases was 95.8% for PCI and 93.8% for community hospital fibrinolytic therapy (relative risk 1.021 with a number needed to treat of 50); however, when PCI was compared to best-case community hospital fibrinolytic therapy there was relative risk of 0.980 with a number needed to harm of 50. It is difficult to know the exact value of bypass based on this study, but it brings the practice into some question. In a 2009 study out of Toronto Gladstone et al evaluated the effect of HB on the administration of tPA to stroke patients. The authors noted that an HB protocol coupled with a prehospital stroke notification system led to an increase in patient arrival within the treatment window (they used 2.4 hours) from 35.1% to 49.2% which was accompanied by an increase in percentage of stroke patients who received tPA from 9.5% up to 23.4%.[21] This resulted in what the authors state was one of the highest tPA treatment rates in North America. If tPA is truly beneficial therapy, then this may be a significant improvement in EMS system function, however, there is a question of whether this particular initiative represents an improvement in more than just the time of arrival. There was no comparison of outcome between the groups, only the statement that the postinitiative

TABLE 11-1	Some Important References on Ambulance Diversion

1990	*Lagoe RJ, Jastremski MS. Relieving overcrowded emergency departments through ambulance diversion. Hospital Topics. 1990;68(3):23.*
	– First paper to describe successful us of diversion as a novel way to decompress ED
	– Originally described for patients with "relatively minor injuries"
	– Used criteria to initiate AD
	  1. ≥10 admitted patients were awaiting inpatient beds or all inpatient monitors were in use
	  2. 3/4 hospitals on diversion—send to outlying hospitals
	– Limited effect—lasting only 4 months

1994	*Neely KW, Norton RL, Young GP. The effect of hospital resource unavailability and ambulance diversions on the EMS system. Prehospital Disaster Medicine. 1994;9(3):172-177.* – Five-month prospective study – 9-1-1 diversions compared to 5% random sample of nondiversions – Mean transport time nondiverted 11.5 vs 16.5 minutes ($P < 0.002$) – Distance to intended destination 1.3 to 4.6 miles further for diverted – Suggested was related to unavailability of specialty services – Recommended research into outcome differences
1994	*Redelmeier, et al. No place to unload: a preliminary analysis of the prevalence, risk factors, and consequences of ambulance diversion. Annals of EM. 1994;23(1):43-47.* – Observational cohort study over a 4-year period – 153,167 total transports; 5% diverted – Longer transport time during diversion: 13.3 (±7.5) vs 11.6 minutes (±6.9); $P < 0.005$ – No difference in rate of transport associated death

2003	*Lagoe RJ, et al. Reducing ambulance diversion: a multihospital approach. Prehospital Emergency Care. 2003; 7(1):99-108.*
	– Retrospective review of procedures for reducing diversion
	  • System-wide exchange of information on diversion status
	  • Hospital commitment to providing resources needed to reduce diversion
	  • Individual hospitals spot checking by management level personnel
	– Between 2000 and 2001 hours on diversion were reduced by 33.3%
	– Previous paper (2002) by Lagoe et al. showed 51% time on diversion

2004	*Vilke GM, et al. Community trial to decrease ambulance diversion hours: the San Diego County patient destination trial. Ann EM. 2004; 44 (4): 295-303.*
	– Retrospective study postimplementation of a diversion protocol
	– Authorization of diversion required ED attending and charge nurse. After 3 hours then authorization by hospital administrator
	  • Decreased hours on diversion
	    – Pretrial = 4007/during trial = 1079/posttrial = 1774
	  • Decreased number of patients diverted
	    – Pretrial = 1320/during trial = 322/posttrial = 499
	    – 75% reduction of diversion away from requested ED

2007	*Carter AJE, Grierson R. The impact of ambulance diversion on EMS resource availability. Prehospital emergency care. 2007;11(4):421-426.* – Retrospective study of periods on diversion vs periods off diversion – Only one hospital in system on diversion at a time – Diversion could last up to 1 h with extension granted by health department – Results: no difference in response time, on-scene time, transport time, hospital turnaround time, out-of-service time

TABLE 11-1	Some Important References on Ambulance Diversion *(continued)*

2011	*Shen YC, Hsia RY. Association between ambulance diversion and survival among patients with acute myocardial infarction. JAMA. 2011 Jun 15;305(23):2440-2447.*
	– exposure to <6, 6 to <12, and ≥12 h of diversion
	– <12 h of diversion = no difference
	– >12 or more hours of diversion were associated with higher 30-day mortality (392 patients [19%] vs 545 patients [15%])
	  • higher 90-day mortality (537 patients [26%] vs 762 patients [22%])
	  • higher 9-month mortality (680 patients [33%] vs 980 patients [28%])
	  • higher 1-year mortality (731 patients [35%] vs 1034 patients [29%])

tPA group had a Rankin score of <2 28% of the time. In the case of trauma patients, there have been studies reporting significant mortality and morbidity benefits to HB to a tertiary trauma center.[22,23] However, a systematic review from 2011 questions the benefit due to a lack of significant outcome differences and a more recent review from 2013 showed mixed results and the authors concluded that there was inconclusive evidence to either support or refute the benefit of HB with direct transport to a level 1 or level 2 trauma center.[24,25] Conversely, a study from 2006 showed a significant clinical outcome benefit to direct transport of traumatic brain injury patients to a level 1 or 2 trauma center and a recent study also showed that patients with prolonged transport times did not deteriorate to a greater extent while being transported to the trauma center directly.[26,27] It is likely that the heterogeneity of different EMS systems and geographic variability confounds generalization of current available studies. Therefore, EMS system medical directors must consider reviewing available literature and comparing local outcomes before making decisions concerning institution of HB. Significant political and financial implications also exist, and therefore, ideally there should be a documentable patient outcome benefit prior to instituting change. Destination decision making is discussed in more detail in Chapter 53.

PATIENT DEMAND

A number of factors may be involved when destination decision making occurs. PD has been cited as the one of the most influential components in this process. This is an important factor, as in many jurisdictions, the patient or family can "trump" the provider when destination is concerned. In a 2011 study of trauma patients, PD was found to be the deciding factor in 52.2% of transports, and was as high as 78% for nontrauma patients.[28] In a more recent study from 2013, the factor effecting transport destination was determined to be PD in 50.6% of cases.[29] Other cited factors included proximity to a facility (20.7%) and status of the hospital as a specialty resource center (15.2%).

AMBULANCE OFFLOAD DELAY

AOD is an important benchmark time interval because it represents a delay in patient care. In some states EMS providers are not allowed to care for patients inside the hospital, and therefore AOD represents a time when the hospital staff and the EMS providers are not rendering care to the patient. Patient satisfaction and privacy are also at risk during AOD because the stretchers are often lined up in the ED hallway. Communications from the Centers for Medicare & Medicaid Services (CMS) have revealed that EMTALA is in opposition to AOD[30,31] As additional attention is paid to AOD it is likely that it will be considered for incorporation into standards by accrediting organizations like The Joint Commission and DNV. With only a few studies to evaluate it may be difficult to initially determine where to set the bar for AOD. Current studies are aimed at establishing a baseline, evaluating the risk, and determining a reasonable a goal or benchmark. Currently the available data and expert opinion suggest that an AOD of <15 minute (90% of the time) should be considered high-quality

Box 11-1	
Ambulance Offload Delay Benchmarks	
<15 minutes (90% of the time)	High quality
15-30 minutes (90% of the time)	Moderate quality
30-60 minutes (90% of the time)	Low quality
>60 minutes (90% of the time)	Unacceptable
> 60 minutes (per event)	Reportable incident

performance, 15-30 minutes should be considered acceptable, and an AOD episode of >60 minutes should be considered a reportable incident and should trigger a root cause analysis (**Box 11-1**).

REDUCTION IN AOD

Offload nurses/providers are one option to improve AOD. Traditional ED staffing models typically provide for nursing coverage based on the physical rooms or patient care areas in the ED. This leaves "no staffing" to allow for patients in the hallway with EMS. The offload nurse/provider takes responsibility for these patients and can care for them and move them to stretchers/chairs, allowing EMS providers to leave the ED and prevent the negative effects of AOD on the EMS system. A prehospital dashboard of system hospital capability and status can lead to improved destination decision making by allowing prehospital providers to more accurately gauge and compare factors that may indicate potential for AOD at different hospitals.[32,33] Another solution to reducing mean AOD is to utilize a "bed ahead" process for assigning and ED bed for ambulance patients prior to arrival, based on radio report (or electronic prearrival clearance). Keeping the ED from becoming unnecessarily crowded is a key factor in preventing AOD. Throughput initiatives that allow for additional ED staffing during high demand, improved discharge processes on the hospital floors and in the ED, streamlined ED-to-floor patient transfer processes, provider in triage models, and a variety of other strategies may significantly impact crowding, and therefore effect AOD. The NEDOCS score may be beneficial in triggering surge capacity relief during EDC. Sending additional staff, giving increased priority to ED patient labs and imaging, and placing the hospital on AD can be linked to a specific NEDOCS score. This type of surge response allows for more flexible operating parameters while allowing for management of unexpected crowding.

EVALUATING THE COST OF AOD

The cost of AOD is multifaceted when considering the entire system. The most obvious cost to the system is that of the burden it places on the EMS system. As crews wait in the ED they are unavailable to respond to the next emergency call. This means that another unit must answer this call. As more AOD is added to the EMS system, more units are needed to answer the same number of calls. The UHU of the system then declines, leading to a higher cost per transport. There is a cost to the ED/hospital when attempting to address AOD. If throughput measures are not the focus, and additional capacity becomes the focus, there is likely to be an unfavorable return on investment. As the ED and staffing grows the demand for inpatient beds will not decline, and therefore the bottleneck does not decrease. AOD is tied to EDC, and EDC is tied to throughput. Most important, however, is the cost of AOD to the patient. Delays in care are frequently tied to increases in morbidity and mortality. Nothing indicated that AOD should be any different than other delays. In addition, patient satisfaction and privacy are also lost during the AOD, which can then also affect the ED/hospital.

FUTURE STUDY

Future studies will be focused on identifying risk factors related to increased AOD. An association with NEDOCS scoring (EDC) has been noted and may offer additional insight, or possibly show evidence for using NEDOCS scores as triggers for diversion or to inform providers

and patients prior to destination decision making. When evaluating the cause of AOD, it is important to attempt to determine causative factors (eg, patient specific, staffing, facility type). It is also important to further quantify specific effects on the EMS system (eg, UHU, response times, provider satisfaction / attrition). **Table 11-2** highlights some important references on AOD.

TABLE 11-2	Important References on Ambulance Offload Delay
2005	*Schwartz B, et al. Improving access to emergency services: a system commitment. Report to the Ministry of Health and Long-term care, Government of Ontario, Canada. 2005.*
	– Commitment from all stakeholders is the fundamental requirement for improvement in emergency department overcrowding and ambulance offload delay.
	Cannot focus solely on the emergency department
	EDC is a symptom of systemic issues, not the source of the problem
	– Stakeholders must be held accountable
	– Principal cause of offload time is lack of capacity to treat hospital inpatients
	– Solution to problem must look at inpatient capacity
	– Set goal of 30 minutes for offload
2007	*CMS. EMTALA Issues related to emergency transport services. April 27, 2007. [Clarification of 7/13/06 letter].*
	– EMTALA responsibility of hospital begins when an individual arrives and not when the hospital "accepts" the individual from the gurney
	– Hospital has an obligation to provide appropriate medical screening examination and necessary stabilization
	– Failure to meet these requirements constitutes a violation of EMTALA
	– Exception to immediate offload may be in times of extreme demand (multiple trauma/critical care patients arriving)
	– Hospital must triage the patient's condition immediately upon arrival to ensure that an emergent intervention is not required and the EMS providers can care for the patient
2008	*Asamoah OK, et al. A novel diversion protocol dramatically reduces diversion hours. Am J EM. 2008; 26 (6):670-675.*
	– Retrospective study of a countywide diversion protocol
	– Hospital could go on divert for 1 hour only and then off diversion for next 8 hours
	– Outcomes: number of hours on diversion and drop-off times for diversion periods compared to nondiversion periods
	Protocol decreased diversion by 82%
	Increased drop-off time (ie, offload delay) = 1.66 minutes/month (95% CI 0.33-2.98) (increase of 32%)
	Increased unit time = 178 hours/month (95% CI 74-283) (Unit time = [90% drop-off time – 15 minutes] × no of transports]/60 minutes)
	Little effect on EDC
2011	*Cooney DR, et al. Ambulance diversion and emergency department offload delay: resource document for the National Association of EMS Physicians position statement. Prehosp Emerg Care. 2011 Oct-Dec;15(4):555-561.*
	– Reviewed literature and noted lack of data supporting specific need to use or lose concept of diversion
	– Noted possible significant patient care impact of offload delay
	– Supported NAEMSP position
	– Recommended AOD be tracked by EM and EMS administrators
2013	*Cooney DR, et al. Evaluation of ambulance offload delay at a university hospital emergency department. Int J Emerg Med. 2013 May 10;6(1):15.*
	– Mean offload delay was around 11 minutes
	– Significant variation with notable outliers
	– NEDOCS score was associated with AOD

ALTERNATIVE DESTINATIONS

One particularly interesting concepts in management of EDC, AD, and AOD is the potential utilization of alternative destinations for ambulance transport of individuals who do not require emergency department care. Modern EMS systems provide transport to a number of patients who are not felt to have emergency conditions and who might be better served by a visit to an urgent care of primary care office.[34] Some research has been done to evaluate the potential for EMS providers to utilize alternative destinations.[35,36] The advantages of this type of system could be significant and the goal of reallocating emergency care resources to those most in need could be better realized. Unfortunately, at this time there is not enough available data to adequately support the use of prehospital provider determination of acuity to the level of denying transport of a patient to the ED that has called with report of an emergency.[37] It is likely that successful determination to decline transport and/or to utilize transport to alternative destination is currently being performed in a safe and effective manner with appropriate education and CQI in some EMS systems. Future studies are indicated and may show more favorable results.

KEY POINTS

- Despite this common practice, and the commitment of EMS system resources, HB may, or may not, influence patient outcomes in patients being transported to stroke, PCI, and trauma centers. Local studies may be needed to determine the value of this practice in each EMS system.
- AOD is an evolving marker of ED patient care quality.
- AOD and AD are interrelated and hospital throughput is a key causative factor.
- AOD represents a real and potential delay in patient care in the ED and in the prehospital environment.
- AD may be a useful tool if utilized judicially and in context with hospital throughput initiatives and surge capacity planning.
- Further study is needed to identify best practices in hospital throughput, AD, and AOD reduction.

REFERENCES

1. Appleby J. ER conditions critical. *USA Today*. 2000:A01.
2. Lee C. Crowded ERs raise concerns on readiness. *Washington Post*. 2006:A11.
3. Lagoe RJ, Jastremski MS. Relieving overcrowded emergency departments thorough ambulance diversion. *Hosp Top*. 1990;68:23-27.
4. Lagoe RJ Hunt RC, Nadle PA, Kohlbrenner JC. Utilization and impact of ambulance diversion at the community level. *Prehosp Emerg Care*. 2002;6:191-198.
5. Andrulis DP, Kellermann A, Hintz EA, Hackman BB, Weslowski VB. Emergency departments and crowding in United States teaching hospitals. *Ann Emerg Med*. 1991;20:980-986.
6. Burt CW, McCaig LF, Valverde RH. Analysis of ambulance transports and diversion among US emergency departments. *Ann Emerg Med*. 2006;47:317-326.
7. Derlet RW, Richards JR. Overcrowding in the nation's emergency departments: complex causes and disturbing effects. *Ann Emerg Med*. 2000;35:63-68.
8. Schull MJ, Szalai JP, Schwartz B, Redelmeier DA. Emergency Department overcrowding following systemic hospital restructuring: trends at twenty hospitals over ten years. *Acad Emerg Med*. 2001;8:1037-1043.
9. Asplin BR. Does ambulance diversion matter? *Ann Emerg Med*. 2003;41(4):477-480.
10. Schull MJ, Morrison LJ, Vermeulen M, Redelmeier DA. Emergency department gridlock and out-of-hospital delays for cardiac patients. *Acad. Emerg Med*. 2003; 10(7):709-716.
11. Hwang U, Richardson LD, Sonuyi TO, Morrison RS. The effect of emergency department crowding on the management of pain in older adults with hip fracture. *J Am Geriatric Soc*. 2006;54(2):270-275.
12. Pham JC, Patel R, Millin MG, Kirsch TD, Chanmugam A. The effects of ambulance diversion: a comprehensive review. *Acad Emerg Med*. 13(11):1220-1227.
13. Carter AJ, Grierson R. The impact of ambulance diversion on EMS resource availability. *Prehosp Emerg Care*. 11(4):421-426.
14. Schull MJ, Morrison LJ. Emergency department gridlock and out-of-hospital delays for cardiac patients. *Acad Emerg Med*. 2003;10:709-716.
15. Redelmeier DA, Blair PJ, Collins WE. No place to unload: a preliminary analysis of the prevalence, risk factors, and consequences of ambulance diversion. *Ann Emerg Med*. 1994; 23:43-47.
16. Roth R, Stewart RD, Rogers K, Cannon GM. Out-of-hospital cardiac arrest: factors associated with survival. *Ann Emerg Med*. 1984; 13:237-243.
17. Cummings RD, Eisenberg MS, Hallstrom AP, Litwin PE. Survival of out-of-hospital cardiac arrest with early initiation of cardiopulmonary resuscitation. *Am J Emerg Med*. 1985;3:114-118.
18. Asamoah OK, Weiss SJ, Ernst AA, Richards M, Sklar DP. A novel diversion protocol dramatically reduces diversion hours. *Am J of Emerg Med*. 2008;26:670-675.
19. Vilke GM, Castillo EM, Metz MA, et al. Community trial to decrease diversion hours: the San Diego county patient destination trial. *Ann Emerg Med*. 2004 44(4):295-303.
20. Wang HE, Marroquin OC, Smith KJ. Direct paramedic transport of acute myocardial infarction patients to percutaneous coronary intervention centers: a decision analysis. *Ann Emerg Med*. 2009 Feb;53(2):233-240.
21. Gladstone DJ, Rodan LH, Sahlas DJ, et al. A citywide prehospital protocol increases access to stroke thrombolysis in Toronto. *Stroke*. December 2009;40(12):3841-3844.
22. Sampalis JS, Denis R, Fréchette P, Brown R, Fleiszer D, Mulder D. Direct transport to tertiary trauma centers versus transfer from lower level facilities: impact on mortality and morbidity among patients with major trauma. *J Trauma*. August 1997;43(2):288-295.
23. Sampalis JS, Denis R, Lavoie A, et al. Trauma care regionalization: a process-outcome evaluation. *J Trauma*. April 1999;46(4):565-579.
24. Hill AD, Fowler RA, Nathens AB. Impact of interhospital transfer on outcomes for trauma patients: a systematic review. *J Trauma*. Decemebr 2011;71(6):1885-1900.
25. Williams T, Finn J, Fatovich D, Jacobs I. Outcomes of different health care contexts for direct transport to a trauma center versus initial secondary center care: a systematic review and meta-analysis. *Prehosp Emerg Care*. October-December 2013;17(4):442-457.
26. Härtl R, Gerber LM, Iacono L, Ni Q, Lyons K, Ghajar J. Direct transport within an organized state trauma system reduces mortality in patients with severe traumatic brain injury. *J Trauma*. June 2006;60(6):1250-1256.
27. Fuller G, Woodford M, Lawrence T, Coats T, Lecky F. Do prolonged primary transport times for traumatic brain injury patients result in deteriorating physiology? A cohort study. *Prehosp Emerg Care*. January-March 2014,18(1):60-67.
28. Newgard CD, Nelson MJ, Kampp M, et al. Out-of-hospital decision making and factors influencing the regional distribution of injured patients in a trauma system. *J Trauma*. June 2011;70(6):1345-1353.
29. Newgard CD, Mann NC, Hsia RY, et al. Patient choice in the selection of hospitals by 9-1-1 emergency medical services providers in trauma systems. *Acad Emerg Med*. September 2013;20(9):911-919.

30. Wright D, ed. *Memorandum to All Region VI Hospital Associations.* Baltimore, MD: Centers for Medicare & Medicaid Services; 2002.

31. Centers for Medicare & Medicaid Services. *Final Report of the Emergency Medical Treatment and Labor Act Technical Advisory Group to the Secretary of Health and Human Services.* Baltimore, MD: Centers for Medicare & Medicaid Services; 2008.

32. McLeod B, Zaver F, Avery C, et al. Matching capacity to demand: a regional dashboard reduces ambulance avoidance and improves accessibility of receiving hospitals. *Acad Emerg Med.* 2010 Dec;17(12): 1383-1389.

33. Sprivulis P, Gerrard B. Internet-accessible emergency department workload information reduces ambulance diversion. *Prehosp Emerg Care.* July-September 2005;9(3):285-291.

34. Richards JR, Ferrall SJ. Inappropriate use of emergency medical services transport: comparison of provider and patient perspectives. *Acad Emerg Med.* January 1999;6(1):14-20.

35. Schaefer RA, Rea TD, Plorde M, Peiguss K, Goldberg P, Murray JA. An emergency medical services program of alternate destination of patient care. *Prehosp Emerg Care.* July-September 2002;6(3): 309-314.

36. Challen K, Walter D. Physiological scoring: an aid to emergency medical services transport decisions? *Prehosp Disaster Med.* July-August 2010;25(4):320-323.

37. Brown LH, Hubble MW, Cone DC, et al. Paramedic determinations of medical necessity: a meta-analysis. *Prehosp Emerg Care.* October-December 2009;13(4):516-527.

CHAPTER

12

EMS System Design

Jeremy T. Cushman

INTRODUCTION

The emergency medical services (EMS) system is a complex combination of various providers and facilities that provide three basic medical functions: stabilization, evacuation, and redistribution. Although organizational structures and resources vary worldwide, the fundamental components of any EMS system are essentially the same. This chapter will provide the EMS physician with a vital understanding of the organization of EMS systems and how such design considerations provide challenges and opportunities for patient-centered emergency medical care.

OBJECTIVES

- Define the EMS system in terms of the overall medical response to emergencies.
- List the original 14 components of an EMS system.
- List and describe the components of an EMS system as defined by NHTSA.
- Describe the basic types of emergency medical service agencies.
- Describe the main differences between urban and rural EMS systems.
- Discuss how community groups, corporations/businesses, patient advocacy groups, and health care facilities affect EMS system design.
- Define mutual aid and describe how it is employed in EMS system design.
- Discuss state, regional, and local EMS councils and/or administrations.
- Discuss state, regional, and local medical oversight committees.

PATIENT FLOW WITHIN AN EMS SYSTEM

The entry of a patient into the emergency health care system brings with it a complex cascade of events, with a number of possible outcomes. **Figure 12-1** displays a simplified look at the emergency health care system from the time of entry to the time of exit. Most striking to this flow diagram is its serial nature, and therefore, input to one process is limited by its output. This input-throughput-output conceptual model of the emergency health system is essential to consider as one examines the design of EMS systems, as an output limitation such as unstaffed ambulances or hospital crowding will progressively limit the system's ability to function and respond to the demands placed on it.[1,2]

The majority of patients who enter the emergency health care system do so by making a telephone call to the 9-1-1 system. The Medical Priority Dispatch System (MPDS) or the Association of Public-Safety Communications Officials (APCO) Emergency Medical Dispatch Program are specifically designed to abstract this caller information through a question-driven protocol and direct appropriate resources based on that information. Although a complete discussion of Emergency Medical Dispatch will be covered in Chapter 15, it is important to recognize that nearly all public safety answering points (PSAPs) are able to begin rendering care for the patient over the phone by using prescripted, postdispatch, and prearrival instructions.[3-6] The instructions could include directing a bystander to perform CPR, assist with the delivery of a newborn, or direct self-care such as hemorrhage control or aspirin administration. Further, the prioritization of requests for EMS service through any call-taking program based on call severity is essential to the underlying mission of getting the right equipment to the right patient at the right time.

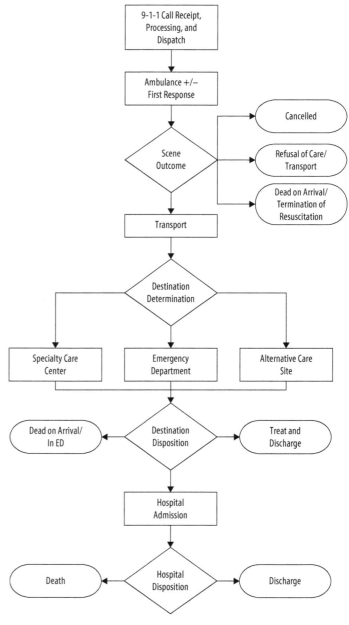

FIGURE 12-1. Patient flow within the emergency health care system.

SYSTEM RESPONSE

The standard response to a request for service includes sending an ambulance. There are limited circumstances in some systems whereby based on caller interrogation the requestor may be directed to alternative sources of care (eg, a poison control center for an accidental ingestion without any symptoms) or attended to by first responders without transport capability (eg, a request for lifting assistance). Depending on system design, the ambulance that is dispatched could be able to provide care at the BLS level, the ALS level, or in some systems may utilize a BLS ambulance with an ALS intercept (paramedic engine, paramedic "fly-car," etc). In systems that do not send ALS resources on every request for service, the use of an EMD program often allows differentiating those requests for service that are most likely to require ALS from those most likely to require BLS, and therefore assign resources accordingly. Determining which types of calls get which types of resources is often the responsibility of the 9-1-1 center or the system's medical director.

First responders are essential to the EMS system, particularly for cases of imminent life-threatening conditions such as choking, respiratory arrest, or cardiac arrest. Various systems employ a myriad of first-response deployment models. This could include fire department or law enforcement, and be trained and able to provide care anywhere from the first responder to the paramedic level. Further, depending on the historical influences on system design, these first responders could be dispatched on everything from no EMS requests for service to all of them.

There should exist in the EMS system a careful balance of the type of ambulance response (ALS or BLS), rapidity of response (lights/sirens or not), and necessity of first response. The facilitation of such balance is often the job of the system's medical director and is best determined based on patient outcome data from that system being weighed with the contractual obligations (if any) of the system and tempered by the inherent risks of over- and underresponse.

TRANSPORT DECISION MAKING

Once on scene, there are generally four possible outcomes. In most systems, anywhere between 20% and 30% of EMS calls result in no transport: Being cancelled on scene or prior to arrival; finding the patient dead on arrival or electing to terminate resuscitative efforts prior to transport; and having the patient refuse transport and/or treatment are the outcomes expected, resulting in no transport. For the majority of requests for service, however, the patient is transported to a destination to provide additional care. Most often, this destination is a local emergency department and that selection is often based on geography, patient preference, and continuity of care.[7] In an ever-increasing number of circumstances, local protocol may dictate transport to a specialty care destination. Often emergency departments, these specialty care centers are able to provide advanced care in trauma, burn, stroke, pediatric, cardiac care, or other specialized disciplines. In some communities, the option exists to transport the patient to an alternative care site such as an urgent care center or community health clinic. Although an important destination for EMS during disasters, these alternative care sites are unique opportunities to create a parallel care track in the decidedly serial nature of the EMS system to move patients more efficiently through the health care system. There are challenges to this approach and a more detailed discussion can be found in Chapter 11.

TRANSPORT OUT OF A HOSPITAL

Once at the destination, most commonly an emergency department, there are generally three outcomes. In some cases, the patient may be transferred from that ED to another hospital for specialty care or because of bed availability. Both of these outcomes may affect the EMS system as transfers almost universally result in the use of EMS resources, and in some cases, specialized resources and/or teams. If admitted to the hospital and subsequently discharged, this may be to home, a rehabilitation facility, or a long-term care facility. The latter two may also impact the EMS system as these patients are often transported by EMS due to their continued health care needs and/or inability to safely ambulate or transfer.

EMS system design must take into consideration not only the emergency requests for service, but also the nonemergency and interfacility transport requests. Efficiently utilizing limited and often costly resources in a linear and flow-constricted system is the challenge of EMS system managers, and the role of the EMS physician to ensure the system meets its primary mission of patient care should not be underestimated.

THE COMPONENTS OF AN EMS SYSTEM

Prior to 1973, the components of an EMS system were as varied as the EMS systems themselves and consisted of transportation, not necessarily treatment. When published in 1966, *Accidental Death and Disability: The Neglected Disease of Modern Society* began focusing on the inadequacies of emergency care in general, and prehospital care in particular.[8] In great part prompted by *Accidental Death and Disability*, and a demonstration project by the newly established Robert Wood Johnson Program, in 1973 Congress passed and President Nixon signed the EMS Systems Act.[9]

The Act called for a lead agency under the Department of Health, Education, and Welfare and identified 15 components to assist planners with the design of EMS systems stimulated by federal funding from this Act to over 300 regions nationwide. The original 15 components of the EMS Systems Act are included in **Table 12-1** and notably lack concepts such as medical direction, financing, performance expectations, or a legal framework within which to operate.[9] Although established to promote regionalization, the Act set into motion dozens of differently structured EMS systems that facilitated isolation, without planting the important seed of establishing initiatives to continually fund EMS at the local, regional, or even federal level.

The EMS Systems Act did not put the patient at the center of the system, nor did it promote the importance of clinical care as the primary driver of system design. In essence, the Act merely promulgated the pre-1973 concept that EMS systems were merely specialized transportation systems. By the early 1990s, greater interest in the clinical care of patients led to the 1996 National Highway Transportation Administration's release of the *EMS Agenda for the Future*.[5] This document made an important contribution by outlining the following 14 essential components that form the basis for current system design[10]:

Integration of health care service: As a component of the health care system, the care interaction with EMS should not occur in isolation and should be integrated with other community health resources within the health care system.

TABLE 12-1 EMS Systems Act Components of System Design[9]
Ensure adequate personnel
Establish recruitment, initial training, and continuing education programs
Ensure centralized communication
Ensure adequate transportation vehicles (air, water, and land)
Establish facilities that can continuously operate in coordination with each other and do not duplicate
Provide access to specialized critical medical care units
Provide for effective utilization of public safety agencies
Allow for community participation
Provide emergency care without prior inquiry as to ability to pay
Provide for transfer of patients to appropriate follow-up and rehabilitation care
Provide for standard record keeping
Provide public education programs
Provide for periodic, comprehensive, and independent review and evaluation
Ensure care provision during mass casualties or disasters
Provide for reciprocal services (mutual aid)

EMS research: Research is essential to improve care and allocate resources by determining the efficacy, effectiveness, and efficiency of prehospital care.

Legislation and regulation: Affecting EMS funding, system design, provider credentialing and scope of practice, enabling legislation and its associated regulations significantly affect how all aspects of prehospital care are provided.

System finance: In order to continuously provide essential public safety services, EMS systems, whether public or private, must be financially viable and built upon a strong financial foundation.

Human resources: The most valuable asset to EMS patients, the human resource, must be composed of a dedicated team with complementary skills and expertise that provide qualified, competent, and compassionate care.

Medical direction: Involving the delegation of authority and acceptance of responsibility, medical direction ensures the standards of medical practice are upheld to ensure optimal care for patients.

Education systems: To meet the evolving standard of care, EMS education systems must meet the cognitive, psychomotor, and technological needs of new and seasoned EMS professionals.

Public education: The EMS system has a responsibility to foster health promotion.

Prevention: The EMS system has a responsibility to promote prevention activities that reduce human morbidity and mortality.

Public access: Prompt and appropriate EMS care must be provided regardless of socioeconomic status, age, or special need.

Communications: Robust systems that allow accurate and timely transfer of information are essential to system success.

Clinical care: Mobility and immediate availability to the entire population distinguishes EMS in its ability to provide medical care to those with perceived need and provide transport to, from, and between health care facilities.

Information systems: Collecting, transmitting, and analyzing valid, reliable, and accurate data are essential to system improvement and integration within the health care system.

Evaluation: System and continuous evaluation is essential to assess the quality of system performance and identify strategies for improvement.

SYSTEM PERFORMANCE

Although system design should take into account the 14 aforementioned components, system performance can, and should, be measured frequently by a variety of different metrics. Early proponents of measuring system performance as a means of optimizing system design included Jack Stout, who was long involved in designing and implementing EMS systems and as early as 1983 promulgated his "10 Standards of Excellence" (**Table 12-2**), which closely mirror the NHTSA components published 13 years later.[11] Stout's "standards" have been replaced in the last decade with accreditation which is often used as a means to measure a system's performance against a set of standards, many of which have a basis derived from the goals and expectations of the *Agenda for the Future*. The Commission on Accreditation of Ambulance Services (CAAS), the Commission on Accreditation of Medical Transport Systems (CAMTS), and the Joint Commission International (JCI) are all well-established accreditation entities. CAAS is more widely known in the ambulance industry and provides a comprehensive set of standards designed to promote quality patient care.[12] CAMTS concentrates on patient care and provider safety and primarily accredits air medical services and ground interfacility services.[13] The JCI provide criteria used by international health care organizations to measure performance against a set of expectations and patient care benchmarks.[14] Other accreditation entities include the National Academies of Emergency Medical Dispatch which offer accreditation for Emergency Medical Dispatch Programs,[15]

TABLE 12-2 Jack Stout's 10 Standards of Excellence

Clinical performance

Medical accountability

Dispatching and system status management

Access, first responder, and citizen CPR

Disaster capability

Personnel management practices

Stability, reliability, and fail-safes

Pricing policies, billing, and collection practices

Response time performance

Public accountability

Reproduced with permission from Jack Stout (www.jackstout.com). From Stout J. Measuring your system: Jack Stout's ten standards of excellence. *JEMS*. 1983 Jan;8(1):84-91.

and the Commission on Fire Service Accreditation International for fire-based EMS operations.[16] Although accreditation is a means to accomplish the introspection of system analysis, it is clear that every aspect of the EMS system should be regularly reviewed and measured against the agency's goals. This allows shortfalls to be addressed and either patient outcome or system efficiency to be enhanced.

TYPES OF EMS SYSTEMS

The types of EMS systems are as numerous as the systems themselves. Since current system design evolved from the political, historical, and funding influences of the 1960s and 1970s, they offer varying clinical sophistication provided by a myriad of organizational structures. The following are the more common EMS system designs found in the United States:

VOLUNTEER

Volunteer systems, despite the decline in volunteerism, still provide a significant source of EMS in primarily suburban and rural communities. Challenges include volunteer recruitment and retention; limited funding streams whether from local taxes, fund-raising, or billing for services; and assembling highly qualified staff that can maintain the ever-increasing training requirements and be able to meet the demand for services during peak times, often during the day. Most agencies provide only 9-1-1 service and rarely provide interfacility or scheduled service. Many volunteer agencies have moved to supplemental paid staffing to meet call demand, and there tends to be greater dependence on mutual aid in volunteer systems. Due to the intensive training requirements for ALS providers, it is becoming increasingly rare to find volunteer paramedics and thus meet the local demand for ALS services, often requiring another agency or paid staff to provide ALS.

FIRE BASED

The number of fire-based EMS systems continues to increase and there may be some benefits seen in optimizing the first response and transport roles when organized in such a structure. Funded primarily from local government, many fire departments are also able to bill for service, providing a rare source of income to a public safety entity. However, legislative and/or regulatory restrictions, such as those found in New York, prohibit most fire departments from billing for services, thus providing an example of how state legislation can significantly affect system design. Similar to volunteer systems, fire-based EMS often provides only 9-1-1 service and rarely provides interfacility or scheduled service.

HOSPITAL BASED

Despite being one of the first providers of EMS in the United States in as early as the 1860s, hospital-based providers are not nearly as common as in the past. Such systems are often able to allow prehospital personnel to work in the hospital setting, providing outstanding opportunities to maintain skill sets, particularly with regard to interfacility transfers with critical patients. Some of these systems provide only interfacility transports, others also provide 9-1-1 service. Similar to fire-based EMS, legislative and/or regulatory restrictions in some states either foster or discourage hospital-based EMS systems.

■ PRIVATE

Private EMS companies, whether for-profit or not-for-profit, often operate under a contract with a municipality to provide 9-1-1 services. Many also provide interfacility and nonemergency transport services and first response is typically delegated to the fire department. Private companies will bill the patient or third party for the majority of their revenue. In some cases, these agencies may receive a subsidy from the municipality, or the municipality is paid (a so-called franchise fee) for the right of sole proprietor following a public bid process. More commonly contractual obligations are built into the service agreement between the private company and the municipality to encourage a predefined performance level. These are often penalty based and result in fines paid back to the municipality if certain performance standards (response time, call coverage, clinical performance measures, etc) are not met.

■ THIRD SERVICE

The *third-service model* is whereby EMS is provided by a governmental department or authority much like law enforcement or fire service is provided. There are multiple variations based on the deployment model (fixed "station" versus system-status management), funding (tax subsidies, billing for service, and combinations of the two), ability to provide first-response capabilities, and ability to provide interfacility transports.

■ PUBLIC UTILITY AND FRANCHISE

In this model, an EMS agency or authority is overseen by a board of directors and often independent medical oversight. This group establishes the expectations of service delivery, from response time to clinical performance and then contracts with a private company. In the *public utility model*, the agency or authority owns all assets, determines billing rates and collects revenue, and pays the contractor a set fee. The contractor is then responsible for managing the system to meet the performance standards for the lowest cost in order to realize a profit. The *franchise model* allows the contractor to collect revenue, but the agency or authority has specific controls over the contractor's assets.

SYSTEM PERFORMANCE CONSIDERATIONS

All of the system types mentioned must manage limited resources in order to provide quality clinical care at the lowest possible cost. A number of techniques are used to accomplish this, and although a complete understanding of system design and performance is beyond the scope of this chapter, the following terms and concepts may be useful for the EMS physician.

The *response time reliability* (RTR) is a key metric in most systems. RTR may be parsed by geographic area, BLS vs ALS, dispatch priority, etc, and is measured most often in fractiles and not means, often at the 90th fractile. For example, a contract may state that City X is divided into eight geographic zones and each zone must maintain an RTR of 8:59 or less, 90% of the time. Failure to do so may result in fines which are designed to enforce the RTR of the contractor. These fines must be large enough to make it more cost effective to cover the 90th fractile than simply not staffing, and therefore, not meeting the contractual (or community) expectation of service delivery.

In order to meet the RTR, the EMS agency will often need to maximize the efficiency of their EMS units by deploying the number of units required to meet the historical demand, and positioning (and repositioning) them to minimize the response time. Systems generally position their resources in two ways: Static deployment is most often seen in fire-based and volunteer EMS systems whereby an ambulance is located in a station and responds to calls in its primary response area. When the call is

completed, it returns to that station but during the time it is not available, that response area remains "uncovered" and requires the use of another resource either from the same agency located at a different station or a different agency (mutual aid) to cover the request in the response area. This leads to often lengthier response times. *System status management* (SSM) is a technique whereby units are generally not statically deployed but rather are actively moved around the service area based on their use, traffic patterns, and other factors in order to minimize response time in the service area and therefore maximize RTR performance.

The *unit hour* (UH) and *unit hour utilization ratio* (UH/U) are two additional key metrics in most systems. The UH is simply 1 hour of a staffed, available ambulance. Thus, an agency that staffs one unit, 24 hours a day, has 24 UHs per day or 154 UHs per week. The UH/U is a fraction of the amount of time a unit (ambulance) is loaded with a patient and being used to generate revenue divided by the number of UHs. A UH/U of 1.0 would mean that the unit is always "loaded" with a patient and therefore doing "work" or generating revenue. The lower the UH/U, the less efficient a system is; thus, a UH/U of 0.1 means that the available units are only generating revenue 10% of the time. This may be allowable in a rural system that must maintain service availability despite a low call volume, but may not be realistic for an urban system with short transport times and large volume. The challenge of system designers and administrators is to maximize the UH/U, while meeting the RTR of the community (or of the contract). Thus, although it is possible to have an RTR in a large city of 3:59, 90% of the time, the number of UHs required to meet that are financially unsustainable.

To maximize UH/U while achieving the call coverage expected of the community, many systems will perform a demand analysis to temporally identify where the demand lies. This can be as simple as graphing the number of calls for each hour of the day for each day of the week. This allows the administrator to add UHs when the demand is there (days and perhaps early evenings) and decrease the UHs during lower demand (overnights, perhaps weekends). Adding or removing UHs requires adjustments in staffing, and subsequently a "peak-load staffing plan" may be developed to staff the units during the hours they are needed as personnel costs are the largest expense for nearly all systems. The process of performing a demand analysis to determine UHs and system status plan necessary to meet the RTR of the system, and developing a peak-load staffing plan to meet the UH needs, then optimizes the UH/U which ultimately results in a more efficient and financially viable system, irrespective of the system type.

EXTERNAL EFFECTS ON SYSTEM DESIGN

There are a number of factors independent of the type of EMS system that affects how EMS is provided within the system. The most obvious is geography. Urban areas typically have a large enough call volume and demand for services, that many different service delivery models can exist, most often fire-based, private, or public utility/franchise models. Urban environments more often than not have response time performance expectations in the case of an external contractor that provides such service. Challenges faced within these systems include the sheer volume of calls in a relatively small geographic area resulting in rapid call turnover, the violence and safety risks inherent to some urban environments, and thus, the physical and emotional fatigue placed on the EMS provider. This can result in high employee turnover which can limit the clinical experience of the workforce. This urban environment also offers challenges and great opportunities in the realm of public health interventions (eg Public Access Defibrillation programs, community CPR training, car seat checks, bicycle safety), as well as disaster preparedness for all types of chemical, biological, radiological, nuclear, and explosive hazards. This may mean additional opportunities for the EMS system to engage in specialty teams such as tactical, urban search and rescue, and other special operations disciplines.

Rural areas have unique challenges as well. Although the 9-1-1 system reaches more than 98% of the US population, it is disproportionately absent in rural settings, making access more difficult.[17] Further, the robust communications infrastructure taken for granted in the urban and suburban setting may limit the coordination and use of resources common in other settings. The robust first-response systems found in most urban and suburban areas are often lacking, simply because of the extremely sparse population, making response time performance measures that are standard in the urban and suburban environment impossible in the rural areas. Due to the lower volume over a higher area, the challenges of skills retention and ensuring adequate clinical experience place higher reliance on continuing education which, although facilitated by distance learning technology, may not meet the needs of the provider. Often critically ill patients must be transported significant distances and perhaps even further if requiring specialty care not available at a local or critical access hospital. Funding such rural systems often requires significant tax subsidy to offset a lower call volume and payer mix. Rural areas are disproportionately served by volunteer agencies, thus the challenges of the volunteer agency type add to those caused by geography. There is generally an increase in use of air medical transport services, which may in fact be the primary source of ALS in the rural and wilderness community. Aside from system design, many of these factors also require the EMS medical director to adjust scope of practice or medical protocols to account for the unique nature of the rural or wilderness environment.

Irrespective of the geography, there are other external factors that may affect system design, its performance, and its administrative and medical oversight. The most obvious is the often state-specific enabling legislation that may limit the operating territory and type of ambulance service, require determination of public need through a certificate of need process in order to operate, define the levels of care provided or minimum equipment required, or establish state-wide or regional standards of medical care. Elected officials such as mayors, city councils, and county/parish executives may affect system design through influences on contracts for ambulance services. In some cases, business and industry may have direct influences on system design (eg, a large industrial facility having its own fire and ambulance service), or may influence indirectly by promoting the use of certain products or equipment that may or may not have medical evidence to support their use but are often associated with increased cost (eg, disposable medical equipment or patient carrying equipment). In some cases, health care facilities can have significant influence on the system. The most obvious are those systems that are hospital based, but more subtle influences may exist through interfacility contract agreements or other service contracts.

In some cases, community groups may exert pressure on elected officials to advocate for a certain delivery system or more likely the expectations of that system. For example, with the right subsidy, almost any jurisdiction can achieve an ALS response on every request for service in less than 5 minutes from the time of call. Most communities do not wish to provide the (very large) subsidy required to meet the aforementioned response time requirement, even if there is little evidence to support ALS on every EMS call and a 5-minute response time to every request for service. Community expectations, such as response time, tax levies, services provided, etc, can have significant influences on the type of system. Further, patient advocacy groups may not directly influence system design, but they may influence the scope of practice within that system. For example, a patient advocacy group may lobby the local, regional, or state EMS oversight bodies to add a certain medication or training to the scope of practice. In some cases, that may represent a minuscule number of EMS contacts per year, and so the balance of medication cost and rotation, along with training, may not be cost-effective in every system.

MUTUAL AID

Although most EMS systems are designed to accommodate the majority of the demand for service, no system can afford the excess capacity in order to meet every request for service, all of the time, particularly in circumstances of excess demand due to mass casualty incident or epidemic. Mutual aid is an important component of any system design, and its reliance to ensure uninterrupted service varies, often due to system type (eg, generally more often utilized in volunteer systems than commercial

ones), and may be an infrequent occurrence or a daily one. Often defined in enabling legislation or intermunicipal agreement, mutual aid has three essential components: they are formal agreements; the resources are coming from "outside" the system; and they are reciprocal. One of the earliest definitions of mutual aid can be found in the EMS Systems Act whereby mutual aid is defined as an agreement that provides "for the establishment of appropriate arrangements with emergency medical services (EMS) systems or similar entities serving neighboring areas for the provision of EMS on a reciprocal basis where access to such services would be more appropriate and effective in terms of the services available, time, and distance." Although it is essential that every system has a process for sending and receiving mutual aid, the frequency of use may be indicative of the challenges faced by the system itself.

ADMINISTRATIVE OVERSIGHT OF EMS SYSTEMS

EMS systems generally have two different types of oversight: administrative and medical. At the state level, there is typically a lead agency such as a State EMS Office or Bureau of EMS that has administrative oversight of the state EMS system. In most states, this lead agency is under the State Department of Health, while the remainder often houses it in a State Department of Homeland Security, Department of Public Safety, Department of Transportation, or as a stand-alone department. The lead agency is often managed by a state EMS director who provides administrative direction for the lead agency and is often a nonphysician. Approximately a third of states have a regulatory board, while two-thirds have an advisory board that work in concert with the state EMS director. The roles and responsibilities of the lead agency vary tremendously in role and function as a result of the empowering legislation. Generally the lead agency will have a regulatory role, a leadership role, and a facilitator role.

The *regulatory role* may include establishing minimum standards for training and equipment carried by EMS personnel and processing, verifying, and awarding certification or licensure to EMS providers, agencies, or vehicles. The lead agency may establish regional or local oversight and may also designate EMS receiving facilities such as emergency departments, alternative destinations, or specialty care such as stroke, cardiac, or trauma centers.[18]

The *leadership role* may include providing model policies, procedures, or protocols to EMS services within the state, or facilitating the creation of those through advisory boards or medical oversight boards. The state has an important leadership role in system planning, particularly with regard to disaster and public health preparedness, as well as communications infrastructures. Injury prevention and emergency medical services for children programs are often administered by the lead state agency. Lastly, the state often serves as a main repository for data collection and tracking and in some cases, defines how that data will be collected and processed, or provides the very system that is used for field data entry.

Equally important to the regulatory and leadership roles, the state has an important *facilitator role* with other state departments, such as Fire, Homeland Security, Health, Narcotics Enforcement, and so on, which have important effects on how the EMS system in the state is able to practice—particularly with regard to scope of practice and enabling legislation. The state agency is also vital for facilitating the state mutual aid plan and interacting with the state emergency management office as well as ensuring strong working relationships with neighboring states.

Based largely from the EMS Systems Act of 1973, many states have some form of regional administrative oversight that work in concert with the lead state agency. Generally, the use of a regional structure is authorized by the empowering legislation for the EMS system. These regional oversight bodies may be defined by hospital catchment area, political jurisdiction (county or legislative boundaries) or be completely arbitrary. Generally composed of regional "councils" or "coordinating entities," they may be appointed by the governor, state EMS director, or defined for autonomous appointment by the enabling legislation. These regional councils often advise lead EMS agencies on policy direction and act as EMS advocates. Depending on the state, these bodies may establish standards or coordinate care by recruiting and credentialing providers, providing training, establishing operating authority for EMS agencies, establishing protocols and policies for patient care, and providing for regional quality assurance programs.

Local administrative oversight is generally limited to county or municipality issues. This typically relates to any local ordinances that regulate the provision of emergency services. In those jurisdictions with private, public utility, or franchise model EMS systems, the local administrative oversight may be significant in the form of developing performance standards, awarding contracts, and ensuring contract performance. The local administrative oversight often coordinates inter- and intracounty (or parish) mutual aid as well as coordinating with the State Department of Health or Emergency Management during disaster declarations. Local communications systems to include both radio and data communications, as well as public safety answering points, may fall under local administrative oversight as well.

MEDICAL OVERSIGHT OF EMS SYSTEMS

Similar to the administrative oversight of EMS systems, medical oversight may have state, regional, and agency levels. At the state level, the *state medical director* may be the same position as the state EMS director, may be the chair of an advisory or regulatory council, or may be a separate position entirely. The responsibility of the state medical director often includes overall state level medical supervision particularly with regard to protocol development and scope of practice consideration. The state EMS medical director often has an important liaison role with medical professional organizations and regional/local medical directors. A joint position statement on the role of state EMS medical directors from NAEMSP and ACEP is an important resource and reference document.[19]

A *regional medical director* may establish and uphold/oversee standards, if delegated from the state. This may include the regional credentialing of providers, the training of those providers, the creation of protocols and policies, and most often the regional quality assurance program. The responsibilities and authority of the regional medical director most often are codified in the enabling legislation and regulation.

The *agency medical director* is responsible for the clinical care provided by the EMS service and establishes and oversees internal, or agency-specific medical policies, provider credentialing, and quality assurance at a minimum. Section 2 in this text provides a more thorough overview of *medical oversight*, but it is important to recognize that in most states there are at least two, if not more levels of medical oversight and the responsibilities of each may be different, but equally important in ensuring strong clinical care. An important resource for all EMS physicians is the joint NAEMSP and ACEP position statement on the role of an agency EMS medical director which outlines the many roles the medical director may have depending on the type of system.[20]

At the state, regional, or local level, medical oversight committees may work with, or in place of, appointed medical directors to facilitate the medical oversight of the EMS system. These committees or councils are often composed of physicians representing various constituents and users of EMS. For example, a local or regional medical oversight committee may be composed of physicians from the local hospitals, whereas a state medical oversight committee may be composed of physicians from various regions around the state. The powers of such a body are often defined in enabling legislation and may include approving protocols, identifying the scope of practice, or defining the education requirements of EMS providers. In many cases, these committees or councils ensure appropriate checks and balances in the oversight of such EMS systems to ensure that the needs of the community are met.

CONCLUSION

The design, administration, and medical oversight of an EMS system are complex and rooted in the history of the EMS system. It is important that the EMS physician familiarize themselves with the different system designs, challenges, and opportunities that each provide, as well as review the enabling legislation, administrative, and medical oversight that is unique to each state to understand the many roles for EMS physicians and how to ensure that the system is meeting its intent to provide high-quality, evidence-based medical care and transportation.

- Patient flow within the EMS system is generally linear with key inputs and outputs which affect system design and efficiency.
- The EMS Agenda for the Future identified 14 essential components that form the basis for current EMS system design.
- The types of EMS systems are as numerous as the systems themselves and generally include volunteer, fire-based, hospital-based, private, third-service, public utility, and franchise systems.
- A basic EMS system performance characteristic is response time reliability, which can be optimized by utilizing system status management along with peak load staffing plans to efficiently deploy the unit hours needed to achieve performance goals.
- The EMS system can be affected by a number of factors including geography, enabling legislation, elected officials, and consumer groups.
- Mutual aid is an important component of system designs and its reliance to ensure uninterrupted service varies often due to system type.
- Administrative oversight of EMS systems may be provided by a director and councils or committees and include regulatory, leadership, and facilitator roles.
- Medical oversight of EMS systems often has layers at the state, regional, and local levels and may be provided by a single physician working with a medical oversight committee or council.

REFERENCES

1. Asplin BR, Magid DJ, Rhodes KV, et al. A conceptual model of emergency department crowding. *Ann Emerg Med.* 2003;42:173-180.
2. Hoot NR, Aronsky, D. Systematic review of emergency department crowding: causes, effects, and solutions. *Ann Emerg Med.* 2008; 52:126-136.
3. Rawshani A, Larsson A, Gelang C, et al. Characteristics and outcome among patients who dial for the EMS due to chest pain. *Int J Cardiol.* October 20, 2014;176(3):859-865.
4. Painter I, Chavez DE, Ike BR, et al. Changes to DA-CPR instructions: can we reduce time to first compression and improve quality of bystander CPR? *Resuscitation.* September 2014;85(9):1169-1173.
5. Hardeland C, Olasveengen TM, Lawrence R, et al. Comparison of Medical Priority Dispatch (MPD) and Criteria Based Dispatch (CBD) relating to cardiac arrest calls. *Resuscitation.* May 2014;85(5): 612-616.
6. Fessler SJ, Simon HK, Yancey AH 2nd, Colman M, Hirsh DA. How well do General EMS 911 dispatch protocols predict ED resource utilization for pediatric patients? *Am J Emerg Med.* March 2014;32(3):199-202.
7. Moss C, Cowden CS, Atterton LM, et al. Accuracy of EMS trauma transport destination plans in North Carolina. *Prehosp Emerg Care.* 2015;19(1):53-60.
8. National Academy of Sciences (US) and National Research Council (US) Committee on Trauma, National Academy of Sciences (US) and National Research Council (US) Committee on Shock. *Accidental Death and Disability: The Neglected Disease of Modern Society.* Washington (DC): National Academies Press (US); 1966.
9. Public Health Law 93-154. EMS Systems Act of 1973. Washington, DC; 1973.

10. National Highway Traffic Safety Administration. *EMS Agenda for the Future*. Washington, DC; 1996.

11. Stout J. Measuring your system: Jack Stout's ten standards of excellence. *JEMS*. January 1983;2(1): 84-91.

12. Commission on Accreditation of Ambulance Services. CAAS Standards for the Accreditation of Ambulance Services, Version 3.0. Glenview, IL. 2009. www.caas.org.

13. Commission on Accreditation of Medical Transport Systems. Accreditation Standards of the Commission on Accreditation of Medical Transportation Systems, 8th Edition. Anderson, SC. 2010. http:/www.camts.org.

14. Joint Commission International. Joint Commission International Accreditation Standards for Medical Transport Organizations, 1st Edition. Oak Brook, IL. 2003. www.jointcommissioninternational. org/Medical-Transport/.

15. International Academy of Emergency Dispatch. Accreditation/ Re-Accreditation Application and Self-Assessment. Version 12.0. Salt Lake City, UT. 2010. www.emergencydispatch.org/Accreditation.

16. Center for Public Safety Excellence. Commission on Fire Accreditation International. Chantilly, VA. 2011. www.publicsafetyexcellence.org/ agency-accreditation/about-accreditation-cfai.aspx.

17. Personal Communication. National Emergency Number Association. July 12, 2011.

18. Carr BG, Matthew Edwards J, Martinez R. Academic emergency medicine consensus conference, beyond regionalization: integrated networks of care. Regionalized care for time-critical conditions: lessons learned from existing networks. *Acad Emerg Med*. December 2010;17(12):1354-1358.

19. American College of Emergency Physicians, National Association of State EMS Officers, National Association of EMS Physicians. Role of the state EMS medical director. February 2009. http:// www.naemsp.org/Documents/Position%20Papers/POSITION%20 RoleofStateMedDir-NASEMSO.pdf.

20. Alonso-Serra H, Blanton D, O'Connor RE. Physician medical direction in EMS. *Prehosp Emerg Care*. 1998;2(2):153-157. www.naemsp. org/pdf/physicianmedical.pdf.

CHAPTER 13

EMS Personnel

Christian C. Knutsen

INTRODUCTION

Individual states regulate the education, certification, and licensure of their EMS providers. Historically, the federal government has support EMS development at the state, regional, and local levels. The EMS Systems Act passed by Congress in 1973 created a categorical grant program to support developing state and regional EMS systems and led to the distribution of more than $300 million for EMS research, planning, operations, and improvement.[1] While the act identified 15 essential elements of EMS systems (communications, training, manpower, mutual aid, transportation, accessibility, facilities, critical care units, transfer of care, consumer participation, public education, public safety agencies, medical records, independent review and evaluation, and disaster linkage), it did not set national standards how these elements were to be enacted. In 1974, the Robert Wood Johnson Foundation contributed an additional $15 million to 44 regional EMS project, marking one of the largest private grants for EMS. Without a unified EMS model, states' EMS systems became significantly different from each other and customized to their needs.

OBJECTIVES

- Discuss common types of providers within EMS systems, including firefighters and first responders, EMTs, flight nurses, physician assistants, and physicians.

- Discuss national standard EMS provider certifications, as well as regional and state-specific designations (eg, EMT-D, EMT-I99, EMT-CC, licensed paramedic, critical care paramedic).

- Discuss types of other medical personnel involved in prehospital care and transport.

- Discuss state versus NREMT certification and reciprocity issues.

- Discuss some occupational health concerns for EMS providers.

The Omnibus Budget Reconciliation Act of 1981 folded federal EMS funding with preventative health block grants to states.[2] States determined how these grants were divided and distributed, leading to a significant reduction in total funding for EMS across the Unites States. Differences between licensure levels and scopes of practice persisted. In 1996, a minimum of 44 levels of EMS certifications existed across the United States.[3] In 2005, a survey of 30 states found 39 different licensure levels still existed.[4] Even with the same title, providers' scopes of practice varied between states. This disparity created four specific obstacles for EMS personnel:

1. Public confusion

2. Reciprocity challenges

3. Limited professional mobility

4. Decreased efficiency due to duplication of efforts

In 1996, the NHTSA and HRSA published a consensus document, the EMS Agenda for the Future, outlining a vision of EMS fully integrated with health care and supporting the health of their communities.[3] Designed to help all levels of government guide planning, decision making, and policy regarding EMS, the Agenda addressed 14 attributes requiring improvement including education.

Building on the Agenda, the EMS Education Agenda for the Future: A Systems Approach released in 2000 by the NHTSA proposed a nationally consistent system of education, certification, and licensure for all levels of EMS professionals.[5] The Educational Agenda outlined five primary

components: national EMS core content, national EMS scope of practice, national EMS educational standards, national EMS education program accreditation, and national EMS certification.

In 2004, the National EMS Core Content defined the domain of out-of-hospital care.[6] In 2005, the National Scope of Practice Model recommended dividing the core content into four levels of EMS providers: emergency medical responders (EMRs), emergency medical technicians (EMTs), advanced EMTs (AEMTs), and paramedics.[4] In addition, the Scope outlined the minimum education preparation and designated the appropriate psychomotor skills for each licensure level. While the Scope had no regulatory authority, it provided a framework that states could use to model their licensure levels and to facilitate a national consistency for EMS personnel between states. Adopting this national structure offered states' EMS systems and personnel several benefits:

1. National standards for the minimum psychomotor skills and knowledge of EMS personnel

2. Consistency among states' scopes of practice

3. Facilitation of reciprocity

4. Improved professional mobility

5. Consistency of EMS personnel titles

6. Better name recognition and public understanding of EMS personnel

Even if all states adopted the recommendations in the Scope, some variation in scopes of practice and skills for each licensure level would remain. States require the flexibility to expand or customize their EMS providers' scopes of practice to address unique local needs. While states may add to each licensure level, states are urged not to fall below its recommended scopes of practice.

Scope of practice is a legal description of the distinction between licensed health care personnel and the lay public and between different licensed health care professionals. Scopes of practice, defined by individual states, establish the activities and procedures that are illegal if performed without a license and what level of licensure is required to perform them. A standard of care is not the same as scope of practice. A standard of care is defined by what should be done in a given situation. Scope of practice defines what activities and procedures a licensed provider may do.

PREHOSPITAL PERSONNEL

There are a number of different types of prehospital personnel operating in the field. These include firefighters (with first aid, CPR, and AED skills), certified first responders, EMT (basic), advanced EMTs, paramedics, critical care/flight paramedics, nurses, and physicians. There are still a number of locations that have other types of providers that fit somewhere in-between the various EMT types (eg, EMT-CC, EMT-I99). National standards exist that are now widely recognized and are discussed below. Almost every state provides providers with a document that allows EMS providers (nonnurse, nonphysician) to perform their skills. Many states refer to this as EMS provider certification. However, certification should only refer to a certificate stating completion of a course or qualification in a certain set of skills. When a state provides a document that allows an individual to do something that would otherwise be illegal, that state has provided that individual with a license. Therefore, the distinction between certification and licensure needs to be recognized by the medical director of any EMS agency or system.

Each state has its own requirements for obtaining and maintaining licensure. In the case of "certified providers," states may consider allowing for reciprocity from another state, or from the National Registry of EMTs. This acknowledgment of like qualifications is strictly a matter of the states and their regulatory structure for EMS. At the time of this writing, the National Registry certification is accepted as proof of initial qualifications and/or continued certification in 46 states in the United States (nonregistry states include Illinois, New York, North Carolina, and Wyoming) (**Figure 13-1**).

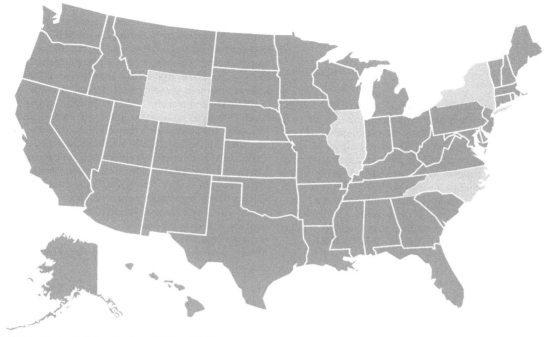

Green = recognizes National Registry of EMTs certification

FIGURE 13-1. National registry states. Highlighted states recognize National Registry of EMTs certification.

OTHER PERSONNEL IN THE PREHOSPITAL CARE SYSTEM

Nurse practitioners, physician assistants, respiratory therapists, nurses, and physicians who are not EMS trained may also be found working in the prehospital environment, as part of either a disaster relief effort or an interfacility transport effort.[7,8] Those who serve on a specialty transport service team are typically trained and supported in their specific role on the team. There is no universal standard or training curriculum that covers these providers specifically. Each program and/or system typically provides this training.

NATIONAL STANDARDS FOR EMS PROVIDERS

A significant amount of effort is needed for every licensure level to develop national educational, accreditation, and certification standards and material and the means of maintaining competency. Therefore, only a limited number of licensure levels are reasonable. In *the Scope*, licensure levels are substantially different from other levels based on skills, practice environment, knowledge, qualifications, services provided, risk, levels of supervisory responsibility, amount of autonomy, and critical thinking and decision-making requirements. Below are the descriptions, scopes of practice, and psychomotor skills for each licensure level outline in *the Scope*.[4]

EMERGENCY MEDICAL RESPONDER

EMRs focus is on immediate lifesaving care to critical patients. They possess the basic knowledge and skills necessary to provide lifesaving interventions while awaiting additional EMS support and to assist higher level personnel at the scene and during transport. EMRs perform basic interventions with minimal equipment.

Scope of Practice In many communities, EMRs provide a mechanism to increase the likelihood that trained personnel and lifesaving equipment can be rapidly delivered to serious emergencies. Their goal is to minimize the morbidity and mortality associated with acute out-of-hospital medical and traumatic emergencies. Additionally, the EMR

provides care designed to minimize secondary injury and to comfort the patient and family while awaiting additional EMS resources.

EMRs are the first part of a tiered response system. EMRs work alongside other EMS and health care professionals as an integral part of the emergency care team. A major difference between the lay person and the EMR is the "duty to act" as part of an organized EMS response. After initiating care, the EMR transfers care to higher level personnel. The EMR serves as part of an EMS response system that ensures a progressive increase in the level of assessment and care.

EMRs may serve as a part of the crew on a transporting EMS unit. However, the EMR cannot be the highest level caregiver and must function with higher level personnel during transportation of emergency patients.

Psychomotor Skills The following are the minimum psychomotor skills of the EMR:

- Airway and breathing
- Insertion of airway adjuncts intended to go into the oropharynx
  - Use of positive pressure ventilation devices such as the bag-valve mask.
  - Suction of the upper airway.
- Supplemental oxygen therapy
  - Pharmacological interventions.
  - Use of unit dose autoinjectors for the administration of lifesaving medications.
  - Intended for self- or peer rescue in hazardous materials situations (MARK I, etc).
  - Medical/cardiac care.
  - Use of an automated external defibrillator.
  - Trauma care.
  - Manual stabilization of suspected cervical spine injuries.
  - Manual stabilization of extremity fractures.
  - Bleeding control.
  - Emergency moves.

EMERGENCY MEDICAL TECHNICIAN

EMTs provide basic emergency medical care and transportation for critical and emergent medical and trauma patients. This individual possesses the basic knowledge and skills necessary to provide patient care and transportation. EMTs perform interventions with the basic equipment typically found on an ambulance.

Scope of Practice The EMT's scope of practice includes basic skills focused on the acute management and transportation of critical and emergent patients including basic, noninvasive interventions to reduce the morbidity and mortality associated with acute out-of-hospital medical and traumatic emergencies. Additionally, EMTs provide care to minimize secondary injury and provide comfort to the patient and family while transporting the patient to an emergency care facility. Their work may occur at an emergency scene until transportation resources arrive, from an emergency scene to a health care facility, between health care facilities, or in other health care settings. In many communities and especially in rural areas, EMTs provide a large portion of the out-of-hospital care.

An EMT's knowledge, skills, and abilities are acquired through formal education and training. The EMT has the knowledge of, and is expected to be competent in, all of the skills of the EMR. A major difference between the EMR and the EMT is the knowledge and skills necessary to provide medical transportation of emergency patients.

The EMT level is the minimum licensure level for personnel transporting patients in ambulances. The EMT transports all emergency patients to an appropriate medical facility. The EMT is not prepared to make decisions independently regarding the appropriate disposition of patients and must consult with medical oversight for destination selection. The principal disposition of the patient encounter will result in the direct delivery of the patient to an acute care facility. In addition to emergency response, EMTs can perform medical transport services of patients requiring care within their scope of practice.

Psychomotor Skills The following are the minimum psychomotor skills of the EMT:

- Airway and breathing
  - Insertion of airway adjuncts intended to go into the oropharynx or nasopharynx.
  - Use of positive pressure ventilation devices such as manually triggered ventilators and automatic transport ventilators.
- Pharmacological interventions
  - Assist patients in taking their own prescribed medications.
  - Administration of the following over-the-counter medications with appropriate medical oversight:
    - Oral glucose for suspected hypoglycemia
    - Aspirin for chest pain of suspected ischemic origin
- Trauma care

ADVANCED EMERGENCY MEDICAL TECHNICIAN

The AEMT provides basic and limited advanced emergency medical care and transportation for critical and emergent patients. AEMTs possess the basic knowledge and skills necessary to provide patient care and transportation. AEMTs perform interventions with the basic and advanced equipment typically found on an ambulance. The AEMT is a link from the scene to the emergency health care system.

Scope of Practice The AEMT's scope of practice builds on the EMT's scope of practice by including basic, limited advanced airway and pharmacological interventions to reduce the morbidity and mortality associated with acute out-of-hospital medical and traumatic emergencies.

The AEMT's knowledge, skills, and abilities are acquired through formal education and training. The AEMT has the knowledge associated with, and is expected to be competent in, all of the skills of the EMR and

EMT. The major difference between the AEMT and the EMT is the ability to perform limited advanced skills and provide pharmacological interventions to emergency patients. The AEMT is the minimum licensure level for patients requiring limited advanced care at the scene or during transportation. The scope of practice model is limited to lower risk, high-benefit advanced skills that are effective and can be performed safely in an out-of-hospital setting with medical oversight and limited training.

For many communities, AEMTs provide an option to provide high-benefit, lower risk advanced skills for systems that cannot support or justify paramedic level care. This is frequently the case in rural and volunteer systems. In some regions, AEMTs are the highest level of out-of-hospital care.

The AEMT transports all emergency patients to an appropriate medical facility. The AEMT transports all emergency patients to an appropriate medical facility. The AEMT is not prepared to make decisions independently regarding the appropriate disposition of patients and must consult with medical oversight for destination selection. The principal disposition of the patient encounter will result in the direct delivery of the patient to an acute care facility. In addition to emergency response, AEMTs often perform medical transport services of patients requiring care within their scope of practice.

Psychomotor Skills The following are the minimum psychomotor skills of the AEMT:

- Airway and breathing
  - Insertion of airways that are *not* intended to be placed into the trachea.
  - Tracheobronchial suctioning of an already intubated patient.
- Pharmacological interventions
  - Establish and maintain peripheral intravenous access.
  - Establish and maintain intraosseous access in a pediatric patient.
  - Administer (nonmedicated) intravenous fluid therapy.
  - Administer sublingual nitroglycerine to a patient experiencing chest pain of suspected ischemic origin.
  - Administer subcutaneous or intramuscular epinephrine to a patient in anaphylaxis.
  - Administer glucagon to a hypoglycemic patient.
  - Administer intravenous D50 to a hypoglycemic patient.
  - Administer inhaled β-agonists to a patient experiencing difficulty breathing and wheezing.
  - Administer a narcotic antagonist to a patient suspected of narcotic overdose.
  - Administer nitrous oxide for pain relief.

PARAMEDIC

The paramedic's primary focus is the advanced emergency medical care for critical and emergent patients. This individual possesses the complex knowledge and skills necessary to provide patient care and transportation. Paramedics perform interventions with the basic and advanced equipment typically found on an ambulance.

Scope of Practice The paramedic's scope of practice includes basic and advanced skills focused on the acute management and transportation of the broad range of patients who access the emergency medical system. As part of a tiered EMS response system, paramedics represent the highest level of out-of-hospital care. Their scope of practice includes invasive and pharmacological interventions to reduce the morbidity and mortality associated with acute out-of-hospital medical and traumatic emergencies. Emergency care is based on an advanced assessment and the formulation of a field impression.

The paramedic has knowledge, skills, and abilities developed by appropriate formal education and training. The paramedic has the knowledge associated with, and is expected to be competent in, all of the skills of the EMR, EMT, and AEMT. The major difference between the paramedic and the AEMT is the ability to perform a broader range of advanced skills. These skills carry a greater risk for the patient if improperly or inappropriately performed, are more difficult to attain and maintain competency in, and require significant background knowledge in basic and applied sciences.

The paramedic transports all emergency patients to an appropriate medical facility. The paramedic may make destination decisions in collaboration with medical oversight. The principal disposition of the patient encounter will result in the direct delivery of the patient to an acute care facility. In addition to emergency response, paramedics often perform medical transport services of patients requiring care within their scope of practice.

Psychomotor Skills The following are the minimum psychomotor skills of the paramedic:

- Airway and breathing
  - Perform endotracheal intubation.
  - Perform percutaneous cricothyrotomy1.
  - Decompress the pleural space.
  - Perform gastric decompression.
- Pharmacological interventions
  - Insert an intraosseous cannula.
  - Enteral and parenteral administration of approved prescription medications.
  - Access indwelling catheters and implanted central IV ports for fluid and medication administration.
  - Administer medications by IV infusion.
  - Maintain an infusion of blood or blood products.
- One percutaneous means access via needle puncture (or other approved puncture device) and DOES
- *Not* include "surgical" access using a scalpel
- Medical/cardiac care
  - Perform cardioversion, manual defibrillation, and transcutaneous pacing.

OCCUPATIONAL HEALTH CONCERNS

A variety of health and safety concerns are present in the prehospital environment.[9] Due to the fact that the Bureau of Labor Statistics does not define EMS providers as a specific industry or occupational code it is difficult to know the true and accurate scope of provider injury and death.[10] Based on available data in the publication by Maguire et al, there were a total of 114 fatalities from 1992 to 1997. These included those associated with ground transportation, air ambulance crash, cardiovascular, assault homicide, and other (**Table 13-1**).[10] Although some

standards exist designed to protect providers from a general workplace standpoint and from the National Association of Pire Protection (NFPA), there is still a lack of consistent application of policies and standards aimed at protecting EMS providers from death and injury. Some medical directors have sought to apply NAFPA 1582 (*Standard on Comprehensive Occupational Medical Program for Fire Departments*), 1583 (*Standard on Health-Related Fitness Programs for Fire Department Members*), and 1584 (*Standard on the Rehabilitation Process for Members During Emergency Operations and Training Exercises*), universally for the protection of their system's providers. This is a significant challenge and further work in this area is being done. Future guidelines and application strategies will likely lead to greater recognition of this important threat to the future of EMS.

- Each state determines the levels and qualifications of prehospital providers within their jurisdiction and provides them licensure.
- The National Highway Traffic Safety Administration's National Scope of Practice Model lays out a potential national standard for all systems to potentially adopt.
- The National Registry of Emergency Medical Technicians, now recognized in 46 states, provided a basis for national certification and the potential for a nationalized reciprocity between states.
- Prehospital provider health and safety is a growing concern requiring significant attention from EMS system and agency medical directors.

REFERENCES

1. Emergency Medical Services Systems Act of 1973. Public Law 93-154, Title XII of the Public Health Services Act. Washington, DC; 1973.
2. The Omnibus Budget Reconciliation Act of 1981. Public Law 97-3982. Washington, DC; 1981.
3. National Highway Traffic Safety Administration. *EMS Agenda for the Future*. Washington, DC: US Department of Transportation; 1996.
4. National Highway Traffic Safety Administration. *National EMS Scope of Practice Model*. Washington, DC: US Department of Transportation; 2005.
5. National Highway Traffic Safety Administration. *EMS Education Agenda for the Future: A Systems Approach*. Washington, DC: US Department of Transportation; 2000.
6. National Highway Traffic Safety Administration. *National EMS Core Content. #DOT HS 809 989*. Washington, DC: US Department of Transportation; 2005.
7. Davis C. 'Care in the air': the role of in-flight staff. *Emerg Nurse*. March 2012;19(10):12-15.
8. Wisborg T, Bjerkan B. Air ambulance nurses as expert supplement to local emergency services. *Air Med J*. January-February 2014;33(1):40-43.
9. Bigham BL, Jensen JL, Tavares W, et al. Paramedic self-reported exposure to violence in the emergency medical services (EMS) workplace: a mixed-methods cross-sectional survey. *Prehosp Emerg Care*. October-December 2014;18(4):489-494.
10. Maguire BJ, Hunting KL, Smith GS, Levick NR. Occupational fatalities in emergency medical services: a hidden crisis. *Ann Emerg Med*. December 2002;40(6):625-632.

TABLE 13-1 EMS Provider Fatalities (1992-1997)

Cause	Total[a]	Percentage
Ground transport	67	58.8%
Air ambulance crash	19	16.7%
Cardiovascular	13	11.4%
Assault homicide	10	8.8%
Other	5	4.4%

[a]Estimates based on data from Maguire BJ, Hunting KL, Smith GS, Levick NR. Occupational fatalities in emergency medical services: a hidden crisis. *Ann Emerg Med*. December 2002;40(6):625-632.

David P. Thomson

INTRODUCTION

The goal of any medical service is to provide the patient with the right resources at the right time. For many in our society any wait for anything is too long, hence the concept of a "Starbucks on every corner."[1] Although it is arguable that there is a greater need for emergency medical services (EMS) than for coffee, very few EMS agencies could afford to place an ambulance on every corner. Because of this EMS have used various deployment strategies to meet their patient care goals.

Deployment, according to one definition from the Free Dictionary, means, "To distribute (persons or forces) systematically or strategically."[2] Historically, ambulances were dispatched from fixed bases, most commonly from fire stations or funeral homes, depending on the local model. These stations were usually cited based on political subdivisions that have little or nothing to do with the needs of the community. In many areas, this practice continues today. In rural areas, and areas served by volunteer agencies, basing the ambulance at a station is the only system that makes sense. In urban areas, however, it is better to site equipment based on patient demand, rather than provider convenience. In these areas, as Overton and Gunderson have noted, the pattern of EMS usage resembles that of a police, rather than a fire department.[3] Because of this, many high-volume urban organizations have adopted plans where ambulances are dispersed to predetermined "posts" around the service area. These posts may be a specific corner or perhaps a mall parking lot; in some cases the ambulance crew is given a general geographic area in which they are to be located. EMS agencies using this model of dynamic deployment are often described as "high performance" although this term may be a misnomer.

OBJECTIVES

- Define deployment and posting.
- Describe the phases of ambulance response.
- Describe how red-lights-and-siren responses affect the ambulance response.
- Define system status management.
- Describe the basic research concepts behind SSM.
- Describe how technologies have changed SSM.

AMBULANCE RESPONSE

EMS systems have historically been designed to address two major problems: cardiac arrest and motor vehicle trauma. Spaite et al note that cardiac arrest accounts for a very small number of ambulance responses, and that there is no good data on the effects of EMS system components on trauma. He contends, "...Most prehospital trauma research has emphasized the wrong issues, asked the wrong questions, and used the wrong methods."[4] An attempt to rectify the lack of information on trauma patients demonstrated that there was no evidence supporting time sensitivity for trauma mortality.[5] The problem, according to Spaite and his colleagues, is that EMS research has historically emphasized individual diseases and interventions, rather than system issues.

Many EMS agencies have a response standard written into their contract. Commonly such a clause says that the service must respond to a call within a specified number of minutes. Frequently the clause says that such a response is expected 90% to 95% of the time. There may be monetary penalties associated with failure to meet these expectations.

Eight minutes, 90% of the time, is frequently used as a standard. These standards are usually based on data for cardiac arrest survival.[6] Other services may have expectations that there will be a BLS response within 4 minutes and an ALS response within 8 minutes, 90% of the time. These standards are based on the National Fire Protection Association's (NFPA) 2010 response standards (NFPA 1710).[7] These specify that the service shall provide an AED response within 240 seconds of travel, following 60 seconds of "turnout" time. Aside from Spaite's contention that the basis for this standard is a very small part of the EMS realm,[4] it also may not take into account all of the pieces that need to fall into place to access the patient, care for the patient, and transfer them to the hospital. A recent publication by the United Kingdom's National Audit Office reflects this concern, stating, "Performance over the last decade has been driven by response time targets and not outcomes.... Its existence in isolation from more direct measures of patient outcomes has, however, created a narrow view of what constitutes 'good' performance, and skewed the ambulance services' approach to performance measurement and management."[8]

The University of Arizona group tried to bring some of this science into the medical realm in a 1993 article in which they defined and validated a model for the time intervals in an EMS response.[9] This article defined 10 intervals between the event and the return to service. This granularity allows EMS to more appropriately address the problems that may occur as EMS agencies try to provide care to patients in a timely fashion. For example, many providers report that they are "on scene" when they park their vehicle at the patient's residence. This would be a useful basis for comparison if everyone were in a single floor, single family dwelling, and there was a standard way to label dwellings. Unfortunately, most areas have a mix of single family and multiple family dwellings. The time to access a patient in a single-family ranch is very different than the time to locate a patient in a 20-story urban high rise. Understanding the difference between the response interval and the patient access interval is important for EMS managers looking to improve their systems. It is also important to clinicians and politicians who may be trying to explain why their survival statistics are not as good as other agencies' numbers.

Most systems do not use this level of detail. Instead they employ several strategies to minimize the response and transport intervals, paying little attention to the other eight intervals. The most common method to minimize the response and transport intervals is through the use of fast driving, facilitated by the use of red lights and a siren. Although this is how the public sees EMS,[10,11] it is unclear whether such use produces significant time savings. Ho and his group noted the use of red lights and sirens in both urban[12] and rural[13] environments saved time. A group from East Carolina University attempted to match the route taken by an ambulance and found very little difference between emergency response and routine traffic.[14] O'Brien et al in Louisville employed a similar technique. They found that there was a time saving associated with the use of red lights and siren (RLS), but that the time savings did not translate into any clinically important interventions upon arrival at the hospital.[15] Others have reported a similar experience.[16] A UK study suggests that EMS providers feel that the current performance standards place them at jeopardy.[17] Blackwell and Kaufman noted that in his system in Mecklenburg County, North Carolina, unless patients could be reached within 5 minutes there was no evidence that there would be a survival improvement.[11] A study of the use of RLS in pediatric patients showed that over 1/3 of the pediatric patients were unnecessarily subjected to an emergency response.[18] In addition to the questionable efficacy from the use of RLS transport, there are concerns that care of the patient within the vehicle may suffer. Although ambulances are being designed to keep the caregiver restrained while performing patient care, it is still difficult to perform even basic procedures with the rapid stops and quick starts that often accompany RLS transports. The risk involved with these emergency responses is substantial. A group from Milwaukee found that over an 11-year period most of the crashes and fatalities in ambulances occurred during an emergency response.[19] "Wake effect" crashes, which occur due to the distraction produced by the emergency vehicle's passage, further compound the problems caused by this response.[20] Current and future work on reduction of response times will likely focus on prediction algorithms and the concepts of dynamic posting and system status management.[21,22]

SYSTEM STATUS MANAGEMENT

The concept of the high-performance EMS system using system status management (SSM) is commonly attributed to Jack Stout, an economist. He looked at the EMS system using tools usually applied to industry and developed these concepts along with the public utility model for EMS.[23] Stout reveals his background when he says that the purpose of SSM is to match supply and demand.[24] He notes that SSM does not require that ambulances be moved around, describing roving ambulances as "a waste [of] human energy, fuel, and money." The primary difference between the systems that Stout describes and the historical fixed base model is that Stout advocates placing bases or posts based on patient need, not political subdivisions. This typically involves basing positioning of ambulances and staffing on historical geographical call data with variance in time, day of the week, and seasons. This strategy may also take into consideration types of calls, key locations, highway access, traffic patterns, and weather issues.

Bledsoe has criticized SSM, saying, "I was surprised that there was no scientific evidence to support the practice," and claiming that it "increases work stress" and "causes an increase in vehicle maintenance and miles traveled."[25] As his references Dr Bledsoe refers to a single study of one EMS system, and concludes by saying that, "I can't document the following statement with science just with experience and emotion. I believe that employee satisfaction, morale and pay are generally lower in systems that use SSM, while employee turnover, stress and physical ailments are higher." Fortunately, there is a solid basis for SSM.

Most of the information regarding SSM is derived from the operations management literature. The classic use of SSM has been in the area of industrial transportation and in manufacturing plant design. ReVelle and his colleagues explained this problem as having the, "objective of maximizing some measure of utility to the owners while at the same time satisfying constraints on demands and other conditions."[26] Clearly this fits the description of an EMS system as well as it fits a manufacturing operation.

One of the things that makes EMS deployment complex is the nature of the service. EMS can, however, be looked at in a manner similar to other service industries. The consumer can control the demand for some goods. The provider may schedule other services. **Table 14-1** provides examples of this.

The basic problem for EMS is therefore the unpredictability of customer demand. Other issues, such as traffic and weather, as well as the variable nature and severity of the patient's complaint further complicate this model. Although the geographic distribution of calls and their nature seem completely random, there are ways to predict these incidents and use this information to appropriately distribute EMS resources (**Figure 14-1**).

This literature is vastly different from the usual EMS literature. These articles range from very descriptive papers to some which require an understanding of high-level mathematics. Goldberg has made an attempt to bring some of this literature into the realm of EMS.[27]

An early attempt to address the problems of emergency services was made by Toregas and his colleagues in 1971.[28] Their work mathematically modeled a system that minimized the travel time from a fixed base to the site of need. This model emphasized the ability for a vehicle to cover a set of geographic points. To some extent their model was limited by the computing power available to them. Additionally, they focused on fire services, as EMS was then in its infancy. These models are known as static models because the model assumes a fixed site for both the responder and the patient. Later models, taking advantage of the increase in computing power, incorporated more stochastic[29] systems.[30]

Marianov and ReVelle, two pioneers in this field, took advantage of this increase in power with their development of the "maximal availability location problem."[31] This model built on the Toregas model, designed to find the least number of ambulances to cover an area, and some other work by ReVelle, which incorporated time and distance standards. The problem, as Marianov points out, is that these models did not take into account "congestion," or the possibility that an ambulance in a given node would already be busy when the next call came in. In order to account for congestion, they employ queuing theory, which allows them to better model how coverage might be provided by ambulances located in adjacent cells. This is more typical of a real-world mutual aid system.

Queuing theory is an important concept in our society, because it not only explains how an EMS system might function, but it also explains how networks, be they road or communications networks, behave. The basic concept for queuing theory is known as Little theorem, which is written: $N = \lambda T$, where N is the number of customers served, lambda (λ) is the average customer arrival rate, and T is the average time required to serve the customer.[32] A recent article about ED observation units has a nice explanation of this law.[33] Those readers who wish a more detailed, mathematical description of this phenomenon are referred to Bassamboo and Randhawa's description of fluid models of queuing theory.[34]

An example of how this type of work might apply to a real-world EMS system is a paper by Rajagopalan and his colleagues.[35] They created a mathematical model of an EMS coverage system, and then used a reactive tabu search algorithm, which they wrote in Java on a desktop personal computer. They applied this to a hypothetical city to test the capabilities of the algorithm. Once they found it worked they applied it to Mecklenburg County, North Carolina, an EMS system with accurate up-to-date call data. Their system broke the county down into 2 × 2 mile blocks and into time intervals of 3 hours each. They ran a simulation using their data and compared it to actual run data. Their model was able to provide coverage for the calls, but was able to do it with fewer vehicles. The authors suggest that using models like this would allow EMS to modify their shift and coverage to improve their efficiency or to provide additional rigs for nonemergency transports.

Another model that has been applied to a real EMS system is the hypercube model.[36] The hypercube model assumes that each node will have independent demand characteristics. This is another step closer to the real world, where each call, and its location, is completely independent of any other call. This group then applied their model to the Edmonton, Alberta, EMS system, and they were able to use it to predict improved coverage patterns.

A group from Cornell University has taken a different approach to the Edmonton data, using the Erlang loss function,[37] a concept developed for the communications industry. They assumed a fixed base (static) system, but their model takes into account the sharing of resources between bases. Their model provides another tool for EMS managers to use when

TABLE 14-1	Demand and Capacity Management		
		Can the service preschedule individual customers?	
		Yes	No
Can customers control the timing of their demand?	Yes	Airlines	Utilities
		Hotels	Package/postal services
		Transportation	Travel agencies
		Professional services	Retailing
		School classes	Public transportation
		Sporting events	Restaurants
	No	Court appearances	*Emergency services*
			Walk-in clinics
			Insurance claims
			Funeral homes

Adapted from Klassen KJ, Rohleder TR. Demand and capacity management decisions in services: how they impact on one another. *Int J Oper Prod Man.* 2002;26(5/6):527-548.

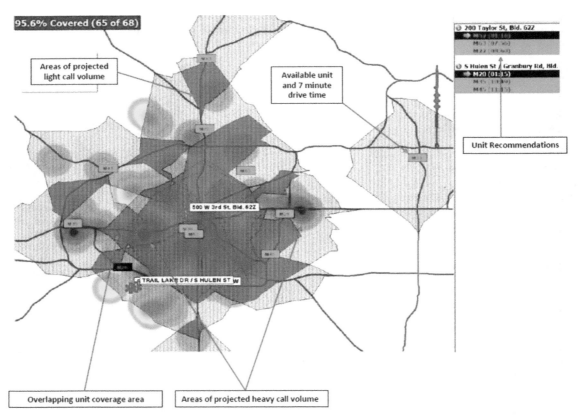

FIGURE 14-1. Digital call map. (From MedStar9-1-1 Web site. http://www.medstar911.org/Websites/medstar911/Blog/666201/New%20Deployment%20Monitor.pdf. Accessed October 1, 2013. Reproduced with permission.)

deciding on how to distribute fixed base ambulances around a city. However, they do note that when there is a multiple casualty incident, this model may not work.[38]

It is important to also consider that there may be political as well as operational considerations in the basing or posting of ambulances. The authors of one study of EMS service distribution considered this a matter of equity between high- and low-use areas in a city, and so constructed their model to account for this.[39] They applied their analysis to the Huntsville, Alabama, system, suggesting deployment schemes that would decrease response times. They also point out that their model would allow a system to alter its basing depending on the historical clinical experience. That is, based on history, ambulances might be better deployed to areas with a higher likelihood of cardiac arrest than leg fractures, the former being more time sensitive than the latter.

Models have been used to assess the EMS in other locations, including Riyadh, Saudi Arabia,[40] East Aurora, New York,[41] and Greenville, South Carolina.[42] This literature is extensive, and much of it is outside the usual EMS journals. Medical directors who wish to explore this science may wish to contact the operations management faculty of their local business school.

NEW TECHNOLOGIES AND SSM

DISPATCHING PRIORITIES

Even the best systems take a few minutes to arrive at the patient's side. Often there are several simultaneous requests for service, so triage is as important for EMS as it is for an emergency department. The purpose of EMS dispatch, in the words of Dr Jeff Clawson, is, "... sending the right resources to the right person, at the right time, in the right way, and doing the right things until help arrives."[43] This is accomplished

through the use of a trained emergency medical dispatcher (EMD) and a system of questions and instructions the EMD uses to elicit information from, and provide instruction to, the caller. Through a series of scripted questions the dispatcher ascertains the nature of the call and, if necessary, provides the caller with information on how to provide care to the patient. At the same time the dispatcher determines the medical resources that are needed for the call, and sends them to the patient. These scripts, and the decisions they prompt, are usually contained on a series of cards or a sequence of computer screens. The dispatcher determines whether the problem requires an immediate response or can be placed in a queue awaiting an available vehicle. In systems using both BLS and ALS responses, the dispatcher may determine the level of response through these questions.

At one time dispatching was provided by whoever picked up the telephone at a station. Clawson says that in Salt Lake City in the 1970s, dispatchers had less than 1 hour of medical training. Today organizations such as the National Academies of Emergency Dispatch (www.naemd.org) provide certification for dispatchers and accreditation of dispatch centers.

Several studies have looked at the use of trained dispatchers and their effects on the EMS response. An Oregon study from the late 1990s indicated that dispatchers in the Portland, Oregon, area were unable to identify patients who had what they described as, "important clinical field findings."[44] The communications center in this study used a locally created dispatching algorithm. Bailey, O'Connor, and Ross, from Delaware, were able to demonstrate that the use of Medical Priority Dispatch System (MPDS) (www.naemd.org) resulted in a decrease in the overutilization of ALS resources in their system.[45] A University of Rochester group found that they were able to reliably identify low-acuity patients using MPDS.[46] These findings were later validated by a study in the Wake County, North Carolina, EMS system.[47]

Computer-Aided Dispatch Historically, calls have been allocated to the appropriate vehicle based on districts. The call was simply given to the vehicle in the caller's district. If that vehicle was unavailable, dispatchers would consult a grid to see who was assigned to provide a backup, and they would send that vehicle. Such a search function is a natural fit for computerization. In a system with mobile posts, it is an absolute necessity. In addition to determining the nearest appropriate vehicle for the call, computer-aided dispatch (CAD) systems provide services with better information about the location and nature of calls. These data can then be used to improve the posting strategy. In a busy center, calls could potentially be lost or dropped, and the use of computers helps dispatchers remain aware of the callers who are waiting. When combined with caller identification technology, the CAD can help dispatchers reconnect with those callers who have been waiting for a response.[48]

Although the concept of having a computer assist the dispatcher in finding the nearest appropriate vehicle sounds like a simple concept, the programming involved has the potential to become very complex, as the system must account for various types of calls, varieties of road conditions, and differing vehicle availabilities. Designing a program unique to each area could be prohibitively expensive, especially when the system has to be extremely reliable. Fortunately there are some generic programs that allow the local conditions to be overlaid in a simple and inexpensive fashion.[49]

In addition to just assisting the dispatcher in locating a call and creating a queue of calls, CAD systems have a number of functions:

- Incident information
- E9-1-1 Interface
- Location verification
- Information files
- Incident display
- Unit display
- Incident dispatch
- Timestamping
- Special features
- Report generation
- External links
- Mapping
- Maintenance
- Security[50]

GPS Systems The development of GPS technology has affected dispatching systems in multiple ways. Original 9-1-1 systems required the caller to be able to tell the dispatcher their location. Later systems were able to identify the caller's telephone number with a function known as *automatic number identification* (ANI). This is more familiar to the public as caller ID. Advances in software allowed the number to be linked to a specific address, providing *automatic location identification* (ALI). While this worked fine for wired telephones, the explosion of mobile telephones initially presented a problem, since there was no easy way to determine the caller's location. The refinement of GPS technology has allowed *public safety answering points* (PSAPS) the ability to acquire ANI and ALI information from these devices (more properly named since most provide more than a telephone capability).

GPS is also being used to determine vehicle location. Prior to the development of these systems knowing a vehicle's location often required frequent calls from the dispatcher. If a vehicle was traveling to or from a post the dispatcher might not know their exact location, resulting in delays as other vehicles responded. Or, if a general broadcast was made for "units in the vicinity of…" there might be too many ambulances coming to a single call. With GPS technology dispatchers know the exact location of an ambulance, allowing them to dispatch the closest appropriate vehicle.

SUMMARY

The placement of EMS vehicles plays a significant role in the ability of systems to respond to calls. Whether the system employs fixed bases or uses a high-performance SSM posting algorithm, it is important for EMS physicians to understand the limitations of their system. Although much of the science for these systems is outside what many might consider medical literature, there is nevertheless a scientific basis for how they work.

Fast driving is no substitute for proper deployment. EMS physicians must use their influence to make their EMS and public safety colleagues understand the risks (great) and benefits (few, if any) of responding with red lights and sirens. The public also has an expectation, so it is important that the public understand the limitations of this intervention, just as physicians often have to explain the limitations of CT and MRI scans.

EMS physicians who wish to further understand how these deployment systems work may find that there are professors in their local business schools who are interested in this particular part of what is generically called "operations management." In addition to the references cited in the bibliography, there are several important resources that EMS physicians may use.

- *Principles of Emergency Medical Dispatch*, by Clawson et al is currently in its 4th edition.[51] This is the textbook commonly used by personnel studying for their Emergency Medical Dispatcher certification.
- "Operations Research Models for the Deployment of Emergency Services Vehicles," by Goldberg.[28] This article attempts to bridge the gap between the science of operations management and the world of EMS management.
- For an overview of operations management topics, including location analysis as well as other topics that may be of use to EMS physicians, such as Six Sigma and schedule management, readers may find Meredith and Shafer's *Operations Management for MBAs*, 3rd edition useful.[52]

- EMS response intervals need to be analyzed individually in order to improve response times.
- EMS systems may use fixed bases or mobile posts; the proper configuration depends on the local conditions.
- System status management is a well-researched way to properly deploy emergency response assets.
- The use of red-lights-and-siren responses or fast driving is no substitute for appropriate deployment strategies.
- Priority dispatching systems can improve EMS deployment by making sure the correct resources are sent to the call.

REFERENCES

1. Associated Press. A Starbucks on every corner? October 25, 2006. MSN Money. http://articles.moneycentral.msn.com/News/AStarbucksOnEveryCorner.aspx. Accessed June 12, 2011.
2. Farlex. Deployment. The Free Dictionary. 2009. http://www.thefreedictionary.com/deployment. Accessed June 12, 2011.
3. Overton J, Gunderson M. System design. In: Delbridge TR, Cone DC, O'Connor RE, Fowler RL, eds. *Emergency Medical Services: Clinical Practice and System Oversight*. Vol 2. Dubuque, IA: Kendall-Hunt Professional; 2009.

4. Spaite DW, Criss EA, Valenzuela TD, Guisto J. Emergency medical service systems research: problems of the past, challenges of the future. *Ann Emerg Med*. 1995;26(2):146-152.

5. Newgard CD, Schmicker RH, Hedges JR, et al. Emergency medical services intervals and survival in trauma: assessment of the "Golden Hour" in a North American prospective cohort. *Ann Emerg Med*. 2010;55(3):235-246.

6. Ludwig GG. EMS response time standards. . EMS World. April 1, 2004. http://www.emsworld.com/article/article.jsp?id=2255. Accessed July 16, 2011.

7. National Fire Protection Association. NFPA® 1710. Standard for the Organization and Deployment of Fire Suppression Operations, Emergency Medical Operations, and Special Operations to the Public by Career Fire Departments. International Association of Fire Fighters. 2009. www.iaff.org/et/pdf/NFPA_1710_10.pdf. Accessed July 16, 2011.

8. Hughes G. Transforming NHS ambulance services. *Emerg Med J. 2011*, Sep; 28(9): 734.

9. Spaite DW, Valenzuela TD, Meislin HW, Criss EA, Hinsberg P. Prospective validation of a new model for evaluating emergency medical services systems by in-field observation of specific time intervals in prehospital care. *Ann Emerg Med*. 1993;22(4):638-645.

10. Harvey AL, Gerard WC, Rice GF, Finch H. Actual vs. perceived EMS response time. *Prehosp Emerg Care*. 1999;3(1):11-14.

11. Blackwell TH, Kaufman JS. Response time effectiveness: comparison of response time and survival in an urban emergency medical services system. *Acad Emerg Med*. 2002;9:288-295.

12. Ho J, Casey B. Time saved with the use of emergency warning lights and sirens during response to requests for emergency medical aid in an urban environment. *Ann Emerg Med*. 1998;32(5):585-588.

13. Ho J, Lindquist M. Time saved with the use of emergency warning lights and siren while responding to requests for emergency medical aid in a rural environment. *Prehosp Emerg Care*. 2001; 5(2):159-162.

14. Hunt RC, Brown LH, Cabinum ES, et al. Is ambulance transport time with lights and siren faster than without? *Ann Emerg Med*. 1995;25(4):507-511.

15. O'Brien DJ, Price TG, Adams P. Effectiveness of lights and siren use during ambulance transport by paramedics. *Prehosp Emerg Care*. 1999;3(2):127-130.

16. Wydro GC, Kruus LK, Yeh EC, Hatala KM. Utilization of emergency lights and sirens by urban paramedics: analysis of indications for their use. *Ann Emerg Med*. 2007;50(3):S81.

17. Price L. Treating the clock and not the patient: ambulance response times and risk. *Qual Saf Health Care*. 2006;15:127-130.

18. Lacher ME, Bausher JC. Lights and siren in pediatric 911 ambulance transports: are they being misused? *Ann Emerg Med*. 1997;29(2):223-227.

19. Kahn CA, Pirrallo RG, Kuhn EM. Characteristics of fatal ambulance crashes in the United States: An 11-year retrospective analysis. *Prehosp Emerg Care*. 2001;5(3):261-269.

20. Clawson JJ, Martin RL, Cady GA, Maio RF. The wake effect: Emergency vehicle-related collisions. National Association for Emergency Dispatch. 1997. http://www.emergencydispatch.org/articles/wakeeffect1.htm. Accessed July 17, 2011.

21. Wei Lam SS, Zhang ZC, Oh HC, et al. Reducing ambulance response times using discrete event simulation. *Prehosp Emerg Care*. April-June 2014;18(2):207-216.

22. Tanaka Y, Yamada H, Tamasaku S, Inaba H. The fast emergency vehicle pre-emption system improved the outcomes of out-of-hospital cardiac arrest. *Am J Emerg Med*. October 2013;31(10):1466-1471.

23. Stout T. About Jack. Jack Stout. n.d. www.jackstout.com. Accessed June 20, 2011.

24. Stout J. System status management: the fact is, it's everywhere. *Jems*, Vol 14(4) April 1989.

25. Bledsoe BE. EMS Myth #7: System status management lowers response times and enhances patient care. EMS World. January 12, 2011. http://www.emsworld.com/article/article.jsp?id=2030&siteSection=8. Accessed June 23, 2011.

26. ReVelle C, Marks D, Liebman JC. An analysis of private and public sector location models. *Manag Sci*. 1970;16(11):692-707.

27. Goldberg JB. Operations research models for the deployment of emergency services vehicles. *EMS Manage J*. 2004;1(1):20-39.

28. Toregas C, Swain R, ReVelle C, Bergman L. The location of emergency service facilities. *Oper Res*. 1971;19(6):1363-1373.

29. Merriam-Webster. Stochastic: involving chance or probability. n.d. http://www.merriam-webster.com/dictionary/stochastic. Accessed July 17, 2011.

30. Brotcorne L, Laporte G, Semet F. Ambulance location and relocation models. *Eur J Oper Res*. 2003;147:451-463.

31. Marianov V, ReVelle C. The queueing maximal availability location problem: A model for the siting of emergency vehicles. *Eur J Oper Res*. 1996;93:110-120.

32. EventHelix.com. Queueing theory basics. 2011. http://www.eventhelix.com/realtimemantra/congestioncontrol/queueing_theory.htm. Accessed June 15, 2011.

33. Lovejoy WS, Desmond JS. Little's law analysis of observation unit impact and sizing. *Acad Emerg Med*. 2011;18(2):183-189.

34. Bassamboo A, Randhawa RS. On the accuracy of fluid models for capacity sizing in queueing systems with impatient customers. *Operations Research*. 2010;58(5):1398-1413.

35. Rajagopalan HK, Saydam C, Xiao J. A multiperiod set covering location model for dynamic redeployment of ambulances. *Comput Oper Res*. 2008;35:814-826.

36. Erkut E, Ingolfsson A, Sim T, Erdogan G. Computational comparison of five maximal covering models for locating ambulances. *Geogr Anal*. 2009;41:43-65.

37. Jagerman, DL. Some properties of the Erlang Loss Function. *Bell System Technical Journal*. Blackwell Publishing Ltd., 53(3): 1538-7305.

38. Restrepo M, Henderson SG, Topaloglu H. Erlang loss models for the static deployment of ambulances. *Health Care Manag Sci*. 2009;12:67-79.

39. Fortenberry JC, Mitra A, Willis RD. A multi-criteria approach to optimal emergency vehicle location analysis. *Comput Ind Eng*. 1989;16(2):339-347.

40. Alsalloum OI, Rand GK. Extensions to emergency vehicle location models. *Comput Oper Res*. 2006;33:2725-2743.

41. Simpson N. Modeling of residential structure fire response: exploring the hyper-project. *J Oper Manag*. 2006;24:530-541.

42. Budge S, Ingolfsson A, Erkut E. Approximating vehicle dispatch probabilities for emergency service systems with location-specific service times and multiple units per location. *Oper Res*. 2009; 57(1):251-255.

43. Clawson JJ. Emergency medical dispatch and prioritizing response. In: Cone DC, O'Connor RE, Fowler RL, eds. *Emergency Medical Services: Clinical Practice and Systems Oversight*. Vol. 2. Dubuque, IA: Kendall-Hunt Professional; 2009; 554-589.

44. Neely KW, Norton RL, Schmidt TA. The strength of specific EMS dispatcher questions for identifying patients with important clinical field findings. *Prehosp Emerg Care*. 2000;4(4):322-326.

45. Bailey ED, O'Connor RE, Ross RW. The use of emergency medical dispatch protocols to reduce the number of inappropriate scene responses made by advanced life support personnel. *Prehosp Emerg Care*. 2000;4:186-189.

46. Shah MN, Bishop P, Lerner EB, Fairbanks RJ, Davis EA. Validation of using EMS dispatch codes to identify low-acuity patients. *Prehosp Emerg Care*. 2005;9(1):24-31.

47. Hinchey P, Myers B, Zalkin J, Lewis R, Garner JD. Low acuity EMS dispatch criteria can reliably identify patients without high-acuity illness or injury. *Prehosp Emerg Care*. 2007;11(1):42-48.

48. Nesbary D. The acquisition of computer-aided dispatch systems: administrative and political considerations. *Soc Sci Comput Rev*. 2001;19(3):348-356.

49. Sun J, Dong JS, Jarzabek S, Wang H. Computer-aided dispatch system family architecture and verification: an integrated formal approach. *IEE P-Softw*. 2006;153(3):102-112.

50. Allen G. Computer aided dispatch software resources. DISPATCH Magazine On-Line. n.d. http://www.911dispatch.com/info/cad/index.html. Accessed August 28, 2011.

51. Clawson JJ, Dernocoeur KB, Rose BH. *Principles of Emergency Medical Dispatch*. 4th ed. Salt Lake City, UT: NAEMD; 2009.

52. Meredith JR, Shafer SM. *Operations Management for MBAs*. 3rd ed. Hoboken, NJ: John Wiley & Sons; 2007.

CHAPTER 15

Communications and Dispatching

Karl A. Sporer

Prasanthi Govindarajan

INTRODUCTION

Emergency medical services (EMS) systems were developed in the early 1970s when federal resources were made available to provide for creation of the prehospital system infrastructure.[1] A few years following the development of the EMS systems, NHTSA with the assistance from NASEMSD (National Association of State EMS Directors) developed a two-tiered statewide communication plan which was adapted to satisfy communication needs within EMS systems while also providing for compatibility and interoperability with other EMS components.[2] Although the need for creating a communication infrastructure was recognized early and the system-level elements are well understood by the planning committee members, the various components of EMS communications are less understood by providers of emergency care systems. The common misconception related to emergency communication is that it is thought to involve exchange of information for medical control purposes when in fact, the actual process includes any exchange of the information between providers or between providers and the public or between emergency care providers and public safety agencies.

OBJECTIVES

- Describe the usual events involved in the dispatching of an EMS agency for an emergency call.
- Describe modes of response related to dispatching.
- Describe computer-assisted dispatching.
- Describe the common types of radio communication and frequencies.
- Describe common types of "radio speak," including signals, codes, and plain speak.
- Discuss why plain profession radio speak is considered superior to signals and codes.
- Describe common terms used in radio communication to communicate the status of a unit.
- Describe an emergency department base station and list types of individuals who may be answering the call.
- Describe the types of "calls" that EMS providers make to the EMS base station.
- Detail the essential components of base-station training.
- Describe alternatives to radio for communications.
- Discuss new technology, including the transmission of ECGs, real-time telemetry, and video streaming from the field.

COMMUNICATIONS

Until fairly recently, there was no a comprehensive network of emergency communication centers, even in the United States. The evolution of the existence of "9-1-1" centers has led to a convenient and accessible way for the public to call for emergency assistance. There are a few components of the communication chain that illustrates how this system functions (**Figure 15-1**).

▨ INITIAL CALL FROM PUBLIC, LANDLINE, CELL PHONE, VOIP

Emergency services are an important element of health care system and immediate, reliable, and easy access to this system is provided to the community through activation of 9-1-1 system. Common ways of accessing this system include the landline phones, mobile phones, vehicle-based access using automatic crash notification (ACN), and commercial voice-over-Internet protocol (VoIP) service, which refers to

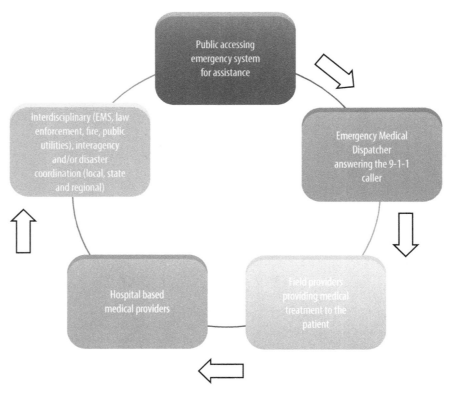

FIGURE 15-1. Communication chain.

communication using the Internet rather than the public switched telephone network providers. ACN is a system that alerts EMS systems when a crash occurs and information obtained using this system helps determine severity and location of the collision as well as notify and create a communication link with EMS providers and the crash victim.[3] Once emergency care systems are activated through any of these pathways, the system recognizes the need for the emergency service, leading to identification of the caller/communication device, dispatch to the site of event, and transport to an appropriate or closest emergency care facility.

ROLE OF PUBLIC SERVICE ANSWERING POINTS (FUNCTION OF ALI/ANI INFORMATION AND LOCATION VIA CELL TOWERS)

9-1-1 call centers or public service answering points (PSAPs) are the first line of contact for the public with the emergency care systems (**Figure 15-2**). PSAPs can be integrated with the dispatch center or be an autonomous agency established to receive calls. They are of four types and are designated as direct if the field teams are directly dispatched by the agency after the call is received and interrogated by the PSAP. The other types include centers which transfer the call to the agency to allow direct communication between the dispatching agency and the caller (secondary PSAP) or a relay model in which the information is collected by the PSAP and is given to the dispatching agency which does not directly communicate with the caller. Referral models are the least recommended approach in which the information is taken from the caller who is then given the appropriate number to call the emergency medical dispatcher: The next element in the communication chain is the emergency medical dispatch center. Emergency medical dispatchers are personnel with skill in basic telecommunications who serve as a link between the public and the field teams. They receive the information from the public, monitor the field teams, as well as direct and dispatch them to the scene. Enhanced features of the 9-1-1 system used to contact PSAPs/dispatch center are able to selectively route the call to the center based on the caller location and also display of the caller phone number (automatic number identification) and location (automatic location identification) in the dispatch screen.[3] These features significantly improve the reliability of response even when the caller is unable to provide information on their location. The various modes of communication available for EMDs include one-way paging or "alert dispatching" which helps simultaneously communicate with many units or communicate with field providers and other public safety agencies (law, enforcement, fire) during mass casualty incidents, using radio systems. Other methods of communication may involve direct telephone communication with other public safety agencies and/or the medical facilities.

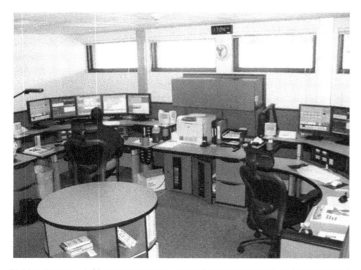

FIGURE 15-2. Public service answering point. (By en:User:Coldcaffeine [Public domain], via Wikimedia Commons.)

MEDICAL CONTROL COMMUNICATION

Another important component of the communication chain includes medical providers in the hospitals. The teams providing care on scene need to communicate with the receiving hospital for notification of the time of arrival, patient medical condition, and transmission of data such as ECG or telemetry.

INTERAGENCY COMMUNICATION

This involves communication using radio equipment with other public safety agencies. This link involves local coordination using mobile and portable radios with multiple mutual aid responding units and/or regional coordination in disaster situations that require large-scale coordination between EMS resources as well as communication with public safety agencies as determined by on-scene needs of the responding unit.

BACK-UP COMMUNICATION

This involves a mechanism for communication between medical control, dispatch, and interagency coordination in the event of outages of primary dispatch, base hospital or during disaster scenarios.[4]

Communication Equipment The exchange of information between the different components of the communication network is facilitated using a basic unit consisting of transmitter and receiver units. The radio communication equipment which is used in one-way communication such as paging or alerts involve a receiver and transmitter unit tuned to the same frequency within the radio range of each other. For two-way communication, a receiver and transmitter is usually placed at both sites. A *simplex* communication involves one frequency channel for communication and involves transfer of information both ways by provider taking turns on a single frequency channel (**Figure 15-3**). By using two different frequencies it is possible for the providers to interrupt each other during a communication in a *duplex* system. A duplex communication system can also be modified to have a duplex setup at one end and a simplex at the other end. This provides for the physician to interrupt the field provider communication during patient care to provide medical direction whereas a field provider would not be able to break a physician communication. A duplex system designed to automatically retransmit what is relayed is called a mobile relay system, for example, an incoming information on frequency 1 from a mobile unit is automatically connected and relayed to another mobile unit or ambulance on frequency 2.[5]

EMERGENCY MEDICAL RADIO SERVICE FREQUENCIES FOR PROVIDER COMMUNICATION

In 1993, Under the Federal Communication Commission (FCC) established the emergency *medical radio service* (EMRS). This *public safety radio service* (PSRS) was created to improve the reliability of communications in an emergency setting by providing specific frequencies to life support–related communication. Advanced and basic life support providers were eligible to use these channels of communication when providing basic or advanced life support services.[6]

EMRS frequencies available for EMS communications are in the VHF "high band" (150-173 MHz), the UHF "ultrahigh frequency" band (453-465 MHz), the 220-MHz band, and the 800-MHz band (**Table 15-1**). Also, while no 800-MHz band frequencies are allocated to EMS, all EMRS eligible entities are allowed to license 800-MHz frequencies allocated for public safety agencies and also use SERS (*specialized emergency radio service*) channels for essential nonemergency communication with other entities.

800-MHz PUBLIC SAFETY SPECTRUM

Radio systems used by public safety officers, that is, police, firefighters, and emergency medical technicians operate in multiple sections of the 800-MHz band which consists of spectrum at 806 to 824 MHz paired with spectrum at 851-869 MHz.[6] Under guidelines provided by

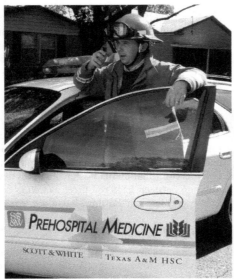
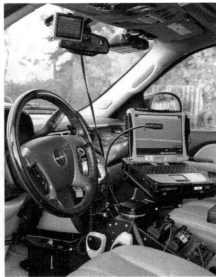

FIGURE 15-3. EMS physician on a two-way radio (simplex). Interior on the right is of EMS physician SUV with radios, mobile data terminal (MDT). and GPS. (Photo by Dr. John Lyng, North Memorial Ambulance, Minneapolis, MN.)

the National Public Safety Planning Advisory Committee (NPSPAC), a 6-MHz spectrum in this band has been provided for exclusive use of public safety agencies. However, since the 800-MHz band is also used by commercial wireless carriers and private radio systems, FCC reconfigured the band plan in 2004 to separate the commercial users from the public safety agencies using cellular architecture. However, some of the problems faced by providers and agencies include the lack of compatibility between service areas due to differences in architecture of the communication equipment, not being able to use vehicle repeaters limiting communication within closed settings like homes and limited frequency range limiting communication particularly in rural regions.[7]

VHF RADIO SYSTEMS

Rural and suburban agencies use the VHF radio systems due to the properties of the radio waves that are suited for the flat terrain of the rural areas. VHF systems are simplex and have a range of 15 miles without repeaters, for communication. Repeaters receive signals on one frequency and retransmit on the other frequency and can overcome problems with range limitations and distance but are not permitted for use by EMS systems in the low frequency range, by FCC.[8]

UHF RADIO SYSTEMS

Urban systems use the UHF radio systems that have the properties for use in heavily population regions. Unlike the VHF systems, UHF systems are usually duplex systems and have 10 channels dedicated by FCC for use by the EMS agencies. When using UHF radio systems, EMS agencies can also use special features such as squelch which limit the communication from being shared by other agencies.

OTHER METHODS OF COMMUNICATION

Trunking Trunking technology creates a dedicated communication line between two sites and uses a small number of trunks for a large number of users. This method of communication is based on the probability that not all users will simultaneously use the trunk lines. The major advantage of this system includes the availability of open channels, secure connection, and lack of interference while some of the problems related to this technology include the cost of the infrastructure, dependence on the computer infrastructure, and automated call switching.[9]

Microwave Relays Microwave relays work by converting radio frequencies into telephone/microwave frequencies and back to radio frequencies on the receiving end and extend the range of communication manyfold. Microwave systems can accommodate state and local emergency services radio systems and also systems used by nonemergency responders such as highway maintenance crews.[8]

2.4- to 5.9-GHz Systems and Fiberoptic Connections Wireless "hot spot"–based ("mesh") systems evolving in urban areas and along major highways offer the advantage of both voice and data communications. However, they require a "line of sight" between the device and the connection, making this extremely expensive in nonurbanized areas. Other concerns with these systems include open access model to any user, which suggests potential interference, reduced data transfer speed due to bogging, and security issues. Although these systems may start up well they do get impeded as public use of the system increases. However, the use of 4.9-GHz band (4940-4990 MHz) is licensed strictly for public safety uses including EMS and is coordinated by regional users. The benefits of this system in addition to the existing advantages of the 2.4-GHz system are communication security and lack of interference.[8]

TABLE 15-1	Range and Properties of the Frequencies Used for EMS Communication			
	VHF—High Band	VHF—Low Band	UHF	800 Band
Radio frequency spectrum	30-50 MHz	138-174 MHz	406-470 MHz	806-940 MHz
Properties	Structures-like leaves may interfere with transmission of low frequencies		Overall, higher frequencies bounce off building structures and well suited for transmission in areas with high-rise buildings	
			UHF have less atmospheric interference and suited for long distance transmissions	
Uses	Rural and suburban areas		Urban areas	

TABLE 15-2	Code Language Versus Plain Language Used in EMS Communication				
	Agency 1	Agency 2	Agency 3	Agency 4	Agency 5
Signal Codes					
Signal 5	N/A	N/A	Jail	Traffic contact	Go to control
Signal 32	Accident with fatality	N/A	Check records	Drive-by shooting	N/A
Signal 99	Need assistance	Structure fire	Structure fire	N/A	N/A
10-Codes					
10-12	No available units	On portable	Bystanders present	Subject present	Standby
10-97	Arrived at scene	Test tone	N/A	Arrived at scene	Check signal
10-100	Send all available units	Taking a personnel break	N/A	Stage units	N/A
Response Code					
Known life threat (lights and siren)	Priority 1	Code 1	Code 1	Red	Priority 1
Possible life threat (lights and siren)	Priority 2	Code 2	Code 2	Red	Priority 2
Emergency (no lights and sirens)	Priority 3	Code 3	Code 3	White	Priority 3
No need for additional units	Status all-set	Code 4	Code 4	Hold with units on scene	Code 4

Land Mobile Satellite Communications This method of communication has been described as an alternate method of communication for remote rural regions and the technology uses satellites positioned in low orbits or geostationary orbits.

Cellular Telephones and Digital Technology The benefits of cellular technology include the ability to operate in radio dead spots and also use additional features such as image transmission and ease of use. However, while these options are available to systems to help with their communication needs, cost of replacing systems with digital technology and operational difficulties in disaster situations and interagency communication for cellular phone users may limit exclusive use of these technologies nationwide.

700-MHz Public Safety spectrum FCC has made available 34 MHz of mixed narrowband and broadband spectrum for use by public safety in the 700-MHz range since February 2009.[10] The spectrum allocation is in the upper 700-MHz spectrum and includes 6 MHz of narrowband for each mobile and base radio communications (12 MHz total) and 5 MHz each of broadband for mobile and base communications with a 1 MHz each of "guard band" in each mobile and base spectrum to separate the narrowband and broadband uses. This spectrum has been licensed by FCC to a single national licensee (Public Safety Spectrum Trust [PSST]) with a 10-MHz spectrum licensed to a private entity which will also be available for public safety when needed. The advantages of this system is that it will cover 99% of the US population by 2019 and can be used to transmit voice and data such as multivital sign telemetry (ECG, capnography, pulse, video images) for EMS systems who are planning on developing advanced communication systems.

Future Technologies In the near future, emergency communications may include "hotspot"-based technology at 5.9 MHz and or community fiberoptic system application for rural areas.[11] The first methodology envisions hotspots that can communicate with a vehicle at 5.9 GHz along the roadway, which then connects to communication systems. In rural areas, providers can also link to fiber-optic system using the hotspots or wireline access located at the facilities.

PROVIDER AND INTERAGENCY COMMUNICATION

EMS provider communication involves use of code language and plain language. The code system was developed by law enforcement officials to keep the two-way communications secure and also reduce the volume of traffic. Other opinions stated by emergency providers in favor of coded language include protecting the officer as well as the nature of information being communicated to the provider. On the contrary, some of the problems recognized by providers using the code language were lack of interoperability due to uniqueness of the code language to each jurisdiction (**Table 15-2**) and ability of the nonemergency provider community to decipher the meaning of the codes used.[12,13]

In addition to the lack of clear benefits for code language, the known benefit of using plain language was the simplicity of the communication which did not impede communication between providers from different agencies. This has led states like Virginia to use plain language for day-to-day activities. However, use of coded language is permitted under certain circumstances, such as communicating sensitive information about subjects who are in close proximity, taking a subject into custody who may offer resistance, or if the emergency responder needs assistance or is in immediate danger.[13] For systems transitioning from use of 10 codes to plain language is not a simple single-step process and requires planning of implementation strategies like computer-assisted dispatch reprogramming and training of emergency responders.

Communication between emergency providers and hospitals is important for patient care and is usually simple, direct, and standardized. Official titles are reported followed by estimated time of arrival, patient status (stable or unstable vital signs), age, chief compliant, relevant history, standing orders that were completed and request for medical orders. Usually the medical orders are repeated to make sure there is no error in communication. An example of a communication between the field provider and the hospital and radio terms used to provide the status of a responding unit are shown in **Table 15-3**.

TABLE 15-3	Radio Terms Used by EMS Providers When Communicating With the Destination Hospital or Other Units
Responding	Unit en route to scene
On scene	Unit has arrived at scene
Transporting	Unit transporting a patient to destination
Arrived	Unit transporting a patient arrived at destination
Available	Unit available for response
On the air	Unit available and monitoring dispatch
Scene secure	The scene has been deemed safe for public safety agencies
Emergency traffic	Channel is available for emergency communication
On Scene—investigating	Investigating circumstances on scene

EMERGENCY MEDICAL DISPATCH

Emergency medical dispatch (EMD) is a system of categorizing medical 9-1-1 calls into discrete groups in order to send an appropriate medical response in a timely fashion. One of its goals is to differentiate those calls that have a high likelihood of requiring a time-dependent treatment such as defibrillation from those that are less time sensitive.[14] It also attempts to assign a need for *basic life support or advanced life support* assessment and its timeliness. EMD has been demonstrated to improve response times to urgent calls and the general ability to differentiate between predicted needed levels of service.[1-4,15-22] Prior studies in differing EMS configurations have used a variety of EMD programs with both health and nonhealth trained dispatchers as well as different clinical measures to gauge success.[15-18,23-29]

Some calls may be safely handled without sending a response. These are commonly called that can be handled by a poison control center and those patients with obvious or expected death. The United Kingdom is currently experimenting with redirecting some select calls to nurse advice centers directly (telephone redirection) and after evaluation and treatment by paramedics (postevaluation redirection).[30,31] Similar pilot projects are being started in various US cities.

More recently, the EMD systems have evolved to have the dispatcher instruct the caller with early first aid.[32-35] The instruction in performing bystander CPR has been best studied and has demonstrated improved survival. These studies have also demonstrated that dispatch-assisted CPR with chest compressions only has a better success rate than attempting to teach both ventilation and chest compressions.[36-39] Other types of prearrival instructions include early administration of aspirin in chest pain patients, performance of the Heimlich maneuver, AED instructions,[40] as well as assisting in eminent childbirth.

The need for a rapid response to those patients in cardiac arrest drives the organization of most systems. A recent study examined the effect of the timing of EMS arrival and they demonstrated that survival among patients in cardiac arrest declined by 5.2% per minute between 5 and 10 minutes.[41] As the treatment of cardiac arrest evolves toward more BLS care, the rapid response of an automatic defibrillator and someone who is trained perform CPR can be accomplished by dispatching fire engines, police, or more recently citizens via social media.[42]

The diagnostic accuracy of dispatchers for prehospital cardiac arrest patients ranged from 51% to 86% in several studies with most in the 50% range.[33,43-45] The introduction of an EMD system versus no system with nonclinician dispatchers demonstrated an improvement in recognition of cardiac arrest from 15% to 50%.[46]

There is very modest evidence that trained paramedics may be better than nonclinician dispatchers at recognizing cardiac arrest patients.[44] The agonal respirations commonly seen in early cardiac arrest can be confusing to many reporting callers and refining of the questions posed or actually measuring the respiratory rate in questionable cases may improve this rate.[47] The accurate recognition is important because in one modest study the survival rate among those patients with a witnessed ventricular fibrillation cardiac arrest was significantly higher in those cases correctly diagnosed.[48]

The great majority of calls with cardiac arrest are dispatched with a lights-and-sirens response (along with other categories such as respiratory distress, seizure, or unconscious) but a 6% to 10% are not.[17,21,22,44,46,47,49] The ability of an EMD system to predict the diagnosis of a stroke has been well studied and ranges from 42% to 48%.[50-52]

The *medical priority dispatch system* is a proprietary EMD system that is used by 71% of major US cities and is also commonly used internationally.[53] This system has been studied the most and has either a card-based system or a fully computerized program. This system uses callers' responses to categorize cases into one of 33 possible standardized, complaint-based categories, which are further generally classified as Alfa (BLS cold [no lights and siren]), Bravo (BLS hot [lights and siren]), Charlie (ALS cold), Delta (ALS hot), or Echo (ALS hot with AED support). The computerized system has an added advantage of full documentation of the decisions made by the dispatcher as well as a robust quality improvement process. Individual dispatch centers who meet exacting standards can qualify as a "center of excellence."

Criteria-based dispatch is another commonly used system that was designed by the EMS system in Kings County and Seattle.[54] A number of large cities (Houston, NYC, Phoenix, Chicago, and Portland) use an EMD system that they have developed locally. Only a few communities use a system developed by the Association of Public Safety Communication Officers.[55]

Any EMD system will benefit from an active quality improvement system.[56] This commonly involves having someone review selected calls for compliance and accuracy. This can be accomplished by selecting a percentage of calls by dispatchers or more focused audits. These commonly include the review of calls with the need for prearrival instructions, those with a cold response and a hot return to the hospital, as well as certain problem categories such as calls from medical facilities.

■ COMPUTER-AIDED DISPATCH

Any modern medical dispatch system will be heavily dependent on a fully functioning computer-aided dispatch (CAD) software. This complex system will need to be integrated with a large number of other information sources. These can include inputs from various alarms, ALI/ANI information, cell phone location, output to various mobile data systems, time synchronization sources, records management systems, hospital diversion data, multicasualty incident tracking software, and if integrated with law enforcement, various criminal justice databases. For those systems with a dynamic deployment of prehospital resources, there is often some type of real-time decision making software that allows for the optimal deployment of ambulances based on historical call volume by location and time of day. The record-keeping function as well as a consistent measurement of various times for dispatch, response, and arrival at scene are invaluable for recreating the sequence of events for any sentinel investigations. There are over a dozen commonly used proprietary versions of CAD available.[57]

Most EMS systems send out some type of text information about the call using either pagers, cell phone texting, or dedicated mobile data terminals. These systems decrease radio traffic and avoid confusion about numeric addresses. Many systems also use Web-based data systems that are commonly used to monitor the diversion status of local area hospitals and other receiving facilities and for providing information in both directions during multicasualty incidents.

Many systems have developed some method of transmitting electrocardiograms in the setting of suspected STEMI. There have also been some novel uses of technology to transmit real-time telemetry, vital signs, end-tidal carbon dioxide, and photos of the accident scene. Some have used video streaming from the field to assist in medical decisions and in one area for the supervision of video laryngoscopy.

BASE STATION (ONLINE MEDICAL CONTROL)

Most EMS systems have some method of providing real-time oversight and advice, most commonly through an EMS base station. These are most commonly designated hospitals' emergency departments with specially trained personnel but in larger cities can be a clinician solely dedicated to this function. These trained personnel can be either nurses (commonly referred to as mobile intensive care nurse [MICN]) or emergency physicians. In past decades, most procedures or administration of medications required base station approval but the current trend has been toward more permissive clinical protocols that allow the paramedic greater clinical latitude. These types of calls that prehospital providers may make to the base station are listed in **Table 15-4**. The indication for each of these depends greatly on local clinical policies and procedures.

The essential component of base station training include

- Knowledge of local scope of practice for prehospital providers
- Knowledge of local clinical protocols
- Legal underpinning of medical control
- Understanding of AMA issues

TABLE 15-4	Provider Calls to Medical Control
Notification (impending patient)	Informing the hospital of the arrival of a specific patient, which needs hospital preparation; this can be especially useful for the trauma or stroke patient
Medication order	Useful for infrequently used drugs or higher than normal dosing
Procedure orders	Systems may require base hospital contact for specific low-frequency, high-risk procedures
Clarification of protocols	Situations that are not fully addressed by protocols
Hospital destination issues	May meet criteria for specialty center care, but destination decision making is otherwise complex
Patient refusal (against medical advice)	This is commonly used to enlist the ED physician in discussing medical issues with a reluctant patient
Termination of resuscitation	Many systems require the approval of the base hospital to terminate cardiac arrest efforts. There are many unclear DNR situations that can be guided by the base station.
Need for additional resources	Providers my encounter need for additional resources that the base station can activate (EMS physician, emergency management)
Multiple casualty incident notification	The potential for patient surge should be communicated
Hospital diversion issues	In some specific cases, diversion could be directly detrimental to a specific patient requiring specific specialty services, or in whom immediate stabilization would be significantly delayed

- Local destination requirements (trauma center, STEMI, stroke centers)
- Ability to make patient-centered decisions that deviate from written protocols

Most base stations also commonly require that their personnel take part in the training of paramedics and EMTs as well as regular prehospital field observation.

KEY POINTS

- Emergency medical dispatch (EMD) is a system of categorizing medical 9-1-1 calls into discrete groups in order to send an appropriate medical response in a timely fashion.
- EMS identifies most but not all urgent calls with a considerable degree of overtriage.
- Prearrival instructions such as dispatch-directed CPR have been demonstrated to increase survival in cardiac arrest patients.
- The diagnostic accuracy of EMD ranges around 50% but with 90% dispatched with lights and sirens.
- Computer-aided dispatch (CAD) is an integral part of any EMS system and allows for dynamic deployment, rapid assignment of appropriate calls, and record keeping of various response times.
- Base stations with specifically trained clinicians provide real-time consultation for field personnel for a variety of clinical situations.
- EMS communication begins with the initial call to the public service answering points and the various components of the communication network include the dispatch center, field providers, hospital command center, and other public safety agency providers.
- EMS providers communicate using plain language and code language. Code language was developed to keep the communication secure and plain language is preferred for its simplicity of communication.
- Communication can be one way such as in paging alerts or bidirectional. Two-way communication types can be simplex or duplex or modified duplex in nature.

REFERENCES

1. Committee on the Future of Emergency Care in the United States Health System. History and Current State of EMS. Emergency Medical Services At the Crossroads. 2007. http://www.iom.edu/Reports/2006/Emergency-Medical-Services-At-the-Crossroads.aspx. Accessed April 2014.
2. The National Association of State Emergency Medical Services Directors. Planning Emergency Medical Communications. State Level Planning Guide. Volume 1. 1995. http://www.nasemso.org/NewsAndPublications/News/documents/NASEMSD_VOLUME1.pdf. Accessed August 29, 2011.
3. Hunt RC. Emerging communication technologies in emergency medical services. *Prehosp Emerg Care*. 2002;6:131-136.
4. Back- Up Communications. Wisconsin Emergency Medical Services Communications Plan. 2006. https://www.dhs.wisconsin.gov/publications/p0/p00342.pdf. Accessed April, 2015.
5. Private Land Mobile Radio Services. Telecommunication. 2015. http://edocket.access.gpo.gov/cfr_2006/octqtr/47cfr90.7.htm. Accessed August 29, 2011.
6. Public Safety and Homeland Security Bureau. 800 MHz public safety spectrum. 2011. http://transition.fcc.gov/pshs/public-safety-spectrum/800-MHz/. Accessed August 29, 2011.
7. Augustine JJ. Communications. In: Kuehl AE, ed. *Prehospital Systems and Medical Oversight. Vol* 3rd ed. Dubuque, IA: Kendall/Hunt Publishing Company; 2002.
8. EMSCOM. Radio communications user manual. www.nmems.org/Communications/EMSCOM%20Manual%20809.pdf. Accessed August 29, 2011.
9. National Association of State EMS Officials. Guide to Emergency Medical Services Information Communications Technology (ICT) Systems For EMS Officials. Falls Church, VA. August, 2008. http://www.nasemso.org/Projects/CommunicationsTechnology/index.asp. Accessed August 29, 2011.
10. Careless J. Public safety gets the D block—what it means for EMS. How can we harness the potential of 700 MHz for the provider in the field? *EMS World*. July 2012;41(7):71-73.
11. Erich J. Big plans for broadband. *EMS World*. June 2013;42(6):27-30.
12. Plain Language Guide. Making the transition from ten codes to plain language. http://www.safecomprogram.gov/default.aspx. Accessed August 29, 2011.
13. Virginia's Common Language Protocol. http://www.interoperability.virginia.gov/pdfs/LLIS_CommonLanguageProtocol.pdf. Accessed August 29, 2011.
14. Hardeland C, Olasveengen TM, Lawrence R, et al. Comparison of medical priority dispatch (MPD) and criteria based dispatch (CBD) relating to cardiac arrest calls. *Resuscitation*. May 2014;85(5):612-616.
15. Palumbo L, Kubincanek J, Emerman C, Jouriles N, Cydulka R, Shade B. Performance of a system to determine EMS dispatch priorities. *Am J Emerg Med*. July 1996;14(4):388-390.
16. Neely KW, Eldurkar JA, Drake ME. Do emergency medical services dispatch nature and severity codes agree with paramedic field findings? *Acad Emerg Med*. February 2000;7(2):174-180.
17. Feldman MJ, Verbeek PR, Lyons DG, Chad SJ, Craig AM, Schwartz B. Comparison of the medical priority dispatch system to an out-of-hospital patient acuity score. *Acad Emerg Med*. September 2006;13(9):954-960.
18. Craig A, Schwartz B, Feldman M. Development of evidence-based dispatch response plans to optimize ALS paramedic response in an urban EMS system (abstract). *Prehosp Emerg Care*. 2006;10(1):114.
19. Neely KW, Eldurkar J, Drake ME. Can current EMS dispatch protocols identify layperson-reported sentinel conditions? *Prehosp Emerg Care*. July-September 2000;4(3):238-244.
20. Calle P, Houbrechts H, Lagaert L, Buylaert W. How to evaluate an emergency medical dispatch system: a Belgian perspective. *Eur J Emerg Med*. September 1995;2(3):128-135.
21. Clawson J, Olola C, Heward A, Patterson B. Cardiac arrest predictability in seizure patients based on emergency medical dispatcher

identification of previous seizure or epilepsy history. *Resuscitation.* November 2007;75(2):298-304.

22. Clawson J, Olola C, Heward A, Patterson B, Scott G. The Medical Priority Dispatch System's ability to predict cardiac arrest outcomes and high acuity pre-hospital alerts in chest pain patients presenting to 9-9-9. *Resuscitation.* June 16, 2008;78(3):298-306.

23. Bailey ED, O'Connor RE, Ross RW. The use of emergency medical dispatch protocols to reduce the number of inappropriate scene responses made by advanced life support personnel. *Prehosp Emerg Care.* April-June 2000;4(2):186-189.

24. Flynn J, Archer F, Morgans A. Sensitivity and specificity of the Medical Priority Dispatch System in detecting cardiac arrest emergency calls in Melbourne. *Prehosp Disaster Med.* 2006;21(2):72-76.

25. Shah MN, Bishop P, Lerner EB, Czapranski T, Davis EA. Derivation of emergency medical services dispatch codes associated with low-acuity patients. *Prehosp Emerg Care.* October-December 2003;7(4): 434-439.

26. Myers JB, Hinchey P, Zalkin J, Lewis R, Garner DG. EMS dispatch triage criteria can accurately identify patients without high-acuity illness or injury. *Prehosp Emerg Care.* 2005;9:119.

27. Shah MN, Bishop P, Lerner EB, Fairbanks RJ, Davis EA. Validation of EMD dispatch codes associated with low-acuity patients. *Prehosp Emerg Care.* January-March 2005;9(1):24-31.

28. Michael GE, Sporer KA. Validation of low-acuity emergency medical services dispatch codes. *Prehosp Emerg Care.* October-December 2005;9(4):429-433.

29. Sporer KA, Youngblood GM, Rodriguez RM. The ability of emergency medical dispatch codes of medical complaints to predict ALS prehospital interventions. *Prehosp Emerg Care.* Apr-Jun 2007;11(2): 192-198.

30. Gray JT, Walker A. AMPDS categories: are they an appropriate method to select cases for extended role ambulance practitioners? *Emerg Med J.* September 2008;25(9):601-603.

31. Gray JT, Walker A. Avoiding admissions from the ambulance service: a review of elderly patients with falls and patients with breathing difficulties seen by emergency care practitioners in South Yorkshire. *Emerg Med J.* March 2008;25(3):168-171.

32. Hallstrom A, Cobb L, Johnson E, Copass M. Cardiopulmonary resuscitation by chest compression alone or with mouth-to-mouth ventilation. *N Engl J Med.* May 25, 2000;342(21):1546-1553.

33. Hallstrom AP. Dispatcher-assisted "phone" cardiopulmonary resuscitation by chest compression alone or with mouth-to-mouth ventilation. *Crit Care Med.* November 2000;28(11 suppl):N190-N192.

34. Idris AH, Roppolo L. Barriers to dispatcher-assisted telephone cardiopulmonary resuscitation. *Ann Emerg Med.* December 2003;42 (6):738-740.

35. Rea TD, Eisenberg MS, Culley LL, Becker L. Dispatcher-assisted cardiopulmonary resuscitation and survival in cardiac arrest. *Circulation.* November 20, 2001;104(21):2513-2516.

36. Roppolo LP, Pepe PE, Cimon N, et al. Modified cardiopulmonary resuscitation (CPR) instruction protocols for emergency medical dispatchers: rationale and recommendations. *Resuscitation.* May 2005;65(2):203-210.

37. Woollard M, Smith A, Whitfield R, et al. To blow or not to blow: a randomised controlled trial of compression-only and standard telephone CPR instructions in simulated cardiac arrest. *Resuscitation.* October 2003;59(1):123-131.

38. van Tulder R, Roth D, Havel C, et al. "Push as hard as you can" instruction for telephone cardiopulmonary resuscitation: a randomized simulation study. *J Emerg Med.* March 2014;46(3):363-370.

39. Clegg GR, Lyon RM, James S, Branigan HP, Bard EG, Egan GJ. Dispatch-assisted CPR: where are the hold-ups during calls to emergency dispatchers? A preliminary analysis of caller-dispatcher interactions during out-of-hospital cardiac arrest using a novel call transcription technique. *Resuscitation.* January 2014;85(1):49-52.

40. Ecker R, Rea TD, Meischke H, Schaeffer SM, Kudenchuk P, Eisenberg MS. Dispatcher assistance and automated external defibrillator performance among elders. *Acad Emerg Med.* October 2001;8(10):968-973.

41. Gold LS, Fahrenbruch CE, Rea TD, Eisenberg MS. The relationship between time to arrival of emergency medical services (EMS) and survival from out-of-hospital ventricular fibrillation cardiac arrest. *Resuscitation.* May 2010;81(5):622-625.

42. Rea T, Blackwood J, Damon S, Phelps R, Eisenberg M. A link between emergency dispatch and public access AEDs: Potential implications for early defibrillation. *Resuscitation.* August 2011;82(8):995-998.

43. Clark JJ, Culley L, Eisenberg M, Henwood DK. Accuracy of determining cardiac arrest by emergency medical dispatchers. *Ann Emerg Med.* May 1994;23(5):1022-1026.

44. Garza AG, Gratton MC, Chen JJ, Carlson B. The accuracy of predicting cardiac arrest by emergency medical services dispatchers: the calling party effect. *Acad Emerg Med.* September 2003;10(9): 955-960.

45. Johnson NJ, Sporer KA. How many emergency dispatches occurred per cardiac arrest? *Resuscitation.* November 2010;81(11):1499-1504.

46. Heward A, Damiani M, Hartley-Sharpe C. Does the use of the Advanced Medical Priority Dispatch System affect cardiac arrest detection? *Emerg Med J.* January 2004;21(1):115-118.

47. Bang A, Herlitz J, Martinell S. Interaction between emergency medical dispatcher and caller in suspected out-of-hospital cardiac arrest calls with focus on agonal breathing. A review of 100 tape recordings of true cardiac arrest cases. *Resuscitation.* January 2003;56(1):25-34.

48. Kuisma M, Boyd J, Vayrynen T, Repo J, Nousila-Wiik M, Holmstrom P. Emergency call processing and survival from out-of-hospital ventricular fibrillation. *Resuscitation.* October 2005;67(1):89-93.

49. Merchant RM, Kurz MM, Gupta R, et al. Identification of cardiac arrest by emergency dispatch. *Acad Emerg Med.* 2005;12 (5 suppl):457.

50. Ramanujam P, Guluma KZ, Castillo EM, et al. Accuracy of stroke recognition by emergency medical dispatchers and paramedics-san diego experience. *Prehosp Emerg Care.* July-September 2008;12(3): 307-313.

51. Buck BH, Starkman S, Eckstein M, et al. Dispatcher recognition of stroke using the National Academy Medical Priority Dispatch System. *Stroke.* June 2009;40(6):2027-2030.

52. Deakin CD, Alasaad M, King P, Thompson F. Is ambulance telephone triage using advanced medical priority dispatch protocols able to identify patients with acute stroke correctly? *Emerg Med J.* June 2009;26(6):442-445.

53. Cady G. The medical priority dispatch system-a system and product overview http://www.naemd.org/articles/ArticleMPDS(Cady).html. Accessed August 24, 2011.

54. Criteria Based Dispatch. 2011. http://www.emsonline.net/assets/ CriteriaBasedDispatchGuidelines-Rev2010.pdf. Accessed August 24, 2011.

55. Association of Public Safety Communication Officers. 2011. http:// www.apco911.org/. Accessed August 26, 2011.

56. Clawson JJ, Cady GA, Martin RL, Sinclair R. Effect of a comprehensive quality management process on compliance with protocol in an emergency medical dispatch center. *Ann Emerg Med.* November 1998;32(5):578-584.

57. Computer-Aided Dispatch Software Resources. 2011. http://www. 911dispatch.com/computer-aided-dispatch-resources/. Accessed April, 2015.

CHAPTER 16

Interfacility Transport
Deb Funk

INTRODUCTION

Over the past several decades, advancements in medical care and technology have led to significant specialization in medical practice in many areas. These specialized services are often offered only at tertiary care centers where the resources exist to support the practice. In much the same way as trauma center designation occurred several decades ago, designation of specialized centers for stroke and cardiac care is seen in many areas.[1-4] Even when a formal designation process is not in place, consolidation of advanced services for many conditions is evident within regions and hospital systems. Smaller hospitals have taken on the role of identification and stabilization of conditions that require more advanced resources for definitive management.[5] Once such a condition has been identified and the patient appropriately stabilized, transfer to the facility capable of providing definitive care is necessary.

Since the 1970s the emergency medical services (EMS) system has developed and evolved to meet the needs of patients requiring transport to the hospital from a prehospital environment. EMS providers have been trained to efficiently assess patients and provide stabilizing care and safe transport to the most appropriate facility. This ability to provide safe and expeditious transport makes the EMS system the most logical means to move a patient from one hospital to another in an emergent situation.

It may be obvious to some that the needs of a patient being moved from the scene of an accident to a hospital are significantly different than the needs of a patient who has been assessed and stabilized at a hospital and requires transport to a tertiary care center for further care. The hospitalized patient often will have a specific diagnosis and have advanced interventions in place at the time of transfer. Traditional training for EMS providers is focused on identification of symptoms and rapid stabilizing care during transport to the closest appropriate hospital. With rare exception, the ongoing management of specific diagnoses has not been addressed in standard EMS training.

EMS systems have begun to evolve to meet the needs of this new patient population. While there are recently published national guidelines for interfacility transfer (IFT), many areas are still evolving to meet the needs of this patient population.[6] The involvement of a physician who understands the EMS system as well as the needs of the IFT patient is crucial in the development and management of a comprehensive IFT program. This chapter will review the history of interfacility transfers and discuss the different aspects of the system that the EMS physician must be familiar with.

OBJECTIVES

- Define *interfacility transport*.
- Describe indications for patients to be transferred by EMS to other health care institutions.
- Discuss how COBRA and EMTALA impact interfacility transfers.
- Describe the development of interfacility transport specific protocols.
- Discuss the role of advanced and ancillary medical providers used in specialty transport operations.
- Discuss the role of the EMS physician with regard to interfacility transfers.
- Discuss different modes of transport, including air versus ground units.
- Describe specialty transport teams.

EMERGENCY MEDICAL TREATMENT AND ACTIVE LABOR ACT

In the early 1980s it was not unusual for transfers to be motivated by not only the need for a higher level of care, but also for financial reasons. Hospitals might arrange a transfer of a patient with less ability to pay simply to avoid expending the resources when compensation was not likely. These hospitals may have had the resources to handle the patient's medical needs, but recommended transfer for purely economic reasons. This practice was often referred to as "dumping" and was obviously not in the best interests of the patient's medical needs in most cases.

In response to accumulating evidence of this economically driven denial of care throughout the country, in 1985 Congress enacted a law that was intended to prevent this unethical practice. The Emergency Medical Treatment and Active Labor Act (EMTALA) was a part of the Consolidated Omnibus Budget Reconciliation Act (COBRA), and while it has been amended a number of times it remains the most significant regulation ever enacted related to the emergency care and transfer of patients in the United States. It was the first law that provided a right to emergency medical care for every citizen.

The law defines a hospital's responsibility to provide emergency care to anyone presenting with a request for help. It details the obligations of the hospital with regard to initial evaluation and management as well as with regard to transfer arrangements. Hospitals are obligated to obey these guidelines under penalty of hefty fines.

Shortly after this law was enacted that mandated the emergency care of any patient requesting such, a new problem emerged. The original language of EMTALA mandated the care that must be provided at the hospital to which the patient presents but did not address the responsibilities of higher level centers to which patients might be transferred. When hospitals attempted to transfer patients they felt were in need of care at another facility, they encountered difficulty in getting acceptance of these patients. This problem also appeared to have financial motivation in some cases. This is sometimes referred to as "reverse dumping" and is just as big an ethical issue as the original problem.

In 1989, EMTALA was amended to include language that required higher level hospitals to accept patients in transfer when they had the ability to manage the patients' condition. The details of the many amendments of these laws are rather confusing; therefore, interpretive guidelines have been issued over the years clarifying hospitals' responsibilities under the law.[7]

▨ SENDING HOSPITAL OBLIGATIONS

Screen and Stabilize The law requires that every hospital provide an appropriate screening examination to any patient who requests examination or treatment. This screening cannot be delayed for financially motivated reasons. If the screening examination reveals an emergency medical condition, the hospital is obligated to stabilize the patient, or if this is not possible, transfer the patient to a hospital that can. The interpretive guidelines issued over the years are extensive and have clarified many of the details regarding these responsibilities.

Affect an Appropriate Transfer There are a number of requirements for sending hospitals when arranging the transfer of an unstable patient. First is the certification of medically necessity. The documentation of this may take many forms but must include a definition of the medical benefits expected from transfer as well as the risks that can reasonably be expected by the transfer. The sending facility must certify that the expected benefits outweigh the potential risks of the transfer.

Consent for transfer must always be obtained, whether directly from the patient or family member or implied under the emergency doctrine. This consent must be in writing and is often included as a part of the certification of risks and benefits.

The sending hospital has an obligation of arrange an "appropriate" transfer. There are five components to this outlined in the law:

1. The hospital must provide treatment within their capacity to minimize the risks of transfer. This might range anywhere from initiating

IV access to intubation or chest tube placement if it is felt that these interventions would reduce the risk of the transfer.

2. Arrangements must be made for another hospital to accept the patient in transfer. Simply transferring a patient without having another hospital identified that it is willing and able to accept the patient would constitute a violation of the law.

3. It is a legal obligation for the sending facility to ensure that relevant data be sent with the patient for use by the receiving staff in continuation of care. This includes documentation of care and radiographic studies performed.

4. The transfer must be affected through qualified personnel and transportation equipment. It is important to recognize that the needs of the patient are not just what the patient needs at the time of the transfer, but has to include potential needs if the situation changes during the move. This must be based on the treating physician's best estimate of what the patient may need during transfer. For example, if a patient with an acute coronary syndrome is being transferred, there is a good possibility that they may experience an arrhythmia during transport. The team chosen to complete that transfer must be qualified and have the equipment necessary (ie, medications and defibrillator) to effectively manage arrhythmias. Similarly, a patient with an acute stroke may deteriorate and require intubation during transport. The team accompanying the patient should be qualified and have appropriate equipment to offer this intervention if needed.

The vehicle utilized should be that which is determined to be most appropriate for the patient's condition at the judgment of the sending physician.

5. It is also crucial to consider that the sending facility is legally responsible for the patient until care is assumed by the receiving facility. This includes the care provided by the transport agency. It seems imperative for the sending facility to have a proper understanding of the capabilities of the transport team. There should be prior communication and preplanning between hospitals and transport agencies in order to facilitate safe transport of these patients.

It is important to remember that the EMTALA regulations regarding transfers relate to *unstable* patients, those whose conditions have not been stabilized. Once a patient has been stabilized, these regulations do not apply and transfers can be arranged for economic reasons if desired. EMTALA defines "stabilized" as when it is determined that a patient will not likely deteriorate during transfer. An appropriate level of care for the patient's current needs is obviously still required.

RECEIVING HOSPITAL OBLIGATIONS

Hospitals that offer specialized services have an obligation under EMTALA to accept patients in transfer if they have the ability and capacity to manage that patient's condition at that time. This must be done without any consideration of the patient's ability to pay for such care. Refusal to accept transfers is one of the largest areas of EMTALA violation investigations. This has led to very complicated algorithms in some hospitals to determine the hospital's capacity at any given time for managing any given condition. If a hospital determines that it does not have the ability or capacity to manage a patient for whom transfer is requested, they can refuse without being in violation of the law. This would seem to be very reasonable, as it would not be safe to bring an unstable patient to a hospital that did not have the ability to safely manage their condition. In today's age of hospital overcrowding, overfull emergency departments and lack of hospital beds may result in interfacility transfers that bypass one or more institutions that would have otherwise been able to manage a patient's condition. This translates into what may be very long transport times for the IFT team.

TRANSPORT PROVIDER OBLIGATIONS

While the practice of an EMS provider during interfacility transfer is not directly detailed in this regulation, it is helpful to understand the background behind the details of the transfer process. It is clear that there

are legal obligations for the transport agency and providers to affect a medically appropriate patient transport in the safest manner possible; however, they are not detailed under EMTALA. These regulations may differ from state to state and the EMS physician involved with a transport team should be familiar with the relevant local regulation.

It certainly makes sense for a transport service to meet with local hospitals for purposes of preplanning regarding IFT needs. The transport service should educate the hospital regarding the capabilities of the transport team and equipment. This knowledge will enable the facility to make appropriate decisions regarding staffing during a transfer. There may be times when it is necessary for hospital staff to accompany a patient during transfer. It is helpful to have some sort of collaborative training prior to this occurrence that enables the hospital staff to function safely in the transport vehicle. Clarification of the roles and responsibilities of each of the providers staffing the transport in this case is helpful.

CURRENT PRACTICE

In the United States today, EMS systems have evolved to accommodate the needs of the patients they encounter. The presence of technology assisted patients in the community has led to increased specialized training for EMS providers who will be called upon to transport them if the need arises. In much the same way, as hospitals within a community consolidate specific services to one regional center, the type of patient that requires transport between facilities will change. An EMS system should be aware of such changes within their region and take steps to ensure that the needs of the IFT patient are adequately met during transport. This may require additional training and equipment for EMS providers or it may require the development of a more advanced team that involves hospital-based resources. EMS systems around the country are widely disparate in their preparation for the IFT patient. Some systems are well tied in with regional hospitals and have advanced training and credentialing programs for providers while other systems offer less specific preparation to their providers. There are many factors to consider when developing an IFT program. The ultimate goal is to match patient need with appropriate knowledge, skills, equipment, and an infrastructure to enable safe, effective, and efficient IFT.[6]

THE PATIENT

Patients require transfer for any one of a number of reasons. These might include a need for specialized services not available at the original institution, desire for care by a particular physician or in a particular locale, or a need to move to a facility where a physical bed is available. Depending on the patient condition and reason for transfer, several categories of transfers should be discussed.

STABILIZED VERSUS NOT STABILIZED

As previously discussed, every hospital has a federal obligation to assess a patient who presents with a request for medical care. If the assessment reveals that the patient has an emergency medical condition, stabilization is required. A patient can be considered to be stabilized if they have been treated to a point where deterioration is felt to be unlikely during transfer. Depending on the patient's condition and specific needs, the hospital may not have the ability to stabilize their condition, making transfer in an unstable condition necessary. The hospital has an obligation to do everything they can to make the patient as safe as possible for transfer.

Not Stabilized The patient who remains unstable by definition has the possibility of deterioration during transport. The providers staffing the transport must have the training, equipment, and protocols to allow them to manage the deterioration that is predicted. An example of an unstable patient requiring transfer might be a patient with a ruptured abdominal aortic aneurysm who is at a hospital that does not have a vascular surgeon. This patient can be markedly unstable; however, despite that instability, transfer is necessary to offer definitive management. In this case, adequate intravenous access might be the necessary treatment provided by the hospital in order to best prepare the patient for emergent transfer. The transport team should have the ability to manage deterioration in this patient's condition to include advanced airway management, additional intravenous access, administration of crystalloid, and blood products where necessary.

CONDITIONS REQUIRING TRANSFER

There are many conditions that might require a patient to be transferred from one facility to another. This will be largely depending on the resources available at the local hospital. Some common emergency conditions often requiring transfer from community hospitals to larger institutions are listed in **Table 16-1**.

NEEDS DURING TRANSFER

Depending on the patient condition, the EMS provider may be required to perform different interventions during the course of the transfer. It is imperative that the provider be appropriately trained, and have the necessary equipment and guidelines to perform any skill that might be required during a patient transport.

THE TEAM

In order to appropriately match the transport team to the patient, several factors must be considered. These relate to the urgency of the patient's condition, the distance between facilities, and the interventions needed during the transfer.

TOTAL TIME

If the patient's outcome is dependent on how quickly they have a particular intervention performed, then everything should be done to decrease the time it takes to get to that intervention. An obvious example of this would be a ruptured abdominal aortic aneurysm. This patient needs surgical intervention quickly for the best outcome. This type of surgery is often only offered at specialized vascular centers. This requires any patient who presents to a hospital that does not have that capability be transferred for definitive care. In this case, the most appropriate transfer arrangement would be that which allowed the shortest total time to the operating room at the receiving facility while still allowing for proper care during the transport. Total time is important in conditions of a very time-sensitive nature where an intervention will be performed immediately upon arrival at the receiving center.

OUT-OF-HOSPITAL TIME

Some patients would be better off with less time spent out of the hospital even if it means extended time in the sending facility awaiting the transport team. Conditions that may fall into this category would include preterm

labor, neonatal emergencies, patients with hemodynamic instability, and other conditions that have increased risk of decompensation during the transport phase. In these situations air medical transport may offer the desired decreased out-of-hospital time and be justifiable. The sending physician must make this decision with knowledge of the time and distance involved as well as the available transport resources in the region.

LEVEL OF CARE

In general, the staffing required for an IFT should be determined based on the expected needs of the patient during the transport. There may be local regulation that specifies what type of provider must staff a given transport. The American College of Emergency Physicians specifies that a patient's condition and the potential for complications should dictate the level of services available during IFT.[8] In some systems, EMS leaders have provided guidance concerning this issue and communicate this in formal documents for providers to review.[9] The Santa Clara County document includes tables with drugs and interventions listed by provider type.

As in any hospital environment, the level of training required of the caregivers for a particular patient will depend on that patient's illness, the complexity of the interventions, and the frequency with which reassessments and changes in care are expected. For example, a patient who does not require ventilatory or hemodynamic support and whose condition is stable enough to not require reassessment more than every few hours might be appropriately situated on a nonintensive care unit of a hospital. The training level of the nursing staff is not at the critical care level and the ratio of patients to nurses is high. Similarly, the patient who is more unstable, who has need of reassessment more frequently or has interventions in place that require advanced training, will require an intensive care unit bed. Typically, the nursing staff on an ICU are credentialed by the hospital to perform additional advanced skills and the ratio of patients to nurses is much lower than on a non-ICU floor. This allows for the more unstable patients to be given more attention as their condition mandates. Ultimately, the level of care a patient receives in a hospital should be maintained during the transport, which then also dictates the level of IFT provider and type of equipment needed.

TRADITIONAL EMS

The majority of interfacility transports are completed by EMS providers who hold a standard certification with no additional training specific to IFT. Most patients who require transport from one hospital to another do not have needs that go beyond what a traditionally trained EMS provider is capable of handling. A small percentage of patients will have more extensive needs during transport. In this case, the options include providing additional training to the EMS provider or adding additional specially or alternatively trained staff to the transport team.

ADDITIONALLY TRAINED PROVIDERS

Knowing that traditional EMS training focuses on scene response, some may argue that an EMT at any level who intends to staff an IFT should have some form of additional training to prepare them for this new environment and patient population. This will likely be regulated at the state or local level. Some states, such as Maine, have formal programs for educating paramedics for this area of prehospital medicine, while other states allow a "critical care paramedic" designation to be given based on an agency medical director's determination of advanced education and skill. Currently, the Board for Critical Care Transport Paramedic Certification (BCCTPC) has developed standard credentialing examinations, and the International Association of Flight Paramedics (IAFP) has provided recommendations for training these personnel.

BASIC LIFE SUPPORT

Oxygen administration, CPR, and automatic defibrillation are included in the skill set of the EMT (EMT-basic). The EMT who staffs an IFT should have some basic knowledge of the laws surrounding the

TABLE 16-1	Specific Conditions That May Be Encountered in Interfacility Transfer		
Trauma	Nontrauma	Pediatric	Obstetrical
Traumatic brain injury	Acute coronary syndrome	Epiglottitis	Preterm labor
Spinal cord injury	Acute stroke	Reactive airway disease	Premature rupture of membranes
Vascular injury	Status epilepticus	Sepsis	Preeclampsia/eclampsia
Thoracic injuries	Respiratory failure	Diabetic ketoacidosis	Placental abruption
Intraabdominal injuries	Endocrine emergencies	Traumatic Injuries	Trauma during pregnancy
Orthopedic injuries	Aneurysms, dissections, or vascular occlusions		

movement of patients between hospitals. The scope of practice and any relevant policies regarding the EMT's responsibilities during an IFT are clearly of importance. Basic knowledge of the common conditions likely to be seen during IFT would be helpful to the EMT whose training is classically symptom based rather than diagnosis based. Finally, the EMT should have an understanding of the more common medical devices seen during these types of transports. These might include indwelling urinary catheters, nasogastric or gastrostomy tubes, and nonmedicated intravenous access devices. Depending on local training and policy, EMTs may be asked to move patients with these devices in place, yet not have received training in their management. This can present a safety hazard and can be alleviated by preplanning and training providers for the situations they are expected to see.

ADVANCED LIFE SUPPORT

As with the EMT at the basic level, the advanced EMT (AEMT) should also have an awareness of the relevant laws and policies regarding IFT in the local area. Knowing that the original AEMT training is meant to prepare the student to provide the initial assessment and management of a given symptom complex, the AEMT would also likely benefit from some additional training regarding management of the hospitalized patient. Once again, a patient with an actual diagnosis rather than an undifferentiated complaint is managed differently. A good example is that the patient who has chest pain and is diagnosed with an acute thoracic aortic dissection. Standard AEMT training and protocols would guide the administration of certain medications that might be contraindicated in this specific condition. Understanding the need for specific care guidelines based on the hospital diagnosis is important.

While the AEMT will have a broad knowledge base regarding pharmacology in a traditional training program, there are medications commonly used during IFT that are not usually seen during scene response. These medications deserve review for the AEMT staffing an IFT. Some common examples might be nitroglycerin or heparin infusions or administration of electrolytes or antibiotics.

Similarly, an AEMT has knowledge of anatomy and physiology that would enable understanding of common interventions utilized in hospitalized patients. Specific training regarding these devices would not likely have happened in the original training but would be important to have prior to an IFT in which it may be encountered. Some examples might include thoracostomy drainage tubes, ventilators, Swan-Ganz catheters, and intra-aortic balloon pumps.

SPECIALTY CARE TRANSPORT

The advent of the National Medicare Ambulance Fee Schedule on April 1, 2002, defined a separate category of reimbursement for IFT patients requiring specialized interventions beyond the scope of practice of EMT-paramedic. This level of reimbursement was labeled *specialty care transport* (SCT). These interventions were to be provided by professionals with appropriate training such as emergency or cardiovascular physicians, nurses, respiratory technicians, or paramedics with additional training.[10] While the billing schedule coined the term, it should be clear to the medical community that there was a need for a class of provider that had special training to care for critically ill patients during interfacility transfer.

Some might argue that the most appropriate staff to accompany a critically ill patient during IFT would be those credentialed by the hospital to manage their condition. However, hospital staff are not trained to practice in the out-of-hospital environment and would not typically be best suited for it. With this in mind, one might conclude that the ideal transport team would include both hospital-trained staff as well as EMS-trained staff. Some transport agencies' staff nurses and paramedics for this reason. Another alternative might be to have a nurse from the sending facility accompany the paramedic from the transport agency to the receiving facility. This is done in a number of areas and may serve to offer both levels of expertise to the patient. It is important to recognize that the hospital-trained nurses should have some specialized training to be best equipped to provide care in this nontraditional setting.

There is another option which is becoming more common as hospitals are experiencing nursing shortages and the training of paramedics is being expanded in several areas to serve local needs. This involves expanding the scope of practice of the paramedic to specifically enable them to care for critically ill patients during IFT. These paramedics are provided training beyond the standard curriculum specifically meant to prepare them to care for the critically ill patient during IFT. Ideally this training is accompanied by clinical training in a hospital. In keeping with the CMS terminology that was introduced in 2001, this level of care might be called *specialty care*.

PARAMEDIC WITH ADDITIONAL TRAINING

The scope of practice is the extent to which a health care provider is permitted to perform medical procedures. This is defined differently from state to state and might be based on the educational curriculum, protocols, or a stand-alone document detailing the procedures allowed. The EMS physician should be familiar with the prescribed scope of practice for the region in which he or she practices. To ask an EMS provider to perform procedures beyond that scope of practice would not be appropriate without specific guidelines to allow it and training to support it.[11]

A paramedic who is provided with additional training in a defined area has an expanded scope of practice. This should be clearly defined so that the provider knows to what level he may practice. This expanded scope of practice should be defined by the governing body or regulatory agency with authority over EMS providers in that locale. It is important to recognize that simply attending additional training or obtaining advanced certification by an accrediting organization (ie, BCCTPC) does not necessarily enable the provider to perform these interventions. If the intervention goes beyond the usual scope of practice for that provider, an expanded scope of practice should be defined. In jurisdictions that recognize critical care paramedics, these personnel should be utilized when IFT dictates this higher level of care. These personnel should be coupled with appropriate hospital staff when specialty drugs, equipment, or other interventions are being employed that are beyond the scope of the EMS provider performing the transport. Other types of critical care transport specialists include specially trained physicians, nurses, and respiratory therapists, and are typically assigned based on activation of specialty transport teams or as part of a specific critical care transport team or agency. Critical care paramedics are key members of these teams in some areas of the country.

HOSPITAL STAFF

It is not uncommon for a hospital staff member such as a nurse, respiratory therapist, or perfusionist to accompany a patient during an IFT. It is important to remember that even though providers may be caring for a critically ill patient in the hospital, they are often doing so under the supervision and guidance of a physician, following physician orders in a controlled hospital environment. For these reasons, hospital staff should have additional training if they are to be a part of a transport team. This training must address safety in a transport vehicle as well as the priorities associated with care of a patient in the transport environment. Independent practice is sometimes required especially in rural situations where online medical control may not be available. Written orders or guidelines must account for the inability to reach a physician during the transport phase.

An EMS system should work with their local hospitals to facilitate safety training for hospital staff that may have occasion to provide care in an ambulance during IFT.

SPECIALTY TEAM

Some hospitals with specialized services provide a team that will go to outlying hospitals and provide care during transport back to the tertiary care center. It is not uncommon for an EMS provider to accompany that

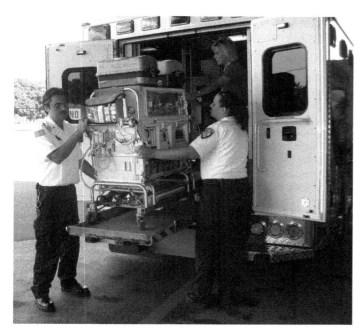

FIGURE 16-1. Pediatric and neonatal specialty teams offer specialized care to specific patient populations during IFT.

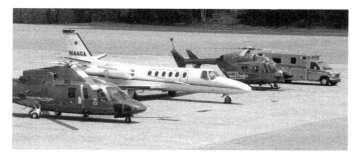

FIGURE 16-2. The transport vehicle is chosen based upon the needs of the patient.

team to assist them with patient movement and ensure their safety in the EMS vehicle. Pediatric and neonatal teams are probably the most common specialty teams encountered (**Figure 16-1**).

The utilization and benefits of specialized neonatal and pediatric teams have been well described and studied in this country.[12] The success of such teams has led in many areas to the development of other types of specialized teams such as obstetrical or cardiovascular teams. The EMS physician should be a part of the development of specialty transport teams to ensure appropriate integration within the existing EMS and transport systems. In some locales specialty teams are formed to support all types of critically ill patients and are part of the EMS system, in contrast to some hospital-based teams. Many of these teams are equally prepared to be deployed by ground or air medical transport. The participation of members that are cross-trained, licensed, and certified, such as nurse paramedics, may cause some regulatory issues if this is not adequately addressed relative to the existing laws, regulations, and policies of the particular locale.

THE VEHICLE

The type of vehicle used to move a patient during an IFT will be dependent on the patient's condition, the distance to the receiving center, and the staffing configurations of local services(**Figure 16-2**).

▧ GROUND AMBULANCE

Most IFT are completed by ground ambulance. The vehicle utilized must be large enough to accommodate the needed devices and staff and must be equipped with the necessary equipment for the patient's needs.

It should be intuitive, but is worth a reminder that all personnel and equipment must be secured in the back of the vehicle when the vehicle is in motion. The illness of a patient should never prompt a provider to make an unsafe decision for himself or herself or his or her team. On the same token, road conditions must be factored into the decision-making process when determining the safest mode of transport for a given patient. Poor road conditions may make the risk of transfer too great and a delay or alternative means of transport might be more acceptable.

▧ ROTOR WING

Patients who are in need of transfer from one facility to another may benefit from the use of rotor wing aircraft in several circumstances. The most obvious would relate to the speed of travel. This should be thought of in two circumstances. First, if the overall time to the receiving center can be minimized by use of a helicopter for transport it should be considered. This is especially relevant in time-dependent conditions in which a crucial therapy awaits the patient at the destination facility. Second, the out–of-hospital time can almost always be shortened by helicopter transport when compared with ground travel. This can be extremely important in patients who are unstable or whose conditions would not benefit from prolonged time in a moving vehicle.

Perhaps more commonly, air medical services are requested to transport patients between facilities for reasons related to the level of care that they offer. Increasingly, hospitals are beginning advanced therapies as they work to stabilize patients prior to transfer. These therapies require trained hands to manage during the transport. The presence of a team with advanced capabilities in the transport vehicle is necessary. In many areas, the most advanced teams are found on helicopters. Some areas do have ground-based critical care transport teams as well and those should be considered if the travel time is less of an issue.[13] Regardless of the vehicle used, it is imperative to realize that the level of care for the patient must be maintained from the sending to the receiving hospital.[14] Care during transport is an important, yet often forgotten phase of a patient's care.

Given the relative paucity of helicopters when compared with ground units, it is imperative that the helicopters be utilized only in circumstances in which they are felt to offer the most benefit. While every state and region should have guidelines to assist local providers with this determination, the Air Medical Physician Association has put forth its own "medical condition list and appropriate use of air medical transport."[15] This document can be considered to be a national standard and can be utilized when creating local guidelines.

▧ FIXED WING

In cases where the distance is greater than the range of a rotor wing service, fixed wing transport might be considered. While fixed wing transport is often more economically feasible than rotor wing, the additional time required to organize and complete a transport and the availability of such a service might preclude its use in a given locale. The team configuration of a fixed wing service is dependent on the operator. The EMS physician should be familiar with services offering fixed wing transport to his or her region.

EMS PHYSICIAN ROLE

▧ TEAM MEMBER

While in the minority, there are a few transport programs that staff a physician as a part of the transport team. While it may seem intuitively better to have this highly trained provider on board the ambulance, there does not seem to be that much of a difference in the interventions they offer or in the ultimate outcome of the patient. Some feel that appropriately trained nurses, paramedics, or respiratory therapists can accomplish the same task at a fraction of the cost.[16] If a physician is to be a member of a transport team, it is imperative that he or she receive training specific to the safety and priorities of interfacility transport.

MEDICAL DIRECTOR

A more common role for the EMS physician in the realm of IFT would be as the program or system medical director. Involvement of an appropriately knowledgeable physician in every aspect of a transport system is crucial. The physician who is charged with oversight of a transport team should have input into hiring, training, credentialing, protocol development, and quality assurance and should be counted on as an advocate for the team members as well as the IFT patient.[17]

The EMS physician is uniquely qualified to understand the key components of a transport program. Knowledge of the scope of practice of the EMS providers, capabilities of different vehicle types, safety factors surrounding out-of-hospital care, as well as inhospital priorities for management of critical patients make the EMS physician an ideal component of a development team for an IFT program.

Understanding the level of training and competence already achieved by the EMS providers in their region, an EMS physician should participate in the educational process for transport team members. Supplementing existing education or in some cases presenting previously learned material from a different perspective to enhance the providers understanding of the hospitalized patient's needs is a useful component to the training of a transport team.

Protocols to guide the practice of the transport team should be based on the known patient types and expected mission of the team. Conditions that are expected to be seen should be addressed sufficiently in both protocols and training. As advances in medical knowledge and practice occur within hospitals, the mission profile of the transport agency may change as well. Updates to protocols and training are necessary on an annual basis and should be based on changes in local practice and current literature. The program medical director should oversee this annual review.

As with any medical practice, the quality of a transport team must continually be reviewed through a total quality management program. Reviewing the care provided by team members and addressing any perceived issues through an established educational process is within the responsibilities of the medical director.

FUTURE DIRECTIONS

REGULATION

While EMTALA does not specifically address the responsibility of a transport team or the EMS system, many states have enacted regulation or offered guidance to this issue. Being in the position to understand the difference between standard prehospital provider education and the training required for members of an IFT team, the EMS physician should participate in development of such guidelines where none exist.

It is incumbent upon an EMS system to ensure that it is adequately prepared to care for all patients in all circumstances, whether prehospital or interhospital. The EMS physician is a critical component to that preparation.

While the organization of the EMS system in each state differs, it is clearly beneficial to have guidance from the appropriate governing bodies and regulatory agencies that will ensure that the goal of matching every patient with the team that has the appropriate knowledge, skills, and equipment is met. Given the sometimes vast differences in the available resources from one region to another, standardization of training and credentialing for providers may be difficult at a state level but may be more appropriately accomplished at a regional level with guidance from the overseeing state body. The EMS physician should always advocate for transport team members and patients by ensuring that appropriate regulations are in place and that protocols, training, and equipment are all sufficient to allow for the interfacility transport of all patients within the system to be accomplished in the safest manner possible.

SPECIALIZATION OF EMS PROVIDER

As hospital systems continue to regionalize and consolidate services, increasing numbers of patients are being transported between facilities in order to receive definitive care for their condition. In many areas, the complexity of the patient care is increasing with advancing technology. EMS providers are called upon to care for patients during IFT that their original training has not prepared them for. It is becoming increasingly common for EMS providers to participate in advanced training programs that supplement their knowledge regarding this sometimes complicated patient population. While the original intent of the EMS system may not have been to care for patients being moved from one intensive care unit to another, the creative flexibility unique to the EMS environment has led to increasing specialization of the EMS provider to meet the needs of their community. The field of interfacility transport offers a potential career path for EMS providers.

IFT EMS PHYSICIAN TRAINING

The EMS physician who will be tasked with providing oversight to an IFT team should ensure that he or she is knowledgeable regarding the patient conditions that are likely to be cared for by his team. This may necessitate seeking training outside his usual specialty, often emergency medicine. There are a significant number of patients that require transport between facilities that have interventions in place that are not commonly utilized in an emergency department. Colleagues in other specialties such as critical care, obstetrics, and neonatology may be called upon by the *program medical director* to offer assistance with additional training and development of protocols specific to their patient populations. It may also be useful to call upon these physicians for quality assurance review of cases that are specific to their specialty. A strong working relationship between the *transport team medical director* and receiving specialty physicians is useful in supplementing his or her area of expertise and in keeping up to date on changes in practice within each area.

SUMMARY

Patients being moved between facilities have specific needs, sometimes quite complex in nature. The providers tasked with caring for them during the transport must be adequately trained, equipped, and empowered to offer the most appropriate level of care. The EMS physician is uniquely qualified to develop and oversee such a team and should play a key role in development of regulation and guidance to ensure the safety and standardization of interfacility transport in their region.

KEY POINTS

- Interfacility transport is the movement of a patient from one health care facility to another, most often accomplished by EMS providers.
- Patients are often transferred between facilities in order to obtain care not available at the original hospital.
- The Emergency Medical Treatment and Active Labor Act defines the responsibilities of the sending and receiving facilities and specifies that any transport must be medically appropriate.
- An EMS system should establish protocols to guide providers staffing interfacility transports.
- Emergency medical technicians and paramedics will often obtain additional training in order to be best equipped to manage patients during IFT. If the patient requires a level of care beyond that of the available EMS providers, appropriately credentialed hospital personnel may join the transport team.

- The EMS physician has an important role in oversight of an interfacility transport program.
- The vehicle used for transport should be chosen based on the patient's needs and local resources.
- Dedicated teams may provide interfacility transport care for specialized patient types such as neonatal, pediatric, or obstetrical patients.

REFERENCES

1. Cooper G, Laskowski-Jones L. Development of trauma care systems. *Prehosp Emerg Care.* July-September 2006;10(3):328-331.
2. Alberts MJ, Latchaw RE, Selman WR, et al. Recommendations for comprehensive stroke centers: a consensus statement form the brain attack coalition. *Stroke.* July 2005;36(7):1597-616.
3. Kereiakes DJ. Specialized centers and systems for heart attack care. *Am Heart Hosp J.* Winter 2008;6(1):14-20.
4. Mechem CC, Goodloe JM, Richmond NJ, et al. Resuscitation center designation: recommendations for emergency medical services practices. *Prehosp Emerg Care.* January-March 2010;14(1):51-61.
5. Chen WL, Ma HP, Wu CH, et al. Clinical research of mortality in emergency air medical transport. *Biomed Res Int.* 2014;2014:767402.
6. NHTSA guide for interfacility patient transfer. http://www.nhtsa.gov/people/injury/ems/Interfacility/. Accessed May 15, 2015.
7. Bitterman RA. Providing Emergency Care under Federal Law; EMTALA. American College of Emergency Physicians, Irving, TX, 2000.
8. Interfacility Transportation of the Critical Care Patient and its Medical Direction. ACEP Board of Directors, September 2005. https://www.acep.org/Clinical-Practice-Management/Interfacility-Transportation-of-the-Critical-Care-Patient-and-Its-Medical-Direction/. Accessed May 15, 2015.
9. Santa Clara County Emergency Medical Services Agency. Interfacility transfer by ground or air ambulance. Reference EMS-808. http://www.sccgov.org/sites/ems/Documents/pcm800/808.pdf. Accessed May 15, 2015.
10. Centers for Medicare and Medicaid Services. January-December 31, 2015 Ambulance Fee Schedule. Baltimore, MD. November 2011.
11. Kupas DF, Wang HE. Critical care paramedics—a missing component for safe interfacility transport in the United States. *Ann Emerg Med.* July 2014;64(1):17-18.
12. Orr RA, Felmet KA, Han Y, et al. Pediatric specialized transport teams are associated with improved outcomes. *Pediatrics.* July 2009;124(1):40-48.
13. Borst GM, Davies SW, Waibel BH, et al. When birds can't fly: an analysis of interfacility ground transport using advanced life support when helicopter emergency medical service is unavailable. *J Trauma Acute Care Surg.* August 2014;77(2):331-336.
14. Guidelines for the transfer of critically ill patients. Guidelines Committee, American College of Critical Care Medicine, Society of Critical Care Medicine and the Transfer Guidelines Task Force. *Am J Crit Care.* May 1993;2(30):189-195.
15. Air Medical Physician Association. Medical condition list and appropriate use of air medical transport. *Air Med J.* May-June 2003;22(3):14-19.
16. King BR, King TM, Foster RL, McCans KM. Pediatric and neonatal transport teams with and without a physician: a comparison of outcomes and interventions. *Pediatr Emerg Care.* February 2007;23(2):77-82.
17. Shelton SL, Swor RA, Domeier RM, Lucas R. Medical direction of interfacility transports. *Prehosp Emerg Care.* October-December 2000;4(4):361-364.

INTRODUCTION

Our colleagues in pediatrics often remind us that children "are not just little adults." In much the same way, rural EMS is not just "little" EMS. Rural EMS departments not only face the same issues as their urban counterparts, but also must cope with challenges specific to rural areas, such as limited local resources and geographic isolation.[1] Because of these differences, rural EMS requires more than just downsizing an urban system to be successful. This chapter will highlight some of the challenges unique to rural EMS systems, and allow the reader to begin to develop an approach to rural medical direction.

OBJECTIVES

- Describe the unique challenges to providing emergency response and EMS care in rural locations.
- Describe differences in volunteer/paid status, provider certification, experience level, and burnout rates when compared to urban EMS.
- Discuss how resource utilization may be different in rural areas.
- Discuss unique injury types and safety concerns in rural areas.
- Describe challenges in EMS agency finance.

DEFINITIONS

The term *rural* brings to mind low population density, few resources spread over a large area, and perhaps a harsh or austere natural environment. The US Census defines "rural" as all areas that are not urban, with "urban" defined as areas having at least 2500 people.[2] Based on this definition, about 72% of land in the United States is considered rural, and about 14s% of the US population, or around 46.2 million people, live there.[3] The term *frontier* has also been used to classify locations of even smaller population density, and is generally defined as a population of six or fewer people per square mile, and a certain traveling distance from key services such as hospitals.[4,5] According to this definition, about 56% of total land area in the United States is frontier, and about 3% of the population resides there.[6] For this chapter, unless specifically stated, the term *rural* will serve to represent both rural and frontier areas (**Figure 17-1**).

RURAL DEMOGRAPHICS

As difficult as it is to define rural areas, it is also difficult to make generalizations about the characteristics of rural populations in the United States. Sometimes, there is more variation between rural areas in different regions of the country than between rural and urban areas in the same region. Looking at census data from across the United States, a greater proportion of the rural population is older than 65 and white, fewer have graduated from college, and there is a lower mean household income as well as a higher poverty rate. In terms of health-related measures, there is no significant difference in health insurance coverage between rural and urban areas, although this varies by region. On a self-reported survey, more rural adults are current smokers, are obese, and more have hypertension, heart disease, cancer, or have had a stroke. Disparities exist in many areas of health care as well. There are proportionately fewer primary care physicians, with about 5 to 6 per 10,000 population in rural areas versus 9 per 10,000 in urban areas as well as far fewer specialists.[7]

Despite a general decline of age-adjusted mortality over the years in both rural and urban areas across the country, the rate of decline has become less in rural areas, leading to a rural "mortality penalty." The cause

of this remains unclear, but is present in cardiac disease, cancer, and stroke, the three leading causes of death in adults in the United States.[8,9] Theories include difficulty initiating appropriate interventions in a timely manner for patients with time-sensitive medical conditions, such as acute myocardial infarction or stroke, and the difficulty of small hospitals in implementing advances in medical care. Although not specifically studied, it stands to reason that a lack of robust EMS systems in many rural parts of the country may contribute to this mortality penalty for rural residents. This highlights the need for improvements in all aspects of rural health care, including EMS, and the importance of active medical direction.

The challenges for rural EMS systems to help combat the mortality penalty are highlighted in some of the major medical emergencies faced by EMS on a daily basis. ST-elevation myocardial infarction (STEMI) is well established as a time-sensitive medical condition with the traditional goal of PCI being achieved within 90 minutes from arrival at the hospital ("door-to-balloon" time). However, since many patients have the diagnosis of STEMI first made on initial evaluation by EMS, emphasis is now being placed on EMS-to-balloon time, with the same goal of 90 minutes.[10] However, it is estimated that 43.6 million adults in the United States live more than 60 minutes from a PCI-capable facility.[11] This makes early recognition of STEMI by rural EMS providers especially important through symptom recognition and early prehospital ECG acquisition.[12-14] Combined with prearrival notification of the cardiac catheterization lab team, and development of protocols to bypass closer but non-PCI capable facilities, rural EMS can help reduce delays and improve outcomes.[10,15]

Studies also suggest worse outcomes for stroke patients presenting to rural hospitals. Barriers to stroke care include lack of neurology specialists and designated stroke teams, lack of 24-hour CT access, and decreased comfort of providers in giving thrombolytics. Furthermore, standards of stroke care tend to be developed at large urban medical centers with extensive resources; implementation of the same standards in small rural hospitals may be impractical.[16] Prehospital care of the stroke patient begins with recognition of the signs and symptoms of an acute stroke, determination of the time of onset of symptoms, and prearrival notification of the nearest appropriate facility.[17] Unfortunately, it has been shown that EMS can have difficulty in stroke assessment. In response to some deficiencies in rural stroke care, the Montana Stroke Initiative sought to provide stroke education to communities, prehospital care providers, and rural hospitals.[18] This and similar training programs are available to EMS providers and may help improve rural stroke care.

In addition to the challenges of rural cardiac and stroke care, multiple studies have shown a higher rate of mortality for rural versus urban trauma victims, for all causes of trauma.[19-22] The cause of this disparity is still unclear, but factors specific to rural environments, such as distance from the scene to definitive medical care, higher speed limits on rural roads, decreased seat belt use, alcohol intoxication, and transport to local hospitals versus trauma centers may all play a role. Studies have reached conflicting conclusions as to the role EMS time intervals (activation, on scene, and transport times) play in mortality in trauma.[19,20,22] Intuitively, shortening the time it takes to reach a hospital would improve survival; studies show IV placement en route rather than on scene achieves a shorter time, while demonstrating a higher success rate.[23,24] However, other studies have shown improved survival for patients with longer EMS contact time, possibly due, in part, to transporting directly to a trauma center and bypassing smaller, less equipped hospitals.[22] Providers may be uncomfortable transporting potentially critical patients past a local hospital to a regional stroke, cardiac or trauma center; however, medical directors should work with EMS agencies and the local and regional health care systems to develop the most appropriate approach for the area.

UNIQUE INJURY TYPES AND SAFETY CONCERNS

In addition to the everyday call types of all EMS agencies, there are some illnesses and injuries unique to rural areas. Farm equipment such as tractors, augers, corn huskers, combines, and thrashers all have multiple

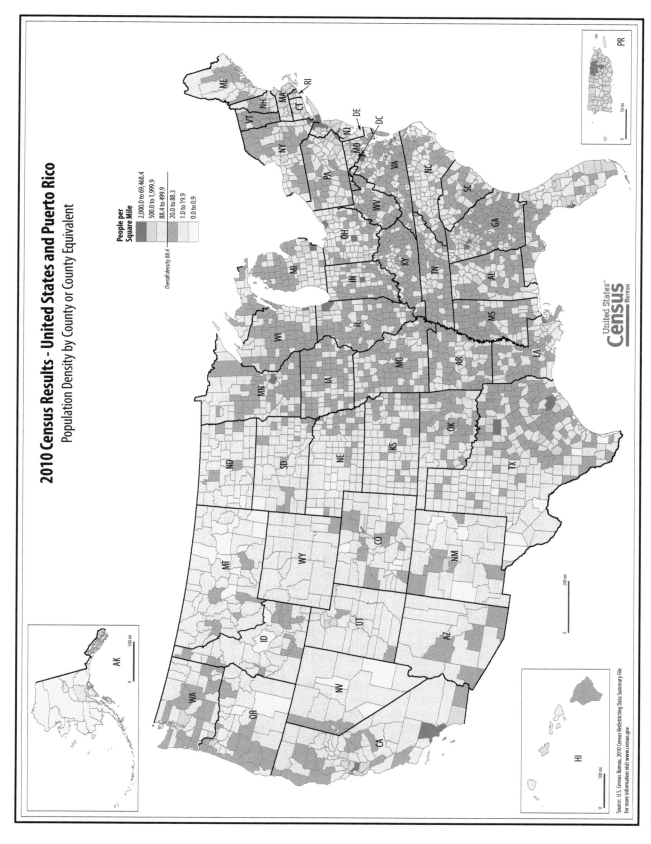

2010 Census Results - United States and Puerto Rico
Population Density by County or County Equivalent

People per Square Mile

- 2,000.0 to 69,468.4
- 500.0 to 1,999.9
- 88.4 to 499.9
- 20.0 to 88.3
- 1.0 to 19.9
- 0.0 to 0.9

Overall density 88.4

United States Census Bureau

Source: U.S. Census Bureau, 2010 Census Redistricting Data Summary File
For more information visit www.census.gov.

FIGURE 17-1. 2010 Population distribution in the United States and Puerto Rico.

dangerous moving parts capable of trapping, crushing, or amputating body parts. In addition, typical EMS rescue tools may not be effective on farming equipment and their use may inflict further injury to the victim.[25] Although most new farming implements come with warning labels and safety mechanisms to help prevent injuries, older equipment may not have these, or workers may intentionally disable safety features to ease access for maintenance. Farm workers may also routinely come into contact with various fuels, solvents, pesticides, and herbicides, which can result in life-threatening exposures and potential exposure to responders. Furthermore, many locations, such as grain silos and livestock pens can pose unique challenges for patient access. Programs, such as the FARMEDIC program begun in the early 1980s in New York State, can help train rural EMS providers to deal with these unique situations, and may be a valuable addition to standard EMS training.[25]

In addition to chemical exposures on farms, large agribusiness or other industrial plants may pose significant HAZMAT risks for the surrounding area. It should not be assumed that the facility's response plan to an event is adequate or accurately estimates the capability of the local EMS agencies. Frank and open discussions with facility safety personnel by local EMS agency staff, including the medical director, can help both sides understand the potential risks and develop response plans for any possible event. In addition to fixed sites, rural EMS agencies and systems must prepare for potential HAZMAT events occurring while dangerous materials are in transit through the area. There may be particular hazards for a specific region based on rail lines and transport routes. Familiarity with HAZMAT procedures as they pertain to EMS response is important for medical directors, and is covered in detail in other chapters.

UNIQUE POPULATIONS

Rural areas are home to many unique and sometimes socially independent populations. Native American reservations are found in many rural areas, and may have independent medical care, but also utilize local EMS. Other unique populations include isolated religious groups, such as the Amish, and other independent-minded individuals, who may have nontraditional attitudes toward modern medicine. For example, the Amish do not object to modern medical care; however, vaccination and prenatal care may not be routine, and they often do not purchase health insurance.[26] Therefore, the cost of medical services is paid out-of-pocket from the entire community, and is a consideration when outside medical care is sought. This can result in more serious presentations of disease not routinely seen by EMS personnel, particularly with trauma, obstetrical, and pediatric emergencies.[27]

Beyond the atypical patient presentations, rural EMS agencies may also face wide variation in the size of the population being served. The population surge may be over days to weeks in the case of county fairs, rodeos, and sporting events, or over weeks to months in the case of seasonal attractions, such as ski resorts and national parks. Seasonal migrant workers may also expand the population at various times of the year. In some cases, the population surges are impressive.[28] The Black Hills Motorcycle Rally in Sturgis, South Dakota, adds 500,000 to 750,000 additional motorcyclists to the usual population of around 6000 almost overnight. Yellowstone National Park attracts about 3 million visitors each year, above the state population of 493,000. These massive surges are particularly challenging in rural areas where resources are already very limited. Defined events such as festivals may require weeks of planning, and may require coordination between multiple agencies, and possibly contracting with additional commercial ground and air medical services to fully prepare. When EMS agencies are working together, it may be necessary to modify protocols or grant temporary credentials for providers working under a different system. In addition, providers and medical directors should plan for the demographics of the expected population surge, and the expected illness or injury patterns. Trauma is to be expected at ski resorts and motorcycle rallies. In addition, however, visitors to parks and festivals may have multiple comorbidities, leading to complicated presentations to EMS.

RURAL EMS PROVIDERS

Many of the challenges with rural EMS medical direction rise from the unique characteristics and differences in both providers and agencies compared to urban systems. Rural providers are more likely to be volunteers, older, EMT-B level providers, and often have less access to training programs and continuing education opportunities.[29-31] Recruitment and retention is especially difficult in rural areas. Many rural EMS providers choose to volunteer; however, demands of work, family, and other activities, coupled with the significant time commitment of EMS and lack of appropriate pay, mean that rural agencies have a harder time filling vacancies. Rural agencies have attempted to solve these problems in unique ways. One volunteer BLS agency encourages members with a $20 per shift stipend. Another rural area uses a paid ALS agency to cover a large area, and maintains a volunteer BLS agency as backup. After their local ER closed, one hospital provided and staffed an ALS intercept vehicle to help rural BLS agencies. Unfortunately, not every rural EMS agency has this ability and recruitment and retention remains a major issue.[32]

Even if an individual is willing and able to serve, becoming certified and maintaining that certification can be very challenging. EMS students may have to travel long distances several times a week for EMT classes and clinical rotations, making it even more difficult for rural providers to attain advanced certification. In addition, once certified, maintaining certification and skills retention can be daunting in many areas due to lack of education resources. Some of this can be accomplished through computer programs and distance learning programs, and/or teleconferencing to provide training and continuing education to EMS personnel who live far from education centers.[33] In addition, a rural EMS medical director must take the time to hold regular training sessions to ensure continued competency of the providers operating under his or her license.[34] This can be difficult if the medical director does not live or work locally or provides direction for multiple agencies. However, creative solutions such as meeting with multiple small agencies at once or utilizing regional resources to provide some educational materials and supplies may help.

PROTOCOL DEVELOPMENT

Protocol development is another area of rural EMS medical direction that requires understanding of the unique issues in the rural setting. As highlighted in the chapter, a paradox exists that the farther away from medical care a patient is, the more likely a higher level of prehospital care needed, but is least likely to be available.[35] Protocols are one way to help address this issue.[36] There are multiple models of EMS protocols, from statewide or regional protocols to local community or agency-specific protocols. All of these approaches have advocates and detractors and no approach is perfect. A rural medical director must work within state and regional regulations to develop the best approach for his or her agency. Not every agency can support ALS operations and smaller agencies may only have one or two advanced providers. A medical director must discuss with agency leaders if the training and costs of drugs and supplies, along with meeting various regulations and quality measures, are worth having for the occasional advanced response capability. One solution can be to incorporate multiple small agencies in a general geographic area to work together and share resources, training, and even personnel. Regardless of whether an agency's protocols are simplified or highly aggressive, involved medical direction is critical during development and implementation.

RURAL EMS AGENCIES

It has been said that "if you've seen one EMS system, you have seen one EMS system." This certainly holds true for rural EMS agencies, and there is wide variability in the types of agencies found across the country. An agency may be paid, volunteer, or a mix of both. It may be fire department, municipal, or hospital based, a freestanding EMS agency, or commercially owned, or it may be a hybrid of multiple models. A geographic area may be covered by one larger agency or multiple smaller agencies. They may be transporting or nontransporting. For a rural EMS medical director, it is important to understand the different capabilities and response plans for not only his or her agency or agencies, but for surrounding agencies as well.

Funding can be a challenge for all EMS systems, and is more difficult for those in rural areas. Every EMS agency, no matter what the size, has a set of fixed costs, including ambulances and other response vehicles, fuel, equipment, supplies, and buildings.[35] With economies of scale, the more calls run, the lower the percentage of costs that are fixed. One way this is typically measured in EMS is *unit hour utilization* (UHU). The typical calculation for the UHU ratio is to divide the number of transports by *unit hours*. A unit hour is typically defined as a fully staffed and equipped ambulance for 1 hour. This calculation, done at the system level, can help indicate the efficiency of the EMS system and provide a way to determine if changes are beneficial or not. UHU can be affected by percentage of transports versus patient "sign-offs", and transport time. A busy urban system with multiple hospitals and short transport times can obtain a UHU greater than 0.5, and small adjustments in staffing or procedures may produce noticeable improvements in UHU. Unfortunately, even in strong and well-organized rural EMS systems, the low call volume, long transport time, and rural patient demographics with possible increased "sign-offs" have a negative effect on UHU, sometimes producing numbers well below 0.1. However, it must be emphasized that when considering rural EMS systems, improved UHU does not necessarily correlate with better patient outcomes or quality of care, but is simply a tool that tracks utilization of resources. Although UHU can be a potential tool for rural agencies, it must be balanced with other evaluation benchmarks to justify budgets for resources and should not be the only metric utilized.

Another ongoing challenge for rural agency funding is being able to collect for services. The process of billing for services with multiple payers and ever changing regulations is complicated, and many small agencies simply do not have the qualified personnel to bill effectively for services, leading to lost potential revenue. In addition to income from patient transports, EMS agencies often rely on funding from local taxes, local hospital support, fundraising, and various types of local, state, or federal grants, all of which can be highly variable and dependent on overall economic health and priorities for the funding agencies. Medical directors can serve an important role by working with agencies to educate local funding sources in the importance of the EMS system and help justify continued financial support. Specifically, medical directors should work with agencies to find ways to lower costs, through local hospital pharmaceutical exchange programs, grants designed for rural areas, and protocols adjusted to use alternate and less expensive drugs or equipment. Finally, there are several different types of resources for rural EMS grants that may not come from the traditional local resources. These can come from states, federal agencies, or private institutions and a simple Web search is a good place to start. Although not a complete list, **Table 17-1** provides some resource types and specific Web resources that could be useful for rural agencies.

ENVIRONMENTAL

The terrain itself can also challenge rural and frontier systems. Even when addresses are organized and well marked, being able to locate the patient may be difficult in rural settings. The first challenge is simply determining where the call is coming from. Advanced, or "E9-1-1", allows the call taker to see the number of the caller and the location of the call while on the line with the caller. Although E9-1-1 is common in urban areas, there are still large rural areas of the country not covered. "Wireless E9-1-1", which uses cell tower locations to triangulate the location of the caller, is even less likely to be available in rural areas.[37] Without this service, those calling 9-1-1 from mobile phones must know their location, which may be difficult for visitors to these isolated areas.

TABLE 17-1	Sources of Grant Funding	
Type	Examples	Notes
Government	Department of Health Department of Emergency Services Department of Homeland Security FEMA HRSA CDC NHTSA	• Often originate from federal programs and distributed locally • Local branches may manage grant funds from several sources and can be good resources
Professional organizations	NAEMSP ACEP AAEM NAEMT NVFC RAC	• Consider fire and police organizations as well as EMS • Good source of grants for scholarships/training
Commercial	EMS/medical supply companies Local businesses	• Businesses may have community support or grant programs
Nonprofits	Memorial foundations Health care–related nonprofits (ie, United Way)	• Not necessarily EMS specific • May need to "think outside the box" to relate grants from these sources to EMS • Includes foundations in honor of victims of illness or injury that may provide funds or grants
Other	www.federalgrantswire.com www.ems1.com/grants/ www.emsgrantshelp.com	• Free and fee-based resources for grants

After obtaining the location of the patient, the next challenge is to reach that location. Directions to a rural call may include a lengthy set of instructions including landmarks and statements such as "turn just past the site of the big barn fire last year." Rural areas often may not have coordinated address systems, and maps may not have been updated in years. Even when officials develop a new system, it must have acceptance by the community, and funding to replace signs and maps. In one successful project in rural Colorado, a revised addressing system was developed that led to the renaming of roads and changing of addresses throughout the county, including standardized, highly visible address markers. Although a success, it did take almost 9 years to finish the project in all the communities, in part due to logistical and political problems.[38]

Rural roads are not often in a simple grid pattern and may follow rivers, lakes, or mountains (**Figure 17-2**). Even when the location is known, determining the fastest route may be difficult and misleading using maps alone. One of the most useful technologies to come to EMS in some time, particularly for rural and frontier agencies, are small and affordable GPS units. While providers who live in the area they serve may feel they are adequately familiar with local roads, GPS has been shown to significantly decrease response times.[39] However, it should be kept in mind that a GPS unit is not perfect and standard maps should always be available as a backup. Nonetheless, GPS can help overcome some of the difficulty with rural EMS response.[40]

All this should highlight the importance of coordinated dispatch centers with personnel training in call interrogation techniques for rural communities. Communications and dispatch is covered in other chapters, but rural medical directors should become familiar with these topics and educate local leaders about the importance of E-9-1-1 systems, centralized dispatch with call interrogation, and GPS units for response vehicles.

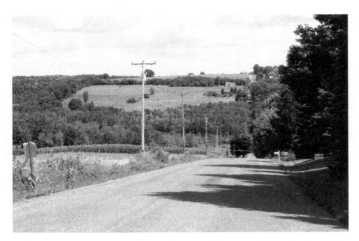

FIGURE 17-2. Rural road: roads in rural areas may be narrow, winding, and poorly lit at night. (Reproduced with permission from Stephen Dreher.)

After the location of the patient is found, access may still be a significant barrier in rural and frontier areas. Victims may be miles away, or thousands of feet up or down from the nearest access point. Wilderness search and rescue can often be part of the responsibilities of a rural EMS agency, either independently or as part of a much larger operation. Wilderness medicine is covered in more detail in a separate chapter, and the rural medical director should be somewhat familiar with the risks and requirements of search and rescue operations in which his or her providers will be involved. Prior planning for such events, and educating providers on good hygiene practices and on-scene rehabilitation for rescuers involved, can help minimize injuries and optimize the response capability.

Besides the dangers of rural and frontier terrain, the particular risks of extreme climate should be kept in mind. Flash floods, electrical storms, tornados, and blizzards can all occur with little warning and turn a routine call into a dangerous situation for patients and providers. Even when the weather is known, the challenges for EMS and search and rescue are significant due to extreme temperatures and other weather elements. Medical director involvement in training and decisions about when and how to respond in certain situations is paramount to ensure provider safety.

RESPONSE

Due to the lack of resources in most rural locations, different EMS agencies need to work closely together to provide adequate response for the areas they cover. This can be a particular challenge for several reasons. Rural areas may have old or outdated municipal and fire districts, which no longer represent current population distribution. There may also be fire or EMS agencies that persist for historical and sentimental reasons, despite redundancy, or inability for consistent and effective response. In the past, local agencies could be very territorial, not "allowing" a neighboring EMS unit to respond, even if closer to the location. Fortunately, much of this territorialism is gone due to changing attitudes and the reality of modern EMS. Nonetheless, it is important that the rural EMS medical director takes the time to learn about the history of area departments and their boundaries, and be sensitive to local customs in this regard if any attempt to implement change is to be successful.

Again, most EMS agencies today do work with each other as needed to provide EMS response for a given area. Rural EMS agencies will often have mutual aid agreements with nearby agencies to allow cross coverage if the primary agency cannot respond, or provide additional resources if needed. These agreements can involve neighboring agencies, or additional resources from city, county, state, or federal agencies, such as national parks. Despite the willingness to work together, the cooperating

agencies involved may have different staffing and may operate under different protocols, especially when agencies are responding from different regions, or even states.

Another way that rural areas have addressed EMS response is through the use of tiered systems. This may be especially vital for BLS or nontransporting agencies. ALS units may respond from a commercial, municipal, or hospital-based agencies, and may be automatically dispatched based on call type, or be requested by the BLS responding unit after patient contact is made. Either approach may be appropriate depending on the area's needs, but active medical direction is necessary to help optimize the system.

Air medical EMS is covered in detail elsewhere, but it plays a particularly important role in rural areas, providing faster transport to definitive care, and sometimes providing the first advanced life support to a patient. Furthermore, air medical services can significantly decrease transport time to definitive care for patients with time-sensitive medical conditions such as stroke or major traumatic injuries. Unfortunately, the need does not always correspond with the available coverage. Air medical units are very expensive to operate. This combined with difficult terrain and variable weather conditions means that while rural areas have a distinct need for air medical support, coverage in these areas may be variable and limited (**Figure 17-3**). It is also important for ground EMS personnel to be trained in the appropriate use of air medical services and not simply call for the helicopter because it is there. Various triage tools[41] and training programs for the ground ambulance crews can be used to aid in these decisions.

The decision of where to transport can have an even greater significance in rural areas, where transport to a larger regional center instead of the local hospital can mean a difference of hours. In areas with limited resources to begin with, this additional time can translate into lack of coverage for a district, and significantly increase costs. Although miles can be billed, the unit will still be out of service for an extended period of time and may leave part of their district uncovered, straining neighboring mutual aid agencies. Although transporting to regional centers may add significant time, patients should ideally be taken to the most appropriate facility. The agency medical director must navigate local tendencies and politics that can influence transport decisions toward either the local hospital to avoid long transport times or routinely bypassing the local hospital because of perception of hospital capabilities. Working with all stakeholders, the rural medical director can help create a system in which patients are transported to the correct facility efficiently.

EXPANDED SCOPE EMS

Given the frequent lack of medical resources, some rural communities have turned to EMS to provide medical services beyond their usual scope of practice. This seems like an attractive option; EMS providers have a certain amount of medical training and experience, and may have a relatively small call volume. The communities frequently lack adequate health care resources, including primary physicians, and visiting nursing care. In addition, there may be significant physical barriers in the natural environment, such as in the case of island communities, to obtaining frequent medical care. The use of EMS for medical care beyond their usual scope of practice has been referred to by several names, including expanded scope EMS, community paramedicine, or mobile integrated health care.[42-46]

Projects have ranged from simple safety screenings to training paramedics to staff a community health clinic, with varying success. One program in a rural community in New York State developed a brief questionnaire for elderly patients, including a screening for fall risk, depression, and medication safety, including referral to appropriate resources if indicated.[47] Two isolated island communities in Nova Scotia developed protocols for expanded scope of practice for paramedics, in conjunction with a nurse practitioner on the islands. This included wound care, blood pressure and diabetic checks, and phlebotomy services, as well as safety education. An ambitious project in rural New Mexico established a clinic staffed by expanded scope EMS providers, after training

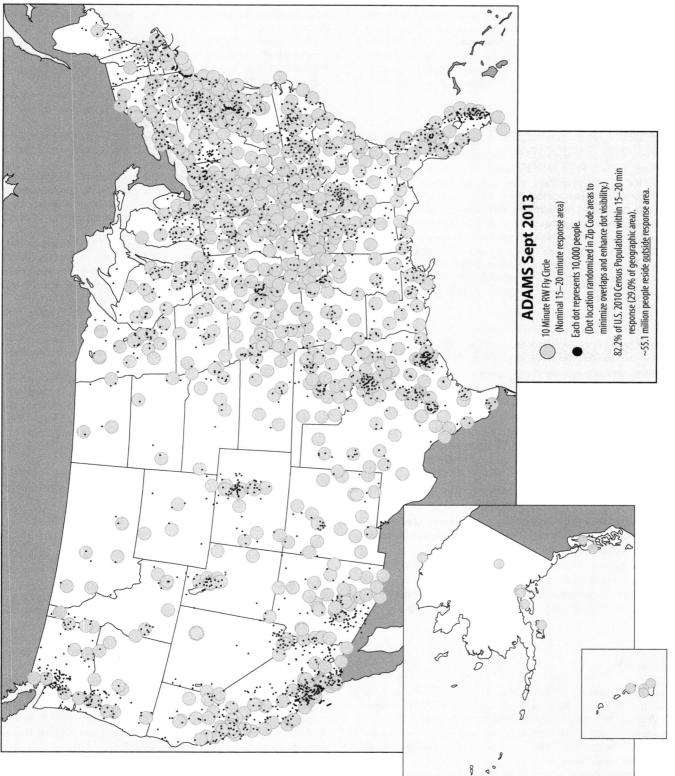

FIGURE 17-3. 2010 Air medical coverage in the United States; air medical base locations with 10-minute fly circles. Reproduced from the Atlas and Database of Air Medical Services (ADAMS), 11th ed. 2013, with permission from CUBRC and the Association of Air Medical Services (AAMS).

and protocol development for the treatment of some acute medical problems, as well as chronic disease surveillance and preventive medicine. Protocols allowed for minimal medicine administration and basic wound suturing and wound care. Unfortunately the program voluntarily closed after review, which showed poor record keeping, and high incidence of protocol violation, including care provided beyond the scope of practice. Other problems included competition with local health care providers, high rate of EEMS provider turnover, and lack of strict oversight.[48] While it may seem tempting to allow providers to operate beyond their training when there is no other medical care available in the community, success seems to depend on strict protocols and oversight of any expanded scope practice.

CONCLUSION

In addition to the typical issues faced by EMS agencies in all locations, rural EMS agencies face many unique challenges, making an active and involved medical director even more important. Rural medical directors should review other sections of this book for greater detail on many of the subjects discussed. Furthermore, there are numerous national, state, and local agencies and programs that may be beneficial resources in training and funding for rural EMS agencies and should be investigated for help with a specific EMS agency. Rural EMS medical direction has many challenges, but by better understanding rural providers and agencies, medical directors can provide valuable insight and educational opportunities, helping to improve emergency medical care in the communities they serve.

KEY POINTS

- Large coverage areas and local geography can lead to difficulty locating patients. This also extends response and transport times, leading to patients missing standard time benchmarks for conditions such as STEMI and CVA.

- Due to multiple factors, rural residents face a "mortality penalty" compared to their urban counterparts. Furthermore, population surges and unique injury and illness patterns can severely stress a rural EMS system already strained by limited resources.

- Recruitment and retention can be adversely affected by limited access to training and continuing education.

- Rural providers are more likely to be volunteers and changes in attitudes surrounding volunteerism in rural communities has decreased the number of people even willing to serve.

- Rural EMS medical directors need to be actively involved with all aspects of a rural EMS agency. Training opportunities, protocol development, and advocacy for EMS providers and agencies should all be priorities for any rural EMS medical director.

REFERENCES

1. Whiteman C, Shaver E, Doerr R, et al. Trauma patient access: the role of the emergency medical services system in North-Central West Virginia. *W V Med J*. May-June 2014;110(3):30-35.
2. US Census Bureau. 2010 Census urban and rural classification and urban area criteria. 2010. http://www.census.gov/geo/www/ua/2010urbanruralclass.html.
3. USDA Economic Research Service. Rural population and migration. 2009. http://www.ers.usda.gov/topics/rural-economy-population/population-migration/shifting-geography-of-population-change.aspx. Accessed May, 2015.
4. Rural Assistance Center. Frontier frequently asked questions. 2011. http://www.raconline.org/info_guides/frontier/frontierfaq.php#definition.
5. National Center for Frontier Communities. Consensus definition- 2007 Update. 2007. http://frontierus.org/wp-content/uploads/2007/01/consensus-definition-2007-update.pdf. Accessed May, 2015.
6. National Center for Frontier Communities. Update: frontier counties in the United States. 2000. http://frontierus.org/wp-content/uploads/2014/12/map-2000-frontier-counties-50-states.pdf. Accessed May, 2015.
7. United States Department of Agriculture, Economic Research Service. Health status and health care access of farm and rural populations. 2009. http://www.ers.usda.gov/media/155453/eib57_1_.pdf. Accessed May, 2015.
8. Cosby AG, Neaves TT, Cossman RE, et al. Preliminary evidence for an emerging nonmetropolitan mortality penalty in the United States. *Am J Public Health*. 2008;98:1470.
9. Cossman JS, James WL, Cosby AG, Cossman RE. Underlying causes of the emerging nonmetropolitan mortality penalty. *Am J Public Health*. 2010;100:1417.
10. Rezaee ME, Conley SM, Anderson TA, Brown JR, Yanofsky NN, Niles NW. Primary percutaneous coronary intervention for patients presenting with ST-elevation myocardial infarction: process improvements in rural prehospital care delivered by emergency medical services. *Prog Cardiovasc Dis*. 2010;53:210.
11. Nallamothu BK, Bates ER, Wang Y, Bradley EH, Krumholz HM. Driving times and distances to hospitals with percutaneous coronary intervention in the United States: implications for prehospital triage of patients with ST-elevation myocardial infarction. *Circulation*. 2006;113:1189.
12. Brooks SC, Allan KS, Welsford M, Verbeek PR, Arntz HR, Morrison LJ. Prehospital triage and direct transport of patients with ST-elevation myocardial infarction to primary percutaneous coronary intervention centres: a systematic review and meta-analysis. *CJEM*. September 2009;11(5):481-492.
13. Brunetti ND, Di Pietro G, Aquilino A, et al. Pre-hospital electrocardiogram triage with tele-cardiology support is associated with shorter time-to-balloon and higher rates of timely reperfusion even in rural areas: data from the Bari- Barletta/Andria/Trani public emergency medical service 118 registry on primary angioplasty in ST-elevation myocardial infarction. *Eur Heart J Acute Cardiovasc Care*. September 2014;3(3):204-213.
14. O'Connor RE, Nichol G, Gonzales L, et al. Emergency medical services management of ST-segment elevation myocardial infarction in the United States—a report from the American Heart Association Mission: Lifeline Program. *Am J Emerg Med*. August 2014;32(8):856-863.
15. Cone DC, Lee CH, Van Gelder C. EMS activation of the cardiac catheterization laboratory is associated with process improvements in the care of myocardial infarction patients. *Prehosp Emerg Care*. July-September 2013;17(3):293-298.
16. Leira EC, Hess DC, Torner JC, Adams HP Jr. Rural-urban differences in acute stroke management practices: a modifiable disparity. *Arch Neurol*. 2008;65:887.
17. McNamara MJ, Oser C, Gohdes D, et al. Stroke knowledge among urban and frontier first responders and emergency medical technicians in Montana. *J Rural Health*. 2008;24:189.
18. Oser CS, McNamara MJ, Fogle CC, Gohdes D, Helgerson SD, Harwell TS. Educational outreach to improve emergency medical services systems of care for stroke in Montana. *Prehosp Emerg Care*. 2010;14:259.
19. Gonzalez RP, Cummings G, Mulekar M, Rodning CB. Increased mortality in rural vehicular trauma: identifying contributing factors through data linkage. *J Trauma*. 2006;61:404.
20. Gonzalez RP, Cummings GR, Phelan HA, Mulekar MS, Rodning CB. Does increased emergency medical services prehospital time affect patient mortality in rural motor vehicle crashes? A statewide analysis. *Am J Surg*. 2009;197:30.
21. Muelleman RL, Wadman MC, Tran TP, Ullrich F, Anderson JR. Rural motor vehicle crash risk of death is higher after controlling for injury severity. *J Trauma*. 2007;62:221.

22. Newgard CD, Schmicker RH, Hedges JR, et al. Emergency medical services intervals and survival in trauma: assessment of the "golden hour" in a North American prospective cohort. *Ann Emerg Med.* 2010;5:235.

23. Gonzalez RP, Cummings GR, Phelan HA, Mulekar MS, Rodning CB. On-scene intravenous line insertion adversely impacts prehospital time in rural vehicular trauma. *Am Surg.* 2008;74:1083.

24. Gonzalez RP, Cummings GR, Rodning CB. Rural EMS en route IV insertion improves IV insertion success rates and EMS scene time. *Am J Surg.* 2011;201:344.

25. National Farmedic Training Program. 2007. www.farmedic.com.

26. Bledsoe BE. Simple way of life: EMS in Amish country. *JEMS.* March 2012;37(3):42-44, 46.

27. Vitale MA, Rzucidlo S, Shaffer ML, Ceneviva GD, Thomas NJ. The impact of pediatric trauma in the Amish community. *J Pediatr.* 2006;148:359.

28. National Center for Frontier Communities. Seasonal population fluctuations in rural and frontier areas. 2003. http://frontierus.org/wp-content/uploads/2003/01/Seasonal-pop-fluctuations-Report2003.pdf. Accessed May, 2015.

29. Larry Gamm LH, Dabney B, Dorsey A. Rural healthy people 2010. 2010. http://www.srph.tamhsc.edu/centers/rhp2010/Volume1preface.pdf.

30. Freeman VA, Slifkin RT, Patterson PD. Recruitment and retention in rural and urban EMS: results from a national survey of local EMS directors. *J Public Health Manag Pract.* 2009;15:246.

31. EMS workforce for the 21st century. A national assessment. 2008. http://krhis.kdhe.state.ks.us/olrh/Notices.nsf/16a37e057485808986256c060074399d/ee8654b1c604ed6b862574670059ab11/$FILE/EMS%20WorkforceReport.pdf.

32. National Rural Health Association. Rural and frontier emergency medical services agenda for the future. Kansas City, MO. 2004. https://www.ruralcenter.org/sites/default/files/rfemsagenda.pdf. Accessed May, 2015.

33. Hubble MW, Richards ME. Paramedic student performance: comparison of online with on-campus lecture delivery methods. *Prehosp Disaster Med.* 2006;21:261.

34. Slifkin RT, Freeman VA, Patterson PD. Designated medical directors for emergency medical services: recruitment and roles. *J Rural Health.* 2009;25:392.

35. Rowley T. Solving the paramedic paradox. *Rural Health News.* 2001. http://ircp.info/Portals/11/Downloads/General%20Articles/RHNfall01.pdf. Accessed May, 2015.

36. Bradley JS, Billows GL, Olinger ML, Boha SP, Cordell WH, Nelson DR. Prehospital oral endotracheal intubation by rural basic emergency medical technicians. *Ann Emerg Med.* 1998;32:26.

37. Hatfield D. A report on technical and operational issues impacting the provision of wireless enhanced 911 services. Tech. Rep. 2002: Federal Communications Commission.

38. Lohmeyer H. "OC Mayor Addresses the Issue of Addresses." Delta County Independent 8 Dec. 2010. Print. http://www.deltacountyindependent.com. Accessed May, 2015.

39. Gonzalez RP, Cummings GR, Mulekar MS, Harlan SM, Rodning CB. Improving rural emergency medical service response time with global positioning system navigation. *J Trauma.* 2009;67:899.

40. Gonzalez RP, Cummings GR, Mulekar MS, Harlan SM, Rodning CB. Improving rural emergency medical service response time with global positioning system navigation. *J Trauma.* 2009 Nov;67(5):899-902.

41. Purtill MA, Benedict K, Hernandez-Boussard T, et al. Validation of a prehospital trauma triage tool: a 10-year perspective. *J Trauma.* 2008;65:1253.

42. Heightman AJ. Mobile integrated healthcare. *JEMS.* July 2014; 39(7):14, 16.

43. Weber MJ. Policy & how to change it. To realize the potential of EMS in mobile integrated healthcare, we must know how to shape the playing field. *EMS World.* August 2014 ;43(8):42-45.

44. Community paramedics fill gaps, take load off EDs. *ED Manag.* March 2014;26(3):30-34.

45. Bigham BL, Kennedy SM, Drennan I, Morrison LJ. Expanding paramedic scope of practice in the community: a systematic review of the literature. *Prehosp Emerg Care.* July-September 2013;17(3):361-372.

46. Misner D. Community paramedicine: part of an integrated healthcare system. *Emerg Med Serv.* April 2005;34(4):89-90.

47. Shah MN, Caprio TV, Swanson P, et al. A novel emergency medical services-based program to identify and assist older adults in a rural community. *J Am Geriatr Soc.* 2010;58:2205.

48. Hauswald M, Raynovich W, Brainard AH. Expanded emergency medical services: the failure of an experimental community health program. *Prehosp Emerg Care.* 2005;9:250.

CHAPTER 18

Air Medical Transport

Jesse L. Hatfield
Stephen H. Thomas

INTRODUCTION

The growing air medical transport sector represents a highly visible concentration of resources. A 2007 publication estimated that in the United States, 753 helicopters (and 150 dedicated fixed-wing aircraft) were in EMS service, providing about 3% of all ambulance transports.[1] By 2011, the Association of Air Medical Services (AAMS) placed the number of rotor-wing (ie, helicopter) transport vehicles at about 900. Individual helicopter EMS (HEMS) programs' mission profiles and crew configurations vary widely. Varying programs have varying mission breakdowns (as well as differing aircraft and crew configurations), but a typical US HEMS program performs 54% interfacility transports, 33% scene runs, and 13% "other" mission types (eg, neonatal, pediatric, transplant related).[2]

OBJECTIVES

- Discuss the utilization and integration of air medical services in field response.
- Discuss the unique role of air medical transport for interfacility transfers.
- Describe the physiologic changes and medical limitations associated with air medical transport.
- Describe the utilization of fixed-wing versus rotor-wing transport.
- Discuss different rotor-wing aircraft types and give specific examples.
- Discuss unique safety considerations.
- Describe operations for establishing an LZ and for safe landing/take-off of rotor-wing aircraft in the field and at the hospital.
- List governmental and professional agencies that set standards for aircraft and air medical operations.
- Discuss the licensure and certification implications of operations across state boundaries.

UTILIZATION AND INTEGRATION OF AIR MEDICAL SERVICES IN FIELD RESPONSE

While there is occasional utility in HEMS deployment for nontrauma situations (eg, time-critical diagnoses such as stroke),[5,6] most of the applicable use and evidence for scene response deals with HEMS dispatch for injured patients. The availability of rotor-wing response is variable throughout the country based on the location of air bases in relation to populations they serve (**Figure 18-1**).

EVIDENCE SUPPORTING INCORPORATION OF AIR MEDICAL ASSETS INTO SYSTEM SCENE RESPONSE

An independent 2007 review of all studies dating from the year 2000, conducted by the Institute of Health Economics for the Canadian health ministry in Alberta, concluded: "Overall, patients transported by helicopter showed a benefit in terms of survival, time interval to reach the healthcare facility, time interval to definite treatment, better results, or a benefit in general."[7] This finding was endorsed in a recent review of the worldwide HEMS scene response literature.[8] Since the landmark 1983 *JAMA* paper from Baxt and Moody,[9] which suggested roughly 50% mortality improvement with HEMS, the preponderance of subsequent evidence has identified lesser—but significant—outcomes improvement in the range of 20% to 30% better survival.[11-15] As outlined elsewhere,[11-15] evidence supporting HEMS use varies in methodology and quality, but the overall state of the data support a benefit when HEMS is properly used.

POSSIBLE MECHANISMS BY WHICH HEMS SCENE RESPONSE MAY IMPROVE OUTCOME

Analysis of over 250,000 scene trauma transports from the National Trauma Data Bank (NTDB)[19] found that HEMS (as compared to ground EMS) reduced mortality by 22%. However, methodology did not focus on mechanism for benefit, leaving this question open. Several different proposed characteristics may explain this benefit (**Box 18-1**).

EARLIER ARRIVAL OF ADVANCED-LEVEL PREHOSPITAL CARE

It is both fashionable and foolish to dismiss the idea that, at least occasionally, HEMS benefit is in its speed. In some situations there is undoubtedly an important time advantage. Particularly in rural regions, the only readily available ground prehospital care may be BLS level.[2] Data focusing on patients with severe trauma including head injuries suggest that the HEMS crews' early provisions of ALS-level airway and hemodynamic support (ie, intravenous access and fluid management) are the mechanism for improved overall outcome and better neurological function.[20] Better functional outcome in HEMS near-drowning patients has been theorized as explainable by deployment of HEMS to areas lacking ALS coverage (by ground EMS).[21]

STREAMLINED PREHOSPITAL TIMES AND DIRECT TRANSPORT TO HIGH-LEVEL CARE

Studies conducted from regions as disparate as California and the Netherlands clearly demonstrate HEMS mortality benefit, yet often find similar scene-to-trauma center times for ground and HEMS transports.[31,32] Authors focusing on logistics support the notion that time to definitive care (ie, arrival of advanced crew on scene) is an appropriate primary endpoint, writing that "correlation between length of time to definitive care and outcome has been well established in the literature, so the premise that faster transport is better seems justifiable."[35] For areas in which there is no trauma center, air medical scene response for direct transport of injured patients to the trauma center is often the best course.[37] On the nontrauma front, suggestion of potentially growing indications for HEMS "scene" transports of noninjured patients is provided by an evolving literature consisting of both case series (eg, for primary percutaneous intervention) and sporadic reports (eg, scene transport to neurological centers for lytic therapy for ischemic stroke).[5,38,39]

EXTENSION OF ADVANCED LEVEL OF CARE THROUGHOUT A REGION

HEMS may allow an EMS system to provide for early ALS in isolated and/or difficult-to-reach areas which otherwise would be poorly covered. In pointing out that HEMS can cover roughly the geographic area of seven ground ALS ambulances, Hankins[2] has written that: "This kind of coverage, in many areas of the country, provides advanced care where it is not otherwise available." Others considering the US trauma system as a whole have agreed that at least in some areas of the United States the extension of trauma regional care provided by HEMS is critical.[19]

AIR MEDICAL SERVICES AND INTERFACILITY TRANSPORTS

As compared to scene response, there are fewer data directly addressing outcomes benefits associated with interfacility air medical transport. This section discusses secondary missions.

EVIDENCE SUPPORTING INCORPORATION OF AIR MEDICAL ASSETS INTO SYSTEM INTERFACILITY TRANSPORT

Reports outlining extension of percutaneous coronary intervention (PCI) to community hospitals include incorporation of HEMS into systems planning as a necessary backup in cases where urgent CABG is required.[44] It is increasingly well known that time savings can be helpful: each 30 minutes' additional ischemia time increases mortality by 8% to

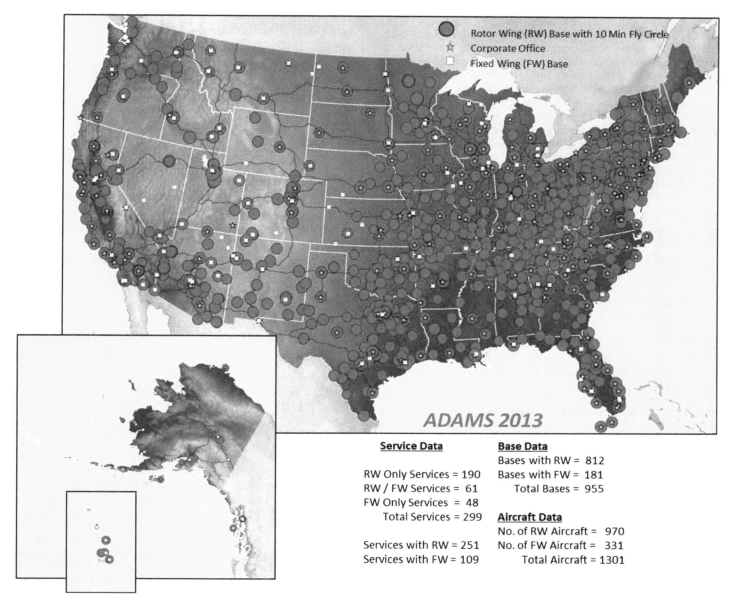

FIGURE 18-1. US rotor-wing airbases (per ADAMS). (Reproduced from the Atlas and Database of Air Medical Services [ADAMS], 11th ed. 2013, with permission from CUBRC and the Association of Air Medical Services [AAMS].)

10%.[45] Similar to the situation with integration of HEMS into cardiac care systems is the rapidly solidifying role for air transport in stroke care. NAEMSP recommends air transport of stroke patients if the closest fibrinolytic-capable facility is more than an hour away by ground.[47] The American Stroke Association Task Force on Development of Stroke Systems[48] identified HEMS as an important part of stroke systems, with helicopters to be used to streamline times. There are data addressing interfacility HEMS trauma transport. Brown et al identified a significant benefit for secondary HEMS trauma transport when Injury Severity Score (ISS) exceeded 15.[52] A Canadian study, notable for its similarity in

---

BOX 18-1

Benefit of Air Medical Transport in Field Response

• Earlier arrival of advanced-level prehospital care

• Streamlined prehospital times and direct transport to high-level care

• Extension of advanced level of care throughout a region

---

acuity between air and ground transport cohorts (ground patients were those in whom HEMS was requested but was unavailable), also found that air transport significantly improved mortality.[54]

POSSIBLE MECHANISMS BY WHICH HEMS INTERFACILITY RESPONSE MAY IMPROVE OUTCOME

Many of the putative mechanisms for air transport's salutary outcomes effects in scene patients are reproduced for interfacility transports. HEMS crews may in fact have more comfort with high-acuity patients than even physicians at a referring hospital.[2,34] Furthermore, data demonstrate HEMS utility for time savings (and mortality advantage) in interfacility trauma transport.[52] Loss of HEMS availability has been recognized as a potentially important factor causing increased trauma mortality in patients presenting to non-Level I centers.[55] A logistics study from the University of Wisconsin[49] demonstrated the importance of time savings accrued by HEMS for interfacility transports of patients with time-critical cardiac or neurological conditions. In assessing average transport times from their 20-hospital network, the investigators found that for all hospitals, the *average* HEMS total transport time over the study period was at least as good as the *best* ground transport time—this finding occurred despite the fact that for many hospitals ground EMS was on-site at the time of transport request. The Wisconsin group found clinically significant time savings for all institutions: patients at close-by hospitals accrued an average of 10 minutes' savings, while those from further-out hospitals' HEMS transport times were up to 45 minutes shorter than those achievable by ground. For interfacility transfers, an additional time interval of "out-of-hospital" time is reduced. Obstetrics transports serve as an excellent example of a situation in which out-of-hospital time is best minimized. HEMS has also long been known to allow for fetal/maternal outcome benefits occurring when HEMS or fixed-wing aircraft allow high-risk obstetrics transports that simply would not have occurred (due to prolonged transport times) in the absence of air transport.[56]

APPROPRIATE UTILIZATION OF AIR MEDICAL RESOURCES

Since even the harshest critics of air transport acknowledge its potential for occasional benefit, the question of "appropriate utilization" forms the crux of the HEMS debate. (Probably because of its use in situations in which ground EMS is simply not an option, fixed-wing utilization tends to garner less attention.)

▦ TRIAGE AND APPROPRIATE UTILIZATION

Whether indications relate to chance for patient improvement or time-distance factors and "protection" of ALS coverage for a given region, HEMS dispatch should occur only when there is potential advantage over alternatives. No guidelines for dispatch are ideal, and authorities on the subject recognize the inevitability—and necessity—of some degree of HEMS overtriage.[7] Some have identified gross deficiencies (eg, regions lacking HEMS triage guidelines)[65] and others have identified low ISS and high rates of early hospital discharge.[66] However, the most recent nationwide data (assessing over 250,000 ground and air scene responses) find that HEMS patients are in fact far more acutely injured, and require far more hospital resources, than ground EMS patients.[19] The triage question has to incorporate distance, since rural regions may have fewer non-HEMS options for transport of injured patients. Even the ISS question seems to be related to distance; while 57% of HEMS patients in the nationwide NTDB study had ISS <15, this average ISS fell below this critical value only for those patients with transport times of over 2 hours.[19]

Some authors suggest that ground transport times of at least 30 minutes are consistent with need for HEMS transport for head trauma patients[71]; others recommend using 45 miles[72] or 110 km (62 miles).[73] Although there is not likely a uniform exact distance relating to proven patient benefit, the range of approximately 45 miles from the trauma center is endorsed by those executing large-scale studies of HEMS trauma scene response.[19] Logistics decisions are also informed by the consideration that depending on the specific aircraft, HEMS units can cover a radius of roughly 150 to 200 miles from their base. Another approach uses time rather than mileage. One group has suggested that HEMS be reserved for cases where ground transport to appropriate trauma centers exceeds 45 minutes.[74] This group pointed out that time benefits of air transport are optimal only if the referring and receiving hospitals have ready access to helipads.[75,76]

The authors of one discussion addressing triage[74] conclude that: "The decision to use a helicopter is not straightforward, and a number of important geographical, physiological, and pathological factors need to be considered." The question is how to use prospectively available information, rather than retrospectively calculated scores (such as ISS) to maximize triage sensitivity while maintaining acceptable positive predictive value. The many previous studies of field triage have been overviewed in a review by Lerner.[70] Highlights of the literature include consistent findings that, to achieve sensitivity in the 95% or higher range, positive predictive value falls to under 10%.[86] In an air transported population, the ACS triage criteria were associated with an admirable 97% sensitivity—but at a cost of specificity of 8%.[87] In Australia, a study

found that even the most seasoned paramedics (air crews) were able to achieve acceptable triage sensitivities only with high levels of overtriage.[69] Until trauma triage is better understood, HEMS will be fraught with overtriage.

Although many studies use an ISS cutoff of 15 to define "major" injury, there is not uniform agreement on what ISS defines the possible need for HEMS.[65] Since data have shown HEMS-associated outcomes improvement (W of 8.8, or about 9 lives saved per 100 transports) with air transport use for ISS at least 11,[89] setting the cutoff for HEMS appropriateness at an ISS of 15 is suboptimal. There is solid evidence on some points: (1) rapid transport to trauma centers saves lives[92]; (2) much of the US population can *only* reach Level I centers in timely fashion by HEMS[36,49]; and (3) trauma transport decision making is heterogeneous and inconsistent even when physicians (at community/rural hospitals) are doing the triage.[55,93] Both sides of the HEMS debate agree that future research efforts should focus on refinement of triage.[66,94] Until such ideal triage data exist, those involved in HEMS have a duty to utilize whatever data are available to generate sensible guidelines for helicopter dispatch. Though any system of guidelines will have flaws, the alternative (of haphazard HEMS dispatch without regional cooperative planning) is clearly an inferior option. NAEMSP generated updated Guidelines for Air Medical Dispatch in 2003.[95] These guidelines have also been endorsed by the Air Medical Physician Association (AMPA) and the Association of Air Medical Services (AAMS), as well as the American Academy of Emergency Medicine (AAEM) (**BOX 18-2**).

UTILIZATION REVIEW

The a posteriori follow-up of HEMS utilization is critical to determining whether the ongoing utilization of HEMS in a particular region is optimal. After criteria have been generated and implemented, ongoing air medical optimization must take into account that regions will have varying degrees of compliance with "agreed-upon" protocols for air transport. Broad variability in HEMS use, in areas operating under the same triage guidelines, has been demonstrated in many areas.[63,97] Well-executed studies reporting years of experience demonstrate that the correct use of these triage guidelines, even in the most rural settings, can result in optimal HEMS triage even without requiring base station contact.[98] There can be little doubt that when viewed from a large-sample, post-transport perspective, HEMS overutilization is rampant *if* overutilization is defined as execution of missions for which transport mode appears retrospectively to have had no impact on outcome. In fact, this definition, though often used, is flawed: post hoc determination that air transport did not impact outcome is a *necessary*, but not *sufficient*, requirement for defining a flight as unnecessary. On a case-by-case basis, HEMS overtriage should be defined as occurring when the aircraft use offered insufficient potential advantage (logistical, clinical, etc) to justify resource expenditure.

COST-EFFECTIVENESS

Exploration of the broader "regional coverage view" has resulted in at least one economic study concluding that HEMS is *less* expensive than same-area coverage through development of a wide-ranging fleet of ground EMS vehicles.[99] Unfortunately, the job of assessing HEMS' incremental (as compared to ground transport) cost-effectiveness is made difficult by the limited amount of information on cost-effectiveness of ground EMS itself.[100]

SYSTEM-BASED DATA ASSESSING HEMS COST-EFFECTIVENESS

One study, calculating cost -benefit for the entire spectrum of HEMS transports in Norway, concluded: "The analysis indicates that the benefits of ambulance missions flown by helicopters exceeds the costs by a factor of almost six."[101] Another group estimates that HEMS contributes to the cost-effectiveness of primary PCI.[102] In a study conducted in Finland, authors calculated that the cost of HEMS, per beneficial mission, was roughly $30,000.[103] In a report of the British Department of Health,[104] HEMS' cost per QALY (quality adjusted life year) was $10,000 to $30,000, within the UK's "acceptance threshold" of about $35,000. In the Netherlands, HEMS' cost-effectiveness (depending on models) was $10,000 to $50,000 per QALY.[34,105]

COST-EFFECTIVENESS FOCUSING ON NONTRAUMA TRANSPORTS

Though most extant information addresses use of HEMS for trauma, it should be pointed out that cost-effectiveness calculations are increasingly being applied to other patient populations. One of the studies is that of Silbergleit et al,[108] who demonstrate HEMS cost-effectiveness for patients with acute ischemic stroke (for thrombolytic therapy). Cardiac patients may be the next population for HEMS cost-effectiveness studies. A 2010 study revealed that centralization of cardiac catheterization resources, with appropriate buildup of EMS transfer systems, is significantly more cost-effective than construction of multiple cardiac catheterization centers; the relevance of this to the HEMS issue is emphasized when the same authors note that 20% of Americans live more than an hour away (by ground) from a cardiac catheterization center.[109]

AIR TRANSPORT PHYSIOLOGY AND IN-AIRCRAFT MEDICAL LIMITATIONS

Parameters of altitude interest include elevation above mean sea level (MSL—Denver is much higher at "ground altitude" than is Boston), pressurization level for fixed-wing aircraft (which rarely pressurize to MSL), and equipment in use on a given transport.

GAS LAWS

Perhaps the most important of the gas laws is *Boyle's law*, which states that a gas' volume is inversely proportional to the pressure exerted upon it. As altitude increases (and atmospheric pressure decreases), the molecules of gas move farther apart and the gas volume expands. Expansion and contraction of gases within the body can occur with altitude changes. "Squeeze" on descent, and "reverse squeeze" on ascent occur when decrease in ambient barometric pressure leads to an increased volume of

the air trapped within physiologic spaces. Depending on the particular space in the body, exertion of pressure on adjacent structures may cause, for example, sinus pain or enlargement of a pneumothorax. Medical equipment containing closed air spaces (eg, tubes for balloon tamponade of bleeding from esophageal varices) can also be affected. Intravenous flow rates, the pressure in air splints and in pneumatic antishock garment suits, and endotracheal tube cuff volumes may be altered with altitude.[110]

Charles' law follows from the volume effects of Boyle's law, and states that temperature and volume of a gas are directly related. Molecular dispersion seen with increases in gas volume at altitude means there is less heat produced from the naturally occurring molecular collisions—thus temperature decreases as altitude increases. The maintenance of desired patient temperatures is sometimes challenging in the air transport environment, and attention must be paid to proper provision of insulating blankets when hypothermia is a risk. Furthermore, absolute humidity decrease associated with low temperatures can cause problems with thickening of respiratory secretions. Hydration should be paid particular attention during air transport.

Dalton's law states that the total barometric pressure at any given altitude equals the sum of the partial pressures of gases in the mixture. This accounts for the decrease in partial arterial oxygen tension as altitude increases. Since patients are usually on supplemental oxygen, Dalton's law ramifications are crew focused (ie, need for occasional supplemental oxygen).

Henry's law states that the mass of gas absorbed by a liquid is directly proportional to the partial pressure of the gas above the liquid. This has particular application to dive medicine, where decompression sickness results from rapid ascent (gases to come out of solution into the bloodstream). In general, this is not an issue with air transport, although sudden decompression at altitude can cause the same dysbarism seen in too-rapid ascent when diving.

ENVIRONMENTAL LIMITATIONS IN AIR TRANSPORT

In-cabin care challenges are surmountable with appropriate education, training, and preparation. These are mentioned here, in order to emphasize the unique nature of in-transport care. Early concerns about vibrations and their possible ramifications with respect to bleeding after thrombolytic therapy have not been borne out for either cardiac or stroke patients.[111,112] Vibrations may contribute to crew fatigue; there is no evidence they pose a risk to patients. Larger-scale movements of the aircraft may result in motion sickness, both for crew and patients. In some cases (eg, trauma patients with cervical spine immobilization), intratransport emesis can be problematic and prophylactic antiemetics may be wise. The helicopter cabin is loud. Crew and patients should have hearing protection, and crew may not be able to auscultate effectively.[113] Most crew members have learned to use other physical examination or related clues (eg, ventilator pressures) to mitigate the information loss from auscultation, but esophageal stethoscopy may be useful on occasion.[114] The physical size and layout of aircraft cabins differ widely with varying HEMS vehicles (**Table 18-1**) (**Figure 18-2**). Ergonomic issues include possible impairment of performance of advanced medical tasks such as intubation and chest compressions.[115,116]

FIXED-WING TRANSPORT CONSIDERATIONS

Many of the same issues mentioned for rotor-wing aircraft apply to fixed-wing airplanes. A full outlining of the specifics of fixed-wing transport is outside this chapter's scope, but this section will highlight some noteworthy subject areas.

OUTCOMES LITERATURE

While data are sparse, the available evidence suggests desirability of incorporation of fixed-wing aircraft into regionalized care systems. Fixed-wing transport allows for long-distance transfer of complicated patients (eg, those on extracorporeal membrane oxygenation[119,120]) to centers of excellence. In rural areas, fixed-wing assets allow for air transports that would be nonfeasible by alternative means of transport.[121]

TABLE 18-1	Aviation Characteristics of Selected Helicopters[a]		
	Cruise Speed	Cruise Range	Approx Cabin Volume
EC-130 AStar	130 knots (150 mph)	300 nautical miles (379 miles)	120 cubic feet
EC-135	137 knots (158 mph)	342 nautical miles (394 miles)	175 cubic feet
EC-145	133 knots (153 mph)	370 nautical miles (426 miles)	170 cubic feet
BK-117	120 knots (138 mph)	292 nautical miles (336 miles)	180 cubic feet
BO-105	110 knots (127 mph)	310 nautical miles (357 miles)	85 cubic feet
S-76	145 knots (167 mph)	360 nautical miles (414 miles)	200 cubic feet
Bell Longranger	115 knots (132 mph)	350 nautical miles (403 miles)	80 cubic feet
Bell 407	133 knots (152 mph)	324 nautical miles (372 miles)	85 cubic feet
AS-365			
Dauphin	150 knots (173 mph)	375 nautical miles (432 miles)	180 cubic feet
S76 C++			
Sikorsky	155 knots (178 mph)	411 nautical miles (473 miles)	204 cubic feet
AW-139 AgustaWestland	165 knots (190 mph)	675 nautical miles (1250 miles)	222 cubic feet

[a]There can be significant variations between models within the same aircraft type.

TRIAGE

The NAEMSP Guidelines for Air Medical Dispatch include relevant recommendations for fixed-wing transport.[123] Advantages of airplanes include long range (hundreds or even thousands of miles). Fixed-wing aircraft require airports, and incur an extra set of transfers (ie, to and from the airport), but as distance increases these time costs are offset by rapidity of transport. Airplanes may often be utilized when weather renders HEMS unsafe. Unlike helicopters, fixed-wing planes cannot easily divert while in-transport; patients with potential to require emergent care beyond the capability of flight crews are usually poor candidates for fixed-wing transport.

AIRCRAFT ISSUES

Just as triage issues will depend significantly on the specific logistics of the transport and airplane being used, the environmental in-cabin situation is far different for varying airplanes (see **Figure 18-3**). The 400+ mph cruise speed and 1500-mile range of the CitationJet II in Figure 18-3B is far different from the speed and range characteristics of a turboprop (Figure 18-3A). The gas laws and physiology of altitude also vary with fixed-wing aircraft. Like larger commercial airline flights, air medical transports by fixed-wing are usually executed with effective in-cabin altitudes thousands of feet above MSL (eg, 5000-8000 feet is a common pressurization altitude for commercial flights). The ability of an aircraft to maintain cabin pressure is limited to some degree by the altitude at which it is operating. Thus, "pressurized" cabins in fixed-wing aircraft do not obviate the need to pay attention to altitude-related issues as previously outlined.

SAFETY AND LANDING ZONE (LZ) CONSIDERATIONS

In recent years, safety in air medical operations has rightfully garnered significant attention. The issues of safety revolve around both patient safety as considered from a medical perspective, and also patient and crew safety as considered from the aviation perspective.

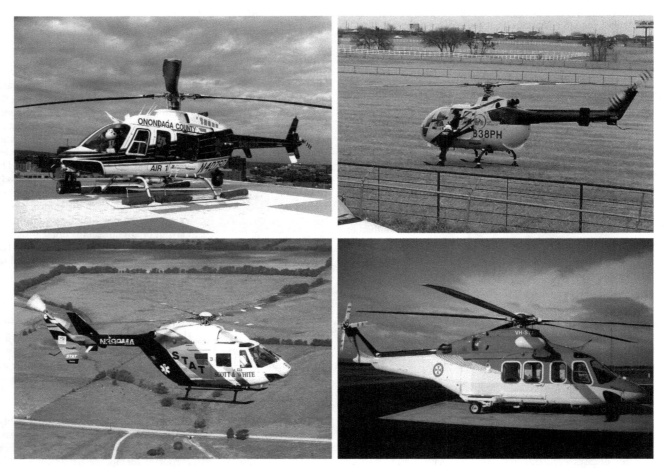

FIGURE 18-2. Different rotor-wing aircraft examples. **A:** Bell 407 (Onondaga County Sheriff Air-1). Permission granted by the photographer, Dr. Chris Fullagar. **B:** BO-105 (Stat-Air/PHI Air Medical). **C:** BK-117 (Stat-Air/Scott & White Memorial Hospital). **D:** AW-139 (Ambulance Service of New South Wales, Australia). All photos reproduced with permission.

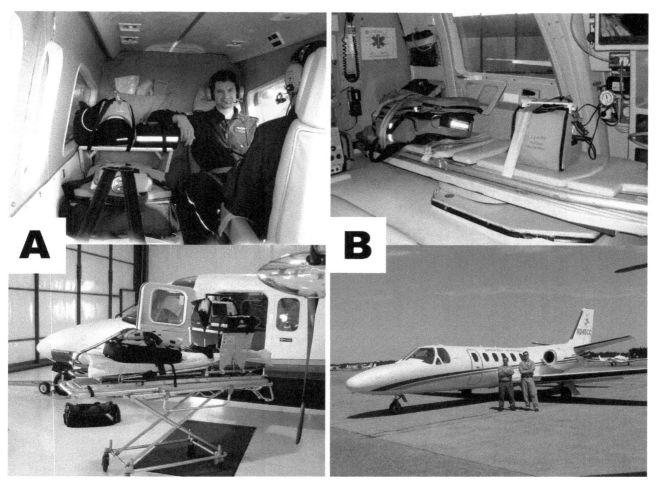

FIGURE 18-3. Different fixed-wing examples. **A:** Mercy Flight Central, New York (turboprop). **B:** Boston Med Flight, Massachusetts (jet). All photos reproduced with permission.

PATIENT SAFETY FROM THE MEDICAL PERSPECTIVE

Although previously cited data demonstrate that breath sounds are often not auscultatable in helicopters,[113] large multicenter series of air medical intubation data reveal near-zero rates of unrecognized esophageal intubation.[124] Patient safety issues that were postulated to result from vibrations, electrical interference, or other transport-mediated phenomena (eg, catecholamine surge) have also gone undemonstrated in patient safety studies.[111,112,125,126] Some specific medical safety issues do arise during HEMS or fixed-wing flight that warrant mention. Example situations include transport of combative patients (paralysis and intubation are usually indicated due to risk of patients' causing aviation problems) and transport of patients with issues susceptible to impact from altitude changes (eg, patients with significant pneumothoraces may develop tension pathology with ascent).

PATIENT AND CREW SAFETY FROM THE AVIATION PERSPECTIVE—AIR TRANSPORT CRASHES

While transport itself, even intrahospital transport, is long known to engender risks ranging from inadvertent extubation to equipment failure,[76,129] concerns with HEMS (and fixed-wing transport) center on crash risk. Some important safety concepts will be introduced here. HEMS safety is a critical issue, and is the industry's self-identified number one priority. Air medical transport safety has clearly deserved the attention it has gotten in recent years, from experts (eg, Dr Ira Blumen of the University of Chicago) who have led the way in addressing the air medical safety issue.[130] The fact that the *rate* of problems (eg, fatalities per 100,000 flight hours) is generally on the decline since the HEMS'

worst period of the 1980s is only a partial consolation when considered against some of the preventable accidents of recent years. Air transport must strive to be 100% safe, but it should be kept in mind that the surface transport alternative is not risk free. A recent report from the UK overviewed 5 years (1999-2004) of road and helicopter ambulance fatalities: there were zero HEMS-associated fatalities and 40 fatalities in accidents involving ground EMS vehicles.[133] One US group provides what may be the best perspective, noting that the 6500+ ambulance crashes (and 32+ deaths) per year does not mean that ground EMS is unsafe—but it does mean that a rational examination of HEMS safety risks and benefits should include consideration of risks with alternative transport.

SPECIFIC AIR TRANSPORT SAFETY AND AVIATION ISSUES— HELIPADS AND LANDING ZONES

The main point to be made regarding helipads is that if a hospital uses the helicopter with any frequency, an on-site helipad is best for patients. This position, endorsed by NAEMSP and other air transport groups, has been outlined in detail elsewhere.[76,135] In short, access to on-site helipad LZs eliminates the time and risk costs associated with the additional transfer steps. Available data demonstrate there is no aviation safety-related risk to hospital-sited LZs.[76] Some details for LZ setup will depend on the particular aircraft and situation. For example, larger aircraft may require larger LZs, and some services have preidentified, Global Positioning System–sited LZs for many possible landing areas in their service radius. These and other factors may impact the size and nature of the LZ setup for a given transport.

Any LZ should be cleared of debris such as trash cans, cones, etc. Obstructions such as wires should be relayed to the helicopter crew.

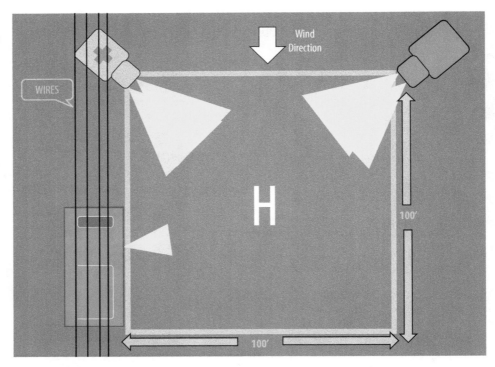

FIGURE 18-4. Setting up a landing zone (LZ).

During a night landing, no lights should be pointed skywards, and emergency lights should be on to help locate the LZ (two vehicles may be stationed at corners to create an "X" with their headlights). Obstructions should be illuminated at night. Since an increasing number of air crews are using night vision goggles (NVGs), ground personnel should be ready to switch off certain lights such as flashing emergency lights. As the helicopter approaches, the process of preparing for its landing should be executed. Communication must exist between the air crew and ground personnel in order to identify the LZ and clear the area. Highway and open field landings are the most common LZs, and night landings are the most common dangerous occurrences; in all cases, communications and vigilance are paramount. Training of out-of-hospital providers to clear LZs is an important part of HEMS outreach. An example of an LZ setup is shown in **Figure 18-4**. In some HEMS scene response situations, using a nearby hospital's helipad as a rendezvous point is beneficial in terms of safety. This practice is not (as judged by the Centers for Medicare and Medicaid Services) a violation of the Emergency Medical Treatment and Active Labor Act (EMTALA).[136]

Regardless of LZ placement, ground personnel should monitor the area around the LZ while the aircraft approaches. Ground personnel should be reminded to keep the area secure for security and safety reasons, while the aircraft is at the LZ. Aircraft engines will usually, but not always, be running (rotors may or may not be turning). At no time should anyone approach the aircraft without permission from, and optimally accompanied by, flight crew. In the usual case of patient loading, air crew will assign up to four individuals from the ground support personnel to assist in stretcher carrying. The crew will brief those personnel—who should have optimally had prior training in helicopter operations by the HEMS service—on procedures for safe patient loading. Chinstraps should be secured, and unsecured hats should be removed. Potential foreign object debris (FOD) should have been removed prior to initial helicopter approach, but the area should be policed again prior to liftoff to ensure lack of hazards.

Patient loading (**Figure 18-5**) approaches depend on the aircraft; patients are loaded from the side or the rear. Helicopters should be approached from the 3-o'clock or 9-o'clock positions, so that the crew can guide personnel and tail rotors can be avoided.

■ OTHER SAFETY ISSUES

There are other issues that arise, with respect to the safety conversation about HEMS. Some highlights will be noted, and readers are referred to external sites (eg, the Association of Air Medical Services' Web site, www.aams.org) for further information. Weather is one of the most

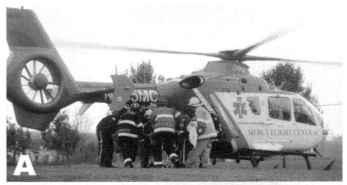

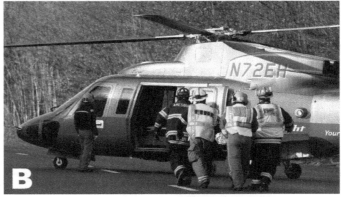

FIGURE 18-5. Approach to patient loading in rotor-wing aircraft. **A:** rear-loading clamshell (EC-135—Mercy Flight Central). **B:** Side loading (Sikorsky S76 C++ – Boston MedFlight). Both photos reproduced with permission.

important, and predictable, issues impacting safe helicopter operations. One step that can be taken to optimize safe weather-related practices is the blinding of mission-acceptance decision makers (ie, pilots) from patient information that can cloud objective assessment as to whether a flight should be attempted.

Related to the weather issue is the question of whether aircraft and pilots should be set up for *visual flight rules* (VFR) or *instrument flight rules* (IFR) operations. Unplanned encountering of *instrument meteorological conditions* (IMC) poses obvious risks for VFR-only aircraft. Although data are sparse, some programs use aircraft with increased capability for either single- or dual-pilot IFR. Of course, adding two pilots on a mission—like using an aircraft with two engines instead of one—increases comfort levels at a significant monetary cost. Some of the interventions that optimize safety have to do with crew. The best intratransport care is provided by experienced crew members who are trained in the practice of air medicine. Surprisingly, one of the methods to optimize safety is to "slow down." Upon receipt of a call, the process of mission consideration, dispatch, and aircraft entry and takeoff should occur at a professional, unhurried pace. Response should be fast, but not rushed.

GOVERNMENT AND REGULATORY ISSUES

Issues surrounding regulation of air transport tend to focus on safety and monetary issues. As noted by air medical transport expert Dan Hankins of Mayo Clinic, as recently as 2011, there is still no strong central oversight over the medical aspects of critical care transport (eg, triage, what constitutes a "critical care flight crew").[137]

AVIATION AND SAFETY

The Federal Aviation Administration (FAA) is responsible for establishing and ensuring compliance with myriad rules regarding safe aviation operations. The pertinent regulations are as numerous as they are important, and address everything from pilot training to aircraft modifications. Information relevant to HEMS and fixed-wing operations can be found at www.faa.gov. Aviation crashes are investigated by an independent federal agency, the National Transportation Safety Board (NTSB, www.ntsb.gov). The NTSB is charged with assessing the causes for a given crash, and also is tasked with making recommendations for future improvements in safety. Until just recently, HEMS safety was on the list of highest-priority items for the NTSB. Information from the NTSB relevant to HEMS safety can be found at their Web site (www.ntsb.gov), which provides links to documents such as the 2009 NTSB special report on HEMS safety (http://www.ntsb.gov/doclib/speeches/sumwalt/ACEP-10052009.pdf) that endorsed night vision goggle use among other changes in HEMS.

UTILIZATION AND REIMBURSEMENT

The NTSB has communicated with the Department of Homeland Security Federal Interagency Committee on Emergency Medical Services (FICEMS). After the 2009 hearings (prompted by the fact that 2008 was the deadliest year on record for HEMS), the NTSB recommended the FICEMS develop national guidelines for the use and availability of HEMS. In response to that request, the National Highway Traffic Safety Administration (NHTSA) and the Centers for Disease Control and Prevention (CDC) are collaborating on an expert panel approach to generate guidelines for appropriate air medical utilization. The panel, which includes this chapter's senior author, is early in its work but is taking the approach of adapting HEMS into the previously published CDC National Field Triage Guidelines.[138] A special case in reimbursement occurs when HEMS services cross state lines in responding or transporting patients. There are nearly always mechanisms for some reimbursement for these interstate transfers. In the authors' state, for example, there is a process for trauma transport reimbursement for HEMS services that is aimed primarily at those services licensed to perform transports in Oklahoma (including those services that may be based in neighboring states).

HEMS units that fly Oklahoma may apply for reimbursement from this fund, but if they perform interstate response with any frequency the Oklahoma State Department of Health asks those services to obtain Oklahoma licensure.

There are areas for future investigation and regulation in the air transport arena. While fixed-wing services are generally paid for "up front" (by conversations pretransport, with insurers), it is not rare for HEMS operators to encounter payment issues. For instance, rotor-wing transport operators are rarely (if ever) reimbursed when they do not transport patients. Furthermore, in many states HEMS services are licensed as ambulances, and therefore must respond (and transport) when called. Future work in the regulatory arena will focus on whether these sorts of rules are in the best interests of a regional system of care. Hopefully, the continuing evolution of the air medical triage and utilization literature will allow for evidence-based development of guidelines for both HEMS and fixed-wing use.

ADDITIONAL RESOURCES

Some additional resources are recommended to cover information that space requirements preclude from inclusion in this chapter. An annotated bibliography of English-language peer-reviewed HEMS outcomes studies since 1980 is found at www.cctcore.org. The National Association of EMS Physicians (NAEMSP, www.naemsp.org) Web site offers free access to position papers on flight crew and medical director training as well as HEMS dispatch.[3,4]

KEY POINTS

- Air medical EMS includes transport of patients from a scene or during interfacility transfer by both helicopter and fixed-wing aircraft.

- Benefits of air medical transport include earlier arrival of advanced-level prehospital care and more rapid transport of certain patients to destination facilities, although both benefits may not always be realized in tandem.

- EMS physicians should be knowledgeable about specific clinical aspects of air medical transport including altitude physiology.

- The Federal Aviation Administration (FAA) governs the aviation operations of air medical EMS services, but does not govern the patient care provided by such services.

- Appropriate utilization review is an important component of air medical EMS agency quality review practices.

- The National Highway Traffic Safety Administration (NHTSA) and the Centers for Disease Control and Prevention (CDC) are collaborating on an expert panel approach to generate guidelines for appropriate air medical utilization.

REFERENCES

1. McGinnis KK, Judge T, Nemitz B, et al. Air medical services: future development as an integrated component of the emergency medical services (EMS) system. *Prehosp Emerg Care.* 2007;11:353-368.
2. Hankins DG. Air medical transport of trauma patients. *Prehosp Emerg Care.* 2006;10:324-327.
3. Thomas SH, Williams KA. Flight physician training program—core content. *Prehosp Emerg Care.* 2002;6:458-460.
4. Thomas SH, Williams KA, Claypool DW. Medical director for air medical transport programs. *Prehosp Emerg Care.* 2002;6:455-457.
5. Thomas S, Schwamm L, Lev M. A 72-year-old woman admitted to the emergency department because of a sudden change in mental status. *New Eng J Med.* 2006;354(21):2263-2271.

6. Silliman S, Quinn B, Huggett V, Merino J. Use of a field-to-stroke-center helicopter transport program to extend thrombolytic therapy to rural residents. *Stroke*. 2003;34:729-733.

7. Moga C, Harstall C. *Air Ambulance Transportation With Capabilities to Provide Advanced Life Support: IHE Report to the Ministry of Health*. Calgary, Alberta, Canada: Institute of Health Economics; 2007.

8. Ringburg AN, Thomas SH, Steyerberg EW, van Lieshout EM, Patka P, Schipper IB. Lives saved by helicopter emergency medical services: an overview of literature. *Air Med J*. 2009;28:298-302.

9. Baxt W, Moody P. The impact of a rotorcraft aeromedical transport emergency care service on trauma mortality. *JAMA*. 1983;249:3047-3051.

10. Baxt W, Moody P, Cleveland H. Hospital-based rotorcraft aeromedical emergency care services and trauma mortality: a multicenter study. *Ann Emerg Med*. 1985:859-864.

11. Thomas S. Helicopter emergency medical services transport outcomes literature: annotated review of articles published 2004-2006. *Prehosp Emerg Care*. 2007;11:477-488.

12. Thomas S, Biddinger P. Helicopter EMS and trauma outcomes. *Curr Opin Anesth*. 2003;153-158.

13. Thomas SH. Helicopter emergency medical services transport outcomes literature: annotated review of articles published 2000-2003. *Prehosp Emerg Care*. 2004;8:322-333.

14. Brown B, Pogue K, Swenton C, Thomas S. Helicopter EMS transport outcomes literature: annotated review of articles published 2007-2009. 2010. wwwcctcoreorg. Accessed May 1, 2011.

15. Brown B, Pogue K, Williams E, Hatfield J, Kaufman J, Thomas S. Helicopter EMS transport outcomes literature: annotated review of articles published. 2010. wwwcctcoreorg. Accessed May 1, 2011.

16. Wang H, Peitzman A, Cassidy L, Adelson P, Yealy D. Out-of-hospital endotracheal intubation and outcome after traumatic brain injury. *Ann Emerg Med*. 2004;44:439-450.

17. Zink B, Maio R. Out-of-hospital endotracheal intubation in traumatic brain injury: outcomes research provides us with an unexpected outcome. *Ann Emerg Med*. 2004;44:451-453.

18. Cudnik MT, Newgard CD, Wang H, Bangs C, Herrington Rt. Distance impacts mortality in trauma patients with an intubation attempt. *Prehosp Emerg Care*. 2008;12:459-466.

19. Brown JB, Stassen NA, Bankey PE, Sangosanya AT, Cheng JD, Gestring ML. Helicopters and the civilian trauma system: national utilization patterns demonstrate improved outcomes after traumatic injury. *J Trauma*. 2010;69:1030-1034; discussion 4-6.

20. Berlot G, La Fata C, Bacer B, et al. Influence of prehospital treatment on the outcome of patients with severe blunt traumatic brain injury: a single-centre study. *Eur J Emerg Med*. 2009;16:312-317.

21. Barbieri S, Feltracco P, Delantone M, et al. Helicopter rescue and prehospital care for drowning children: two summer season case studies. *Minerva Anestesiol*. 2008;74:703-707.

22. Cocanour CS, Fischer RP, Ursic CM. Are scene flights for penetrating trauma justified? *J Trauma*. 1997;43:83-86; discussion 6-8.

23. Gausche-Hill M, Lewis R, Stratton S. Effect of out-of-hospital pediatric endotracheal intubation on survival and neurological outcome: a controlled clinical trial. *JAMA*. 2000;283:783-790.

24. Davis D, Dunford J, Ochs M, Heister R, Hoyt D. Ventilation patterns following paramedic rapid sequence intubation of patients with severe traumatic brain injury. *Neurocrit Care*. 2005;2:2.

25. Davis DP, Douglas DJ, Koenig W, Carrison D. Buono C, Dunford JV. Hyperventilation following aero-medical rapid sequence intubation may be a deliberate response to hypoxemia. *Resuscitation*. 2007;73(3):354-361.

26. Davis D, Dunford J, Hoyt D, Ochs M, Holbrook T, Fortlage D. The impact of hypoxia and hyperventilation on outcome following paramedic rapid sequence intubation of patients with severe traumatic brain injury. *J Trauma*. 2004;57:1-10.

27. Davis D, Peay J, Serrano J, Buono C, Vilke G. The impact of aeromedical response to patients with moderate to severe traumatic brain injury. *Ann Emerg Med*. 2005;46:115-122.

28. Davis D, Stern J, Ochs M. A follow-up analysis of factors associated with head-injury mortality after paramedic rapid sequence intubation. *J Trauma*. 2005;59:486-490.

29. Harrison T, Thomas S, Wedel S. Success rates of pediatric intubation by a nonphysician-staffed critical care transport service. *Pediatr Emerg Care*. 2004;20(2):101-107.

30. Tiamfook-Morgan TO, Harrison TH, Thomas SH. What happens to SpO2 during air medical crew intubations? *Prehosp Emerg Care*. 2006;10:363-368.

31. Frankema S, Ringburg A, Steyerberg E, Schipper MEI, Vugt Av. Beneficial effect of helicopter emergency medical services on survival of severely injured patients. *Br J Surg*. 2004;91:1520-1526.

32. Davis DP, Peay J, Sise MJ, et al. The impact of prehospital endotracheal intubation on outcome in moderate to severe traumatic brain injury. *J Trauma*. 2005;58:933-939.

33. Ringburg AN, Spanjersberg WR, Frankema SP, Steyerberg EW, Patka P, Schipper IB. Helicopter Emergency Medical Services (HEMS): impact on scene times. *J Trauma*. 2007;63:258-262.

34. Ringburg A. *Helicopter Emergency Medical Services: Effects, Costs, and Benefits*. Rotterdam, the Netherlands: Erasmus University (Trauma Surgery); 2009.

35. Karanicolas PJ, Bhatia P, Williamson J, et al. The fastest route between two points is not always a straight line: an analysis of air and land transfer of nonpenetrating trauma patients. *J Trauma*. 2006;61:396-403.

36. Branas C, MacKenzie E, Williams J, Teter CSH. Access to trauma centers in the United States. *JAMA*. 2005;293:2626-2633.

37. Salomone JP. Prehospital triage of trauma patients: a trauma surgeon's perspective. *Prehosp Emerg Care*. 2006;10:311-313.

38. Hata N, Kobayashi N, Imaizumi T, et al. Use of an air ambulance system improves time to treatment of patients with acute myocardial infarction. *Intern Med*. 2006;45:45-50.

39. Imaizumi T, Hata N, Kobayashi N, et al. Early access to patients with life-threatening cardiovascular disease by an air ambulance service. *J Nippon Med Sch*. 2004;71:352-356.

40. Hyde R, Kociszewski C, Thomas S, Wedel S, Brennan P. Prehospital STEMI diagnosis and early helicopter dispatch to expedite interfacility transfer reduces time to reperfusion (abstract). *Prehosp Emerg Care*. 2008;12:107.

41. Candelise L, Gattinoni M, Bersano A, Micieli G, Sterzi R, Morabito A. Stroke-unit care for acute stroke patients: an observational follow-up study. *Lancet*. 2007;369:299-305.

42. Slater H, O'Mara M, Goldfarb I. Helicopter transportation of burn patients. *Burns*. 2002;28:70-72.

43. Varon J, Fromm R, Marik P. Hearts in the air. *Chest*. 2003;124:1636-1637.

44. Frutkin AD, Mehta SK, Patel T, et al. Outcomes of 1,090 consecutive, elective, nonselected percutaneous coronary interventions at a community hospital without onsite cardiac surgery. *Am J Cardiol*. 2008;101:53-57.

45. Pinto DS, Kirtane AJ, Nallamothu BK, et al. Hospital delays in reperfusion for ST-elevation myocardial infarction: implications when selecting a reperfusion strategy. *Circulation*. 2006;114:2019-2025.

46. Cantor WJ, Fitchett D, Borgundvaag B, et al. Routine early angioplasty after fibrinolysis for acute myocardial infarction. *N Engl J Med*. 2009;360:2705-2718.

47. Crocco TJ, Grotta JC, Jauch EC, et al. EMS management of acute stroke—prehospital triage (resource document to NAEMSP position statement). *Prehosp Emerg Care*. 2007;11:313-317.

48. Schwamm L, Pancioli A, Acker J. Recommendations for the establishment of stroke systems of care. *Stroke*. 2004;36:1-14.

49. Svenson J, O'Connor J, Lindsay M. Is air transport faster? A comparison of air versus ground transport times for interfacility transfers in a regional referral system. *Air Med J*. 2006;24:170-172.

50. Konstantopoulos WM, Pliakas J, Hong C, et al. Helicopter emergency medical services and stroke care regionalization: measuring performance in a maturing system. *Am J Emerg Med*. 2007;25:158-163.

51. Hacke W, Donnan G, Fieschi C, et al. Association of outcome with early stroke treatment: pooled analysis of ATLANTIS, ECASS, and NINDS rt-PA stroke trials. *Lancet.* 2004;363:768-774.

52. Brown JB, Stassen NA, Bankey PE, Sangosanya AT, Cheng JD, Gestring ML. Helicopters improve survival in seriously injured patients requiring interfacility transfer for definitive care. *J Trauma.* 2011;70:310-314.

53. Mann N, Pinkney K, Price D. Injury mortality following the loss of air medical support for rural interhospital transport. *Acad Emerg Med.* 2002;9:694-698.

54. McVey J, Petrie DA, Tallon JM. Air versus ground transport of the major trauma patient: a natural experiment. *Prehosp Emerg Care.* 2010;14:45-50.

55. O'Connor RE. Specialty coverage at non-tertiary care centers. *Prehosp Emerg Care.* 2006;10:343-346.

56. Elliott J, O'Keeffe D, Freeman R. Helicopter transportation of patients with obstetric emergencies in an urban area. *Am J Obstet Gynecol.* 1982;143:157-162.

57. Ohara M, Shimizu Y, Satoh H, et al. Safety and usefulness of emergency maternal transport using helicopter. *J Obstet Gynaecol Res.* 2008;34:189-194.

58. Thomas SH, Harrison T, Wedel SK, Thomas DP. Helicopter emergency medical services roles in disaster operations. *Prehosp Emerg Care.* 2000;4:338-344.

59. Assa A, Landau DA, Barenboim E, Goldstein L. Role of air-medical evacuation in mass-casualty incidents—a train collision experience. *Prehosp Disaster Med.* 2009;24:271-276.

60. Ringburg A, de Ronde G, Thomas SH, Van Lieshout EMM, Patka P, Schipper IB. Validity of Helicopter Emergency Medical Services dispatch criteria for traumatic injuries: a systematic review. *Prehosp Emerg Care.* 2009;13:28-36.

61. Champion H. New tools to reduce deaths and disabilities by improving emergency care: Urgency software, occult injury warnings, and air medical services database. In: NHTSA, ed. *Proceedings of the 19th International Technical Conference on Enhanced Safety of Vehicles (NHTSA sponsored)*, June 6-9, 2005. Washington, DC: US Department of Transportation; 2005.

62. Moront M, Gotschall C, Eichelberger M. Helicopter transport of injured children: system effectiveness and triage criteria. *J Pediatr Surg.* 1996;31:1183-1188.

63. Tiamfook-Morgan T, Browne C, Barclay D, Wedel S, Thomas S. Helicopter scene response: regional variation in compliance with air medical triage guidelines. *Prehosp Emerg Care.* 2008;12(4):443-450.

64. Thomas S, Harrison T, Buras W, Wedel S. Helicopter transport and blunt trauma outcome. *J Trauma.* 2002;52:136-145.

65. Shatney C, Homan J, Sherck J, Ho C-C. The utility of helicopter transport of trauma patients from the injury scene in an urban trauma system. *J Trauma.* 2002;53:817-822.

66. Bledsoe BE, Wesley AK, Eckstein M, Dunn TM, O'Keefe MF. Helicopter scene transport of trauma patients with nonlife-threatening injuries: a meta-analysis. *J Trauma.* 2006;60:1257-1265; discussion 65-66.

67. American College of Surgeons Committee on Trauma. *Resources for Optimal Care of the Injured Patient.* Chicago, IL: American College of Surgeons; 1999.

68. Mango N, Garthe E. Statewide tracking of crash victims' medical system utilization and outcomes. *J Trauma.* 2007;62:436-460.

69. Mulholland SA, Cameron PA, Gabbe BJ, et al. Prehospital prediction of the severity of blunt anatomic injury. *J Trauma.* 2008;64:754-760.

70. Lerner EB. Studies evaluating current field triage: 1966-2005. *Prehosp Emerg Care.* 2006;10:303-306.

71. Caldow SJ, Parke TR, Graham CA, Munro PT. Aeromedical retrieval to a university hospital emergency department in Scotland. *Emerg Med J.* 2005;22:53-55.

72. Diaz M, Hendey G, Bivens H. When is the helicopter faster? A comparison of helicopter and ground ambulance transport times. *J Trauma.* 2005;58:148-153.

73. Shepherd MV, Trethewy CE, Kennedy J, Davis L. Helicopter use in rural trauma. *Emerg Med Australas.* 2008;20:494-499.

74. Black J, Ward M, Lockey D. Appropriate use of helicopters to transport trauma patients from incident scene to hospital in the United Kingdom: an algorithm. *Emerg Med J.* 2004;21:355-361.

75. Burany B, Rudas L. [Interhospital transport of acute coronary syndrome patients from Bacs-Kiskun county]. *Orv Hetil.* 2005;146:1819-1825.

76. Thomas SH. On-site hospital helipads: resource document for the NAEMSP position paper on on-site hospital helipads. *Prehosp Emerg Care.* 2009;13:398-401.

77. Kaufmanh M, Moser B, Lederer W. Changes in injury patterns and severity in a helicopter air-rescue system over a 6-year period. *Wilderness Environ Med.* 2006;17:8-14.

78. Henry MC. Trauma triage: New York experience. *Prehosp Emerg Care.* 2006;10:295-302.

79. Hedges JR, Newgard CD, Mullins R. Emergency Medical Treatment and Active Labor Act and trauma triage. *Prehosp Emerg Care.* 2006;10:332-339.

80. Eichelberger M, Gotscholl C, Sacco W, Bowman L, Mangubat E, Lowenstein A. A comparison of the trauma score, the revised trauma score, and the pediatric trauma score. *Ann Emerg Med.* 1989;18:1053-1058.

81. Kaufmann C, Maier R, Rivara F, Carrico C. Evaluation of the pediatric trauma score. *JAMA.* 1990;263:69-72.

82. Engum S, Mitchell M, Scherer L, et al. Prehospital triage in the injured pediatric patient. *J Pediatr Surg.* 2000;35:82-87.

83. Cottington E, Young J, Shufflebarger C, Kyes F, Peterson F, Diamond D. The utility of physiologic status, injury site, and injury mechanism in identifying patients with major trauma. *J Trauma.* 1988;28:305-311.

84. Long W, Bachulis B, Hynes G. Accuracy and relationship of mechanisms of injury, trauma score, and injury severity score in identifying major trauma. *Am J Surg.* 1986;151:581-584.

85. Newgard CD, Lewis RJ, jolly B. Use of out-of-hospital variables to predict severity of injury in pediatric patients involved in motor vehicle crashes. *Ann Emerg Med.* 2002;39:481-491.

86. Norcross E, Ford D, Cooper M, Zone-Smith L, Byrne T, Yarbrough D. Application of the American College of Surgeons' field triage guidelines by prehospital personnel. *J Am Coll Surg.* 1995;181:539-544.

87. Wuerz R, Taylor J, Smith J. Accuracy of trauma triage guidelines in patients transported by helicopter. *Air Med J.* 1996;15:168-170.

88. Gearhart PA, Wuerz R, Localio AR. Cost-effectiveness analysis of helicopter EMS for trauma patients. *Ann Emerg Med.* 1997;30:500-506.

89. Mitchell AD, Tallon JM, Sealy B. Air versus ground transport of major trauma patients to a tertiary trauma centre: a province-wide comparison using TRISS analysis. *Can J Surg.* 2007;50:129-133.

90. Harrison T, Thomas S, Wedel S. Interhospital aeromedical transports: delayed air medical activation in adult and pediatric trauma patients. *Am J Emerg Med.* 1997;15:122-124.

91. Mackersie RC. History of trauma field triage development and the American College of Surgeons criteria. *Prehosp Emerg Care.* 2006;10:287-294.

92. MacKenzie EJ, Rivara FP, Jurkovich GJ, et al. A national evaluation of the effect of trauma-center care on mortality. *N Engl J Med.* 2006;354:366-378.

93. Newgard CD, McConnell KJ, Hedges JR. Variability of trauma transfer practices among non-tertiary care hospital emergency departments. *Acad Emerg Med.* 2006;13:746-754.

94. Fallon W. Editorial comment following Bledsoe BE, Smith MG: medical helicopter accidents in the US. *J Trauma.* 2004;56:1325-1329.

95. Thomson D, Thomas S. Guidelines for air medical dispatch [position statement for National Association of EMS Physicians]. *Prehosp Emerg Care.* 2003;7:265-271.

96. Mackersie RC. Field triage, and the fragile supply of "optimal resources" for the care of the injured patient. *Prehosp Emerg Care.* 2006;10:347-350.

97. Lemson J, van Grunsven PM, Schipper IB, et al. [Helicopter-mobile medical teams in the Netherlands: significant differences in deployment frequencies between different emergency room regions]. *Ned Tijdschr Geneeskd*. 2008;152:1106-1112.

98. Purtill MA, Benedict K, Hernandez-Boussard T, et al. Validation of a prehospital trauma triage tool: a 10-year perspective. *J Trauma*. 2008;65:1253-1257.

99. Bruhn J, Williams K, Aghababian R. True costs of air medical vs. ground ambulance systems. *Air Med J*. 1993;12:262-268.

100. Lerner EB, Maio RF, Garrison HG, Spaite DW, Nichol G. Economic value of out-of-hospital emergency care: a structured literature review. *Ann Emerg Med*. 2006;47:515-524.

101. Elvik R. Cost-benefit analysis of ambulance and rescue helicopters in Norway: reflections on assigning a monetary value to saving a human life. *Appl Health Econ Health Policy*. 2002;1:55-63.

102. Selmer R, Halvorsen S, Myhre KI, Wisloff TF, Kristiansen IS. Cost-effectiveness of primary percutaneous coronary intervention versus thrombolytic therapy for acute myocardial infarction. *Scand Cardiovasc J*. 2005;39:276-285.

103. Kurola J, Wangel M, Uusaro A, Ruokonen E. Paramedic helicopter emergency service in rural Finland - Do benefits justify the cost? *Acta Anaesthesiol Scand*. 2002;46:771-778.

104. Nicholl J, Turner J, Stevens K, et al. A review of the costs and benefits of helicopter emergency ambulance services in England and Wales: report to the Department of Health. In; 07/03/2003.

105. Hubner B. Evaluation of the immediate effects of preclinical treatment of severely injured trauma patients by Helicopter Trauma Team in the Netherlands. Vrije Universititeit Amsterdam (thesis). 1999.

106. Cummings G, O'Keefe G. Scene disposition and mode of transport following rural trauma: a prospective cohort study comparing patient costs. *J Emerg Med*. 2000;18:349-354.

107. Thomas SH, Orf J, Peterson C, Wedel SK. Frequency and costs of laboratory and radiograph repetition in trauma patients undergoing interfacility transfer. *Am J Emerg Med*. 2000;18:156-158.

108. Silbergleit R, Scott P, Lowell M, Silbergleit R. Cost-effectiveness of helicopter transport of stroke patients for thrombolysis. *Acad Emerg Med*. 2003;10:966-972.

109. Concannon TW, Kent DM, Normand SL, et al. Comparative effectiveness of ST-segment-elevation myocardial infarction regionalization strategies. *Circ Cardiovasc Qual Outcomes*. 2010;3(5):506-513.

110. Bassi M, Zuercher M, Erne JJ, Ummenhofer W. Endotracheal tube intracuff pressure during helicopter transport. *Ann Emerg Med*. 2010;56:89-93. e1.

111. Conroy M, Rodriguez S, Kimmel S, Kasner S. Helicopter transfer offers benefit to patients with acute stroke. *Stroke*. 1999;30:2580-2584.

112. Fromm R, Hoskins E, Cronin L. Bleeding complications following initiation of thrombolytic therapy for acute myocardial infarction: a comparison of helicopter-transported and nontransported patients. *Ann Emerg Med*. 1991;20:892-895.

113. Hunt R, Bryan D, Brinkley V. Inability to assess breath sounds during air medical transports by helicopter. *JAMA*. 1991;265:1982-1984.

114. Stone C, Stimson A, Thomas S. The effectiveness of esophageal stethoscopy in a simulated in-flight setting. *Air Med J*. 1995;14:219-221.

115. Thomas SH, Farkas A, Wedel SK. Cabin configuration and prolonged oral endotracheal intubation in the AS365N2 Dauphin EMS helicopter. *Air Med J*. 1996;15:65-68.

116. Thomas SH, Stone CK, Bryan-Berge D. The ability to perform closed chest compressions in helicopters. *Am J Emerg Med*. 1994;12:296-298.

117. Stone CK, Thomas SH. Can correct closed-chest compressions be performed during prehospital transport? *Prehosp Disaster Med*. 1995;10:121-123.

118. Hightower DP, Thomas SH, Stone CK, Brinkley S, Brown DF. Red cabin lights impair air medical crew performance of color-dependent tasks. *Air Med J*. 1995;14:75-78.

119. Coppola CP, Tyree M, Larry K, DiGeronimo R. A 22-year experience in global transport extracorporeal membrane oxygenation. *J Pediatr Surg*. 2008;43:46-52; discussion.

120. Foley DS, Pranikoff T, Younger JG, et al. A review of 100 patients transported on extracorporeal life support. *ASAIO J*. 2002;48:612-619.

121. Tintinalli J, Lisse E, Begley A, Campbell C. Emergency care in Namibia. *Ann Emerg Med*. 1998;32:373-376.

122. Harrison TH, Thomas SH, Wedel SK. Success rates of pediatric intubation by a non-physician-staffed critical care transport service. *Pediatr Emerg Care*. 2004;20:101-107.

123. Thomson DP, Thomas SH. Guidelines for air medical dispatch. *Prehosp Emerg Care*. 2003;7:265-271.

124. Thomas S, Judge T, Lowell MJ, et al. Airway management success and hypoxemia rates in air and ground critical care transport: a prospective multicenter study. *Prehosp Emerg Care*. 2010;14:283.

125. Fromm R, Taylor D, Cronin L, McCallum W, Levine R. The incidence of pacemaker dysfunction during helicopter air medical transport. *Am J Emerg Med*. 1992;10:333-335.

126. Hon K, Olsen H, Totapally B, Leung T. Air verus ground transportation of artificially ventilated neonates: comparative differences in selected cardiopulmonary parameters. *Pediatr Emerg Care*. 2006;22:107-112.

127. Orf J, Thomas SH, Ahmed W, et al. Appropriateness of endotracheal tube size and insertion depth in children undergoing air medical transport. *Pediatr Emerg Care*. 2000;16:321-327.

128. MacDonald RD, Banks BA, Morrison M. Epidemiology of adverse events in air medical transport. *Acad Emerg Med*. 2008;15:923-931.

129. Braman S, Dunn S, Amico C, Millman R. Complications of intrahospital transport in critically ill patients. *Ann Intern Med*. 1987;107:469-473.

130. Blumen I. *A Safety Review and Risk Assessment in Air Medical Transport*. Salt Lake City, UT: Air Medical Physician Association; 2002.

131. Holland J, Cooksley D. Safety of helicopter aeromedical transport in Australia: a retrospective study. *Med J Aust*. 2005;182:17-19.

132. Hinkelbein J, Dambier M, Viergutz T, Genzwurker H. A 6-year analysis of German emergency medical services helicopter crashes. *J Trauma*. 2008;64:204-210.

133. Lutman D, Montgomery M, Ramnarayan P, Petros A. Ambulance and aeromedical accident rates during emergency retrieval in Great Britain. *Emerg Med J*. 2008;25:301-302.

134. Sanddal ND, Albert S, Hansen JD, Kupas DF. Contributing factors and issues associated with rural ambulance crashes: literature review and annotated bibliography. *Prehosp Emerg Care*. 2008;12:257-267.

135. On-site hospital helipads: joint position statement of the National Association of EMS Physicians and the Association of Air Medical Services (approved 8/27/06). 2006. http://www.naemsp.org/position.html. Accessed October 16, 2008.

136. Centers for Medicare and Medicaid Services. Revised EMTALA interpretive guidelines. 2004. http://www.cms.gov/SurveyCertification GenInfo/downloads/SCLetter04-34.pdf. Accessed July 25, 2011.

137. Hankins D. The safety net at risk. *Air Med J*. 2011;30:125.

138. Sasser SM, Hunt RC, Sullivent EE, et al. Guidelines for field triage of injured patients. Recommendations of the National Expert Panel on Field Triage. *MMWR Recomm Rep*. 2009;58:1-35.

CHAPTER 19

Emergency Management

Jean B. Bail

Steven J. Parrillo

INTRODUCTION

Put simply, emergency management deals with risk and risk avoidance.[1] This simple phrase turns into a complex, comprehensive discipline and field of study considering all hazards, all phases, all impacts, and all stakeholders.[2] All hazards include the many possible natural (earthquake, hurricane, tornado, flood, climate issues) or man-made (domestic/ international terrorism, cyber) threats that create risk and vulnerability to an organization, community, or region. Using the phases of prevention, preparedness, mitigation, response and recovery, emergency management forms a management paradigm that prepares the organization to be disaster resistant and disaster resilient. All impacts include assessing the effects on population, human services, the economy, and infrastructures. Stakeholders include the individual, community, organization, business, hospital and the government as well as the collaboration between public, private, and governmental agencies. Emergency managers exist at all levels and function to coordinate and mobilize the right people, right agreements, and right policies and procedures when needed in an incident. The EMS physician is in a perfect position to assume a leadership or supportive role in many emergency management functions.

OBJECTIVES

- Define the role of emergency management organizations.
- Discuss the relationship between emergency management and EMS, fire and law enforcement.
- List the major communications modalities with advantages and disadvantages for each.
- Define the roles of relevant Emergency Support Functions as well as the role the EM/EMS physician might play in each.
- Discuss the role of EMS physicians as part of the Emergency Management system.

HISTORY OF EMERGENCY MANAGEMENT

Emergency management is the coordination and integration of all activities necessary to build, sustain, and improve the capability to prepare for, protect against, respond to, recover from, or mitigate against threatened or actual natural disasters, acts of terrorism, or other manmade disasters. The US development of emergency management began as a reactive model to a New Hampshire town destroyed by fire in 1803 when the government authorized dollars to rebuild. Under Franklin Roosevelt in the 1930s, the Reconstruction Finance Corporation and the Bureau of Public Roads led the effort to rebuild public facilities after disasters through loans. Flooding was an issue evidenced by the Tennessee Valley Authority projects and the Flood Control Act of 1934 leading to increased use and authority of the US Army Corps of Engineers to design and build flood control projects. Beginning in the 1950s, the focus shifted to the potential effects of nuclear war and the Cold War era began. Civil Defense programs were in place in every community and the familiar "Duck and Cover" program was taught in the schools and fallout shelter signs were common. During this time emergency preparedness was embedded in the Office of Defense Mobilization before being combined with Civil Defense into to the *Office of Civil Defense and Mobilization*. Natural disaster events such as Hurricanes Hazel and Audrey were dealt with in the previous reactive model of post event funding for recovery of the affected regions.

President Kennedy changed the federal structure when he created the Office of Emergency Preparedness to deal with natural disaster events while maintaining the Office of Civil Defense in the Department of Defense to deal with Cold War issues. During the 1960s, many events occurred that caused tremendous damage and lives lost which, although handled in the reactive post event funding model, set the stage for changes in the 1970s. Over 100 different agencies had involvement in disaster preparedness and response, leading to confusion and fragmentation of services. Efforts began to grow to consolidate federal emergency management activities into a centralized agency and gained momentum after issues arose in the response to the Three Mile Island nuclear power plant accident in 1979. Under President Carter, *Federal Emergency Management Agency (FEMA)* was created merging many disaster-related functions under one structure. Under this new agency, an Integrated Emergency Management System was developed combining natural disasters and civil defense into an all hazards approach. The 1980s and early 1990s were turbulent, controversial times for FEMA based on poorly handled responses to events such as Hurricanes Hugo, Andrew and Iniki, the Loma Prieta earthquake, political issues and unpopular decisions until President Clinton appointed James Lee Witt as director in 1993.

Under Witt's leadership, FEMA developed into a more functional and responsive agency with a new emphasis on disaster preparedness, mitigation, and customer service. As the first director with state emergency management experience, Witt was able to build relationships, focus on customer service, embed technology and build community disaster resilient programs. During Witt's tenure as director many natural disaster incidents occurred as well as the Oklahoma City bombing. The success of FEMA's response to all of these events created the platform for emergency management's growth as a profession and as an international model of resilience, mitigation, and response. During this time the *Federal Response Plan* (FRP) was enacted to coordinate federal assistance and resources to states and local governments overwhelmed by a major disaster, supporting implementation of the *Robert T. Stafford Disaster Relief and Emergency Assistance Act*.

After September 11, 2001 the attention turned to terrorism with the majority of resources being directed through the newly created small Office of Homeland Security which evolved within a year to the *Department of Homeland Security*. Combining 22 agencies, budgets, and personnel with the mission of protecting the nation, reducing the vulnerability to terrorist attacks, and reducing damages from all incidents man made or natural led to sweeping changes. With the focus on terrorism, less attention was spent on mitigation and preparedness of natural disasters until the impact of Hurricane Katrina was realized in 2005. Due to the inefficient response to Katrina, the Post Katrina Emergency Management Reform Act was passed in 2006, realigning functions within the Department of Homeland Security including elements of FEMA.

As a profession Emergency Management embraces the management principles necessary to build an effective organization—one that is able to build resilience based on the core principles of emergency management:

1. **Comprehensive**—Emergency managers consider and take into account all hazards, all phases, all stakeholders, and all impacts relevant to disasters.
2. **Progressive**—Emergency managers anticipate future disasters and take preventive and preparatory measures to build disaster-resistant and disaster-resilient communities.
3. **Risk-driven**—Emergency managers use sound risk management principles (hazard identification, risk analysis, and impact analysis) in assigning priorities and resources.
4. **Integrated**—Emergency managers ensure unity of effort among all levels of government and all elements of a community.
5. **Collaborative**—Emergency managers create and sustain broad and sincere relationships among individuals and organizations to encourage trust, advocate a team atmosphere, build consensus, and facilitate communication.
6. **Coordinated**—Emergency managers synchronize the activities of all relevant stakeholders to achieve a common purpose.

7. **Flexible**—Emergency managers use creative and innovative approaches in solving disaster challenges.

8. **Professional**—Emergency managers value a science and knowledge-based approach based on education, training, experience, ethical practice, public stewardship, and continuous improvement.[2]

FRAMEWORK IN US—NATIONAL RESPONSE FRAMEWORK

The current US model, the National Response Framework, was created out of the earlier models to guide the interagency response of communities, tribes, States, the Federal government, private, and nongovernmental partners in a coordinated national response. It defines the principles, roles, and structure that organize how the response to any event is organized into an effective approach using best practices. Coming out of the *Homeland Security Act of 2003*, Homeland Security Presidential Directives 5, 7, and 8 strengthened US preparation for domestic incident response, including incidents from terrorism, pandemics, to natural disasters. Built on the concepts of engagement and collaboration, tiered response, a scalable, flexible, and adaptable capability, and unity of command all support a readiness to act from the individual or community level all the way to the federal government.

National Incident Management System (NIMS) is the country's process for organizing disaster management. It is a comprehensive, multiagency plan to improve communications, coordination, command, and control across all elements involved in a systematic response.[3] Using a common framework provides for a standardized but flexible response that every responding agency can apply with an understandable structure and terminology. The *Incident Command System* (ICS) is the most visible aspect of NIMS, developed out of the need to add organization to events where multiple people and groups come together to deal with a disaster situation. These situations most often call for response services from multiple jurisdictions and types of response agencies to converge on a specific location to address incident needs. Bringing responders together that have different internal command structures, protocols, communication systems, and expectations usually resulted in chaos. Firefighting Resources of Southern California Organized for Potential Emergencies (FIRESCOPE) developed from the California wildfire experience and created the Incident Command System management model to begin to organize command, control and communications across multiple organizations platforms.

Organization can occur across responding units by building a common structure of responsibilities and reporting. Functionality can be capitalized upon to provide an organized response to the event. Using common language and reporting structures allows responding units to avoid interpretation errors and to be placed in settings to perform the needed tasks. Using this command management system every day, paid and volunteer staff become acclimated to the structure, command and control, reporting mechanisms, and paperwork. The ICS structure has five primary components: *command, operations, planning, logistics, and finance/administration*. Additional elements are incorporated based on the situation and technical expertise necessary.

APPLICATION OF THE ICS MANAGEMENT FRAMEWORK IN EVENTS

■ UNIFIED COMMAND

The concept of unified command speaks to the way different jurisdictional response agencies relate to each other, respecting the integrity of each agency's internal chain of command while creating a mechanism of coordination across jurisdictions.[4] With the goal of organizing and maximizing the skills of each agency and still having an effective command structure, unified command brings this expertise into a single command function.[5,6] In this function a single set of incident objectives and collaborative strategies are created. Duplication of resources is minimized and communications enhanced.

■ COMMUNICATIONS

Communication is often the Achilles heel of disaster response. Plans often foolishly assume that normal modalities will work in all situations. For many reasons, that will not be the case in a disaster. Infrastructure damage may limit some modalities. Sheer volume may overwhelm others. One goal of NIMS is to ensure that the systems necessary for emergency management are in place. Time should not be lost devising a plan to deal with a failure that could have been avoided. Poor interoperability may make it impossible for one responding agency to communicate with another. The keys to communications success are preparation and redundancy.

In addition to the hardware listed below, the word "communications" also refers to interpersonal dialogue. Planning and mitigation involve discussion among key stakeholders. The hospital EOP, for example, should be the product of all those from whom buy-in is required. That includes not only those who directly provide health care, but also ancillary services, facilities management, human resources, and others. Many hospital EMCs wisely ask guidance from local EMS representatives. It is also critical to remember that the media will be the major entity getting information to the public. Emergency management officials need to speak with the media and must name and train a Public Information Officer (PIO). That role is critical. The PIO is part of the Command Staff. (See Chapter 74 for a more thorough description of this ICS position.)

There is no doubt that the cell phone—especially the "smart phone"—is the most popular and arguably the most useful communication device in the setting of a disaster. The device is ubiquitous in the US. It is so popular that the landline phone industry has declined significantly. Many individuals no longer own a land line phone. Most cellular carriers scale operations to handle only a fraction of system capacity. In a disaster cellular use increases markedly, sometimes enough to overwhelm capacity. During the August 2011 east coast 5.8 Richter earthquake that caused no real damage and generated no injuries, most could not use their cell phones for several hours. There are ways, however, for providers to increase capacity. Carriers can send trailers into the congested area with antennas, repeaters, generators. Additionally, some carriers can provide predesignated emergency workers priority, though there is no legal requirement that they do so.[7] That does not guarantee that a call will go through, but makes it more likely that the worker will get a connection. Additionally, most phones have the capacity to send text messages. Thankfully, the texting function works even when cellular capacity is overwhelmed. Finally, the Department of Homeland Security allows key disaster responders to obtain an enhanced cellular signal using the National Communications System "Government Emergency Telecommunications Service" or GETS card. The license is usually given to a facility or service which then requests a specific number of GETS cards. That card must be surrendered when an individual leaves the facility or the emergency management service position within that facility.

Notification of key personnel is critically important during an MCI or disaster. Until recently such notification was most likely to be done by telephone, often using call algorithms specific to a department or service. Mass notification systems such as Lynx, MIR3, E2Campus, and others have been in existence for years, but their use increased markedly after the 2007 Virginia Tech shooting. Many universities, hospitals, and emergency services use such a system. Most allow for simultaneous notification of all subscribers to their cell phones, home and work e-mails, desktop and laptop computers, and other mobile communication platforms. For the EMS physician, such a system allows simple, instantaneous communication of need at the hospital, response service, DMAT, and other important resources. Usually only a few people have the administrative ability to initiate a call.

Although more expensive than the cellular phone, the satellite phone has come into its own. The phone is now roughly the size of a laptop and service is available for approximately $1 per minute.[7] Some services now allow for a subscriber to purchase time only when needed, rather than paying for time plus a monthly fee. Most can now maintain a line of sight to a satellite even while moving. Reliability is a plus.

Many EMS providers are very accustomed to mobile communication vehicles. Available devices can include radio, satellite phone, Internet connection, fax machine, and scanners. Most are generator powered—a clear advantage in a disaster situation. Radio communication is still standard in EMS systems and even hospital emergency management. Popular push-to-talk systems are now available from a number of carriers that also supply cellular service. Standard radios use a variety of frequencies. High frequency (HF) is good for long distance but may be adversely affected by environmental conditions. Very high frequency (VHF) requires line of sight. Although it is less susceptible to environmental "noise," land features may block transmission. Ultra high frequency (UHF) requires line of sight and penetrates manmade and land features well. Super high frequency—also called microwave—is the most reliable. This frequency penetrates land features and passes readily through the atmosphere.[7] Many hospital EOPs call for the physician in the ED to receive a radio for use during an event. The EMS physician needs to know the uses and limitations of his or her equipment. Additionally, he or she should seek to provide input into the choice of new systems.

Tablet computers are the latest addition to the communication armamentarium. These powerful devices can instantly provide rapid communication among members of a given group. Internet connection is reliable even away from "hot spots." Many can serve as cellular phones as well and users can readily access news information services. Users have instant access to pre-loaded data such as a facility's EOP and ICS/HICS positions. Because they are Internet capable, users can access mass information systems being used among multiple entities. For example, in several eastern Pennsylvania counties, emergency management, EMS, law enforcement and hospitals subscribe to a service called Knowledge Center. Each subscriber has a unique access code, but information that is facility specific can be shared with all users. Bed availability can be updated as needed. Names are typed into ICS/HICS positions and changed for each operational period. The information stored can be used to produce ICS/NIMS forms filled in with pertinent data and is valuable when the after action report must be written. The available store of useful "aps" is exhaustive and grows regularly. One of the challenges is to choose and use only a small number of useful applications.

Regardless of the modality used by the EMS physician, one of the first duties is to communicate pertinent information about the disaster/MCE site to appropriate agencies. Data regarding the nature of the event, an estimate of victim number and injury severity, the need for services such as law enforcement, fire, search, and rescue, or HAZMAT help authorities make educated decisions about allocation of resources. Effective communication should help with appropriate distribution of victims. The physician (or lead medic at the scene) might also relay information about establishment of an ICS.[8]

In addition to one manager or responder speaking to another, it is critical to remember that the media will be the major entity getting information to the public. Emergency management officials need to speak with the media and must name and train a Public Information Officer (PIO). That role is critical. The PIO is part of the Command Staff. (See Chapter 74 for a more thorough description of this ICS position.)

Various early warning systems complete the discussion of communication in disasters. Federal and state modalities seek to provide authorities that a biologic agent may be in the area. Such information may allow for significant mitigation. Examples include the CDC's National Electronic Disease Surveillance System (NEDSS) and Health Alert Network (HAN) and others.[9,10]

EMERGENCY SUPPORT FUNCTIONS

FEMA Emergency Support Functions (ESF) provide a concept of operations, procedures, and structures to achieve needed coordination of essential functions and response objectives in an incident. Developed into 15 categories that align governmental and private sector agencies

that provide specific services, a lead agency is designated for each. There are several ESFs that apply to emergency management for the EMS physician. Each is listed below with a brief description.

FEMA can deploy assets and capabilities through ESFs into an area in anticipation of an approaching storm or event that is expected to cause a significant impact and result. This coordination through ESFs allows FEMA to position Federal support for a quick response, though actual assistance cannot normally be provided until the Governor requests and receives a Presidential major disaster or emergency declaration. This "leaning forward" or prepositioning of assets is now the model for predicted events.

ESF 4—FIREFIGHTING

ESF 4 "provides Federal support for the detection and suppression of wildland, rural, and urban fires resulting from or occurring coincidentally with an incident requiring a coordinated Federal response."[11] The Department of Agriculture/Forest Service is the lead agency, supported by the Departments of Commerce, Defense, Homeland Security, Interior, State and the Environmental Protection Agency. The physician role has several foci: medical clearance for service, provider rehabilitation, and hazardous materials threat assessment and chemical impact from an incident. Understanding the Incident Command System is essential since this is the management model of the fire service. Many types of technical rescue teams that benefit from physician involvement are provided out of the fire service. Confined space, high angle, building collapse, urban search and rescue, and hazardous materials are several; medical oversight and on-scene support are critical components for safe, effective operations. Anticipating the high heat, high stress, variable weather conditions, hazards and the impact upon personnel, victims, and the community places the physician at the heart of medical preparedness.

Understanding the National Fire Protection Agency (NFPA) 1600 Standards on Disaster/Emergency Management and Business Continuity Programs[12] combine both the clinical care aspects of the physician role with the management understanding of the larger picture of emergency management. Adopted by the Department of Homeland Security as the national preparedness standard, NFPA 1600 established a common set of criteria for disaster, emergency management, and business continuity programs in both public and private sectors.

ESF 6—MASS CARE, EMERGENCY ASSISTANCE, HOUSING, AND HUMAN SERVICES

ESF 6 "coordinates the delivery of Federal mass care, emergency assistance, housing and human services when local, tribal, and State response and recovery needs exceed their capability."[13]

DHS/FEMA is the ESF coordinator as well as the lead agency. Every state designates a lead agency; that agency works with the governor. Supporting Federal agencies include the Departments of Agriculture, Defense, Health and Human Services, Housing and Urban Development, Interior, Justice, Labor, Transportation, Treasury, Veterans Affairs, as well as the Social Security Administration, Small Business Administration, US Postal Service, American Red Cross, and several other NGOs.

Of the four ESF six components, the EMS physician is most likely to be involved in "mass care." That portion includes emergency first aid for victims as well as sheltering, feeding, and collecting/distribution of information on victims to family members. The Annex specifically mentions that the sheltering and medical needs of special needs populations are included. Health care providers may also be called upon to provide ongoing care for those in the shelters. Although the EM/EMS physician probably will not be involved in the evacuation of nursing home patients, he or she may be one of the medical care providers for them before or after they are relocated. The physician may be requested to coordinate and provide input on process and resource needs and use during these events. Understanding the mutual aid agreements and assistance plans regionally, intrastate, and interstate is very helpful when managing evacuation and sheltering needs.

ESF 8 - PUBLIC HEALTH AND MEDICAL SERVICES

This is the largest of the ESFs that are likely to involve the EMS physician. The purpose includes "responding to medical needs associated with mental health, behavioral health, and substance abuse considerations of incident victims and response workers." It also covers "the medical needs of members of the 'at risk' or 'special needs' population described in the Pandemic and All-Hazards Preparedness Act and in the National Response Framework (NRF) Glossary, respectively."[14] The Department of Health and Human Services (HHS) serves as both ESF Coordinator and Primary Agency. HHS does this through the *Office of the Assistant Secretary for Preparedness and Response* (ASPR). Supporting agencies include the Departments of Agriculture, Commerce, Defense, Energy, Homeland Security, Interior, Justice, State, Transportation and Veterans Affairs as well as the Environmental Protection Agency, General Services Administration, US Postal Service, and American Red Cross.

EMS physicians and Emergency Medicine physicians who serve in a military reserve unit may find themselves as part of a Department of Defense deployment for casualty clearing, staging, and treatment. Likewise, those who are members of the Medical Reserve Corps may be called upon to assist State, tribal, and local public health and other medical personnel. EM physicians on staff at NDMS-affiliated hospitals may be part of emergency department receiving teams for disaster victims transported to their areas. Emergency physicians with training in psychological first aid or critical incident stress management could assist if HHS asks for assistance from partner organizations. Finally, ESF 8 can deploy National Medical Response Teams to assist with victim decontamination, surge response, etc. Emergency medicine physicians are often part of those teams. For more about the potential for physician involvement, see "Roles of EM / EMS Physician in Emergency Management" below.

ESF 9—SEARCH AND RESCUE (SAR)

The purpose of ESF 9 is to rapidly deploy "Federal SAR resources to provide lifesaving assistance to State, tribal and local authorities, to include local SAR Coordinators and Mission Coordinators, when there is an actual or anticipated request for Federal SAR assistance."[15]

Operational involvement may involve structural collapse, maritime/coastal/waterborne or land scenarios. FEMA is the ESF Coordinator. Other primary agencies include the US Coast Guard, the Department of the Interior/National Park Service, and the Department of Defense. Support agencies include the Departments of Agriculture, Commerce, Health and Human Services, Justice, Labor, Transportation as well as NASA and the US Agency for International Development.

The primary agency for each type of SAR depends on the setting. DHS/FEMA takes the lead for structural collapse urban search and rescue—US&R. DHS/US Coast Guard is responsible for maritime/coastal/waterborne events. For land SAR, responsibility resides with the Department of the Interior/National Park Service and Department of Defense.

Currently there are 28 US&R task forces distributed throughout the US. The goal is 6 hours from notification of need to departure. All teams are prepared to be self-sufficient at the site for 3 days. Personnel categories include search, rescue, medical, and technical.[16] Nationwide, many EMS physicians serve on urban search and rescue teams as medical providers in support of other team members who find and rescue victims. They provide care both for team members and patients.

ESF 11—AGRICULTURAL

ESF 11 may not seem to impact the health and medical community until it is viewed in these terms: "nutrition assistance, response to animal/plant diseases and pests, safety of meat, poultry, and egg products, protection of natural and cultural resources and historic properties and the safety and well-being of household pets."[17] The EMS physician may become involved with response teams that use search dogs, shelters where pets are being cared for as well as people, or events involving the consumption of contaminated meat or foods. It is important to note that the epidemiology of these events may be a shared public health, Federal Bureau of Investigation, and Department of Agriculture function.

ESF 13 PUBLIC SAFETY AND SECURITY

ESF 13 includes "force and critical infrastructure protection, security planning and technical assistance, technology support, general law enforcement assistance to both pre-incident and post-incident situations.[18] The Department of Justice (DOJ) is the ESF #13 coordinator and primary agency supported by the Bureau of Alcohol, Tobacco, Firearms and Explosives, the Drug Enforcement Administration, Federal Bureau of Investigation, Office of Justice Programs, and the U.S. Marshals Service. Other support agencies include Department of Commerce, Environmental Protection Agency (Hazardous Materials evidence response teams), and the Department of Energy (nuclear/radiological incident response).

The EMS physician may become involved with tactical medicine in support of law enforcement and SWAT functions and in support of detection and investigation of chemical, biological, and radiological incidents. A primary role will be facilitating operations from the health standpoint: evaluating occupational and environmental health needs, responder safety and health, logistics and operational needs coordinated with those section chiefs, and continued training and exercises where the process of ICS is refined, strengths and weaknesses identified and addressed and specific unit objectives achieved. In some areas, the tactical physician will be cross trained in the police academy.

ROLES OF EM/EMS PHYSICIAN IN EMERGENCY MANAGEMENT

The primary focus of this chapter is the physician's actual role in a disaster or MCI whether or not that physician serves as an emergency manager. Although it will of course vary depending on the circumstances surrounding the event, the manager is primarily the one in charge of logistics. The reasons are stated above, but essentially depend in his knowledge of the community, hospital, etc. Often the physician with this responsibility is thought of as "the disaster guy" by colleagues and coworkers in the hospital. They assume that this person will take over. Most of them have very little knowledge of what managing an MCI actually involves. They depend on "the disaster guy."

For most settings in which an EMS or EM physician is involved as the manager, someone else is the IC or Operations Chief. In a hospital-based event, he/she may be in the Emergency Operations Center (EOC) serving as a technical medical specialist or assistant to the IC. If the physician is in the ED when the event occurs, he or she may serve in an operations position until relieved by another EM physician, allowing him to move to the EOC. For the EMS physician in the field, the role will depend on the personnel with him at the time. The EMS physician who is not an emergency manager plays an equally important role. He is an expert in areas that are critically important to the successful management of a disaster. Many use mobile command centers and can offer that assistance to be included in an Emergency Operations Plan (EOP). Most know MOUs and MOAs well enough to advise others how to write them, incorporate them into an EOP, and execute them when the time comes. Part of the EMS physician's job is to know what equipment might be needed in a disaster and how to obtain that equipment—knowledge that can be imparted to a person charged with logistics. These physicians can serve as consultants/subject matter experts, reviewing an entity's mass casualty response plan, and making recommendations to make that plan complete and practical.

Although many assume that EM residencies prepare their residents to deal with disasters and MCIs, that is not the case. In 2010, the Society for Academic Emergency Medicine EMS Interest Group surveyed residencies to determine how many included training in disaster medicine. (Personal communication, Chris Martin-Gill, 2011) Only 57% of the responding residencies stated that training is mandatory. The training is available but optional in 38%. In those programs where training is optional, only 20% of residents participate. Authorities such as Subbarao are trying to change that by proposing an educational framework and competency set for disaster medicine and public health professionals.[19]

The American College of Osteopathic Emergency Physicians proposed an emergency medicine residency Disaster Medicine Curriculum to the American Osteopathic Association on July 16, 2011.[20]

The American College of Emergency Physicians (ACEP) encourages emergency physicians to be actively involved in disaster planning and response.[21] ACEP also has a Disaster Medicine Section. In 2010 the American College of Osteopathic Emergency Physicians (ACOEP) started a section of the World Association of Disaster and Emergency Medicine (WADEM) for its members. Several emergency medicine physicians have served on the WADEM Board. The National Association of EMS Physicians also affirms that such clinicians should take a lead role in disaster/MCI preparedness and response.[22] The basic process of learning emergency management begins with completing the online courses from FEMA. There are multiple independent study (IS) courses that create a common structure and language. Supporting the independent learning courses are several in-class, regionally delivered course on advanced ICS that provide more skills in a collaborative model.[23]

Although not universal, many hospitals have emergency physicians either as members or Chairs of their Emergency Management Committees (EMC). Doing so goes a long way toward integrating the hospital into local, regional, and even statewide emergency management. By training and expertise, this physician is uniquely qualified to serve on that committee. EMS physicians are especially suited to serve. By training, these physicians have learned and use mass casualty management and Incident Command Systems. They are in a unique position to initiate HICS—the Hospital Incident Command System. Many EM physicians have also written about hospital and alternate facility surge.[24,25] The physician leader helps his department comply with emergency preparedness requirements from regulatory agencies such as The Joint Commission and state departments of health. The EMS physician and the EM phsycian accepts a 24/7/365 existence as a fact of life. Most work nights, weekends, and holidays. They live and work in communities. From day to day practice and involvement in hospital EMCs as well as local and regional emergency planning councils and other emergency management entities, EM physicians and EMS physicians understand things like mutual aid agreements and memoranda of understanding. Those important documents may help guide local and regional assistance in the areas of patient movement and allocation of human and material resources. They have probably given thought to how another agency would bring equipment to the hospital and considered that area hospitals would also be competing for the same resources. No one understands the triage process like an EMS physician. That expertise can be shared with those who may be involved locally and regionally in response efforts.

Many look for opportunities to help in the Medical Reserve Corps, DMAT, or search and rescue team. The excitement of helping out in a mass casualty event (MCE) intrigues many from this discipline in a way that doctors from other specialties may not understand. MCE care is much like a day in the ED on a grand scale but without the unlimited resources. They have made decisions about allocation of those resources (like ICU beds) that are not unlimited and have learned from those decisions. Treating "all comers" - adults, children, elderly, pregnant – is part of the job.

It is important for EMS physicians seek out opportunities to advance their knowledge of emergency management. There are numerous online and traditional training programs that allow motivated physicians to obtain masters level education in all aspects of emergency management. For example, the Disaster Medicine and Management (DMM) Masters at Philadelphia University has trained and graduated several EMS physicians as well as paramedics, physician assistants, and registered nurses. All EMS/Disaster Fellows at Einstein Healthcare Network in Philadelphia register for this Masters as part of the fellowship. Most DMM graduates use their education either as part of their medical/EMS positions or in support of an emergency management career. Other educational programs at the masters or doctoral level are offered through universities such as North Dakota State University and St Louis University.

EMS physicians often provide care at the scene along with their EMTs and paramedics. While most such incidents involve only one patient, the potential exists for mass casualty events of various sizes. In that case, the physician would initiate an ICS response at the scene and could serve in a variety of capacities including Incident Commander, Operations Chief, Triage Leader, Treatment Team Leader, or even Transportation Officer. Many require that their prehospital providers use ICS for even small events such as an MVC with several victims in order to maintain proficiency. That MCE can then be evaluated at a later time by the Medical Director and other EMS leadership.

As mentioned under ESF 9, many EMS physicians serve on SAR teams. EMS physicians and Emergency Medicine physicians are often part of mass gathering medical care. Such gatherings present logistical challenges that are "routine" in emergency management. Professionals who understand and actively practice the principles of ICS and acute care are prepared to meet those challenges.[26,27]

SUMMARY

Emergency Medicine and EMS physicians are in a unique position to assume leadership in emergency management. By training and expertise through regular use, no other medical disciplines routinely practice the Incident Command System and the principles of prevention, preparedness, mitigation, response, and recovery. The opportunities to serve and have a positive impact are extensive.

KEY POINTS

- There are five phases of Emergency Management: Prevention, Preparedness, Mitigation, Response, and Recovery.
- The core principles of Emergency Management include practices that are: Comprehensive, Progressive, Risk driven, Integrated, Collaborative, Coordinated, Flexible, and Professional.
- FEMA was created during the Carter Administration following the events at 3-mile Island.
- The Federal Response Plan was enacted to coordinate federal assistance and resources to states and local governments overwhelmed by a major disaster and supported implementation of the Robert T. Stafford Disaster Relief and Emergency Assistance Act.
- The Department of Homeland Security (DHS) was created following the attacks on September 11, 2001, and combined 22 separate agencies with the mission of protecting the nation, reducing vulnerability to terrorist attacks, and reducing damages from both man-made and natural incidents.
- The Homeland Security Act of 2003 established Homeland Security Presidential Directives (HSPD). HSPD 5, 7, and 8 are of particular importance to EMS physicians.
- There are 15 categories of Emergency Support Functions (ESF), of which ESF 4, 6, 8, 9, 11, and 13 are most applicable to EMS and EMS physicians

REFERENCES

1. Haddow GD, Bullock JA, Coppola DP. *Introduction to Emergency Management.* 3rd ed. Boston: Elsevier; 2008.
2. Blanchard BW. Principles of emergency management. Federal Emergency Management Agency. 2007. http://training.fema.gov/EMIWeb/edu/emprinciples.asp. Accessed May, 2015.
3. Glow SD, Colucci VJ, Allington DR, Noonan CW, Hall EC. Managing multiple-casualty incidents: a rural medical preparedness training assessment. *Prehosp Disaster Med.* August 2013;28(4):334-341. doi: 10.1017/S1049023X13000423. Epub 2013 Apr 18.
4. Department of Homeland Security: National Response Framework. January 2008. http://www.fema.gov/emergency/nrf/.

5. Coordination and control. *Scand J Public Health*. May 2014;42(14 suppl):56-75.

6. Deal KE, Synovitz CK, Goodloe JM, King B, Stewart CE. Tulsa oklahoma oktoberfest tent collapse report. *Emerg Med Int*. 2012;2012:729-795.

7. Budd C. Informatics and telecommunications in disasters. In: Ciottone GR, Darling RG, Anderson PD, Auf der Heide E, Jacoby I, Noji E, Suner S, eds. *Disaster Medicine*. Philadelphia, PA: Elsevier Mosby; 2006:130-138.

8. Miller KT. Emergency management services scene management. In: Koenig KL, Schultz CH, eds. *Koenig and Schultz's Disaster Medicine: Comprehensive Principles and Practices*. New York: Cambridge University Press; 2010:275-284.

9. Centers for Disease Control and Prevention. National Electronic Disease Surveillance System (NEDSS). Bethesda, MD. 2011. http://www.ncbi.nlm.gov/pubmed/1171375.

10. Centers for Disease Control and Prevention. Health Alert Network. Bethesda, MD. 2011. http://www.bt.cdc.gov/HAN/.

11. Federal Emergency Management Agency. IS-804: Emergency Support Function (ESF) #4—Firefighting. January 2008. http://www.training.fema.gov/EMIWeb/IS/IS804.asp. Accessed May, 2015.

12. NFPA 1600. Standards on Disaster/Emergency Management and Business Continuity Programs. 2009 ed. Quincy, MA: National Fire Protection Association; 2009.

13. Federal Emergency Management Agency. IS-806: Emergency Support Function (ESF) #6—Mass Care, Emergency Assistance, Housing and Human Services Annex. January 2008. http://training.fema.gov/EMIWeb/IS/IS806.asp.

14. Federal Emergency Management Agency. IS-808: Emergency Support Function (ESF) #8—Public Health and Medical Services. January 2008. http://training.fema.gov/EMIWeb/IS/IS808.asp.

15. Federal Emergency Management Agency. IS–809: Emergency Support Function (ESF) #9—Search and Rescue. February 2011. http://training.fema.gov/EMIWeb/IS/IS809.asp. Accessed May, 2015.

16. Ciottone G. Urban search and rescue in disaster medicine. In: Ciottone GR, Darling RG, Anderson PD, Auf der Heide E, Jacoby I, Noji E, Suner S, eds. *Disaster Medicine*. Philadelphia, PA: Elsevier Mosby; 2006:269.

17. Federal Emergency Management Agency. IS-811: Emergency Support Function (ESF) #11—Agriculture and Natural Resources Instructor Guide. February 2009. http://training.fema.gov/emiweb/is/is811/instructor%20guide.pdf. Accessed May, 2015.

18. Federal Emergency Management Agency. IS-813: Emergency Support Function (ESF) #13—Public Safety and Security Instructor Guide. February 2009. http://training.fema.gov/emiweb/is/is813/instructor%20guide.pdf. Accessed May, 2015.

19. Subbarao I. A consensus-based educational framework and competency set for the discipline of disaster medicine and public health preparedness. *Disaster Med Public Health Prep*. 2008;2(1):57-68.

20. American Osteopathic Association. American Osteopathic Association supports implementing disaster response training at osteopathic medical Schools. Chicago. 2011. http://www.osteopathic.org/inside-aoa/events/annual-business-meeting/house-resolutions/Documents/A2011-HOD-Resolution-Roster-200-SERIES.pdf. Accessed May, 2015.

21. Board of Directors, American College of Emergency Physicians. Disaster planning and response. Dallas, 2008. http://www.acep.org/Clinical-Practice-Management/Disaster-Planning-and-Response/. Accessed May, 2015.

22. Catlett CL, Jenkins JL, Millin MG. Role of emergency medical services in disaster response: resource document for the National Association of EMS Physicians position statement. *Prehosp Emerg Care*. July-September 2011;15(3):420-425.

23. Jones J, Staub J, Seymore A, Scott LA. Securing the second front: achieving first receiver safety and security through competency-based tools. *Prehosp Disaster Med*. October 14, 2014:1-5.

24. Glassman E, Parrillo SJ. Use of alternate healthcare facilities as alternate transport destinations during a mass casualty incident. *Prehosp Dis Med*. 2010;25(2):175-180.

25. Hick JL, Barbera J, Kelen G. Refining surge capacity: conventional, contingency and crisis capacity. *Dis Med Pub Health Prep*. 2009;3(2S):S59-S67.

26. Jaslow D, Yancey A, Milsten A. Position Paper—NAEMSP—mass gathering medical care. *Prehosp Emerg Care*. 2000;4(4):359-360.

27. Parrillo SJ. Mass gathering medical care. In: Hogan DE, Burstein JL, eds. *Disaster Medicine*. 2nd ed. Philadelphia, PA: Williams and Wilkins; 2007:326-330.

CHAPTER 20

Community Paramedicine and Mobile Integrated Health Care

Kevin G. Munjal
Hugh H. Chapin

INTRODUCTION

Whereas traditional EMS largely focuses on the provision of emergency care and the stabilization and management of patients during transport, out-of-hospital care agencies have long been interested in alternative frameworks of providing care that could expand the role and increase the value of EMS systems to the community, to patients, and to the health care system.[1,2] The *EMS Agenda for the Future* published in 1996 envisions EMS treatment to be a part "of a complete health care program," with "finances…linked to value."[3] In 1997, Neely et al. articulated the *multiple option decision point* model which allows for an EMS call to be responded to with a variety of transportation options and to a variety of destinations.[4] In recent years, these ideas have become embodied within the term *community paramedicine* (CP), also known as *mobile integrated health care*.

OBJECTIVES

- Define community paramedicine and mobile integrated health care.
- Discuss integration with the health care network.
- Discuss medical direction considerations.
- Describe examples of existing programs.

While the precise definitions of these two terms are not entirely agreed upon, we will use the terms interchangeably to describe a model of care in which the roles of EMTs, paramedics, and EMS systems are expanded to allow for greater flexibility and patient centeredness in emergencies, better clinical integration with hospital and health care systems, or for the prevention of emergencies before they begin. Any individual EMS agency might serve in a variety of different expanded roles depending on the needs of their community. We categorize these roles into three areas:

1. *Patient-centered emergency response*: Making 9-1-1 more flexible and adaptable to meet the needs of the patient including transporting to alternate destinations (primary care office, dialysis centers, urgent care centers, etc) and "treat and release" protocols.

2. *Integration with coordinated health care systems*: Extending a hospital's or health system's care model into the community through proactive out-of-hospital care programs and improved clinical coordination of care, including innovations in telemedicine. Adding value to routine patient interactions during non-9-1-1, interfacility, and discharge-associated ambulance transports.

3. *Integration with the community and public health*: Integrating out-of-hospital care systems into the public health infrastructure of a community. Vaccination programs, personal preparedness training, fall risk reduction are just a few of the ways that EMS can serve as the foot soldiers of the public health system.

EARLY US PROGRAMS AND INTERNATIONAL EXPERIENCE

Early community paramedicine programs were largely based in rural settings to help fill the gaps created by a scarcity of primary care and other health care resources. The state of Alaska has been implementing community paramedicine, with trained professionals called community health aides/ practitioners (CHA/Ps), since the 1950s in order to meet the health needs of those living in remote villages. In the mid-1990s, paramedics in New Mexico participated in the Red-River project in which they were trained to provide a range of primary care skills. The program successfully reduced emergency call volume but was discontinued due to concerns over inadequate supervision. Unlike modern CP initiatives in the United States, these programs both involved a change in the scope of practice.[5]

CP programs have also been successfully implemented in Canada, Australia, and the United Kingdom in a variety of different models. Canada has a range of pilot programs ongoing including emergency response models with the option to transport to non-ED destinations, programs like the Community Referrals by EMS (CREMS) program in Toronto where EMS has an enhanced ability to connect patients to social services, and programs like the one in Nova Scotia where EMS providers bridge the gap with primary care by offering more complex care. In the United Kingdom, the most well-known program is a specialized *emergency care practitioner* (ECP) model with certain advanced skills which are utilized in both urban and rural settings with the goal of treatment of minor conditions in the field.[5] A study of Australian programs identified three service delivery models: the primary health care model, the substitution model, and the community coordination model.[6]

HEALTH REFORM AND THE US COMMUNITY PARAMEDICINE MOVEMENT

While the concept of community paramedicine and expanded roles for EMS has been around for well over a decade, little progress had been made in the United States largely due to a combination of regulatory and financial barriers. Most notably, current Medicare and private payer reimbursement policies require an EMS agency to transport a patient to an emergency department (ED) for a service claim to be paid.[7] This fee-for-service model creates a perverse incentive for agencies to transport patients to the hospital ED, even if this is not what a patient needs or wants, and even if other alternatives might be better, less expensive, or more patient centered.[8] As the 2007 Institute of Medicine Report points out, changes to the current system are urgently needed due to ED overcrowding and increasing rates of utilization by people seeking treatment for nonurgent conditions.

In the last few years, health care is beginning to move away from fee-for-service medicine and toward the triple aims of improving access, improving quality, and lowering costs through a realignment of incentives with value and efficiency.[9] These recent trends have been facilitated and accelerated by the passage of the American Recovery and Reinvestment Act (ARRA) of 2009 which incentivized hospitals and physicians to adopt electronic medical records, and the Patient Protection and Affordable Care Act (ACA) of 2010 which authorized numerous demonstration projects within Medicare including the accountable care organization (ACO). The culmination of these changes and innovations in the health care system is an environment less focused on inhospital care and more conducive to experimentation with new approaches to patient care and population health management. Community Paramedicine, an innovative model in which existing health care resources are being redeployed to better meet patient needs, is thus very much in line with the goals of the ACA and is now beginning to attract the attention from health care systems, payers, and providers beyond the EMS community.

Some of the more recent pioneers in the current, ever-changing health care environment include the MedStar Mobile Integrated Health Care program in Texas, the Transitional Response Vehicle program in Arizona, the Supporting Public Health with Emergency Responders (SPHERE) program in Seattle and Wake County, NC, and the well-established CP program at Western Eagle County Ambulance District in Colorado.[2] Some pilot programs are being funded internally, others through governmental grants and in some cases by insurance companies. Three programs involving community paramedicine were funded during the initial offering of Health Care Innovation Challenge Awards offered through the Center for Medicare and Medicaid Innovation.

One CP program is already getting reimbursed for their services. North Memorial Medical Center in Minneapolis, Minnesota, was successful in getting state legislation passed that allows reimbursement for CP home services such as health assessments, immunizations and vaccinations, collection of lab specimens, follow-up after hospital discharge, monitoring/educating patients with chronic disease, minor medical procedures approved by the medical director, and medication compliance checks.

As this health care model gains momentum and popularity, new programs are being created faster and faster. The success of these programs, the current era of change in the health care laws, and the need to fill the gaps in our health care delivery model indicate that CP will only grow in the future.

EDUCATION

An important and unresolved question is how much education and training are needed for CP and how should it be structured? Should CP be its own level of certification above that of a paramedic with a basic and uniform level of education required before a provider can perform any new or innovative services within an EMS system (the all or none approach)? Or should individual EMS agencies craft short just-in-time training programs specific to a program or service being implemented within a single agency or community (the modular approach)?

Although a few curriculums are already in place, there is little consensus as to the best approach. In the United Kingdom, ECPs are trained alongside emergency room RNs to fill the niche created by a decrease in resident physician hours in 2009 through university-based curriculums that "add on" to the skill-set of health care workers with experience in ambulatory care.[10] Colleges in the state of Minnesota have used a similar model and are recruiting paramedics into college credit bearing programs with a curriculum that combines live didactics, online modules, and clinical training experiences. Others such as Medstar in Fort Worth, Texas, have an internally developed educational program with oversight and credentialing through the medical director. Future considerations also need to include developing a robust continuing medical education standard for the CP community analogous to most other careers in health care.

MEDICAL DIRECTION

There is little written about or agreed upon regarding the role of the medical director in community paramedicine or mobile integrated health care, but many of the models being developed were initiated by or had significant involvement from not only the EMS medical director, but primary physicians as well. Although the scope of practice is not being expanded in most US programs, broadening the role of EMS from strictly stabilize and transport to outreach, education, follow-up, and more will likely require a greater degree of involvement in terms of protocol and policy development, building relationships with other community-based providers, quality assurance and for real-time clinical consultation. As a nationwide model, CP is still in its infancy and the exact role of the medical director is being molded. Important questions remain, such as will the physician's knowledge base need to be expanded? How will the medical director share responsibility and oversight with other physicians in the community, such as the medical director of a patient-centered medical home or a primary care physician?

DATA, PERFORMANCE IMPROVEMENT, AND OUTCOME EVALUATION

If the community paramedicine model or expanded roles for EMS providers and systems are to become widespread, there will need to be sufficient evidence to justify regulatory change and reimbursement reform. There are a number of sophisticated pilot studies and demonstration projects currently underway and the EMS community is eagerly awaiting reporting and publication of the results of these projects.

There will also need to be a set of metrics by which community paramedicine programs can be compared and best practices can be identified so that patients may benefit from the best quality care available. The US Department of Health and Human Services published the first major effort at developing measures and metrics in its 2012 Community Paramedicine Evaluation Tool. It described CP as "…an emerging field in health care" and the document's purpose as an "assessment tool… designed to allow existing programs to conduct self-assessments…" and "…a potential framework to guide in the development of new community paramedicine programs."[11]

CONCLUSION

By using emergency medical technicians (EMT) and paramedics who are already a part of our communities, community paramedicine (or mobile integrated health care) promises to fill in gaps in the current system, divert unnecessary repeat emergency room (ER) visits, and prevent emergencies in the community before they begin. By altering the financial incentives and in some cases the legal restrictions around EMS activity, it is possible that prehospital providers might be able to serve as an extension of the physician or hospital network as the name "paramedicine" implies.

KEY POINTS

- Community paramedicine may hold many future advantages related to health care reform.
- EMS physicians may require significant additional education to meet the challenges of providing medical direction to providers with a broader preventative and public health scope.
- The US Department of Health and Human Services published the first major effort at developing measures and metrics in its 2012 Community Paramedicine Evaluation Tool.

REFERENCES

1. Pasquier F. *Health Care Access: Innovative Programs Using Non-physicians.* Washington, DC: United States Government Accountability Office; 1993. Report No.: 93-128.
2. Joint Committee on Rural Emergency Care (JCREC), National Association of State Emergency Medical Services Officials, National Organization of State Offices of Rural Health. Discussion Paper on Development of Community Paramedic Programs; 2010. https://www.nasemso.org/Projects/RuralEMS/documents/CPDiscussionPaper.pdf. Accessed October, 2013.
3. Delbridge TR, Bailey B, Chew JL Jr, et al. EMS agenda for the future: where we are … where we want to be. EMS Agenda for the Future Steering Committee. *Ann Emerg Med.* 1998;31:251-263.
4. Neely K. Demand management: the new view of EMS? *Prehosp Emerg Care.* 1997;1:114-118.
5. Wang H. Community paramedicine: summary of evidence. International Roundtable on Community Paramedicine. 2011. http://ircp.info/Portals/11/Downloads/Research/Community%20Paramedicine%20Summary%20of%20Evidence%20-%20Hui%20Wang%20%202011%20January%2028.pdf. Accessed May, 2015.

6. Natalie Blacker LP, Walker T. Redesigning paramedic models of care to meet rural and remote community needs. 10th Annual Rural Health Conference, Cairns, Australia, May 17-19, 2009. http://www.ruralhealth.org.au/10thNRHC/10thnrhc.ruralhealth.org.au/papers/docs/Blacker_Natalie_D4.pdf. Accessed May, 2015.

7. Centers for Medicare & Medicaid Services. *Ambulance Billing Guide December 2012*. Hingham, MA: NHIC Corp; 2010.

8. Munjal K, Carr B. Realigning reimbursement policy and financial incentives to support patient-centered out-of-hospital care. *JAMA*. 2013;309:667-668.

9. Berwick DM, Nolan TW, Whittington J. The triple aim: care, health, and cost. *Health Aff (Millwood)*. 2008;27:759-769.

10. Emergency care practice BSc. Northumbria University - Newcastle. 2013. http://www.northumbria.ac.uk/?view=CourseDetail&code=DUPECP1. Accessed October 16, 2013.

11. Health Resources and Services Administration. U.S. Department of Health & Human Services. Community paramedicine: an evaluation tool. 2012. http://www.hrsa.gov/ruralhealth/pdf/paramedicevaltool.pdf. Accessed May, 2015.

CHAPTER

21

Legal Parameters of EMS

Abigail R. Williams

INTRODUCTION

There are two areas of legal concern for EMS practitioners:

- First, what is the legal structure under which EMS is practiced?
- Second, what are the legal liabilities faced by EMS practitioners and their physician medical directors?

Both of these concerns are addressed in this chapter. First, we will review the structure of the legal system and discuss areas of legal liability. Then, the chapter outlines the government regulation of EMS in the United States and discusses several important areas of consideration, including patient transfer, and end-of-life issues.

OBJECTIVES

- Discuss "duty to act" for EMS personnel.
- Discuss "due regard for public safety" as it applies to EMS operations.
- Discuss legal aspects of out-of-hospital DNR, advance directives, and living wills.
- Discuss EMS provider role when aiding law enforcement (eg, blood draw for blood alcohol levels).
- Describe federal legislation that defined EMS systems and provided the initial funding opportunities for states to develop them.
- Define COBRA and EMTALA.

STRUCTURE OF THE US LEGAL SYSTEM

Although describing the legal system in a few paragraphs is an oversimplification, as it would be for medicine, a brief outline is warranted. There are three general categories of law in our system: criminal law, civil law, and administrative law.

▒ CRIMINAL LAW

In criminal law, the aggrieved party is the government and the defendant is charged with a crime. Penalties include incarceration, fines, and other severe limitations. A relevant example would be fraudulent billing by an ambulance company where fictitious patient transports were submitted for payment. The responsible party or parties would be charged with a crime, insurance fraud, and if convicted would be penalized with fines and/or jail time. Since the penalty is severe, the legal standard is that the defendant must be found guilty beyond a reasonable doubt. Guilt is determined by a finding that the defendant violated the law without a reasonable defense or explanation. Just as rules in medicine have exceptions, laws often have exceptions and circumstances that may be used as a defense. For example, murder (the killing of one by another) is against the law, but self-defense, military engagement, and police actions may be exceptions depending on the circumstances. It is said that our need for attorneys depends more on the exceptions than on the laws.

Attorneys advocate for the party that they represent, trying to convince the judge and jury that interpretation of the law, legal precedent established through the resolution of prior similar cases (case law), and the special circumstances of the particular case should result in a decision in favor of their client (government or defendant). In most cases, a jury is involved in deciding criminal cases, but some criminal matters are handled by judges or other means.

Criminal liability involving EMS usually involves one of the following circumstances:

1. Criminal conviction of an EMS provider with resultant license action. For example, an EMS provider convicted of child pornography may be required to surrender his or her license.

2. Crimes involving misuse of or diversion of controlled substances. Physician medical directors may be responsible for the entire system that acquires, inventories, stores, distributes, uses, and replaces controlled substances within an EMS system. If a provider is found to be diverting controlled substances, or if an audit discovers discrepancies, the involved provider and physician may be liable for criminal or civil penalties depending on the infraction.

3. Criminal conviction of an EMS provider related to an on-duty action. Vehicular homicide, assault and battery, and other criminal charges may ensue after negligent vehicle operation, assault of a patient or bystander, or other similar acts.

4. Fraud involving billing. Filing of false insurance claims and other billing fraud may lead to criminal charges against the involved parties.

5. Crimes involving sexual harassment, boundary violations, discrimination, and other illegal behavior in the workplace. These charges may involve supervisory personnel as well as the individual or individuals accused of the illegal behavior if the workplace fails to provide adequate safeguards and measures to provide a proper work environment.

▒ CIVIL LAW

Civil law resolves disputes between the parties. The plaintiff charges the defendant with a civil violation such as medical malpractice, breach of contract, or defamation of character. The plaintiff must prove that the defendant, more probably than not, (a less stringent test than for criminal cases) met four tests for guilt in a civil matter. These are:

1. Duty
2. Breach
3. Causation
4. Damages

Generally, these four tests mean that the defendant had an obligation to behave toward the plaintiff in a certain manner (duty), failed to meet that obligation (breach), that the plaintiff suffered some harm (damage), and that the breach of the defendant caused the damage (causation). The fact that a civil matter reaches the courtroom is evidence that it was not resolved in some more amicable manner. Therefore, some people assert that there is actually a fifth element in civil cases: anger. Without anger, the plaintiff would not proceed to file legal charges against the defendant. This is the basis for approaches that embrace honesty, transparency, and apology in the etiquette of medical error management; acknowledgment of human frailty in a setting where diligent efforts were made to provide good care is often accepted by otherwise angry potential plaintiffs. While many civil disputes are decided by juries or at bench trials where the judge also serves as a finder of fact (the jury's role in a jury trial, where the judge oversees the legal proceedings but does not decide which evidence is factual), alternative dispute resolution such as mediation or arbitration may be used to resolve civil cases, and many civil cases are settled through negotiation. The penalty in civil cases is most often a financial payment, although there may be specific performance required, such as judicial orders to improve training, staffing, or some other aspect of care. Due to difficulties with assuring compliance (the court system is ill equipped to inspect such aspects of the health care system), specific performance is more often a part of a settlement or mediation agreement than a judicial order.

■ DUTY

Duty attaches for most professionals when a clearly defined relationship is established with a client. For example, when a physician specialist evaluates a patient during a scheduled office visit, or when an attorney signs a contract with the client seeking professional services to craft a will. In EMS, however, duty may attach before the individual EMS provider is near any particular patient. Depending upon what services the agency holds itself out to perform or what contracts have been signed, duty may attach to the entire population of an area (*duty to the public or public duty*), to a person in peril, or to a specific patient (*special duty*) who has requested aid, even though none has yet arrived. For example, some disaster relief agencies hold themselves out to be prepared to respond to disaster circumstances and able to provide relief within particular jurisdictions or for particular problems. In some circumstances, it could be argued that they owe a duty to persons in those jurisdictions should a disaster arise, or for victims of the particular problem they claim to be capable of handling (cave rescue, urban search and rescue, earthquake relief, etc) Another example is an agency contracted to provide emergency EMS response for a particular jurisdiction which has promised (by contract) to provide timely and excellent EMS care for the citizens of that area. Again, in some circumstances, it could be argued that they then owe a duty to someone in peril within that jurisdiction, and that they certainly owe a duty to a specific patient who has requested aid. Of course, it is clear that EMS providers owe a duty to patients they touch, evaluate, and transport. However, they also owe a duty to those patients who refuse transport, and (if allowed) to patients the EMS providers refuse to transport.

EMS providers also owe a duty to persons other than the patient they are caring for and transporting.

Public Duty of EMS Providers (and Other Emergency Services)

- The agency and its providers have a duty to provide emergency response to a community that they are designated to serve. This includes ensuring readiness and provision of the appropriate response when activated.

- They owe a duty to others on or near the route of response or transport to operate the responding vehicle or ambulance with *due regard for public safety*. Ambulance operations involve the risk of injury to persons in the vehicle, pedestrians, and occupants of other vehicles. Operation of an ambulance in a manner that increases these risks often occurs when warning lights and sirens are used because the ambulance may be violating (legally) standard vehicle operating laws and practices. However, unsafe operation does not require the use of lights and sirens. Likewise, lights and sirens operation can be carried out safely and effectively.

- They also owe a duty to other responders to perform their job in a safe and coordinated manner so as to prevent injury and illness and others. In addition to vehicle operations, the use of rescue equipment, sharp medical equipment, contaminated medical supplies, and patient movement equipment can all be managed in a manner that either protects or risks harm to other responders.

- They owe a duty to their employer and/or supervisor to practice within the bounds of their training, jurisdictional regulations and protocols,

and agency policies and procedures. Failure to follow these rules places both the individual provider and their superiors at legal risk.

- Some would argue that they also owe a duty to the next patient, as yet unknown, and therefore should timely and efficiently complete care of the current patient so they can return to availability. Unwarranted delay and deception to avoid the appearance of the availability (eg, failing to notify a dispatcher of availability in order to relax, chat, etc) may result in response delay and thereby harm to subsequent patients.

Special Duty of EMS Providers (and EMS Physicians)

- When a specific individual can be identified as the one in need of care or emergency services the provider then takes on special duty to provide an appropriate response. Special duty may be simple to define, such as when the EMS physician is on scene and has interacted with a specific patient, given orders, and supervised their care. In this case, the EMS physician has a similar duty to the patient as the EMS provider on scene.

- When a provider calls for online medical control with specific information and a request for direction, it may be considered that the EMS physician, or medical control physician, now has the same special duty requirements.

Once a duty exists, there is an expectation that the professional will provide *due care*. Negligence is care less than that which would be provided by a like trained person in like circumstances, and due care is treatment at or above the level of ordinary care which would be provided by a like trained person and like circumstances. The standard of care is the dividing line between negligent care and due care. It is determined by the testimony of experts, who are typically professionals with training and experience similar to the defendant. In civil litigation, the plaintiff has claimed that the defendant has *breached* their duty by practicing negligently, that is, below the standard of care. The defense may include arguments to the contrary, or offer other reasons why the defendant should not be found guilty.

One common defense used by EMS providers is that of *immunity*. All states have some form of "Good Samaritan" legislation, enacted to encourage volunteerism and community assistance for those in need. Typically, this legislation provides immunity for responders by raising the standard for negligence if the care rendered is done so in good faith. Common elevated standards include gross and willful misconduct, willful and wanton misconduct, intentional harm, and similar terms; there are variations from state to state. In other words, a plaintiff claiming a breach of duty to provide ordinary care may find the defendant successfully arguing Good Samaritan protection by showing that the care provided, although not optimal, was not so negligent as to constitute gross and willful misconduct. However, recent case law has often successfully shown that Good Samaritan immunity should not be applied to those who hold themselves out as scheduled, uniformed, trained, and often compensated EMS providers. In other words, courts are now finding that EMS providers are professionals, and should not be shielded by Good Samaritan immunity while practicing their profession. When off duty, however, Good Samaritan immunity typically still applies.

In civil law, there are claimed *damages*. Damages may be physical, emotional, or occasionally financial. In order to be convincing to a jury, they must be substantial and permanent. Temporary discomfort caused by spinal immobilization, for example, may not be as convincing as permanent paralysis resulting from failure to immobilize the spine when indicated.

Causation is an unbroken and logical link between the alleged breach and the claimed damages. For example, if a surgeon incorrectly identifies the operative site and amputates the incorrect leg, the damage would be loss of a leg and the cause would be the surgeon's negligent failure to identify the correct leg.

Liability for EMS providers involving civil law takes the form of suits filed against the provider, their supervisory staff and medical director, and their EMS agency. The suits may allege negligent care, personal injury from use of poorly maintained or faulty equipment, negligence in training, hiring, or supervision, negligent operation of vehicles and other transport equipment, or other charges. EMS providers should be familiar with the involved legal principles, be competent and current in their medical care, follow all relevant laws, regulations, protocols, policies and procedures, and participate in quality improvement and customer service efforts in order to minimize their exposure to civil suits. In addition, adequate liability insurance is a requirement. EMS providers and physician medical directors should ask specifically about coverage provided by their agency or employer to be certain that it covers their scope of practice.

■ ADMINISTRATIVE

Administrative, or regulatory, law is the final category found in our legal system. In many ways, it is the most complicated. While general laws may empower an agency or government department to regulate an activity such as EMS, the resulting regulations, guidelines, treatment protocols, and individual interpretations and decisions made by government officials may result in an amazingly complex bureaucracy. The legislation forming the basis for administrative law tends to be general, and sometimes purposefully vague. It is the job of regulations, guidelines, policies, protocols, and procedures to specify the bounds and exact nature desired. For example, in Rhode Island, the empowering legislation notes that it is supportive of any EMS scheme that will save lives and promote healing.[1] (See **Box 21-1**). From that legislation, regulations are promulgated by the Department of Health and subsequently protocols, which are more specific about the actions of EMS providers. Failure to follow the standards of EMS practice or the specifications of these protocols and regulations can result in action against the license of an EMS provider or ambulance service. In some jurisdictions, penalties may also include fines. In many cases concerns about EMS performance results in a negotiated settlement where the provider or service promises certain specific performance such as retraining, probationary supervision, and other measures. Although details vary significantly from state to state, in general, there are federal, state, and local sources of administrative law regulating EMS.

Given this general overview of our legal system, we will now discuss some circumstances where EMS providers should be familiar with the law—patient transfer and end-of-life issues, and then discuss some of the specifics involved in legal regulation of EMS. This description is organized by jurisdiction starting with international and federal laws and regulations, and ending with a description of state and local variations.

LEGAL ISSUES INVOLVING PATIENT TRANSFER

The health care system in the United States is pressured by the need to serve both charitable purposes and to be financially successful. While financial success can come from government funding, donation, research grants, and other sources external to the care of a particular patient, in many cases financial survival for a hospital or medical practice/facility depends on collecting reimbursement for individual patient care from the patient or an insurance provider. The need to be financially successful can conflict with the moral obligation to provide care for patients in need. In many circumstances within our health care system, this conflict is shielded by the need for patients to secure referrals and appointments before access to medical practices or facilities. Although one could argue that this is a superficial and artificial insulation, it is currently common in our health care system. Patients cannot simply walk into the office of a medical specialist, a rehabilitation facility, or an independent urgent care center and demand care with the expectation that it will be provided without reimbursement.

However, this is no longer true for hospital facilities, including clinics and ambulance services owned by hospitals. After years, where it was common for hospitals to refuse care to the uninsured, those without a particular insurance, those without a physician on staff at the hospital, or on the basis of some other discrimination, federal legislation and regulation have now repeatedly required that hospitals offering emergency services see all persons presenting for emergency care without discrimination. In 1946, the Hill Burton act required that hospitals provide

care for persons residing in the territory of the hospital if the hospital accepted federal funds.[2] While this requirement was generally ignored, there was little impact in areas where emergency department volume was low. However, as emergency department volume increased during the 1950s and 1960s, a series of civil cases established several legal theories under which patients could successfully sue hospitals for refusing care. These included the theory of detrimental reliance, whereby a person could rely, to their detriment, on the promise of emergency care when a hospital advertised emergency services, and then denied them to that person, negligence theory, where delayed or partial care for particular classes or groups of patients was found to be below the standard of care, and the beneficence of public policies that argue for nondiscriminatory access to care at hospitals receiving public funds.

There were slow improvements in some areas, but the 1959 case of 4-month-old Darien Manlove[3] is illustrative. His parents had been bringing him to his private physician for several days due to fever, diarrhea, and inability to sleep. On a Wednesday, when the doctor's office was closed and the infant appeared worse, his parents brought him to Wilmington General Hospital in Delaware. There, he was not examined by a nurse on duty in the emergency ward, "she never got up from her chair," and refused access to and treatment from the intern physician on duty even though "there were no other patients in the emergency ward" because he was already under the treatment of a private physician. Unable to contact the private physician, the nurse recommended that the parents bring their ill baby to the pediatric clinic the next day, but Darien died that night. His parents brought suit against the hospital, and in their defense, the hospital claimed that they had no duty to provide care because they were a private institution and no "frank emergency" existed, and filed for summary judgment. When the judge found that the parents could proceed with their case, denying the motion for summary judgment, the case was appealed by the hospital.[4] In his opinion, the appeals judge set the legal stage for several important concepts regarding the rights of emergency patients.

Evaluation to Determine the Presence of an Emergency Condition: The Screening Examination After clarifying that *Manlove* did not revolve around negligent treatment, but in fact around refusal of treatment, the appellate judge found:

> But this is not a case in which the hospital assumed to treat the patient. The claim is that it should have treated him, and that the nurse was negligent in failing to have the infant examined by the interne on duty, because an apparent emergency existed.
>
> This leads to the inquiry: What is the duty of a nurse to one applying for admission as an emergency case? Obviously, if an emergency is claimed, someone on behalf of the hospital must make a *prima facie* decision whether it exists. The hospital cannot reasonably be expected to station an interne at all times in the receiving room. It therefore keeps a nurse on duty. If the nurse makes an honest decision that there is no unmistakable indication of an emergency, and that decision is not clearly unreasonable in the light of the nurse's training, how can there be any liability on the part of the hospital?

This finding sets forth the legal precedent later amplified in the 1986 antidumping legislation whereby the hospital has an obligation to screen persons presenting for emergency care in a regular and professional manner to determine if an emergency exists, and has the right to deny care if they reasonably find that there is no such emergency, but an obligation to provide care if there is an emergency condition present.

▨ DETRIMENTAL RELIANCE

After reversing the lower court and finding that Wilmington General had not become "public" through receipt of public funds, and noting that the alleged "rule" of the hospital to refuse aid to those already under the care of a private physician (due to the risk of conflicting treatments) was not substantiated by any production of a written rule, or even any testimony that detailed the alleged "rule," the appellate judge found:

> It may be conceded that a private hospital is under no legal obligation to the public to maintain an emergency ward, or, for that matter, a public clinic.... But the maintenance of such a ward to render first-aid to injured persons has become a well-established adjunct to the main business of a hospital. If a person, seriously hurt, applies for such aid at an emergency ward, relying on the established custom to render it, is it still the right of the hospital to turn him away without any reason? In such a case, it seems to us, such a refusal might well result in worsening the condition of the injured person, because of the time lost in a useless attempt to obtain medical aid.

There was no difference, therefore, between public and private hospitals, only that an emergency ward was maintained. After *Manlove*, additional challenges arose as the population became increasingly mobile and as managed health care plans and health maintenance organizations appeared. In response to continued concerns about patient dumping (refusal of care, or improper transfer after inadequate care), the federal government passed antidumping legislation as part of the Consolidated Omnibus Budget Reconciliation Act (COBRA) of 1986.[5] The section of COBRA that applied to patient dumping was called the Emergency Medical Treatment and Active Labor Act (EMTALA), and went into effect in 1990. It has since been modified by several releases of regulations and by case law. The importance of EMTALA to EMS revolves around the following provisions (although the law includes others):

1. A person presenting to the hospital for care must be offered a screening evaluation to determine if an emergency exists. Presentation to the hospital includes presentation to hospital-operated clinics and other facilities, including ambulance services. However, regulatory clarification states that these patients may receive their care at other hospitals within an organized system of care. In other words, EMTALA does not require that a hospital-owned ambulance or helicopter bring all patients to the base hospital for evaluation. However, it does require that persons on the hospital premises requesting emergency care be offered that care, and this may include persons in parking lots or on other property who require EMS transport in order to receive an evaluation. It is permissible for patients to pass through a hospital, for example, between an emergency ambulance entrance and a rooftop helipad, without such a screening examination if there is no intent for the patient to seek care at that facility.

2. A patient may not be transferred inappropriately. An appropriate transfer includes one that is requested by the patient, or one where the treating physician certifies that the medical benefits of transfer outweigh the risks, and where treatment to minimize risk is provided. This includes ensuring that the receiving facility has accepted the patient and has capacity for treatment, that all pertinent records are transferred to the receiving facility, and that the transferring EMS process includes qualified personnel, vehicle, and equipment.

3. Regional specialty receiving centers cannot discriminate against transfer patients, and must accept appropriate patients referred for specialty care if they have capacity to provide that care.

EMTALA requirements for appropriate transfer do not apply once the patient is admitted to the hospital, if the patient is found to be stable, and if the patient either requests or refuses transfer.

END-OF-LIFE LEGAL ISSUES

In general, patients have the right to consent to, or refuse, any offered medical therapy. As with other areas of medicine and law, issues about consent and end-of-life decisions involve a variety of complex decisions and exceptions to this rule. It is unlikely that a patient experiencing a critical medical emergency has the capacity to properly consent to or refuse medical therapy. Likewise, there are circumstances under which the patient's competence for decision making is inadequate to make these decisions. Therefore, the medical system has adopted a number of measures to improve this decision-making process:

1. *Futility*: There are circumstances under which the application of certain medical therapies is futile, meaning that there is no reasonable hope of improving a patient's condition with the therapy. Most EMS systems contain a description of circumstances under which EMS providers may consider resuscitation efforts, and other care futile. The circumstances often include massively disruptive trauma, evidence of long-standing death, and significant challenges to transportation, such as cardiac arrest in a remote wilderness area. In many systems, recognizing that hospital therapy for sudden death or death caused by blunt trauma adds little to the capabilities of an advanced EMS system, transportation of such patients unless resuscitation efforts are successful is considered futile and they are presumed dead after care at the scene. As the predictive capabilities of noninvasive monitoring, and other resuscitation research advance, it may be possible to better predict when further EMS efforts are futile.

2. *Advance directives*: Advance directives are statements made in advance of need by the patient or an authorized surrogate such as a living will, durable power of attorney, or a health care proxy. These directives do not necessarily limit care; they may be limited to naming a person or persons authorized to make health care decisions when the patient is incapacitated. Typically, a living will specifically addresses wishes for care, while a durable power of attorney or health care proxy is a means for the patient to identify a person or persons who can express their wishes. If they limit care, it is important that they use plain and simple language and avoid terms such as *heroic measures* and *terminal condition*. Such advance directives may be memorialized in the health care system through physician orders that limit care, such as "do not resuscitate," "comfort measures only," or "allow natural death" orders. Recent efforts to make patient wishes known across the health care system have resulted in many states adopting portable orders regarding life-sustaining treatment, known a *physician* (or *portable*) orders

for life-sustaining treatment. These documents are recognized across multiple facilities, and travel with the patient. In addition, many states and EMS systems have developed protocols and identification methods that ease in recognition of the patient's wishes. These systems typically include a bracelet or other identifier that makes the patient's wishes for limited resuscitation efforts immediately clear.

KEY POINTS

- EMS providers should be familiar with criminal, civil, and administrative sources of law.

- EMS providers should be familiar with local legal requirements, and be certain to have adequate liability insurance.

- There are three elements of law: criminal, civil, and administrative.

- Guilt is defined differently depending on the applicable law.

  - Criminal law requires proof beyond a reasonable doubt. Civil law requires "proof" that the defendant is guilty "more probably than not."

- There are four tests of civil liability: duty, breach, causation, and damages.

- Negligence is defined as care less than that which would be provided by a like provider in similar circumstances.

- Due care is defined as treatment at or above the level of ordinary care provided by a like trained person and under like circumstances.

- Standard of care is determined by the testimony of experts and defines the dividing line between negligence and due care.

- Good Samaritan immunity is not applicable to scheduled, uniformed, trained, and/or compensated EMS providers per case law.

- Public duty refers to the duty to provide emergency response to the community, whereas special duty is to an individual patient.

- The EMS physician should be especially aware of the risk for legal issues related to vehicle operations, mismanagement of controlled substances, improper workplace actions, refusal of care, negligent care, advanced health care directives, and patient transfers.

REFERENCES

1. Title 23. Health and Safety. http://webserver.rilin.state.ri.us/Statutes/title23/23-4.1/23-4.1-1.HTM. Accessed May, 2015.
2. Hill Burton, 42 U.S.C.A. sec. 0 (1988 & Supp. II 1990).
3. Find A Case. http://de.findacase.com/research/wfrmDocViewer.aspx/xq/fac.19610321_0001.DE.htm/qx. Accessed May, 2015.
4. Wilmington General v. Manlove, 54 Del 15 (1961).
5. Centers for Medicare & Medicaid Services, HHS. http://edocket.access.gpo.gov/cfr_2004/octqtr/pdf/42cfr489.24.pdf. Accessed May, 2015.

CHAPTER 22

Government Regulation of EMS

Abigail R. Williams

INTRODUCTION

Regulatory oversight of emergency medical services occurs primarily at the state level based on the provision laid out in the Emergency Medical Services (EMS) Systems Act of 1973. Despite this fact various levels of regulation exist at various levels of government in order to address the needs of the overall system. In addition to governmental agencies, some nongovernmental entities have produced standards that have been adopted by many jurisdictions (federal and state), making them de facto parts of the regulatory structure, despite their lack of regulatory authority.

OBJECTIVES

- Discuss federal regulations that directly and indirectly impact EMS systems.

- Discuss the states' provision of EMS and give examples of different state EMS organizational systems.

- Give examples of local, regional, state, and federal regulatory organizations that govern/oversee EMS systems.

- Discuss how no governmental organizations influence regulation of EMS.

INTERNATIONAL REGULATION OF EMS

While the laws, regulations, and policies that regulate EMS within the United States flow from our federal government for EMS operations within our borders, some EMS agencies transport across these borders. International operations, such as fixed-wing aircraft EMS, must be aware of and in compliance with a variety of international laws and regulations. In particular, transport of controlled substances, licensing of providers, and operation of aircraft outside of the United States require particular attention. Any international EMS operation, including disaster relief, repatriation via commercial aircraft, and any cross-border ambulance transport should enquire about these issues prior to initiating operations.

FEDERAL REGULATION OF EMS

The history of federally regulated EMS in the United States dates from the 1960s, when physicians returning from the Vietnam War noted differences between military medicine and civilian EMS. In 1966, the Institute of Medicine published *Accidental Death and Disability, the Neglected Disease of Modern Society*, also known as the EMS White Paper.[1] This report argued effectively that the lack of civilian EMS and trauma care was leading to many avoidable disabilities and deaths. Congress followed by funding regional EMS system development in 1973 with addition of the *Emergency Medical Services (EMS) Systems Act of 1973 (42 U.S.C. 300d)* to the *Public Health Service Act*. This empowering legislation provided funding for states to establish EMS systems. Subsequent funding, including specific funding for EMS for children efforts, has aided in further development and regulation of EMS in the United States.

In addition, specific federal legislation, such as that regulating transfer of patients between facilities, reimbursement of healthcare providers, release of medical information, control of pathogens, and other topics are of particular importance to EMS. While not an inclusive list, the outline below describes in brief several federal agencies and other organizations that act at a national level to regulate EMS in the United States.

■ DOT NHTSA EMS

The Department of Transportation, National Highway Traffic Safety Administration, EMS Division, or DOT NHTSA EMS is the federal home for EMS in the United States.[2] NHTSA is the origin of a variety of educational and funding initiatives, including the EMS Agenda for the Future, the National Scope of Practice Model, and National EMS Core Content. Their office acknowledges a variety of other federal agencies that are involved in leadership for a comprehensive national EMS system, ranging from the Office of Rural Health Policy to the Centers for Disease Control and Prevention. (See **Box 22-1**.) NHTSA EMS provides coordinating leadership and funding that substantially controls the curriculum for EMT training in the United States, the scope of practice generally accepted for EMTs at various levels, and interstate coordination and cooperation of EMS systems.

■ DEA

The US Drug Enforcement Administration (DEA)[3] is a branch of the US Department of Justice, and enforces the laws and regulations of the United States relating to controlled substances. When EMS agencies use controlled substances, such as narcotics and benzodiazepines, they must comply with DEA regulations. Typically, this involves a physician medical director or physician acting with similar authority who prescribes or orders these controlled substances for the ambulance service, and then a series of policies and procedures, which provide control over access to use of and inventory of these drugs. Failure to properly comply with these regulations and/or discovery of drug diversion may constitute significant legal and regulatory concern for the involved physician.

■ FAA

The Federal Aviation Administration (FAA) is the federal agency that controls the operation of aircraft and the licensing of aircrew in the United States. Therefore, it is involved in helicopter and fixed-wing aircraft EMS operations.[4] While operation of an aircraft and EMS medical care may seem like clearly distinct areas, there is overlap and controversy. It appears that the FAA is attempting to clarify that its authority is limited to operation of the aircraft and the qualifications of the crew, and that the medical system determines whether there is need for patient transport by aircraft. However, controversies include decisions about federal versus state regulatory authority, the safety of medical helicopter operations, and the aviation qualifications of medical flight crew.[5] For example, does the FAA or a state EMS agency have the authority to control whether a helicopter ambulance can respond to certain types of patient problems, where it can land, and what equipment and capabilities are available in

---

Box 22-1

Federal Agencies with EMS Responsibilities in Addition to DOT/NHTSA

Department of Health and Human Services

- Office of the Assistant Secretary for Preparedness and Response

- Agency for Healthcare Research & Quality (AHRQ)

- Emergency Medical Services for Children (EMSC)

- Indian Health Service

- Centers for Disease Control and Prevention (CDC)

Department of Homeland Security

- Office of Health Affairs

- U.S. Fire Administration

  - National Fire Academy

Federal Communications Commission

- Public Safety and Homeland Security Bureau

the patient compartment? Are the medical crew, often EMTs and/or nurses, subject to FAA aircrew regulations, including duty work hours and drug testing? These and other controversies are currently under discussion (2011).

GSA

The US General Services Administration (GSA), among many other activities, offers minimum requirements to meet federal specifications for patient transport ambulances.[6] These specifications, known as KKK-1822, are updated every 5 years, and are currently in revision F.[7] As can be seen in **Box 22-2**, the GSA specifications refer to a number of laws and specifications from other agencies and organizations. In addition, the National Fire Protection Administration (NFPA) has developed a standard for ambulance construction as well. This standard, NFPA 1917, went into effect in 2012 and will likely be merged with the KKK specifications in the future.[8]

DMAT/NDMS/DHHS

Disaster Medical Assistance Teams (DMATs) are federal assets organized as part of the National Response Framework (NRF) under the Department of Health and Human Services.[9] DMATs include EMS professionals and others, and respond when requested to mass casualty and disaster events, where they provide emergency care, field hospital and similar support, and generally augment whatever medical system is functioning during the event. EMS professionals affiliated with DMATs may be providing care far from their "home" system, and do so as federal employees during deployments. In addition to the DMAT system, there are numerous other federal and state EMS assets and teams, including mortuary teams (DMORTs), Urban Search and Rescue teams (USART), Medical Reserve Corps (MRCs), and others that may respond to a request for aid. The process for requesting aid involves state government and federal liaison, and brings with it a significant system of regulatory, administrative, and legal arrangements to authorize, fund, coordinate, and deploy the indicated assets.

NASEMSO

The National Association of State EMS Officials (NASEMSO)[10] is an association representing state government EMS regulators. It works to improve cooperation and collaboration between the federal government and state regulators, and between states. They promulgate guidelines and policy statements, and offer professional conferences, and other educational opportunities. To the extent that their activities influence federal and state EMS supervision, they can be seen as a source of administrative law. The majority of its membership consists of state EMS regulators who are the source of significant regulatory and administrative law, in the form of guidelines, regulations, and protocols at the state level.

NAEMSP

The National Association of EMS Physicians (NAEMSP),[11] is a group of physicians and other professionals collaborating to provide leadership and excellence in EMS. They promulgate guidelines and policy statements, and offer professional conferences, and other educational opportunities. To the extent that their activities influence federal and state EMS supervision, they can be seen as a source of administrative law. Many of their members service physician medical directors for EMS agencies, regions, or states and therefore participate in the development of regulations and protocols.

AMPA

The Air Medical Physician Association (AMPA)[12] is the largest professional association dedicated to helicopter and fixed-wing air medical transport and ground critical care transport. They promulgate guidelines and policy statements, and offer professional conferences, and other educational opportunities. To the extent that their activities influence federal and state EMS supervision, they can be seen as a source of administrative law. Most members of AMPA are physician medical directors of air medical or ground critical care transport programs and participate in the development of operational protocols.

STATE REGULATION OF EMS

Due in part to the overall structure of our government and the power of states, and due in part to funding legislation passed in the 1970s, every state and territory in the United States has some authority over EMS operations within its borders. However, this distributed authority has led to a wide variety of EMS system models and regulatory structures. Common themes are some degree of control over the licensing (or equivalent) of ambulances and EMS providers and their scope of practice. This structure worked reasonably well when EMS was commonly provided at a local level by local providers. Over the past 20 years, a number of regional and national EMS providers have developed. Some of these providers offer services in many states, often using centralized coordination and dispatch centers and standardized fleets of ambulances. The obvious advantages of standardization in provider and vehicle licensing conflict with varying local, regional, and state requirements. In many jurisdictions, additional common issues such as interjurisdictional licensing conflicts, medical control and protocol variations, and scope of practice variations raise additional concerns. For example, there are frequently at least three levels of EMS provider licensed (or similarly authorized by measures such as certificate, authority to practice under a physician's license, or other method–all referred to as licensing for the purposes of this chapter) in each state. However, EMS providers with the same title often have different training and scope of practice when compared with their neighbors.

Ambulances providing mutual aid to other states in situations such as major incidents or disasters often arrive with different level providers, different equipment and medications, and different communication systems than the local services. The potential for confusion and patient harm in these situations is obvious. In addition, many air and ground ambulance agencies routinely operate across state borders, requiring multijurisdictional licensing, written or unwritten permission to provide "mutual aid," or other authority to practice. The need for an EMS provider to ask the pilot or driver "Where am I?" before administering a medication or performing a procedure in order to determine if the necessary authority exists is both absurd and dangerous.

These developments have complicated an already richly diverse system. Therefore, there are significant current efforts to understand these issues and develop common standards and operating parameters. These efforts are important for patient care, for the individual EMS provider, and for the EMS agencies, as well as for regulatory authorities.

Given the complexity and diversity of state and regional EMS regulation, it is important for the reader to thoroughly research and understand the system or systems in which they are working. While this section focuses on state and territorial authority, it should be recognized that there are a substantial number of EMS providers in the United States who practice under federal authority. These include providers in the military, various federal agencies such as the Border Patrol and Secret Service, and other federal employees, either full or part time (such as DMATs), who provide EMS care. In general, the categories of regulatory and administrative authority that exist in most systems, both federal and state, include training, licensing, and authority to practice.

EMS PROVIDER TRAINING, LICENSING, AND AUTHORITY TO PRACTICE

Many states and federal agencies recognize the National Registry of EMTs,[13] an organization that provides standardized testing and continuing competency assurance. The National Registry is careful to remind users of its services that national certification does not

Box 22-2

GSA KKK-1822F Referenced Standards and Regulations*

The following standards and regulations form a part of this specification, to the extent specified or required by law. Unless a specific issue of a standard or regulation is identified, the issue in effect, on the date the ambulance is contracted for, shall apply.

FEDERAL SPECIFICATIONS:

- RR-C-901C—CYLINDERS, COMPRESSED GAS: HIGH PRESSURE, STEEL DOT 3AA AND ALUMINUM APPLICATIONS

FEDERAL STANDARDS:

- Federal Standard No. 297—Rustproofing of Commercial (Nontactical) Vehicles

MILITARY STANDARDS:

- MIL-STD-461 Requirements for the Control of Electromagnetic Interference Characteristics of Subsystems and Equipment.
- MIL-STD-1223 Non-tactical Wheeled Vehicles, Painting, Identification Marking, and Data Plate Standards.

LAWS AND REGULATIONS:

- 29 CFR 1910.1030: Blood borne Pathogens
- 29 CFR 1910.7 Definition and Requirements for a Nationally Recognized Testing Laboratory
- 21 CFR 820: Quality System Regulation
- 40 CFR 86: Control of Air Pollution from New Motor Vehicles and New Motor Vehicle Engines.
- 47 CFR, PART 90: Public Safety Radio Services (FCC)
- 49 CFR 393: Federal Motor Carrier Safety Regulations (FMCSR)
- 49 CFR 571: Federal Motor Vehicle Safety Standards (FMVSS)

2.2 OTHER PUBLICATIONS.

The following documents form a part of this specification to the extent specified. Unless a specific issue is identified, the issue in effect, on the date the ambulance is contracted for, shall apply.

THE TIRE AND RIM ASSOCIATION, INC.

- Yearbook

NATIONAL FIRE PROTECTION ASSOCIATION

- 70—National Electric Code
- 1901—Standard for Automotive Fire Apparatus

2. APPLICABLE DOCUMENTSSOCIETY OF AUTOMOTIVE ENGINEERS (SAE), INC., STANDARDS, AND RECOMMENDED PRACTICES:

- J163 Low Tension Wiring and Cable Terminals and Splice Clips
- J537 Storage Batteries
- J541 Voltage Drop for Starting Motor Circuits
- J553 Circuit Breakers
- J561 Electrical Terminals, Eyelet, and Spade Type
- J575 Tests for Motor Vehicle Lighting Devices & Components
- J576 Plastic Materials, For Use In Optical Parts Such As Lenses and Reflectors of Motor Vehicle
- Lighting Devices
- J578 Color Specification for Electric Signal Lighting Devices
- J595 Flashing Warning Lamps for Authorized Emergency, Maintenance, and Service Vehicles
- J638 Test Procedure and Ratings for Hot Water Heaters for Motor Vehicles
- J639 Safety Practices for Mechanical Vapor Compression Refrigeration Equipment or Systems Used
- To Cool Passenger Compartment of Motor Vehicles
- J689 Approach, Departure, and Ramp Break over Angles
- J682 Rear Wheel Splash and Stone Throw Protection
- J683 Tire Chain Clearance
- J858 Electrical Terminals, Blade Type
- J928 Electrical Terminals, Pin, and Receptacle Type
- J994 Backup Alarms, Performance Test and Application
- J1054 Warning Lamp, Alternating Flashers
- J1127 Battery Cable
- J1128 Low Tension Primary Cable
- J1292 Automobile, Truck, Truck-Tractor, Trailer, and Motor Coach Wiring
- J1349 Engine Power Test Code, Spark Ignition and Diesel
- J1318 Strobe Warning Lights
- J2498 Minimum Performance of the Warning Light System Used on Emergency Vehicles

NATIONAL TRUCK EQUIPMENT ASSOCIATION / AMD:

- AMD STANDARD 001—AMBULANCE BODY STRUCTURE STATIC LOAD TEST
- AMD STANDARD 002—BODY DOOR RETENTION COMPONENTS TEST
- AMD STANDARD 003—OXYGEN TANK RETENTION SYSTEM STATIC TEST
- AMD STANDARD 004—LITTER RETENTION SYSTEM STATIC TEST
- AMD STANDARD 005—12-VOLT DC ELECTRICAL SYSTEM TEST
- AMD STANDARD 006—PATIENT COMPARTMENT SOUND LEVEL TEST
- AMD STANDARD 007—PATIENT COMPARTMENT CARBON MONOXIDE LEVEL TEST
- AMD STANDARD 008—PATIENT COMPARTMENT GRAB RAIL STATIC LOAD TEST
- AMD STANDARD 009—125V AC ELECTRICAL SYSTEMS TEST
- AMD STANDARD 010—WATER SPRAY TEST
- AMD STANDARD 011—EQUIPMENT TEMPERATURE TEST
- AMD STANDARD 012—INTERIOR CLIMATE CONTROL TEST
- AMD STANDARD 013—WEIGHT DISTRIBUTION GUIDELINES
- AMD STANDARD 014—ENGINE COOLING SYSTEM TEST
- AMD STANDARD 015—AMBULANCE MAIN OXYGEN SYSTEM TEST
- AMD STANDARD 016—PATIENT COMPARTMENT LIGHTING LEVEL TEST
- AMD STANDARD 017—ROAD TEST
- 4AMD STANDARD 018—REAR STEP AND BUMPER STATIC LOAD TEST
- AMD STANDARD 019—MEASURING GUIDELINES: CABINETS & COMPARTMENTS
- AMD STANDARD 020—FLOOR DISTRIBUTED LOAD TEST
- AMD STANDARD 021—ASPIRATOR SYSTEM TEST, PRIMARY PATIENT
- AMD STANDARD 022—COLD ENGINE START TEST
- AMD STANDARD 023—SIREN PERFORMANCE TEST
- AMD STANDARD 024—PERIMETER ILLUMINATION TEST
- AMD STANDARD 025—MEASURING GUIDELINES: OCCUPANT HEAD CLEARANCE ZONES

AMERICAN COLLEGE OF EMERGENCY PHYSICIANS (ACEP):

- Guidelines for Ambulance Equipment

AMERICAN SOCIETY FOR TESTING AND MATERIALS (ASTM) STANDARDS:

- F 920 Standard Specification for Minimum Performance and Safety Requirements for
- Resuscitators Intended for Use with Humans
- F 960 Standard Specification for Medical and Surgical Suction and Drainage Systems
- D 4956 Standard Specification for Retroreflective Sheeting for Traffic Control
- D6210 Standard Specification for Fully-Formulated Glycol Base Engine Coolant for
- Heavy-Duty Engines
- B117 Standard Practice for Operating Salt Spray (Fog) Apparatus
- IPC-610D Acceptability of Electronic Assemblies

NATIONAL EMSC (EMERGENCY MEDICAL SERVICES FOR CHILDREN) RESOURCE ALLIANCE:

COMMITTEE ON AMBULANCE EQUIPMENT AND SUPPLIES

- Guidelines for pediatric equipment and supplies for Basic and Advanced life support ambulances

AUTOMOTIVE MANUFACTURERS EQUIPMENT COMPLIANCE AGENCY (AMECA):

- Approval of Motor Vehicle Safety Equipment (emergency lights and sirens)

AMERICAN NATIONAL STANDARDS INSTITUTE (ANSI):

- Z535.1 American National Standard for Safety Colors

For assistance in obtaining the referenced documents, contact the Department of Commerce, National Technical Information Service (NTIS).

*From http://www.deltaveh.com/f.pdf. Accessed May, 2015.

constitute a license to practice in any particular jurisdiction. Some states and many federal agencies administer their own EMS provider training and testing. Many states also provide a system for reciprocity licensing with other states.

The legal structure of the EMS provider licensing varies significantly. In some states, EMS providers are considered extenders of physician medical directors, and therefore their authority to practice flows from the physician's license. In other states, EMS providers hold a truly independent licensed to practice, but their scope is limited by regulation and protocol that may be directed by physicians. In still other states, EMS providers require both a state and a regional or local authority or to practice once they have certain satisfied certain requirements. Once state authority to practice is determined in some way, then a county, regional, or local authority, such as a medical director or "base hospital," may further control or limit the provider's scope or ability to practice. For example, in some jurisdictions, an EMS provider trained and licensed (or the equivalent) at an advanced level by state authority is limited to practice at a more basic level by their employer, system, or medical director. This may occur because the EMS provider is working for an agency that holds a basic-level service license, because it is the design of a particular system to limit the number of advanced practice providers, or because there is particular concern raised about the individuals' ability to practice at a higher level until certain competency is ensured.

In addition to initial provider licensing, most jurisdictions require some method of ensuring continuing education and competency. This may take a variety of forms, including attestation by a medical director, refresher courses, successful passage of competency tests, attendance at continuing education events, distance-learning courses, and others.

In addition to legislation, regulations and protocols specific to EMS operations, providers must also be aware of laws and regulations that may require action on the part of EMS providers. These may include the required reporting of certain circumstances, such as child abuse or elder abuse and neglect, knowledge of or contact with certain infectious diseases or conditions, awareness of impairment of drivers, peers or other healthcare professionals, concern about the adequacy of health care facility capabilities, etc. EMS providers should also be aware of regulations regarding the restraint, care (including testing such as drawing blood for legal purposes) and transport of patients in circumstances such as psychiatric impairment, court order, or incarceration by police. There is considerable variation from state to state and even within states regarding these requirements, and therefore the EMS provider should research local requirements.

AMBULANCE LICENSING AND EQUIPMENT

It is common for states to regulate the level of service provided by ambulance agencies, such as basic or advanced, to regulate certain aspects of the ambulance vehicle (such as meeting KKK specifications or other standards), and to specify the equipment carried, including medical equipment, equipment used for rescue and access, safety equipment, and communications devices. The degree of specification may vary from exact requirements to use a specific brand and model of equipment (for example, in order to provide data for a specific quality assurance effort) or it may generally require that a capability be provided without specifying the exact nature of the brand or model to be used (for example, cardiac monitoring and defibrillation).

Some jurisdictions allow individual EMS providers to personally carry equipment that would be authorized for their level of practice even when they are not in an ambulance. This allows these providers to render aid when they are the first responder to an incident and when they are posted at an event without an ambulance nearby (such as "coverage" at a high school football game), which increases the system capability to respond to a mass casualty event. However, regulation and inspection of this equipment is a concern. One solution is that

the equipment be a responsibility of both the individual provider and an affiliated agency that is subject to inspection and regulation by the proper authorities.

EMS PROVIDER SCOPE OF PRACTICE

Regulation of the scope of practice appears in many parts of the EMS system. It may be specified in law, flow from standards of training and practice, be controlled by licensing requirements for both providers and ambulance services, or be outlined in protocol, policy, and procedure. In some jurisdictions, there is a single controlling authority, such as a state EMS office, that sets forth the different EMS provider levels of practice and a scope of practice for each. In other models, a state authority sets a range of acceptable practice, including minimum and maximum procedural and medication limits, but leaves individual ambulance agency and provider scope to a county, regional, local, or even individual service level.

DISCIPLINARY PROCESS

Ultimately, the agency that issues the EMS provider or ambulance service license (or equivalent process) to practice or offer services has authority to take action against that license if necessary. Across the United States, this authority typically exists at the state level, although local and regional structures may exist to investigate, gather preliminary data, and make recommendations to the licensing authority. There should be clearly defined due process rules for the disciplinary process that allow the EMS provider to tell their side of the story, present witnesses, and be heard by the licensing authority.

KEY POINTS

- The practice of EMS medicine across international borders raises important concerns of regulation of controlled substances, licensing, and vehicle/aircraft operation.
- Multiple federal agencies regulate different aspects of the EMS system including the DOT NHTSA EMS, DHHS, DEA, FAA, and GSA, among others.
- State regulations vary greatly and affect training, licensing, scope of practice, controlled substances, and operation of emergency vehicles.

REFERENCES

1. Committe on Trauma and Committee on Shock, Division of Medical Sciences, National Academy of Sciences, National Research Council. Accidental death and disability: the neglected disease of modern society. http://www.ems.gov/pdf/1997-reproduction-accidentaldeath dissability.pdf. Accessed May, 2015.
2. EMS. http://www.ems.gov/. Accessed May, 2015.
3. DEA. http://www.justice.gov/dea/index.htm. Accessed May, 2015.
4. Federal Aviation Administration. Fact Sheet – FAA Initiatives to Improve Helicopter Air Ambulance Safety. February 20, 2014. http://www.faa.gov/news/fact_sheets/news_story.cfm?newsId=15794. Accessed May, 2015.
5. Kreindler & Kreindler LLP. Aviation law emergency helicopter safety crisis, federal preemption. http://www.kreindler.com/Publications/Aviation-Law-Emergency-Helicopter-Safety-Crisis-Federal-Preemption.shtml. Accessed May, 2015.
6. GSA. Ambulances. http://www.gsa.gov/portal/content/100721. Accessed May, 2015.

7. GSA. Federal Specification for the Star-of-Life Ambulance. KKK-A-1822F. August 1, 2007. http://www.deltaveh.com/f.pdf. Accessed May 16, 2015.

8. National EMS Management Association. NFPA 1917 Standard for Automative Ambulances. Past, present, and future. http://www.nasemso.org/documents/NASEMSONFPA1917.pdf. Accessed May, 2015.

9. Public Health Emergency. Disaster medical assistance team (DMAT). http://www.phe.gov/Preparedness/responders/ndms/teams/Pages/dmat.aspx. Accessed May, 2015.

10. National Association of State EMS Officials. www.nasemso.org. Accessed May, 2015.

11. National Association of EMS Physicians. www.naemsp.org. Accessed May, 2015.

12. AMPA. Advancing Air & Ground Critical Care Transport Medicine. www.ampa.org. Accessed May, 2015.

13. National Registry of Emergency Medical Technicians. http://www.nremt.org/. Accessed May, 2015.

Physician-Patient Relationships in EMS

Bradley M. Pinsky

INTRODUCTION

Medical directors play an integral role in the care of patients in the pre-hospital setting. Along with the ability to have a positive impact on the care of the patient goes the responsibility to strive for the best possible outcome. Medical directors must ensure that they carry out their roles with the due care which the law will impose on them. The failure to carefully carry out their roles may not only result in harm to the patient, but also to liability of the physician and the physician's employer.

OBJECTIVES

- Define the circumstances which must be present in order to form a physician-patient relationship.
- List the components of the physician-patient relationship.
- Identify whether a physician-patient relationship has been formed given a set of facts.
- Discuss the nature of the physician-patient relationship when a physician responds to the field to assist with treatment.
- Identify potential liability issues when a physician provides online and off-line medical direction.
- Explain the roles of the physician in providing off-line medical direction
- Describe ways in which EMS agencies can obtain useful feedback and detail a method for handling complaints.

DEFINE THE STANDARD MEANING OF PHYSICIAN-PATIENT RELATIONSHIP

In the United States, the physician-patient relationship is defined on a state-by-state basis through either judge made case law or state statute. As a result, the definition of this relationship varies from state to state. Physicians are generally not obligated to treat a patient unless they choose to do so or have assumed a duty to do so, although there are certainly exceptions to this rule. A patient-physician relationship is formed when a physician affirmatively acts on behalf of a patient by examining, diagnosing, or treating the patient or by agreeing to do so. Once the physician consensually enters into a relationship with a patient in any of these ways, a legal contract is frequently formed in which the physician owes a duty to that patient to continue to treat the patient until the relationship is actually and properly terminated.

The American Medical Association has commented on the physician-patient relationship as follows:

> The practice of medicine, and its embodiment in the clinical encounter between a patient and a physician, is fundamentally a moral activity that arises from the imperative to care for patients and to alleviate suffering.
>
> A patient-physician relationship exists when a physician serves a patient's medical needs, generally by mutual consent between physician and patient (or surrogate). In some instances the agreement is implied, such as in emergency care or when physicians provide services at the request of the treating physician. In rare instances, treatment without consent may be provided under court order…. Nevertheless, the physician's obligations to the patient remain intact.
>
> The relationship between patient and physician is based on trust and gives rise to physicians' ethical obligations to place patients' welfare above their own self-interest and above obligations to other groups, and to advocate for their patients' welfare.

> Within the patient-physician relationship, a physician is ethically required to use sound medical judgment, holding the best interests of the patient as paramount….

OPINION OF THE AMERICAN MEDICAL ASSOCIATION, E-10.015 (2001)

Attorneys may look at this relationship a bit differently. The physician-patient relationship is most often formed voluntarily with the mutual consent of the physician and the patient. The relationship involves an explicit or implied set of expectations between an individual and a physician which has reasonably imposed a duty of care on the physician to diagnose and/or treat the patient within the standard of care of the practice of medicine. The relationship relies on the actual or implied trust of the patient in the knowledge and/or skills of the physician. The formation of the relationship dictates that a physician has or should have the expectation that the patient is relying on the physician for present and/or future diagnosis, treatment, and/or evaluation.

The physician-patient relationship, once formed, imposes a duty on a physician to diagnose and treat a patient within the standard of care. The resulting relationship is one where a patient either explicitly or implicitly desires the physician to provide medical diagnosis and/or treatment. The goal of the relationship usually is for the physician to provide diagnoses of a condition, an answer to a question and a solution to a medical and/or health concern and issue. The relationship is based on the patient's trust in the physician to provide timely and accurate answers and/or solutions. Although not all medical conditions are capable of being treated to the point of remission or healing, the physician-patient relationship is one of an expectation by the patient that the physician is knowledgeable in the subject matter or will if necessary refer the patient to a physician capable of performing such a diagnosis and/or treatment.

However, a relationship is not formed simply because a patient has an expectation that the physician has become obligated to diagnose and/or treat the physician. The patient's expectations must be based on a reasonable set of circumstances which bind the physician to become bound to a duty of care to the patient. In determining whether a physician-patient relationship has been formed, courts frequently wrestle with the underlying facts of the alleged relationship between the physician and the individual.

Although in most instances determining whether such a relationship has been formed is not difficult, persons who have come in contact with a physician in some manner frequently allege that they have earned a duty for care from a physician to be treated as a patient. Not all physicians will agree that the level of contact they have had with an individual resulted in a duty of care owed to that individual as a patient.

Certain state statutes and judge made law impose only limited physician-patient relationships in various instances, such as when a physician is required to evaluate a patient's medical condition in order for the court to make certain findings on the patient's physical or mental well-being or when an individual is required to have a physical and/or mental examination prior to employment. These situations are discussed more in detail below.

Numerous courts have engaged in fact-finding missions of whether a physician's contact with an individual rose to the level of a physician-patient relationship.

Questions which could arise in the emergency medical services industry are ever abundant. Some potentially common situations are as follows:

- A physician provides medical control over the phone or radio, instructing or confirming the administration of a treatment or medication to a patient in an ambulance.
- A physician responds directly to a scene of an accident to assist with the treatment of a patient, such as by removing a limb in order to extricate the patient from a vehicle.
- A member of a fire department or ambulance services asks what seems like an innocuous medical question of their medical director as to the member's own medical or health issues.

- A paramedic is permitted to operate "under the license" or "under the supervision" of a physician, and the physician oversees the competency of the paramedic.
- A physician reviews the care of emergency medical service providers under quality control, and permits the providers to operate in the field, having deemed them "competent" providers with adequate knowledge and skills.
- A physician in his or her off time happens upon the scene of an accident or medical emergency, and (a) provides advice to the emergency medical service provider, (b) actually provides instructions to the emergency medical service provider, or (c) actually treats the patient.

Although the creation of a physician-patient relationship is generally easy to determine, as the patient usually seeks out the physician, and the physician then accepts the patient as a client, the relationship is not always clearly established. More difficult questions of whether such a relationship has been formed are, for example:

- A physician with no relationship to the emergency medical service happens upon a scene of a medical emergency and asks a paramedic if he or she needs assistance with treating a patient, and the paramedic refuses assistance or alternatively accepts assistance.
- A physician offers advice to a treating paramedic, which the paramedic utilizes in its treatment.
- A physician with no relationship to the emergency medical service happens upon a scene of an accident, but offers no medical advice to the patient or the paramedic, but simply assists the paramedic in carrying out a manual task such as intubation or application of a splint.
- A physician directly treats the patient, but the patient is unconscious and unaware of the treatment.

As stated above, the relationship is often a voluntary relationship where the physician can choose to accept the individual as a patient or choose not to do so. Most frequently, physicians can refuse to accept an individual as a patient for almost any nondiscriminatory reason (such as gender, race, sexual preference).

In some instances, physicians have waived the right to accept patients, such as physicians who work in emergency rooms and are presented with patients in potentially emergency situations, or physicians who are under a contract with a private or government insurance program to accept patients.

Additionally, some states impose duties of care on all individuals to take reasonable action, for example, Minnesota, Vermont, Hawaii, Rhode Island, and Wisconsin. What defines an action to be reasonable or unreasonable is a matter of case law. In these few states, however, the failure of a physician or emergency medical technician to render care within the scope of their authorized practice may be deemed a violation of the state statutes.

Physicians may choose to refuse to take on individuals as patients for a variety of reasons, including but not limited to:

- *The treatment request is beyond the physician's competence.*
- *The treatment request is scientifically or medically invalid or unnecessary.*
- *The treatment request is incompatible with the physician's personal beliefs.*

PHYSICIAN-PATIENT RELATIONSHIP IN CLINICAL AND HOSPITAL PRACTICES

As stated, states vary in how they define a patient-physician relationship. However, a patient-physician relationship is generally formed when a physician affirmatively acts in a patient's case by examining, diagnosing, treating, or agreeing to do so. Once the physician enters into a relationship with a patient by providing an examination, diagnosis, and/or treatment, or simply agrees to do any of these actions, a legal contract is likely formed in which the physician owes a duty to that patient to continue to treat or properly terminate the relationship.

Broken into its parts, the relationship frequently requires the following components:

- A request, either expressly or implicitly, by the individual to the physician to provide a diagnosis and/or treatment
- An acceptance by the physician or a preexisting legal obligation of the physician diagnose and/or treat the physician

Not all states require that there be an actual agreement between the physician and the patient in every instance. In Oregon a court held that "in the absence of an express agreement by the physician to treat a patient, a physician's assent to a physician-patient relationship can be inferred when the physician takes an affirmative action with regard to the care of the patient." A patient-physician relationship was formed because the physician took an affirmative action in rendering an opinion on the course of the patient's care.[1]

States commonly recognize that a physician who actually treats a patient has a duty of care toward that patient.[2] In limited situations, courts have held that diagnosing patients does not necessarily create a physician-patient relationship.

Even though physicians may not form a physician-patient relationship with certain individuals, the physician may still owe the individual a limited duty of care.

For example, physicians also engage persons in other situations, such as to perform preemployment screening or "fit for duty" evaluations. Courts have generally held that no physician-patient relationship exists when a physician merely examines a patient on behalf of the patient's employer. However, if the physician treats the patient for any condition, such a relationship has been formed (see article for cases).

Courts have found that a physician has a limited duty to a patient to conduct the diagnostic tests accurately.

Although a physician-patient relationship might not exist in certain circumstances, a physician may still acquire a legal duty to a patient to advise the patient of a dangerous health situation discovered during an examination. For example, if a blood test reveals that an individual he or she examines is HIV positive or has a life-threatening heart condition, the physician may be deemed to owe the individual a limited duty to advise him or her of the condition. Some states have enacted statutes and/or regulations requiring such disclosure by the physician.

In hospital settings, the relationship is often formed in ways different from that of a private office setting.

■ THE EMERGENCY ROOM PATIENT

The Emergency Medical Treatment and Labor Act (EMTALA) was first enacted in June 1994. EMTALA applies to all hospitals which accept Medicare (so, almost all hospitals except Shriners Hospitals). The purpose of EMTALA is to prevent hospitals from rejecting patients, refusing to treat them, or transferring them to "charity hospitals" or "county hospitals" because they are unable to pay or are covered under the Medicare or Medicaid programs. It is therefore called the Antidumping Act.

EMTALA requires that no patient who presents to a hospital with an emergency medical condition and who is unable to pay may be treated differently than patients who are covered by health insurance. Any patient who "comes to the emergency department" requesting "examination or treatment for a medical condition" must be provided with "an appropriate medical screening examination" to determine if he or she is suffering from an "emergency medical condition." If so, then the hospital is obligated to either provide the patient with treatment until the patient is stable or to transfer patient to another hospital in conformance with EMTALA's directives.

EMTALA imposes an obligation on the part of the hospital to provide an appropriate medical screening examination within the capabilities of the emergency department for the purpose of determining whether an "emergency medical condition" exists. EMTALA further imposes an obligation upon the hospital to institute treatment if an "emergency medical condition" does exist. The statute further imposes restrictions on transfers of persons who exhibit an "emergency medical condition or are in active labor". One critical restriction is that the decision to transfer may not be made based upon the patient's ability to pay or the source of their income. A pregnant woman who presents in active labor must be admitted and treated until delivery is completed, unless a transfer under the statute is appropriate. The statute explicitly provides that this must include delivery of the placenta.

EMTALA applies to all persons entering the hospital campus within 250 yards of the emergency room. The 250-yard rule comes from the definition of "campus," which is generally defined as the physical area immediately adjacent to the provider's main buildings, and other areas and structures that are not strictly contiguous to the main buildings but are located within 250 yards of the main buildings.

If the patient does not have an "emergency medical condition," the statute imposes no further obligation on the hospital.

In the event that the hospital owns and operates its own ambulance service, the patient has been deemed to have entered the emergency room as soon as they are placed in the care of the emergency medical technicians staffing such ambulance. However, if the ambulance transports the patient to a different hospital pursuant to community-wide policies which direct the patient to a different hospital, the patient will be deemed the patient of that receiving hospital. Of course, while the patient is within that ambulance, the medical director of such ambulance (and its employer) may still remain liable for all acts and omissions of the emergency medical technicians.

PHYSICIAN-PATIENT RELATIONSHIP WHEN A PHYSICIAN RESPONDS TO THE FIELD

Physicians have become integral components of the emergency medical services industry. Physicians are no longer confined to the internal boundaries of a hospital setting, and instead are often called upon to respond to the location of a patient. In these instances, it is not a patient who requests the services of a physician, but is more frequently an emergency medical technician or fire chief who requests the presence of the physician at the scene. This scenario presents very complex questions on whether a physician-patient relationship has been formed. Since the questions are based on state case law or statute, the answers could vary. However, important factors which will be considered by a court are as follows:

- Did the physician actively treat the patient, provide advice or orders to an emergency medical technician, or diagnose the patient?

  - The more involvement by the physician with the patient's treatment will increase the creation of the physician-patient relationship.

- Did the physician communicate with the patient? Did the physician give the patient a reason to rely on the physician? Did the physician ask questions of the patient in order to be able to diagnose and/or treat the patient?

- Did the physician advise the patient to continue seeing the physician at a later date?

A court has stated that "a physician is not to be held liable for arbitrarily refusing to respond to a call of a person even urgently in need of medical…assistance provided that the relation of physician and patient does not exist."[3]

VARIATIONS IN LIABILITY ASSOCIATED WITH FIELD CARE BY A PHYSICIAN (GOOD SAMARITAN, VOLUNTEER VERSUS PAID, DUTY TO ACT)

Many states have created laws which are designed to encourage physicians and other emergency care providers to provide assistance in unanticipated emergency situations. The laws can generally be divided into two categories: those that impose a duty to act and those that protect an individual when they have voluntarily acted.

Some states require that a person, including a physician, provide assistance to those in an emergency. The statutes stop short of imposing a burden to provide medical assistance, but do require "reasonable care."

These statutes create numerous issues in their applications, such as determining what a "reasonable" action is for a physician.

Some state statutes provide protection specifically for medical directors who volunteer their time with an emergency medical service agency, but limit their protection to medical directors who receive no remuneration for their services. Medical directors should evaluate whether the compensation they receive is worth the loss of protection they might receive. Alternatively, prospective medical directors should demand that the ambulance service indemnify them for their acts and/or omissions. Of course, providing this indemnification imposes a burden on the emergency medical service agency to ensure that the medical director is diligently performing its own duties. The contract with the medical director should ensure that the medical director's responsibilities are stated clearly.

"Good Samaritan" statutes provides varying degrees of immunity for physicians when they choose to provide medical assistance outside their scope of employment. Most commonly, these statutes require that the medical assistance is not offered in exchange for any type of remuneration. The law then provides either a full immunity or a partial immunity, called "qualified immunity." Full immunity provides absolute protection to a physician for their acts and omissions. This is less typical.

More common is that a statute provides a qualified immunity to the physician for any negligent care, being care that does not meet the standard of care. The limit on the immunity is that no immunity is extended to the physician for assistance rendered in an intentionally harmful way or a manner which is reckless or is likely to cause injury.

The patient must not have already assumed a duty to the patient through another means, such as performing such services through their employment requirement.

Under these statutes, the physician is not required to render any specific amount of care or advice, but is simply encouraged to do so with the grant of the limited immunity.

One problem that may exist for the physician is that of insurance and defense coverage. Many insurance policies only insure the physician for acts performed within the scope of his or her employment. Some employment agreements limit the scope of employment to within the physical boundaries of the workplace, thereby excluding coverage to the physician when acting in an emergency situation. Thus, some physicians may be immune or partially immune from liability for their acts and omissions, but will not have insurance coverage to provide them costs for attorneys to defend them, or insurance coverage in case they lose a lawsuit. Thus, whether such a statute actually encourages someone to become involved in an emergency situation is questionable.

It is important to note that Good Samaritan laws do not always provide absolute protection for an emergency medical service or a physician. Although these statutes frequently provide absolute or partial immunity for negligent care, their immunities do not always extend to negligent supervision or training of the emergency medical service providers. Said another way, while an emergency medical service may successfully defend a lawsuit for its negligent treatment, it may lose the same lawsuit on the theory that the treatment would not have been negligent had the medical director ensured that each provider was properly trained, evaluated, and supervised.

ONLINE MEDICAL DIRECTION

As discussed above, a physician-patient relationship is most commonly formed when a physician assumes a duty to act on behalf of a patient and provides medical treatment as opposed to simply a diagnosis. Both situations occur with online medical control. In the online medical control situation, a patient does not request the assistance of a physician. At best, a patient or a third party called 9-1-1 and requested an ambulance. The patient has no relationship with the physician and in fact may never meet the physician providing medical control.

In some instances, the patient will be brought to the hospital at which the physician is employed. In other instances the physician is at another location separate and apart from the receiving facility.

The physician becomes directly involved with the diagnosis and treatment of the patient through the words and acts of another, being the paramedic or emergency medical technician.

OFF-LINE MEDICAL DIRECTION

Off-line medical direction generally occurs when a physician issues standing orders to an emergency medical services provider to utilize a drug or procedure in the field without the direct supervision of the physician and without having to make a request of the physician. The standing orders are only initiated upon the determination that a condition exists which warrants the use of such drugs or procedure.

In some states, the medical directors do not issue the list of drugs which may be administered or the care that may be rendered while in others the medical directors have more control over these decisions. Frequently, the medical director "signs-off" on the use of such drugs and skills by the agency, even limiting the rights which are granted by the state or region.

Generally, an agency which receives permission from a physician to provide advanced emergency medical care is viewed to be working "under the license" of the medical director. Thus, the medical director becomes obligated to review the skills of the emergency medical service providers and to ensure that they are properly trained in the use of such drugs and procedures. Without the permission of the medical director, the agency may not utilize such drugs and/or procedures. This oversight creates a duty of supervision and thus it is more accurate to state that the EMS providers are providing care "under the supervision of the licensed physician." (A discussion on EMS provider certification versus licensure is detailed in Chapter 21.)

The liability from off-line medical direction arises from the supervisory relationship between the physician and the emergency medical service provider. The physician is responsible for ensuring that clear and medically appropriate advanced medical orders are issued to the provider, and that the provider possesses the knowledge and skills to carry out the advance orders in the appropriate medical situations. If an injury was caused by the improper administration of the drug or procedure, or the failure to utilize such drug or procedure, the lawsuit may focus on the acts and/or omissions of the medical director in training, supervising, and evaluating the skills of each of the emergency medical service providers. Medical directors are not always required to directly train, evaluate, and supervise each provider, but they must be involved in the evaluation and administration of the program used to do so. The lack of medical oversight by the physician may lead to a determination of negligence on the part of the emergency medical service or the agency itself.

In one filed lawsuit in Washington, DC, the mother of a deceased 2-year old sued on behalf of her child who died after EMTs failed to transport the child. The EMTs advised the mother to place the child in a steaming shower, instead of transporting the child to the hospital. The mother called back a few hours later, but it was too late to save the child. The lawsuit alleges that, among other reasons alleging liability, the ambulance corps failed to properly train and supervise the EMTs and that such lack of training and supervision leads to the negligent decisions of the EMT.[4] In Washington, DC, a state statute imposes liability on the medical director personally if the liability results from the gross negligence of the medical director.

LIABILITY CONCERNS FOR TRANSFERRING AND ACCEPTING PHYSICIANS, AND INTERFACILITY TRANSPORT PROGRAMS

Emergency room physicians are governed by the Emergency Medical Treatment and Labor Act with regard to their actions of and consequences for accepting, evaluating, and transferring patients from the emergency room. A more complete discussion of this federal law appears above.

Generally, physicians cannot discharge or transfer a patient unless they are stable. EMTALA was designed to prevent "patient dumping"

when the hospital did not want to care for the patient due to payment concerns.

That said, there are certainly times when a patient has to be transferred simply because the transferring hospital cannot adequately treat the patient. For example, some hospitals may not be able to perform the necessary surgery on a patient that came into their care. So long as the patient understands the risks of being transferred and is adequately advised of such risks, and so long as the patient is stabilized as much as possible, the transferring physician should not encounter actual liability for harm encountered by the patient during transfer.

The receiving physician must have agreed to accept the patient and must agree to offer the necessary care. A transfer cannot be safely undertaken without such an agreement. "Blind transfers" will no doubt lead to violations of EMTALA and are simply unsafe for the patient.

LAWSUITS AGAINST EMS MEDICAL DIRECTORS

Lawsuits against medical directors are less common then lawsuits against the emergency medical service itself. Common allegations against the medical director involve:

- Negligent diagnosis of the patient, either directly on-scene or through the questioning of the emergency medical technicians
- Negligent treatment of the patient, either directly on-scene or by giving harmful instructions and/or orders to the emergency medical technicians
- Negligent supervision and/or training of the emergency medical service providers

Since many states or governing municipalities provide standing orders to paramedics and emergency medical technicians for the drugs and procedures they can render, physicians are not always directly involved in the actual care provided.

However, medical directors are frequently tied into the lawsuit through the allegation that the medical director failed to properly supervise and/or train the care providers. These lawsuits allege that the medical director failed to carry out his or her role. Thus, the question of what role the medical director was required to play is important. The role of the medical director can be defined by state law, a local municipal law, or a contract between the emergency medical service agency and the physician.

In the event that a lawsuit directly or indirectly implicates the acts or omissions of the medical director, the medical director must evaluate his or her exposure and course of action. If the medical director was an employee of the agency, the medical director will likely be defended and indemnified by the ambulance service. However, if the medical director was an independent contractor, the medical director may be sued directly by the patient or even brought in by the emergency medical service itself. In either event, the medical director will want to notify his or her insurance carrier.

There should always be some sort of agreement between a medical director and an emergency medical service agency which addresses at least the following:

- The roles and responsibilities of the medical director
- Which party is responsible for providing insurance coverage
- Whether the medical director and/or the agency will defend and/or indemnify the other

MANAGING COMPLAINTS

Emergency medical services agencies will always be targets for lawsuits. Common lawsuits against EMS agencies involve allegations of more than negligent care and treatment, but also negligent hiring, training, and supervision, as well as many other underlying allegations.

Some lawsuits may be prevented by addressing concerns of patients and their families. Addressing a patient/family complaint may prevent the same issue from reoccurring in the future and may uncover provider issues which might lead to a lawsuit in the future with a different patient. Thus, EMS agencies need to provide a method to receive, address, and resolve complaints. At the same time, EMS agencies maintain valid concerns to protect themselves from potential lawsuits.

One important step that an emergency medical service can take to uncover problems and address concerns is to solicit and receive patient feedback. Unfortunately, agencies frequently do not view themselves as a "customer service." However, patients and their families have unique views of the actions of emergency medical care providers.

Consider this scenario: Ambulance service responds to a combative patient. The family states that the patient is disoriented and has a history of low blood sugar. The patient flails its arms at the emergency medical service providers. In an attempt to start to administer medications through an IV, the emergency medical technicians restrain the patient for his own safety. The EMS provider misses the vein initially, and continues with the struggling patient, resulting in black and blue marks on the patient's arm. There is no other harm to the patient.

What the family believes occurred may be quite different from the view of the emergency medical service providers. The patient's family saw two individuals physically restrain their loved one and repeatedly plunge a large needle in his harm, causing black and blue marks. The family was scared for their loved one and did not know what was occurring. Instead of having any contact with the emergency medical service to express their concerns or obtain an explanation, they turn to the television lawyer soliciting clients of medical abuse. The attorney, having no better understanding of what occurred than the family, turns to the courts to receive an explanation and compensation for the alleged assault.

Some emergency medical services mistakenly believe that if the patient or their family had a concern, they would simply pick up the phone and call. That attitude only further exacerbates the situation and causes the patient's concerns to escalate.

Emergency medical service agencies should consider providing an easy method of reaching out to the patient and soliciting their feedback. There are numerous methods of communicating with a patient, including:

- Providing a form to the patient to return to the agency after they are released from the hospital
- Providing a Web site with a survey page
- Mailing a follow-up card to the patient

Feedback should also be solicited from employees, as well as from entities such as nursing homes and hospitals, whose staff had the opportunity to observe the attitudes and treatment rendered by the emergency medical providers.

Sometimes, asking "how did we do" is enough to prevent the patient from increasing their anger over what they believe may have occurred. For-profit services always stand a better chance of maintaining contracts with nursing homes, hospitals, and other facilities by requesting feedback about their service.

More important, however, is that receiving, evaluating, and addressing complaints provide a method to uncover problematic caregivers. Repeated complaints by multiple patients about the attitude or care of an emergency medical technician could permit the agency to correct a problem before a more serious issue arises.

The feedback solicited should track the core values of the emergency medical service agency. The patient can evaluate whether the agency is achieving its mission and adhering to its core values.

Questions which can be asked include, but are not limited to:

- Do you have any questions or concerns about the treatment rendered?
- Are you satisfied by the care received?
- Were the staff members courteous?
- Would you like a call back from a member of the emergency medical service?

Like all customer-based businesses, soliciting feedback also provides employees with an incentive to be careful of their actions and attitudes, as they know that the employer is requesting feedback about them.

Emergency room physicians and nurses are frequently the source of the more significant reports of misconduct and negligence. Hospitals should easily be able to report such concerns to the ambulance company, and should be given direct access to a supervisor to quickly and easily make such a report. Otherwise, the hospital staff may contact the municipal agency which oversees the licensing of the ambulance service or discuss its concerns with the patient's family.

Emergency medical service agencies must understand that hospitals and physicians also have a need to protect themselves. Thus, ensuring that the blame for a poor outcome lies with the correct provider may be of vital concern to the hospital. Open lines of communication with a hospital are simply paramount to running a successful EMS program.

Of course, providers should also be a direct source of reports. Providers will not want to report their own errors, but they must be instructed that the failure to report a potential or actual issue can result in discipline to them. They should also be comforted that the self-reporting of an error will may be met with additional training and oversight in lieu of discipline whereas covering up such acts or omissions will be dealt with harshly. Partners and supervisors should also be encouraged to make reports, even if the report could result in bad relations with the other provider.

The routine method of monitoring the quality of care, being Quality Improvement and Quality Assurance programs, is only part of a comprehensive program to detect quality issues. Coupled with the above programs, however, a QI/QA program can be effective.

EMS agencies should be aware that not all quality assurance and quality improvement (QA/QI) proceedings are confidential. For example, in New York State, although the QI/QA process is generally protected from disclosure in lawsuits and public information inquiries, New York State law provides that if a person who is or later becomes a defendant in a lawsuit, the individual's testimony before the QA/QI process is discoverable.

An emergency medical service agency should openly solicit and address feedback on the care provided to patients. Such programs will pay significant dividends by not only addressing concerns after they occur, but preventing systemic problems before they cause real harm to a patient and the agency itself.

KEY POINTS

- The establishment of a physician-patient relationship for EMS physicians may be less clear in legal terms than that of hospital-based physicians.
- Liability for EMS physicians/medical directors lies primarily in three potential areas: negligent diagnosis/assessment, negligent treatment, and negligent supervision or training of prehospital providers.
- Three potential ways to gather important patient feedback include providing a feedback form, offering a Web site with survey page, mailing out a follow-up card.
- Feedback on quality of care should also include self-assessment and peer review.

REFERENCES

1. *Mead v Adler*, 231 Or App 451, 220 P3d 118 (Or 2009).
2. *Dallas-Stephenson v. Waisman*, 39 A.D.3d 303, 307, 833 N.Y.S.2d 89 (1st Dep't 2007).
3. *Childs v Weis*, 440 SW2d 104 (Ct Civ App Tx 1969).
4. *Stephanie Stephens v. Geoffrey Mount-Varner, MD.*

CHAPTER 24

Capacity and Refusal of Care

Shannon D. O'Keefe

Lori L. Harrington

INTRODUCTION

Due to the difficulty in addressing the ethics and science of determining a patient's ability to participate in important medical decision making, it is important to review basic medical ethics principles. In order for these principles to be more fully understood, this chapter includes a number of clinical vignettes that are used to introduce principles and discuss their implementation in the prehospital environment.

A 45-year-old man calls 9-1-1 after experiencing 15 minutes of substernal chest pain. On your arrival to the patient, he denies any complaints and his chest pain has subsided without intervention. You assess the patient and find he has an elevated blood pressure 200/100 and an ECG reveals NSR without ischemic changes. The patient reports feeling well and refuses further intervention or transport to the hospital. You feel the patient is at high risk for cardiac disease and believe he should be treated and transported. What do you do?

OBJECTIVES

- Describe the principles of assessing a patient's capacity as defined by Applebaum and Grisso.
- Discuss the prehospital assessment of capacity.
- Discuss the basis for the right to refuse care.
- Describe key elements of documentation during a patient refusal.
- Describe indications for calling for law enforcement assistance.
- Discuss state differences in laws regarding providing involuntary psychiatric treatment in the field.
- Give examples of appropriate and inappropriate refusals.

INFORMED CONSENT

The medical legal concept of patient consent to medical treatment dates back to 1912 US case law in which Justice Cardoza writes: "Every human being of adult years and sound mind has a right to determine what shall be done with his own body."[1] This concept is further refined as *informed consent* by 1957 US case law with the addition of the duty to disclose information.[2] This doctrine of informed consent relies on the principle of autonomy in which an individual has the right to self-determination, even if it results in harm. Although the medical, legal, and ethical principles of informed consent, medical decision-making capacity, and refusal of care have their foundation in medical care provided by physicians, they apply as well, and often with greater challenge, to prehospital providers: first responders, EMTs, and paramedics.

In order for medical personnel to provide medical care, including assessment, evaluation, and transport of that patient by a prehospital provider, the patient must first consent to have that care provided. Many may assume the principle of informed consent does not apply to emergency medical services (EMS) because the care being provided is assumed to be in the case of an emergency, and therefore this exception to informed consent would apply. This idea of implied or emergent consent is often used by EMS but can only be assumed in a situation in which the care must be given to prevent death or serious injury. This emergency situation is not always the case in the emergency room or prehospital setting because not all circumstances are true emergencies and may not require immediate life-saving intervention. If there is enough time to discuss the treatment options with the patient and obtain informed consent,

then the emergency exception does not apply.[3] Therefore, for situations in which the provider is caring for a non-life-threatening emergency, the concept of informed consent applies and must be understood. There are three fundamental elements of valid informed consent.[3-5] The patient: (1) must have capacity to make the medical decision, (2) must be given sufficient information to make an informed decision, and (3) make the decision voluntarily without coercion or duress from the provider or other family or friends.

DETERMINING CAPACITY

In general, determining a patient's medical decision-making capacity occurs as an inherent part of a patient's assessment; the provider, as well as the law,[6] assumes a patient has capacity unless the patient's decisions are called into questions. The vast majority of persons are capable of making their own decisions.[5] The question of a patient's capacity usually arises when the patient refuses care that the provider feels is indicated. There are generally three categories of patients in regard to capacity. It is easy to determine capacity in the majority of patients, with the general assumption being those who are seeking care have capacity. There are also patients in whom it is easily determined that they lack capacity, for example, those who are profoundly mentally handicapped, comatose, or acutely psychotic. The challenging group is the many patients who fall in between these two categories, those with psychiatric illness, substance abuse, delirium, dementia, head trauma, or other underlying illnesses that may cause change in mental status. There are many underlying medical, psychological, developmental, and toxicologic diagnoses which may impair a patient's capacity to make a medical decision.

In order for a patient to consent to and accept medical treatment or to refuse that treatment, it is essential that the providers assess if the patient has capacity to make that decision. The terms capacity and competence are often used interchangeably in both medical and legal literature. Generally, competence is a legal determination, enforced by a judge's ruling and is usually a global decision of a person's general ability to make decisions.[4] Persons who are determined to be incompetent lose their right to consent to or refuse treatment and instead have a legal guardian appointed to make those decisions for them. Medical decision-making capacity, however, refers to the ability to make a decision applicable to a specific medical event. Because medical situations vary from benign, low-risk, uncomplicated interventions, to highly complex, high-risk situations, a patient's level of capacity may vary depending on the individual and the situation. Some individuals may have medical decision-making capacity for low acuity, basic medical decisions, but may not have capacity in more complex situations. Applebaum and Grisso[5,6] describe four essential skills a patient must possess in order to have medical decision-making capacity (**Box 24-1**).

In order for a provider to assess a patient as having capacity, the patient must be able to *understand* the relevant information given to them. If they do not understand what they have been told, they do not have the capacity to make a decision based on that information. The patient must have the attention span and memory to remember the information given to them, and the ability to comprehend it. The EMT might ask the patient to restate the information provided regarding their illness to ensure they have the memory to retain it, but more importantly to ask them to restate it in their own words to determine that the patient actually understood the information. The patient must *appreciate* the significance

---

Box 24-1

Applebaum and Grisso's Determination of Capacity

1. Understand relevant information.

2. Appreciate the situation and consequences.

3. Reason about treatment options.

4. Communicate a choice.

and implication of the illness, and the consequences of a treatment decision, including the risks and benefits of treatment or not being treated. The patient must have insight into actually having a medical illness. They might be asked to describe their illness, the proposed treatment, and the likely outcome of being treated or not. The patient must be able to *reason* through the process of balancing the treatment options based on the relevant information. This rational manipulation of information involves the ability of weighing each choice and making a logically consistent conclusion based on those weighted choices. The patient can be asked to compare treatment options and their consequences and to give a reason to their decision. Finally the patient must be able to *communicate* a choice of the preferred treatment option, and maintain that choice long enough for that plan of care to be implemented.

There are vast challenges to determining a patient's capacity in the field: initial patient assessment can occur in very austere environments; unlike ongoing medical care by physicians, emergency medical personnel do not have a preexisting relationship with the patient to rely on, nor do they have much time to make this assessment. Other challenges include language barriers without the help of translators, cultural differences, and often the lack of supporting players such as family members who may assist the patient in their decision making. Explicit extensive assessment of patient's capacity is often not feasible in the field. Although there are a number of quantitative tools, which can be used in hospital, such as the mini-mental status examination or MacArthur Competence Assessment Tool for Treatment, these tools are not applicable to the field provider given the length of time and additional skill needed to implement them. They are beyond the scope of practice of the field provider.

Despite all these limitations the field provider will frequently have to determine if a patient has capacity, usually in the setting of a patient who refuses medical aid and/or transport. One study showed that among ethical dilemmas encountered, EMTs stated that those regarding patient refusal of care occurred most frequently.[7] Another study showed that when ethical conflict did arise in the prehospital setting, 17% of the time it involved patient competence.[8] In these circumstances, it is important that the field provider is informed of the above criteria and of their services', state's, or regional protocol for determining capacity, and should use these as guidance to determine if a patient has capacity to refuse that treatment. Unfortunately, there is no single, simple measure of a patient's decision-making capacity.[3] A basic approach for the field provider should include determining if the patient understands and appreciates the specific situation at hand, including risks and benefits, that the patient has sufficient information to reason through the potential treatment choices, and that the patient is able to make a choice, and that choice is made voluntarily. The field provider should also be able to determine if there is a basic underlying condition interfering with the patient's capacity including, for example, change in mental status from hypoglycemia, intoxication, seizure, or psychiatric illness. The provider should use other resources that may be present or accessible such as family, medic alert tags, or available medical information to aid in their assessment of the patients' capacity. The field provider may also rely on other members of the service such as command or supervisory staff or online medical control to help assess the situation when necessary.

Consider, for example, a patient for whom a third-party called 9-1-1, after the patient was noted to fall while walking on the sidewalk. On arrival to the scene, the EMS crew finds a well-dressed, middle-aged man sitting comfortably on the sidewalk leaning against a wall, with an obvious contusion and laceration to his forehead. The patient is otherwise in no distress. On further assessment the patient is alert, oriented to self only, not to the situation, or to purpose of the interaction. He has an obvious odor of alcohol. He is unable to give any history surrounding the events of the evening, does not know how he arrived at this place or situation. He tells the crew that he is fine and will find his way to his car. He declines assistance by EMS. He is perseverative, repeating over and over that he is just fine. This situation is a common one encountered by prehospital providers. The patient is clearly not oriented, and he does not have the ability to understand the situation given that he is unable to relay the circumstances surrounding it. He clearly does not have medical decision-making capacity to refuse the medical care and transport. It would be appropriate for the crew to transport this patient to the hospital.

EXCEPTIONS TO INFORMED CONSENT

There are few exceptions to providing care without a patient's informed consent. If a patient is assessed and determined to lack the capacity to make a decision, the prehospital provider should seek guidance from a substitute decision maker such as the patient's next of kin to obtain informed consent for care. As already discussed, in an emergency situation an exception to informed consent exists and the prehospital provider can provide appropriate emergent care under the presumption that a reasonable person would have consented to such treatment to prevent death or serious harm, or the presumption that if this patient were able to consent he would do so to preserve life. There are other circumstances in which a patient is determined to have capacity to consent to treatment, but abdicates the decision to someone else, usually a family member, to make decisions on their behalf. This waiver of consent allows another person to make the decision for a patient and should be respected by the field provider.

REFUSAL OF CARE

A competent adult has the legal right to refuse care as described by 1957 case law[2]; however, assessment of their capacity must be pursued prior to allowing refusal of care. The most salient legal liabilities revolving around refusal of care are negligence and abandonment.[9] These comprise the majority of all lawsuits involving EMS.[10] Negligence is multifaceted and requires: (1) that an act or an omission was committed, (2) there was a legal duty, (3) the act or omission resulted in damages, and (4) there was a breach in the professional standard of care.[11] Abandonment refers to the intentional stopping of medical care without legal excuse, justification, or the patient's consent, and includes transfer of care to someone of lesser training when higher level of training is needed to provide adequate care.[12] Most authorities conclude that abandonment is based on the principles of negligence, and identify these patients who may lack capacity to decline medical treatment as a specific area of concern. In contrast, treating a competent patient without their consent could be interpreted as assault and battery. Concerns about medicolegal implications and patient outcomes have prompted most EMS systems to implement prehospital protocols and policies regarding refusal of care and transport. One survey showed that 91% of responding agencies utilized formal refusal-of-transport policies, with 81% requiring determination of capacity first.[13]

Refusal of care is a common entity and one that prehospital providers will encounter with regularity. Most studies cite an overall refusal of transport rate of 5% to 10%; however, one study reported a rate as high as 30%.[14-18] These studies have also sought to describe the demographics of patients who typically decline care. Most patients involved in refusal of transport are young (18-64 years of age), whereas those older than 65 are least likely to reject transport. There is relatively even gender distribution. The most common chief complaints associated with refusal of care are motor vehicle accidents, falls, hypoglycemia, chest pain, and seizures. In one study, approximately 11% of patients received some treatment prior to their refusal, most commonly dextrose, naloxone, or albuterol.[15,16]

Among patients who decline transport and medical care, reliable outcome data are limited in the literature due to difficulty obtaining follow-up data on these patients, and findings are variable. Most studies report that approximately 40% to 55% of adult patients who initially decline transport ultimately seek additional medical care within 1 week of their initial call.[19,20] It is more difficult to surmise how many patients needed emergency transport during their initial visit as it is recognized that some patients may request an ambulance in the absence of alternate means of transportation. However, one study reports a rate of almost 70% of patients not transported who later sought medical attention and required a change in medical care.[21] Overall admission rates for patients who were not transported ranges from 6% to 12% in the literature.[17,20-22] A very small percentage (0.05%) of patients in one study died.[21] It is also important to note that although elderly patients less frequently refuse transport, they have the highest rates of hospitalization and death after refusal of EMS care.[15]

As health care professionals, prehospital providers must balance patient autonomy with protection of patients from harm due to illness and injury. Because a substantial number of lawsuits involving EMS providers involve issues surrounding negligence and abandonment, online medical control has been examined as a possible mitigating factor. Multiple studies have demonstrated significant benefit both in terms of improved transport rates as well as more robust documentation at the time of refusal, with the use of online medical control.[23-26] One study documented a transport rate of only 3% among patients who had initially refused when a more persuasive attempt made by EMS was the sole intervention; however, this increased to 35% when online medical control was utilized.[27] These findings were confirmed in other studies which demonstrated similarly large increases in the numbers of patients who were agreeable to transport after discussion with online medical control.[24-26] Implementation of online medical control may help identify and intervene upon patients needing further care earlier in their clinical course.

Two categories of patient nontransports are generally recognized: patient initiated refusal, and EMS provider initiated refusal. Patient initiated refusals are far more common, and thought to be multifactorial. Patients may decline transport in situations where bystanders may have called ambulances such as in the setting of motor vehicle accidents or seizure, they may feel that they do not need transport because their medical condition is resolved, such as in hypoglycemia, or they may have concerns about drug or alcohol use, or the cost and inconvenience associated with transport and hospitalization.

Alternatively, some states and EMS agencies may allow EMS providers to make a determination at the scene regarding the need for emergent transport. Because of the medicolegal risk involved with EMS provider initiated nontransport, this is infrequent and often prohibited by the state or EMS agency, or involves mandatory consultation with online medical control. Studies show similar rates of patients seeking additional medical care and requiring an intervention or change in medical care, regardless of whether it was the patient or EMS provider who initiated the refusal.[21] These findings suggest that it may be difficult for EMS providers to accurately predict which patients need further medical care. A review of the published literature suggests a number of high-risk criteria for adverse medical outcomes be considered for mandatory transport, including psychiatric complaints, dementia, abnormal pulse (<50 or >110 beats/min), abnormal systolic blood pressure (<90 or >200 mm Hg), head injury, and age >55 years.[21,27,28] Those studies suggest that had these criteria been utilized, it would have resulted in transportation of the vast majority of the EMS initiated refusals that resulted in hospital admission.

Given the inherent risks involved with patient refusal of transport, many EMS agencies have developed a standard protocol that must

be followed in order for a patient to decline transport. The American College of Emergency Physicians (ACEP) as well as the National Association of EMS Physicians (NAEMSP) recommend that all EMS providers develop medically directed protocols regarding these patients, and feel that refusal can occur only in the setting of direct medical guidance or detailed off-line protocols.[29] There are a number of key elements that should be integrated into these plans. First, patients must have medical decision-making capacity. Components of this determination include assessment of orientation, intoxication, head injury, comprehension of condition, and understanding the risk of refusal. Some EMS include additional components such as presence of clear speech, age-appropriate behavior, emotional control, and finger stick glucose to further aid in the determination of decision-making capacity. New York, for example, requires a patient to be alert and fully oriented, and understand the consequences of refusal of medical care. Online medical control is required to complete the refusal process. ACEP also recommends the development of patient education materials that can be given to patients who refuse transport. EMS and online medical control providers must take care to ensure that decisions are made in the best interest of the patient, not the providers. Finally, performance improvement programs should be implemented to follow the outcomes of patients who decline transport, and to monitor compliance with the assessment of decision-making capacity.

Detailed documentation on these patients is essential, and minimal documentation should include a complete set of vitals, assessment of capacity, and a signature of the patient. Further documentation could also include history and reason for EMS activation, pertinent medical history, description from scene (if relevant), and on-scene treatment provided. Online medical control has been shown to significantly improve documentation for medicolegal purposes. One study reviewed records from patient initiated refusal of transport cases, and found missing documentation from almost half of all the reports.[23] These documentation deficiencies included primarily missing vital signs and physical examination findings, including mental status and orientation, which is a key component in the determination of decision-making capacity. With the addition of online medical control, no deficiencies were noted between the combined paramedic and online medical control physician documentation. Improved documentation has the potential to substantially reduce medicolegal liability in the case of a poor patient outcome (**Figure 24-1**).

Consider the situation of a patient with change in mental status, for example. The girlfriend of the patient calls 9-1-1 because he is unable to speak except for incomprehensible sounds and is unable to get up off the couch. On arrival the EMS crew finds the patient alert with eyes open, with garbled speech. He is able to follow some simple commands. He is protecting his own airway. He is diaphoretic, slightly tachypneic, and tachycardic. On further history, the girlfriend states the patient is a known diabetic. He had taken his insulin earlier in the morning but they had not yet eaten breakfast. The crew checks the patient's blood glucose and finds it to be 21 mg/dL. The patient is given a tube of oral glucose with good effect. His skin dries up. He becomes oriented to self and the situation. Shortly after receiving the glucose, he is able to relay specifics of the situation that he

---

[X]—Patient oriented to Person, Place and Time.

[X]—Patient DOES NOT appear to be under the influence of drugs or alcohol.

[X]—Patient DOES NOT exhibits signs and/or symptoms of head trauma.

[X]—Patient has been directed to call 9-1-1 back if they change their mind or the condition worsens.

[X]—Patient answering questions appropriately.

[X]—Patient is at least 18 years old, or in the case of a minor, is the Parent or Legal Guardian present and meets all of the above criteria.

[X]—Patient DID NOT lose consciousness.

[X]—Patient expresses understanding of the risk of refusal of treatment and/or transport by EMS.

[X]—Patient answers all questions with clear speech (to patient's known baseline).

[X]—NO potential life/limb threatening condition exists (e.g., CP, SOB, major trauma, etc).

[X]—Patient has been advised of the potential consequences of refusing treatment/transport, including worsening of condition.

FIGURE 24-1. Example of patient refusal documentation checklist from electronic patient care record.

had taken his insulin but had not eaten. He makes himself a sandwich, which he begins to eat. He expresses thanks to the crew for their treatment but declines transport to the hospital. The crew discusses with the patient the risk of not going to the hospital for further monitoring and treatment, including recurrent hypoglycemia, permanent disability, and death from untreated hypoglycemia. The patient is alert and oriented, is able to understand the risks associated with refusal, and can paraphrase what was told to him. He is able to weigh the choice of staying home with accepting transport to the hospital and still declines transport. The crew contacts online medical control, which is their agency's protocol with patient refusals, and the online physician agrees with the patient refusal. Prior to completing the call, the crew documents the patient's vital signs and examination including mental status, his pre- and posttreatment glucose, which is normal, the online physician's discussion, and the patient and crew sign the documentation. Although initially this patient did not have capacity, after treatment and a short time he clearly improved and had capacity to refuse care. The crew appropriately followed their internal policy for patient refusal and completion of refusal documentation.

PATIENT RESTRAINT

When it is determined that a patient is unable to decline medical care for any reason, and transport against the will of the patient is indicated, it may be difficult and even dangerous for EMS providers, as these patients may become combative and violent. EMS providers are never required to enter into situations that pose a threat of physical harm to themselves. Law enforcement should be involved with any patient who is a threat to themselves or others. Police may also be of assistance if a patient requires restraints. If a patient is to remain handcuffed during transport, a law enforcement officer must accompany the patient.

Physical restraints may be appropriate if reasonable belief exists that the person is an imminent risk of self-injury or injury to EMS personnel, and may allow for more timely treatment and transport to an appropriate facility for medical evaluation.[30] Restraints are most useful when violent behavior is the result of a medical condition, or if determination of the cause of the behavior is not possible in the prehospital setting. Types of physical restraints available to EMS providers vary by EMS agency including soft restraints, hard restraints or handcuffs, and chemical restraints. Chemical restraint may be an option in special circumstances, however, almost always requires online medical direction prior to its use. Some principles that apply to all restraints include use of the least invasive or restrictive possible method of restraint to accomplish patient and provider safety, never utilizing prone positioning, and avoiding placement of anything restrictive over the face, head, or neck of the patient. The patient should be closely monitored for development of any adverse outcomes related to the restraints.

SPECIAL POPULATIONS

There are a number of special populations with regard to the subject of consent and refusal of care. Under US common law, parental consent is generally required for the medical treatment of minors under age 18.[31] There are, however, several exceptions to this, which are applicable to situations that frequently occur in the emergency setting. Four general categories of exceptions are commonly recognized. First, minors may seek care without parental or guardian consent in situations requiring emergent or urgent medical attention. Second, emancipated minors are exempt from this requirement. Emancipated minors are self-reliant or independent, and include individuals who are married, serving in the military, court emancipated, or financially independent and living apart from parents. In some states, minors may be considered emancipated if they are in college, pregnant, a runaway, or a minor mother. A third category of minors not requiring parental consent are those that are considered "mature," generally thought of as a minor over the age of 14 years who possesses the intelligence to understand and appreciate the risks, benefits, and alternatives of the proposed treatment, and is able to make

a voluntary and rational choice. Some consideration must be made on the part of the treating provider as to the nature and complexity of the disease process and proposed treatment. The mature minor is not recognized by the US Supreme Court; however, many states have recognized this doctrine. Finally, minors who do not fall into any of the aforementioned categories may seek treatment without parental consent for some specific medical conditions including mental health services, pregnancy, contraception, testing and/or treatment for HIV or AIDS, sexually transmitted diseases, substance abuse, or care for a crime-related injury.

Generally, the law supports parental control over basic matters affecting their children; however, if parental actions result in inadequate medical care, there is a departure from this standard doctrine. If there is no life threat, and no potential for serious impairment, the parents' refusal may be respected; however, a parent does not have the authority to forbid saving their child's life. Parental refusals require that one or both parents have normal mental status, are not under the influence of drugs or alcohol, and understand the risks of refusal. These facts should be well documented and include parental signatures. Ultimately it is most important to keep the welfare of the child at the forefront.

The concept of parental refusals can become significantly more complicated when there is a suspicion of child abuse or neglect. EMS providers have a legal and ethical duty to report and intervene in this case, regardless of the child or parent's desire for evaluation. Each state has unique laws governing child abuse and protective custody, and EMS providers are always considered a compulsory reporter. Massachusetts, for example, uses law 51A to mandate EMS providers, in their professional capacity as a provider of medical services, to report cases of suspected physical, emotional, or sexual abuse, neglect, or malnutrition. Violation of that law could result not only in a monetary fine, but also adverse outcomes for the child or other children involved. It is important to recognize the signs of child abuse, and take care not to make accusations as this may delay transport. If parents refuse transport in the setting of suspected child abuse, law enforcement should be involved.

Far fewer studies exist which focus on pediatric patients and parents who refuse transport; however, Seltzer et al investigated this in a 2001 study looking at outcomes of children who were not transported to the hospital after EMS activation.[32] In this study, parents sought some form of medical care for their child in 84% of cases which is significantly higher than the adult population. Most care was obtained from an emergency department (ED) or primary care physician's office, and transport was most commonly a private vehicle. This study reports a 10% admission rate, which is similar to general population studies, all of which were related to cardiac or respiratory complaints. Most care was sought on the same day as the EMS activation. It is somewhat unclear what causes parents to decline transport. One plausible theory is that parents are less likely to trust a provider they and their children are not familiar with, or fear about unnecessary testing in the ED. Again, online medical control may be helpful in these situations, or if there is concern for an emergent medical condition or abuse, it is appropriate to transport the child without parental consent.

A man calls 9-1-1 after he is involved in a motor vehicle accident. He is the passenger in the vehicle, which struck a telephone pole in a rainstorm. The driver, his wife, appears injured. She was not wearing her seatbelt, and she struck her head on the windshield. In the backseat is the couples' 4-year old daughter. She had not been restrained in a booster seat or a seat belt. The scene is as described on arrival. The man appears uninjured and is in the backseat trying to extricate his child. The wife is boarded and collared by first responders. As you try to assess the child who is still in the back seat, the father refuses for you to touch his daughter. From outside the vehicle you can see that she is crying and holding her arm. She appears to have a deformity of her wrist with an open fracture. She also appears to have an abrasion on her forehead. Despite explaining the severity of these injuries to the father, he continues to decline that you care for his daughter citing that he does not trust anyone with his child. You understand the legalities of a parent's right to refuse care for his child, but you also understand your obligation to care for a child with an emergent medical condition. You call for a supervisor and law enforcement for assistance. With some police assistance, you are able to care for the child and transport her to the hospital with her mother.

Patients in custody represent another special population with respect to refusal of medical care. During incarceration, prisoners lose a variety of basic rights and freedoms; however, the Supreme Court has noted that prisoners retain a constitutional right to health care as deprivation of these would constitute "cruel and inhuman" punishment.[33] Specifically, prisoners should be allowed to retain rights consistent both with their values, and with penological objectives; however, there have been varying decisions about a prisoner's right to refuse medical care. Two salient examples represent this struggle between basic constitutional rights and the principles of imprisonment. In *Commissioner of Corrections v Myers* (1979) the Supreme Judicial Court of Massachusetts prevented a prisoner from refusing hemodialysis, citing that prison order and security could be threatened by the state's failure to prevent a death of an inmate.[34] In contrast, in *Thor v Superior Court* (1993), the Supreme Court of California allowed a quadriplegic prisoner to refuse food and medication, stating that he has the same right to refuse unwanted life-sustaining treatment as did patients outside of a prison setting.[35] These court cases support a modified right of refusal of medical care in the case of prisoners, that their rights may be limited by "legitimate penological interests" such as overall prison security and health.[3] While these cases do not specifically address EMS transport, or even emergency care in general, they do highlight some issues that may be pertinent to prehospital providers; prisoners may be allowed to refuse treatment in certain circumstances; however, the security and health of other prisoners may also determine their overall right to refuse.

One of the recurring themes in refusal of transport and care is the topic of psychiatric care. It is widely recognized that patients who suffer from many different types of mental illness including severe depression, psychosis, paranoia, or suicidal/homicidal ideation may not have decision-making capacity, and cannot refuse care or transport. Each state is unique; however, each has laws that address involuntary commitment of psychiatric patients, for example, the Massachusetts Section 12, California 5150, and Maine Blue Paper. In general, these laws all require that an individual be an immediate danger to him/herself, usually in the case of suicidal ideation, an immediate threat to the safety of another individual, or gravely disabled. Patients who are considered gravely disabled are unable to provide themselves with food, clothing, or shelter as a result of their psychiatric condition. This is generally determined by a physician, psychologist, or qualified clinical mental health provider, and allows for a 48- to 72-hour involuntary hold depending on the state. If one of these clinical providers is not available, which is usually the case in the prehospital setting, a police officer is also usually allowed to make this involuntary commitment as well in order to get them to a medical or psychiatric facility for evaluation by a qualified provider. Use of law enforcement may be necessary to transport these patients against their will for the safety of the patient and EMS personnel.

You are called to the apartment of a patient who is known to you from his frequent use of the EMS system. He is known to be a psychiatric patient who lives independently, but is quite eccentric. When you arrive on scene, the neighbors state that the patient is acting bizarrely, banging on the walls, and shouting profanities. You are able to gain access to the apartment through the open front door. You encounter a slightly disheveled naked man, who seems to recognize you from your multiple prior encounters. He becomes more calm and cooperative with you. You are able to perform vital signs, which are within normal. Your further physical assessment is unremarkable. During the assessment, the patient is rambling on about how he is going to save the world by ridding it of evil spirits like his neighbors who called. As you try and direct him toward the exit to go to the ambulance, he refuses to go with you saying you are one of the evil spirits as well and he will not go with you. Despite extensive time trying to convince the patient that you are just trying to help, he continues to refuse, becoming more and more agitated. You decide to allow the patient to stay because he seemed calm prior and leave without him. He does not sign a refusal. The care of acutely ill psychiatric patients can be very challenging. However, it is essential that with all patients, the provider must first determine if the

patient has capacity to refuse care. In this situation, the patient is unable to understand the situation. He does not understand the provider is there to help and is not able to communicate this to the provider. The provider should not allow this patient to refuse care as he does not have medical decision-making capacity, as well as he appears to be a danger to others. This situation is one in which law enforcement or further help may be necessary to assist in transport of the patient.

As the overall age of our population increases, EMS providers will invariably be faced with increasing numbers of individuals with advance directives. This poses another set of challenges for prehospital providers to address as they prepare for transport, on-scene medical care, and manage refusals of care and transport. A patient's end-of-life wishes must also be balanced with family member disagreement and grief in a time of high emotion. Multiple types of advance directives exist, including living wills, appointment of a health care proxy, and comfort care/do not resuscitate (DNR) orders. A DNR order is executed by a physician, nurse practitioner, or physician assistant, and is valid in out-of-hospital settings to avoid unwanted life-saving measures. In order to recognize a valid DNR order, the original form must be located and presented at the time of patient contact. In this setting, it is appropriate for EMS providers to perform any measures consistent with comfort care and palliation, including airway clearance and suctioning, oxygen (no positive pressure ventilation), placing patient in a position of comfort, application of splints, stopping bleeding, pain control per protocol, and giving emotional support to family. Transport depends on the situation, and it may be reasonable under some circumstances to allow refusal of transport in consult with online medical direction. A living will is a written statement of a patient's wishes for medical treatment and end-of-life care in the event that they are unable to make health care decisions or communicate them directly. Many states do not recognize the living will as a legally binding document for medical care; however, if a health care proxy is appointed, a living will is evidence of a patient's end-of-life wishes. If EMS is activated and the patient has only a living will or durable power of attorney, the patient must legally be transported. Finally, a health care proxy is an appointed individual who makes medical decisions on behalf of the patient based on what the patient would have wanted, or if that is unknown, in the patient's best interest. DNR orders can be revoked at any time by the patient, the attending physician, or a legal surrogate. It is recommended that documentation of events surrounding EMS activation in the setting of preexisting DNR orders include documentation of a valid DNR order, an indication of why EMS was activated, and documentation of contact with medical control, the patient's physician, or the medical examiner.

Capacity and refusal of care are important and complex issues that prehospital providers are confronted with daily. They are responsible for the majority of lawsuits involving EMS personnel, and oftentimes contrast patient self-determination with their well-being, creating ethical and legal dilemmas. There are a number of challenges of informed consent and capacity assessment that are unique to the prehospital setting, and can be further complicated by special populations. It is essential to understand the state-specific regulations, as well as ensure utilization of all available resources including family, online medical control physicians, and law enforcement officers to achieve the difficult balance of patient independence and safety.

- In order for a patient to receive medical care, the patient must give informed consent. The patient must have capacity, must be given appropriate information, and must make a decision to receive care voluntarily in order for consent to be valid.
- A patient must be determined to have medical decision-making capacity to give consent or refuse care. In order to have decision-making capacity a patient must understand and appreciate the situation, reason through options, and communicate their decision.

- If a patient has capacity, he/she has the right to refuse medical care and transport from prehospital providers. Patient refusals must be considered high-risk interactions and providers must follow written protocols, and complete accurate documentation of the patient interaction.

  - The EMS physician should understand the differences between *capacity* and *competence*.

  - The EMS physician should understand reasons for exception to parental consent for a minor.

REFERENCES

1. *Schloendorff v New York Hospital*, 149 App. Div. 915 (March 1, 1912).
2. *Salgo v Leland Standford Jr. University Board of Trustees*, 317 P.2d 170 (1957).
3. Moskop JC. Informed consent and refusal of treatment: challenges for emergency physicians. *Emerg Med Clin N Am.* 2006;24:605-618.
4. Moskop JC. Informed consent in the emergency department. *Emerg Med Clin N Am.* 1999;17:327-340.
5. Applebaum P. Assessment of patients' competence to consent to treatment. *N Engl J Med.* 2007;357:1834-1840.
6. Applebaum P, Grisso T. Assessing patients' capacity to consent to treatment. *N Engl J Med.* 1988;319:1625-1628.
7. Heilicser B, Stocking C, Siegler M. Ethical dilemmas in emergency medical services: the perspective of the emergency medical technician. *Ann Emerg Med.* 1996;27:239-243.
8. Adams JG, Arnold R, Siminoff L, Wolfson AB. Ethical conflicts in the prehospital setting. *Ann Emerg Med.* October 1992;21(10):1259-1265.
9. Nower RW, Collopy KT, Kivlehan SM, Snyder SR. Processing the patient refusal. *EMS World.* December 2011;40(12):32, 34-6, 38-43.
10. Soler JM, Montes MF, Egol EB, et al. The ten-year malpractice experience of a large urban EMS system. *Ann Emerg Med.* 1985;14:982-985.
11. Vukmir RB. Medical malpractice: managing the risk. *Med Law.* 2004;23(3):495-513.
12. Maggiore WA. Patient abandonment: what it is—and isn't. *JEMS.* October 4, 2007. http://www.jems.com/article/industry-news/patient-abandonment-what-it-an. Accessed August 29, 2011.
13. Weaver J, Brinsfield KH, Dalphond D. Prehospital refusal-of-transport policies: adequate legal protection? *Prehosp Emerg Care.* 2000;4(1):53-56.
14. Hipskind JE, Gren JM, Barr DJ. Patients who refuse transportation by ambulance: a case series. *Prehosp Disaster Med.* 1997;12:278-283.
15. Moss ST, Chan TC, Buchanan J, Dunford JV, Vilke GM. Outcome study of prehospital patients signed out against medical advice by field paramedics. *Ann Emerg Med.* 1998;31(2):247-250.
16. Wampler DA, Molina DK, McManus J, Laws P, Manifold CA. No deaths associated with patient refusal of transport after naloxone-reversed opioid overdose. *Prehosp Emerg Care.* July-September 2011;15(3):320-324.

17. Sucov A, Verdile VP, Garettson D, Paris PM. The outcome of patients refusing prehospital transportation. *Prehosp Disaster Med.* 1992;7:365-371.
18. Knight S, Olson LM, Cook LJ, Mann NC, Corneli HM, Dean JM. Against all advice: an analysis of out-of-hospital refusals of care. *Ann Emerg Med.* 2003;42(5):689-696.
19. Zachariah BS, Bryan D, Pepe PE, Griffin M. Follow-up and outcome of patients who decline or are denied transport by EMS. *Prehosp Disaster Med.* 1992;7:359-363.
20. Burstein JL, Henry MC, Alicandro J, Gentile D, Thode HC, Hollander JE. Outcome of patients who refused out-of-hospital medical assistance. *Am J Emerg Med.* 1996;14:23-26.
21. Pringle RP, Carden DL, Xiao F, Graham DD. Outcomes of patients not transported after calling 911. *J Emerg Med.* 2005;28(4):449-454.
22. Vilke GM, Sardar W, Fisher R, Dunford JD, Chan TC. Follow-up of elderly patients who refuse transport after accessing 9-1-1. *Prehosp Emerg Care.* 2002;6(4):391-395.
23. Cone DC, Kim DT, Davidson SJ. Patient-initiated refusals of prehospital care: ambulance call report documentation, patient outcome, and on-line medical command. *Prehosp Disaster Med.* 1995;10(1):3-9.
24. Stuhmiller DFE, Cudnick MT, Sundhein SM, Threlkeld MS, Collins TE. Adequacy of online medical command communication and emergency medical services documentation of informed refusals. *Acad Emerg Med.* 2005;12(10):970-977.
25. Burstein JL, Hollander JE, Delagi R, Gold M, Henry MC, Alicandro JM. Refusal of out-of-hospital medical care: effect of medical-control physician assertiveness on transport rate. *Acad Emerg Med.* 1998;5(1):4-8.
26. Hoyt BT, Norton RL. Online medical control and initial refusal of care: does it help to talk with the patient? *Acad Emerg Med.* 2001;8(7):725-730.
27. Alicandro J, Hollander JE, Henry MC, Sciammarella J, Stapleton E, Gentile D. Impact of interventions for patients refusing emergency medical services transport. *Acad Emerg Med.* 1995;2:480-485.
28. Burstein JL, Hollander JE, Henry MC, Delagi R, Thode HC Jr. Association of out-of-hospital criteria with need for hospital admission. *Acad Emerg Med.* 1995;2:863-866.
29. ACEP. Refusal of Medical Aid Policy Statement. 2007. https://www.acep.org/Clinical-Practice-Management/Refusal-of-Medical-Aid-%28RMA%29. Accessed May, 2015.
30. Hopple JP. Teaching 'restraint'. Improper technique risks injury and lawsuits. *JEMS.* February 2011;36(2):24, 26.
31. American Academy of Pediatrics Policy Statement. Consent for emergency medical services for children and adolescents. *Pediatrics.* 2003;111(3):703-706.
32. Seltzer AG, Vilke GM, Chan TC, Fisher R, Dunford JV. Outcome study of minors after parental refusal of paramedic transport. *Prehosp Emerg Care.* 2001;5(3):278-283.
33. *Estelle v Gamble*, 429 US 97 (1976).
34. *Commissioner of Corrections v Myers*, 379 Mass. 255, 399 NW 2d 452 (1979).
35. *Thor v Superior Court*, 5 Cal. 4th 725, 855 P.2d 375, 21 Cal. Rptr. 2d 357 (1993).

Business Practices and Management

CHAPTER

25

EMS Finance

Naveen B. Seth

Jeffrey M. Goodloe

INTRODUCTION

One of the biggest challenges involved in providing superior prehospital care is obtaining the appropriate funding to pay for it. Funding is needed for salaries, equipment, as well as ongoing training. It seems that there is a disproportionate amount of money available for fire services, but these funds tend not to be as readily obtainable by emergency medical services (EMS). There are, of course, many models for EMS, all of which vary in their funding structure, but rarely does any model rely on a single revenue source. Similarly, each model has different requirements and often a different focus. For example, whereas a paid municipal department may rely heavily on tax revenues and government funding to pay for their employees and benefits, a private volunteer agency may receive no public funding and have minimal if any costs associated with payroll. However, both agencies would likely look to other funding sources such as private businesses, donations, state and federal grants, etc, to ensure the reliable delivery of high-quality care.

There is also variance among agencies regarding the level of service they are willing and able to provide, which may be a direct result of financial concerns. For example, some agencies choose to staff *advanced life support* ambulances only. Others choose to staff a mix of *basic and advanced life support*. Some choose to staff multiple ambulances to try to ensure their agency is the one providing timely service in the district, while others staff only a single ambulance, relying on surrounding agencies to cover their district when the primary agency is unavailable. These decisions of how to staff and the level of service to provide are often based on cost and resources but are key to strategic planning.

Another important aspect of EMS finance that varies among agencies is reimbursement. Serving a relatively poor population can be quite expensive, particularly if it is busy. Despite the high volume, low reimbursement rates and inability to collect on self-pay patients can lead to high losses. These agencies often are dependent on funding from the municipality as a public service. Conversely, serving an affluent area with patients carrying excellent insurance can be very lucrative, even with relatively low volume. Location near an institution with a large number of paid transfers can also be extremely lucrative. Regardless, finding funding sources to offset low reimbursements is critical to viability as is the ability to collect on bills. Variances in reimbursement vary not only locally, but regionally as well and these differences must all be considered when developing a budget and business strategy.

OBJECTIVES

- Describe sources of funding for EMS agencies.
- Discuss levels of reimbursement for EMS.
- Detail CMS (Centers for Medicare & Medicaid Services) criteria for reimbursement and discuss regional variability for reimbursement.
- Define "payor mix" and discuss the financial impact of regional variability on EMS agencies.

- Describe mileage as a modifier to reimbursement.
- Describe "medical necessity" and preauthorization for interfacility transport calls.
- Describe how electronic PCR (patient care record) may improve reimbursement.
- Describe tax districts and discuss municipal funding.
- Describe EMS district contracts.
- Describe grant writing as a method to obtain needed equipment and training.

EMS FUNDING SOURCES

The National Academy of Sciences-National Research Council's *Accidental Death and Disability: The Neglected Disease of Modern Society* and subsequent Highway Safety Act of 1966 contended that prehospital care had been terribly neglected. One of the tenets of the Highway Safety Act was to establish the Department of Transportation (DOT) and in doing so, gave the DOT authority and funding to try to improve EMS. This was essentially the first federal funding for EMS. Unfortunately, while somewhat helpful initially, these funds led to solutions that lacked sustainability despite extensions of funding in 1976 and 1979 and the bulk of the burden of funding fell to individual states and individual agencies to maintain financial viability—part of the reason why there is such variability in financial stability among EMS agencies.

Today, funding comes from a myriad of sources including various taxes, special contracts, direct patient billing, grants, private funding, fund-raising, and subscription services to name a few.[1] We will examine each of these potential revenue streams.

▦ TAX REVENUE

Taxes are one of the most common means of raising money for EMS systems. These can include property taxes, sales taxes, real estate taxes, or other "special taxes." Property taxes are among the most common. These taxes vary with property values and may or may not increase depending on assessed values, leading to the potential for variability. For better or for worse, it also follows that areas that are more affluent often generate more revenue with this type of system whereas poorer areas do not, and hence may not collect adequate funds. Sales taxes are another type of tax and can be used in different ways depending on the location. For example, a simple sales tax addition would net revenue for sales of all goods. However, in areas in which there is a large transient population or tourist population, a more specific sales tax may help offset some of the burden on the local population. This might include a hotel tax, restaurant tax, or other "tourist" tax.

In addition to property taxes, special real estate taxes can be added to real estate sales. These can be very lucrative but are most effective in areas where single-family homes are bought and sold as opposed to areas with many homes and apartments that are simply rented. Other special taxes may be instituted that are simply for the generation of fire/EMS funds. Most commonly the level of these types of taxes are based on dwelling size, fire-fighting measures (sprinklers), materials, etc. These taxes tend to be more often linked to fire prevention and therefore aid municipal fire service-based agencies far more than private/volunteer agencies.

CONTRACTS

Exclusive contracts are often an effective way to secure part of the market. These contracts are made between an agency and a municipality, a fire department, or a specific facility. With municipalities, in return for a sum of money and/or other considerations, a guarantee regarding certain services is given. This usually involves guarantees of response time, level of service, and availability. In some areas, contracts may be made between the fire district and an ambulance agency, and in others, the fire chief can simply decree that a certain agency will be called first for calls in the fire district and only if that agency is unavailable will a second agency be called. This type of exclusivity ensures a certain revenue stream despite where and how competitors may be positioning themselves. Contracts can also be made between agencies and facilities. This can be for transports into or out of that facility. Often specialty centers such as pediatric hospitals, burn centers, trauma centers, etc, contract with an agency for their many transfers of patients. Securing such a contract may be particularly lucrative as these transfers often carry a premium and commonly have a higher reimbursement rate than a typical emergency call.

The most intuitively obvious way to get paid for providing prehospital care is by billing the patient. Paradoxically, this is often the most complicated due to varying reimbursement schemes, which are discussed later. In general, reimbursement occurs via billing to Medicare, Medicaid, private/commercial insurance, or self-pay. Obviously not only is there wide variation based on the area of the country, but even within a local region there may be variance in payor mix between a relatively affluent area of young professionals and an area of poor seniors, both of which may be served by the same ambulance service.

GRANTS AND LOANS

Grants are another way in which EMS systems may earn revenue, although the availability of these grants by far favors fire agencies over EMS agencies. EMS agencies that are fire based may share in some of these funds depending on the precise wording and appropriation of the monies, but often are still left working with old and outdated equipment while their fire colleagues enjoy new vehicles, safety gear, and other critical apparatus necessary to their mission. Initially, these grants were often federal, beginning in 1966 and continuing through 1981 with some focus on self-sustainability. However, much of the grant money shifted from federal grants to state grants, which also left EMS competing for funds with other state public health initiatives. In very rare occasions, local grants may be available, but generally any grant money to be found must be located at the state and federal levels.

State funds are often available in the form of low-interest loans for capital improvements or state taxes or assessments related to driver licenses fees and fines. These are often only meager as they are generally distributed across the entire state. States may also become involved in special purpose grants designed for very specific reasons, but which then can have benefits beyond the original stated purpose. State grants may also be in the form of matching grants, in which case an agency must demonstrate that they can match the state dollars or at least some predetermined percentage of those dollars in order to receive them. Again, these funds tend to favor fire agencies far more often than they do EMS agencies, but occasionally these dollars do become available. Federal grant money is available, but rarely directly to an individual agency. Rather, these funds are most often dispensed through state agencies.

Private funding is another potential revenue stream that is available to a few agencies that often have the good fortune of being located in close proximity to large, national corporations with significant presence in an area and/or that have a large number of employees who live in a certain area. These corporations often support public services as a demonstration of goodwill and being a good neighbor, as well as for the obvious public relation benefit and tax benefits they may enjoy. Nonetheless, this type of funding is often available when sought out. Smaller corporate neighbors often can also contribute on a smaller scale and are happy to do so. Corporations may also sponsor employee donation matches, and in doing so, support their own employees as well as the organizations

that they personally care about. Outside of the local community, there are also various foundations locally or nationally that may have funding available for EMS. These, again, tend to favor fire agencies over EMS, but in the age of current technology, Web sites such as http://foundationcenter.org help agencies locate foundations that may be of potential benefit to them. These foundations are often nonprofit organizations that exist expressly for supporting various causes. These are usually independent foundations. There are also corporate foundations that are formed as a vehicle for corporations to conduct their charitable contributions. Lastly, there are sometimes local foundations that tend to be more community based, focusing on aiding a specific area.

FUND-RAISING

Many agencies participate in some type of public fund-raising efforts. Those may include bake sales, car washes, boot drives, or simple direct-mail fund-raisers. Some popular fund-raisers that are often held at meetings or gatherings are 50/50 raffles, where the winner wins half and the other half goes to the sponsoring agency. The best type of fund-raiser may vary from area to area and with different demographics. These are decisions that must be made carefully, as while the funds do need to be raised, pragmatic concerns such as safety, the relative affluence of the community, etc, may impact which type of fund-raiser would be best received by the community and how frequently fund-raisers should be held.

One of the newer means of raising funds involves a "subscription service." As opposed to a fire-based subscription service, which is often based on an annual fee per square foot with modifications for fire prevention measures, EMS programs usually charge an annual fee per address, which would cover either any and all EMS provided that year or the portion that is not covered by the patients' health insurance. In this way, subscribers need not worry about calling the ambulance and significant expense for transportation. Conversely, the ambulance agencies may collect an annual "premium" without needing to provide any services at all. Nonsubscribers are billed in the traditional method and unaffected by this service. This type of program is obviously somewhat involved to implement and manage and requires due diligence be performed to ensure that the time and money invested by the agency in such a program does, in fact, yield a net benefit, but can be helpful to both the agency and the community.

REIMBURSEMENT FOR EMS

The simplest way to understand EMS reimbursement is to recognize the use of the HCPCS (Healthcare Common Procedure Coding System) for billing by CMS (Centers for Medicare & Medicaid Services). These codes are used so that the appropriate level of payment is billed based on the services provided. In EMS, they range from AO425 to AO436, each with a slightly different code description, reflective of the various levels of service (**Table 25-1**).

The following definitions for the services above are provided by Chapter 10 of the *Medicare Benefit Policy Manual*:

ALS1 (advanced life support, level 1): Transportation by ground ambulance providing supplies and services including an ALS assessment or at least one ALS intervention. For these purposes, ALS is defined as an individual trained above the level of a Basic EMT. An ALS intervention is one that requires higher training than an EMT Basic and is deemed medically necessary.

ALS1-emergency (advanced life support, level 1-emergency): This is the same as an ALS1 response, but in the context of an emergency response. That is, one which requires an immediate response. In most systems, this would constitute a priority 1 or 2 response, a "hot" response, or a lights and sirens response. The type of response is determined by the dispatch protocol for that type of complaint.

BLS (basic life support): Transportation by ground ambulance, staffed by at least one EMT-basic

HCPCS Code	Code Description
TABLE 25-1	**EMS Reimbursement Codes**
A0425	Ground mileage, per statute mile
A0426	Ambulance service, advanced life support, nonemergency transport, level 1 (ALS1)
A0427	Ambulance service, advanced life support, emergency transport, level 1 (ALS1-emergency)
A0428	Ambulance service, basic life support, nonemergency transport (BLS)
A0429	Ambulance service, basic life support, emergency transport (BLS-emergency)
A0430	Ambulance service, conventional air services, transport, one way (fixed wing)
A0431	Ambulance service, conventional air services, transport, one way (rotary wing)
A0432	Paramedic intercept (PI), rural area, transport furnished by a volunteer ambulance company which is prohibited by state law from billing third-party payers
A0433	Advanced life support, level 2 (ALS2)
A0434	Specialty care transport (SCT)
A0435	Fixed-wing air mileage, per statute mile
A0436	Rotary-wing air mileage, per statute mile

BLS-emergency (basic life support-emergency): Like ALS1, this is the same as a BLS response, but in the context of an emergency response as described above.

Paramedic intercept: These are ALS services that are provided without the ambulance transport. Usually this is in the context of an agency with BLS services being dispatched to transport a patient, but requiring advanced ALS services and so an ALS provider meets the ambulance on the way to the hospital. There are only limited situations in which this code can be used, as the services must be in a rural area, with a contract with a volunteer agency.[2] The volunteer agency must be prohibited from billing anyone for their services, and the ALS service must bill all patients who receive services from them, regardless of whether they are Medicare beneficiaries. As of 2008, New York is the only state in which these services are covered.

ALS2 (advanced life support, level 2): This is ALS service by ground ambulance that requires at least three separate administrations of one or more intravenous medications or the performance of at least one of several advanced procedures such as defibrillation, endotracheal intubation, chest decompression, etc.

SCT (specialty care transport): This is an interfacility transport by ground ambulance that requires a level of service above that that can be provided by a paramedic. Often this may require a nurse or physician to provide a higher level of care or monitoring of medications that are beyond the scope of the paramedic.

SCT transports are particularly lucrative because the *relative value units* (RVUs) for an SCT are 3.25 compared with 2.75 for the ALS2, 1.90 for the ALS1-emergency, and 1.20 for ALS1. This is interesting given that while SCTs often may involve the critically ill patient, there is a higher level of care available that may often provide whatever increased level of care is required.

In addition to the level of service that provides a reimbursement rate, there are also mileage modifiers to take into account the distance traveled with a patient aboard the ambulance. So, for example, an ALS1-emergency service would be reimbursed at the rate of the ALS1 rate plus the distance in miles traveled multiplied by the ground mileage rate. This aids agencies that have longer transports to facilities.

Air ambulance services, regardless of fixed wing or rotary wing, differ from ground ambulance coding in that the patient must meet certain requirements to determine whether reimbursement at the air ambulance rate will be approved. As with ground service, the service must be both "necessary and reasonable." The air ambulance rates are much greater than ground to account for the much higher costs associated with providing such services. To qualify for this reimbursement rate though, a patient must meet certain requirements that make ground service inappropriate, which include such requirements as:

- The patient requires immediate and rapid ambulance transportation that could not have been otherwise provided by ground.
- The point of pickup is inaccessible by ground.
- Great distances or obstacles are involved in getting the patient to the nearest appropriate hospital.

Medical reasonableness may be determined when time is a significant factor that puts the patient's health at severe risk. Conditions that may meet this requirement include intracranial hemorrhage, life-threatening trauma, emergent need for a hyperbaric oxygen chamber, etc. When time is a significant factor and that time by ground is excessive, air ambulance transport may also be appropriate.

CMS CRITERIA FOR REIMBURSEMENT

In brief, the criteria for reimbursement are based on the codes as described above and the necessity of the services that are provided. Presuming that reimbursement is appropriate, over the past two decades, various adjustments have been made to the fee schedule to help account for differences in rural versus urban transports. In 1997, this began with the Balanced Budget Act which implemented the national fee schedule. Then the Medicare Prescription Drug, Improvement and Modernization Act of 2003 made adjustments that allowed for a regional fee schedule as well as a bonus on the mileage for transports over 50 miles. It also increased the base pay for ground ambulance transports originating in certain rural areas when the point of pickup was in a group of designated ZIP codes. Finally, a temporary increase in payments for rural areas (2% increase) and urban areas (1%) between 2004 and 2007 was approved. In 2008, the Medicare Improvements for Patients and Providers Act extended these increases through 2009 and increased them to 3% for rural and 2% for urban. Base payment rate for ground ambulance trips from the most rural areas based on population density was increased in 2010 with the Patient Protections and Affordable Care Act of 2010, unofficially referred to as the "super-rural" bonus. Rural and urban increases were extended through 2010 with this act and then again through 2011 with the Medicare and Medicaid Extenders Act of 2010 and through 2012 with the Temporary Payroll Tax Cut Continuation Act of 2011 and the Middle Class Tax Relief and Job Creation Act of 2012. The current legislation, the American Taxpayer Relief Act of 2012, extends the increases once again through 2013 along with the "super-rural" bonus.

The current payment structure is exceedingly complicated and open for change on a yearly basis. In addition to the various adjustments for rural and super-rural ZIP codes, there is also an adjustment based on the Geographic Practice Cost Index (GPCI), which adjusts for regional cost differences. For example, West Virginia has a GPCI of 0.828, while the areas that are classified in San Francisco, CA, have a GPCI of 1.360. When the full calculation is performed, for a rural ground base rate, the calculation is $(RVU \times (0.3 + (0.7 \times GPCI))) \times$ base rate $\times 1.03 +$ base rate $\times 1.03$, and then for those in the super-rural areas in the lowest quartile of all rural populations by density, the base rate is then multiplied by 1.226, and for the first 17 miles of rural mileage by ground, the rural mileage rate is 1.5 times the base rural mileage rate.[3]

IMPACT OF PAYOR MIX ON REIMBURSEMENT

Reimbursement can be very highly variable based on demographics. While across the board, according to the Government Accountability Office Survey of Ambulance Services, nationally, a typical payor mix consists of approximately 40% to 45% Medicare, 15% to 20% Medicaid, 15% to 20% private/commercial insurance, and about 25% private pay, these numbers can vary drastically. What this means for an individual agency is that if the majority of their patients are uninsured or self-pay patients, they may have an extremely difficult time collecting any of their charges. Conversely, if the demographic mix is biased toward the Medicare population, the agency may be able to count on the complicated fee structure described previously, but may not be able to collect much more than that. If an agency has the good fortune of being located in an area that is relatively affluent or even primarily working middle class with private insurance, they may do very well with collecting charges and being a solvent agency while an agency with similar volume across town struggles to make ends meet. The GPCI mentioned above helps take these differences into account and adjust for them. While it may not completely solve the problem of agencies being able to collect charges from self-pay patients, at least it will ensure they will be able to recover monies from the Medicare and private insurance patients to help subsidize the other patients.

MILEAGE REIMBURSEMENT

As previously discussed, the mileage reimbursement factor can also make a significant impact on a fee. These rates can be substantial, as exemplified by the state of Georgia, which gives an example from the 2009 rules in which the base BLS-emergency rate for a rural 44-mile transport is $540.34, but the mileage component from a rural area adds another $11.26 per mile, nearly doubling the reimbursement.[3] There are also mileage bonuses that are designed to help rural services that perform only very few transports (rural adjustment factor or RAF). For rural ground mileage in which the point of pickup is from a certain ZIP code, miles 1 to 17 are reimbursed at 150% of the rural mileage rate, even further increasing this valuable factor.

The definition of a "rural" area for the purposes of reimbursement, except for a paramedic intercept, is any ZIP code located outside of either a Metropolitan Statistical Area (MSA) (**Figure 25-1**) or in New England, a New England County Metropolitan Area (NECMA). There are also the rural areas which exist within an MSA or NECMA that are categorized as rural under the Goldsmith modification. This was described by Harold Goldsmith, Dena Puskin, and Dianne Stiles in 1993 to account for sparsely populated areas within very large metropolitan ZIP codes that necessitate long transports to appropriate health services. There are also the "super-rural" areas, in which they are in a rural ZIP code that is among the lowest quartile of all rural ZIP codes based on population density. For transports that originate from the super-rural ZIP codes, the base payment for ground ambulance transports increases by 22.6%. Everything that is neither rural nor super-rural is classified as "urban," though it may hardly be a typical large, bustling metropolis.

One of the caveats to the mileage reimbursement rate is that mileage is reimbursed only up to the mileage for the closest appropriate facility. Bypassing an appropriate facility to travel to one with comparable services farther away is not generally covered. However, as long as the origin of the transport is within the same "locality" as that of another that might be receiving the patient, then the mileage to either of the facilities is covered. Locality is defined as "the service area surrounding the institution to which individuals normally travel or are expected to travel to receive hospital or skilled nursing services." The *Medicare Benefit Policy Manual* explains that despite having a hospital closer to a patient's home, if there are other hospitals that are farther away, but routinely provide services to members of that patient's community, then the community is

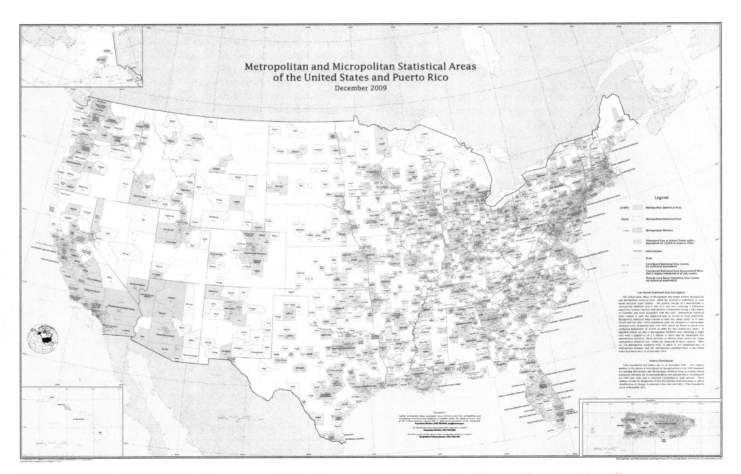

FIGURE 25-1. Metropolitan Statistical Areas. (From census.gov. http://www2.census.gov/geo/maps/metroarea/us_wall/Dec_2009/cbsa_us_1209_large.gif.)

considered to be within the "locality" of those other hospitals and ambulance service to any of these hospitals should be covered.

MEDICAL NECESSITY

One of the requirements for reimbursement of services is to demonstrate medical necessity of services. Necessity is defined as "when the patient's condition is such that use of any other method of transportation is contraindicated." It is irrelevant as to whether those other methods of transportation are actually available, but if the patient does not *need* an ambulance, payment may not be made. Those alternatives may include such options as wheelchair van, taxi, bus, or even privately owned vehicle. Additionally, the transport must be for a medically necessary reason. This would include both transport to, or return from receiving a Medicare covered service. The *Medicare Benefit Policy Manual* includes a fairly complete list of the circumstances under which necessity is covered, but some of the more common reasons include bed confinement, oxygen dependency, need for restraints, need for stretcher, or transport in an emergent situation.

In the scenario in which a patient is transferred from one facility to another facility because the first facility lacked the appropriate or necessary resources to care for the patient, this transfer is generally a covered service. Any emergent transport, interfacility or otherwise, is a covered service. However, when services are deemed to be nonemergent, proof of the necessity of an ambulance is often required and cannot be met simply by a physician's order. The proof is demonstrated via the prior authorization process. This is generally required for nonemergent repetitive scheduled transports, nonemergent nonrepetitive scheduled transports, and some nonemergency, nonscheduled transports. An example of the nonemergency repetitive scheduled transports would be routine dialysis. To meet the "repetitive" requirement, a transport must be required at least weekly for 3 weeks or at least three times within 10 days. Nonemergent, nonrepetitive scheduled transports might include transport for a scheduled doctor visit for which the patient requires an ambulance as opposed to some other means of transportation. "Scheduled" means when the transport is scheduled more than 24 hours prior to the time of transports, while "nonscheduled" transports occur within 24 hours of scheduling.

ELECTRONIC PATIENT CARE REPORT

For years, ambulance agencies have been using the *patient care report* (PCR) as a means of both medical documentation and for billing purposes. Historically, this has been a handwritten document of widely variable utility based on legibility, incompleteness, inaccuracy, and variation in practice, not to mention susceptibility to being lost. As technology has moved forward, electronic PCRs have come to market, which have had a tremendous impact on billing, reimbursement, and general operations. Now, rather than having to be mailed, faxed, or otherwise sent into billing agencies, literally at the click of a mouse, the electronic patient care report (ePCR) can immediately be sent to billing, the state for research, the agency archives, and almost anywhere else that it is needed. The impact that the ePCR has had on reimbursement through decreased time, better legibility, autopopulating of fields, and compliance with completion of mandatory fields has been impressive. In addition, these ePCRs can be linked directly to third-party billers as well as supply software, to help streamline both the billing process and the inventory process without duplicating work.

There is still great debate in the EMS community about the actual time savings that an ePCR brings. For an individual call, completing the documentation may be more tedious with the ePCR than it once was. However, many users are comparing their current ePCRs to the shoddy handwritten documentation that they had been allowed to get away with. The ePCRs do have many time-saving features for the user, but they do mandate certain fields, sometimes have limited options from a drop-down box, and are prone to technological glitches that can prove extremely frustrating.

Nobody can deny the impact of ePCR on legibility, and with the aid of spell check, documentation is often much clearer than it had been using the traditional PCR. However, not all providers have entirely embraced this technology as it has required them to learn some basic typing skills, and some of the programs can be quite tedious with multiple pages and many data elements to capture. Nonetheless, the legibility aspect has greatly improved the PCR as a true communication tool. Physicians in the emergency department can now read and understand a PCR much more easily; billing companies can similarly appreciate what was done and why.

One feature of many ePCRs is the ability to autopopulate certain fields. For example, certain demographic information on patients such as address details can autopopulate when used with a certain CAD device (AmbuPro EMS and TriTech IMC CAD). In other programs such as ESO ePCR, fields such as City, County, and State can be automatically filled in when the ZIP code is entered. Similarly, for common pickup points or destinations, simply selecting the name of the location can autopopulate the entire address field. For patients for whom prior calls have been made, medication lists, allergies, past medical history, etc, can be retrieved. This can save a tremendous amount of time with documentation, and instead of starting from scratch, the provider can simply verify this information and make updates as needed. Alternatively, in a critical patient who cannot give much history, this may prove useful in gathering additional information about the patient.

Electronic PCRs can often check for mandated fields required for reimbursement, or reporting purposes. If they do not hold up processing of the chart, at the very least they can prompt the user to fill in these required fields. This can decrease delays in reimbursement and in fact has allowed the reimbursement process to begin sometimes before the crew even returns from the call through wireless submission of the ePCR. Many states and regions maintain databases such as the National EMS Information System (NEMSIS) that require certain information about each patient. Similarly, there are some required data fields needed for billing. With paper PCRs, these fields can easily be bypassed, but ePCR not only can force the user to fill out those fields, but can allow administrators to customize mandatory fields.

Many of the ePCRs on the market further enhance the billing process by electronically connecting the PCR with third-party billing companies. Again, at the click of the mouse, the information is sent electronically via secure server to the billing company, allowing more rapid and accurate billing and hence, reimbursement. Several of the ePCR solutions available on the market are more robust than others, offering features to further streamline operations such as either directly linking with existing inventory software or offering their own inventory software that links with the ePCR software. In this way, when the PCR is completed, indicating what resources were utilized, the inventory is automatically updated to reflect this, reducing redundancy of data entry and ensuring proper updating of the inventory and reconciliation with the PCRs.

DISTRICT CONTRACTS

The delivery of ambulance services can come in many varieties, all of which must not only provide appropriate care, but be financially responsible. Some communities operate only municipal ambulances—that is, the ambulance service is provided by the local government and local taxpayers. Other communities contract with commercial services such as Rural/Metro Ambulance Service or American Medical Response, two of the largest companies in the United States. Still other communities contract with somewhat smaller, local agencies to ensure that while the daily management responsibilities and cost of running an ambulance service are not the municipality's, significant resources are put forth to ensure that its citizens are afforded excellent and timely care. An agency that is able to secure a contract of this type may help ensure that even if another ambulance agency holds a Certificate of Need that encompasses that district, they should get the first call for calls in the district. On the other hand, if circumstances change and the contract needs to be dissolved or withdrawn, as a standard item, the contracts generally have details that outline this process and under what circumstances this is allowed. For example, failing to meet the response time parameters, failing to keep the ambulance staffed as per the contract, or failing to meet other performance measures that are written into the contract may all result in dissolution of the contract and subsequent withdrawal.

Contracts with agencies can vary widely in content and structure. Often there is a certain level of service that is specified, such as ALS or BLS, with certain response time during certain hours. For example, a municipality may contract with an agency that for their district, they expect one ALS ambulance and one BLS ambulance during the day, dropping down to one ALS ambulance overnight. Similarly, a contract may specify that at all times, a minimum of two BLS ambulances will be in service. Obviously, these decisions are best made with recommendations by the agency itself based on historical data, but these type of stipulations may be written directly into the contract. Another requirement of the contract may be response time. For example, within EMS, there has long been a standard that responses should be within 8 minutes 90% of the time. While this standard has persevered for years, it may not be applicable or practical to all areas. In particular, more rural areas or even areas in which there is not 24-hour coverage would likely find it impossible to meet this standard. Regardless of whether the 8-minute standard is clinically significant or not, these types of timing standards are often incorporated into district contracts.

GRANT WRITING

There are grants available for EMS at every level, from local to state to federal, although as previously discussed, these grants often favor fire agencies and availability is much more variable at the local level. The US Fire Administration published their Funding Alternatives for Emergency Medical and Fire Services report in April 2012 that outlines many of the options for EMS funding and provides a starting point for finding many of the state and federal grants. It also provides information and resources on how to write a better grant proposal and other places to find assistance. EMSgrantshelp.com is another Web site that helps agencies, though generally fire, locate relevant grants that are available. These types of resources are only the starting point for locating grants and ones that are a bit harder to find may be less competitive and potentially easier to obtain.

Local grants may be available through philanthropic foundations, local corporations, small businesses, etc. Some national companies will try to ensure that each of their stores or franchises will support the local community through small local grants. While these may not be tremendously lucrative, they do tighten the bonds within the community and may help a small agency significantly.

State grants may include such items as surplus state vehicles, matching grants for capital equipment purchases, training, etc. Other types of state grants address state-specific problems. For example, Alaska has vast territory with very rural landscape, so one of the state grants (Code Blue) helps fund equipment for rural EMS in that state. California has specific state grants available to assist with wildfire education and safety, given their high risk of such events.

Finally, there are the federal grants which are available, but sought after by many agencies. There tend to be several ways in which federal grant money can be provided. The easiest is through a block grant, which essentially allows the federal government to give individual states money fairly and equally based on a formula. These monies are then filtered down to the state agencies and/or down to local government for distribution. The more well-known type of grants are project grants that fund specific programs and agencies or organizations compete for limited dollars, equipment, etc. Much more controversial are funds that are granted through federal legislation, earmarking certain funds for projects, but with highly political tactics used to obtain these funds.

Specific federal departments will also fund grants. For example, the US Department of Transportation funds the Hazardous Materials Grant Program, which has three main grants within it, one of which is the Hazardous Materials Emergency Preparedness Grants. In 2012, this comprised over $21 million that was distributed to the states, territories, and Native American tribal councils, and then filtered to local EMS agencies.

The National Highway Traffic Safety Administration has also served as a source of funding for EMS systems. In 2009, the NHTSA helped develop and administer a grant program to help 9-1-1 centers upgrade to enhanced 9-1-1, providing the caller's location information automatically. The NHTSA has also sponsored a half million dollar safety grant for a National EMS "Culture of Safety" Conference and development of a national strategy to address EMS safety. In addition, the NHTSA has co-sponsored a number of other grants with other governmental agencies to aid EMS agencies at the state and local levels.

One of the agencies with which the NHTSA has worked closely is the Department of Health and Human Services. In 2013, the DHHS announced the Emergency Medical Services for Children (EMSC): Targeted Issues Demonstration grant to enhance pediatric emergency medicine. This is just one of several efforts that the EMSC has been involved in, including the very important Pediatric Emergency Care Applied Research Network (PECARN) project. The Office of Rural Health Policy is a specific office within the Health Resources and Services Administration that addresses health care issues for rural areas at the local and state levels. One of its many responsibilities is to administer grant programs that help with upgrades in EMS such as through the Medicare Rural Hospital Flexibility Grant Program (Flex).

The National Institute of Health has also been actively involved in grants that apply to EMS, such as Research on Emergency Medical Services for Children. While NIH grants such as this are often very broad, encompassing everything from prehospital care to in-patient care, demonstration of applicability to the overall goals of improving pediatric emergency care may give eligibility to agencies. The EMSC is a national initiative to reduce pediatric injury and illness. In Arizona, for example, funds have been used to support pediatric specific education. In Maryland, the EMSC Program develops "state guidelines and resources for pediatric care (and) review of pediatric emergency care and facility regulations." In addition, grants for EMS biomedical and bioengineering research are also available through the NIH.

The Centers for Disease Control and Prevention has recognized trauma as a disease and promotes health "through information dissemination, preparedness, prevention, research, and surveillance." While they annually award around $7 billion in grants and contracts, these funds are generally available to large organizations with a broad outreach. There have been some block grants through the CDC, such as the Preventive Health and Health Services Block Grant, which help provide EMS to states, excluding equipment purchases. For example, in Massachusetts, these funds were used to help set standards for EMT training.

Even the US Department of Housing and Urban Development offers grants and aid to EMS providers, in a somewhat different manner from other federal agencies. The HUD Good Neighbor Next Door Program offers full-time emergency services providers the opportunity to buy a HUD-owned home at 50% off the market value. More traditionally, to promote areas of lower socioeconomic status and ensure public safety, the HUD has Community Block Development Grants that have been used by some cities to purchase new vehicles and renovate old buildings or build new structures used for public safety.

CORRELATION OF EMS SYSTEM COST STRUCTURE TO REVENUE SOURCE(S)

The basic design of an EMS system typically carries closely associated mechanisms for generation of revenue to fund ongoing and future EMS system needs and capabilities. Revenue models commonly differ between fire department (or other city agency administrated systems) and those conducted by public utility or privately held organizations. In fire service led agencies, EMS operational revenue generally is allocated from the fire department's overall annual budget. This, in turn, is most often funded from city, township, village, county, or fire district governmental authority general operating budget monies, also known as the "general fund" for that authority. General funds are most commonly enabled through tax revenue resulting from collection of sales taxes, property taxes, and in some areas, specifically identified fire service taxes. In local government agency–administered EMS systems in which the fire service may provide initial response and treatment, but does not transport, operational revenue is largely collected via the same mechanism(s) and then allocated to that government's so-called "third-service" EMS agency (the other two public safety services being the police and fire agencies).

In contrast, public utility model and privately owned EMS agencies rarely derive whole or majority percentages of operating revenue from geographical-related taxation.[4] Important, though minority percentages, of EMS agency financing may be obtained via governmental area subsidy. For example, a city may contract with a private provider of ambulance service, giving the agency a set amount of money upfront per annum to partially offset the provider's anticipated operating costs in that city. Typically, the subsidy is far less than the income realized by the agency through billing for its medical care services directly to patients or indirectly via their health insurance companies.

Additional mechanisms of revenue more commonly affiliated with public utility model and privately owned EMS agencies are utility fee assessments for EMS and agency-specific service subscription programs. In the utility fee model, citizens in a served area may be assessed a set fee per month of utility service, typically water based, but any provided utility could be coupled for EMS revenue generation based on local government regulatory preferences. The concept in this model is straightforward: spreading EMS system operating costs among as many potential patients as possible increases funding stability while simultaneously keeping costs per potential patient reasonably low in most locales. Local governments generally allow citizens to "opt out" of such assessments, but commonly structure such preference to require active communication from the citizen to either the local government or the EMS agency directly. In the utility fee assessment model, while the participating population percentages will vary based on the individual agency and/or location served, a significant majority of the population usually participates. Some utility fee funding programs have enjoyed widespread acceptance by allowing participants to utilize EMS without additional billing beyond their health insurance covered charges.

In lieu of utility-linked fees, EMS subscription fee models exist to leverage revenue generation against the same concept. Even in communities utilizing a utility-linked fee, residents of rental property, multi-unit dwellings, retirement facilities, or extended care facilities may not be eligible to participate based on the involved utilities being billed to property owner entities, individual, or corporate. In these situations, the subscription program allows individuals to pay on a set schedule, most often in advance and yearly, for EMS at reduced or no out-of-pocket costs at the time of actual service. Given the purposeful action that must be undertaken, and repeated at least annually, to participate in these subscription programs, EMS agencies often prefer the utility fee-related funding mechanism when given the option by its affiliated governmental authority. Either method can provide some financial certainty to EMS agencies that, solely due to system design, cannot access general fund taxation revenues.

USER COSTS

The charges to the users of EMS may be established at agency or local governmental level. The actual costs paid by patients or their representative vary substantially depending on billing methodology. In EMS systems fully funded by one or more of the mechanisms discussed above, no further charges are generated. In these situations, the costs of care rendered have essentially been "prepaid" usually by the larger populace in taxation or utility-linked assessments or occasionally by the individual through a subscription program. Complete cost of care coverage is rare in subscription programs due to a more limited pool of participating subscribers.

Insured individuals are commonly provided EMS care with subsequent agency billing to their insurance carriers, health care oriented, or, in the specific instances of motor vehicle-involved injuries, automotive coverage oriented. Depending on local, state, and federal allowable practices, many EMS agencies negotiate reimbursement charges and rates with prominent insurance providers for the care delivered to their covered parties. This is the same concept utilized by hospitals and individual medical practitioners in establishing their payment schedules with the same insurers. Some areas allow EMS systems to bill insured patients any charges not paid by their insurers. This practice is commonly referred to as "balance billing" the patient. Other locales specifically prohibit this practice by local or state regulation.

In EMS systems that generate bills for services, patients that are uninsured/self-pay can expect to receive an invoice for charges set by the agency or its governing body. An EMS system may choose to utilize this billing practice for all users, with the insured individuals subsequently responsible for getting paid back by their own insurance company. This latter practice is relatively uncommon due to efficiency of payment channels that can be established directly between EMS agencies and insurance providers, depending on an individual agencies billing infrastructure.

AGENCY BILLING

Agencies that generate bills for individual service do so through two primary billing structures—in-house or contracted. "In-house" billing refers to local government or an EMS agency directly employing billing professionals and handling all aspects of its billing, from negotiating reimbursement rates and charges with insurance companies to the accounting related to individual payments. Given the complexity of health care financing and insurance reimbursement practices today, many governmental authorities and EMS organizations choose to subcontract billing services to a specialized financial firm. These billing companies are paid either by flat fee or percentage of billable dollars depending on their contract with the EMS system. While structuring the subcontract payment in percentage of billable dollars terms can provide motivation to bill and collect maximum allowable charges, this same motivation can be the genesis for questionable billing practices unless strict adherence to ethical billing is maintained.

The responsibility for ethical billing rests with the EMS agency, or in the case of governmental body-provided EMS, that local governmental body. This "ownership" of billing practices remains with the EMS even when contracting for billing services. Examples are evident in the lay press of the veracity of this principle. While billing service vendor deliberations are rarely part of an EMS physician's duties, the EMS system's adherence to appropriate stewardship of trust extended to it in all forms by its served citizens has clear benefit in fostering and protecting a reputation for quality clinical care.

PATIENT PAYOR MIX

Regardless of billing structure, financial viability of an EMS agency is directly impacted by its patient payor mix. Systems with a majority of patients covered by government programs, namely Medicare, Medicaid, and/or Tricare, are substantially impacted by subtle changes in reimbursement rates or timetables in these programs.[5] Systems with significant portions of patients covered by commercial health insurance may also be affected by the aforementioned government programs, as some private insurers often index their payment rates to one of these same programs. With a multitude of options available in the commercial health insurance market, an EMS system that serves a community with diverse industry and administrative services may well find no one insurer has prominent effect on its revenue projections (**Figure 25-2**). EMS systems serving a preponderance of uninsured or underinsured patients may find increasingly difficult financial realities. As the practice of EMS medicine involves increasing technology-assisted therapies and emerging pharmaceuticals, costs of clinical care provision, regardless of insured status, rise for all patients.

In light of difficult economies over the last several years in the United States, many patients once insured, are now without health care

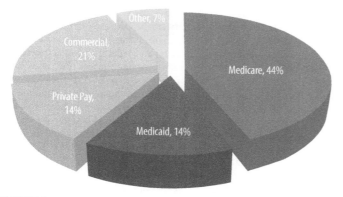

FIGURE 25-2. EMS payor mix. (Based on data from the National EMS Advisory Council EMS System Performance-based Funding and Reimbursement Model May 23, 2012.)

underwriting. These patients may find particular value in EMS systems that do not charge individuals, offer relatively small utility-linked service fees, or encourage participation in subscription programs as previously discussed in this chapter. Although many clinical and administrative EMS personnel view "self-pay" status as equivalent to "no pay," realities in many communities prove a number of patients view financial obligations to EMS systems seriously, arranging individual payment plans for services they have received.

No single mix of patient payor sources is optimal. In fact, nearly every EMS system finds on such analysis that just as it serves the full spectrum of the human condition, it is compensated by the full spectrum of payors. Accurate appraisal of payor sources and percentages of such sources is important for individual EMS system financial planning, particularly in regard to needed billing resources and efforts in collections.

▓ BILLING PERFORMANCE

Detailed discussions and advisements concerning formal contractual arrangements and performance stipulations for billing services are beyond the intent and the scope of this text. However, general concepts can be discussed with a solely educational objective. A major focus, at least in some billing service marketing materials and in comparing in-house billing activities with potential outsourcing options, involves the percentage of billable dollars collected, especially those ultimately placed into the EMS agency's operating funds. Many large, urban EMS systems in America that do bill individual patients realize less than 50% of billable dollars in return. Obviously, assuming proper ethical practices and financial efficiencies, the closer to 100% of billable dollars collected, the more favorable impact on future fiscal abilities in an EMS system.

Percentage collections of billable accounts may often trend with percentage collections of billable dollars, but this is a distinctly separate measure of billing efficacy. This performance measure evaluates the thoroughness of billing collection across the spectrum of payor mix. Even in the best of EMS systems with thorough care documentation and diligent billing efforts, insurers may deny payment for a variety of reasons and uninsured accounts may convert to unpaid accounts. Thus, while 100% of billable accounts reflecting collections would promote highly desirable service revenue, this is unlikely to be approached in nearly all EMS systems serving populous communities.

Both percentage of billable dollars collected and percentage collections of billable accounts are subject to view in timeliness of collections. "Aging" of an account refers to the length of time between invoicing and collecting revenue for services. For example, a bill for services sent March 1 and unpaid on May 10, would place that account in a 60- to 90-day "age" profile. Due attention should be paid to account aging in calculating usable revenue abilities in an EMS system. Theoretically, a billing operation could recognize close to 100% collection of billable dollars and billable accounts, but its affiliated EMS agency could be in financial ruin if the typical aging of accounts necessitated aging in years, not days.

As with any administrative service, the costs of billing operations will vary depending on multiple factors. Business overhead of operational space, computers, communications, numbers of full-time and part-time employees, employer-provided employee benefits, professional insurance, and ongoing professional continuing education are just a few of the factors impacting the finances of financial services. These costs of billing, particularly if outsourced, may be expressed to an EMS agency in an agreed upon total, or fixed, cost. Alternatively, a billing service may take its revenue as an agreed upon percentage of dollars billed on behalf of the EMS agency. At least one positive and one pitfall to such arrangement have been reviewed above.

There are no such EMS industry "standards" in either fixed costs or percent dollars billed costs. The astute EMS administrative leader must carefully evaluate costs of in-house billing operations against suitable outsourcing options and make a decision in the EMS agency's best financial interests.

▓ BILLABLE CHARGES

Regardless of billing service infrastructure, the actual allowable charges for EMS have changed over time. Throughout the 1980s and the 1990s, EMS agencies were allowed to itemize bill for equipment and personnel utilized in the clinical care rendered an individual payment. Translated to a real example, the billing for a cardiac arrest resuscitation might include the following: bag-valve-mask device, oral airway, oxygen at 25 minutes use, endotracheal tube stylet, endotracheal tube, 10-cc syringe, electrocardiogram monitor/defibrillator supplies (electrodes, tracing paper, defibrillation pads), intravenous (IV) catheter, IV start kit, four epinephrine 1:10,000 prefilled syringes, two lidocaine 2% prefilled syringes, paramedic attendant, mileage from scene of cardiac arrest to hospital rounded up to nearest whole mile. Simply summed, the more equipment and procedures involved, the higher the bill. Other allowable billing options included: (1) one inclusive charge, reflecting supplies, service, and mileage; (2) two charges, one for supplies and service with a companion charge for mileage; and (3) two charges, one for service and mileage with a companion charge for supplies. With any of these four allowable billing calculations, once a Medicare beneficiary had paid their deductible costs, the beneficiary remained responsible for 20% of Medicare paid fees. Medicare also allowed for EMS agencies to directly bill the beneficiary for charges above those paid by Medicare. This process is known as balance billing.

Significant change in allowable billing structure occurred with the Medicare ambulance fee schedule implemented April 1, 2002. While overall Medicare spending for EMS-related services was forecast to slightly decrease, an individual agency's Medicare revenue could vary widely under the new schedule depending on prior billing practices, particularly attention to detail in itemized billing. The new, and current, Medicare ambulance fee schedule is based on two primary components: level of clinical care provided and distance of patient transportation. Additional monies are paid to EMS agencies initiating transports in classified rural areas.

Medicare now requires a signature from hospital personnel to certify EMS transport. Further, EMS billings must be filed using specified diagnosis and procedure coding. Based on Medicare review of the EMS documentation of patient condition, payment on behalf of its beneficiaries are made using the following nine levels of ambulance service: basic life support (BLS)-nonemergency; BLS-emergency; advanced life support, level 1 (ALS1)-nonemergency; ALS1-emergency; ALS, level 2 (ALS2); specialty care transport (SCT); paramedic intercept (PI) services; fixed-wing (FW) air ambulance; and rotary-wing (RW) air ambulance.[6] Emergency designators apply to EMS agencies responding in immediate means to calls placed via 9-1-1 communications or an equivalent in areas without such systems. The clinician reader of this text may question the inclusion of even cursory details of current Medicare payment structures. The Medicare allowable payments translate into significant clinical ability impacts.

As mentioned earlier, many private insurance allowable payments closely follow those for Medicare beneficiaries. Additionally, in Medicare's billing structure since April 2002, itemized billing for used supplies is notably absent. Thus, when an EMS medical director discusses a new assessment technology, a new therapeutic device, or a new pharmaceutical for inclusion in an EMS agency's standards of care, the financial reality is that the direct costs of implementing that standard of care cannot be transferred in billings as an itemized component. Simple summation with current Medicare allowable charges is the more equipment and procedures involved, the less likely the EMS agency is to have its true costs of service reimbursed.

The clinician reader is directed to their local administrative EMS leaders and relevant health insurer ambulance service reimbursement materials for further study as may be warranted.

EXPENSE EVALUATION: LABOR

Like most service professions, EMS expenses are significantly comprised by costs of labor.[7] Many EMS agencies, particularly those serving populous suburban and urban areas, find human-related costs far exceed capital and disposable equipment expenditures. Salaries and benefits have variability on nearly any geographic scale, to an extent that a multitude of related factors must be considered by prospective EMS employees. It is not unusual in many areas of the United States for a single ambulance, staffed at a paramedic level, and placed available for continuous service to be budgeted exceeding $300,000 per year, exclusive of medical equipment.

CAPITAL EQUIPMENT

Durable medical devices prove integral in support of advancing the standards of EMS medical care. The EMS medical oversight physician must work cooperatively with operational and financial leaders to plan clinical advances with fiscal responsibility. Electrocardiographic (ECG) monitor/defibrillators have progressed tremendously over the past 15 to 20 years, now featuring multiple modality monitoring, such as automatic blood pressure determination, waveform capnography, and core temperature measurement. Prominent in clinical care support, these devices are equally prominent in capital equipment budgeting. Many urban EMS are now faced with a literally multimillion dollar decision when purchasing these newest generation monitors.

Mechanical chest compression devices, transport ventilators, battery-powered lift-assist stretchers, and self-loading and unloading stretchers are several other higher expense items increasingly encountered by EMS agencies. While each example can be advocated by medical and marketing literature, none can be obtained cheaply. Technology advances, pure and simple.

These higher dollar devices are by design or necessity often placed in multiyear purchasing plans for EMS agencies. Rarely does a sizeable EMS agency have capital equipment reserves or budgets to outfit an entire fleet upgrade by single purchase. The EMS oversight physician must always be a patient advocate, though a financial realist simultaneously.

A litany of other capital medical equipment is involved, but easily to overlook. Oxygen tanks, oxygen regulators, wall-mounted suction units, medical equipment carrying devices (backpacks, kits, bags), and portable communications, including Internet access, phones, and radios must be considered.

All of the previously mentioned capital equipment can be useful, but particularly so when placed on an ambulance for mobility of care provision. While ambulances may prove the ultimate expense in capital equipment budgeting for an EMS agency, the collective costs of durable and disposable medical equipment usually far exceed the base vehicle cost. It is certainly not cheap to buy a new ambulance; it is not cheaper to medically provision it in most situations.

Ambulance purchasing is typically the domain of an EMS executive or applicable government official. While respecting the authority of such, EMS medical oversight physicians should also clearly communicate clinical needs to assist in the proper specification of new vehicles. One current example involves periresuscitation therapeutic hypothermia. Cooling of normal saline to 4°C can be reliably achieved and maintained, but dedicated refrigeration or cooling devices are needed in planning ambulance design, preferably prior to construction of the involved vehicles.

DISPOSABLE EQUIPMENT

Variety of disposable equipment options dwarfs that of capital equipment options. While many disposable items common in the delivery of EMS care costs fractions of a US dollar, those fractions often compound to surprising amounts in a year's budget. Conscientious EMS leaders, clinical and administrative, want to ensure needed equipment is reliably available. Often supply "cushions" create snowball effects in physical space and fiscal impacts. The sage supply officer may begin to question traditional practices common throughout the spectrum of medical supply stocking and ask: "Are we stocking what we stock by tradition? Or … are we stocking what we really use?" Accurate and timely data are essential in evaluating supply and demand answers for an EMS agency. The bottom line is increasingly the bottom (financial) line in stocking. Many answers to efficiency in ordering and inventory of EMS supplies now exist in commercially available software and hardware.

TRAINING COSTS

Financing education for EMS professionals becomes increasingly important once considering the ever-increasing clinical standards of care available. Some EMS agencies fund initial certification training for personnel either joining the organization or for established employees advancing in scope of practice level. Within these EMS systems, a few agencies directly conduct initial education programs using educators they employ full time for this purpose. Nearly all EMS organizations sponsor or contribute to some form of continuing education for their affiliated personnel, volunteer or paid. Costs of training go far beyond the educators involved. Training schedules can have significant impact on the costs for the delivery of information. Many EMS agencies choose to conduct ongoing training for only on-duty personnel to eliminate overtime labor costs. Depending on whether collective bargaining is involved in local EMS labor agreements, the duty status of personnel during continuing education may be additionally regulated. Textbooks, Internet accessed materials, tuition for packaged programs, and training materials such as manikins, disposable medical equipment, and capital equipment dedicated to training roles must be considered and budgeted. EMS medical oversight physicians will need to consider the training schedules and costs associated with new standards of care to promote their successful delivery.

INSURANCE COSTS

Financial protection for all aspects of the EMS system previously discussed in this chapter must be seriously considered, and in many cases, is required by local statute or regulation. While medical liability and vehicle insurance premiums are quick to identify as necessary costs, additional suggested policies are numerous and include employee benefit insurance premium portions paid by the employer, durable medical equipment damage protection costs, and directors' and officers' policies for administrative leaders of the EMS system, just to name a few. Some systems also cover the costs for EMS physician policies that cover medical malpractice and administrative liability claims as part of the medical oversight professional services contract.

In sum, considerable attention is due to the expense evaluation of an EMS system given the multitude of required expenses and the variability that exists not only within those cost centers, but additionally those driven by additional standards of administrative and clinical capabilities. The future of EMS funding is likely to prove dynamic. As physician reimbursement is being viewed in bundling models with hospitals under accountable care organizations (ACOs), EMS may well prove inclusive in several of the ACO proposals.

FUTURE CHANGES

In the current environment of health care finance and delivery restructuring, it is unclear how EMS will be funded in the future. Opportunities to contract with *accountable care organizations* and the possibility of a change from the current reimbursement scheme to one that pays for care rendered without transport are actively developing at the time of the writing of this text. The further development of community paramedicine and the desire for hospitals and health care systems to prevent avertable admissions and nonemergency visits to the emergency department may drive this new EMS finance landscape. EMS agency administrators and medical directors will need to meet these new challenges together in order to ensure solvency and to avoid disruption in delivery of emergency medical care services due to denial of payment or other preventable budgetary shortfalls.

- District contracts are a means to secure an arrangement in a certain area for EMS to be provided, assuming they meet certain criteria often spelled out in the contract. These contracts provide assurances to both parties and should include dissolution terms if the need to separate should arise.

- Grants are another means to secure funding and are available at the local, state, and federal levels. While local grants may be easier to obtain once identified, state and federal grants can have a large impact on many people.

KEY POINTS

- Funding in EMS may come from taxes, special contracts, direct patient billing, grants, private funding, fund-raising, and subscription services

- Reimbursement for EMS utilizes a complex formula based on the level and type of service provided and miles transported, with many special considerations to rural areas and especially poorly populated rural areas.

- CMS criteria for reimbursement include proof of the level of service and mileage traveled as well as demonstration of necessity.

- Payor mix can play a critical role in the ability to collect bills and financial dependence on outside sources, such as a municipality to provide appropriate services.

- Mileage modifiers play a tremendous impact on reimbursement and can significantly increase the charges on long transports as are common in rural areas. Along with the rural modifiers, this can help offset the reduced volume that rural agencies often experience.

- Medical necessity essentially is the proof that an ambulance is required as opposed to other means of transportation as defined by Medicare. A physician's order is insufficient to meet this requirement.

- Electronic PCRs have had tremendous impact on ability to capture data, reduce time for billing, and improve the utility of the PCR as a communication tool.

REFERENCES

1. FEMA/USFA. *Funding Alternatives for Fire and Emergency Services.* Emmitsburg, MD: Federal Emergency Management Agency, United States Fire Administration; 1999

2. National EMS Advisory Council. EMS system performance-based funding and reimbursement model. May 23, 2012. http://www.ems. gov/pdf/nemsac/may2012/Finance_Committee_Interim_Advisory-Performance-Based_Reimbursement.pdf.

3. Harold F. Goldsmith, Dena S. Puskin, Dianne J. Stiles. Improving the operational definition of "rural areas" for federal programs. Rockville, MD: U.S. Department of Health and Human Services, Health Resource and Services Administration, Office of Rural Health Policy; 1993:11. http://www.raconline.org/pdf/improving-the-operational-definition-of-rural-areas.pdf. Accessed May, 2015.

4. Narad R. Emergency medical services system design. *Emerg Med Clin N Am.* 1990;8:1-8.

5. United States Government Accountability Office. Ambulance Services: Changes Needed to Improve Medicare Payment Policies and Coverage Decisions. Report to Congressional Committees. GAO-02-244T. Washington, DC; November 2001. http://www.gao.gov/assets/110/109068.pdf. Accessed May, 2015.

6. Centers for Medicare and Medicaid Services. 42 CFR parts 410 and 414: Medicare program; fee schedule for payment of ambulance services and revisions to the physician certification requirements for coverage of nonemergency ambulance services; final rule. *Fed Regist.* 2002;67(39):9100-9135.

7. Key C. Operational issues in EMS. *Emerg Med Clin N Am.* 2002; 20:913-927.

INTRODUCTION

Computer-aided dispatch (CAD), electronic patient care records (ePCR), patient satisfaction surveys, billing systems, medical devices, etc as data collection have become more prevalent in EMS agencies, so does the opportunity to use that data to more effectively manage the organization. Understanding the types of data available, and how that data are best used to measure performance, is essential to the success of an EMS agency.

The majority of efforts in measuring EMS performance fall into three categories: clinical, operational, and financial. EMS leaders find it increasingly necessary to balance these categories in order to maintain a healthy organization. In addition to maintaining equilibrium among these areas, many of the measures described in this chapter have some level of correlation to other measures. One can easily see that poor financial performance might lead to an inability to fund clinical advancements, or that longer response times might impact the survival rate of out-of-hospital cardiac arrest (OHCA) patients. The more we study EMS performance measures, the more we see new examples of not only correlation, but in some cases direct causal relationships. Although clinical measures may be the area that the medical director is called upon for more guidance, it is important for anyone in that position to understand all measures used to manage an EMS agency and how they relate to the overall success of the organization.

OBJECTIVES

- Define key terminology used in EMS performance measures.
- Describe the value of monitoring EMS performance measures as related to the strength of an EMS agency.
- Outline the most commonly used clinical performance measures in EMS.
- Describe the components of response time compliance monitoring.
- Describe the unit hour utilization formula, and its use.
- Describe the demand analysis process used to match staffing levels with EMS call volume.
- Describe the concept of developing and utilizing a vehicle deployment plan.
- Outline common safety related performance measures.

DEFINING PERFORMANCE MEASUREMENT

Terminology used in EMS performance measurement can vary from one source to another. For the purposes of understanding the contents of this chapter, as well as understanding performance measures shared among EMS agencies, the following is offered as a clarification.

Key performance indicators (KPIs) are specific areas of measurement determined to be valuable to monitor. This is the "what" in terms of measuring EMS Performance Measurement. Medication errors, response time reporting, and cash collections are examples of clinical, operational, and financial components of KPIs. Specific examples of the most commonly used clinical and operational KPIs in EMS will be the focus of this chapter.

A *benchmark* may be used to describe one of two things. More commonly, the term benchmark is used to define a goal to aim for, or a level to try to achieve. This use of the term is often derived from identifying best practices, or a measure that has been recognized as being done well in another similar circumstance. The second use of the term benchmark would be to simply set a point of measurement that can be used for future comparison. This is often the current state, documented prior to efforts undertaken to improve measured results of a specific item.

Where monitoring ambulance response times for certain types of calls may be the KPI, a benchmark may be to achieve 90% compliance within a certain time standard defined for that type of call.

Worth mentioning, but outside the scope of this chapter are two other areas of using EMS data to measure performance and ultimately benefit the EMS agency and or/system.

First is the use of data to answer individual questions that arise outside of regular KPI measures. The more the EMS agency uses and understands their data, the more opportunities they will discover to use it for nontraditional benefit. An example would be a police agency looking to determine if there is value to adding naloxone to their patrol cars. Analyzing patient care report and CAD data to determine the amount of times an EMS agency utilizes Naloxone on calls where police arrived first on scene would be a valuable piece of information to provide the decision makers.

Second is the practice of data mining, or predictive analytics. This practice is gaining attention in the EMS industry. Essentially, data mining is the process of analyzing large quantities of data to look for patterns or relationships that might otherwise go unnoticed. Being able to discover and predict these patterns and relationships is the reward. As large data collections begin to emerge, such as the National EMS Information System, the idea of data mining in EMS becomes much more feasible.

CLINICAL PERFORMANCE MEASURES

SKILL SUCCESS RATES

One of the more common performance measures involves the monitoring and tallying of clinical skills. Endotracheal intubation, IV, intra osseous, and other common skills are measured by displaying successful attempts versus total attempts. Although often an indicator for areas where training may need to be enhanced, these measures are falling out of favor in many areas as EMS leaders gain a better understanding of both the number of variables that go into the success of a particular skill attempt and the acceptable alternatives for many skills, such as alternative airway devices available for patients who may be difficult to intubate. Large quantities of aggregate data can provide a picture of system performance, while reviewing data for individual providers needs to be done with caution and full consideration of the number of things that may impact those numbers.

PROTOCOL COMPLIANCE

For many reasons, not the least of which involves the delegated medical practice within EMS systems, adherence to specific medical protocols is of value to monitor and review for the EMS medical director and all EMS leaders. With the growing number of EMS agencies using electronic patient care reports, automated reporting of variances from medical protocol is becoming the norm. Specific examples include:

- Percentage of chest pain patients of a particular age group that received NTG and or ASA within a certain time of arrival at the scene.
- Percentage of chest pain patients of a particular age group that received a 12-lead ECG.
- Medication administration matching all protocol components.
- Time spent on scene for major trauma
- Transport to designated specialty hospitals. What percentage of the time are patients delivered to designated specialty hospitals when indicated? STEMI, stroke, trauma, and burn designations are common examples.

Additionally, reporting on recently updated medical protocols can also be set up to provide an opportunity for the medical director to view all cases in a particular area, looking to see if the changes made to a protocol had the desired impact.

TIME TO FIRST DEFIBRILLATION

In out-of-hospital cardiac arrest, where defibrillation is performed on the presenting rhythm, many agencies measure the time from activation of the EMS system (caller contacting PSAP) until the first defibrillation. This is used to determine the overall effectiveness of the EMS system response to cardiac arrest.

PAIN RELIEF

This measure is used to display how pain has increased, decreased, or remains the same from first recorded EMS measurement to final recorded EMS measurement on an event. This is viewed by many agencies as an area that EMS is able to make a measurable difference to patients.

MEDICAL ERRORS

Monitoring all reported medication errors, flagged either through the protocol compliance review process or otherwise, is a critical component of measuring EMS performance. As with most EMS performance measures, this is one is of particular importance to monitor for provider and/or system-wide trends. Timely reporting of issues, with a historical review of any similar issues, will help the agency quickly devise a plan to prevent future recurrences. Medication errors and unrecognized esophageal intubations are the most common to be reviewed.

UTSTEIN STYLE UNIFORM REPORTING OF OHCA DATA

One of the earlier forms of standardizing EMS data definitions and reporting measures, the Utstein-style cardiac arrest definitions and reporting template, is widely used by EMS agencies as a means to measure their impact on cardiac arrest patients.

OPERATIONAL PERFORMANCE MEASURES

RESPONSE TIME PERFORMANCE

Compliance to a particular response time standard is among the most widely used EMS performance measures. In a typical system, a response time benchmark is established for different categories of calls. The performance measure process widely accepted in EMS is to measure how reliably an agency meets that benchmark. For example, a system may have a goal to have 90% compliance with an 8 minute 59 second total response time standard for top priority call types. Reporting is usually done to display the percent of time that an agency meets this time standard. The time standard remains constant in the reporting, while the compliance percentage varies from one reporting period to the next. Typical response time reporting periods include weekly, monthly, and annual summary reports. Trends are identified, reported, and remeasured to determine the effectiveness of system changes made. Common examples of system changes made to address response time compliance issues include altering EMS provider schedules and changing vehicle deployment plans.

RESPONSE TIME INTERVALS

With the commonness of measuring time stamps for the various components of an EMS response, most systems review the various intervals for trends and potential opportunities to improve. Typical intervals measured are:

- Call processing time: the interval from the time of call intake (answering phone) to the time EMS resources are notified of the call.
- Out-of-chute time (also known as Turnout time): the interval from the time EMS resources were notified of a call to the time the EMS vehicle is physically moving toward the scene.
- En route time (also known as travel time): the interval from the time the EMS vehicle begins moving toward the scene to the time the EMS vehicle is placed in park at the scene.

- Total response time: Call Processing Time + Out of Chute Time + En route Time. In other words, the interval from time of call intake to the time the EMS vehicle is placed in park at the scene.

"At patient side" is another time used in some systems to add an additional interval—the time the EMS vehicle was placed in park at the scene until the EMS providers are physically at the patient's side.

Worth noting is the growing debate over response time standards. At the time of this writing, little clinical data are available to validate the standards set in most systems. Historical information about timely defibrillation in OHCA patients is what often drives these standards. Yet to be resolved in most systems is the way to set response time standards that are based on true clinical outcome impact, along with the expectations of the public for a rapid response.

UNIT HOUR UTILIZATION

Regardless of EMS agency infrastructure, essentially all EMS mission–oriented organizations routinely analyze the number of service requests to which a response was made. These reports may be generated in multiple formats, in hourly to yearly intervals. The types of responses are commonly classified using at least two delineations: (1) red lights and sirens (RLS) utilized versus non-RLS travel and (2) primary service mission type (eg, medical, rescue, fire suppression, scheduled event standby). Beyond the basic calculations of numbers and types of responses, a wealth of operational analysis tools exists in EMS. Many evaluation measures are credited to a pioneer in EMS operational analysis, Jack Stout. Mr Stout advanced the concept of the public utility model of EMS in the late 1970s with measurement standards such as unit hour and unit hour utilization. Regardless of system architecture, these measurement standards and others such as unit cost and cost per patient transport can be used in evaluation of operational efficiencies.

Unit A unit is an emergency response vehicle, specifically as applied to EMS, staffed by certified EMS professionals per jurisdictional requirements and equipped to provide medical standards of care per applicable treatment guidelines or protocols.

Unit Hour A *unit hour* is defined as a 60-minute time period with a staffed and equipped vehicle (a unit, as defined above) able to respond to incidents, or actually assigned to an incident. If a unit is taken out of service for any reason other than an incident (such as a training, mechanical repair, etc), unit hours do not accrue in those situations. A simple example serves to make the calculation of an agency's daily unit hours. Let us say that Anytown Ambulance operates three ambulances, each staffed 24 hours a day. Assuming personnel and ambulances are not taken out of service, Anytown Ambulance utilizes 72 unit hours daily in serving its geographical response area. Comparisons to other agencies can easily be calculated by unit hour totals on a daily or weekly basis, but alone, the measure does not allow for evaluations of efficiency.

Unit hour utilization (UHU) is a calculated number that represents a snapshot of an agency's call volume compared to available resources for a given period of time, originally meant to define a level of efficiency. In the simplest form, it is often used to describe "how busy" EMS crews are. The measure is used frequently to benchmark an agency against their past performance, and sometimes used to compare an agency to other similar sized EMS agencies. Using the recent example of Anytown Ambulance, consider the UHU determination for this organization if 24 patients are transported on the day of analysis. The UHU calculation looks like this: 24 transports/72 unit hours = 0.33 UHU.

A *unit* as an emergency response vehicle, specifically as applied to EMS, staffed by certified EMS professionals per jurisdictional requirements and equipped to provide medical standards of care per applicable treatment guidelines or protocols.

There are a few standard variations on the UHU calculation:

- Call UHU: the number of calls (requests for service) divided by the number of unit hours for the same period of time. Look at an example of a day where 25 calls came into the EMS agency, and they had two fully staffed 24 hour vehicles, and an additional 10 out day vehicle,

TABLE 26-1	Unit Hour Utilization Benchmarks
.55-.45—optimal	
.45-.35—above Average	
.35-.25—average	
.25-.15—below average	
.15-.01—poor	

the calculation would be 25/58, with a resulting UHU value of 0.431. **Table 26-1** shows some UHU benchmarks that are sometimes used to assess performance.[1]

- *Transport UHU*: the number of patient transports divided by the number of unit hours. Using the scenario above, but where 21 of those calls ended up with patients being transported. The transport UHU in this case would be 21/58, or 0.362.

- *Weighted UHU*: This is the same calculation as either one of the above, multiplied by the average total task time, in hours, for the same time period. Task time being defined as the amount of time it takes a vehicle and crew to complete an entire EMS call from start to finish. More systems are beginning to look at this model, as the previous two calculations are based on an assumption that most EMS calls are not only the same length of time, but equal to about 1 hour. The weighted transport UHU in the above example, if the average time to complete an EMS call is 72 minutes, would be 0.362 × 1.2 (72/60), or 0.434

Figure 26-1 reflects how a year's daily UHU evaluation could be displayed. The UHU determination in this example uses patient transports alone in the numerator. The example reflects an EMS system with an average daily UHU of 0.35 and average daily transports of 183 over the course of the year analyzed. The chart reflects a system in which the transport volume and UHU are closely correlated, indicating unit hours supplied are distinctly influenced by anticipated and realized patient transport volumes. **Figure 26-2** is a control chart showing in more visible detail the daily variation in UHU. The middle horizontal bar reflects the averaged UHU of 0.35. There can be a rating assigned to ranges of UHU to describe the utilization of a particular agency (Table 26-1).

UHU can be impacted through several factors, including staffing models and crew configurations, fixed versus system status management deployments, response obligations, and duty status of personnel in training. For instance, fixed deployment models may require more units to meet desirable response times. System status management, a system in which emergency vehicles are dynamically deployed based on prior call location models, could promote response time capabilities using a slightly smaller fleet. In such situation, the overall unit hours are reduced, and thus, an increase in UHU could be expected for any applicable amount of transports or responses, depending on the chosen numerator paradigm.

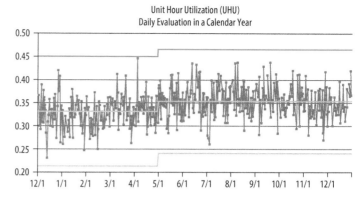

FIGURE 26-2. Example daily variation in UHU.

Additional metrics related to unit hours include the production of unit hours and the distribution of unit hours. These two measurements, viewed as "megaprocesses," were termed "key processes" of EMS field operations by Jack Stout in 1997 and are unit hour production and unit hour distribution.

Unit Hour Production Unit hour production is determined by any activity incumbent on creating a staffed and equipped emergency response vehicle. Examples of necessary activities toward unit hour production include personnel recruiting, training, and scheduling, as well as vehicle purchasing, equipping, and maintaining. One measure of unit hour production capability is comparing the number of produced unit hours to the number of scheduled unit hours for a given time period. **Figure 26-3** reflects just such a comparison in control chart format. The middle horizontal bar reflects produced unit hours at 101% of those scheduled in the first half of the calendar year being evaluated. In the last half of the year, produced unit hours drop to 98% of those scheduled. Produced unit hours exceeding the upper control limit could be reflections of situations in which additional unit hours were purposefully added over typical schedules to compensate for special events, severe weather, or seasonal illness/injury patterns. Produced unit hours falling below the lower control limit could be reflections of situations in which personnel were unable to fulfill work obligations due to personal sickness or situations in which scheduled hours were reduced in anticipation of low call volumes (eg, Christmas Day in some locales).

Unit Hour Distribution Unit hour distribution is based on emergency vehicle location assignments, dispatches to requests for service, and all activities that prepare the system to respond to the next request for service. Unit hour distribution effectiveness is primarily measured in compliance with response time standards or goals. Many systems use a simple calculation that divides the number of responses to calls

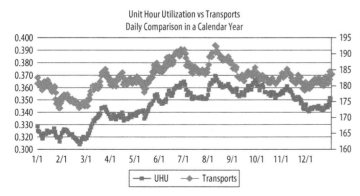

FIGURE 26-1. Example unit hour utilization versus transports.

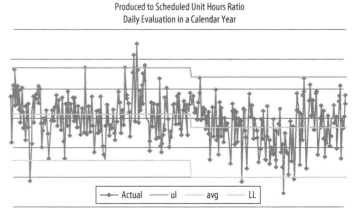

FIGURE 26-3. Example produced hours versus scheduled hours.

within the indicated response time benchmark by the total number of call responses. Often, EMS agencies are required to meet time parameters at a 90% compliance standard by their local government regulations. A common standard in EMS over the past 30 years has been response within 7 minutes 59 seconds to cardiac arrests. This standard was derived from early analysis in cardiac arrest, suggesting a 10% decrease in survival per minute of cardiac arrest. Based on interim scientific work, response time standards for EMS now reflect significant variability across the United States. Compliance may be required on daily, weekly, monthly, quarterly, or yearly intervals depending on local expectations and regulations.

Merging financial and operational benchmarks, two additional measures can be calculated in evaluating the efficiency of an EMS agency: unit cost and cost per transport. Relatively self-explanatory, unit cost is simply the summation of all costs necessary to place that unit in service for its specified interval, be it a 24-hour daily shift or peak demand determined interval. Cost per transport specifically takes the discussed summation of costs and divides those by the transports provided by that specific unit, or entire fleet if evaluating macroscale economies of the agency.

DEMAND ANALYSIS

Of critical importance for any EMS agency's mission is to match supply of resources with demand for service. Nearly all EMS systems have some variance in demand for service (call volume) by time of day, day of week, and in many cases seasonally. An EMS demand analysis is a specific performance measuring process by which EMS leaders graphically show their trended call demand along with their planned scheduling of resources. By reviewing the data graphically, one can note areas where it may be advisable to shift resources from a time of low call volume to a time of high call volume. Traditionally accepted methods for a demand analysis involve looking at 20 weeks' worth of historical call data, plotted out by each of the 168 hours in a week.[2] The more sophisticated models take into account the amount of time spent on an EMS call (task time), as all EMS calls do not equal 60 minutes in length and therefore do not plot entirely accurately on an hour-by-hour graph.

Although no one can predict when an individual call for help will come in, patterns and trends to aggregate data are usually fairly easy to identify. Staffing plans adjusted to meet predicted demand allow for improvements in clinical, operational, and financial components of an EMS agency. EMS leaders also evaluate the consistency of these patterns (standard deviation) when making decisions about the required level of staffing to meet system demands. A time with greater variability will require a higher level of additional resources to meet future demand than a time with more consistent predictability.

The demand analysis tool is one that when used effectively, can have a direct impact on many other performance measures, including response time compliance, unit hour utilization, and calls requiring assistance from mutual aid plans.

Because this tool is such an important one for EMS leaders to understand and use, it is equally important to be aware of other issues that may impact staffing needs outside of the call volume arena. Unplanned periods with excessive offload times in emergency departments can quickly turn a scientifically planned staffing model into a vulnerable EMS System. EMS leaders will work to define variables like offload times, unfilled staffing openings, EMS provider sickouts, weather events, and other variables, in order to bring more reliable predictability to the demand analysis.

DEPLOYMENT PLANNING

Along with the demand analysis process, which yields the appropriate number of vehicles needed in a system, many EMS leaders follow up with a deployment plan designed to place these vehicles strategically in the response territory. By analyzing areas with the largest call volume demand, along with travel times, and areas that may need attention with response time compliance, a deployment plan is developed to best cover the response area with whatever number of resources remain available to do calls. If there are 20 vehicles available to respond to calls, the

deployment plan will outline the best location for each of the vehicles to be placed. Likewise, if the system is extremely busy, and there is only one available vehicle left to respond to the next call, the deployment plan specifies the best place for that vehicle to be placed.

EMS VEHICLE CRASHES

Although each crash is to be reviewed on a case-by-case basis for cause and prevention identification, many EMS agencies report their vehicle crashes as a ratio of crashes per 1000 EMS responses as a means to compare to other systems and the note changes to trends within their organization.

EMS PROVIDER INJURIES

Similar to the measurement of vehicle crashes, each injury is reviewed individually for cause and prevention identification, as well as compiling information that can be used to identify any trends.

PATIENT SAFETY EVENTS

In addition to medical errors, events such as stretcher drops, ambulatory patients falling, and other such incidents are measured and reported.

Of note in each of the three safety categories above, EMS agencies will commonly tally and report "near-miss" events for the purposes of identifying opportunities for improvement.

CRITICAL VEHICLE AND EQUIPMENT FAILURES

Commonly defined as any vehicle or equipment failure that occurred during an EMS event (as opposed to other times like vehicle checks), these events are measured and tallied, with or without impact on the patient or provider. Systems often report these numbers as days between critical failures.

SATISFACTION SURVEYS

Patients, other response agencies, and hospitals are all viewed as key customers and partners that are in a position to form an opinion about the quality of service provided by an EMS agency. As such, EMS agencies will routinely solicit feedback to identify areas that are perceived as needing improvement.

KEY POINTS

- Today's EMS agencies are more effectively managed by utilizing various data sources to develop and monitor key performance indicators.
- The three main categories of EMS performance measures are intertwined—clinical, operational, and financial.
- Benchmarks are measurement points used by EMS agencies to compare current states to past measures or goals.
- Clinical performance measures, such as skill success rates, protocol compliance, monitoring for medical errors, and others are increasingly automated based on electronic medical record use.
- Routine statistical review of call volume, staffing patterns, response times, and resource deployment plans allow the modern EMS agency to operate at high levels of efficiency.

REFERENCES

1. Calculating Your EMS Service's Average Cost of Service and Unit Hour Analysis. J.R. Henry Consulting. 2011. http://www.emscon sult.org/images/Unit_Hour_Analysis_with_instructions.pdf. Accessed May, 2015.
2. Brown LH, Lerner EB, Larmon B, LeGassick T, Taigman M. Are EMS call volume predictions based on demand pattern analysis accurate? *Prehosp Emerg Care.* April-June 2007;11(2):199-203.

CHAPTER 27
Human Resources and Employee Relations

Brian M. Clemency

Adin J. Bradley

INTRODUCTION

Human resources (HR) deal with the hiring, training, compensating, managing, and unfortunately, at times the disciplining or terminating of employees. Human resources managers are expected to have expansive knowledge of these fields. However, all individuals in supervisory roles must have a basic understanding of the agency's HR framework. Physician medical directors bring extensive medical knowledge to an organization, but often have minimal business training or experience. Unlike their counterparts in dentistry or chiropractic medicine, physicians are given little, if any, education in the business world. While all of these functions do not fall directly under the purview of medical direction, an astute medical director should have an understanding of their role within an organization's human resources structure.

Emergency medical services is a unique profession, straddling the worlds of public safety and allied health. Like other public safety professionals, prehospital care providers respond to emergency calls from the community 24 hours a day, 7 days a week. Providers often feel a special kinship with the firefighters and police officers alongside whom they work. However, the medical education they must possess distinguishes them from these colleagues and aligns them more closely with nurses and other health care professionals. Limited resources exist for dealing specifically with human resources issues in emergency medical services. By examining allied health and public safety references, one can better navigate these minimally charted waters.

OBJECTIVES

- Define the role of the medical director as a part of the EMS or fire agency administration.
- Contrast the HR/ER roles of the medical director against those of the agency director or fire chief.
- Contrast the terms *remediation* and *discipline* as they relate to a response to EMS provider performance issues.
- Describe the proper method for instituting remediation, probation, and suspension of privileges.
- Describe liability issues for medical directors related to labor laws.
- Give examples of pitfalls related to the handling of HR/ER issues.

THE MEDICAL DIRECTOR'S RELATIONSHIP TO THE AGENCY

There are various models for the relationship between medical directors and the agencies they oversee. These models may alter the expectations, functions, and protection of the medical director. In an employee relationship, the medical director serves as a member of the agency's management team. He or she, like any other manager, may be hired or fired based on relevant employment law. The medical director's status as an employee may afford him or her a degree of liability protection. As independent contractors, however, medical directors may not have these same protections. The scope of their authority, protection, and subsequent liability will vary greatly based on their contracts.

A medical director may also provide oversight for an agency as an employee of a third party. Hospitals, physician groups, or academic programs may contract with outside organizations to provide medical direction. In these cases, the medical director has some degree of employee protection, but not from the EMS organization he or she is overseeing.

Many medical directors provide uncompensated services to the agencies they oversee. In general, organizations expect, and get, less support from uncompensated medical directors. This is a common model for volunteer and other smaller agencies. In some cases, this lack of compensation may offer additional protection to the medical director. In New York State, noncompensated medical directors are protected from liability by New York State Public Health Law: Article 30 Section 3013, which states that

> …any physician who voluntarily and without the expectation of monetary compensation provides indirect medical control, shall not be liable for damages for injuries or death alleged to have been sustained by any person as a result of such medical direction unless it is established that such injuries or death were caused by gross negligence on the part of such physician.

INTERFACING OPERATIONS AND MEDICAL OVERSIGHT

Medical director involvement varies widely among agencies. Some medical directors provide little more than a signature on a page, while others are a full-time presence at their agency. The more involved a medical director becomes, the more important it is to define his or her role within the agency's overall structure. This should be defined early in the relationship to avoid potential problems. Medical directors can be very influential, but they rarely have any direct subordinates. The role is frequently depicted as an offset box below the agency's CEO (**Figure 27-1**). There may be many actual or implied dotted lines representing influence over clinical personnel, education, CQI, and other relevant departments.

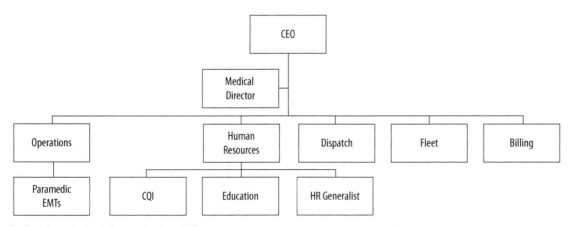

FIGURE 27-1. Condensed organizational diagram of a private EMS agency.

As the chief medical officer of the organization, ensuring quality patient care and employee safety should be the medical director's primary role. The agency's CEO, on the other hand, must balance a litany of concerns, including financing, staffing, external politics, and, in some agencies, fire suppression. Ideally, the medical director will serve as a strong advocate, while still respecting the CEO's other concerns. By understanding these other concerns, the medical director can advocate for his or her goals within the broader organizational goals. A collegial relationship between the medical director and the CEO is valuable for the smooth operation of the agency.

Medical directors who respond to calls should also understand their field rank. Field rank refers to their role in the on-scene Incident Command System. Medical directors may respond to the scene as part of the agency, part of another agency, or on their own. Issuing a medical director a response vehicle may not always be practical, but an agency may provide their medical director with a radio and call sign at a negligible cost. While on scene, the physician medical director has the final say on any patient care decision in the form of online (on-scene) medical control. However, based on field rank, he or she may defer to another on-scene incident commander for control of the scene and other big-picture issues.

EMPLOYEE HIRING/REVIEW/PROMOTIONS

Hiring new employees is arguably the most important HR role in any organization. Hiring clinical personnel can be challenging, and is further complicated when the hiring pool is limited to already certified (or licensed) individuals. By limiting the pool of applicants to those who have already completed certification, agencies may miss potential employees who would excel in the long term. A company limiting itself to personnel already certified will often look for potential employees who are either currently employed by a competitor, trained but working in another field (this is often true of volunteers), or perhaps unemployed with existing certification.

In a municipal system, new civil service employees are typically put through a formal examination process. In some regions, a single civil service test may feed new applicants into multiple municipal agencies. Initial qualification standards may include a high school diploma, college credits or degrees, residency or the ability to obtain residency, a driver's license, specialized training or certification. While the core of this process is a written examination, follow-up testing and additional points for qualifications such as experience or residency shape the final pool of potential hires. These secondary steps are useful for weeding out applicants who are strong tests takers, but poor fits for the position. Unfortunately, due to the nature of the process, it can be difficult to hire those who are poor test takers but would be good fits for the position.

CREDENTIALING EMPLOYEES

Once hired, employees must be credentialed prior to beginning work. An orientation and training period before new employees are able to function at their appropriate level of care is common. Ideally, the hiring process screens out employees who will ultimately not be able to be credentialed. Training employees who cannot be utilized can be costly for agencies. Nationally, 28% of paramedics meet with their medical director as part of this process.[1]

PERFORMANCE REVIEWS

Clinically and nonclinically minded managers may have different opinions when it comes time for reviewing an employee. An agency's best workers may not be their best clinicians. The best workers are employees who are team players, rarely call in sick, have no disciplinary actions, and always obtain complete billing information. The best clinicians rarely have QA issues, are constantly working to grow their practice base, and consistently provide superb patient care. Unfortunately, while attendance, billing compliance, and bad patient care are often easy to quantify, excellent patient care is often very difficult. The absence of clinical

disaster does not always equate to excellent care. The ideal employee excels in both areas. Depending on the job in mind, the relative importance of these qualities may vary. It is important that these issues be critiqued separately to give a fair portrayal of the employee's work and of the areas needing improvement.

RECOMMENDATIONS FOR PROMOTION

The most important promotion in EMS is the step between EMT and paramedic. Companies may incentivize this training by covering enrollment costs, paying employees while attending school, or extending them full-time benefits while taking course work full time and working part time. Factors that improve a provider's chance of success on the NREMT-paramedic exam include EMT-basic exam score and length of time as an EMTbasic.[2] Nonclinical personnel, such as dispatchers, billers, or supply techs, may apply for clinical positions. Promoting a well-known employee from a nonclinical to a clinical position may be less risky than hiring a new employee. The medical director can serve an important role in advocating for the clinical side of the position in relation to the relative importance of that new job role.

EMPLOYEE TRAINING

In order to obtain and maintain certification/licensure, minimum training standards must be followed. These standards may include national "alphabet soup courses" such as ACLS, PALS, CPR, ITLS, etc. Larger operations often offer these courses to their employees. Employers may pay for, and in some circumstances pay employees to take, these courses. Additional medical training beyond the minimum standards offers further opportunities for provider development. Beyond medical training, education in emergency driving, patient maneuvering, and company policies round out the new employee's education. The cost of training a new employee can be significant, making employee retention an important goal of any organization.

EMPLOYEE COMPENSATION

Companies must find a balance of offering employees an attractive compensation package, while still remaining fiscally responsible. If a company can do this successfully and can increase the percentage of payroll dollars allocated, it will be a strong recruitment tool for the best and brightest providers.

Salary is the most basic form of compensation, and varies among region, job type, and provider model. The Bureau of Labor Statistics has the nation's most comprehensive employee database; however, in the case of EMS, its data are muddied because they does not distinguish between paramedics and EMTs. The annual Salary and Workplace Survey by Fitch and Associates, published in the *Journal of Emergency Medical Services*, makes this distinction. When corrected for a 40-hour work week, the 2010 survey revealed higher average compensation in the east coast regions compared to the rest of the country. However, while correcting the data for a fixed work week is useful for comparison, the mandatory or expected overtime built into many providers' schedules becomes part of what they consider as their base pay.[1] Municipal positions tend to have higher salary and compensation packages, often including pensions, compared to the private sector.[3]

The EMS industry has a high risk of injury, particularly back, neck, and joint injuries. As a result, worker compensation is a significant non-wage payroll expense for agencies. In addition, as with any time off, not only is there a cost of paying the employee that is away from work, but also the cost of the replacement worker that must fill the schedule.

RETIREMENT

The physical demands of prehospital care limit the number of years an employee can continue to practice. As a result, employees are well served to consider their options for retirement savings early in their career. Young employees may not fully appreciate the value of retirement income, instead preferring to receive more money up front. The most stable retirement option is the defined benefit program (pension), seen predominantly in municipal systems. In the absence of a pension, employers can promote retirement savings by offering 401K plans and matching contributions. An employee's retirement plan, regardless of the system, is a crucial part of the overall compensation package.

EMPLOYEE REMEDIATION AND DISCIPLINE

Employee remediation and discipline is a reality in any organization. When faced with any adverse event, the medical director must first determine if there is a clinical component to the incident. Nonclinical incidents are not the purview of most medical directors. Driving, attendance, and uniforms are typically operational issues that fall outside of the medical director's jurisdiction. Medication, treatment, or other clinical error fall well within the scope of the medical director's authority. Other topics such as patient drops, medication/equipment theft, and patient information disclosure represent gray areas that may vary by organization or event.

Honest clinical errors should be viewed as an opportunity for professional growth. Medical directors should work to cultivate an organizational culture where providers feel comfortable disclosing their potential errors. Fear of discipline may lead employees to not disclose their shortcomings, and, in doing so, they miss an opportunity for growth. Once an issue or event is deemed to be clinical, the next step is to determine whether the event represents a provider error. Separating the employee's action from the outcome is often difficult. Critical errors may occur without a bad outcome, just as morbidity and mortality may occur in the absence of provider error. That said, there may be an opportunity for education and clinical improvement even in cases where the standard of care has been met. Not all clinical issues will rise to the level of the medical director. Minor events may be handled by supervisors or quality assurance staff. For this reason, it is crucial that the medical director set the tone for the way minor issues should be handled and which issues should be referred to the medical director. The Commission on Accreditation of Ambulance Services (CAAS) requires agencies to maintain a list of triggers for medical director notification.

In most cases, discipline for clinical issues should be reserved for intentional or overt acts, the most serious of which may result in the withdrawal of a provider's privileges. There are many levels of discipline warnings; verbal or written constitute the lowest levels of discipline. Suspensions or termination represent more severe levels. In progressive discipline, a step-wise approach is taken with successive events (**Figure 27-2**). Disciplinary actions should not occur to the exclusion of remediation. Withdrawing privileges may also be necessary if a provider is unwilling or unable to be remediated. Organizations may terminate an employee, making this step unnecessary. Alternatively, an employee being decredentialed may lead an organization to terminate that employee.

EMPLOYEE SCHEDULING

Scheduling will continue to remain a challenge for the EMS industry, as the nature of the industry requires 24/7 coverage. Depending on which type of market is served, call demand fluctuates by day, week, month,

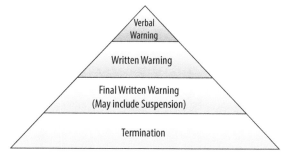

FIGURE 27-2. Example of progressive discipline steps.

Sun	Mon	Tue	Wed	Thu	Fri	Sat
				1 8a - 6p	2 8a – 6p	3
4 8a – 6p	5 8a – 6p	6	7	8 8a – 6p	9 8a – 6p	10
11 8a – 6p	12 8a – 6p	13	14	15 8a – 6p	16 8a – 6p	17
18 8a – 6p	19 8a – 6p	20	21	22 8a – 6p	23 8a – 6p	24
25 8a – 6p	26 8a – 6p	27	28	29 8a – 6p	30 8a - 6p	

FIGURE 27-3. Example of fixed schedule.

and season. A valuable tool used today is a *demand analysis*, which plots historical call data to best assess when call volume is at its highest and lowest points, as well as all points in between. Staffing templates are then designed in order to best meet the demands of the company, which in turn meets the demand of the community it serves.

The goal of scheduling is to meet the needs of the agency, as well as the employee. This is a very difficult balancing act at times. The EMS industry has long struggled with staffing appropriately outside of traditional business hours. Fixed schedules (ie, the employee works every Monday, Wednesday, and Saturday) allows a level of stability in an employee's schedule. Knowing that an employee will be working, for instance, every Saturday, is the strength and the weakness of this model (**Figure 27-3**). Many, especially including the fire service, utilize rotational shifts (**Figures 27-4** and **27-5**). The length and patterns of the shifts must be considered when creating a rotational schedule. By publishing shift calendars in advance, an agency can help employees and their families plan for their work obligations. By utilizing a hybrid of fixed and rotational schedules, agencies can account for standard response obligations and predictable variations in volume.

The most difficult times to cover are weekends and holidays. The dichotomy we experience here is that the call volume in a 9-1-1 system generally "spikes" during these times. In order to ensure coverage, many EMS companies employ an escalated pay scale during these times,

Sun	Mon	Tue	Wed	Thu	Fri	Sat
				1 24 hours	2	3
4 24 hours	5	6	7 24 hours	8	9	10 24 hours
11	12	13 24 hours	14	15	16 24 hours	17
18	19 24 hours	20	21	22 24 hours	23	24
25 24 hours	26	27	28 24 hours	29	30	

FIGURE 27-4. Example of rotational schedule with 24 hour shifts, 1 day on/2 days off schedule. Most frequently seen in fire service.

Sun	Mon	Tue	Wed	Thu	Fri	Sat
				1 Day	2 Day	2 Night
4 Night	5	6	7	8	9 Day	10 Day
11 Night	12 Night	13	14	15	16	17 Day
18 Day	19 Night	20 Night	21	22	23	24
25 Day	26 Day	27 Night	28 Night	29	30	

FIGURE 27-5. Example of 2 days, 2 nights/4 off rotational schedule. Shifts may all be 12 hours, or may be varying lengths—for example, 8-hour day shifts and 14-hour night shifts.

whether a "holiday" pay scale or shift differentials, which pay a premium for hard-to-fill shifts. There have been times where it has been necessary to invoke a "mandation" schedule. This allows the company the ability to force employees to work to meet schedule needs. This comes at a very high price; not only are employees paid double time, but they also suffer stress and anxiety. This practice should be reserved as a last resort.

Along with call demand, historical behavior of employees is considered when determining the proper schedule. Agencies often add or delete shifts dependent on the historical data of employee absences and late arrivals. They also build in a buffer to ensure that enough extra shifts are available for employees desiring overtime. This again becomes an expense to the company, as the absent employee usually has paid time off available and so is being paid for the absence, while a premium is required to pay his or her replacement. While this has always been a cost of providing good service, agencies attempt to limit the opportunities for unscheduled time off.

EMPLOYEE MORALE

Employee morale can be influenced by many factors, some of which the medical director may have influence over. In any profession, morale is tied strongly to job satisfaction. In the case of emergency medical services, job satisfaction can be bolstered by providing support to an employee in providing superior care. Educational opportunities, cutting edge protocols, and feedback all contribute to a provider's professional growth. The value of positive feedback, including case follow-up, cannot be overestimated. The use of employee feedback and advisory committees serve the dual role of improving operations and giving employees the satisfaction of knowing their voices are being heard.

OCCUPATIONAL HEALTH AND EMPLOYEE SAFETY

Preemployment physical evaluations are important for both the provider and the agency.[4-6] From the provider's prospective, physical evaluations ensure the provider will be able to perform the basic functions of the job without undue risk to themselves or others. From the agency's perspective, it is important to determine whether the potential employee is able to meet the physical rigors of the job. Making this determination early minimizes the cost of training an individual who will ultimately not be able to be utilized.

The first step in physical evaluation is to determine which physical qualifications are necessary for the job. Creating standards which are substantiated and applied consistently minimizes the agency's liability

of job discrimination claims. Many states provide guidance on provider fitness. Utah requires new EMTs to fulfill 12 criteria, including mobility, self-care, hearing, visual, and tactile.[7] Agencies may use these criteria to create their own policies for physical assessments.

According to the DOT National Standard Curriculum, "Aptitudes required for work of this nature are good physical stamina, endurance, and body condition which would not be adversely affected by lifting, carrying, and balancing at times, patients in excess of 125 pounds (250, with assistance). EMT-Basics must be able to work twenty-four-hour continuous shifts. Motor coordination is necessary for the well-being of the patient, the EMT-B, and co-worker over uneven terrain."[8] The 125-pound lift is a common criterion, with the 250-pound lift born from the fact that EMS providers commonly work in two-person teams. Individuals who cannot adequately lift put their patients, their partners, and themselves at risk for physical injury, and their agency at risk for liability. An analysis of back problems among EMS providers showed that employee fitness and satisfaction with their assignment were negatively correlated with a new self-reported back problem.[9] Some preemployment fitness-for-duty evaluations include a set of stations designed to test the applicant's ability to safely participate in occupational activities prior to initiating the hiring process. This is referred to as a work skills assessment, physical abilities test, or essential function test (**Table 27-1**). Some agencies will use a more job-specific test, with EMS tests and equipment in every station.[10]

Right to Know is the legal principle that an individual has the right to know about chemicals they are exposed to in the workplace. EMS agencies need to ensure they have material data safety sheets (MSDSs) for all potentially harmful agents in the workplace. Examples of potential harmful substances include medications, cleaning supplies, and vehicle fluids. A hazard communication program should be established to effectively communicate to all employees the identified agents within their workplace, as well as the location of and how to read and use all the MSDSs in the organization.

In caring for patients, providers are often exposed to patients' acute and chronic conditions. Prehospital providers, like all health care providers, are potentially exposed to blood borne pathogens such as hepatitis B, hepatitis C, and HIV. Fortunately, most exposures do not result in infection. Agencies should have policies regarding employee reporting and agency response to such exposures. Based on the exposure, the response may include risk stratification, postexposure prophylaxis, and/or employee and source testing.[11]

TABLE 27-1 Example of Basic Essential Function Test Components

Cardiovascular	
Single-Stage (Ebbeling) Treadmill Test	
Flexibility/Postural Tolerance	
Tolerances for crouching, squatting, stooping, kneeling, sitting-reaching, reaching overhead	Must meet unlimited level
Forward bend at the waist	10 times in 14 seconds
Strength	
Dynamic lift	
Modified lumbar Progressive Isoinertial Lifting Evaluation (PILE)	100 lb
Dynamic carry	
Carry 50 ft	50 lb
One hand carry 50 ft	35 lb
Dynamic push/pull	
Push 50 ft	200 lb
Pull 50 ft	200 lb
Grip test	
Right and left hand grip	Normal for age and gender

Best practices include preemployment and interval PPD tests, offering hepatitis vaccines or checking titers and providing tetanus shots. The availability of personal protective equipment such as masks, goggles, gloves, and gowns is an important part of an occupational health program. Safety devices and supervisors who emphasize safe behaviors have been shown to minimize the frequency of needle sticks.[12] These potential dangers such as motor vehicle collisions and attack by patients further contribute to the dangerous work environment that EMS providers face.[13,14]

Emergency physicians are typically well versed in these occupational health issues. The medical director's role in providing basic occupational health services is a source of debate. Some providers feel that performing both functions blurs the lines of their role. When two different physicians are used, it should be clearly delineated whose responsibility it is to take a provider off the street, as well as the reasons for doing so. Others do not see a conflict, and use the occupational health program to further interact with their providers. In some cases, physicians provide "free" medical direction to the agencies by which they are paid to provide occupational health services.

COLLECTIVE BARGAINING/UNIONS

Collective bargaining unions represent 27% of paid EMS providers.[3] Union membership is higher among paramedics (37%) and providers in fire-based agencies (67%), many of whom are also firefighters.[15] Many are not represented by unions that specialize in EMS. Many belong to unions that represent the trucking and freight industries, and to communications and service employees' unions. Organizations that are represented by unions that represent other EMS or firefighter unions may have a greater understanding of the issues that face both employees and management. The unionization of a company may alter the dynamic between the company and its employees, and may lead to a more confrontations between the union and the company.

The Teamsters, a large national union, typically collect 2 to 2.5 times a member's hourly salary per month in dues.[16] In exchange for their dues, employees expect the union will obtain improved compensation and protection for them, including collective agreements on working conditions, benefits, PTO, and wages. Improved compensation may take the form of increased wages, retirement plans, insurance, and/or time off. Unionized NREMT-basics and NREMT-Ps have greater earnings than their nonunionized counterparts ($32,094 vs $14,535 and $40,506 vs $31,386, respectively). This relationship remains significant even after controlling for factors like experience, gender, type of service, and type of organization.[15] Improved protections may come from worker safety measures and job protections. Unions will represent their employees in grievances including discipline and termination. This protection may make it more difficult to discipline or terminate weaker employees. It may also lead a company to deal with a good employee more harshly than they would like to in order to demonstrate consistency.

In "union security states," employees may be required to pay union dues, even if they do not wish to have union membership. A "closed shop" refers to an organization where all employees are forced to pay union dues as a condition of employment. In "right to work states," union membership and fees are options. Not surprisingly, unions tend to be less influential in right to work states.

The medical director is best served taking a neutral or no position on issues between the agency and the union. The medical director's absolute ability to decredential employees should not be limited by an organizational policy or collective bargaining agreement. Ideally, a union contract should specifically carve out medical director's actions as nongrievable and nonreviewable.

MEDICAL DIRECTOR LIABILITY

In our increasingly litigious society, medical directors must understand their risk. As discussed earlier in the chapter, the medical director's role and subsequent liability vary greatly based on his or her relationship with the agency. Potential medical director liability comes in various forms. The most obvious is medical malpractice liability. Most emergency physicians serving as medical directors have existing malpractice insurance covering their actions in the emergency department. Medical directors should check specifically with their carriers to ensure that their prehospital care is covered under their existing insurance. The provision of online medical direction is well established as part of the emergency physician's role within the emergency department. Off-line medical direction, as well as physician's actions in providing direct prehospital care, should also be covered, but medical directors are best served to clarify the extent of their coverage with their carrier.

General liability and *employee practice liability* are also potential pitfalls for a medical director. The implications for medical directors in regard to these nonmedical liabilities are still poorly defined. However, the limited number of cases in which medical directors have been named suggest they are perceived to have limited liability in these areas. Allegations of sexual harassment (by the medical director or his or her subordinates), unfair termination, or other employment actions are not covered by standard medical malpractice policies. Medical directors should understand their liabilities and protections in these areas. Protection from nonmedical claims may take the form of contractual indemnifications, municipal protections, director's and officer's insurance, or specific EMS medical director insurance policies.

- Medical directors should have an understanding of their role within an organization's human resources structure.
- As the chief medical officer of the organization, ensuring quality patient care and employee safety should be the medical director's primary role.
- The goal of scheduling is to meet the needs of the agency, as well as the employee.
- Medical directors may assume medical and nonmedical liability. Human resources issues are a potential source of nonmedical liability.

REFERENCES

1. Greene M, Williams DM. Jems 2010 salary and workplace survey: an employee's journey. *JEMS*. 2010;35(10):38-47.
2. Ferandez A, Studnek J, Cone D. The association between emergency medical technician-basic (EMT-B) exam score, length of EMT-B certification and success on the National paramedic certification exam. *Acad Emerg Med*. 2009;16(9):881-886.
3. Bureau of Labor Statistics. Emergency Medical Technician and Paramedics. *Occupational Outlook Handbook*, 2010–11 Edition. Washington, DC: US Department of Labor; 2010.
4. Collopy KT, Kivlehan SM, Snyder SR. Preventing back injuries in EMS. What's the best approach to avoiding harm to providers? *EMS World*. May 2014;43(5):23-4, 26-31.
5. Evanoff A, Sabbath EL, Carton M, et al. Does obesity modify the relationship between exposure to occupational factors and musculoskeletal pain in men? Results from the GAZEL cohort study. *PLoS One*. October 17, 2014;9(10).
6. Poston WS, Haddock CK, Jahnke SA, Jitnarin N, Day RS. An examination of the benefits of health promotion programs for the national fire service. *BMC Public Health*. September 5, 2013;13:805.
7. Bureau of Emergency Medical Services, Utah Department of Health. Technical, academic and physical standards for the emergency medical technician-basic. 2011. http://health.utah.gov/ems/certification/. Accessed May, 2015.

8. United States Department of Transportation. Functional Job Analysis. *EMT-Basic: National Standard Curriculum.* National Highway Traffic Safety Administration. Washington, DC; 1994.

9. Studnek J, Crawford J. Factors associated with back problems among emergency medical technicians. *Am J Ind Med.* 2007;50:464-469.

10. EMS Medic Field Physical Ability Course. Austin-Travis County Emergency Medical Services. http://www.austintexas.gov/page/ems-medic-i-field-physical-ability-course. Accessed May 5, 2014.

11. Exposure to Blood: What Healthcare Personnel Need to Know. Centers for Disease Control and Prevention (CDC), National Center for Infectious Diseases, 2003. http://www.cdc.gov/HAI/pdfs/bbp/Exp_to_Blood.pdf. Accessed May, 2015.

12. Leiss J. Management practices and risk of occupational blood exposure in U.S. paramedics: needlesticks. *Am J Ind Med.* 2010;53:866-874.

13. Maguire BJ, Levick NR, Hunting KL, Smith GS. Occupational fatalities in emergency medical services: a hidden crisis. *Ann Emerg Med.* 2002;40(6):625-632.

14. Maguire BJ, Smith GS, Hunting KL, Guidotti TL. Occupational injuries among emergency medical services personnel. *Prehosp Emerg Care.* 2005;9(4):405-411.

15. Brown W, Dawson D, Levine R. Compensation, benefits and satisfaction: the Longitudinal Emergency Medical Technician Demographic Study (LEADS) Project. *Prehosp Emerg Care.* July 2003;7(3): 357-362.

16. International Brotherhood of Teamsters (IBT), Frequently asked questions. 2011. http://www.teamster.org/content/frequently-asked-questions-faq#faq05. Accessed May, 2015.

CHAPTER 28

Ethical Practices

David M. Landsberg

Derek R. Cooney

INTRODUCTION

There can be no greater calling or higher standard for ethical behavior than that assumed by the physician. Our obligation to our patients is paramount and society expects that we conduct ourselves within this standard. We enjoy great privilege as part of our maintenance of these standards and likewise we are held emphatically to these expectations as well. There is little room for lenience among us when these standards are compromised. This is appropriate as the effect on patients, colleagues, and entire organizations can be profound. Public trust and decades of ethical investment may be compromised by the actions of a single transgressor.

The importance of these standards cannot be overstated. This is reflected in the innumerable organizational codes of ethical behavior as well as in federal, state, and local statutes. As physicians the most generally applicable reference is the American Medical Association's Code of Medical Ethics.[1] In keeping with the focused nature of this text we will constrain our discussion to how these principles affect the ethical management and oversight of EMS organizations.

OBJECTIVES

- Discuss principles of ethical management and medical oversight (honesty, responsible mentoring, maintaining objectivity, respect for colleagues, integrity, social responsibility, carefulness, nondiscrimination, openness, competence, legality, respect for intellectual property, confidentiality, human subjects' protection, responsible publication).

- Define *fiduciary responsibility*, and discuss how this relates to EMS administrators and medical directors.

- Describe work place harassment and how it affects individuals and an agency as a whole.

- Describe the duty to report, as it relates to illegal acts, unethical conduct, and impaired providers.

MEDICAL ETHICS

EMS physicians have the same ethical obligations as other health care providers. These are applied in a wide variety of circumstances, including during individual patient encounters, mass casualty incidences, and in management of medical oversight of an EMS system. Adhering to the expected medical code of conduct requires personal attention and a keen attention to EMS provider education. The protocol-driven nature of much of prehospital medical care can lead to unintentional violations of ethical standards.

Nonmaleficence: (*Primum non nocere*) "first do no harm." Acting in a way as to minimize risk to the patient rather than focusing on therapeutic interventions. It is important to emphasize this concept when considering protocol and procedure development. Some protocols and dogmatic approaches to clinical situations may lead to unnecessary interventions if too general of an approach is advocated or prescribed in the protocol. Routine placement of IV catheters may be an example of a potentially harmful intervention that could be overly prescribed based on wording of a protocol.

Beneficence: acting in a manner that in one's best judgment will benefit the patient. This concept is core to all areas of health care and must be constantly reinforced as the driving principle behind every act by every physician and EMS provider in the system.

Autonomy: the right to make one's own decisions, using one's own value system, and act on those decisions, without undue coercion from other people or influences. This is an important ethical concern that is sometimes difficult to instill in emergency responders who have been trained to act and respond to certain emergencies by protocol. It is important for medical directors to actively review policies and procedures relating to respecting patient autonomy and provide education on an ongoing basis relative to refusal of care and transport in the field.

Justice: attempting to maintain a fair distribution of resources, while assessing competing needs, rights and obligations, and potential conflicts with established legislation. It is important to ensure that emergency resources are appropriately distributed based on medical needs of the system. An EMS medical director should avoid advocating for positioning of EMS assets based on real or perceived financial or political gain.

ETHICAL PRINCIPLES

Medical ethics and codes of conduct commonly refer to a set of guiding ethical principles. One specific set of principles is shown in **Table 28-1**.

■ HONESTY

Honesty is a cornerstone in all relationships. It is endemic to any good work environment.[1] The consistent prioritization of honesty in the workplace is the foundation by which we meet many of our ethical responsibilities. Honesty demands accurate evaluation of employee performance and leads to responsible mentoring. It also fosters constructive employee feedback to their supervisors.[2] It supports openness of communication and the unfettered ability to maintain objective two-way communication. An environment that prioritizes honesty allows all members of the community to be heard without fear of reprisal and is absolutely indispensible to effect needed change as it allows for the objective identification of areas for improvement.

Honesty, including being honest with one's self, allows for the maintenance of objectivity. Objectivity is crucial when supervising others and leads to productive supervisory interventions rather than ones undermined by the showing of emotion or lapses that reveal more visceral responses. The constant application of objectivity demonstrates respect for your colleagues and peers and will only lead to enhanced effectiveness on your part. In your role as an EMS medical director, it is hoped that you will support scholarly pursuits for the advancement of the field at large and the professional advancement of your employees, your peers, and yourself. Honesty again plays an important role here with the respect of others' intellectual property. This includes the highest ethical standards in citing the work of others. Whether this is appropriate citation of other indexed works or balanced representation of authorship of scholarly works the same principles apply.

TABLE 28-1	Ethical Principles in Medicine
- Honesty	
- Responsible mentorship	
- Objectivity	
- Respect for colleagues	
- Integrity	
- Social responsibility	
- Carefulness	
- Nondiscrimination	
- Openness	
- Competence	
- Legality	
- Respect for intellectual property	
- Confidentiality	
- Protection of human subjects	
- Responsible publication	

Honesty again guides us when we are confronted with our colleagues' lapses in professional behavior. We have an ethical and often legal responsibility to report certain acts.[3] While we are expected to report illegal and unethical behavior, this is not always the case.[4] By not reporting such behavior you become an accessory to it and open yourself to significant consequences. We should always remember that when our colleagues act outside the rules, and do so in a way that we have become aware of it, they have selfishly jeopardized us and, in the author's view, enjoy no obligation from us to protect them. This, of course, includes the reporting of impaired providers as covered in detail in Chapter 8.

RESPONSIBLE MENTORSHIP

One of the most important roles of the EMS physician is mentorship. Ensuring success of colleagues (other physicians, EMS providers, agency/system administrators, community partners) leads to greater safety for patients and the public. Because of the public nature of emergency services, there can be temptation to withhold advice, support, and/or other forms of mentorship when political or financial gain may be considered at stake. Academic advancement may also influence EMS physicians in university-based systems and lead to concerns over credit for publications, research, and service or citizenship at the institution. Responsible and honest mentorship is key to contemporary and future success of an EMS system and therefore EMS physicians should seek and provide mentorship where appropriate.

OBJECTIVITY

Ensuring objectivity can be difficult when evaluating resource allocation, system and provider performance, and personal effectiveness. All these areas are crucial for success of the system. Maintaining objectiveness may require external review and utilization of multisource evaluations and national performance benchmarks. Maintaining objectivity is sometime threatened by concerns over poor performance evaluations and subsequent financial and/or professional consequences. Setting goals and reviewing benchmarks and trends may aid in maintaining objectivity while limiting the risk to individuals within the agency/system.

RESPECT FOR COLLEAGUES

In order for patient care and safety to remain the primary concern of all providers throughout the phases of care, all members of the health care team must show respect for each other at all times. Prehospital providers, physicians, nurses, technicians, clerks, and other staff must all share this important philosophy. One of the key components of ensuring cohesiveness is for all members of the team to acknowledge to roles, responsibilities, skills, and contributions of all the other members. Unnecessary criticism, negative comments, and unprofessional behavior all endanger this component of ethical medical practice.

INTEGRITY

The concept maintaining professional integrity is linked to all aspects of care and carer development. Ensuring accuracy in reporting medical information, clinical interventions, outcomes, and research data are examples of integrity. Conflicts of interest arise frequently when considering medical errors and coding and billing practices, but they may also arise in industry relationships. Choosing a particular medical device (eg, monitor/defibrillator) due to familiarity or friendship with the sales representative may even be considered a lack of integrity on the part of the decision maker because the foremost consideration should be patient care and provider and patient safety. Altering or manipulating system outcome data or research data is also a significant threat to professional integrity, even when the manipulation is not altering the information, but rather simply presenting it in a more favorable way.

SOCIAL RESPONSIBILITY

Social responsibility can be framed to incorporate any practice that contributes to the betterment of the community. Although the general focus of EMS is health, some of the activities of EMS systems, agencies, and providers impact other areas, such as happiness and prosperity. When a member of the community is sick or injured and the EMS system is activated there is a significant potential for that individual to not only be suffering a health problem, but inflated cost of health care delivery will impact the patient's bill, potentially to the detriment to their perceived prosperity and happiness. When significant costs are passed on to the community in the form of taxes designed to support emergency services, this can also have a negative impact. In addition to ensuring that provision of emergency care and preventative health initiatives are properly implemented, costs should be considered and efforts made to provide care and services at the most efficient level.

CAREFULNESS

Supporting the practicing carefulness in medical care does not that defensive medical practice should be instituted. Rather, carefulness here means that the provider will exhibit prudence and attention to detail in the assessment and management of their patients. This goes beyond the concept of simply adhering to the standard of care, but rather implies that the duty of the provider extends to also being literally careful in all aspects of caring for their patients. The risks of failure to adhere to this principle include all potential causes of provider fatigue, inattentiveness, and complacency.

NONDISCRIMINATION

Discrimination or profiling of patients, or even other providers, can lead to significant medical errors and emotional harm and cannot be tolerated in the EMS arena. Withholding comfort measures, including pain medication, from patients based on their sex, race, ethnicity, religion, or socioeconomic status can lead to major injustices and poor medical care overall. Discrimination also leads to a hostile work environment that may lead to impairment of a provider. The impact on the individual, the agency, and the system can be significant.

OPENNESS

Openness in health care is typically thought of as a principle necessary to ensure continued trust in a health care provider and the health care system in general. Although it is uncommon for a patient to suffer a poor outcome as a result of a medical error or series of errors, it is important to consider how to effectively, and openly, communicate these facts to the patient and/or family. The perception of a patient or family member later discovering that a provider was not open and potentially withholding this type of information would likely be that there was an intentional deception taking place. This may lead to mistrust of the provider and the system. It is also equally important to communicate realistic expectations to patient and families and to not ignore the need to discuss medical futility when appropriate.

COMPETENCE

In this context competence refers to the skill and correctness of the care provided by a health care provider. In order to ensure competence, initial and continuing education must be adequate, medical knowledge and procedural skills must be tested and verified, and providers must ascribe to up-to-date medical practices. A failure to maintain current medical knowledge and skills or a failure to enhance or adapt one's medical practice to meet current standards of care and medical advances can constitute incompetence. EMS providers and physicians must be dedicated lifelong learners to ensure competence.

LEGALITY

Laws represent societal standards and norms and health care providers are bound to honor these standards as members of society. It is the responsibility of EMS providers and physicians to seek changes to the laws and regulations that may stand in the way of best practices, access to care, and changes or enhancements required to improve the delivery of patient care. Improvements and changes to the system should always be sought through legal means.

RESPECT FOR INTELLECTUAL PROPERTY

During the usual practice of an EMS physician, a significant volume of what can be referred to as intellectual property is utilized. All original documents, presentations, techniques, devices, and business strategies could be considered intellectual property of the individual, group, or corporation that developed or contracted for their development. The medical and scientific communities have been trained on the value of sharing information and technology to advance health care. Although this seems to imply that the most ethical course of action would be to share all these materials and ideas in order to help others improve their system and care of patients, this would ignore another ethical concern. Intellectual property issues relative to medical practice in era of globalization have created a more complex view of this area of ethics.[5] The intellectual labor of individuals, groups, and corporations should be protected as their property. If this were not the case, then there would be a disincentive to invest in advancement and development of new health care strategies. These two seemingly opposed ethical concerns must be carefully respected. In accordance with respect for colleagues it is also important to consider that misrepresenting the origin of materials created by other EMS providers, physicians, and other colleagues violates both ethical principles: respect for colleagues and respect for intellectual property. When protocols, procedures, presentation materials, and other materials developed by others are used by the EMS physician, it should be done with appropriate citation and in some cases express permission should be obtained.

CONFIDENTIALITY

While we are all very familiar with HIPAA there is also widespread misunderstanding of what this means for practice improvement.[12] It was never the intent of HIPPA to constrain quality improvement initiatives. In fact the law specifically allows for "health care operations" as a permitted disclosure.[11,12] Patient's personal data must always be protected but review of that data for the express purpose of call review and quality improvement is absolutely legal. Organizations must have continuous quality improvement initiatives if they are to move forward. Wherever possible patient identification should be protected whenever the situation allows. For example, if a call report is to be reviewed with a group of providers for examples of documentation the name and address should be removed as they do not further the discussion unless that is specifically where the original error occurred. A high-profile call under review should not be hampered by the fact that everyone happens to know who the patient was but all care should be used to keep the discussion among the professionals who can learn from the events and no others. HIPPA compliance allows for sharing of protected health information for the purposes of continuous quality improvement and this right to review outcome data and pertinent medical records is expressly allowed for all "covered entities" which covers almost every EMS agency, provided they transmit any health care information electronically for certain transactions.

PROTECTION OF HUMAN SUBJECTS

As physicians we are always bound to our first duty which is "competent medical care with compassion and respect for human dignity and rights."[1] This fundamental principle is our fallback litmus test for clinical investigations and their impact on human subjects. We must always follow the highest ethical and professional standards when engaging in clinical research. The public trust is at stake and the mere appearance of conflict of interest here can be devastating to an organization. Institutional review boards are an indispensable part of ethical clinical research whose approval is generally required to get any such research published. The US Department of Health and Human Services has a specific Office for Human Research Protections to underscore the extent to which this is a regulated enterprise.

RESPONSIBLE PUBLICATION

Publication of new methods, research findings, and observations is one of the important contributions that can be made by an EMS physician. Maintaining a high standard for medical publication and ensuring the accuracy and validity of published works is a high priority in maintaining an ethical medical practice because inaccurate information published in the medical literature could have a negative impact on patient care. A great deal of trust is involved in the system of peer review for publication and skewing or manipulating findings threatens that system. In addition to ensuring accuracy of data and conclusions included in manuscripts, it is also important to submit unpopular or unexpected findings for publication, even if they are not favorable to the investigator in some way, as withholding this information may also negatively impact the care of future patients.

In sum, if we are always honest and act on behalf of our patient's best interests we will be acting like the physicians we all hope to be. "A physician shall, while caring for a patient, regard responsibility to the patient as paramount."[1]

FIDUCIARY RESPONSIBILITY

A fiduciary duty is a legal duty to act solely in another party's interests.[10] Parties owing this duty are called fiduciaries.[10] The individuals to whom they owe a duty are called principals.[10] Fiduciary responsibility implies the strictest duty of care defined in the US legal system. A fiduciary may only profit from their relationship with the principal if the principal has expressly granted this power. A fiduciary must be free of any conflicts of interest on behalf of their principal including the representation of other principals whose interests may conflict. EMS administrators and medical directors have fiduciary responsibility to their organizations. They must always act to the benefit of the organization. This applies not only to the strictest of financial management and appropriate allocation of agency resources but also applies to behavior. When we act solely in another party's interest it encompasses how we represent that party. Our professional demeanor, statements we make on behalf of the agency, and, in smaller communities, how we act when we are off duty all affect how an organization is viewed by the public. I hurry to include how we drive our emergency vehicles as one of the most visible displays of an EMS organization. Aggressive driving and overuse of sirens may demonstrate a lack of respect for the very community that we are ostensibly so eager to serve. Fiduciary responsibility has no time clock and you cannot punch out as long as the relationship exists. While it is a privilege, it should be recognized for the full-time responsibility that it encompasses.

WORKPLACE HARASSMENT

Workplace harassment is considered a form of discrimination. There are very broad definitions of legally protected characteristics such as age, religion, gender, and sexual orientation whose members when in receipt of unwelcome verbal or physical conduct based on these characteristics can claim workplace harassment.[6-8] The offended party must demonstrate that conduct is sufficient to create a hostile work environment or that when a supervisor has committed the offense it has resulted in change of employment status in the protected party.[9] Beyond the fact that this behavior is illegal, it has caustic effects on the workplace environment. Injecting this negativity in the workplace can only serve to divide workers and fracture morale. It cannot contribute to a shared environment of responsibility and accomplishment. This harassment alienates entire populations and undermines the authority of supervisors who commit it as even those individuals not the target of the harassment lose respect for the offender. When a supervisor is guilty of harassment the entire organization is at risk. The organization at large can only hope to avoid penalties if it acted decisively to correct the situation in a rapid and open manner. As physicians we must be cognizant of our responsibilities here. Whether an EMS physician is a formal member of an organization's administrative team or not they will be seen as such with clear responsibility to intervene both ethically and legally. These kinds of accusations can dramatically impair an agency's reputation with the expected public attention and media coverage. This is not how your EMS agency wants to get on the news. On a practical note be mindful not to unwittingly place yourself at risk for a casual comment in the workplace. An EMS physician must be professional at all times.

- There are 15 guiding ethical principles that all EMS physicians should understand and ascribe to.

- EMS physicians have a duty to their organizations and agencies based on their role as an EMS field provider and/or medical director, but they also have some fiduciary responsibility and a duty to protect intellectual property.

- Working to ensure honesty and respect at all times, and at all levels, is an important role of the EMS physician that can aid in daily operations and in all areas of medical direction.

REFERENCES

1. American Medical Association. Code of Medical Ethics of the American Medical Association: Council on Ethical and Judicial Affairs, Chicago, Il; 2012.

2. Murphy KR. *Honesty in the Workplace. The Cypress Series in Work and Science.* Belmont, CA: Thomson Brooks/Cole publishing; 1993.

3. AMA Council on Ethical and Judicial Affairs. Opinion 9.0305 - Physician Health and Wellness. Code of Medical Ethics of the American Medical Association. Chicago, IL: American Medical Association; 2012-2013.

4. Spickard A, Billings FT. Alcoholism in a medical school faculty. *N Engl J Med.* 1981;305:1646-1648.

5. Shah AK, Warsh J, Kesselheim AS. The ethics of intellectual property rights in an era of globalization. *J Law Med Ethics.* Winter 2013;41(4):841-851.

6. Civil Rights Act 1964, Title VII.

7. The Age Discrimination in Employment Act of 1967.

8. Title I of The Americans with Disabilities Act of 1990.

9. Equal Employment Opportunity Commission Regulations Parts 1600-1699.

10. Legal Information Institute of Cornell University, online 2013. https://www.law.cornell.edu/supremecourt/text/home. Accessed May, 2015.

11. The Health Insurance Portability and Accountability Act of 1996 (HIPAA), Public Law 104-191, enacted on August 21, 1996.

12. Privacy Rule at 45 CFR 164.501. Treatment, Payment & Health Care Operations.

PART II

Clinical Practice

CHAPTER

29

Roles and Responsibilities in the Field

Alvin Wang

Ernest Yeh

Gerald Wydro

INTRODUCTION

Traditional roles for the physician in EMS have involved quality improvement, protocol development, and provider education. In general, physicians do not typically provide routine EMS care in the field setting; however, the role of the EMS physician has been evolving. The National Association of EMS Physicians (NAEMSP) has issued a position statement affirming the role of EMS physicians in the field.[1] The role of the EMS physician is myriad and not well standardized as described in a 2000 field survey of the 125 largest cities in the United States.[2] Many EMS systems now provide mechanisms by which EMS-trained physicians can be called into the field to directly provide and/or coordinate patient care for unusual circumstances. These same EMS physicians can also provide real-time education, quality assurance, and online medical direction on routine calls.[3] In addition, direct exposure to the challenging field environment can help the EMS physician with protocol development and provider education programs. In this chapter, we will provide an overview of the roles and responsibilities of EMS physicians in the field.

OBJECTIVES

- Describe the responsibilities of an EMS physician on the scene of a patient care call.
- Describe the some specific responsibilities of an EMS physician on the scene of an MCI (details covered in Chapter 75), the scene of a fire (details covered in Chapter 65), and on the scene of a tactical operation (details covered in Chapter 66).
- Discuss situations in which the EMS physician should act as a direct, on-scene, provider of patient care.
- Discuss how the EMS physician's on-scene roles and responsibilities affect EMS provider education, CQI, and protocol development.

EMS PHYSICIAN ON THE SCENE

UNDERSTANDING THE CHALLENGES OF THE PREHOSPITAL ENVIRONMENT

Yet another benefit of EMS medical director field response is for the physician to gain a better understanding of the highly unique challenges of prehospital patient care. This level of understanding is crucial in protocol development, planning, and resource allocation. Although many EMS medical directors have had direct EMS experience as an EMS provider prior to becoming a physician, this is not universally the case. As EMS systems advance in complexity, the increased need for EMS medical directors has resulted in many non–EMS-trained physicians being asked to oversee EMS programs. This diversity of experience has proven to be a benefit to the science of EMS medical oversight as increased involvement also brings new energies and ideas to the table.

Moreover, each EMS system poses its own unique set of geographic, political, technical, and financial challenges. It is important for the EMS medical director to be intimately familiar with the challenges of the prehospital system that he or she is tasked to oversee. This degree of technical understanding is necessary to operate effectively as a medical director and can only be gained through the regular interactions with EMS personnel and patients in the field.

ENHANCING PATIENT CARE

Field response of EMS medical directors and EMS physicians may directly enhance patient care through the direct application of advanced skills and procedures that are out of the scope of practice for nonphysician EMS providers.[4] Some examples may include:

- Central-line placement
- Tube thoracostomy
- Field amputation of entangled extremities
- Prehospital ultrasound
- Awake, fiber-optic intubation
- Blood product transfusion
- Procedural sedation
- Prolonged treatment of patients who are unable to be transported in a timely fashion to receiving hospitals (**Figure 29-1**)

However, the presence of an EMS medical director in the field can enhance patient care in situations even without the need to perform these advanced procedures.[5] For example, physicians may be more adept at providing death notifications to family members in cases of

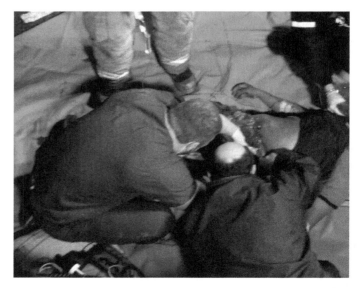

FIGURE 29-1. EMS physician performing damage control interventions after preforming a field amputation to free a severely injured patient who was hopelessly entangled.

field termination of resuscitation. In addition, additional clinical experience may also allow EMS medical directors to counsel EMS providers in making decisions about high risk but infrequently used procedures such as the decision to control an airway in a spontaneously breathing patient via RSI and surgical cricothyrotomy.

■ REAL-TIME EMS EDUCATION

Traditional medical education is built around an apprenticeship model which provides graduated degrees of responsibility and training as experience progresses. In the physician-education model with which physicians are most familiar, medical students progress from the preclinical didactic years to clerkship rotations, internships, and residencies. As medical students and residents progress through these education phases, learner-contact time with physician mentors increases in duration and intensity. In particular, during emergency department residency training, experienced attending physicians are generally required to be present "at the bedside" and/or immediately available to resident physicians.

EMS education programs are modeled in a similar fashion with didactic sessions followed by structured clinical rotations in various settings. Learners are given increased autonomy as their training progresses. Unfortunately, this is where the similarity ends. Unlike the physician education model, EMS students are often supervised by preceptors that are generally seasoned EMS personnel rather than physicians. Although these preceptors are expert field providers, as a generalization, they may lack the depth of clinical knowledge and experience that comes with the thousands of educational hours spent by physicians during medical school and residency. Moreover, because of the relative scarcity of EMS-trained physicians, when EMS students are exposed to physician-led educational experiences (such as emergency department, anesthesia, and ob/gyn rotations), the physician mentors in these settings are rarely EMS-trained physicians. Although non–EMS-trained physicians are unquestionably experts at their particular application(s) of clinical medicine, they may not be as familiar with the practical applications of their clinical knowledge to the myriad of technically challenging environments faced by EMS personnel on a daily basis. Lastly, upon completion of their training program, EMS personnel interaction with physicians may become limited to a few brief moments during ED handoffs, continuing-education refresher lectures, and regularly scheduled skill verification sessions.

Placing EMS physicians in the field can very effectively bring the strengths of the physician education model to the realm of EMS. An experienced, EMS-trained medical director who responds in the field can provide expert real-time guidance to a paramedic student who is preparing to perform their first field intubation. In addition, the direct "bedside" presence of the EMS physician can help guide learners and even seasoned paramedics through critical thinking scenarios such as whether or not a patient requires medication facilitated intubation. Moreover, the EMS physician can assist the EMS provider with high-risk, infrequently performed procedures such as needle thoracostomy, cricothyrotomy, and rapid-sequence induction. At the completion of a call the EMS physician can discuss the call with the provider and answer clinical management questions that will benefit the provider in future encounters (**Figure 29-2**).

■ CONTINUOUS QUALITY IMPROVEMENT FROM THE FIELD

Another role of the EMS physician is to provide real-time feedback and quality assurance. Many states require some form of formal ongoing verification of paramedic skill performance to maintain medical command authorization or licensure. Although there are often established methods of skill verification using patient simulators and procedure training mannequins, there really is no better way to ensure that the EMS providers are delivering high-quality patient care than direct observation in the field. Of course although there may be some degree of "Hawthorne effect," if it serves to increase the overall quality of care that is provided, then the desired result is still achieved. It is important, however, that the EMS physician takes care to ensure that this degree of close field supervision remains well received by the EMS providers. To help accomplish

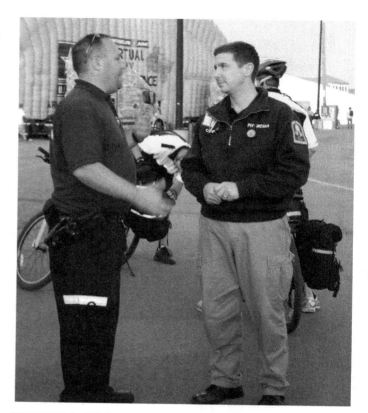

FIGURE 29-2. EMS physician providing real-time education.

this, when in the field, the EMS physician should be especially conscientious of their tone and demeanor. They should present themselves to their EMS providers as an additional resource to provide help rather than "big brother" who is only waiting to catch them making a mistake. Using phrases such as "What can I do to help?" instead of "Why are you doing that?" will help build this rapport. In addition, the EMS physician should strive to offer as much assistance as possible even with nonpatient care tasks such as carrying bags and equipment as well as cleanup and restocking after the call.

For the EMS physician to be directly able to participate in any of these field activities, various logistical concerns must be addressed. Although they can ride along as an additional crew member in an ambulance, the EMS physician is often much more effective when they can respond autonomously. This generally requires that the physician be provided with an emergency response vehicle which is capable of being equipped with, at a bare minimum, the same medication, equipment, and supplies as an ALS ambulance. The EMS physician will also need additional equipment to perform procedures and medications not normally available. In addition, the EMS physician must be able to communicate directly with the ambulances and the dispatch center. Thus, it should also be equipped with mobile data terminals and two-way radio equipment as well.

There are other issues that need to be addressed to ensure that the EMS physician is available for field responses. In some EMS systems there may be direct financial compensation to the physician or the physician's group practice for physician EMS. In other models, indirect compensation may be in the form of adequate protected time for EMS activities.

RESPONSE TO MASS CASUALTY INCIDENTS

Any incident that generates more patients who can be treated and transported by first responding ambulances presents a potential need for field triage. These incidents can be as simple as two patients in a rural area where the nearest backup EMS provider is more than 30 minutes away or as complex as the tragic sequence of events surrounding hurricane Katrina in 2005 which required the triage, treatment, and evacuation of hundreds of thousands of patients over the course of several weeks. Although several triage schemas exist and some debate exists as to which is the most accurate, a common theme among all protocols is that they are designed to be implemented by EMTs and paramedics, and do not mandate physician involvement. It has been suggested that physician involvement in initial triage and subsequent retriage can be beneficial in optimizing patient outcome.[6] Accordingly, traditional teaching is that the most experienced EMS provider (not necessarily the highest trained provider) at the scene should perform triage. Although not impossible, it is unlikely that the EMS physician will be the first arriving EMS responder at the scene of an MCI and initial triage will likely have already been accomplished prior to the arrival of the physician. Depending on the scope and magnitude of the incident and the length of time it will take to transport all patients from the incident to receiving hospitals, there may be a need for the EMS physician to further prioritize treatment and transport priority within triage categories. On the other hand, if all patients are triaged and timely transport is available, the EMS physician may best assist by leading the treatment sector for patients who are awaiting transport to definitive care.

■ NONTRANSPORT OF PATIENTS FROM MCI

In traditional models of MCI management, all patients are eventually transported to designated receiving facilities. However, in certain incidents, there may be a fairly large subset of patients who, although present at the scene of the MCI, may not be injured at all or may only require timely outpatient follow-up rather than an emergent ED visit.[7,8] While many EMS systems do not routinely permit treat and release (vs treat and refusal of transport) due to limitations in the scope of practice of EMTs and paramedics,[9] the on-scene EMS physician can perform a medical screening examination for these patients and subsequently release them directly from the scene (**Figure 29-3**). In this circumstance, the EMS physicians should be careful to provide adequate "discharge" instructions which may include recommendations for outpatient follow-up care.

The presence of an EMS physician at the scene of such an MCI can also be helpful in early mobilization of inhospital resources. Initial reports of patient information received from the scene are often inadequate and may be grossly incorrect. Moreover, the preliminary information from the scene may not contain sufficient detail to assist emergency department personnel in prestaging equipment, supplies, and personnel resources. While one might assume that the inhospital preparations required are the same for all disasters, in reality, the nature of the incident can dramatically alter the resources required. For example, a study found that 42% of the survivors required intubation after two confined-space

bombing incidents in Israel whereas only 7% of survivors required endotracheal intubation after an open-air bombing that occurred the same year.[10] An experienced EMS physician, however, if present on scene at the disaster can act as a liaison with the hospital by identifying these needs and communicating them to inhospital personnel in advance of patient arrival. A review of several studies found that frequently required critical interventions after blast injuries include airway management, tube thoracostomy, and blood transfusion.[11] The EMS physician provides superior medical capabilities and complex medical decision making, but should not be used to provide triage decisions, as there appears to be no benefit to this practice.[12]

EMS PHYSICIAN ON THE FIRE SCENE

Another role for the EMS physician occurs on the fire scene. Federal regulations[13] and industry standards[14] require EMS to be present at the scene of working fires to provide treatment and transport for injured firefighters as well as rehabilitation for firefighters exposed to the severe physiologic stresses of working on the fire scene.[15,16]

Various firefighter rehabilitation protocols exist but none have been proven to be clearly superior. Although all rehab protocols vary slightly, one commonality is that the firefighter must meet various physiologic parameters in order to be discharged from the rehabilitation sector and return to active firefighting duties. Although the rehab sector can be run by EMS without direct physician oversight, there may occasionally be times of conflict where the firefighter and EMS provider disagree upon readiness to return to active duty. In this situation, the presence of the on-scene physician can be very valuable in helping to make the "go/no-go" decision and can act as the mediator or the final decision maker between the two services. Moreover, the EMS physician can help preserve the working relationship between fire and EMS by acting as the "bad guy" when necessary to keep a firefighter in rehab or even encouraging transport to the hospital when necessary for firefighter safety. This authoritative/supervisory position may be more easily assumed if the EMS physician assumes the role of medical sector command under the Incident Command System (**Figure 29-4**).

The fire ground is a common scene for serious medical emergencies in both firefighters and civilians. Medical emergencies can occur as a result of direct firefighting activities and/or exacerbations of chronic medical conditions caused by the physiologic stressors of firefighting operations. The presence of an EMS physician on scene can help ensure that optimum prehospital care is provided in these situations. In addition, in the unfortunate instance of a firefighter death or serious injury, the presence of an EMS physician on scene may help improve morale when

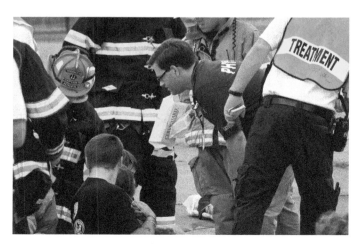

FIGURE 29-3. EMS physician working to help clear victims.

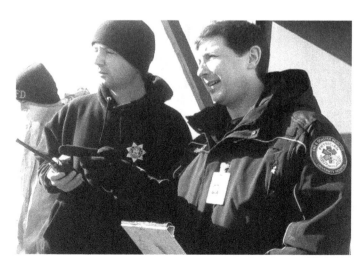

FIGURE 29-4. EMS physician as part of unified command.

firefighters know that their colleague was given every possible chance for successful resuscitation or reduction in morbidity.

EMS PHYSICIAN IN TACTICAL EMS

Yet another role for the EMS physician is to provide special oversight and care on scene of tactical EMS callouts.[17] These callouts are fraught with similar types of high-risk aspects as fire scenes with potential for direct injury to civilians, police officers, and suspects. Moreover, the weight of the body armor and additional gear carried by the tactical team subjects the officers to the same types of environmental and physiological stresses faced by firefighters on the fire ground.

Ideally, the initial involvement of an EMS physician should not be at the site of the SWAT or tactical team deployment. Rather, the EMS physician should be fully involved from the earliest stages of mission planning. They, or a suitably trained designee, should perform a detailed medical threat assessment to include consideration of factors such as environmental conditions, potential hazardous materials exposure, and nature and type of weapons that are anticipated to be encountered. This medical threat assessment should be provided to the mission commander during the planning phase of the operation. In addition, the availability and locations of potentially necessary medical resources such as aircraft for air medical evacuation, trauma centers, burn centers, and closest hospitals should be identified as part of the medical threat assessment. When possible, and only after receiving explicit permission from the mission commander, these resources should be notified and placed on standby prior to starting the operation. In some cases, advance notification may be deemed to be an unacceptable security risk as losing the element of surprise can oftentimes compromise the entire tactical mission.

Once on scene, the role of the EMS physician will vary greatly depending on the arrangements that are unique to each TEMS system. The ideal tactical EMS provider (physician or otherwise) is one who possesses superior tactics and superior medical knowledge and skills. While the EMS physician likely possesses the latter, if they are not afforded the opportunity to train and practice their tactics frequently, it will be difficult for them to maintain tactical superiority. Consequently, the practice model for the EMS physician at a tactical scene varies greatly. Some TEMS systems will have the EMS physician operate as a direct provider of tactical medical care and train and equip them to operate effectively in the "hot" zone. On the other hand, some systems have recognized that EMS physicians may not have the opportunity to maintain full tactical proficiency and thus train them to only operate in the "warm" or even "cold" zones of the combat theatre.

One potentially difficult concept in the area of TEMS is the concept of mission primacy. Although the goal of TEMS is to provide tactical medical care under almost any austere condition, the ultimate responsibility of the mission commander is to accomplish the mission in the safest possible manner. If the threat conditions are so high that the mission commander deems that TEMS operations cannot immediately occur at the time of injury, the EMS physician must recognize the judgment and absolute authority of the mission commander and remain ready to provide medical care as soon as conditions are deemed acceptable rather than rushing into a situation that is insecure and placing additional lives in jeopardy.

The astute tactical physician will recognize that none of the above roles are possible without fully gaining the trust of the officers and commanders of the tactical unit. To this extent, it would be wise to begin building an ongoing relationship with the tactical officers by participating with the team during their training exercises. The tactical physician should consider each of the officers on the team as their long-term patient and work to develop a rapport accordingly. Ideally, they should maintain a comprehensive and secure medical chart for each officer/patient and be able to access that information readily if needed.

In the event that of an officer injury or illness, the tactical EMS physician should, of course, be fully equipped and prepared to provide any necessary prehospital medical care and arrange transport to definitive

care. However, the role of the EMS physician does not end once the patient arrives at the hospital. If tactical operations are still ongoing, the EMS physician still maintains their responsibility to be present on scene if necessary. However, if scene operations are completed, the EMS physician should remain at the hospital with the injured officer to act as a patient advocate. They clearly identify themselves as the team physician and should liaison with the hospital staff caring for the patient and be ready to provide any necessary information regarding the patient's medical history, care rendered in the field, and so on. In addition, the officer's family and friends may have questions relating to patient and the EMS physician should, after consultation with the hospital's treating physicians, help answer these questions when appropriate.

- Field response will allow the EMS physician to develop greater understanding of the field environment, deliver real-time education, conduct in person CQI, and provide physician level services when the scope of the prehospital provider is exceeded.

- During an MCI, the EMS physician will likely be best tasked with providing treatment in the field, resulting in reduction of the transport burden on the system and prevention of some of the overloading of the hospital system.

- On the fire ground, the EMS physician can support medical operations through enforcement of rehab standards and by being present to provide advanced treatment decisions and interventions in cases of severe illness and/or injury.

- Tactical missions can be served by the EMS physician through development of a medical threat assessment, preplanning and arrangements for utilization of clinical resources, care of minor illness and injuries to maintain operator readiness, and provision of advanced trauma care in case of serious injury of an officer.

REFERENCES

1. Alonso-Serra H, Blanton D, O'Conner RE. National Association of EMS Physicians Position Paper: Physician Medical Direction in EMS. Approved by the NAEMSP Board of Directors July 12, 1997.
2. Cone DC, Wydro GC, Mininger CM. Physician field response: a national survey. *Prehosp Emerg Care*. 2000;4:217-221.
3. Catlett CL, Jenkins JL, Millin MG. Role of emergency medical services in disaster response: resource document for the National Association of EMS Physicians position statement. *Prehosp Emerg Care*. 2011 Jul-Sep;15(3):420-425.
4. Raines A, Lees J, Fry W, Parks A, Tuggle D. Field amputation: response planning and legal considerations inspired by three separate amputations. *Am J Disaster Med*. Winter 2014;9(1):53-58.
5. Hagihara A, Hasegawa M, Abe T, Nagata T, Nabeshima Y. Physician presence in an ambulance car is associated with increased survival in out-of-hospital cardiac arrest: a prospective cohort analysis. *PLoS One*. January 8, 2014;9(1):e84424.
6. Catlett CL, Jenkins JL, Millin MG. Role of emergency medical services in disaster response: resource document for the National Association of EMS Physicians position statement. *Prehosp Emerg Care*. 2011;15:420-425.
7. Mallonee S, Shariat S, Stennies G, et al. Physical injuries and fatalities resulting from the Oklahoma City bombing. *JAMA*. 1996;276:382-387.
8. Frykberg ER, Tepas JJ, Alexander RH. The 1983 Beirut airport terrorist bombing: injury patterns and implications for disaster management. *Am Surg*. 1989;55:134-141.

9. Knapp B, Kerns B, Riley I, et al. EMS-initiated refusal of transport: the current state of affairs. *J Emerg Med.* 2009;36(2):157-161.

10. Leibovici D, Gofrit ON, Stein M, et al. Blast injuries—bus versus open-air bombings: a comparative study of injuries in survivors of open-air versus confined-space explosions. *J Trauma.* 1996;41:1030-1035.

11. Halpern P, Tsai M, Arnold J, et al. Mass-casualty, terrorist bombings: implications for emergency department and hospital emergency response (Part II). *Prehosp Diaster Med.* 18(3):235-241.

12. Burén LA, Daugaard M, Larsen JK, Laustrup TK. Visitation by physicians did not improve triage in trauma patients. *Dan Med J.* November 2013;60(11):A4717.

13. Hackman, ME. Hazardous waste operations and emergency response manual and desk reference. McGraw-Hill Professional, 2002.

14. National Fire Protection Association (NFPA) 1500.

15. Farioli A, Yang J, Teehan D, Baur DM, Smith DL, Kales SN. Duty-related risk of sudden cardiac death among young US firefighters. *Occup Med (Lond).* September 2014;64(6):428-435.

16. Kahn SA, Woods J, Rae L. Line of duty firefighter fatalities: an evolving trend over time. *J Burn Care Res.* 2015;36(1):218-224.

17. Young JB, Sena MJ, Galante JM. Physician roles in tactical emergency medical support: the first 20 years. *J Emerg Med.* January 2014;46(1):38-45.

Scene Safety and Size-Up

INTRODUCTION

Practicing emergency medicine in the prehospital setting is rife with opportunities, special considerations, and perils not encountered routinely in the hospital emergency department. EMS physicians transport themselves to the scene, rather than the scene being brought to them as in standard medical practice. They many times initially perform the functions their triage nurse otherwise would, in a deliberate and expedited fashion. Patients in the field are seen at first in parallel rather than in series. The physician is given the opportunity to see the scene as a reflection of the general health of the patient, or as a first-hand account of mechanism of injury. Consequently, the physician is subject to the unique environmental dangers associated with patient care in the field that often contributed to, or are a result of, the patient's injury or illness. A successful EMS physician in active field operations assesses the scene, acts on this assessment, and mitigates danger prior to the provision of any patient care or evaluation.

OBJECTIVES

- Describe the unique dangers inherent to practicing medicine in the prehospital environment and list some specific potential threats.
- Define *size-up* and discuss the various stages.
- Define *staging* and give examples of when it is necessary to stage.
- Discuss potential additional dangers for EMS physicians responding to the scene alone.
- Describe some situational awareness tactics.
- Describe some ways to assist yourself and other providers in escaping a suddenly dangerous scene.
- Describe how to "take cover" on an EMS scene in case of gun fire.

SCENE SIZE-UP

Scene size-up is a multifaceted process that occurs before and immediately upon arrival at the scene, prior to executing any other activities. The purpose of scene size-up is to expeditiously ensure that there is a safe scene on which to provide care, and that the proper resources are summoned to the scene according to the number of patients and their specific care needs. Many scenes evolve even after the first unit has arrived, and various specialty units have different perspectives on the size-up of the same scene. The hazardous materials team will have a different focus and perspective during size-up than the first arriving advanced life support unit. Just as a scene is dynamic, aspects of the size-up should be reevaluated over the course of an incident. The components of scene size-up require simultaneous assessment and include the review of dispatch information, identification of the number of patients, identification of mechanism of injury or nature of illness, resource determination, standard precautions determination, and assessment of scene safety. These components of size-up can initially be assessed from the relatively safety of the emergency response vehicle (**Box 30-1**).

REVIEW DISPATCH INFORMATION

Reviewing and giving consideration to the clues given in the dispatch information should occur en route to the scene. Professional emergency medical dispatchers (EMDs) are trained to extract crucial information from the caller that will help determine response priority, numbers of

---

Box 30-1

Elements of the Scene Size-Up on Arrival

- Evaluate the scene for safety hazards ("the big picture").
- Take the necessary standard precautions for the situation (gloves, helmet, ballistic vest, etc).
- Determine the mechanism of injury versus the nature of illness.
- Establish the number of patients.
- Identify the need for additional resources (police, fire, additional ambulances, helicopter, etc).

Box 30-2

Scene Size-Up Based on Dispatch Information

- Exact location
- Type of occupancy
- Number of patients
- Situation type (mechanism, medical or trauma circumstances)
- Known hazards on scene (HAZMAT, agitated patient, road conditions, animals)

---

units needed, safety concerns, and even what entrance to use to reach the patient most efficiently (**Box 30-2**). They will communicate if there is a known presence of weapons or violent persons. When considering the dispatch information en route to the scene responders should be prepared for the worst case scenario differential diagnosis. The relevant differential based on the dispatch information can provide clues as to what equipment should be brought to the patient, and those pieces that might be left in the vehicle. Dispatch information may prompt the physician to bring specialized equipment such as a mechanical resuscitation device, an obstetrics kit, or a bariatric stretcher with plenty of manpower to utilize it. Dispatch information may also prompt a responder to request certain resources to scene before they even arrive (**Box 30-3**). Many dispatch centers have the capability to dispatch these resources automatically based on call criteria.[1]

Scene physical locations as dispatched can be vitally important in performing a size-up, and forming a mental framework for patient injuries or illness. A motor vehicle crash dispatched as "in front of the post office on Smith Street downtown" may prompt a completely different approach, response level, and injury differential diagnosis as compared to a motor vehicle crash at "mile marker 132 on Interstate 4." A dispatch to a "person down" at a cardiologist's office may evoke different concerns than a "person down" at a pediatrics office or at a drug rehabilitation facility. The location may also be associated with common circumstances and/or patient complaints/conditions. Experienced providers within the system might be able to anticipate these conditions based on the usual *modus operandi* of the patient or persons living there, know the best approach to the scene, and also anticipate specific hazards.

Box 30-3

Additional Resources—Request Based on Scene Information

- Law enforcement—violence or obvious criminal activity
- Heavy rescue—major entrapment or multiple vehicle collision
- Fire department—gain entry or when question of smoke, CO, structural problem, etc.
- Manpower—when MCI is reported
- Hazardous materials team—any time a spill, cloud of gas, or other major risk of exposure
- Utility company—downed power lines, gas leaks

Mobile wireless Internet connectivity and electronic charting permit additional uses of dispatch information in scene size-up. En route to a scene, a savvy emergency medical services provider or EMS physician could search the address in the electronic charting database, and for patients residing or transported from there in the past, the past medical histories, medications, and allergies, as well as prior reasons for emergency response could be immediately available. Scanned ECGs and patterns of emergency medical services utilization may also be available. There may be a different index of suspicion for illness regarding a patient who has been transported numerous times per year to all different area hospitals, as compared to someone who, despite their advanced age, has never before utilized emergency medical services.

Emergency medical dispatchers (or call taker) continue to gather additional information as the caller remains on the line, and will update responders to this pertinent new information. The review of dispatch information, as in all components of scene size-up, is ongoing.

IDENTIFY THE NUMBER OF PATIENTS

Expeditious assessment and reporting of the number of patients at the scene is crucial, as resources from outlying areas may need to be mobilized quickly. Identifying the number of patients and an attempt at quantifying the number requiring advanced life support or basic life support is key.

Keeping a list of patients denoting their approximate age, sex, presenting problem, and START triage designation allocates different resources to patients based on certain physiologic parameters. Various triage algorithms designate patients into four categories: require no acute care, require urgent but not immediate care, require immediate care, and those with no hope for recovery. The first step is to survey the scene from the vehicle, then make a quick walk-through of the scene if there are no obvious hazards. Some scenes may be larger than anticipated, and some patients are not identified until well into the incident. Using clues like mechanism of injury, trajectory of a vehicle, and sounds coming from unexpected locations helps the physician piece together the scene. Utilizing bystanders' knowledge of the number of patients is also a good tactic to estimate the number. It is important to remember that bystanders may have seen the unfolding of events that lead to the emergency, or may have taken some patients away from the scene for their safety. All nonemergency vehicles around a motor vehicle crash scene should be assessed for possible patients, even if it was dispatched as a single car crash. Emergency vehicles that arrived before you may be keeping patients safe. Many bystanders and passersby will take victims into their own vehicles to stay warm and safe. Patients may be scattered around, under, behind, and inside wreckage on the scene of a trauma and even furniture, appliances, and other belongings in their own homes.

More than one patient should be suspected especially in the following scenarios: two car motor vehicle crashes, car seats or diaper bags found in the wreckage, and twin spider webs on the windshields; if no one is inside the car check around the car and in front of it for ejected occupants. Exposures to the elements and environmental toxins often produce multiple patients.

Any scene should be approached with the questions, "Could there be other patients involved in this incident?" and "Are there more patients here than the responding units can transport?" If the answer is yes, multiple casualty protocols need to be initiated. Depending on location and system status, even incidents with just a few patients may require the simultaneous dispatch of units from over an hour travel time from the scene, and can overwhelm a rural emergency medical services system with few resources, or even an urban one which is already operating at full capacity. The term multiple casualty incident has replaced mass casualty incident in many jurisdictions, to encourage incident command processes in all incidents requiring more than one transporting unit, even when there are not dozens of patients. Arrival of multiple units from potentially different directions adds hazard as well as needed assistance and the EMS physician should keep this in mind when maneuvering on the scene.

IDENTIFY THE MECHANISM OF INJURY OR NATURE OF ILLNESS

In order to proceed with the appropriate evaluation and treatment plan, it is necessary to quickly identify the mechanism of the patient's injury or the nature of their illness. Is the patient dispatched as a "man down on the sidewalk" someone who is lying next to a mangled bicycle in a puddle of blood next to a patch of roadway with skid marks, or an older person wearing a jogging head band, MedicAlert tag indicating diabetes, and uninjured at first glance? One patient will require a rapid trauma assessment and law enforcement notification, while the other will require a primary medical survey and workup.

Mechanism of injury has traditionally been taught as an indicator of patient outcome and expected injury patterns. In 2008 in Victoria, Australia, researchers performed a retrospective analysis of 4571 cases which met the established criteria for high-risk traumatic mechanism of injury, but without evidence of injury on initial evaluation.[2] Forty five patients (1%) were considered to have major trauma requiring admission. The authors concluded that mechanism of injury alone is a poor indicator of major trauma, with the exception of entrapment greater than 30 minutes or fall greater than 5 meters. Although its application to patients without obvious signs of injury is questionable, traumatic mechanisms can be evaluated to guide the provider's history and examination.

Upon arrival at a motor vehicle crash scene, attention should be paid to evidence of impacts or rollovers such as bent wheels, blown-out windows, crushed roofs, and damaged trees, telephone poles, and guard rails. Rollovers and airbag deployment can indicate the speed of the crash, as well as the potential for secondary impacts. A bent steering wheel or dashboard may increase suspicion for certain thoracoabdominal injuries, and shattered glass increases the likelihood of bleeding wounds and foreign bodies. Windshield "spider webbing" usually indicates an unrestrained passenger with a head strike on the windshield. Items strewn about the vehicle should be considered projectiles of secondary impact to your patient. Nature of illness is the medical corollary to the traumatic mechanism of injury. Just as the condition of a motor vehicle can suggest an injury pattern in a patient, the scene of a medical patient offers many clues to the disease process before patient contact is even made. Patients may be in extremis or have communication barriers that prevent them from providing you history, but the scene can provide valuable clues.

During each phase of the call certain questions about the scene may be considered: *Is there garbage piling up on the porch, or a driveway that has not been shoveled for days in the dead of a snowy winter? Does the house smell of human waste? Is there a significant odor of tobacco smoke as the door is opened?* These conditions often reflect poor health of the occupants of the dwelling, and a social support structure that is not effective or existent. A home with the windows open in subzero temperatures and human waste in the living space may reflect acute mental illness or delirium. An empty refrigerator or thermostat set where air conditioning and heating are at an absolute minimum might suggest socioeconomic difficulties, which are a reflection of, and contribute to, morbidity. Medications that can foretell medical history might be present in cabinets or in the refrigerator, and drug paraphernalia may be strewn about the house. There may be old hospital wrist bands or bills from hospitals in the home, suggesting recurring illness. The presence of oxygen, nebulizers, and other medical equipment may also paint a picture of the conditions afflicting the patient.

DETERMINATION OF RESOURCES

Many aspects of a scene size-up serve to ensure that the proper resources are summoned according to the needs of the incident. Resource determination is one of the most important components of a scene size-up. Early communication of the number of patients, their mechanism of injury or nature of illness, and any safety barriers will allow for timely arrival of necessary units. Although many basic life support units are capable of transporting multiple patients, these patients need to be family members and have the same destination hospital. Advanced life support units typically transport one patient at a time. Therefore, unless there are related basic life support patients going to the same destination hospital, it is necessary to request as many ambulances as there are patients needing transport.

Air medical units may need to be summoned in situations of prolonged extrication, expected barriers to ground transportation, or long distances (usually 90 minutes' drive or more) to the closest appropriate hospital. At times air medical units are summoned simply for the fact that they are an additional transporting unit when no other ground units are available. Air medical utilization should be judicious, as helicopters are cramped, have limited treatment capabilities, and are associated with safety concerns. In most cases, air medical units carry advanced providers with additional skills, equipment, and medications that are beneficial to the patient or patients on scene. Some air medical units even carry packed red blood cells and other blood products.

Most major motor vehicle crashes will require a heavy rescue unit for stabilization of the vehicle, and sometimes for extrication of the patient. A wrecker is typically summoned as well, and all roadside scenes require traffic control from either law enforcement or the fire department. Asymmetry of utility poles on approach to a scene may indicate downed wires, and thus the need for the utility company to disable the wires. Similarly hazardous materials teams need to be dispatched for the following which are hazardous materials incidents until proven otherwise: motor vehicle crashes with tractor trailers, tanker trucks, alternative fuel vehicles, pesticide vehicles including those used for lawn care, and crashes of vehicles with mounted hazardous materials placards.

Specialized units such as rope and high angle rescue teams, wilderness search and rescue teams, and water rescue teams may need to be requested based on the demands of the scene. These teams may volunteer and require time to assemble and reach the scene. It is essential to declare a multiple casualty incident as soon as one is identified, so that mobile command centers and multiple casualty incident trailers or vehicles can be brought to the scene. These often have extra communications equipment, specialized staff, medical supplies, shelters, and climate control devices not found in a typical ambulance.

DETERMINATION OF NECESSARY PRECAUTIONS

Standard precautions are body substance isolation measures taken to protect health care providers from a patient's body substances, which are conservatively expected to be infectious. Determining the necessary precautionary measures is a component of scene size-up. All patients and care equipment need to be handled with impermeable gloves, and there needs to be anticipation of contact with secretions or respiratory droplets. The need for endotracheal intubation, hemorrhage control, delivering a baby, or exposure to coughing or sneezing patients all necessitate additional protective measures such as a face shield, surgical mask, and even impermeable gown. Standard precautions need to be determined during scene size-up so that the appropriate protective equipment is carried to the scene (**Box 30-4**).

Box 30-4

Personal Protective Equipment

- Head—helmet (rescue), safety glasses, ear plugs (rescue), ballistic helmet (tactical)

- Torso—uniform, coveralls, barrier gown (eg, Tyvek), splash-resistant chemical suit, reflective jacket/vest, ballistic vest (tactical or high-risk operational areas)

- Hands—exam gloves (eg, nitrile), work gloves (rescue)

- Feet—cut, puncture, chemical-resistant footwear with safety toe and shank, splash-resistant shoe covers

- Respiratory—surgical mask, N95 mask, or equivalent protection

---

IDENTIFICATION OF SCENE SAFETY HAZARDS

Surveying the scene for barriers to safety is the most important of all of the elements of scene size-up. The role of the first person on scene is to identify hazards which may include wreckage, hazardous materials, fire, downed wires, slippery conditions, or even violent persons or animals. The goal is to protect patients from unsafe conditions, but also to prevent responders and bystanders from becoming patients and requiring additional scene resources. Traffic is a constant threat on roadsides. Notification to incoming units should be made as soon as possible regarding hazards that are present. The 1994 National EMT Curriculum also advises that the role includes securing the scene, but this should only be done according to your level of training in dealing with hazards. Many EMS physicians will have no capabilities for managing violent persons, downed wires, or unstable wreckage or hazardous materials and may need to retreat from those scenes and await appropriate backup. It is reasonably within the scope of abilities of the physician to initiate the simplest of traffic control measures such as deploying road flares on a scene until other traffic control personnel arrive.

THE DANGERS OF EMS MEDICINE

Comfort, convenience, and safety features of the climate controlled hospital with a multitude of staff members, limited access entry, bright lighting, 24-hour housekeeping, and wheelchair and stretcher access scarcely apply to the prehospital setting. Field medicine many times is initiated in austere environments. Specific, unique, and many times, predictable dangers are faced by prehospital practitioners on a regular basis. Dangers that killed emergency medical services can be tracked and have been reported by the National Emergency Medical Services Memorial Service.[3] These statistics do not include the numerous injuries that occur daily in the provision of emergency medical services, but rather specifically fatalities. Physicians practicing in the field are subject to the same risks.

Routine occupational hazards of emergency medical services most often are related to the physical nature of the work: lifting and carrying bulky equipment and patients over uneven terrain. Analysis of the National Electronic Injury Surveillance System (NEISS-Work) revealed that for emergency medical services workers during the period of 2003 to 2007 the most common nonfatal injury diagnosis was sprains and strains, comprising 38% of all injuries.[4] The most recent year for which NEISS-Work data are available is 2009, with 57% of injuries diagnosed as sprains, strains, contusions, or abrasions. Arm injuries were less prevalent (9%) than injuries of the leg and foot, hand and fingers, upper trunk, and lower trunk which each comprise approximately 20% of injuries. The most common mechanism for these injuries was bodily exertion and motion during the care of a patient.

Bureau of Labor Statistics (BLS) Census of Fatal Occupational Injuries for 2003 to 2007 indicate that 45% of emergency medical services on duty injury-related fatalities were from motor vehicle incidents, and 31% were related to medical aircraft crashes, with these two causes alone accounting for 76% of injury-related fatalities.[4] Analysis of Emergency Medical Services Memorial Service data reveals that over a 10-year period that these two causes account for 77% of all on duty fatalities, with twice as many fatalities accounted by air medical crashes compared to ground motor vehicle crashes. Twenty percent of all on duty fatalities are accounted for by nontraumatic cardiac arrest.[3] The latter may be related to the physical nature of providing emergency medical services, coupled with exposure to night shifts and unhealthy nutritional options that have been linked to increased coronary artery disease, diabetes, and cerebrovascular disease.[5] The stereotypical lifestyle of the emergency medical services provider which involves high levels of stress, sleep deprivation, poor availability of quality nourishment, and night shift work may be as dangerous as any hazard on the scene. The general wellness, lifestyle, and behaviors of the EMS physician are as important in the lifetime before the call as they are during it.

Most fatalities occur getting to and from a scene. Safe travel, due regard, and judicious use of air medical services are crucial. Entering or exiting the response vehicle is a vulnerable time as well, and passersby may be distracted by the flashing lights and not drive cautiously and attentively through a scene: the so-called "rubber necking" phenomenon. Even with traffic control in place, some drivers will navigate around the measures, or fail to slow down at all. Motor vehicle crash scenes are among the most dangerous encountered in routine emergency medical services operations. Traffic remains a major concern, but there is also the risk of fire, exploding fuel, smoke, and toxic fumes.

Care equipment placed on the ground can become a trip point at any scene. The electrical systems of hybrid and electric propulsion vehicles are volatile and a risk to rescuers. Tanker trucks, tractor trailers and trains are prone to their own fuel exploding along with dispersal or incineration of their cargo which may be toxic. Dust from airbags may be irritating to the skin and respiratory tract, and the debris, including shattered glass and the vehicle itself are typically jagged and capable of inflicting injury. Debris itself and uneven or slippery surfaces from precipitation or spilled liquids present a danger of fall as well. Many crashes involve damage and dangers from utilities such as broken fire hydrants and downed electrical wires. Trees or other structures struck in a motor vehicle crash can be unstable following a crash and prone to falling unexpectedly. Response vehicles themselves may become a threat when their undercarriages, hot from a priority response, touch off dry grasses or spilled liquids adjacent to the vehicle.

Absent the calamities of a motor vehicle crash, domestic calls also present risks to the EMS physician. By virtue of medical or mental illness, many homes are not well maintained: cluttered passageways may become trip points, stairs and entrances may not have proper snow and ice removal, and in some cases the structure may be in disrepair to the point that there are sink holes in the flooring or even walls or ceilings that are in danger of collapsing. Stairs are many times steep, uneven, and perhaps not rated for several emergency responders and their heavy equipment. The family dog or other pets may perceive an intruder and attack. Smokers in settings where home oxygen is used, or where supplemental oxygen has been brought to patient by emergency medical services, can become the source of a fire risk and should not be tolerated during emergency medical services operations. Exposure to tobacco smoke second hand is a known health risk, and some scenes may be tainted with elevated levels of carbon monoxide or cyanide, particularly after a fire. Confined spaces such as caves should be considered hazardous spaces that emergency medical services providers without special training and protective equipment should not enter.

Patients themselves and their illnesses present their own dangers to emergency medical services providers. They are by definition, undifferentiated patients, and may expose the provider to communicable disease, or even violence as a result of delirium, intoxication by drug or alcohol, mental illness, or criminal activity. Those in the drug trade often suffer emergencies, and they are associated with large quantities of cash and sometimes weapons. Knives, guns, fists, and any object in reach can be used as weapons. Drug users may carry needles that can cause accidental injury to the emergency medical services provider. EMS physicians are prone to unique dangers. By virtue of a shortage of trained EMS physicians, they often respond alone and can be the first unit arriving on a scene. Their vehicles are typically smaller, less protected, and more prone to roll over than ambulances or fire apparatus. They may have a longer emergency response distance by virtue of covering several ambulance districts, and thus more prone to motor vehicle crashes en route.

First arriving units typically have minimal lighting on scene, and thus there is diminished awareness of hazards. Misrecognition of the EMS physician is of major concern: they typically drive low-profile vehicles that do not resemble an ambulance or fire apparatus, which may appear to be law enforcement vehicles. EMS physicians are not expected on many scenes, and may be mistaken for intruders. Further, many emergency medical services personnel wear uniforms with a badge, double breast pocketed button down uniform shirts, and a name plate that are analogous to law enforcement duty uniforms. This is particularly problematic on violent scenes where law enforcement might be particularly targeted, or where the public may have certain expectations of a public safety person appearing to be a law enforcement officer. There are case reports of the public requesting emergency medical services personnel to intervene in a shooting, mistaking them for law enforcement, perhaps due to their uniforms. Perpetrators of violent acts may still be on scene at the time of arrival, and may mistakenly identify the physician as a law enforcement officer and thus a threat. Also an emergency response vehicle may be thought of as an easy target for carjacking for narcotics, as a hiding spot or as a getaway vehicle. Some may view a physician as a high-value target for hostage taking or a soft target for domestic terrorism or acts of violence.[6,7] Some mentally ill persons call in emergencies for the sole purpose of an emergency response and the opportunity to attack public safety personnel, as evidenced by the December 24, 2012, shootings by sniper that occurred on the scene of a home arson, left two firefighters dead, two wounded, and one police officer wounded in the town of Webster, New York. Emergency medical services status does not offer guaranteed protection from violence, although some states have enacted legislation that makes assault of an emergency medical services provider a high-level felony.

STAGING

One strategy for avoidance of danger is staging. Staging is the intentional placement of public safety resource away from a hazardous scene. Generally, no matter the reason for staging, a staged unit is reasonably close to the scene, but far enough away to accomplish the goals of staging. Typically if a scene is in view of the responder, they are too close and the hazard may be within reach of the provider. A case report describes a law enforcement officer and ambulance crew being put into immediate danger as the ambulance parked close to the scene, someone from the scene saw and approached the ambulance, prompting the officer to attempt to secure the scene immediately rather than waiting for backup as planned. The staging distance from the scene increases on incidents with heightened threat level or congestion on scene.

Staging is indicated at any incident where hazards such violence are predicted. Motor vehicle crashes involving spilled liquids, vehicles that are smoldering, smoking, or on fire all require staging, as do known hazardous materials incidents. It is generally advisable to park several thousand feet upwind of these incidents, but this will vary according to the instructions of the hazardous materials team and incident commander. Any call dispatched as a domestic dispute, injuries from an assault, a suicidal patient, an overdose, or mentally ill patient should involve staging by emergency medical services, should be considered high risk for continued violence, and law enforcement should be utilized to secure the scene first.

Another indication for staging is the organized movement of resources in and out of congested incidents. Large incidents may require a *staging officer* who will coordinate influx of resources from and to a staging area to the scene, to provide for easy egress of patients from congested scenes. Examples might include a school bus wreck with multiple patients on a single lane road, where space for emergency vehicles at the scene is limited, where heavy equipment is being utilized for extrication, and only one ambulance at a time can approach the scene. Staging is also useful on multiple agency incidents where units in the staging area will relieve or supplement units currently at the scene, either as they expend their resources (such as water for firefighting), require rest, or are ready to transport one of multiple patients. Units may proceed into the scene when the scene is declared safe by law enforcement, or under the direction of the incident commander.

SITUATIONAL AWARENESS

Being aware of clues to danger and avoiding dangerous situations are much more effective at evading harm than the best defensive or escape tactics. EMS physicians should be maximally aware of their surrounding at any scene. This usually involves utilizing all the light available: take down lights on the vehicle, interior lights in the home, the vehicle's high beams, a spotlight or a high-intensity flash light held at arm's distance from your body. Lighting will help identify patients, scene hazards including uneven ground, and those in hiding who might attempt to harm responders. Be aware of items on and around the patient that could be used as a weapon in the event that they become agitated. Female patients and bystanders should not be underestimated as potential assailants. Responders must also be cognizant of multiple patients exhibiting similar symptoms: they may have had a toxic exposure, and you may be in the "hot zone" of a hazardous materials incident, and the EMS physicians may need to retreat and have patients decontaminated prior to initiating patient care.

RESIDENCES

Residences provide numerous opportunities for safety awareness. Prior to entry, inspection of the ground, identifying uneven or slippery or unstable surfaces, and checking for potential hazards will help mitigate risk of potential injury to providers. Providers should announce their presence by knocking and standing behind a wall, to the side of the door knob while identifying themselves as "EMS" or "ambulance." Upon entering, quickly identify a primary and secondary exit. The primary exit is typically the route taken into the scene. A secondary exit can be any method of egress: a window, rear door, or fire escape. The display of drugs or weapons, which so often are coincident, should prompt immediate retreat. If encountering lab equipment, large quantities of over-the-counter cold remedies or camping fuel and lye, containers of unexpected chemicals, heating devices or chemical waste, elaborate ventilation or heating devices and glassware, responders should suspect the

presence of a clandestine drug lab. These types of items may also be related to explosives making. Such scenes are not safe, are often booby trapped to evade evidence collection and detection, and need to be cleared by experts.

MOTOR VEHICLES

Scenes involving motor vehicles require special awareness. The first arriving unit should position their vehicle at least 15 feet behind the stopped vehicle, angled 10° to the driver's side, with wheels turned all the way to the left. This vehicle positioning will provide some cover utilizing the vehicle's engine block and wheels should retreat be needed. A properly marked and equipped EMS physician vehicle may help identify you and your role (**Figure 30-1**). After dark high beams and spotlights should be used to illuminate the vehicle, and responders should not walk between the lights and the vehicle, as this will outline their silhouette. The license plate number should be called into dispatch. Holding a flashlight at arm's length away may confuse a would-be assailant about the responders center of mass. The American National Standards Institute and the International Safety Equipment Association (ANSI/ISEA) publishes standards for safety equipment for public safety, and their most recent standard is ANSI 207 for wearable vests which have a specified amount of high-visibility fabric and specified amount of reflective material, yet also provide access to equipment that might be carried on a tool belt.[8] "EMS PHYSICIAN" reflective lettering will serve to identify the physician and their role on the scene to patients, bystanders, and other personnel, and also provide some protection on the roadway (**Figure 30-2**).

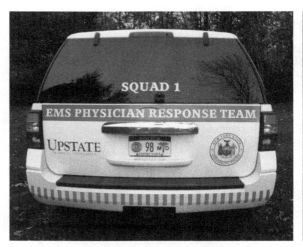
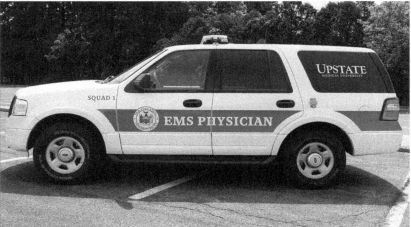
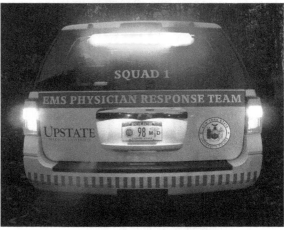
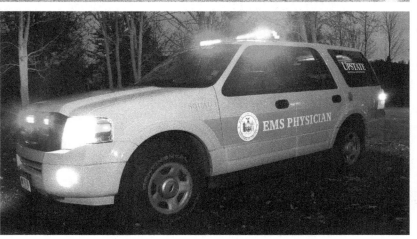

FIGURE 30-1. EMS physician response vehicle with markings and lights.

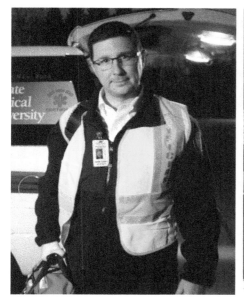 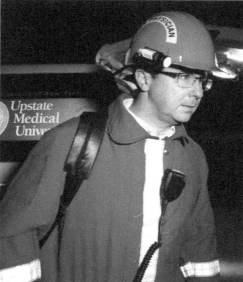 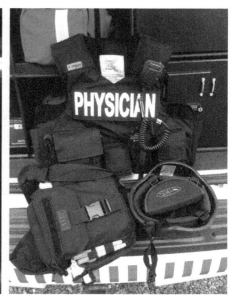

FIGURE 30-2. EMS physician personal protective garments. **A**: Reflective road-side vest. **B**: Flash-resistant Nomex and rescue helmet with light. **C**: Level IIIa ballistic vest and helmet, tactical glasses, and tactical medical support shoulder pack.

If there are multiple responders, only one should approach an unknown vehicle, while others await instructions. They can radio for help and retreat in the event of trouble. The responder approaching the vehicle should approach as close to the passenger's side trunk as possible, front body facing the vehicle; they should then stop at the C post, assess for patients in the rear including positions of their hands, any weapons that might be present, and then if safe to do so, may proceed to the B post to perform the same assessment of the front passengers, prior to initiating care. Vans require careful attention to not being pulled into the van's sliding door. If weapons or drugs are seen, an aggressive stance is taken, or there is an unusual silence or other suspicion about danger, the responder(s) should retreat, stage, and await law enforcement.

ESCAPING A HOSTILE ENVIRONMENT

Many escalating violent or otherwise unsafe scenes will require retreat to a safe location. Retreating from danger should always be the first priority in these cases, as it is the most likely method of avoiding harm, and is the legal expectation in many jurisdictions. Some states stipulate that EMS expend all options of escape and have a duty to retreat before utilizing force. In other states, so-called "Stand Your Ground" statutes apply, in that an individual may be justified in using physical force, including deadly force, if they feel their life is being threatened, they are not engaged in unlawful activity and have a right to be in their current location. Regardless of the law in any practice location, retreat is probably the safest option for all parties involved.

Retreat will become much simpler if the provider has made it habit to keep at least one exit accessible at all times, always has an escape route planned, and has not let the patient or other unknown persons come between the provider and the exit. If in the vehicle, a provider should quickly back away from the scene and call for help, noting the number of aggressors and their descriptions, injuries inflicted, weapons involved, the make, model, license number of any involved vehicles, and their direction of travel. Many radio units are equipped with red or orange "emergency" buttons that will broadcast a distress call to dispatch and other units or will interrupt any other radio traffic in the event of an emergency such as these. These can sometimes be used as "silent alarms" if it is not possible to speak into your radio, and if a

law enforcement response to the scene occurs any time the button is activated.

Throwing the "first in" bag or clipboard at the aggressor has been discussed as a distraction to facilitate escape, although this may further aggravate a would-be assailant. Wedging an ambulance stretcher in a doorway to block an aggressor as well as closing doors during the retreat may afford valuable time to escape. As in a hazardous materials incident, the distance between from a dangerous person significantly decreases the risk of harm. As soon as possible, activate the radio's emergency button and call for help.

CONCEALMENT AND COVER

Escapes are sometimes at least temporarily impossible, and the objective becomes to quickly find cover from danger. The concept of cover is to position an impenetrable (or at least bullet resistant) object between the responder and the assailant. Examples of cover include certain large trees, brick walls, utility poles, steel dumpsters, concrete barriers, vehicle engine blocks, and deep depressions in the ground. Some hardwood furniture and solid appliances provide at least limited cover, and door and window frames tend to be more reinforced than walls. The walls of an ambulance treatment area are not bullet resistant. Typically, only the wheels, and possibly the engine block would provide some cover.

When there is no immediate option for cover, the secondary goal is to achieve concealment, during which the responder would position themself so your assailant's view is obstructed. Concealing objects can be penetrated by bullets, and become shrapnel. Hollow cinder blocks, small trees, and walls provide concealment but not cover. Soft furniture like a sofa or chair, walls, and dark rooms and shadows provide concealment. The objective is to achieve cover as soon as feasible, and that the area with cover takes you further from the hostility, and can be reached without alerting the aggressor to your position. The ambulance treatment area is concealment; however, concealment does not work if the assailant knows you location. Before moving, reassessment of the intended destination and current concealment should occur, then movement should be low to the ground, in a zigzag pattern, and against a structure whenever possible. This will minimize the probability of being hit with a bullet, although ricochet off a wall can still occur.

PROTECTIVE EQUIPMENT AND DEFENSE

Situations may arise where concealment or cover is not an immediate option, or is limited. Sometimes responders may be caught completely by surprise, although situational awareness should minimize this. Ballistic vests may play a role in these situations and are mandated by some emergency medical services, while others allow their providers to wear them if they choose, but may require them to be concealed under a uniform. They are offered in various levels of protection, and typically protect the torso from different types of projectiles. The lightest vests are slash resistant, and increase in weight to produce resistance to small caliber rounds. The heaviest vests incorporate so-called "rifle plates," and increase in weight to nearly 20 pounds to provide protection from large caliber "armor piercing" rounds and high-powered rifles, but are impractical in most EMS operations. Even when successfully employed the vest may not be penetrated by the projectile, but the kinetic energy may still cause injuries due to blunt trauma and secondary impacts from a fall. The vests typically lose their resistance to penetration after successive hits. The legs, extremities, face, and head are still exposed. Further, shrapnel may still cause injury. Ballistic helmets are worn by some tactical emergency medical services units, but are unwieldy for everyday use. Figure 30-2 shows different personal protective garments, including a level IIIa ballistic vent and helmet (right panel).

Faced with a situation where immediate cover or retreat is not possible, the question is whether to resist a potential attacker. Studies on this topic reveal contradictory results. Unarmed resistance to a crime is positively correlated with increased injuries to the victim, and one study showed that during a retail robbery, unarmed store clerks that resisted were 50 times more likely to be killed than those who did not resist. Arming emergency medical services professionals is controversial, and a study published in the *American Journal of Public Health* suggests that people carrying guns were 4.5 times as likely as their unarmed counterparts to be shot, and 4.2 times as likely to be killed.[9] This might be attributed to overconfidence, perceived threat by the aggressor, and decreased likelihood of an expedited retreat. They were also more likely to be shot when given the opportunity to defend themselves. Whether this study of nonpublic safety citizens applies to emergency medical services providers is also debatable. Another study of gun use in resistance to crime shows that armed women were 2.5 times less likely to be injured than their unarmed counterparts, and men were 1.5 times less likely to be injured.[10]

Practicing EMS medicine is particularly rewarding for the physicians who routinely partake in field response; however, the field is uncontrolled and each scene must be approached with the utmost caution. It is only after the scene has been thoroughly assessed, the risks to the EMS physician recognized and evaluated on every call, and the proper steps taken to mitigate danger, that provision of care can commence.

- Scene size-up begins at the time of dispatch and continues through every phase of the call.
- Be cognizant of operational limitations and consider calling for additional resources early.
- Retreat is usually the best option when detecting a threat.
- Personal protective equipment and situational awareness are keys to avoiding foreseeable injury.
- Areas that can provide ballistic cover include large trees, brick walls, dumpsters, and the vehicle engine block.
- EMS physicians should understand the differences and applicability between the concepts of concealment and cover.

REFERENCES

1. Hardeland C, Olasveengen TM, Lawrence R, et al. Comparison of medical priority dispatch (MPD) and criteria based dispatch (CBD) relating to cardiac arrest calls. *Resuscitation.* May 2014;85(5):612-616.
2. Boyle MJ, Smith EC, Archer F. Is mechanism of injury alone a useful predictor of major trauma? *Injury.* September 2008;39(9):986-992.
3. National EMS Memorial Service. Breakdown by cause. National Emergency Medical Services Memorial Service. 2012. http://nemsms.org/press_stats.shtm.
4. Reichard AA, Marsh SM, Moore PH. Fatal and nonfatal injuries among emergency medical technicians and paramedics. *Prehosp Emerg Care.* October-December 2011;15(4):511-517.
5. Scheer FA, Hilton MF, Mantzoros CS, Shea SA. Adverse metabolic and cardiovascular consequences of circadian misalignment. *Proc Natl Acad Sci U S A.* March 17, 2009 17;106(11):4453-4458.
6. Thompson J, Rehn M, Lossius H, Lockey D. Risks to emergency medical responders at terrorist incidents: a narrative review of the medical literature. *Crit Care.* September 24, 2014;18(5):521.
7. Dickinson E. Crosshairs on EMS. Responding to MCIs caused by low-tech terrorism. *JEMS.* September 2013;38(9):46-51.
8. American National Standards Institute, International Safety Equipment Administration. ANSI/ISEA 207-2006 American National Standard for High-Visibility Safety Vests. December 2006.
9. Branas CC, Richmond TS, Culhane DP, Ten Have TR, Wiebe DJ. Investigating the link between gun possession and gun assault. *Am J Public Health.* November 2009;99(11):2034-2040.
10. Kleck G, Gertz M. Armed resistance to crime: the prevalence and nature of self-defense with a gun. *J Crim Law Criminol.* Autumn 1995;86(1):150-187.

CHAPTER 31

Emergency Vehicles

Derek R. Cooney

Jeff Larson

INTRODUCTION

There are a variety of specially designed and equipped vehicles in service as part of the emergency response system in almost every community in North America. These vehicles all serve unique roles and provide benefits, as well as hazards. Some hazards of operation are generalized to the operation of an emergency vehicle and others are specific to different types. EMS physicians must be familiar with these vehicles, their roles, hazards, and capabilities to ensure the physician's maximum safety and effectiveness in the field. Operation of an emergency vehicle is both a privilege and a potentially dangerous activity if care in operation is not observed. This chapter will describe emergency vehicle types and discuss the basics of safe operation. The authors recommend formal training for anyone operating an emergency vehicle.

OBJECTIVES

- Describe common types of emergency service vehicles.
- Discuss the basic principles of safe emergency vehicle operation.
- Describe usual traffic law exceptions and limitations.
- Discuss vehicle placement at the scene and proper parking technique.
- Detail types of emergency vehicle lighting and usual minimum standards for lights and audible warning equipment.
- Discuss the proper use of audible warning equipment during emergency response, and describe the limitations and dangers of their use.
- Discuss some of the common dangers to prehospital providers while operating, and providing care within, emergency vehicles.
- Discuss the merits of nonemergency response for EMS physicians, and other secondary responders.
- Discuss basic vehicle maintenance and out-of-service vehicles.

EMERGENCY VEHICLES

▨ AMBULANCES

Ambulances are emergency vehicles that are specially designed and equipped to provide for medical care and transport of patients typically in the recumbent position. In the United States, these are typically larger vehicles. Three main ambulance design types are prevalent and offer different advantages and disadvantages. Several ambulance standards exist, including those composed by the American Ambulance Association (AAA), the US General Services Administration (GSA): KKK-A-1822F, and the National Fire Protection Association (NFPA): 1917. EMS physicians must understand the differences in the basic ambulance types and should also take the time to review local, state, and federal standards. The ambulance types described below are based on industry common language and not representative of the "typed resources definitions" used by the Federal Emergency Management Agency (FEMA). These are briefly described later in this chapter.

Type I A type I ambulance is built on a truck chassis and the patient compartment typically is shaped like a large rectangular box with a double door on the back and a single side door at the front of the right-hand side of the box (**Figure 31-1**). Because the patient care area is mounted on the truck chassis, there is typically only a very limited pass-through into the driver's compartment. The increased load-bearing capacity of this ambulance type allows for larger patient care areas and makes this

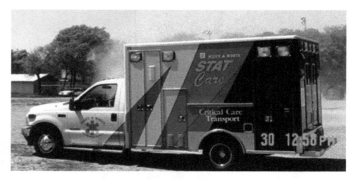

FIGURE 31-1. Type I ambulance. Photo depicts a type I ambulance used for critical care interfacility transport and for scene calls. Note the truck cab front.

type more ideal for complex critical care transport configurations. This type is also sometimes preferred by rural agencies who seek to equip their agency with four-wheel drive units or combination departments with the need to carry additional rescue equipment on their ambulance. The potential downside of the type I ambulance is that it may seem less maneuverable than other types. Some type I ambulances are very large and are based on trucks that more closely resemble construction vehicles rather than pickup trucks. These larger-scale type I ambulances are sometimes referred to as "additional duty" or "medium-duty" (**Figure 31-2**).

Type II A type II ambulance closely resembles a full-size conversion van. Based on the standard full-size utility van, this type typically has an elevated ceiling in the patient care compartment to allow for enough room to load, unload, and provide care en route (**Figure 31-3**). Type II ambulances are relatively maneuverable and more economical. The smaller patient care area may limit their use in interfacility transport and equipment storage can be limited, or at times quite awkward in some configurations. Some systems use them only for basic life support calls.

Type III A type III ambulance is similar in general appearance to a type I ambulance; however, they are based on a large van chassis rather than a truck (**Figure 31-4**). The van cab is maintained but the patient care area is a rectangular box similar to that of the type I. These typically have a lower load-bearing capacity than the type I. The customized patient care area is usually adequate to support all types of standard field and interfacility advanced life support operations. Due to the fact that this type is based on a van chassis, there is usually a larger pass-through into the driver's compartment from the back.

Type IV A type IV ambulance is a term used by some, but not all, members of the EMS industry to refer to ground ambulances that do not conform to the above configurations. These typically mean small motorized (gas or electric) vehicles that have been customized to service in

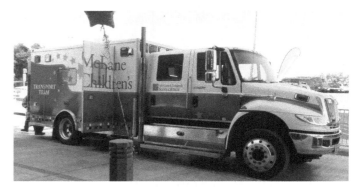

FIGURE 31-2. Type IAD/MD ambulance. Photo depicts a type I ambulance used for pediatric critical care interfacility transport. This unit is based on a larger truck and is of the "additional duty" or "medium duty" class. (Reproduced with permission from Diane Cooney, RN.)

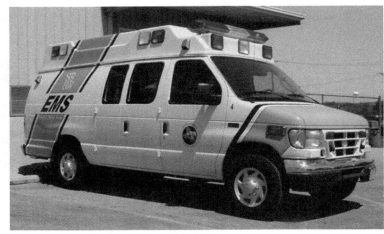
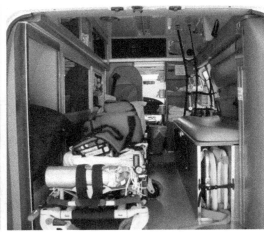

FIGURE 31-3. Type II ambulance. Photo depicts a type II ambulance and the relative constraints of the internal dimensions of the patient care area in this type. Backboards are stored under the bench rather than in an external compartment. (Reproduced with permission from Dr. Derek Cooney.)

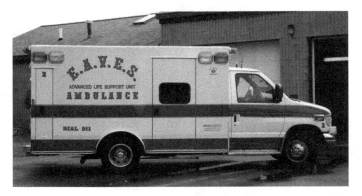

FIGURE 31-4. Type III ambulance. Photo depicts a type II ambulance in service with East Area Volunteer Emergency Services in East Syracuse, New York. Note the cab is that of a van rather than that of a truck. (Reproduced with permission from Dr. Derek Cooney.)

carrying a stretcher and patient. Some examples include golf carts and four- or six-wheel off-road utility vehicles (**Figure 31-5**).

Others Some other examples of vehicles used by EMS providers to reach acutely sick and injured patients include motorcycles and bicycles. Because of their speed and agility motorcycles are employed all over the world to provide various levels of EMS first response. Bicycle response is also an effective tactic to deliver care in crowded areas that are impossible to reach with a standard ambulance (**Figure 31-6**). Bicycle providers are typically utilized in mass gathering events and in heavily populated urban centers with limited roadway access. Bicycles and horseback-mounted providers are also found in remote wilderness locations and in larger public parks. EMS physician vehicles are discussed in a separate chapter on physician field response.

■ FIRE AND RESCUE APPARATUS

There is a wide variety of fire apparatus configurations. Many departments operate custom-designed apparatus that may serve multiple purposes. Knowing the basic types and purposes may help the EMS

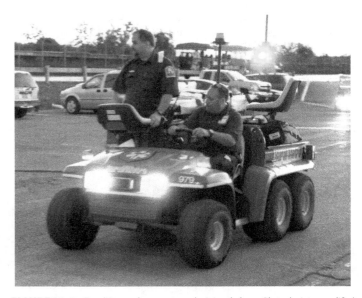

FIGURE 31-5. Type IV example: gas-powered mini-ambulance. Photo depicts a modified six-wheel off-road-capable utility vehicle (the Gator) used by Rural Metro Medical Services of Central New York for event medical coverage. This configuration has two provider positions to allow optimal patient care during transport of a patient on a standard EMS stretcher. (Reproduced with permission from Dr. Norma Cooney.)

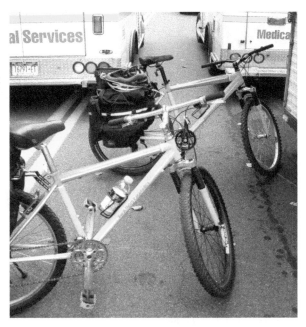

FIGURE 31-6. Bicycles equipped for EMS response. This photo shows "bike team" bicycles used by Rural Metro Medical Services parked at a mass gathering event in Syracuse, New York. These bicycles are equipped for ALS response.

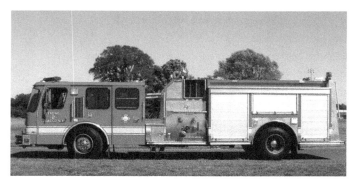

FIGURE 31-7. Fire engine. This engine carries its own hose supply. (Reproduced with permission from the City of Oswego Fire Department, Oswego, New York.)

physician understand on-scene operations better and allow for better placement of the EMS physician vehicle. This basic knowledge is also essential for physicians working with fire-based services.

Engine: The fire engine is the backbone of the fire service and is essentially a vehicle designed to deliver water to the fire scene and access additional water at the scene for the purpose of fighting fire (**Figure 31-7**). These typically carry their own hose and personnel, but may also come in as a single-purpose pump apparatus. Sometimes referred to as a "pumper" the fire engine is specifically not a fire "truck." With reservoirs typically ranging from 500 to 1500 gallons and an outgoing pump capacity of around 120 pounds per square inch, the average engine will be out of water within 5 to 10 minutes and will need to have a supply line established with the hydrant system or portable ponds.

Truck: A fire truck is actually a very valuable utility vehicle that delivers hydraulic pumps and tools, hand tools, power tools, saws, lights, fans, ground ladders, and other rescue operation and fire ground "truck company" equipment and personnel.

Ladder truck: This type of apparatus is a more specific type of truck that carries a large hydraulic latter, or aerial, on top (**Figure 31-8**). These usually have no water, but typically have a waterway that allows for water to be sprayed from the top of the aerial during a rescue operation or fire attack. They come in different forms such as turntable, tower, tiller, hydraulic platform, and aerial ladder platform types. In addition to the "snorkel" ladder on top that may reach around 100 feet, these trucks usually come loaded with many ground ladders. Not all departments can afford to operate this type of apparatus.

Rescue: The rescue type of apparatus is designed to carry and deliver rescue equipment and personnel and may be common to roadway responses. Some rescue vehicles are based on large pickup truck chassis with a custom equipment box and may have hydraulic tools and scene lighting as well as vehicle stabilization equipment. Heavy rescue vehicles are larger and carry more elaborate loadouts. When an engine is configured to provide rescue operations as well, it is often referred to as a "rescue pumper."

HAZMAT/special ops: Specialty vehicles for hazardous materials response, disasters/MCIs, specialized rescue (high angle, swift water, SCUBA, etc) may take the form of a number of different configurations a vehicle types. These are typically large to accommodate the specialty equipment they deliver. Some resemble a heavy rescue while others may be based on a "bread truck" or "moving van"–type vehicle (**Figure 31-9**).

Tanker: Some fire scenes are more rurally located or are in areas of a municipality known to have an aged or less reliable hydrant system. Tankers carry large volumes of water and can typically be drafted from, lay down a portable reservoir, or pond, and in many cases can be used to go on runs to natural water sources to refill and return to dump water into the portable ponds.

Quint: These combination role apparatus are designed to fill the roles of an engine, truck, and ladder truck. The five incorporated elements that make this type a "quint" are the fire pump, water reservoir, hose storage, ground ladders, and an aerial ladder. These are popular in some smaller departments; however, there is significant controversy over their true utility, as they sometimes perform each role to a lesser degree than a dedicated apparatus might. They typically carry the same personnel count and can only engage in one function until additional firefighters arrive.

Wildland truck: This varies in size and configuration, but many times are based on a pickup truck with the ability to "chase" the fire as it moves across a field or other wildland. These vehicles typically care some a small water supply and a coiled hose reel. These are also known as brush truck or grass truck.

Squad: A squad or "mini" is a smaller piece of apparatus and may have almost any function in the department. Some are for delivery of personnel and limited equipment, while others may even be equipped with a smaller fire pump.

Fly cars: A "medic car "or "MICU" may also be designated for first response medical operations. These can take many forms. EMS physician vehicle design is discussed in a separate chapter.

Boats: Some departments have a boat, or marine unit. These can range from inflatable zodiacs for water rescue, to rigid haul craft for operation in larger bodies of water. Some departments also operated pump boats for firefighting. Recently, some departments have begun to use personnel water craft for rescue operations.

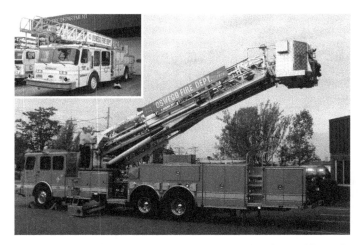

FIGURE 31-8. Ladder Trucks. (Reproduced with permission from the City of Oswego Fire Department, Oswego, New York.)

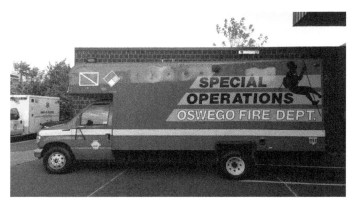

FIGURE 31-9. "Moving van–type" special operations vehicle. This vehicle operated by the City of Oswego Fire Department delivers special operations equipment of a wide variety. (Reproduced with permission from the City of Oswego Fire Department, Oswego, New York.)

▉ AIRCRAFT

Air medical transport is typically broken into aircraft type. Rotor wing refers to helicopter transport and fixed wing refers to airplanes. EMS physicians should be familiar with the safety and operation constraints of these vehicles, even if they do not provide care and transport in an air medical environment. Air medical transport is discussed in a separate chapter.

FEMA TYPED RESOURCE DEFINITIONS

For the purpose of standardization when requesting and organizing resources to respond to a disaster, the National Incident Management System (NIMS) Emergency Support Function (ESF) #8 Public Health and Medical Services Annex defines ambulances by function and capability and assigns them a type. This is not the same as the ambulance types above, because it is not based on design or configuration, but rather is based on functional capacity and services provided.[1] **Table 31-1** is an adaptation of a table from a summary document provided by the United States Fire Administration (USFA).[2]

Of interest is the fact that this document is from 2008 and the new NFPA 1917 standard calls for a single litter patient, thus creating the potential for a resource mismatch based on these guidelines. It is important not to confuse FEMA ambulance typing with industry standard ambulance typing when communicating in disaster planning, communications with government offices, and in publications and educational materials.

OPERATION OF AN EMERGENCY VEHICLE

EMS physicians and medical directors need to have safe and effective means to reach the field in response to scene calls and for the purpose of medical oversight activities. Some still ride with EMS providers in fly cars and ambulances; however, the nature of being on call typically requires a take-home vehicle. Regardless of whether the emergency vehicle is a personally owned vehicle that the physician has equipped or is an agency vehicle, the principles of operation are the same. Before accepting this responsibility, an EMS physician should take an emergency vehicle operators course (EVOC). These are typically offered by government, fire, police, EMS, and insurance agencies, many times at no cost if the student is affiliated with an agency.

▉ TRAFFIC LAW EXCEPTIONS AND LIMITATIONS

Although it may seem that operation under lights and sirens provides immunity to the act of taking exceptions to the usual vehicle and traffic laws, this is not typically the case. Although these laws vary by state, some basic themes exist, and are based on common sense as it applies to providing for the public safety. Many state vehicle and traffic laws authorize exceptions to the usual traffic rules when responding to an

TABLE 31-1	Ground Ambulance EMS Resource Type Definitions—NIMS—ESF#8			
	Type I	Type II	Type III	Type IV
Level of care	ALS	ALS	BLS	BLS
Personnel	One ALS provider	One ALS provider	One EMT	One EMT
	One EMT	One EMT	One EMR	One EMR
	with HAZMAT Ops Capability		with HAZMAT Ops Capability	
Capability	Two litter patients	Two litter patients	Two litter patients	Two litter patients

Adapted from United States Fire Administration. National Fire Academy. EMS resource type definitions. Coffee break training—emergency medical services. No. EMS-2012-2. February 2012. www.usfa.fema.gov/nfa/coffee-break.

TABLE 31-2	Regular Maintenance Tasks
Tires: Check tread wear and tire pressure
Brakes: Test lights and check for uneven breaking, locking, and noises
Warning lights and sirens: Test all lights and the siren
Headlights and running lights: Ensure all are clean and working
Windshield wipers: Check for function and wear and tear
Windows: Ensure they are clean inside and out
Mirrors: Clean and properly positioned
Fluid levels: checked and made nominal
Ensure ease of starting
Check safety equipment (such as fire extinguishers)
Check for general cleanliness and overall condition of vehicle body

List should be checked at every shift change or on a daily basis, whichever is more frequent. Even infrequently used vehicles should be checked weekly.[3]
United States Fire Administration. National Fire Academy. EMS Safety: Techniques and Applications. https://www.usfa.fema.gov/downloads/PDF/publications/fa-144.pdf.

emergency, provided the lights and sirens are used as indicated and the operator maintains and demonstrates due regard for public safety. Some states have specific exceptions and forbid others, so it is important to know the law. In addition to legal constraints, many agencies have rules concerning stopping at intersections and maximum speeds among others.

▉ DUE REGARD FOR PUBLIC SAFETY

The primary concern when operating an emergency vehicle is the safety of the public, the responding personnel, and the patient. Even when taking a legal exception to vehicle and traffic laws during an emergency response with lights and sirens, the driver of an emergency vehicle must still demonstrate due regard for public safety. This means that the driver is still responsible for preventing a motor vehicle collision and any foreseeable risks to persons and property. The lights and sirens do not excuse an arbitrary exercise of the right-of-way privilege or a failure to operate the vehicle in a safe manner. Safe operating speed depends on many factors, including roadway type, location, conditions, visibility, traffic, obstructions, and other factors that may be cause to assume unexpected traffic or obstructions, or the inability of other drivers or pedestrians to be alerted by the audible alert of the siren and the visible warning of the lights. A failure to demonstrate due regard for public safety may result in civil and criminal action, the loss of driver's license, considerations over continuation of your certification and licensure, and the emotional injury associated with causing injury or death to others. Exhibiting due regard also extends to ensuring that the vehicle is properly maintained and ready for service prior to driving and reporting and correcting mechanical failures before continuing to operate the vehicle (**Table 31-2**). In addition to learning safe driving principles, there is also some need for education on how to properly assist the driver from the passenger side. Helping to recognize threats and assess intersections are important "shotgun" position tasks in addition to assisting with operation of the lights, siren, radio, and MDT. When seated up front, all providers have a responsibility to help maintain a proper level of safety during response and scene size-up.

▉ DRIVER TRAINING

Driving an emergency vehicle requires attention to detail and practiced techniques. Avoiding common pitfalls requires awareness and experience. In addition to regular annual driver training with an emergency response agency, EMS physicians should consider formal emergency vehicle driver training. State and local agencies usually offer an emergency vehicle operators course. Commercial EMS agencies and insurance companies are commonly found to provide courses as well. **Table 31-3** shows some

TABLE 31-3	Emergency Vehicle Driver Training Course Examples
CEVO 3	Coaching The Emergency Vehicle Operator 3—Ambulance
EVOC	National Safety Council: http://www.nsc.org
EVDT	Emergency Vehicle Operators Course
	in Case of Emergency Training Programs: http://www.iceems.com
	Emergency Vehicle Driver Training: XTN041
	Texas A&M Engineering Extension Service: http://www.teex.org

examples of different types of courses. Although online courses are offered, these are not recommended as the hands-on driving component is likely a critical factor in retention and application of the material taught in these courses. EMS physicians should also engage in ride-alongs with their agencies in order to learn and observe common practices among their providers and ensure their own familiarity with geography. Safety concerns should always be reported to agency leadership.

SPECIFIC HAZARDS

SPEED

Emergency vehicles typically weigh a great deal more than typical privately owned ones. EMS physicians will likely be operating a "squad" or "fly car" that has been specially outfitted with additional equipment and supplies. A specially configured and fully equipped EMS physician sport utility vehicle can have significant added weight that will change the handling and stopping distance when compared to the stock version. Ambulances and rescue squads are typically built on light axel trucks and configured with significant weight. Weight and road conditions factor into breaking distance. In addition to this function of physics is the human element reflected in perception time and reaction time. Perception time is the time it takes to notice the problem and reaction time is the time it takes for the driver to react to the problem. In addition to the actual distance the breaking event requires there is also a break lag time. This lag time is especially evident in vehicles equipped with air breaks. The stopping distance, therefore, is the sum of the distance covered during the perception time, reaction time, and brake lag, plus the actual breaking distance. Consider that if an alert driver takes 0.75 seconds to perceive a problem and another 0.75 seconds to initiate the braking, the distance traveled at 55 mph before the braking system has been actuated is already 120 feet.[4]

A type I and type III ambulances can weigh around 11,000 pounds and type II ambulances around 9,200 pounds, thus breaking distances will be greater for these vehicles than for cars and SUVs.[5] **Table 31-4** shows some approximate curb weights for some EMS vehicle types. Keeping in mind the physics is important. Limiting speed, while unlikely to make a significant impact on the travel time to the scene, can offer significant safety benefits.

INTERSECTIONS

In one study 42% of all crashes in EMS happen at intersections.[6] Of those crashes 85% happen in what is colloquially referred to as Torpedo Alley. That is the last lane in the intersection of opposing traffic that has the

TABLE 31-4	Emergency Vehicle Approximate Curb Weights
2014 Ford Expedition EL 4×4	6,100 lb
2011 Ford Crown Victoria	4,100 lb
Type I ambulance	11,000 lb
Type II ambulance	9,200 lb
Type III ambulance	11,000 lb
Type IAD/IIIAD (additional/medium Duty)	14,000 lb

Modified with permission from CSGNetwork.com. Vehicle stopping distance and time. http://www.csgnetwork.com/stopdistinfo.html.

green light, and is still going straight through the intersection while you are crossing against the red. When approaching an intersection, operators of an emergency vehicle should observe some basic operational tactics:

1. "Bleed your speed"—the vehicle should be moving slowly when approaching an intersection; covering the brake adds safety; no need to use the accelerator to cross through an intersection.

2. Clearing the intersection early—looking left-right, left-right, and left again; keeping in mind that the first vehicle to meet them will be coming from their left side.

3. Making sure to look through large vehicles with glass—like buses, passenger vans; looking under larger vehicles like semitrailers, SUVs, and buses—these high-profile vehicles will hide many unwanted surprises behind them.

4. Driving in the left hand lane while you are running hot—attempting to "push" traffic into the right lane or berm; jumping from lane to lane may potentially cause confusion with the general public.

5. Changing the siren often—the general public may become "hypnotized" to a single siren tone; during a long run, or in heavy traffic, changing the tone of the siren often is advised.

6. Maintaining a steady speed—speeding up and slowing down in heavy traffic or areas with many intersections may increase response time; the brakes may become too hot for the vehicle, and could potentially result in brake malfunction or failure; considering the concept of "smooth is fast."

ESCORT VEHICLES

At times it may seem like an advantage to follow in behind other emergency vehicles heading to the same call. Other times it may be considered appropriate to use the cover of the lights and sirens of another vehicle when operating an unequipped vehicle. Although these strategies are sometimes practiced, following an emergency vehicle during lights and sirens response can be quite dangerous. The issue is that other drivers typically expect, somewhat instinctively, that there is only one emergency vehicle. Their attention is drawn to that vehicle's warning lights and audible alert and they track it as it passes. Unfortunately, they tend to then proceed without turning their attention back to all directions to check for additional vehicles.

VEHICLE PLACEMENT AT THE SCENE

Emergency vehicle placement at a scene requires insight and knowledge of the type of scene, responding resources, and the role of the unit being operated. For most roadway scenes there will be fire, rescue, EMS, and law enforcement units responding and each must position in a way to provide a safe work area and put the correct resources in position. When operating an EMS physician response vehicle it is likely that there will be other emergency vehicles at the scene around the time of arrival. Typically, EMS physicians should attempt to position their vehicle inside the protection of the work area (typically created by law enforcement and/or fire/rescue vehicles). The vehicle should be parked a safe distance from the scene and should not obstruct other resources, especially fire, rescue, and EMS personnel. The back of the responding ambulance should not be obstructed from the rear and egress for the ambulance should be maintained. If the EMS physician is the first arriving emergency vehicle, then they must position their vehicle upstream from the accident sight with lights left running in order to attempt to protect the accident scene.

PARKING

The general rule is that when not using the vehicle to create the work area it is appropriate to park off of the roadway when practical. Lights should be set to the minimum for safety. The vehicle should be placed at an angle and the wheels turned out to the side (**Figure 31-10**). The goal is to use the vehicle to provide some protection to the scene and to use the angle

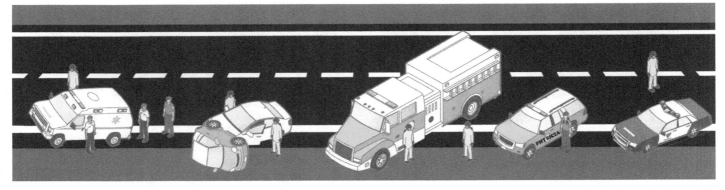

FIGURE 31-10. EMS physician vehicle at the scene. Place the vehicle a safe distance from the scene (50-200 feet) and at an angle with the wheels turned out and the parking break set. This figure is not to scale. The ambulance would be around 100 feet from the accident vehicles and the physician response vehicle would be about 50 to 200 feet from the accident vehicles.

and the turn of the wheels, along with the parking break, to minimize the risk that the vehicle will enter the work area if struck by another vehicle. Before exiting the vehicle, scene size-up should be performed again and the approved roadway safety vest should be donned.

FLARES

If you set flares of reflective markers you should be around 300 feet for traffic traveling at 50 mph and farther for greater speeds. Typically law enforcement and fire will manage traffic patterns on their arrival and the EMS physician will not assume these duties.

USE OF THE VEHICLE FOR PROTECTION

Most emergency vehicles are equipped with passive and active visual warnings. Passive refers to markings on the outside of the vehicle that are meant to make it more visible. Examples include "warning colors," checker patterns, striping, chevrons on the rear, and the use of retro-reflective paint and/or vinyl. The active visual warning system refers to the emergency lighting on the vehicle.[3] Use of lights on the roadside is relatively standard practice; however, there are two caveats to consider. First is that on dark scenes, headlights (especially wig-wag) and the effect of the emergency lighting may be distracting or cause visibility problems for responders working on the scene, and therefore parked vehicles should be set to a more minimal lighting setting. Secondly, there is some concern that certain drivers who are intoxicated may actually swerve or direct their vehicle toward emergency lighting due to their relative incapacitation.

The roadway positioning of emergency vehicles at an angle with outward turned front wheels and applied parking break is thought to offer some protection of downstream responders from oncoming vehicles. This positioning strategy is meant to absorb the force of the oncoming vehicle and minimize the risk that the vehicles would enter the work area.[3]

Scene safety is covered in another chapter; however, it is appropriate to mention here that although ambulance or other emergency vehicle may offer a threatened responder some concealment, only certain parts of a vehicle may resist gun fire. Positioning oneself behind the engine block or behind the wheels of the ambulance or fire apparatus may offer some ballistic protection, whereas the patient care area of the typical ambulance will offer only concealment and likely limited to no real protection from gun fire.

USE OF LIGHTS AND SIRENS

Emergency vehicle lighting usually includes red (or sometimes blue, white, and amber) flashing (or strobing) lights that are visible from all sides of the vehicle. Some state laws only require visibility from the front; however, if active warning lights have value during an emergency response, then they should be equipped in a 360° configuration.

The audible warning should be used during emergency response to alert other roadway users.

CONFIGURATIONS

Many EMS physicians operate vehicles with lights in locations other than the light bar on the roof. Corner lights, side lights, directional sticks, and grill lights are becoming standard, especially since the marketing of newer LED lights. Wig-wag (alternating lighting using the vehicles own headlights and/or tail lights) is becoming less popular because it diminishes the functionality of the headlights and directional signaling of the taillights. Because of these many lighting modules being installed on newer emergency vehicles, the control for these lights may be configured to allow a number of different lighting options from all-on, to rear lights only, to directional stick only, and a number of other possibilities depending on the philosophy of the agency and the operator.

The siren should have multiple modes, including wail and yelp as a minimum and the siren system should comply with some standard. Typically these sirens meet the SAE J1849 standard which is called for in the NFPA 1917 document. The siren should be switched between modes at intersections with preference to the highest signal repeat rate some switching during long stretches of roadway travel should be considered to avoid the potential for

EFFECT

There is an ongoing debate about the use of "code 3" (lights and sirens) response. The time differences to and from the scene have been shown to be relatively clinically insignificant.[7,8] One study showed a difference of 1 minute and 46 seconds in response time.[9] Transport time to the hospital has a difference of around 1 to 4 minutes.[10-13] In the EMS system, emergency medical dispatch has been shown to reduce the usage of this potentially dangerous mode of response.[14,15] Although the medical director may not have any direct authority over standard operating procedures associated with code 3 response, it is part of the medical director's duty to discuss these issues with the individual or group that does. EMS physicians are typically (but not always) responding as a secondary unit or additional asset. It is therefore prudent to consider that unless there are extreme circumstances, the responding physician should respond without taking traffic exceptions and/or the use of lights and sirens. There is likely an enhanced risk of collision when multiple units are responding code 3.[16]

COMMUNICATIONS

Many states now have laws mandating "hands-free" operations for mobile phones while driving a motor vehicle and many have also made it illegal to send text messages while driving. Using pagers, mobile phones, and radios may increase the risk of driver error and motor vehicle collision. Radio and telephonic communication during driving should be minimized to reduce this risk as well and when a second provider is in the vehicle, they should operate the radio whenever possible. EMS physicians should be aware of and minimize potential distractions during driving, especially when using lights and sirens.

EMERGENCY VEHICLE CRASHES

Fire apparatus, police cars, ambulances, and fly cars have all been involved in serious and deadly motor vehicle incidents. It is important for EMS physicians to be aware of these risks even if they are not themselves operating the ambulance or fly car. Data summarized by the Fire Protection Research Foundation show 27,871 ambulance crashes from 1990 to 2009.[17] In this sample of 10 years of crashes, there were 9355 injuries and 265 fatalities. Various causes are found when these crashes are investigated. In addition to other preventable and unpreventable causes, recent concern over something now referred to as "sirencide" has led to additional concerns over dispatch practices and the use of code 3 response.

Sirencide has been defined by the National Transportation Safety Board as "a phenomenon used to describe the emotional reaction of emergency vehicle drivers when they begin to feel a sense of power and urgency that blocks out reason and prudence, leading to reckless operation of the emergency vehicle."[18] There are a number of cases discussed in the lay and professional media that illustrate this problem through a series of cases when bodily harm and death occurred to bystanders and other rescuers seemingly due to reckless operation of an emergency vehicle. One source noted an increase in speed of 10 to 15 mph seemingly in response to the continuous use of the siren.[3] This is an issue that requires research to determine if the issue is the act of employing lights and sirens or rather the emotional effect of being dispatched to a seemingly serious call.

Driver, passenger, and patient restraint systems should be used at all times. For the driver, restraint is not just a safety device in a collision, but also helps keep the driver in position and potentially in control longer.[3] In the case of provider restrain use during patient care, many providers still avoid their use because of a perception that patient care needs preclude their use. One study showed that providers felt that they needed to be unrestrained 41% of the time. Despite this, the same study showed that 18% felt that they could still use their restraint 18% of the time.[19] Some advances in EMS provider restraint systems have occurred since this study was published in 1991; however based on anecdotal observation, many providers and physicians still operate in the patient care area without proper restraint in many cases. In addition, all equipment should be secured and nothing should be placed on the dash of the vehicle that is not secured. These items and equipment may shift and/or become relative projectiles in a collision or adverse driving event and can cause crashes and injury to occupants of the vehicle.[3]

KEY POINTS

- Safe operation of an emergency vehicle is a skill that requires education, training, and experience.
- Parking an emergency vehicle at the scene requires attention to the placement of other vehicles, accident scene, traffic and other hazards, and the use of the minimum emergency lighting setting expected to provide some protection of responders working at the scene.
- Stopping distance is a sum of the distance traveled during the perception time and reaction time (and brake delay) and the actual braking distance.
- Studies evaluating the use of lights and sirens in response and transport have failed to demonstrate a potential clinically significant difference.

- From 1990 to 2009, 27,871 ambulance crashes were recorded with 9355 injuries and 265 fatalities.
- Sirencide is a term that describes the potential emotional stress response that has been suggested leads to poor judgment during Code 3 operation of an emergency vehicle.
- EMS providers as a group have a documented reluctance to wear restraints during patient care activities while transporting.

REFERENCES

1. Federal Emergency Management Agency (FEMA). U.S. Department of Homeland Security. Typed resources definitions: emergency medical services resources. *FEMA* 508-3. March 2009. http://www.fema.gov/media-library-data/20130726-1849-25045-2727/fema_508_3_typed_resource_definitions_emergency_medical_services_resources_2009.pdf. Accessed May, 2015.
2. United States Fire Administration. National Fire Academy. EMS resource type definitions. Coffee break training—emergency medical services. No. EMS-2012-2. February 2012. www.usfa.fema.gov/nfa/coffee-break.
3. United States Fire Administration. National Fire Academy. EMS safety: techniques and applications. https://www.usfa.fema.gov/downloads/pdf/publications/fa-144.pdf. Accessed May, 2015.
4. CSGNetwork.com. Vehicle stopping distance and time. http://www.csgnetwork.com/stopdistinfo.html. Accessed May, 2015.
5. emt-resources. Ambulance types: what is an ambulance. http://www.emt-resources.com/Ambulance-types.html. 2010. Accessed April 2014.
6. Sanddal TL, Sanddal ND, Ward N, Stanley L. Ambulance crash characteristics in the US defined by the popular press: a retrospective analysis. *Emerg Med Int.* 2010.
7. Weiss S, Fullerton L, Oglesbee S, Duerden B, Froman P. Does ambulance response time influence patient condition among patients with specific medical and trauma emergencies? *South Med J.* March 2013;106(3):230-235.
8. Lacher ME, Bausher JC. Lights and siren in pediatric 911 ambulance transports: are they being misused? *Ann Emerg Med.* February 1997;29(2):223-227.
9. Brown LH, Whitney CL, Hunt RC, Addario M, Hogue T. Do warning lights and sirens reduce ambulance response times? *Prehosp Emerg Care.* January-March 2000;4(1):70-74.
10. Dami F, Pasquier M, Carron PN. Use of lights and siren: is there room for improvement? *Eur J Emerg Med.* February 2014;21(1):52-56.
11. Marques-Baptista A, Ohman-Strickland P, Baldino KT, Prasto M, Merlin MA. Utilization of warning lights and siren based on hospital time-critical interventions. *Prehosp Disaster Med.* July-August 201025(4):335-339.
12. O'Brien DJ, Price TG, Adams P. The effectiveness of lights and siren use during ambulance transport by paramedics. *Prehosp Emerg Care.* April-June 1999;3(2):127-130.
13. Hunt RC, Brown LH, Cabinum ES, et al. Is ambulance transport time with lights and siren faster than that without? *Ann Emerg Med.* April 1995;25(4):507-511.
14. Merlin MA, Baldino KT, Lehrfeld DP, et al. Use of a limited lights and siren protocol in the prehospital setting vs standard usage. *Am J Emerg Med.* May 2012;30(4):519-525.
15. Kupas DF, Dula DJ, Pino BJ. Patient outcome using medical protocol to limit "lights and siren" transport. *Prehosp Disaster Med.* October-December 1994;9(4):226-229.
16. Use of warning lights and siren in emergency medical vehicle response and patient transport. National Association of Emergency Medical Services Physicians (NAEMSP) and the National Association

of State EMS Directors (NASEMSD). *Prehosp Disaster Med.* April-June 1994;9(2):133-136.

17. Grant CC, Merrifield D. Analysis of ambulance crash data. The Fire Protection Research Foundation. September 2011. http://www.nfpa.org/~/media/Files/Research/Research%20Foundation/Research%20Foundation%20reports/For%20emergency%20responders/rfambulancecrash.pdf. Accessed May, 2015.

18. Sirencide: the mental state of reckless drivers. EMS Training & Disaster Preparedness Institute. University Hospitals. Case Medical Center. http://www.emsconedonline.com/pdfs/sirencide.pdf. Accessed May, 2015.

19. Cook RT Jr, Meador SA, Buckingham BD, Groff LV. Opportunity for seatbelt usage by ALS providers. *Prehosp Disaster Med.* October-December 1991;6(4):469-484.

INTRODUCTION

Although physicians are not the primary providers of prehospital care in the United States, field response capability is still considered an essential component of a modern EMS system. As discussed in Chapter 29, the EMS physician must be prepared to go to the scene to ensure the quality of the care in the system through direct observation, provide emergency response for mass casualty situations, and provide advanced level care in some infrequent circumstances. In order to perform these various field activities, the EMS physician must first be able to respond to the field. Several methods of transporting the EMS physician to a scene are available. The EMS physician could drive their private vehicle to a scene, or a field supervisor vehicle or law enforcement vehicle could be used to pick up and deliver the EMS physician to a scene. Unfortunately these solutions achieve the task of delivering the EMS physician but do not simultaneously deliver the equipment needed by the EMS physician to perform their mission. A more efficient and effective deployment of the EMS physician can be accomplished by providing the EMS physician with a specially designed, equipped, and dedicated EMS physician response vehicle (PRV). Various EMS systems have implemented such vehicles into their fleet and include the EMS PRV as a deployable asset in many circumstances. The ideal EMS PRV will allow for the safe, rapid, and efficient delivery of the EMS physician and associated specialty equipment to the scene. The development of such an asset must be a careful and thoughtful undertaking, as there are many factors that must be considered as the vehicle is designed, built, and equipped in order to create an end product that meets the needs of the EMS physician and the EMS system.

OBJECTIVES

- Describe the types of physician field response (primary, secondary, and tertiary).
- Describe different types of physician teams and task forces.
- Describe minimum training standards for safe and effective physician field response.
- Give examples of physician field response dispatch criteria.
- Discuss types of advanced interventions provided by EMS physicians in the field.
- Describe the ideal design qualities of an EMS physician response vehicle.
- Discuss specific design details, costs, and benefits.
- Discuss interoperability concerns for EMS physicians relating to communications and radio equipment.
- Describe EMS equipment appropriate for EMS physician response, and discuss when it is appropriate to exclude items known to be carried by local EMS/fire agency vehicles.
- Describe equipment that may be needed to perform EMS physician level interventions.
- Describe the proper storage of controlled substances and other drugs in the vehicle.
- Discuss mobility concerns and limitations to standard EMS bags.
- Describe appropriate PPE levels for various types of operations.
- Discuss the design and deployment of special operations trailers for prolonged events.

PHYSICIAN FIELD RESPONSE

When considering field response it is appropriate to categorize the types of responses and to use this organizational scheme when considering the necessary training and equipment. There are three basic types of responses based on dispatch/notification scenarios: primary, secondary, and tertiary (**Box 32-1**).

▨ PRIMARY

When an EMS physician is notified or dispatched as part of the primary response to an emergency call this is considered a primary field response. Participating in a Primary Emergency Response usually requires the EMS Physician to respond in a fully equipped and legally verified emergency response vehicle. Establishing the infrastructure to allow an EMS Physician to respond in this manner often requires working within specific jurisdictional legal and regulatory parameters, as well as ensuring proper liability insurance has been secured. In some systems an EMS physician may be routinely dispatched to possible cardiac arrests or major trauma incidents. In other systems there may not be routine dispatches of the EMS physician, but the EMS physician may, at their own volition and availability, respond primarily to any type of call in order to perform CQI of system performance measures. These calls might include those requiring routine emergency medical care (cardiac arrest, trauma, seizures, etc). If the physician were first to the scene they may initiate care; however, more than likely they will serve in a supportive/oversight role. These calls allow for CQI and education and require the EMS physician to maintain usual prehospital skills and first response equipment. Suspected mass casualty incidents (MCIs) may also prompt a primary EMS physician response but in most situations does not require that the physician possess extra or specialized equipment or drugs. Training in ICS is important, but advanced knowledge of ICS may not be necessary. EMS physicians are prepared for this level of response, as it does not necessitate much preplanning or maintenance of specialty skills, knowledge, or equipment.

▨ SECONDARY

A secondary response for physicians is usually one that is brought on by recognition of field providers that the physician's presence would be beneficial, or is necessary due to unusual circumstances. Some complex medical decision-making situations are better mitigated by direct field contact rather than over radio communications due to the level of communication required, or in the case where contact with others on scene would significantly change a potential outcome for a particular patient (eg, difficult or confusing refusal situation in which life/limb threats are present and family or law enforcement is not providing expected assistance). In cases of prolonged extrication or in which amputation may be needed in order to free a critically injured patient, providers may call for the EMS physician. Special equipment, medications, and training are required in order to provide these services. Tactical medical support may be called for an active shooter or other active police actions. Proper preplanning, training, and equipment must all be in place in order to ensure maximum effectiveness with minimum risk. Support of fire ground operations and technical rescue requires rehabilitation and medical surveillance of firefighters and rescuers. In order to provide this secondary response the physician must have participated in preplanning, have knowledge of specific policies and procedures, and have access to rehabilitation providers

---

Box 32-1

Types of EMS Physician Field Response

Primary—routine emergency calls, CQI/education, MCI

Secondary—complex medical decision making, advanced field intervention (ie, field surgery), tactical medical support, rehabilitation services for firefighting, and rescue operations

Tertiary—prolonged MCI, prolonged disaster relief, wilderness search and rescue, urban search and rescue

---

and supplies. These requirements mean a higher level of preparation and maintenance of specialty skills, knowledge, and equipment will be necessary for the EMS physician response vehicle/program.

◼ TERTIARY

When a prolonged medical support operation is called for or anticipated, EMS physicians may respond for a prolonged duty cycle. This is very different than other emergency responses and requires consideration of potential unavailability for the other two types of response if the responding physician is the only active physician asset in the system. Prolonged MCIs lead to a need for continued field care and delay of patient transport to the hospital. The EMS physician will provide treatment and likely authorize advanced scope of practice to on-scene EMS providers under their direct supervision. When an event is expected to last greater than 24 hours, then a sustained disaster medical response may be called for. In cases of natural disaster, terrorism acts, wilderness search and rescue, and urban search and rescue operations, the EMS physician team may be tasked with providing or coordinating medical operations. In some circumstances, Medical Reserve Corps (MRC), Disaster Medical Assistance Teams (DMAT), or other medical assistance networks may be engaged and will likely alleviate the need for continued reliance of the local EMS physician(s) once they are fully deployed.

TEAMS AND TASK FORCES

As discussed in Chapter 29, there is no current and meaningful data that quantify and characterize the various types of physician responders and response programs. *Agency medical directors* have provided response to the field for as long as there have been EMS medical directors. This has been done in a number of different forms including ride-alongs, staffing the ambulance or helicopter, and in individual physician vehicles (some emergency vehicles, others not). Field response physicians have ranged in type from fellowship-trained EMS physicians to emergency medicine residents, to surgeons and anesthesiologists.

Although it is clear that organized field response by physicians has been in place in some communities for many years, there exists some variability in the form that this may take. The predominant model that appears to be growing, and will likely be considered the standard in the future, is that of the trained *EMS physician* responding as part of an organized EMS system. This type of responder is many times the medical director of an agency or the system, and has met certain training, equipment, and logistical standards. These physicians are also sometimes part of a system-wide EMS physician response team (eg, Buffalo, NY; New York City, NY; Minneapolis, MN; Philadelphia, PA; Pittsburg, PA; Syracuse, NY; etc). Although there are still systems that allow emergency medicine resident physicians to respond in emergency vehicles with little to no supervision as part of their residency training experience, this is not the recommended model of providing this service to the community. Just as *internal medicine* residents would not perform endoscopy or cardiac catheterizations without supervision, this subspecialty requires training and experience that residents do not yet possess. Residents should be closely supervised in the field due to the unique area of medicine being practiced, procedures required typically being out of their scope of education, and the specific challenges and risks associated with field response. EMS fellows are generally well trained in this area and are given a graded level of responsibility to ensure effectiveness of the field response service with a requirement for levels of supervision that are predefined based on circumstances.

One other model of physician field response is that of the *surgical go team*. Go teams are usually deployed with the notion that the key physician intervention is a surgical procedure that is outside the scope of a prehospital provider, and that hospital-based physicians possess specific skills that are needed in the field. These teams are based out of trauma centers (eg, Baltimore, MD; Columbus, OH) and members of the team must receive training in scene safety, EMS operations, and technical rescue operational awareness. Typically field surgical procedures are not performed in the same way as in the confines of the hospital and variations of the techniques must be taught to these physicians. The advantage of this type of program is that is has a direct connection to the trauma center and members can potentially provide a smooth transition to the hospital trauma services. The disadvantages of this type of program are that: the program does not address any of the other important roles of an EMS physician, there is a potential significant delay mobilizing a hospital-based team versus an on-call EMS physician team that may already be in the field, and the team is reliant on an outside agency to provide transportation to and from the scene. Most of the techniques that would be provided are now considered EMS physician interventions (surgical airway, thoracostomy, amputation, thoracotomy, perimortem C-section, etc), and it is possible that hospital-based teams may not be needed for acute response in the future as EMS-based physician response becomes available in more communities. These surgical go teams may still be very valuable as part of the sustained response to major disasters as part of the effort to care for large numbers of victims in the field until other disaster medical relief assets arrive.

MINIMUM FIELD TRAINING FOR PHYSICIANS

EMS physicians responding to the field should have training in a formal emergency vehicle operators course (EVOC). It is also advisable that all physicians performing field response be educated in basic principles of EMS operations and medical direction due to the nature of their interactions with EMS providers. Most physicians who have not received fellowship training in EMS medicine will benefit significantly from attending a medical director's course (eg, NAEMSP National Medical Directors Course and Practicum, Ohio ACEP EMS Medical Directors' Course, CITF Online Guide for Preparing Medical Directors). Even veteran EMS medical directors and physicians who are previous prehospital providers will benefit from advanced medical director courses and attending EMS medical director symposia. In addition to EVOC, minimum training should include scene safety concepts, ICS and NIMS, hazardous materials awareness, fire ground operations awareness, technical rescue awareness, radio operations, and local protocols and disaster plans.

PHYSICIAN NOTIFICATION AND DISPATCH CRITERIA

One method of providing EMS physician response is for there to always be an EMS physician "on the air" and responding to calls as they come. In almost every system this is impractical and at the best will not ensure comprehensive coverage. Instead, developing a set of criteria for alerting the EMS physician(s) (via text messaging, tone pager, or other means) seems much more practical. In order for this concept to work properly within an EMS system, stakeholders must be involved in the process and understand the implications of physician field response. When setting criteria for use by a dispatch center, two different type of alerts must be considered: notification and dispatch. *Dispatch* implies that the communications center dispatcher has the right and capability to send the EMS physician(s) to a scene and implies that there is no need for confirmation of the need after the criteria have been met. *Notification*, on the other hand, is when an alert is sent, making the physician(s) aware of the situation without the implied automatic response of a dispatch. Although a seemingly insignificant semantically difference on the surface, this concept has operational significance and should be considered based on the availability of the EMS physician resource and the relationship the physicians have to the system. Notification usually requires a call back from the physician to ask for information or to confirm availability and response. Dispatch should be more efficient, in that the implication is that the physician will go en route without the need for confirmation of the details of the call. When the EMS physician is the agency medical director who is in solo practice, this presumes they are on call 365 days/year, 24 hours/day, and a notification-only arrangement may be most appropriate due to

Box 32-2	
Example EMS Physician Notification and Dispatch Criteria	
Onondaga County, NY—Notification Criteria	**City of Pittsburg, PA—Dispatch Criteria**
The physician response team will be notified by the EMS dispatcher on any of the following incidents:	Listed are the guidelines for dispatching the medical command physician:
• Multiple casualty incidents	• Cardiac arrest
• Motor vehicle collisions with significant or hopeless entrapment	• MVA with entrapment
• Hazardous material incidents with multiple patients	• Three alarm fires[a]
• Serious line of duty injury to public safety personnel	• Hostage suicide situations[a]
• Weapons of mass destruction or biological terrorism incident	• HAZMAT incidents with patients[a]
• Three alarm fire or above	• River rescue incidents with potential for injured/ill victims[a]
• Airport alert 2 or 3	• Complicated deliveries at paramedic's request
• Request of any field paramedic, fire chief, or incident commander as deemed necessary	• Cardiac arrhythmia with significant patient compromise
• At the discretion of the 9-1-1 dispatcher	• Shock
	• Severe respiratory distress, arrest, or airway difficulties
	• Multiple casualty incidents
	• Trauma patients with airway compromise[b]
	• Line of duty injury to public safety personnel
	• Request of field paramedic or district chief

[a]Physician to respond to staging area.

[b]Physician to rendezvous with paramedics en route to hospital.

Box 32-3
EMS Physician Field Surgical Procedures
• Surgical airway[a]
• Extremity amputation
• Thoracotomy
• Escharotomy
• Fasciotomy
• Perimortem cesarean section

[a]Discussed in Chapter 59.

The provision of field surgical procedures will require the physician to carry the proper equipment, medications, and supplies needed for these interventions. Field surgery techniques are detailed in Chapter 64. Determining the need for extreme measures requires in-depth understanding of acute critical care medicine and the capabilities and resources available within the EMS and hospital system. By the nature of the critical injuries usually present in such cases, these interventions are potentially time sensitive (**Box 32-3**). In addition to knowing the indications for each procedure, EMS physicians must train to establish proficiency in performance of the procedures themselves, which may require simulation and cadaver lab time to ensure proper instruction and maintenance of skills.

EMS PHYSICIAN VEHICLE DESIGN

The development of an EMS physician field response program requires careful thought, planning, and execution. Most agencies will likely find merit in adopting a project management approach that divides projects into five phases: Project Conception, Project Definition and Planning, Project Execution, Project Progress Monitoring, and Project Completion. **Figure 32-1** applies this phased approach to the process of designing and constructing a PRV program.

■ PROJECT CONCEPTION PHASE

The Project Conception phase of the project management plan is a critical aspect of any EMS PRV program. One of the first tasks that should be addressed is the need to involve and educate the various constituents and stakeholders in the response jurisdictions that will be impacted by the addition of this specialized resource to the community. If proper "buy-in" is not obtained from key representatives or agencies before the PRV is obtained and deployed, the EMS PRV program may not realize its full potential.

Concurrent to establishing these key relationships, a needs assessment and feasibility evaluation of the proposed EMS physician field response program should be completed. Conducting a hazards risk assessment (HRA) to identify the actual and potential events that may occur within a certain response area is an important part of the needs assessment. Upon completion of the HRA, a cascade of questions will follow, as highlighted in **Box 32-4**. The answers to these questions will help guide the development of an EMS physician field response mission framework and will identify the specific intellectual, technical, and capital requirements that must be met to accomplish the field response missions.

Ideally, defining the field response missions will precede the acquisition of the vehicle intended to serve as the PRV. If the missions are focused mainly on responding to routine EMS calls and performing in-field QA in an urban setting, the response vehicle design and equipment needs will differ significantly from the needs required to perform a mission involving advanced extrication techniques or high-angle rescue in a wilderness environment. A *specialty medical response* mission may require the EMS physician to treat conditions like crush syndrome, amputate entrapped limbs, perform a surgical airway, or perform other surgical procedures such as those discussed in Chapters 59 to 64. Additional missions including aspects of technical rescue may obligate

the likely unpredictability of the response. If the EMS physician is on-call as part of a robust, well-staffed, EMS physician response team, it may be more appropriate to use dispatch criteria, especially if the team physicians are under contract to provide this service. In some cases, it may make sense to have a mixture of both, as some situations may necessitate a physician response based on operational design of the system (eg, tactical medical support), whereas other situations may only benefit from the response in some calls of that type. In either situation, having notification and/or dispatch criteria should not inhibit a medical director from responding for CQI and education purposes (without lights and siren) when they have not been sent an alert. Some systems have developed specific criteria for notification and dispatch (**Box 32-2**).

PHYSICIAN-SPECIFIC AND ADVANCED INTERVENTIONS

In addition to augmentation of the clinical care provided by the EMS system providers, physicians can maximize their effect on patient care by coordinating care in unique situations. In mass casualty/disaster response most systems have a mechanism in place by which all components of the EMS protocol are to be treated as standing orders, alleviating some of the need for radio traffic that may not be feasible at the time. In addition, the presence of the EMS physician(s) allows for a greater conversion to standing orders and may lead to situation specific standing orders to be put in place during the event. Providers can then be used in an advanced practice role rather than limiting their care to protocols and standing orders that were designed for routine emergency medical care. This type of coordination of care expands the utility of the physician far beyond their own ability to care directly for patients.

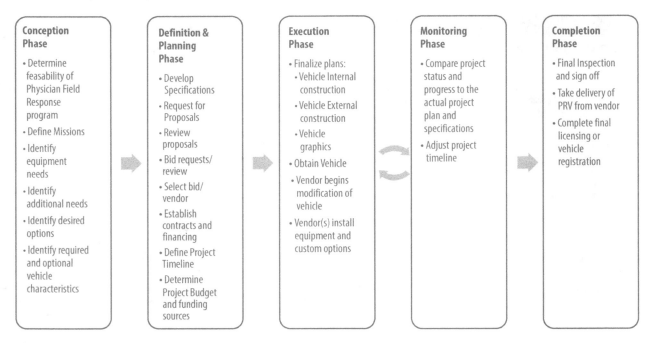

FIGURE 32-1. Project management process.

Box 32-4

Key Questions Triggered by a Hazards Risk Assessment

What type of medical care must the EMS physician be able to provide?

What type of trauma care must the EMS physician be able to provide?

What type of administrative and field leadership support must the EMS physician be able to provide?

What additional services are desired from the EMS physician?

What training does the EMS physician need in order to meet these needs?

What equipment must the EMS physician have available in order to meet these needs?

the response vehicle to carry personal equipment for the physician such as ropes, water rescue gear, or specialty *personal protective equipment* (PPE). The field response missions will define the equipment needed by the EMS physician to perform these missions. Then, the size, shape, quantity, and other characteristics of the EMS physician's equipment will determine certain characteristics of the vehicle that will be used to transport both the equipment and the EMS physician to the field.

In a less ideal order of development, a vehicle may have been acquired before the response missions have been established. In this situation, the characteristics of the vehicle may dictate the type and amount of equipment that is installed or carried, which in turn could limit the capabilities of the EMS physician. Such limitations will affect the missions the EMS physician could potentially execute effectively.

Whether the vehicle intended to serve as the PRV is obtained before or after the field response missions are defined, equipment needs must still be addressed. Regardless of the intended missions, the vehicle must be equipped and designed to allow for an appropriate level of self-reliance. The EMS physician should be able to provide care to any injured or ill patient they may encounter as a single rescuer until additional resources arrive. However, a balance must be established between carrying the equipment needed to be fully prepared for any potential situation and carrying the equipment needed for the most common response situations. The cargo space in the PRV must be viewed as a commodity that must be spent carefully. If more

frequently needed equipment cannot be carried because infrequently used disaster response equipment is taking up space, the cargo capacity of the PRV is perhaps not being spent wisely. It should be recognized that not all EMS physician missions can be accomplished with the equipment that can be carried in a single response vehicle and other deployment strategies may need development. A discussion of equipment and associated deployment strategies will occur later in this chapter.

■ PROJECT DEFINITION AND PLANNING PHASE

After the critical steps of community outreach, education, and relationship building are complete, the EMS physician's missions are defined, the equipment and supplies needed to execute those missions are identified, and vehicle characteristics are identified, the project can transition from the Conception Phase to the Definition and Planning Phase. This second project management phase involves establishing project specifications, researching potential vendors, submitting a request for proposals (RFPs), and requesting and reviewing bids. The RFP, bidding, and vendor selection process will most likely be influenced by the source of project funding, especially if a public funding source will be utilized. Some agencies may have the ability to choose vendors without having to complete a formal project bidding process. In contrast, certain agencies may be mandated to follow specific policies that require projects of this magnitude to be publicly announced and that a formal RFP and bidding process is followed.

After a vendor is chosen, project contracts, financing agreements, and project timelines should be established. An important point that must be discussed with any vendor or subcontractor is whether their work product carries any warranty or guaranty, as well as whether any work performed by the vendor or subcontractors will cause preexisting warranties, such as a vehicle manufacturer's warranty, to become void. Such warranties and guaranties should be established in writing during contract negotiations.

Yet another important part of the Project Definition and Planning phase is establishing a project financing plan with the vendor. A basic project budget is outlined in **Table 32-1**. Down payments, installment amounts and intervals, interest rates, and final payments due upon delivery should be discussed during contract negotiations and should be explicitly defined in the final project contract.

TABLE 32-1	Sample Budget
Vehicle (4 × 4 SUV)	$35,000
After-market conversion package	10,000
Durable and disposable equipment and supplies	15,000
Electronics (communications, mobile data terminal, global positioning or mapping system)	10,000
Total	$70,000

PROJECT EXECUTION PHASE

Once the necessary specifications, contracts, and agreements are established, the project can transition into the Project Execution phase. During this phase the final plans that define the vehicle modifications, the internal and external construction plans, and the vehicle appearance are established. The contracted vendor and subcontractors will then begin construction of the PRV based on the client's specifications.

PROJECT MONITORING PHASE

Shortly after construction begins, the Project Monitoring phase will begin. This phase proceeds in tandem with the Project Execution phase and involves ensuring that the project is proceeding according to the established timeline and that the design specifications are being met. It is possible that modifications to the design plans or project timeline may be needed to ensure that project goals are properly met during the Execution phase.

PROJECT COMPLETION PHASE

The final phase of the project, Project Completion, involves more than simply taking delivery of the completed vehicle. A final vehicle inspection should be conducted by the EMS physician's agency, potentially including the EMS physician, the agency's fleet manager, and other operational or administrative representatives. Steps must be taken in this phase to ensure that before the PRV is placed into service that it is properly licensed and/or registered based on prevailing regulations and that any formal certification inspection is performed by proper governing or regulatory authorities.

EMS PHYSICIAN EQUIPMENT

In a properly designed EMS physician field response program, the EMS physician will bring the skills and equipment to the field that are necessary to augment the level of care that can be provided by the EMS providers that are already present on the scene. Most EMS systems reliably deliver basic supplies like oxygen, intravenous fluids, bandaging supplies, and certain medications to a scene in a standard ambulance. However, many EMS physician missions will require specialized equipment that is not carried by most ambulances.

EQUIPMENT REQUIREMENTS AND OPTIONS

One of the best resources to use to start determining the list of equipment that will be carried on the PRV is to review relevant state or local regulations that establish the minimum standards for the equipment carried on the vehicle. Some states may have several options for licensing or classification of EMS vehicles, and EMS agencies should take care regarding how the PRV is licensed or classified. This decision may have an impact on the equipment that *must* be carried and the equipment that *may* be carried on the PRV because the minimum equipment standards established by associated regulations may be different for each classification of vehicle type depending on how the PRV is licensed or registered. It would be unfortunate for the mission of the PRV to be hobbled because of equipment restrictions that may accompany certain types of vehicle licensure. For example, New York State allows for the registration of nonambulance emergency ambulance support vehicles

(EASV) for nontransport EMS vehicles. To that end, New York has a specific statute that defines "EASV equipment requirements" and dictates the minimum equipment requirements for such an EMS vehicle.[1] The reader is directed to carefully review applicable statutes that govern their respective primary service areas (PSAs) for additional information.

After first considering what equipment must be carried according to applicable statutes, the PRV should be additionally equipped with the patient care equipment similar to that found on advanced life support (ALS) ambulances in the EMS system. This collection of equipment should allow the EMS physician to serve as a first responder in the event they are the first to arrive on scene to care for an ill or injured patient. This self-reliance of the EMS physician must be enabled.

It should be considered though that a one-for-one stocking of equipment between the ALS ambulance and the PRV may result in added expense and unnecessary duplication of equipment resources. **Table 32-2** illustrates examples of PRV equipment substitutions for common pieces of ALS ambulance equipment. Making such equipment substitutions may allow for either a significant cost savings, or redirection of funds toward purchase of other special diagnostic equipment that is not usually carried on an ALS ambulance. Such special items may include cooximeters capable of measuring pulse oximetry, carboxyhemoglobin, and methemoglobin levels or point-of-care blood gas and blood chemistry analyzers, among other devices.

In most cases PRVs are not intended to transport patients, and so large items such as backboards, stokes baskets, or stretchers are probably not necessary to carry in the PRV. Furthermore, space constraints may make carriage of such large items impractical. Fortunately these items are typically available on patient transport units that are responding to the scene. Compact patient carrying devices such as tarps or SKED rescue sleds might be considered as alternatives if there is a need for the PRV to carry a patient movement device.

Although the ability to provide standard ALS care is important, one of the significant values of having an EMS physician respond to the field is that they are capable of bringing a more advanced level of care to the patient's side. Such advanced care may include utilizing paralytic agents during medication assisted airway management, performing field amputation of entrapped or entangled limbs (see also Chapter 52), or performing other field surgical interventions like cricothyrotomy or tube thoracostomy (see also Chapter 64). Obviously if such procedural interventions are within the scope of practice and mission of the EMS physician, then the PRV must carry the equipment needed by the EMS physician to perform those interventions.

INTEROPERABILITY OF EQUIPMENT

Interoperability of the equipment carried on the PRV with other EMS response assets should be a special consideration. This is less of a concern if the EMS physician will only be responding within the PSA of a single EMS agency. However, in many systems the EMS physician may respond to multiple PSAs covered by several different EMS agencies. Accommodating for complete equipment interoperability may be difficult in this case, and may require the physician to carry extra equipment on the PRV to either achieve better interoperability or to achieve greater self-sufficiency. **Table 32-3** lists a suggested PRV equipment supply.

TABLE 32-2	PRV Equipment Substitutes		
ALS Ambulance Equipment	Cost	PRV Equipment Substitute	Cost
Cardiac monitor defibrillator with noninvasive blood pressure (NIBP), pulse oximetry, end-tidal capnography, and 12-lead ECG capability	$13000.00	AED with Lead 2 ECG display	$2500.00
		Manual blood pressure cuff set	$200.00
		Fingertip pulse oximeter	$150.00
		Digital capnometer	$20.00
Compact electric suction unit	$500.00	"turkey baster" bulb suction	$1.00
Total	$13500.00		$2871.00

TABLE 32-3	Suggested PRV Minimum Equipment Supply

Trauma Supplies

4 × 4 gauze pads

Adhesive tape, assorted sizes

Conforming gauze bandage

Elastic (ACE) bandages, assorted sizes

10 × 30 inch universal dressing

5 × 9 inch sterile dressing

Bandage shears

Triangle bandages

Sterile normal saline (0.5 L minimum)

Air occlusive dressing

Sterile burn sheet

Sterile OB kit

CAT tourniquet or similar device

Hemostatic bandages

Needle thoracostomy set

Adhesive Band-Aids

Medications

Oral glucose gel

Analgesics

Sedatives

Paralytics

ACLS medications

IV dextrose

Antihistamines

Specialty medications (Antibiotics, blood products, Tranexamic acid (TXA))

Toxicology (Naloxone, other antidotes, Cyanokit or hydroxycobalamin)

Diagnostic Equipment

Glucometer

AED

Pen light

BP cuff set

Stethoscope

Point-of-care blood assay (iSTAT or similar)

Cooximeter

Vascular Access Supplies

IV catheters

IV tubing

IV normal saline

Intraosseous access device

IV access sundries (alcohol preps, Tegaderm, extension sets, saline flush)

Oxygen and Airway Equipment

BVM (adult, pediatric, and infant sizes)

Oral and nasal airways

Nonrebreather oxygen mask (adult and pediatric sizes)

Nasal cannula (adult and pediatric sizes)

Oxygen cylinder and carrying bag

Portable suction unit

Laryngoscope (traditional, fiberoptic light source)

Laryngoscope blades (Miller and Macintosh, all sizes)

Laryngoscope (video)

McGill forceps (adult and pediatric)

Endotracheal tubes (all sizes)

Supraglottic airway device (all sizes)

Stylettes

Bougies

Surgical Equipment

Cricothyrotomy set

Tube thoracostomy set

Field amputation set (bone saw, Gigli saw, folding camp saw, or cordless reciprocating Sawzall® saw, scalpels, CAT tourniquets, sutures, Kelly clamps)

Suturing set

Skin stapler

Extrication Equipment

Short backboard or KED

Blanket

Cervical collars

Vacuum splint set

Traction splint

Emergency Tool Kit

Hammer

Pliers (adjustable)

Crescent wrench set

Screwdriver (multipurpose, flat, Phillips, and star heads)

Center/window Punch

Jumper cables

Duct tape

Flashlight

Halligan tool

PPE

Nitrile exam gloves

Sharps container

Disinfectant wipes

Alcohol hand sanitizer

N-95 masks

Surgical masks

Eye protection

Ear protection (ear plugs or earmuffs)

Helmet

Bunker gear or extrication jump suit

High visibility vest (ANSI approved)

Extrication gloves

Safety Equipment

Safety flares or reflective roadside triangles

Wheel chocks

5 lb UL ABC fire extinguisher (rated 10BC)

Emergency Response Guidebook (Orange HAZMAT book)

Binoculars

Shovel

Office Supplies

Form holder/clipboard

Pens

Paper

Electronics

Mobile data terminal or laptop computer

Communications radios

Global positioning system or other mapping system

Many of the equipment and supply items in the PRV must be kept in some type of field response bags. However, traditional EMS bags may not be ideally designed for use by an EMS physician. Typical EMS bags are designed like a duffle bag with a shoulder strap and tend to be bulky and heavy, and are potentially difficult to carry. This may be especially true over rough terrain or long distances. It may be advisable to seek out vendors capable of making custom-made equipment bags that can package the EMS physician's supplies in an organized fashion and incorporate ergonomic features into the bag design. Ergonomic features include creating a back-pack style carrying system, reducing the bag's size or weight, or improving item accessibility. Such features should receive special consideration when choosing or designing the bags that will contain the EMS physician's gear. **Figure 32-2** depicts examples of a traditional EMS equipment bag and a more ergonomically designed EMS equipment bag.

In some circumstances, it may be advantageous for the EMS physician to carry the same standard ALS bag that is deployed by their agency. When supplies are used from the bag, it may easily be "swapped out" for a fully stocked bag obtained from the agency's supply and restocking depot. The convenience of restocking with supplies consumed by the EMS physician while performing patient care must be considered.

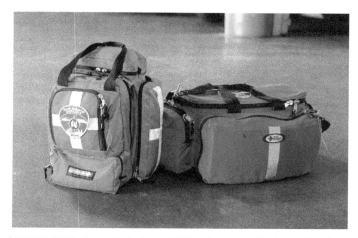

FIGURE 32-2. Ergonomically designed EMS equipment bag. The bag on the left was specially designed for ergonomics and single provider field response.

If there are barriers to efficient restocking, it may be advisable for the PRV to carry additional quantities of commonly used supplies while taking into consideration the space constraints of the PRV.

▓ SPECIALIZED PERSONAL OPERATIONAL AND PROTECTIVE EQUIPMENT

Certain mission environments may necessitate that the PRV carry specialized personal operational equipment for the EMS physician. Items such as high-angle-rescue harnesses and climbing helmets, diving equipment, tactical-law enforcement gear, and SCBAs may allow the EMS physician to perform specific tactical tasks. Depending on the proximity the EMS physician will have to certain hazards while operating in various settings, he or she may require the same PPE as the frontline firefighter or SWAT team officer, or may only need a simple uniform including pants, shirt, and protective footwear. Specialized PPE may include fire and puncture-resistant extrication "jump suits"; Class A-, B-, C-, or D-level HAZMAT or biological suits; "turnout gear"; head, eye, and hearing protection; life jackets and other water safety equipment; cold weather clothing; or bullet-resistant tactical body armor. Accommodations for carrying any of these items must be made when compiling the list of equipment to be stocked in the PRV. Additionally, the response environment may require the EMS physician to be equipped with skis, bicycles, or other terrain-specific equipment that may require specialized racks or carrying devices to be installed on the vehicle in order to carry this equipment into the field.

▓ COMMUNICATIONS EQUIPMENT

In addition to the patient care and operational equipment needed by the EMS physician, the EMS PRV must also be equipped with communications equipment. This equipment must allow for interoperable communications with units from the EMS physician's agency as well as with other EMS agencies, fire departments, law enforcement, air medical units, other public safety personnel, hospitals, and emergency operations centers. Additional discussion regarding interoperable communications and specific types of radio equipment occur in Chapter 15. These concepts must be fully understood when deciding what radio equipment should be installed; however, most decisions will be influenced by the communications equipment that is utilized in the EMS physician's response area.

The selection and installation of interoperable communications equipment will strengthen opportunities for the PRV to serve as the command post for the medical component of emergency and disaster response systems, especially as more systems adopt the practices of establishing a unified command structure (see also Chapters 75 and 76). The inclusion of Internet-capable devices will allow for gathering of information from mapping systems, the media, and, in some cases, electronic medical records, that may be critical to completion of the mission or in providing patient care. Installation of a small printer and laptop computer will provide the capability to print documents from the PRV, further enhancing the communications capabilities of the EMS physician.

VEHICLE CHARACTERISTICS AND SELECTION

Once the EMS physician's field missions have been defined and the necessary equipment has been selected, attention may be turned toward choosing the type of vehicle that will best allow for safe and effective deployment of the EMS physician and their equipment. In addition to the previous discussion points, additional factors that will impact the choice of vehicle that will serve as the PRV include the intended or potential frequency of response; the geography and environmental characteristics of the response area; deployment and dispatch plans; fuel types; two or four wheel drive chassis type; two- or four-door access; vehicle size and maneuverability; and whether a special driver's license such as a CDL is required to operate certain vehicle types. Of course, the vehicle's cost must also be considered as part of the overall project budget.

Various types of vehicles, including sedans, SUVs, pickups, and light-duty rescue trucks have been put into service as PRVs by different types of EMS services. **Figure 32-3** depicts examples of various EMS physician response vehicles. In most cases, these vehicles have been modified from the "standard" model available to the general public. Such modifications include installation of roll cages, more robust braking systems, more powerful engines, and specialized chassis that are necessary to hold up to the physical stresses that are inherent in emergency vehicle operations. Several automobile manufacturers provide emergency vehicle versions of civilian vehicles, such as the Ford "*Police Intercepter*" version of the *Crowne Victoria, Taurus,* and *Explorer* models, the Chevrolet *Caprice* police patrol vehicle (PPV), *Tahoe* PPV and *Tahoe* special services vehicle (SSV), and *Impala* police vehicle, and the Dodge *Charger.*[2]

Although in most cases the PRV will not be utilized to provide patient transport, certain agencies or organizations, including the US General Services Administration Federal Specification KKK-A-1822F and the National Fire Protection Administration (NFPA) Specification 1917, do define the minimum specifications for patient transport ambulances.[3,4] It may be useful to maintain an awareness of such specifications when designing the PRV.

After-market emergency vehicle design and customization vendors can make the required modifications to the power train, vehicle frame, and chassis of stock civilian vehicles. Such "conversion packages" often include construction of specialty equipment storage cabinets, incorporation of climate control devices, and installation of specialty electronics such as communications equipment, mobile data terminals, warning lights, and sirens. These modifications allow for the construction of highly functional PRVs that can be customized to meet the needs of the EMS physician's field response missions.

Many EMS agencies already deploy emergency response vehicles like field supervisor trucks, chief's trucks, quick response vehicles, or ALS fly cars. In these circumstances, it is potentially advisable that the PRV be the same make and model of vehicle as the other vehicles in the fleet. This will allow for uniformity in appearance across the fleet, and, more importantly, will allow for simplified maintenance and repair of the fleet, especially if the agency performs their own vehicle maintenance in-house. Caution should be exercised though, as limiting the vehicle choice for the PRV based on the vehicles that already exist in the fleet may also limit the capability of the PRV to carry the equipment needed to fully realize the EMS physician's unique missions.

VEHICLE INTERIOR DESIGN AND EQUIPMENT CONSIDERATIONS

The interior of the PRV should be carefully designed so as to securely store the physician's equipment but also allow for easy access to the equipment. In some cases it may be desirable to install custom-built cabinetry in the rear of the vehicle where equipment bags and items can be

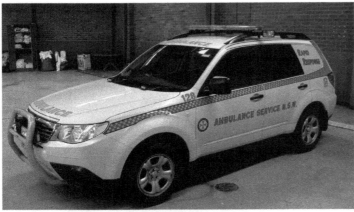
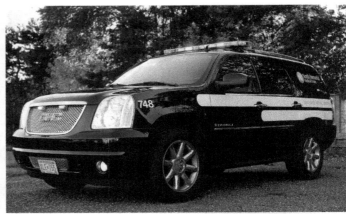
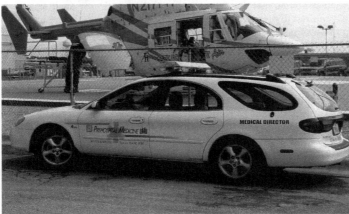
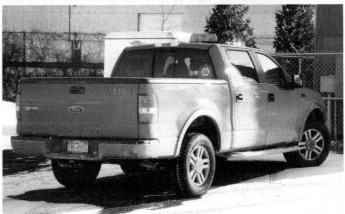

FIGURE 32-3. EMS physician response vehicle examples.

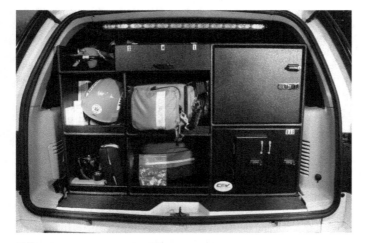

FIGURE 32-4. Custom-built PRV equipment cabinet.

stored. In other cases, it may be more cost efficient to install a reinforced panel or "dog cage" to separate the equipment compartment from the driver's compartment, so as to protect the vehicle occupants from any equipment that might become a projectile in the unfortunate event of a motor vehicle collision involving the PRV. **Figure 32-4** illustrates a physician response vehicle custom-built cabinetry.

One characteristic of the interior of vehicles being considered as the PRV that should receive special focus is the location of the gearshift lever and parking brake. In some vehicle models, these important vehicle operation components occupy space between the front seats of the vehicle or in the center console. In vehicles designed like this, the installation of items like mobile data terminals, communications equipment, or

warning light and siren controls may be difficult or impossible to accomplish while maintaining safe and effective access to vehicle controls. In some cases, third-party vendors may manufacture replacement consoles that will better accommodate installation of after-market electronic equipment items and associated control panels.

Certain equipment carried in the PRV will require electrical service to either maintain battery charges of items like AEDs or monitor/defibrillators, or to provide power for general operation such as for refrigerators used to store certain medications. Installation of electrical current inverters and 120-volt power outlets may be necessary. Depending on the power needed to supply the onboard electronics, modifications to the engine's alternator and fuse or circuit breaker panel may be required. The installation of "shore-line" outlets are often necessary to allow the PRV to be plugged into an external fixed power source to maintain the charge on the engine's battery as well as to provide power to other onboard electrical devices when the vehicle is not in being driven.

■ STORAGE OF CONTROLLED SUBSTANCES AND OTHER MEDICATIONS

It is often cited that controlled substances need to be secured with a double lock. In fact, there are actually no rules or regulations established by the DEA that require a double lock for storage of controlled substances that are used by a practitioner for treating patients in the course of his usual business. However, security of controlled substances is very important. The *DEA Practitioner's Manual: The Code of Federal Regulations Title 21 CFR Section 1301.71(a)* requires that "all registrants provide effective controls and procedures to guard against theft and diversion of controlled substances."[5] Many states also have regulations that contain similar language. For example, the Wisconsin EMS Controlled Substance Management standard states: "Each EMS Service must determine what level of security is necessary. A reasonable minimum is to keep controlled substances secured within a vehicle that is also

---

Box 32-5

Excerpt From New York State Rules and Regulations on Controlled Substances[7]

Any substock of controlled substances in an authorized response vehicle shall be stored as follows:

1. When access to the patient compartment of an ambulance is kept locked at all times, controlled substances shall be secured in a locked cabinet using a key lock different than the patient compartment.

2. When the access to the patient compartment of an ambulance is not kept locked at all times or any other response vehicle is used, controlled substances must be secured in a locked box within a locked stationary cabinet under a two-lock system using different keys.

3. The key(s) to access the cabinet where controlled substances are stored must be maintained under the direct control of a certified and authorized individual.

4. Controlled substances may be maintained in the direct possession and control of a certified and authorized individual at all times while such individual is on duty for the ALS agency; however, at no time shall controlled substances be carried in any personal automobile.

Box 32-6

Opportunities for Improving Emergency Vehicle Visibility and Recognition

- Outline vehicle boundaries with "contour markings" using retroreflective material, especially on large vehicles.

- Concentrate retroreflective material lower on emergency vehicles to optimize interaction with approaching vehicles' headlamps.

- Consider (and allow) the use of fluorescent retroreflective materials in applications where a high degree of day-/night-time visibility is desired.

- Using high-efficiency retroreflective material can improve conspicuity while reducing the amount of vehicle surface area requiring treatment.

- Applying distinctive logos or emblems made with retroreflective material can improve emergency vehicle visibility and recognition.

---

secured or under appropriate surveillance."[6] However, certain states do have more strict standards than the DEA. For example, New York State has enacted a more restrictive standard that is outlined in **Box 32-5**.[7]

It is imperative that EMS physicians be familiar with the controlled substance security and storage standards that exist in their operational jurisdictions. It is also imperative for the PRV design process to ensure that the construction of controlled substance storage areas inside the PRV is compliant with these regulations. If additional "double lock" security is required, as demonstrated in the New York State example, the access control device or locking system should be carefully chosen. Access control devices may include push-button combination locks, rotary dial combination locks, standard keyed locks, or electronic badge reader locks that utilize radio frequency (RF) proximity readers or magnetic strip readers. Ideally the access control device will allow for tracking of personnel who access the cabinet, and, if needed, allow for multiple personnel to securely access the cabinet. This is especially important if multiple physicians on an EMS physician response team will use the PRV.

In addition to ensuring that controlled substances are securely stored, it is also important that temperature sensitive medications are properly stored. This may require the installation of refrigerators, heaters, or special cabinets capable of maintaining a climate-controlled environment. Installation of climate-controlled storage is also critical if the PRV intends to carry blood products.

VEHICLE EXTERNAL DESIGN AND EQUIPMENT CONSIDERATIONS

The external appearance of the PRV is dictated by several factors. In many jurisdictions there are specific regulations that define the external appearance of EMS vehicles. In Virginia, for example, the state administrative code defines three colors that may be used on the external surfaces of nontransport emergency response vehicles, specifies the size of any lettering on the vehicle, that the word EMERGENCY must appear in at least two places, and specifies that the EMS agency name and city, town, or county must appear on two sides of the vehicle.[8] Several other states and jurisdictions have similar regulations.

▓ PASSIVE WARNING DEVICES

Use of passive warning devices and conspicuity markings, including retroreflective graphics and vehicle striping, deserves mention. The US Fire Administration, under FEMA, performed and published the "Emergency Vehicle Visibility and Conspicuity Study" in 2009.[9] Of several key findings, the study identified that "both visibility and recognition are important facets of emergency vehicle conspicuity." The study also identified several

opportunities to improve emergency vehicle visibility, which are described in **Box 32-6** and illustrated in **Figure 32-5**.

There is some science that supports use of certain colors to increase visibility in both daytime and nighttime conditions. *Scotopic vision* refers to the sensitivity of the eye under low light conditions and *photopic vision* refers to the sensitivity of the eye under well-lit conditions. The human retina demonstrates low sensitivity to colors at each end of the visible spectrum like red and violet in both light and dark conditions. However, the retina demonstrates high sensitivity to colors in the middle of the spectrum. In dark conditions the retina is most sensitive to blue-green colors, and in light conditions the retina is most sensitive to green-yellow colors. **Figure 32-6** illustrates the retina's sensitivity to various colors in scotopic and photopic light conditions. In applying this science, it would seem prudent to choose vehicle colors in the midspectrum range. However, the fact that people have been conditioned over time to expect fire trucks to be red, school buses to be yellow, and police cars to be black and white should also be considered when choosing colors for the vehicle's external markings. There is a growing body of literature related to emergency vehicle conspicuity; however further research is needed in order to clearly establish whether particular patterns and color combinations are effective at increasing visibility and recognition, and, more importantly, whether such patterns and colors help reduce or prevent collisions between civilian vehicles and emergency vehicles.

Despite the fact that currently there is no conclusive evidence to support use of specific markings such as a rear chevron, depending on the nature of the EMS agency, use of high-visibility high-efficiency retroreflective side graphics may still be required by certain statutes or guidelines. For example, NFPA Specification 1901 requires that fire apparatus have "retroreflective markings that cover 50 percent of the length of the vehicle sides and 25 percent of the vehicle front."[10] This guideline also requires that "50 percent of the rear-facing vertical surface ... shall be equipped with retroreflective striping in a chevron pattern sloping downward and away from the centerline of the vehicle at an angle of 45 degrees." It is feasible that if the PRV is licensed as a piece of fire apparatus that it could be required to comply with these marking requirements. Several states have adopted legislation that specifies use of retroreflective markings with allowances for use of a rear-facing chevron, but this author is unaware of any states that specifically require use of chevron markings on nonfire apparatus. In Tennessee, *Rule 1200-12-01-.02 Ambulance Safety, Design, and Construction Standards* states that "an ambulance service shall ensure that a minimum of one (1) horizontal solid reflective stripe at least six (6) inches in width shall be displayed on the sides and rear, horizontal to the beltline of the ambulance extending below the window line;" and that "the ambulance service may display a chevron striping pattern in the rear of the vehicle, with a pattern of alternating diagonal elements at least six (6) inches in width. Chevron patterns shall comply with the Manual of Uniform Traffic Control Devices."[11] Many nonfire-based EMS agencies across the country have voluntarily adopted similar visibility marking

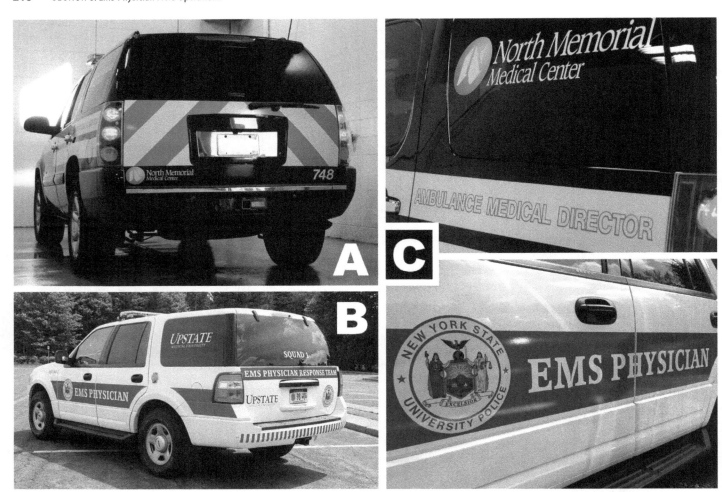

FIGURE 32-5. Conspicuity markings. **A**: Chevrons. **B**: Retroreflective "belt-line." **C**: Reflective emblems.

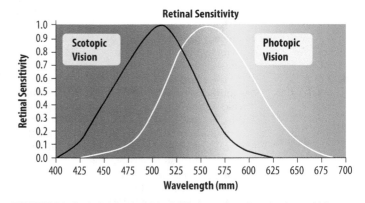

FIGURE 32-6. Optimizing day/night visibility, scotopic vs photopic color sensitivity.

standards for their fleets, even if less stringent legislation exists in their service areas.

ACTIVE WARNING DEVICES

Passive warning devices are only a part of a comprehensive emergency vehicle visibility and recognition plan. These graphics should be paired with certain active warning devices including various types of lights, sirens, and horns. Local regulations may dictate the number, type, location, and color of warning lights displayed on the response vehicle, as well as the type of audible warning devices that can be installed on

emergency vehicles. There is a growing body of literature that evaluates a variety of active warning device characteristics such as siren sounds, warning light color(s), warning light types (LED, halogen, strobe, etc), and optimal placement of warning lights on emergency vehicles. A complete discussion of this topic is outside the scope of this chapter, and the reader is directed to review applicable literature in conjunction with consulting with an emergency vehicle vendor when making decisions about installation of active warning devices on the PRV.

In addition to installation of typical red, white, and/or blue warning lights, it may also be advisable to install amber caution lights such as the "traffic advisor" light bars. Such lighting may potentially enhance roadside visibility and safety. Traffic preempting signals, such as the Opticom traffic signal preemption device by 3M, should also be considered as an installation option depending on local operating environments. Installation of scene-lighting systems may also be necessary depending on the EMS physician's mission and the role of the PRV in on-scene operations.

In many areas, specific approval to operate with "lights and sirens" must be obtained from certain authorizing entities. If the PRV is registered as part of an existing EMS agency or as a government vehicle, it may be simple to obtain approval from governing authorities to operate the vehicle with "lights and sirens." However, if the PRV is being operated by a stand-alone physician response team or as a hospital-based vehicle, it may be more difficult to obtain such approval. Obtaining approval may be especially difficult where PSA laws exist, which restrict the addition of new EMS services in a certain geographic area. Care should be taken to thoroughly research local licensing requirements and options so as to avoid such conflicts when possible.

The PRV design team should also consider whether it will be necessary to install cargo carriers, ski and bicycle racks, towing hitches, winches, or specialty grill guards to allow carriage of large items like Stoke stretchers, ladders, skis, or bicycles or to allow for towing of special operations trailers.

SPECIAL OPERATIONS TRAILERS

It should be realized that not all EMS physician missions can be accomplished with the equipment that can be carried in a single PRV. Missions such as mass casualty support, mass gathering event medical coverage, or other planned and unplanned large-scale events and incidents may require equipment that is too large to be carried in the PRV. Large items like portable shelters, generators, shelter heating and cooling systems, communications systems, medical gas or SCBA cascade refilling systems, collapsible cots, potable water, nonperishable food, decontamination supplies, golf carts or ATVs, portable toilets, and additional quantities of basic medical supplies to support the patient care activities of other responding units are all examples of items that may be needed during a large-scale EMS mission. The ability to support multiple people with shelter, food, water, and toileting facilities must be considered if existing systems do not specifically address these needs for the medical component of the event response structure. Because these items cannot be reasonably carried in the PRV it is much more practical to store such important but bulky and infrequently used equipment in a special operations trailer.

Hazardous materials response implies the on-scene availability of complex personal protection and decontamination equipment. While local resources often include decontamination equipment and the ability to establish hot, warm, and cold zones, there may not be equipment available for additional medical responders who are not already rostered members of the HAZMAT team. In some situations, PPE, HAZMAT resource materials, and perhaps a limited cache of antidotes may be appropriate for the special operations trailer to have in stock.

An important step in developing a special operations trailer is to determine how the trailer will be towed to the scene. If the PRV will be delivering the trailer, then appropriate towing capacity and towing equipment must be factored into the vehicle selection and design process. Because special operations trailers are usually stored at facilities that the EMS physician may be remote from, it may be more practical for some other vehicle in the EMS agency's fleet to be used as the vehicle to tow the special operations trailer to the incident scene.

LEGAL AND OPERATIONAL CONSIDERATIONS

The operation of an EMS physician response vehicle program is more complex than simply putting a physician and certain equipment and supplies into a vehicle and driving to an emergency scene. Just as certain jurisdictions have enacted statutes that govern the equipment carried in ambulances and other emergency vehicles, most jurisdictions have also enacted statutes that govern the operations of emergency vehicles. Such statutes may pertain to vehicle licensure and registration, how and where the vehicle may operate, whether or not the person driving the vehicle must complete an Emergency Vehicle Operations Course or carry a special operator's license, what traffic laws must be obeyed, and even the criminal and administrative offenses associated with unsafe or improper operation of an emergency vehicle. In most jurisdictions, multiple statutes or regulations likely exist and may be found in different sections of the state's administrative rules or constitution or under different individual governing agencies such as the state Department of Transportation, the state Department of Public Safety, or the state Department of Health. The EMS physician should research all of the regulations that exist in their locality and should most certainly read and understand them fully to ensure proper compliance with applicable laws. One resource where EMS physicians can find a searchable database of state-specific regulations is the National Association of State EMS Officials (NASEMSO) State

Legislation Searchable Database: http://www.nasemso.org/legislation/search/Default.aspx.[12]

■ EMERGENCY VEHICLE OPERATIONS CERTIFICATION

Some, but not all, jurisdictions require people who drive emergency vehicles to complete an emergency vehicle operations certification (EVOC) course. Even where not required by law, it is still advisable for the EMS physician to have an awareness of the concepts taught during EVOC, and ideally every EMS physician who operates a PRV would complete an EVOC course. Even when EVOC courses are not required, most jurisdictions have legislation similar to Minnesota Statute 169.17 that explicitly states that legislation defining operations of an emergency vehicle "does not operate to relieve the driver of an authorized emergency vehicle from the duty to drive with due regard for the safety of persons using the highways."[13] The practice of driving with due regard for safety of others is perhaps one of the most important tenets that the EMS physician should be aware of and adhere to. Chapter 31 provides more in-depth discussion regarding EVOC.

SUMMARY

Active field response of EMS physicians is an integral component of many modern EMS systems. The formation and maintenance of an effective PRT ensures the ability of the system to initiate on-scene medical direction, expand the scope of prehospital providers in MCI and disasters, provide in-person assistance on difficult and unusual calls, and provide field surgery when essential to life-saving efforts. The design, development, and deployment of an EMS physician response vehicle is an undertaking that deserves special attention to the details discussed in this chapter. With careful and thoughtful planning, the EMS physician and the equipment and supplies that are carried in the PRV can be established as a valuable asset that will enhance the local, regional, and even the state emergency response system. Providing specialized response capabilities through such a program will add significant value and can significantly augment the existing system resources.

KEY POINTS

- EMS physicians responding to the field should have training in EVOC, scene safety, NIMS/ICS, hazardous materials awareness, fire ground operations awareness, radio operations, and local protocols and disaster plans.
- Relationships with a variety of stakeholders should be established before and during the physician response vehicle project management process to ensure the EMS physician response program is effective in accomplishing its missions and is utilized to its full potential.
- The EMS physician field response missions will define the characteristics of the vehicle and equipment that are deployed with the EMS physician.
- The EMS physician should be aware of the regulations that govern their response jurisdictions with regard to the operations, design, equipment requirements, vehicle appearance, and licensing or registration of an EMS physician response vehicles.
- The EMS physician should be equipped with appropriate personal protective equipment to allow them to operate in environments that may present certain specific risks of injury or risks to personal safety.
- The EMS physician response vehicle, equipment, and equipment bags should be designed with special attention to utility, portability, ergonomics, and appropriateness for the response environment.

- The EMS physician response vehicle should be equipped with the equipment and supplies that are necessary for the EMS physician to accomplish their defined field missions.

- The EMS physician response vehicle should be equipped to allow the EMS physician to operate with an appropriate degree of self-reliance and independent capability.

REFERENCES

1. Chapter VI of Title 10 (Health) of the Official Compilation of Codes, Rules and Regulations State Emergency Medical Services Code Part 800.26-Emergency Ambulance Service Vehicle Equipment Requirements. New York State Department of Health. Effective November 03, 2004.

2. Holmes J. 2012 Ford Explorer police interceptor utility: Ford unveils a police SUV based on the all-new Explorer. Car and Driver. http://www.caranddriver.com/news/ford-explorer-news-2012-ford-police-interceptor-utility. Accessed May, 2015.September 2010.

3. United States General Services Administration. Federal Specification for the Star of Life Ambulance. KKK-A-1822F. www.usfa.fema.gov/downloads/doc/DraftKKK-A-1822FCC.doc. Accessed May, 2015.

4. NFPA 1917: Standard for Automotive Ambulances, 2013 Edition. National Fire Protection Association. 2013. http://www.nfpa.org/codes-and-standards/document-information-pages?mode=code&code=1917. Accessed May, 2015.

5. Code of Federal Regulations. Section 1301.71. Security requirements generally. http://www.deadiversion.usdoj.gov/21cfr/cfr/1301/1301_71.htm. Accessed May, 2015.

6. Wisconsin EMS Controlled Substance Management. October 5, 2010. https://www.dhs.wisconsin.gov/sites/default/files/legacy/ems/system/EMSControlledSubstanceManagement.pdf. Accessed May, 2015.

7. Chapter VI, Title 10 (Health) of the Official Compilation of Codes, Rules and Regulations, Part 80.136. Controlled Substances for Emergency Medical Services. New York State Department of Health. Effective August 04, 1993. http://www.health.ny.gov/professionals/ems/part80.htm.

8. Virginia Administrative Code, Agency 5, Department of Health. Chapter 31: Virginia Emergency Medical Services Regulations. https://www.vdh.virginia.gov/OEMS/Files_Page/regulation/2012EMSRegulations.pdf. Accessed May, 2015.

9. Department of Homeland Security, US Fire Administration. Emergency Vehicle Visibility and Conspicuity Study. FEMA FA-323. August2009.http://www.usfa.fema.gov/downloads/pdf/publications/fa_323.pdf.

10. NFPA 1901: Standard for Automotive Fire Apparatus, 2009 Edition. National Fire Protection Association. 2009. http://www.nfpa.org/codes-and-standards/document-information-pages?mode=code&code=1901. Accessed May, 2015.

11. Tennessee Secretary of State. Tennessee Rule 1200-12-01-.02. Ambulance Safety, Design, and Construction Standards. Effective date 24 August 2010. http://tn.gov/sos/rules_filings/05-22-10.pdf.

12. NASEMSO State Legislation Searchable Database. National Association of State Emergency Medical Services Officials (NASEMSO). http://www.nasemso.org/legislation/search/Default.aspx.

13. Minnesota Statute. Chapter 169: Traffic Regulations. Section 169.17 Emergency Vehicle. 2013. https://www.revisor.mn.gov/statutes/?id=169.17. Accessed May, 2015.

Immediate Life-Threatening Events

CHAPTER
33

Cardiac Arrest

Tanner S. Boyd
Debra G. Perina

INTRODUCTION

EMS medical care provided to cardiac arrest patients has changed dramatically over time. Ambulances initially functioned merely as transport vehicles, while today EMS is an integrated part of the health care system with the ability to provide advanced life support while en route to a hospital. Regional dispatch centers now decide which resources should respond to an emergency call. Dispatchers, trained in emergency medical dispatch (EMD) techniques, have specific protocols to follow to determine whether basic life support (BLS) or advanced life support (ALS) EMS response is required. Prearrival instructions to bystanders can help expedite initial first aid or CPR.[1-4] Recently protocols have expanded the role of EMS providers in treating out-of-hospital cardiac arrest (OCHA) patients ranging from beginning therapeutic hypothermia in the field to bypassing hospitals in favor of a specialized receiving facility.

Historically, much of EMS medical care grew out of traditional practice with little scientific basis. Today EMS practice is influenced by evidence-based medicine concepts as more rigorous studies are completed and systems demand proven benefit prior to the introduction of new procedures, drugs, and adjuncts in prehospital patient care. This is particularly true with OHCA patients where ongoing research is continually investigating the best treatment options. The American Heart Association (AHA) periodically scientifically reviews recent literature and makes recommendations for treatment changes based on the strength and results of these studies. Prehospital resuscitations guidelines often follow the AHA recommendations closely due to the rigorous scientific process utilized in their updates. The most recent AHA update occurred in 2010, and many of the studies and papers reviewed for the most recent guidelines are discussed in this chapter.

OBJECTIVES

- Review the demographics and presentations of out-of-hospital cardiac arrest (OHCA) patients.
- Discuss system access, response types, and processes.
- Discuss current prehospital management of OHCA.
- Review prehospital OHCA outcomes.

DEMOGRAPHICS

The Framingham Heart Study reports that from 1950 to 1999, 48% of sudden cardiac deaths (SCD) and 20% of nonsudden coronary heart disease deaths occurred in patients without previously known coronary artery disease.[5] Rea et al reported that from 1986 to 1994, the overall incidence of cardiac arrest was 1.89 per 1000 subject years, further breaking this down to an incidence of 0.7, 1.91, and 4.1 per 1000 subject years for the age ranges of 50 to 59, 60 to 69, and 70 to 79, respectively. The incidence of cardiac arrest in males was 2.89 compared to 1.04 for females. Compared to other risk factors, a diagnosis of congestive heart failure carried a cardiac arrest incidence of 21.87 per 1000 subject years, while a history of diabetes mellitus, previous MI, smoking, and hypertension produced incidences of 13.8, 13.69, 9.18, and 7.54, respectively.[6] Cardiac arrests, along with myocardial infarction and unstable angina complaints, appear to have a circadian variation with a morning peak shortly after the initiation of daily activities.[7] Lower socioeconomic status is associated with higher incidences of OHCA with a 30% to 80% difference between the highest and lowest socioeconomic quartiles. However, this difference tends to equilibrate in those over 65 years.[8] Another study demonstrated racial differences in OHCA rates with black Americans having a much higher frequency than white or Hispanic Americans.[9]

Initial presenting rhythm in OHCA has been reported to be ventricular tachycardia, ventricular fibrillation, or a shockable rhythm as determined by an AED in approximately 23% of patients. Another 9% had nonshockable rhythms per an AED, 40% had asystole, 20% had PEA, and the final 9% were unknown or not determined. Looking at multiple American and Canadian cities when examined regionally, there appears to be a wide variation in rates of OHCA ranging from 71.8 per 100,000 subject years in Ottawa, Canada, to 159 in Dallas, Texas. Oddly though, variations are often not consistent within geographical regions such as Seattle, Washington's 144 per 100,000 subject years compared to Portland, Oregon, and Vancouver, Canada's 77.5 and 75.9, respectively. Taken together, the overall incidence of OHCA is calculated to be 95 per 100,000 subject years.[10]

Rates of witnessed OHCA and bystander CPR vary widely among localities. Studies in Arizona and New York have reported a 45.1% to 46% incidence of witnessed arrests, respectively.[11,12] A meta-analysis of 79 studies involving 142,740 patients showed 53% of OHCA were witnessed by a bystander with 32% of patients receiving bystander CPR.[13] However, other studies have reported bystander CPR rates as low as 19%.[10] Some of these differences may be due to OHCA location (eg, home, public place, medical facility), but factors such as race and socioeconomic status are important as well. In Los Angeles, only 13% of Black or Latino patients received bystander CPR compared to 24% of white patients.[14] In Arizona, non-Hispanics are more likely to received bystander CPR relative to Hispanics (41.5% vs 32.2%; $P < 0.0001$).[15] Higher socioeconomic groups tend to have higher rates of bystander CPR.[16,17] Knowledge of these disparities can help target certain groups for public education programs as well as strategically placing EMS response units in certain areas to minimize response times.

PRESENTATIONS

The EMS system must be activated for appropriate treatment. Thus, the patient or a bystander must recognize the problem.[18-20] Delays are often frequent as presentations are varied and denial of symptoms can delay summoning help. If a sudden cardiac arrest is witnessed by a bystander or occurs in a public area, EMS is accessed faster than in an unwitnessed event.[21] Arrests outside the home are twice as likely to get bystander CPR compared with residential arrests.[22] A Swedish study reported that a delay of less than 4 minutes from time of cardiac arrest to EMS activation resulted in an increased 1-month survival of 6.9% as opposed to 2.8% ($P < 0.0001$).[23] Quicker EMS response times[24] and shorter delays to CPR initiation increase overall survival. These items can be extrapolated to traumatic cardiac arrests as well.

Delays in recognition and access of care vary in precardiac arrest presentations. One of the largest randomized trials to date addressing delays in treatment to patients experiencing chest pain is the European Myocardial Infarction Project (EMIP).[25] Data were collected from 15 European countries and Canada between 1988 and 1992. This study found the longest delays occurred in female patients, those over age 65 years, those who had experienced chest pain in the previous 24 hours, and those with pulmonary edema. Characteristics of patients with the shortest delay in summoning an ambulance included those with a history of previous myocardial infarction (MI), those in shock, and those experiencing ventricular fibrillation. Numerous smaller studies have also reported similar findings, with the addition of lower socioeconomic status, family member being present at symptom onset, and a belief that symptoms are not severe enough also causing a delay in access of care. Gender differences are not as well defined as some studies point toward increased frequency of atypical symptoms in females, causing a larger delay between symptom onset and access of care,[26] whereas others show no gender difference.[27]

Some populations can present without chest pain at all. Elderly and diabetic patients can have atypical presentations of acute MI with nonspecific symptoms such as dizziness, syncope, malaise, nausea, vomiting, or abdominal pain. Patients experiencing a significant event can also be in congestive heart failure, hypotensive, or in severe respiratory distress. Depending on the significance to the patient, this can cause delays in access of care or even mislead health care personnel in the wrong direction, causing another delay to proper diagnosis and treatment.

A subset of trauma patients can also decline into cardiac arrest. The mechanism of injury can range from blunt injury in car accidents to penetrating insults from stabbings or gunshot wounds. The arrest may be as a result of the traumatic injury or secondary producing a myocardial infarct due to stress. The time to access EMS care varies considerably based on the circumstances surrounding the traumatic event, the ability of the patient to initiate calling for help, and the presence of witnesses willing to intervene.

Public awareness campaigns have been shown to increase bystander CPR rates and recognition of serious symptoms. Frequent public service announcements to inform the public should continue to be encouraged, emphasizing the benefits of bystander CPR, rapid EMS activation, and the importance that time plays in a patient's outcome.[28]

ACCESS

Calling 9-1-1 enters the caller into the system by accessing a public safety answering point (PSAP). Trained dispatchers using prearrival instructions not only dispatch EMS and first responders expeditiously, but also give explicit instructions to bystanders to render care prior to arrival of help. Outcomes are better when dispatchers receive more frequent cardiac arrest calls and when proper units are dispatched faster.[29] Recognition of cardiac arrest is faster when dispatchers query callers regarding the absence of consciousness and quality of breathing.[30] However, any sign of breathing, including agonal breathing, decreases the chances a dispatcher will recognize a cardiac arrest.[31] Teaching dispatchers to recognize agonal breathing increases the detection of cardiac arrests,[32] and also the frequency with which CPR instructions are given.[33] Computer systems have been developed to assist dispatchers in detection of these events. The Medical Priority Dispatch System (MPDS) in Melbourne, Australia, was shown to have a sensitivity of 76.7% and a specificity of 99.2% at detecting a cardiac arrest.[34] Likewise, the Advanced Medical Priority Dispatch System (AMPDS) in London increased the number of people accurately identified as being in cardiac arrest compared to dispatchers alone.[30] While it is clear that these computer systems are helpful, they do miss patients, and there is still room to improve in dispatcher detection of cardiac arrests.

Once a cardiac arrest is identified, a dispatcher can give CPR instructions to a bystander until further help can arrive. Telephone instructions have been shown to increase the rates of bystander CPR[35] and improve outcomes.[29] Using simulation, volunteers who have never been trained to do CPR do compressions just as well with phone instructions as a previously trained person without directions. In any event, any compressions are better than no compressions. Only 2% of witnesses to a cardiac arrest given telephone instructions refuse to do CPR[31] with reasons attributed equally to a person not wanting to do harm to a patient, fear of performing CPR improperly, concern regarding legal consequences, aversion to mouth-to-mouth contact, and being physically unable to perform CPR.[36] When giving instructions, directions to put the phone down during chest compressions do not improve CPR quality.[37] With the advent of cell phones with video streaming capabilities, research in the use of video calls to help dispatchers is currently underway. Dispatchers feel this may help them better assess patients and direct bystanders, but to date there is no evidence supporting the use of this technology.[38]

The elderly have slightly faster times to CPR initiation if given hands-only instructions (ie, no rescue breaths) rather than standard CPR instructions.[39] Given the possibility that compressions-only CPR (COCPR) could increase outcomes, two recent articles in the *New England Journal of Medicine* compared this new technique to standard CPR with breaths. In one study, there was a trend toward increased rates of hospital discharge with COCPR in the subgroups with a cardiac cause of arrest (15.5% vs 12.3%; $P = 0.09$) and a shockable rhythm (31.9% vs 25.7%; $P = 0.09$), but there was no statistical difference between the two groups.[40] In the other study, there was a nonstatistically different trend in hospital discharge (19.1% vs 14.7%; $P = 0.16$) but no change in 30-day mortality (8.7% vs 7.0%; $P = 0.26$).[41] Given the relative ease of guiding someone through these steps, the lack of apparent harm, and the possibility of benefit in giving compressions-only CPR, the American Heart Association in their 2010 guidelines recommends COCPR for untrained laypersons and trained laypersons if they are unable to deliver breathing maneuvers. However, they note that at the present time there is insufficient evidence to support or refute COCPR for trained professional rescuers.[42]

RESPONSE SYSTEMS AND PROCESS

Because of the time sensitivity to first defibrillation, various methods have been developed to decrease the time to defibrillation in a patient with a shockable rhythm. Development of automated external defibrillators (AEDs) has given the lay public access (*public access defibrillation [PAD]*) to easy-to-use machine that can perform this lifesaving intervention.[43-45] Strategically placed in public locations, they can facilitate faster defibrillation of the arresting patient.[46-48] Additionally, law enforcement officers, firefighters, and other first responders often carry AEDs. Approximately 80% of police departments are used as first responders to medical events and of these 39% carry AEDs.[49]

Some EMS agencies have increased overall outcomes using a two-tiered response system in which BLS first responders, with or without defibrillation capabilities, are dispatched at the same time as ALS units. Because there are often more BLS-trained providers in a given region, including firefighters and police, an EMS system can strategically place BLS first responders to minimize response times in a given area to begin care while ALS resources are en route. In one meta-analysis, survival to discharge was greater in two-tiered systems (10.5% vs 5.2%) relative to one-tiered systems.[50] Another study found no statistical difference in outcomes when a BLS squad with defibrillation capabilities arrived prior to ALS. This study reported survival to admission decreased from 26.8% to 19.6% but survival to discharge increased from 8.0% to 8.7%.[51] Cost analysis shows a trend to a two-tiered system being more cost-effective.[52] This study reported that to improve mean response times by 48 seconds through adding more EMS providers, a one-tiered system cost would be $368,000 per quality-adjusted life year (QALY), while a two-tiered system cost would be $53,000 or $159,000/QALY. Changing from a one-tiered to a two-tiered system also has costs with one study reporting $40,000 or $94,000/QALY for pump vehicles or ambulances, respectively.[52] With possible financial and patient outcome benefits, two-tiered EMS systems seem appealing. However, there is no definitive evidence favoring one system over the other. Two-tiered systems if functioning appropriately should at the very least allow for quicker response times and faster times to intervention which are two core measurements of system performance.

In 1979, Eisenberg et al published the landmark paper that defined the 8-minute response interval for cardiac arrest. In this Seattle-based study, if CPR was initiated within 4 minutes and if definitive care was provided within 8 minutes, a survival to discharge rate of 43% among witnessed cardiac arrests patients resulted. Definitive care was defined as defibrillation, intubation, or emergency medication given by paramedics or hospital personnel.[53] From that point forward everyone strove to achieve similar survival rates and thus began the 8-minute response time as a national benchmark of system performance. It is important to remember that this study was done in a selected group of patients (ie, witnessed cardiac arrests), and when paramedic response times were investigated in an unselected population there were benefits if response times were less than 4 minutes, but there was no benefit when times were modeled as a continuous variable or dichotomized at an 8-minute mark.[54] A Scottish study calculated that if response times were decreased from 14 minutes to under 8 minutes or 4 minutes, predicted survival would increase from 6% to 8% or 10% to 11%, respectively.[55]

The race to beat the clock still continues as people try to find novel ways to shave minutes off response times. Compared to using standard maps, GPS units decrease response times from 14.6 to 13.5 minutes.[56] The use of geospatial time analysis can also help strategically place EMS units to decrease overall response times from a median 10.1 to 7.1 minutes.[57] Urban EMS systems have reported that lights and sirens on average reduce response times by 1 minute 46 seconds.[58] However, getting to the scene is only half the problem in urban areas. In New York City 28% of the actual response time was the interval from scene arrival to actually reaching the patient. This interval appears to be able to be decreased by having the dispatcher instruct the caller to send someone as an escort for EMS if the situation allows.[59]

MANAGEMENT OF OHCA

The American Heart Association resuscitation guidelines are the basis for treatment of OHCA. The newest 2010 revisions of the guidelines recommend the following treatment regimens.[60] Once the OHCA patient is reached CPR should be immediately begun and continued while the cardiac rhythm is analyzed using an AED or ECG monitor.[61] The patient should be classified into either a shockable rhythm (ie, ventricular fibrillation or tachycardia) or a nonshockable rhythm (ie, PEA or asystole). If the rhythm is shockable, a single shock should be administered and CPR restarted immediately and continued for 2 minutes prior to another pulse check. If the patient remains in a shockable rhythm, the cycle may be repeated. Drugs may be administered to help increase the odds of a successful resuscitation. Epinephrine 1 mg and amiodarone 300 mg may be given intravenously every 4 to 5 minutes. The first or second dose of epinephrine may be replaced by 40 units of vasopressin if desired. If the rhythm is nonshockable, CPR should be continued with pulse checks every 2 minutes. Epinephrine 1 mg may be given every 4 to 5 minutes, but Atropine is no longer recommended. If the rhythm is PEA/asystole, one should search for a reversible cause. They are easily remembered by the "Hs and Ts" shown in **Box 33-1**. A definitive airway may be necessary for prolonged resuscitations but at the current time there is not enough data to support a specific timing or type of airway.[62]

Resuscitation of OHCA in children is similar to adults but with a greater emphasis on airway management as many cardiac arrests in children are a result of hypoxia. Ventilation using a bag valve mask has been demonstrated to be acceptable especially when transport times are short. Only in prolonged resuscitations or transport should a definite airway be placed with an endotracheal tube. All medications should be weight based in nonobese patients or ideal-body weight based in obese patients. Atropine is still recommended in symptomatic bradycardia, but evidence is insufficient to support or refute the use of atropine or vasopressin in pediatric OHCA. In shockable rhythms, defibrillating with shingle shock algorithms with voltage of 2 to 4 J/kg is recommended.[63]

Various mechanical devices have been created for use in the prehospital setting that are reported to improve the quality of CPR and allow the provider to keep hands free for other activities. *Impedance threshold*

Box 33-1
Major Contributing Factors to Pulseless Arrest (Hs and Ts of ACLS)
5 Hs
Hypovolemia
Hypoxia
Hydrogen ion (acidosis)
Hyper-/hypokalemia
Hypoglycemia
Hypothermia
5 Ts
Toxins
Tamponade (cardiac)
Tension pneumothorax
Trauma
Thrombosis (coronary)
Thrombosis (pulmonary)

devices (ITD) utilize the physiological and mechanical relationships between the respiratory and circulatory systems to take advantage of the negative pressure within the thorax during the release phase of CPR. By limiting air return through the mouth into the chest during the chest wall recoil phase, the ITD lowers the intrathoracic pressure and the enhanced negative pressure results in increasing venous return to the heart, increasing preload and thus the cardiac output on the following compressions. *CPR quality feedback devices*, when placed between the chest and a provider's hands, give real-time feedback regarding the quality of chest compressions. *Load distributing band devices* constrict the thorax using a belt wrapped around the patient's chest. Multiple piston devices place direct anterior-posterior pressure over the sternum, simulating a provider's compressions. Some of these devices attach a suction device to the chest wall to encourage active decompression as well. However, none of these devices have enough evidence to support or refute their use.[60]

Cardiocerebral resuscitation (CCR), introduced in the last decade, strives to improve outcomes by refocusing certain CPR interventions to maximize myocardial and cerebral perfusion. In CCR, chest compressions are started immediately and continued for 200 continuous compressions. During this time, oxygen is given via a noninvasive airway, the rhythm is analyzed, and when appropriate a shock given, this is followed immediately by another interval of 200 compressions without pulse check. Epinephrine is given early, and intubation is delayed until after three rounds of chest compressions.[64] Some support exists for modified CCR by intubating earlier if the initial rhythm is not shockable.[65] While CCR research is ongoing, early data appear favorable. A before and after study in rural Wisconsin reported the total number of patients who survived (47% vs 20%; P = NR) and the total number of patient neurologically intact (39% vs 15%; P = NR) increased with CCR.[65] In another study the overall adjusted odds ratio of survival for CCR was 3.1 (95% CI 1.96-4.76). Some age ranges appeared to benefit more than others, but all age ranges except 70 to 79 years reached significance in confidence intervals.[66] Overall in studies over the past 4 years, CCR showed a survival to hospital discharge increase of 5.4% vs 1.8% (P = NR).[64] Despite promising results this new method of resuscitation will need continued research to determine if it improves long-term outcomes.

Once on scene, the decision to either "stay and play" or "scoop and run" incorporates many factors such as proximity to the closest hospital, public location, initial rhythm, interventions done prior to ALS arrival, and each EMS medical director's personal beliefs. Some medical directors have strong opinions in favor of one option, but most medical directors utilize both approaches allowing EMS providers latitude to make decisions.

If the patient has return of spontaneous circulation, rapid transport to the most appropriate hospital is paramount. However, transport provides its own pitfalls if CPR is ongoing. Studies are variable with respect to the effectiveness of CPR during transport. While compression quality en route was equivalent in one study, hands-off time increased during transport when compared to on scene.[67] Another study showed that efficiency of chest compressions was 95% in a moving ambulance and 86% in a helicopter.[68] Another study noted that the rate and quality of chest compressions increased as the speed of an ambulance increased.[69] When lights and sirens were used during transport, a mean of 2.62 minutes was saved although only 4.5% of patients receiving time-critical interventions.[70] Longer transport times were not associated with increased survival. Data are conflicting regarding bypassing smaller hospitals in favor of a regionally designated resuscitation hospital. More research is necessary.[71,72] Currently patients are most often taken to the closest hospital, stabilized, and then transferred to a larger, specialized hospital. For interfacility transports, specialized critical care ground or air transport is available, providing specialized care options not available in standard ALS units including vasoactive drug administration, blood transfusions, intra-aortic balloon pumps, and ventilator management as the potential for rearrest is present. Approximately 6% of resuscitated cardiac arrest patients rearrest during transported to a tertiary-care facility.[73]

Finally, for those patients with return of circulation, *therapeutic hypothermia* is currently recommended. It is possible to begin cooling the patient with 2 liters of ice-cold isotonic solution which has been shown to decrease the patient's core temperature by an average of 0.8°C.[74] However, this does not appear to improve hospital discharge rates compared to cooling after arrival in the emergency department.

PREHOSPITAL CARDIAC ARREST OUTCOMES

It is estimated that over 1000 patients each day experience cardiac arrest/sudden death. Despite ongoing research efforts to identify effective treatments to increase survival rates, to date few improvements have occurred. Outcomes of OHCA have been difficult to measure due to lack of standardization of variables such as pulse upon arrival to the ED, general return of circulation, patient survival to hospital admission, and survival to discharge with or without being neurologically intact between researchers. In 1995, adoption of uniform definitions, data collection sets, and reporting were standardized with the Utstein criteria allowing better comparison between studies.[75] Despite the criteria, comparison of data is still hampered by EMS system differences, response times, and bystander CPR availability.

Several identified factors appear to be associated with an increased chance of OHCA survival. Bystander CPR, witnessed arrest, initial presenting rhythm of ventricular fibrillation, and short response times to defibrillation are all associated with increased survival rates.[76,77] Eisenburger et al reported having a cardiac arrest in a public place was an independent predictor of improved outcome.[78] Immediate defibrillation of patients in ventricular fibrillation results in a pulse-generating rhythm, with survival to hospital discharge, 56% of the time, but drops to 6% by the third defibrillation. Survival rates appear to be highest if defibrillation occurs within the first 6 minutes of cardiac arrest, leveling off after 11 minutes.[76]

Reported survival ranges for OHCA patients are quite variable and range from 6% to 46%. The largest cumulative meta-analysis study to date documented a mean survival to hospital discharge for all rhythm groups of only 7.6% and a hospital admission rate of 23.8%.[13] Liu et al reported that younger age, nonwhite race, and male gender were associated with outcomes.[79] Time of EMS arrival is linked to higher survival rates, with even a 1-minute decrease in mean response times showing an approximate 1% (0.7%-2.1% range) absolute increase in survival. Decreasing overall pauses in CPR is associated with better results.[80] EMS-witnessed arrests have the best outcomes, followed by bystander-witnessed arrests with bystander CPR, bystander-witnessed arrests without bystander CPR, and unwitnessed arrests, respectively.[81] Presenting rhythm of

ventricular tachycardia or ventricular fibrillation also results in better outcomes.

One of the largest OHCA studies was the Ontario Prehospital Advanced Life Support (OPALS) study which looked at the effects of multiple variables on OHCA survival as ALS care was phased into their area for the first time. In phase one, witnessed arrest, bystander CPR, CPR by fire or police, and short EMS response times were independently associated with survival on multivariate analysis.[82] In phase two, a target of 8-minute response time was set from call receipt to on scene with a defibrillator. Of the 1641 OHCA patients, 90% of calls met the response target with a 33% improvement in survival to discharge in all rhythm groups with an estimated additional 21 lives saved at a cost of $2400 per life.[77] A total of 1391 patients were enrolled in the defibrillation plus BLS phase of the study, and 4247 patients enrolled in the ACLS phase. The ACLS phase had greater return of circulation rates (12.9% vs 18%; $P < 0.001$) and hospital admission rates (10.9% vs 14.6%, $P < 0.001$), but hospital discharge rates were unchanged (5.0% vs 5.1%; $P = 0.83$), leading to an odds ratio of 1.1 for ACLS relative to BLS. This ratio did not compare favorably with the odds ratios for witnessed arrest (4.4), early CPR (3.7), and early defibrillation (3.4), respectively.[83] This is consistent with other studies of ALS care in OHCA without intravenous (IV) medications which reported no difference in return of circulation, hospital admission, or hospital discharge in shockable rhythms. However, if the initial rhythm was PEA or asystole, the IV group had better return of circulation rates (29% vs 11%; $P < 0.001$) and hospital admission (31% vs 16%; $P < 0.001$) but not hospital discharge (2% vs 3%; $P = 0.65$).[84] The lack of change in hospital discharge was not supported in a meta-analysis of 37 articles describing 39 EMS systems and 33,124 patients. When comparing the systems with different capabilities, this study reported a survival to hospital discharge odds ratio of 1.71 for ACLS, 1.47 for a two-tiered system of BLS without defibrillation and ALS, and 2.31 for BLS with defibrillation plus ALS. This study was not sufficiently powered to demonstrate whether one- or two-tiered systems are better, but suggests that either early defibrillation or ALS is more effective than BLS alone.[76]

End-tidal CO_2 (ETCO$_2$) monitoring has become a valuable tool in many EMS systems. Both colormetric and waveform devices are utilized by EMS. Waveform devices are particularly useful for confirmation of airway placement with a sensitivity and specificity of 100%.[85,86] The more commonly used colormetric ETCO$_2$ is useful in conjunction with clinical judgment, but it does not appear to be as sensitive as waveform ETCO$_2$[62] yielding a sensitivity of only 88%.[85] Waveform ETCO$_2$ increased with high-quality CPR and ROSC and thus has some value in OHCA prognostication. High levels appear to correlate with ROSC while levels below 10 to 14.3 mm Hg after 20 minutes of ACLS seem to be a predictor of death.[87,88] This is also consistent in the pediatric population,[63] but more prospective studies are needed before a definitive value as a predictor if death is determined.[62,63] Waveform capnography appears to be a real-time measure of the quality of CPR and the possibility of successful resuscitation.[63]

OHCA outcomes are influenced by hospital destination. Hospital survival rates vary from 29% to 42% with the same prehospital treatment, and outcomes at designated "critical care medical centers" are better.[79,89] Hospitals with cardiac catheterization capability that see at least 40 cardiac arrests per year have better outcomes, regardless of how many beds are in the hospital or whether it is a teaching hospital.[90] OHCA caused by ST-elevation MIs generally do have better outcomes.[91] Surprisingly, higher survival rates are not limited to urban areas as rural locations have documented neurologically intact hospital discharge rates as high as 22%.

Termination of resuscitation efforts in the field is generally accepted practice with only rare problems identified. When to terminate resuscitation efforts is a topic of ongoing debate, with there being a desire to not prolong efforts beyond potential benefit balanced against the desire to not declare death prematurely. Multiple validated rules exist for the termination of prehospital CPR, with the most popular one declaring that only 46% of cardiac arrests need transportation.[92] This rule notes that resuscitation efforts may be terminated if there is no return of spontaneous circulation after three rounds of BLS with defibrillation every

1 to 2 minutes, no shock delivered by an AED, and the cardiac arrest was not witnessed by an EMT or firefighter. This rule has a sensitivity of 57.5% to 64.4%, a specificity of 90.2% to 100%, and a positive predictive value of 99.5% to 100%.[92,93] Furthermore this rule correctly identified 100% of those discharged with good neurological outcome and 36% of those with poor neurologic outcome or without survival.[94] Many EMS agencies no longer routinely transport OHCA patients without return of spontaneous circulation. However, factors that may result in transportation are airway difficulties, persistent ventricular dysrhythmias, excessively public location, family members who are unable to accept field termination, lack of intravenous cannulation, and cultural or language barriers. Additionally, many emergency physicians do not feel comfortable pronouncing a PEA code in the field. Family members generally accept termination of unsuccessful resuscitation efforts in prehospital cardiac arrest.

Prehospital OHCA can be traumatic in origin. These patients have an extremely high mortality rate, and survivors having significant morbidity. The literature suggests that a small subset of such patients can potentially benefit from timely, aggressive treatment while being transported without delay. However, prognosis is dismal in those without signs of life on ED arrival.

SUMMARY

Despite many advances in cardiac arrest resuscitation, long-term outcomes have not changed in nearly three decades and remain dismal.[13] Due to the focus of optimizing each link in the chain of survival, short-term outcomes (eg, return of circulation and hospital admission) are slowly improving. Public education is impacting recognition and early intervention in OHCA. Improvements in EMS dispatch, response times, quicker defibrillation, high-quality CPR, and speedy transport to the most appropriate hospital have slowly positively impacted survival. OHCA research standardization, through the use of the Utstein criteria, have allowed for increasing quality of ongoing research. Continued advancements in ACLS care give hope of further improving outcomes. Additional research to improve each link in the prehospital cardiac arrest chain of survival will continue to bring further advancements.

KEY POINTS

- The incidence of cardiac arrest is higher in males, those with lower socioeconomic status, and black Americans versus white or Hispanic groups.
- Cardiac arrests, along with myocardial infarction and unstable angina complaints, appear to have a circadian variation with a morning peak shortly after the initiation of daily activities.
- System access begins with a 9-1-1 call. Dispatcher telephone instructions have been shown to increase the rates of bystander CPR and improve outcomes.
- Development of automated external defibrillators (AEDs) strategically placed in public locations facilitate faster defibrillation of the cardiac arrest patients.
- Two-tiered response agencies appear more cost-effective and may have better outcomes.
- Shorter time of arrival of EMS is linked to higher survival rates in OHCA.
- Presenting rhythm of ventricular tachycardia or ventricular fibrillation results in better outcomes.
- Despite many advances in OHCA resuscitation, long-term survival has not changed in nearly three decades and remains dismal.
- Reported survival ranges for OHCA patients are quite variable ranging from 6% to 46%.

- Improvements in dispatch, response times, faster defibrillation, high-quality CPR, and rapid transport to the most appropriate hospital may increase survival.
- Cardiac arrest results from a shockable rhythm in approximately 23% of out-of-hospital cardiac arrests.
- Approximately 50% of out-of-hospital cardiac arrests are witnessed.
- Approximately 30% of witnessed out-of-hospital cardiac arrests receive bystander CPR.
- End-tidal CO_2 measurements of <10 mm Hg after 20 minutes of ACLS resuscitation are a predictor of death.

REFERENCES

1. Dameff C, Vadeboncoeur T, Tully J, et al. A standardized template for measuring and reporting telephone pre-arrival cardiopulmonary resuscitation instructions. *Resuscitation*. July 2014;85(7):869-873.
2. Hardeland C, Olasveengen TM, Lawrence R, et al. Comparison of Medical Priority Dispatch (MPD) and Criteria Based Dispatch (CBD) relating to cardiac arrest calls. *Resuscitation*. 2014 May;85(5):612-616.
3. Lerner EB, Sayre MR, Brice JH, et al. Cardiac arrest patients rarely receive chest compressions before ambulance arrival despite the availability of pre-arrival CPR instructions. *Resuscitation*. April 2008;77(1):51-56.
4. Roppolo LP, Pepe PE, Cimon N, et al. Modified cardiopulmonary resuscitation (CPR) instruction protocols for emergency medical dispatchers: rationale and recommendations. *Resuscitation*. May 2005;65(2):203-210.
5. Fox CS, Evans JC, Larson MG, et al. Temporal trends in coronary heart disease mortality and sudden cardiac death from 1950 to 1999: the Framingham heart study. *Circulation*. 2004;110:522-527.
6. Rea TD, Pearce RM, Raghunathan TE, et al. Incidence of out-of-hospital cardiac arrest. *Am J Cardiol*. 2004;93:1455-1460.
7. Muller JE. Circadian variation in cardiovascular events. *Am J Hypertens*. 1999;12:35S-42S.
8. Reinier K, Stecker EC, Vickers C, et al. Incidence of sudden cardiac arrest is higher in areas of low socioeconomic status: a prospective two year study in a large united states community. *Resuscitation*. 2006;70:186-192.
9. Adabag AS, Luepker RV, Roger VL, et al. Sudden cardiac death: epidemiology and risk factors. *Nat Rev Cardiol*. 2010;7:216-225.
10. Nichol G, Thomas E, Callaway CW, et al. Regional variation in out-of-hospital cardiac arrest incidence and outcome. *JAMA*. 2008;300:1423-1431.
11. Bobrow BJ, Spaite DW, Berg RA, et al. Chest compression-only CPR by lay rescuers and survival from out-of-hospital cardiac arrest. *JAMA*. 2010;304:1447-1454.
12. Fairbanks RJ, Shah MN, Lerner EB, et al. Epidemiology and outcomes of out-of-hospital cardiac arrest in Rochester, New York. *Resuscitation*. 2007;72:415-424.
13. Sasson C, Rogers MA, Dahl J, et al. Predictors of survival from out-of-hospital cardiac arrest: A systematic review and meta-analysis. *Circ Cardiovasc Qual Outcomes*. 2010;3:63-81.
14. Benson PC, Eckstein M, McClung CD, et al. Racial/ethnic differences in bystander CPR in Los Angeles, California. *Ethn Dis*. 2009;19:401-406.
15. Vadeboncoeur TF, Richman PB, Darkoh M, et al. Bystander cardiopulmonary resuscitation for out-of-hospital cardiac arrest in the hispanic vs the non-hispanic populations. *Am J Emerg Med*. 2008;26:655-660.
16. Mitchell MJ, Stubbs BA, Eisenberg MS. Socioeconomic status is associated with provision of bystander cardiopulmonary resuscitation. *Prehosp Emerg Care*. 2009;13:478-486.

17. Vaillancourt C, Lui A, De Maio VJ, et al. Socioeconomic status influences bystander CPR and survival rates for out-of-hospital cardiac arrest victims. *Resuscitation.* 2008;79:417-423.

18. Boyce LW, Vliet Vlieland TP, Bosch J, et al. High survival rate of 43% in out-of-hospital cardiac arrest patients in an optimised chain of survival. *Neth Heart J.* 2015;23(1):20-25.

19. Fosbøl EL, Strauss B, Swanson DR, et al. Association of neighborhood characteristics with incidence of out-of-hospital cardiac arrest and rates of bystander-initiated CPR: Implications for community-based education intervention. *Resuscitation.* 2014;85(11):1512-1517.

20. Moon S, Bobrow BJ, Vadeboncoeur TF, et al. Disparities in bystander CPR provision and survival from out-of-hospital cardiac arrest according to neighborhood ethnicity. *Am J Emerg Med.* September 2014;32(9):1041-1045.

21. Swor RA, Compton S, Domeier R, et al. Delay prior to calling 9-1-1 is associated with increased mortality after out-of-hospital cardiac arrest. *Prehosp Emerg Care.* 2008;12:333-338.

22. Vadeboncoeur T, Bobrow BJ, Clark L, et al. The save hearts in Arizona registry and education (SHARE) program: who is performing CPR and where are they doing it? *Resuscitation.* 2007;75:68-75.

23. Herlitz J, Engdahl J, Svensson L, et al. A short delay from out of hospital cardiac arrest to call for ambulance increases survival. *Eur Heart J.* 2003;24:1750-1755.

24. Vukmir RB. Survival from prehospital cardiac arrest is critically dependent upon response time. *Resuscitation.* 2006;69:229-234.

25. Leizorovicz A, Haugh MC, Mercier C, et al. Pre-hospital and hospital time delays in thrombolytic treatment in patients with suspected acute myocardial infarction. analysis of data from the EMIP study. European myocardial infarction project. *Eur Heart J.* 1997;18:248-253.

26. Ottesen MM, Dixen U, Torp-Pedersen C, et al. Prehospital delay in acute coronary syndrome—an analysis of the components of delay. *Int J Cardiol.* 2004;96:97-103.

27. Moser DK, McKinley S, Dracup K, et al. Gender differences in reasons patients delay in seeking treatment for acute myocardial infarction symptoms. *Patient Educ Couns.* 2005;56:45-54.

28. Becker L, Vath J, Eisenberg M, et al. The impact of television public service announcements on the rate of bystander CPR. *Prehosp Emerg Care.* 1999;3:353-356.

29. Kuisma M, Boyd J, Vayrynen T, et al. Emergency call processing and survival from out-of-hospital ventricular fibrillation. *Resuscitation.* 2005;67:89-93.

30. Heward A, Damiani M, Hartley-Sharpe C. Does the use of the advanced medical priority dispatch system affect cardiac arrest detection? *Emerg Med J.* 2004;21:115-118.

31. Bohm K, Rosenqvist M, Hollenberg J, et al. Dispatcher-assisted telephone-guided cardiopulmonary resuscitation: an underused lifesaving system. *Eur J Emerg Med.* 2007;14:256-259.

32. Roppolo LP, Westfall A, Pepe PE, et al. Dispatcher assessments for agonal breathing improve detection of cardiac arrest. *Resuscitation.* 2009;80:769-772.

33. Bohm K, Stalhandske B, Rosenqvist M, et al. Tuition of emergency medical dispatchers in the recognition of agonal respiration increases the use of telephone assisted CPR. *Resuscitation.* 2009;80:1025-1028.

34. Flynn J, Archer F, Morgans A. Sensitivity and specificity of the medical priority dispatch system in detecting cardiac arrest emergency calls in Melbourne. *Prehosp Disaster Med.* 2006;21:72-76.

35. Vaillancourt C, Verma A, Trickett J, et al. Evaluating the effectiveness of dispatch-assisted cardiopulmonary resuscitation instructions. *Acad Emerg Med.* 2007;14:877-883.

36. Coons SJ, Guy MC. Performing bystander CPR for sudden cardiac arrest: behavioral intentions among the general adult population in Arizona. *Resuscitation.* 2009;80:334-340.

37. Brown TB, Saini D, Pepper T, et al. Instructions to "put the phone down" do not improve the quality of bystander initiated dispatcher-assisted cardiopulmonary resuscitation. *Resuscitation.* 2008;76:249-255.

38. Johnsen E, Bolle SR. To see or not to see—better dispatcher-assisted CPR with video-calls? A qualitative study based on simulated trials. *Resuscitation.* 2008;78:320-326.

39. Dorph E, Wik L, Steen PA. Dispatcher-assisted cardiopulmonary resuscitation. An evaluation of efficacy amongst elderly. *Resuscitation.* 2003;56:265-273.

40. Rea TD, Fahrenbruch C, Culley L, et al. CPR with chest compression alone or with rescue breathing. *N Engl J Med.* 2010;363:423-433.

41. Svensson L, Bohm K, Castren M, et al. Compression-only CPR or standard CPR in out-of-hospital cardiac arrest. *N Engl J Med.* 2010;363:434-442.

42. Sayre MR, Koster RW, Botha M, et al. Part 5: Adult basic life support: 2010 international consensus on cardiopulmonary resuscitation and emergency cardiovascular care science with treatment recommendations. *Circulation.* 2010;122:S298-324.

43. Capucci A, Guerra F. Out-of-hospital cardiac arrest and public access defibrillation. *J Cardiovasc Med (Hagerstown).* August 2014; 15(8):624-625.

44. Berger S. Cardiopulmonary resuscitation and public access defibrillation in the current era—can we do better yet? *J Am Heart Assoc.* April 23, 2014;3(2):e000945.

45. Murakami Y, Iwami T, Kitamura T, et al. Outcomes of out-of-hospital cardiac arrest by public location in the public-access defibrillation era. *J Am Heart Assoc.* April 22, 2014;3(2):e000533.

46. Zakaria ND, Ong ME, Gan HN, et al. Implications for public access defibrillation placement by non-traumatic out-of-hospital cardiac arrest occurrence in Singapore. *Emerg Med Australas.* June 2014; 26(3):229-236.

47. Deakin CD, Shewry E, Gray HH. Public access defibrillation remains out of reach for most victims of out-of-hospital sudden cardiac arrest. *Heart.* April 2014;100(8):619-623.

48. Mitani Y, Ohta K, Ichida F, et al. Circumstances and outcomes of out-of-hospital cardiac arrest in elementary and middle school students in the era of public-access defibrillation. *Circ J.* 2014;78(3):701-707.

49. Hawkins SC, Shapiro AH, Sever AE, et al. The role of law enforcement agencies in out-of-hospital emergency care. *Resuscitation.* 2007;72:386-393.

50. Nichol G, Detsky AS, Stiell IG, et al. Effectiveness of emergency medical services for victims of out-of-hospital cardiac arrest: a meta-analysis. *Ann Emerg Med.* 1996;27:700-710.

51. Joyce SM, Davidson LW, Manning KW, et al. Outcomes of sudden cardiac arrest treated with defibrillation by emergency medical technicians (EMT-ds) or paramedics in a two-tiered urban EMS system. *Prehosp Emerg Care.* 1998;2:13-17.

52. Nichol G, Laupacis A, Stiell IG, et al. Cost-effectiveness analysis of potential improvements to emergency medical services for victims of out-of-hospital cardiac arrest. *Ann Emerg Med.* 1996;27:711-720.

53. Eisenberg MS, Bergner L, Hallstrom A. Cardiac resuscitation in the community. Importance of rapid provision and implications for program planning. *JAMA.* 1979;241:1905-1907.

54. Pons PT, Haukoos JS, Bludworth W, et al. Paramedic response time: does it affect patient survival? *Acad Emerg Med.* 2005;12:594-600.

55. Pell JP, Sirel JM, Marsden AK, et al. Effect of reducing ambulance response times on deaths from out of hospital cardiac arrest: cohort study. *BMJ.* 2001;322:1385-1388.

56. Ota FS, Muramatsu RS, Yoshida BH, et al. GPS computer navigators to shorten EMS response and transport times. *Am J Emerg Med.* 2001;19:204-205.

57. Ong ME, Chiam TF, Ng FS, et al. Reducing ambulance response times using geospatial-time analysis of ambulance deployment. *Acad Emerg Med.* 2010;17:951-957.

58. Brown LH, Whitney CL, Hunt RC, et al. Do warning lights and sirens reduce ambulance response times? *Prehosp Emerg Care.* 2000;4:70-74.

59. Silverman RA, Galea S, Blaney S, et al. The "vertical response time": barriers to ambulance response in an urban area. *Acad Emerg Med.* 2007;14:772-778.

60. Shuster M, Lim SH, Deakin CD, et al. Part 7: CPR techniques and devices: 2010 international consensus on cardiopulmonary resuscitation and emergency cardiovascular care science with treatment recommendations. *Circulation.* 2010;122:S338-S344.

61. Morais DA, Carvalho DV, Correa Ados R. Out-of-hospital cardiac arrest: determinant factors for immediate survival after cardiopulmonary resuscitation. *Rev Lat Am Enfermagem.* July 2014;22(4):562-568.

62. Morrison LJ, Deakin CD, Morley PT, et al. Part 8: Advanced life support: 2010 international consensus on cardiopulmonary resuscitation and emergency cardiovascular care science with treatment recommendations. *Circulation.* 2010;122:S345-S421.

63. Kleinman ME, de Caen AR, Chameides L, et al. Part 10: Pediatric basic and advanced life support: 2010 international consensus on cardiopulmonary resuscitation and emergency cardiovascular care science with treatment recommendations. *Circulation.* 2010;122: S466-S515.

64. Bobrow BJ, Clark LL, Ewy GA, et al. Minimally interrupted cardiac resuscitation by emergency medical services for out-of-hospital cardiac arrest. *JAMA.* 2008;299:1158-1165.

65. Kellum MJ, Kennedy KW, Barney R, et al. Cardiocerebral resuscitation improves neurologically intact survival of patients with out-of-hospital cardiac arrest. *Ann Emerg Med.* 2008;52:244-252.

66. Mosier J, Itty A, Sanders A, et al. Cardiocerebral resuscitation is associated with improved survival and neurologic outcome from out-of-hospital cardiac arrest in elders. *Acad Emerg Med.* 2010;17:269-275.

67. Olasveengen TM, Wik L, Steen PA. Quality of cardiopulmonary resuscitation before and during transport in out-of-hospital cardiac arrest. *Resuscitation.* 2008;76:185-190.

68. Havel C, Schreiber W, Trimmel H, et al. Quality of closed chest compression on a manikin in ambulance vehicles and flying helicopters with a real time automated feedback. *Resuscitation.* 2010;81:59-64.

69. Chung TN, Kim SW, Cho YS, et al. Effect of vehicle speed on the quality of closed-chest compression during ambulance transport. *Resuscitation.* 2010;81:841-847.

70. Marques-Baptista A, Ohman-Strickland P, Baldino KT, et al. Utilization of warning lights and siren based on hospital time-critical interventions. *Prehosp Disaster Med.* 2010;25:335-339.

71. Spaite DW, Bobrow BJ, Vadeboncoeur TF, et al. The impact of pre-hospital transport interval on survival in out-of-hospital cardiac arrest: implications for regionalization of post-resuscitation care. *Resuscitation.* 2008;79:61-66.

72. Spaite DW, Stiell IG, Bobrow BJ, et al. Effect of transport interval on out-of-hospital cardiac arrest survival in the OPALS study: implications for triaging patients to specialized cardiac arrest centers. *Ann Emerg Med.* 2009;54:248-255.

73. Hartke A, Mumma BE, Rittenberger JC, et al. Incidence of re-arrest and critical events during prolonged transport of post-cardiac arrest patients. *Resuscitation.* 2010;81:938-942.

74. Bernard SA, Smith K, Cameron P, et al. Induction of therapeutic hypothermia by paramedics after resuscitation from out-of-hospital ventricular fibrillation cardiac arrest: a randomized controlled trial. *Circulation.* 2010;122:737-742.

75. Spaite D, Benoit R, Brown D, et al. Uniform prehospital data elements and definitions: a report from the uniform prehospital emergency medical services data conference. *Ann Emerg Med.* 1995;25:525-534.

76. Nichol G, Stiell IG, Laupacis A, et al. A cumulative meta-analysis of the effectiveness of defibrillator-capable emergency medical services for victims of out-of-hospital cardiac arrest. *Ann Emerg Med.* 1999;34:517-525.

77. Stiell IG, Wells GA, Field BJ, et al. Improved out-of-hospital cardiac arrest survival through the inexpensive optimization of an existing defibrillation program: OPALS study phase II. Ontario prehospital advanced life support. *JAMA.* 1999;281:1175-1181.

78. Eisenburger P, Sterz F, Haugk M, et al. Cardiac arrest in public locations—an independent predictor for better outcome? *Resuscitation.* 2006;70:395-403.

79. Liu JM, Yang Q, Pirrallo RG, et al. Hospital variability of out-of-hospital cardiac arrest survival. *Prehosp Emerg Care.* 2008;12:339-346.

80. Lund-Kordahl I, Olasveengen TM, Lorem T, et al. Improving outcome after out-of-hospital cardiac arrest by strengthening weak links of the local chain of survival; quality of advanced life support and post-resuscitation care. *Resuscitation.* 2010;81:422-426.

81. Hostler D, Thomas EG, Emerson SS, et al. Increased survival after EMS witnessed cardiac arrest. observations from the resuscitation outcomes consortium (ROC) epistry-cardiac arrest. *Resuscitation.* 2010;81:826-830.

82. Stiell IG, Wells GA, DeMaio VJ, et al. Modifiable factors associated with improved cardiac arrest survival in a multicenter basic life support/defibrillation system: OPALS study phase I results. Ontario prehospital advanced life support. *Ann Emerg Med.* 1999;33:44-50.

83. Stiell IG, Wells GA, Field B, et al. Advanced cardiac life support in out-of-hospital cardiac arrest. *N Engl J Med.* 2004;351:647-656.

84. Olasveengen TM, Sunde K, Brunborg C, et al. Intravenous drug administration during out-of-hospital cardiac arrest: a randomized trial. *JAMA.* 2009;302:2222-2229.

85. Grmec S. Comparison of three different methods to confirm tracheal tube placement in emergency intubation. *Intensive Care Med.* 2002;28:701-704.

86. Silvestri S, Ralls GA, Krauss B, et al. The effectiveness of out-of-hospital use of continuous end-tidal carbon dioxide monitoring on the rate of unrecognized misplaced intubation within a regional emergency medical services system. *Ann Emerg Med.* 2005;45: 497-503.

87. Kolar M, Krizmaric M, Klemen P, et al. Partial pressure of end-tidal carbon dioxide successful predicts cardiopulmonary resuscitation in the field: a prospective observational study. *Crit Care.* 2008;12:R115.

88. Levine RL, Wayne MA, Miller CC. End-tidal carbon dioxide and outcome of out-of-hospital cardiac arrest. *N Engl J Med.* 1997;337: 301-306.

89. Kajino K, Iwami T, Daya M, et al. Impact of transport to critical care medical centers on outcomes after out-of-hospital cardiac arrest. *Resuscitation.* 2010;81:549-554.

90. Callaway CW, Schmicker R, Kampmeyer M, et al. Receiving hospital characteristics associated with survival after out-of-hospital cardiac arrest. *Resuscitation.* 2010;81:524-529.

91. Pleskot M, Hazukova R, Stritecka H, et al. Long-term prognosis after out-of-hospital cardiac arrest with/without ST elevation myocardial infarction. *Resuscitation.* 2009;80:795-804.

92. Morrison LJ, Verbeek PR, Zhan C, et al. Validation of a universal prehospital termination of resuscitation clinical prediction rule for advanced and basic life support providers. *Resuscitation.* 2009; 80:324-328.

93. Morrison LJ, Visentin LM, Kiss A, et al. Validation of a rule for termination of resuscitation in out-of-hospital cardiac arrest. *N Engl J Med.* 2006;355:478-487.

94. Ruygrok ML, Byyny RL, Haukoos JS, et al. Validation of 3 termination of resuscitation criteria for good neurologic survival after out-of-hospital cardiac arrest. *Ann Emerg Med.* 2009;54:239-247.

Respiratory Failure and Anaphylaxis

Robert D. Greenberg

Stephen McConnell

INTRODUCTION

Respiratory failure is the inability of the lungs to perform the vital function of gas exchange, and may be caused by an inability to either obtain sufficient oxygen or eliminate carbon dioxide. Numerically, respiratory failure may be defined on arterial blood gas measurement as hypoxemia, with a PaO_2 <60 mmHg, or as hypercarbia, with a $PaCO_2$ >45 mm Hg.[1] Acute respiratory failure may be divided into four types. Type 1 respiratory failure is caused by acute hypoxia, and may be seen in patients with pulmonary edema, pneumonia, pulmonary hemorrhage, or acute respiratory distress syndrome. Type 2 respiratory failure may be seen with hypoventilation and an inability to rid the body of carbon dioxide. Examples of disease processes where this may be seen include central nervous system disorders where the respiratory drive is diminished, neuromuscular disorders where the muscles of respiration are not sufficiently able to produce ventilation, as well as in pulmonary conditions such as pneumothorax, airway obstruction, or pleural effusions. Significant atelectasis is the cause for Type 3 respiratory failure, and is most commonly seen after mechanical ventilation. Type 4 respiratory failure is seen in patients who have hypoperfusion of the muscles of respiration caused by another process, such as shock.[2] Identifying the incidence of acute respiratory failure in the United States is extremely difficult but has been estimated near 140 cases per 100,000 individuals over the age of 5. Of the patients with acute respiratory failure, approximately 36% will not survive to hospital discharge. There seems to be a correlation with increased mortality seen in patients with increase in age, presence of multisystem organ failure, cancer, underlying liver disease, and HIV infection.[3]

OBJECTIVES

1. Describe the causes of respiratory failure and anaphylaxis.

2. Describe interventions used in the prehospital environment to treat respiratory failure and anaphylaxis.

3. Delineate equipment useful in the prehospital management.

4. Outline some easy-to-use mnemonics for airway assessment in the field.

5. Describe unique challenges encountered in the prehospital environment.

6. Delineate medications that are appropriate for use in airway interventions in the prehospital environment.

CAUSES OF ACUTE RESPIRATORY FAILURE

There are many causes of acute respiratory failure, and oftentimes more than one in any given patient. Understanding the underlying disease process may better direct treatment and management of the patient in both the prehospital and hospital environments. Appropriate early interventions may have a significant effect on patient outcome and subsequent management.

▧ NEUROMUSCULAR

Communication from the medullary respiratory center to the muscles of respiration is crucial in the mechanics of respiration. Disruption of neurotransmission may occur by several mechanisms. Severe intoxication or overdoses may decrease the intrinsic capability of the medullary respiratory center to function. Environmental clues may allow for the detection of organophosphate induced respiratory failure, which occurs within the first 4 days of exposure. It is believed that the central nervous action of the organophosphate has a larger role inducing respiratory failure compared to the peripheral effect.[4] Myasthenia gravis, an autoimmune disease with an incidence of approximately 18 individuals out of 1 million,[5] may also present as respiratory distress. Other diseases, such as Guillain-Barre or Eaton-Lambert syndrome may also present with weakness of the respiratory muscles. Trauma may result in damage to the brain or the cervical spinal cord that may also disrupt neurotransmission. A vital capacity less than 20 mL/kg or peak inspiratory pressures greater than −30 cm H_2O combined with bulbar dysfunction are strong predictors of which patients may require mechanical ventilation for neuromuscular dysfunction.[6]

▧ VASCULAR

Gas exchange in the pulmonary vasculature depends on diffusion of both oxygen and carbon dioxide across the alveolar membrane and may be affected by several conditions. Interstitial lung disease, such as pulmonary fibrosis or sarcoidosis in addition to others, may destroy and cause a reduction in capillary-alveolar units. Pulmonary embolism is another vascular process that can lead to respiratory distress and failure, depending on the thrombus location and size. Pulmonary embolism creates a ventilation/perfusion mismatch and can lead to hypoxia, with massive pulmonary embolism creating significant cardiac dysfunction. Additional vascular causes of acute respiratory failure can be related to pulmonary hypertension or iatrogenic interventions secondary to pulmonary artery dissection. This can be seen following catheterization as well as cardiac valve replacement. Other disease processes affecting blood flow through the pulmonary vasculature include right-to-left mechanical shunts and may be found during a workup for another pathological finding, such as an ischemic stroke.

▧ ENVIRONMENTAL AND TOXIC

One of the challenges of prehospital patient care is some of the austere environments that may be encountered. Working in enclosed environments with limited air ventilation, some patients may have exposure to hypoxic environments or be exposed to chemicals which may alter the body's ability to appropriately exchange carbon dioxide and oxygen. Poisoning by carbon monoxide, a byproduct of fossil fuel combustion, may result from intentional or unintentional means. Carbon monoxide with an increased affinity for both hemoglobin and myoglobin, effectively decreases the amount of oxygen available for tissue delivery and can interfere with mitochondrial cytochrome oxidase. Carbon monoxide exposures account for approximately 15,000 emergency department visits and up to 500 deaths annually in the United States.[7] Caring for patients exposed to carbon monoxide should focus on removing the patient from the environment while taking care not to unnecessarily expose prehospital providers. High flow supplemental oxygen should be administered and hyperbaric oxygen therapy, although controversial, may be indicated. Pulse oximetry may not be accurate in patients with carbon monoxide poisoning but an arterial blood gas with cooximetry will give more accurate values. Cyanide poisoning, commonly seen in fire-related injuries, can also result from iatrogenic exposure from prolonged nitroprusside infusion.[8] The primary toxic effect of cyanide is inhibition of mitochondrial cytochrome oxidase.[9] Several antidotes to cyanide toxicity exist, each having a unique mechanism of action and with varying degrees of side-effects from the antidote.[10]

▧ IMPAIRED VENTILATION

Chronic obstructive pulmonary disease (COPD) is increasing in prevalence and incidence throughout the United States and contributes to approximately 5% of deaths annually. Tobacco smoking has been attributed in up to 75% of COPD cases.[11] Airflow obstruction seen in COPD is not completely reversible and is caused by small airway disease as well as parenchymal disease in varying degrees. The hallmark of outpatient management for COPD has remained β-agonist as well as steroid therapy with supplemental oxygen needed in the more severe cases.[12] Approximately 10% of patients with COPD who experience an acute exacerbation will require hospitalization. Etiology of exacerbations may be related to bacterial or viral infections, with *Moraxella catarrhalis*, *Haemophilus influenza*, and *Streptococcus pneumonia* being the most common organisms. Cardiac dysfunction may be seen as a concomitant disease process and may be the underlying process worsening respiratory status. In patients without an explained cause for the acute exacerbation, pneumothorax and pulmonary embolism should be considered, noting that pulmonary embolism may have a prevalence as high as 25% in unexplained exacerbations.[13] Treatment for the acute exacerbation may require an increase in oxygen, inhaled β-agonist and anticholinergic, as well as systemic glucocorticoids, and possibly noninvasive positive pressure ventilation. Reactive airway disease, such as asthma, may affect individuals of any age, but has a higher prevalence among children than adults. Overall, the prevalence in the United States is slightly higher than 8% and increasing.[14] Asthma symptoms occur when the airway diameter is decreased due to smooth muscle contraction, development of bronchial secretions and bronchial wall edema, as well as with vascular congestion. Exacerbations are due to a variety of causes including environmental temperature, exercise, as well as allergens. Management depends on the degree of the disease process, but typically includes short-acting β-agonists, anticholinergics, steroids, noninvasive positive pressure ventilation, and severe acute exacerbations may also include magnesium and/or endotracheal intubation and mechanical ventilation.[15,16]

REDUCED PULMONARY VOLUME

With some patients, an acute presentation of respiratory distress or failure may be caused by a potentially reversible structural cause. For example, a patient with a spontaneous or traumatic pneumothorax may present with chest pain or dyspnea, which may progress rapidly to a tension pneumothorax. Aeromedical transportation is not an absolute contraindication when considering the entire clinical picture. If tension physiology is encountered, emergent thoracostomy is indicated, with some prehospital providers performing both needle and/or tube

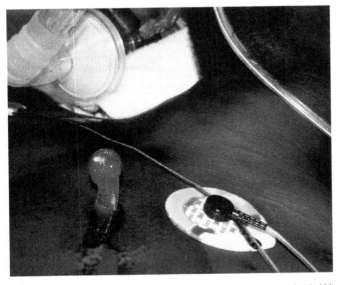

FIGURE 34-1. Needle thoracostomy. Tension pneumothorax with return of air bubbling through blood out of a large-bore IV catheter placed through the anterior chest wall at the second intercostal space, midclavicular line. (Reproduced with permission from Corbett SW, Stack LB, Knoop KJ. Chest and abdomen. In: Knoop KJ, Stack LB, Storrow AB, Thurman R, eds. *The Atlas of Emergency Medicine*. 3rd ed. New York, NY: McGraw-Hill; 2010:chap 7.)

thoracostomy[17] (**Figure 34-1**). Successful placement of a needle thoracostomy depends on several factors including length and physical properties of the catheter. Thoracostomy appears to have more of a role in penetrating thoracic trauma, but can also successfully be employed in blunt trauma.[18,19]

Reduction of the thoracic cavity volume, by either compression from the abdominal cavity as in severe cirrhosis with ascites or extrapulmonary thoracic conditions such as pleural effusions, may result in reduced total lung capacity and cause respiratory distress. Many of these conditions do not develop suddenly, but are more insidious. Understanding the underlying disease process allows for targeted therapy, although procedures such as thoracentesis and paracentesis are not performed in the prehospital environment, knowledge that they may be indicated may direct destination determination. Supportive measures including supplemental oxygen, patient positioning, and noninvasive positive pressure ventilation[20,21] may assist in improving symptoms until definitive care can be obtained.

INFECTION

Pneumonia has the highest overall mortality of any infectious disease in the United States. Annually, approximately 5.5 million cases of community-acquired pneumonia are diagnosed with around 20% requiring hospitalization. *Streptococcus pneumoniae* remains the primary causative organism of bacterial pneumonia. One of the challenges in treating patients with pneumonia is the coinfection with other organisms as well as bacterial drug resistance.[22] Patients with pneumonia may present with cough, sputum production, chest pain, or shortness of breath, with elderly patients having fewer or nonspecific symptoms.[23] Management in the prehospital setting should focus on general supportive measures addressing hemodynamic stability and oxygenation. If the patient shows evidence of shock, appropriate measures should be employed including fluid resuscitation and possibly airway management as indicated.

ANAPHYLAXIS

Anaphylaxis is a Type 1 hypersensitivity immune-mediated reaction based on IgE-mediated effects with multisystem involvement including urticaria, angioedema, hypotension, or bronchospasm. Identified etiologies include food, medications (specifically antibiotics), as well as envenomation.[24] Diagnosis of anaphylaxis is based on clinical presentation and history, with laboratory values having no clinical importance in the immediate treatment phase. Epinephrine administered intramuscular is the emergent intervention of choice with no absolute contraindication. Intravenous resuscitation with isotonic fluids and other medications including antihistamines and corticosteroids may be administered, but definitive treatment still relies on administration of epinephrine. Respiratory failure may be seen in anaphylaxis as a result of bronchospasm, angioedema, or hypotension with a systemic lack of perfusion.[25]

DIAGNOSTIC APPROACH TO ACUTE RESPIRATORY FAILURE

Prompt recognition of patients requiring respiratory support is crucial. Oftentimes, the history obtained from the patient or others will provide the most clues as to how patient care should be approached and which interventions, if any, will help improve symptoms. Identifying the underlying etiology of the respiratory distress may prove more challenging but is of secondary importance. Reviewing a patient's medical history and obtaining an accurate list of medications for review may prove helpful. A patient may have wheezing on examination and review of their medications may show treatments for chronic obstructive pulmonary disease, congestive heart failure, asthma, or other etiologies that could guide management. Sometimes, patients may be in extremis and not able to contribute, but family members present may be able to help significantly. Environmental exposures are also good clues as to the underlying disease process. If the patient is at a chemical plant or found near a pesticide, this could easily direct management and help the prehospital providers take extra precautions so as not to contaminate themselves or anyone else. Removing a patient from an environment may be the simplest intervention needed to improve a patient's symptoms. Clothing may serve as a reservoir for chemical agents, and these should be removed quickly. Physical examination is helpful in evaluating all patients, but especially those who are not able to contribute verbally or answer questions appropriately. Physical examination is not reliable to exclude pneumothorax or hemothorax, as patients still may have breath sounds.[26] Reduced air movement may also not allow for breath sounds to be adequately auscultated. Work of breathing may change in patients who are improving or deteriorating necessitating serial observation and continuous monitoring.

MANAGEMENT OF RESPIRATORY FAILURE IN THE PREHOSPITAL SETTING

Management of respiratory distress, insufficiency, and failure in the prehospital setting may be affected by the uncontrolled environment but has the potential to greatly improve patient outcome. A patient may require anything from supplemental oxygen to aggressive invasive airway control during treatment and transport. Continuous monitoring will allow the provider to determine if an intervention is sufficient or if more support is necessary. Prehospital airway management is an ongoing challenge, which requires close attention from EMS physicians.[27]

▦ OXYGEN

The use of oxygen is widely accepted in a variety of patient conditions. The routine use of pulse oximetry in the prehospital setting allows for identification of patients who are hypoxic and can guide therapy. The use of oxygen in patients with chronic obstructive pulmonary disease is still debated regarding the target oxygenation level with concern related to eliminating the hypoxic respiratory drive and worsening hypercapnia.[28] Waveform capnography is another tool available to the prehospital provider to identify hypercapnia and initiate other treatments such as noninvasive positive pressure ventilation.

▦ NONINVASIVE POSITIVE PRESSURE VENTILATION

Select populations of patients with hypoxemic respiratory failure may benefit by noninvasive positive pressure ventilation (NIPPV) with a reduced intubation rate and decreases in intensive care unit stay and mortality[29] and has been used and advocated for in the prehospital setting.[30,31] NIPPV has been shown to reduce the need for intubation in patients with pulmonary edema, chronic obstructive pulmonary disease, and asthma.[32] Individuals with COPD as well as acute pulmonary edema may benefit from continuous positive airway pressure (CPAP), a form of NIPPV. Utilizing CPAP for patients with severe acute pulmonary edema improves oxygenation,[33] decreases hospital mortality, and decreases need for intubation.[34] Overall hospital length of stay did not significantly decrease, but duration of intensive care unit stay did.[35]

▦ INVASIVE AIRWAY DEVICE

In the event that a patient has decreased mental status, or will not tolerate other forms of airway support, invasive devices may be indicated. The classic airway involves placement of an endotracheal tube by direct laryngoscopy, but multiple other devices are becoming available to the prehospital provider.

▦ BLIND INSERTION AIRWAY DEVICE

Many different manufacturers have created various forms of blind insertion airway devices that are passed through the oropharynx and occlude the esophagus while allowing ventilation to occur. These devices are deployed quickly and can be used as a primary[36] or backup airway device.[37] In the case of cardiac arrest, these devices may be preferred, as placement does not require interruption of chest compressions.[38]

▦ ENDOTRACHEAL INTUBATION

Endotracheal intubation is considered the gold standard for airway management. Prehospital intubation success has been reported with a rate as low as 50% and as high as 98%, with success increased by using rapid sequence algorithms.[39] Video laryngoscopy is also becoming an option for increasing numbers of prehospital providers.[40] There are several different video laryngoscopes available, and some have suggested this as a primary tool in patients with cervical spine injuries or expected difficult airway.[41] Using a video laryngoscope during cardiopulmonary resuscitation with chest compressions may decrease the time needed for definitive airway control.[42]

▦ SURGICAL AIRWAY

Airway management in the prehospital environment is not always easily attainable. In some circumstances, multiple devices may be required to appropriately ventilate a patient. Surgical airway management has primarily been reserved as an option in the failed airway algorithm, and rarely is the primary method for obtaining an airway. A failed airway has been proposed as either the inability to ventilate and oxygenate a patient or three unsuccessful attempts at placement of an endotracheal tube by an experienced operator.[43] It is important to note that in some circumstances proper bag-valve-mask ventilations may provide sufficient oxygenation and ventilation. A number of devices are commercially available to help perform a cricothyroidotomy from surgical kits to those using the Seldinger technique. Providers should be familiar with the technique and equipment available to them to obtain a surgical airway (**Figure 34-2**). Consider transtracheal jet ventilation in children under the age of 10 given anatomic differences between pediatric patients and adults.[44]

INITIAL APPROACH TO AIRWAY MANAGEMENT IN THE PREHOSPITAL SETTING

Many patients who utilize emergency medical services will do so because of respiratory distress and prehospital providers should be ready and capable to respond and care for them. Frequent reassessments should identify if further interventions are required in managing the patient with respiratory distress. Using equipment such as a pulse oximetry, electrocardiogram, end-tidal or waveform capnography may help direct therapy toward the underlying cause of respiratory distress. Evaluating the airway is crucial in managing patients in respiratory distress. If the patient can converse appropriately without distress, the airway is likely intact. If the patient has a muffled voice, one may suspect an obstruction. Stridor may be another physical examination finding that can signal a

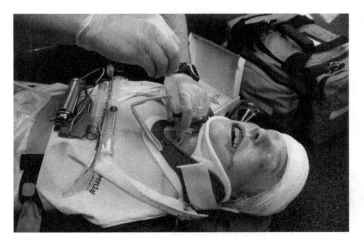

FIGURE 34-2. Percutaneous cricothyroidotomy. One option to obtain a surgical airway is to utilize a percutaneous device such as the QuickTrach®.

patient with potential airway compromise. Auscultation of the lungs may allow the provider to notice abnormal or diminished lung sounds. Medications such as bronchodilators may improve lung sounds as well as the patient's symptoms. Absence of lung sounds, in addition to other physical examination findings, may signify a tension pneumothorax that may necessitate immediate intervention. Anaphylaxis and allergic reactions pose a challenge to prehospital providers. Provider safety is essential but the patient may need to be moved quickly from the environment in which they are found. Anaphylaxis is a true emergency, and when suspected, treatment should not be delayed.

IDENTIFICATION AND APPROACH TO THE DIFFICULT AIRWAY

Identification and preparation for airway management oftentimes will lead to a greater success rate. Understanding the limitations to airway management in the prehospital environment is crucial, as is evaluating the patient and circumstances surrounding the working environment. Several mnemonics[45] have been developed for the rapid evaluation of potential difficulties in bag-valve-mask-assisted ventilations, intubation, blind insertion airway devices, and cricothyroidotomy.

MOANS

All providers should maintain competence in the basic airway technique of bag-valve-mask (BVM) ventilation (**Figure 34-3**). The ability to effectively oxygenate and ventilate a patient using a BVM may be crucial and can be potentially lifesaving. Assist devices such as nasopharyngeal or oropharyngeal airway placement may improve the effectiveness of BVM ventilations. There are several rapid assessment areas that focus on

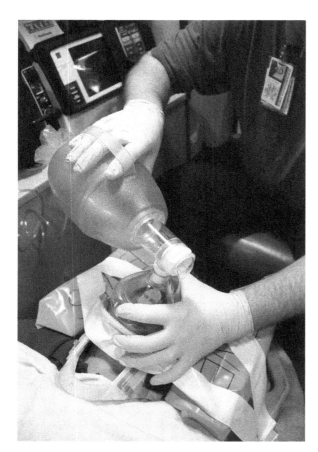

FIGURE 34-3. Bag-valve-mask (BVM) ventilation. Here the classic one-handed "c-hold" helps maintain the seal and allow for BVM ventilation.

setting up for success utilizing a BVM and can be easily remembered by the MOANS mnemonic.

Mask seal. Facial fractures or deformities, either congenital or from prior trauma, may impede the ability to form an airtight seal. Facial hair may also limit the quality of seal that can be obtained. Appropriate mask and bag size selection is also crucial, especially in the pediatric population.

Obesity or **O**bstruction may make ventilation more challenging and not provide for sufficient tidal volumes. Obese individuals have an increase in weight that must be displaced for adequate ventilation and may have redundant pharyngeal tissue that may lead to an airway obstruction. Other factors for consideration include the presence of foreign bodies or anatomical upper airway obstructions.

Age-related factors also need to be taken into account. Both the young and old may have a lack of supporting skeletal structures needed to create a good mask seal. Elderly patients may also lack muscle tone in the upper airway and tend to an obstruction.

No teeth limits the ability to create a good mask seal. If present, leaving dentures in place provides more support to obtain a good seal.

Snoring, **S**tiff lungs, or **S**pinal precautions may also make BVM ventilation more challenging. Individuals who are suspected of having cervical spine injuries are frequently placed in a cervical collar which will limit the ability of the provider to open the airway by mechanical manipulation. Patients with various lung pathology may have reduced pulmonary compliance, while other disease processes may require adjusting the inspiratory to expiratory ratio to prevent air trapping.

RODS

Blind insertion airway devices have become more common in medical practice. Although there are a variety of devices available, the principal design is relatively similar: obstruct entry into the esophagus and allow outflow through the pharynx so ventilation may occur. Placement of these devices depends largely on which device is being used; however, patient evaluation remains similar. Utilizing the RODS mnemonic, one can anticipate which patients will be more challenging for appropriate blind insertion airway device placement.

Restricted mouth opening. This is most commonly caused by a small oral aperture either through the patient's anatomy or injury.

Obstruction of the upper airway either through a foreign body, trauma, or swelling. Consider development of an obstruction or airway dislodgement in a patient who becomes more difficult to ventilate.

Distorted airway anatomy either from trauma, mass effect, or previous surgery may only become evident after attempted placement. These devices work well on normal anatomy, but significant variations may cause the device not to function appropriately.

Spinal precautions and **S**tiff lungs. Elevated airway pressures may reduce the effectiveness of the seal and allow air to enter the stomach or escape from the pharynx. Some devices allow passage of a gastric tube to help reduce the risk of aspiration.

LEMON

Correct placement of an endotracheal tube is still considered the definitive airway device. Many factors combine to make placement of an endotracheal tube successful, and preparation is one of the most important. The LEMON mnemonic was developed to help determine which patients may be more challenging to intubate.

Looking at the external anatomy and features of the patient is paramount. Individuals with significant facial hair may obstruct a provider's view. An abundance of oral secretions or trauma may obscure vocal cord visualization. Patients with prominent incisors may also pose a challenge with direct laryngoscopy.

Evaluate using the 3-3-2 rule will allow for prediction of alignment of the oral, pharyngeal, and laryngeal axis. This is performed by seeing if the patient can open their mouth three fingerbreadths, if there is a distance of three fingerbreadths from the chin to the hyoid bone, and if there is a distance of two fingerbreadths from the hyoid bone to the thyroid.

Mallampati score refers to the four-classification system for ease of visualization of the posterior pharynx (**Figure 34-4**). Class one allows for visualization of the posterior pharynx, soft palate, entire uvula, and tonsil pillars while class two allows for visualization of the soft palate and uvula. Both of these Mallampati classifications should allow for good visualization with direct laryngoscopy. Class three allows for visualization of the soft palate and the base of the uvula while class four allows visualization of the hard palate only. Both class three and four predict a difficult airway. In the prehospital setting, complete Mallampati evaluation is not always appropriate prior to attempting endotracheal intubation.

Obstruction including foreign bodies, soft tissue swelling, and trauma may also pose a challenge to endotracheal intubation. The provider may need to be ready with alternative airway devices or adjuncts in order to secure the airway in patients with suspected obstruction. Patients with pronounced soft tissue swelling may need a smaller diameter endotracheal tube which may allow for smoother passage.

Neck mobility is a concern for all patients requiring airway management in the prehospital setting. Victims of trauma with possible or suspected cervical spine injuries should have cervical spine precautions when feasible. Without the ability to extend the patient's neck, endotracheal intubation may be more challenging. Also consider neck mobility in patients with previous fusion and those with a history of spondyloarthropathies.

■ SHORT

If a patient cannot be intubated, and ventilation cannot occur even with the assistance of BVM or other devices, consideration of a surgical airway such be entertained, specifically cricothyroidotomy. In children, transtracheal ventilation may be a better option depending on the age of the patient. Performing a cricothyroidotomy on a patient with laryngotracheal injuries is a relative contraindication as attempting the procedure

may worsen the injury.[46] There are no absolute contraindications to performing a surgical airway if the patient is in extremis and there are no other means of establishing an airway.

Scars and previous Surgery to the anterior aspect of the neck may interfere with normal anatomy and make the surgical procedure more difficult. Also, the presence of subcutaneous emphysema may signify a disruption to the trachea.

Hematoma formation may be evidence of a vascular injury displacing the trachea from midline and also make the procedure more difficult if active bleeding is ongoing. Obesity will obscure the normal landmarks and oftentimes provide excess subcutaneous tissue to go through before reaching the anterior aspect of the trachea.

Radiation therapy may distort normal anatomy and cause scar tissue formation which may make blunt dissection more difficult.

Tumors and other masses pose an issue in terms of landmark identification, tracheal deviation, and the possibility of bleeding complications if the tumor is violated.

CHALLENGES OF AIRWAY MANAGEMENT IN THE PREHOSPITAL SETTING

There are several challenges when caring for patients in acute respiratory distress or failure. Some of these may be anticipated and prepared for through simulations, continuing education, or experience obtained in an alternative environment such as the operating rooms or cadaver laboratory experiences. Physical obstacles may be encountered in the prehospital environment. Attempting to manage a patient's airway in the controlled environment of the emergency department or operating room is dramatically different than having a patient in a motor vehicle collision or in a small room in a residence. Maintaining cervical spine stabilization during attempted airway management may make the procedure more difficult. Environmental exposures to elements such as rain, extreme heat, and other elements may also provide additional challenges to appropriate airway management.

Equipment available to the prehospital provider may be limited to direct laryngoscopy for placement of an endotracheal tube or a supraglottic airway device. Utilizing a tool such as a gum elastic bougie may increase endotracheal intubation success rates[47] (**Figure 34-5**). With the introduction of video laryngoscopes, some prehospital providers have additional tools to assist with airway management.[48] Supraglottic

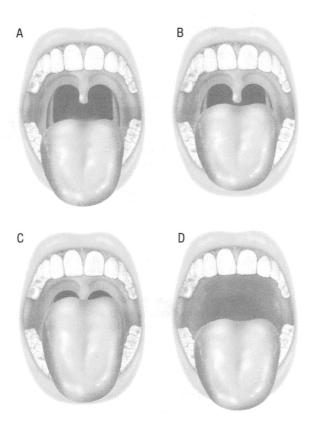

FIGURE 34-4. Mallampati classification. **A**: Class I. **B**: Class II. **C**: Class III. **D**: Class IV. (Reproduced with permission from Reichman EF. Essential anatomy of the airway. In: Reichman EF, ed. *Emergency Medicine Procedures.* 2nd ed. New York, NY: McGraw-Hill; 2013:chap 6.)

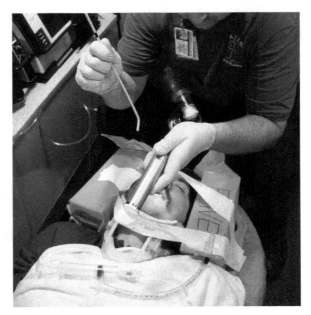

FIGURE 34-5. Limitations in neck mobility may require advanced techniques. The EMS provider is using a bougie to enter the airway due to the use of spinal immobilization.

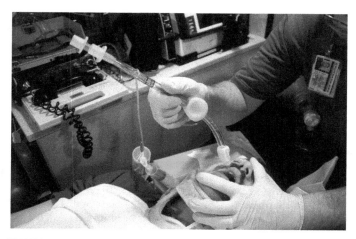

FIGURE 34-6. Supraglottic airway device. The EMS provider is placing a supraglottic airway device (Combitube) as a rescue airway device after failed intubation.

airway devices are also becoming widely used throughout prehospital medicine (**Figure 34-6**). One impetus for this is the low frequency of endotracheal intubations performed by prehospital providers,[49] as well as some studies showing an improvement in time to ventilation with supraglottic devices in patients requiring airway management.[50] In patients with cardiac arrest, reinforcing the importance of early defibrillation and early and high-quality chest compressions remain vital to improved outcomes.[51,52] Utilizing supraglottic airway devices may minimize interruptions to chest compression while performing cardiopulmonary resuscitation.[53] Other equipment challenges encountered in the prehospital environment include lack of backup or supporting devices and personnel.

MEDICATIONS FOR AIRWAY MANAGEMENT IN THE PREHOSPITAL SETTING

Correctly identifying a patient's underlying medical condition will allow prehospital providers to properly choose and implement medications to assist in patient management. Understanding appropriate indications and utilization of these medications in the prehospital environment is paramount in patient safety and outcome. Although the availability of medications may differ depending on the experience of the provider, level of training, and the guidance of the medical director, it is important to understand and be familiar with different medications for managing acute respiratory complaints and respiratory failure.

ADRENERGIC AGONIST

Management of acute bronchospasm, either in the setting of reactive airway disease or another cause continues to rely on the use of short-acting β-adrenergic agonists for dilation of the bronchioles.[54,55] Primarily, this is accomplished through stimulation of the $β_2$ receptor found within the smooth muscle of the bronchioles promoting relaxation of those structures. Several different medications fall into this category and are classified based on their duration of action. Long-acting β-agonists with duration of action over 12 hours, such as formoterol and salmeterol, are used primarily as maintenance medications by individuals who have known chronic obstructive pulmonary disease. The role of these medications in the acute setting is very limited and has been shown in some studies to be harmful. However, short-acting β-agonists such as albuterol and terbutaline, commonly given either through a nebulized solution or via metered-dose inhaler, with onset of action within several minutes and a duration of 4 to 6 hours, are classically used to treat an acute exacerbation of bronchospasm.[56] Albuterol is the most prescribed short-acting β-agonist in the United States.[57] Terbutaline may also be given subcutaneously, but this route of administration is commonly

reserved for patients who do not respond to inhaled therapy or those in extremis.[58] Management of anaphylaxis and anaphylactic shock focuses on early administration of epinephrine.[59] Nonselectively activating both α- and β-adrenergic receptors, epinephrine has many systemic effects including vasoconstriction and increasing cardiac output. Epinephrine also acts to reduce the release of chemical mediators of anaphylaxis.[60] Epinephrine may be given subcutaneously, intramuscularly, or intravenously with the preferred route being intramuscular.[61]

ANTICHOLINERGIC

Anticholinergic agents work by inhibiting muscarinic-mediated bronchoconstriction and mucous production in the central airways and have been used effectively in the maintenance therapy of chronic obstructive pulmonary disease.[62] The synergistic effect seen with the combination of an anticholinergic and a $β_2$ agonist may be related to the effects at both the central (anticholinergic) and peripheral ($β_2$ agonist) airways.[63] The combination has also shown a trend toward improvement in pulmonary function for individuals with both reactive airway disease and COPD.[64] Today, there are both short-acting and long-acting anticholinergic medications available for inhalation with both having low systemic effects.[65] The short-acting anticholinergic ipratropium is also available commercially in combination with albuterol and may be given as either a metered dose inhaler or nebulized solution.

MAGNESIUM

Another agent that is available for the treatment of reactive airway disease or bronchospasm is magnesium. It is believed that giving magnesium will reduce the amount of intracellular calcium in the smooth muscle, reduce contraction, and cause smooth muscle relaxation.[66] Current recommendation for magnesium therapy is limited to those with severe acute asthma[67] or those who have not responded to conventional management. Slow administration via the intravenous route is preferred but some reports of nebulized magnesium do exist.[68]

CORTICOSTEROID

A hallmark of inflammatory disease management has been the administration of corticosteroids and has been used in the treatment of reactive airway disease and chronic obstructive pulmonary disease. In order for corticosteroids to work, they must cross the cellular membrane and combine with intracellular receptors. Following this combination enters the cell nucleus and decreases production of inflammatory mediator proteins. For patients with moderate to severe asthma, administration of systemic corticosteroids within 1 hour of presentation has been shown to reduce hospital admission rates.[69] Small studies have also shown that moving administration to the prehospital environment has a reduction in hospital admission rates as well.[70] Similarly, patients with exacerbations of chronic obstructive pulmonary disease appear to have improved clinical outcomes, improvement in spirometry,[71] and decrease in treatment failure and relapse rates.[72] Corticosteroid management still appears as a treatment option in patients with anaphylaxis although the routine administration of this medication is not supported.[73]

VASODILATOR AND DIURETIC

Nitroglycerin is routinely utilized in the prehospital setting for the treatment of acute coronary syndrome. In the treatment of decompensated congestive heart failure with pulmonary edema, nitroglycerin has also been used, historically administered in combination with other medications including opiates and diuretics. Nitroglycerin is believed to have vasodilatory properties through the relaxation of smooth muscle by the local creation of nitric oxide[74] causing a reduction in preload. When used in the prehospital environment for the treatment of pulmonary edema, nitroglycerin has been shown to improve outcome related to dyspnea and hospital morbidity. As important, if the diagnosis of pulmonary edema is incorrect, which occurs up to 40% of the time, nitroglycerin was not associated with adverse events.[75] Other medications such as angiotensin-converting enzyme (ACE) inhibitors are currently being used in the prehospital setting.[76] Administration of ACE inhibitors has been associated with a decrease of intensive care admissions as well as a decrease in the need for intubation when administered in the emergency department for patients with acute pulmonary edema.[77] Prehospital administration of diuretics such as furosemide is not appropriate. The effects of furosemide are delayed and potentially increase morbidity or mortality if given to a patient with a different disease process such as pneumonia or sepsis.[78]

RAPID SEQUENCE INTUBATION

Performing endotracheal intubation in patients who still maintain protective reflexes, including the gag reflex, may require the administration of a sedative and paralytic to optimize intubating conditions, improve success rates and patient outcome. Classically, positive pressure ventilation is not administered to patients undergoing rapid sequence intubation (RSI) if possible, but is a controversial issue.[79]

▮ PRETREATMENT

Several medications have been administered prior to induction and paralysis in the attempt to blunt the physiologic response to direct laryngoscopy including stimulation of the sympathetic and parasympathetic nerves of the larynx and hypopharynx, increase in intracranial pressure, and bronchospasm. The routine use of some of these medications, usually administered 3 minutes prior to induction, is not well supported.

▮ LIDOCAINE

Lidocaine administration as a pretreatment to patients undergoing RSI due to asthma has been suggested to prevent bronchospasm from direct laryngoscopy and endotracheal tube placement. Studies with patients undergoing general anesthesia have suggested that the addition of lidocaine does not reduce postintubation bronchospasm.[80] Lidocaine has also been suggested to blunt the increase in intracranial pressure which some suggest is mediated by an increase in cardiac output and arterial pressure. Studying lidocaine use in RSI and the effect on intracranial pressure is difficult although some studies in the intensive care unit or elective neurosurgical cases have been performed. Some of the research is limited by confounding issues including other medications administered as well as the clinical setting. It is unclear if the routine use of lidocaine for pretreatment in the setting of acute traumatic head injury reduces intracranial pressure or has a positive effect on patient outcome.[81,82]

▮ FENTANYL

Ultrashort-acting opiates such as fentanyl have been suggested and used as pretreatment medications prior to RSI because they may decrease the sympathetic response seen with direct laryngoscopy. Fentanyl is hemodynamically neutral. When given as a pretreatment medication at 3 μg/kg, fentanyl was able to blunt the hypertension seen with laryngoscopy, but did not have an effect on heart rate.[83,84] In bolus doses higher than those used in RSI, studies have linked fentanyl to an increase in intracranial pressure and a decrease in cerebral perfusion pressure in patients who already have elevated intracranial pressure.[85]

▮ ATROPINE

Atropine administered as part of the pretreatment for a pediatric patient undergoing RSI is still common. The thought is to reduce reflex bradycardia in pediatric patients, but the data are conflicting. Bradycardia has been seen in both patients who do and do not have atropine administered prior to laryngoscopy.[86] Few adverse events have been reported with administration of atropine.

▮ SEDATIVES

As part of RSI, a sedative agent is given prior to neuromuscular blockade. A variety of medications are available for sedation. Understanding the different options for sedation, as well as the appropriate clinical use, is very important. Selecting the appropriate agent may help improve patient outcome, whereas inappropriate sedative agents may have a detrimental effect.

Etomidate Etomidate is an imidazole derivative which has no analgesic properties but is a potent sedative hypnotic agent. The onset of action in induction doses (0.2-0.4 mg/kg) is within 15 seconds with a duration of action up to 15 minutes. Few cardiovascular and respiratory effects are seen after its administration, making it an ideal induction agent. Unlike other induction agents, etomidate reduces intracranial pressure without reducing arterial blood pressure or cerebral perfusion pressure.[87,88] One of the concerns regarding routine use of etomidate for RSI is its potential to cause adrenal suppression. The continuous use of etomidate for sedation is not recommended because of this effect, and the single use for induction in patients has been investigated. Studies suggest that the adrenal suppression is transient and appears to resolve within 12 hours of administration[89] with no significant effect on patient mortality.[90]

Benzodiazepine Benzodiazepines are a class of medication that function through stimulation of the GABA receptors. Of the benzodiazepine agents, midazolam is the most commonly used for induction during RSI. The recommended dose for induction is 0.1 mg/kg to 0.3 mg/kg and may take up to 2 minutes for full effects to occur. When evaluating its use in RSI, midazolam is frequently underdosed in both the pediatric and the adult population.[91] Use of short-acting benzodiazepines, such as midazolam, is limited in part due to the time for effect as well as the dose-dependent decrease in systemic vascular resistance and resultant hypotension.[92]

Barbiturate Ultrashort-acting barbiturates, such as thiopental and methohexital, have been used for induction as part of RSI in patients with suspected elevation of intracranial pressure or with status epilepticus. Barbiturates, similar to benzodiazepines, exert their effect through GABA receptors. Barbiturates have a negative cardiovascular effect and reduce both cardiac output and mean arterial pressure, but appear to have preservation of the cerebral perfusion pressure. Of the ultrashort-acting, methohexital has been reported to be less cardiac depressive. Other negative effects that have been seen with barbiturate administration include laryngeal spasm.[93] Both ultrashort-acting barbiturates have an onset less than 30 seconds and last up to 5 minutes.[94]

Ketamine Ketamine is considered a dissociative anesthetic with analgesic properties although it also causes stimulation of the sympathetic nervous system, resulting in an increase in heart rate, blood pressure, and cardiac output. Other effects of ketamine include bronchial dilation by smooth muscle relaxation. The effects of ketamine work through antagonism of the NMDA receptor.[95] Typical induction dosages of ketamine are 1 to 2 mg/kg when administered intravenously. The use of ketamine has been avoided in patients with suspected head injury due to concern for increase in intracranial pressure, but further research shows that this concern may not be justified.[96]

Propofol Propofol is a sedative hypnotic which also exerts effects by mediating the GABA receptors. Widely used in procedural sedation procedures, propofol has also been used in RSI with dosages of 1.5 to 2.5 mg/kg. Onset of action is approximately 30 seconds with a duration of up to 5 minutes. Propofol has been shown to reduce cerebral blood flow, cerebral oxygen consumption, and decreases intracranial pressure.[97] The role of propofol has been limited in rapid sequence intubation due to the cardiac depressant effect and noted hypotension.

Neuromuscular Blockade With RSI, the administration of a neuromuscular blocking agent assists in optimizing intubation success. There are two different types of neuromuscular blocking medications available currently and differ in the mechanism of action: depolarizing and nondepolarizing. The nondepolarizing neuromuscular blockers may be reversed by administration of acetylcholinesterase inhibitors.

Depolarizing Agents Depolarizing neuromuscular blockers, such as succinylcholine, work by depolarizing the postsynaptic acetylcholine receptors, thus making them resistant to further stimulation by acetylcholine. Succinylcholine has long been used as the neuromuscular blocker of choice in RSI due to the extremely quick time of onset (approximately 30-45 seconds) and its short duration of action (less than 10 minutes). However, there are many relative contraindications which should be well understood by the prehospital provider.

Hyperkalemia has been associated with the administration of succinylcholine with peak increase occurring between 2 and 5 minutes following neuromuscular blockade. The increase in potassium levels has been reported between 0.5 and 1 mEq/L, and is transient over a period of 10 to 15 minutes.[98] It is believed that this increase is caused by an upregulation of the acetylcholine receptor, leading to potassium efflux. Caution should be exercised in patients who may be predisposed to the hyperkalemic side effect of succinylcholine including patients with burns and crush injuries (although in the acute setting, succinylcholine may be administered), chronic peripheral denervation either from stroke or spinal cord injury, severe infections, prolonged immobility with resultant atrophy, certain myopathies, and those who are hyperkalemic or at risk for being hyperkalemic.[99,100]

Succinylcholine has been reported to increase intraocular pressure and it has been propagated that an open globe injury is a contraindication to administration, but there have been no cases of vitreous extrusion or blindness linked to succinylcholine.[101]

Nondepolarizing Agents Nondepolarizing neuromuscular blockers, such as rocuronium and vecuronium, work by blocking the binding of acetylcholine to the postsynaptic receptors in a competitive fashion. There are many different nondepolarizing neuromuscular blockers available, with differing properties in terms of onset as well as duration. Rocuronium has a recommended dosing of 0.6 mg/kg with onset of approximately 1 minute and duration near 1 hour, while vecuronium has a recommended dosing of 0.1 mg/kg with onset of approximately 2 minutes and a duration near 2 hours. Nondepolarizing neuromuscular blockers do not have the same adverse effects as seen in succinylcholine, but the longer onset and duration of action[102] make them less favorable for RSI. Reversal of neuromuscular blockade is possible with acetylcholinesterase inhibitors such as neostigmine, as well as other commercially available medications that are not currently available in the United States, but are currently in use in other countries.[103]

Early comparison studies looking at the difference between success rates of neuromuscular blockade for rapid sequence intubation with succinylcholine compared with rocuronium do not show significant difference.[104]

- Respiratory failure and anaphylaxis are acute life-threatening conditions that can and must be addressed by prehospital providers.
- Causes of respiratory failure and anaphylaxis are numerous and of varied etiologies.
- Treatment options for respiratory failure and anaphylaxis are effective and can range from minimally invasive to invasive.
- Assessment of the airway is important to optimize successful management.
- There are many useful medications and equipment options available to the prehospital provider treating respiratory failure and anaphylaxis.

REFERENCES

1. Lilly C, Ingenito EP, Shapiro SD. Respiratory failure. In: Kasper DL, Braunwald E, Fauci AS, Hauser SL, Longo DL, Jameson JL, eds. *Harrison's Principles of Internal Medicine.* 16th ed. New York, NY: McGraw-Hill, 2005; 1588-1591.
2. Kasper DL, Braunwald E, Fauci AS, Hauser SL, Longo DL, Jameson JL, eds. *Harrison's Manual of Medicine.* New York, NY: McGraw-Hill, 2005; 19-23.
3. Behrendt CE. Acute respiratory failure in the United States: incidence and 31-day survival. *Chest.* 2000;118(4):1100-1105.
4. Tsao TC, Juang YC, Lan RS, et al. Respiratory failure of acute organophosphate and carbamate poisoning. *Chest.* 1990;98(3):631-636.
5. Casetta I, Groppo E, De Gennaro R, et al. Myasthenia gravis: a changing pattern of incidence. *J Neuro.* 2010;257(12):2015-2019.
6. Mehta S. Neuromuscular disease causing acute respiratory failure. *Respir Care.* 2006;51(9):1016-1021.
7. CDC. Carbon monoxide exposures—United States, 2000-2009. *MMWR.* 2011;60:1014-1017.
8. Thomas C, Svehla L, Moffett BS. Sodium-nitroprusside-induced cyanide toxicity in pediatric patients. *Expert Opin Drug Saf.* 2009;8(5):599-602.
9. Leavesley HB, Li L, Mukhopadhyay S, et al. Nitrite-mediated antagonism of cyanide inhibition of cytochrome C oxidase in dopamine neurons. *Toxicol Sci.* 2010;115(2):569-576.
10. Hall AH, Saiers J, Baud F. Which cyanide antidote? *Crit Rev Toxicol.* 2009;39(7):541-542.
11. CDC. Deaths from chronic obstructive pulmonary disease—United States, 2000-2005. *MMWR.* 2008;57(45):1229-1232.
12. Rabe KF, Hurd S, Anzueto A, et al. Global strategy for the diagnosis, management, and prevention of chronic obstructive pulmonary disease: GOLD executive summary. *Am J Respir Crit Care Med.* 2007;176(6):532-555.
13. MacIntyre N, Huang YC. Acute exacerbations and respiratory failure in chronic obstructive pulmonary disease. *Proc Am Thorac Soc.* 2008;5(4):530-535.
14. CDC. Vital signs: asthma prevalence, disease characteristics, and self-management education: United States, 2001-2009. *MMWR;* 60(17):547-552.
15. Agbetile J, Green R. New therapies and management strategies in the treatment of asthma: patient-focused developments. *J Asthma Allergy.* 2011;4:1-12.
16. Beers SL, Abramo TJ, Bracken A, Wiebe RA. Bilevel positive airway pressure in the treatment of status asthmaticus in pediatrics. *Am J Emerg Med.* 2007;25(1):6-9.
17. Davis DP, Pettit K, Rom CD, et al. The safety and efficacy of prehospital needle and tube thoracostomy by aeromedical personnel. *Prehosp Emerg Care.* 2005;9(2):191-197.
18. Ball CG, Wyrzykowski AD, Kirkpatrick AW, et al. Thoracic needle decompression for tension pneumothorax: clinical correlation with catheter length. *Can J Surg.* 2010;53(3):184-188.
19. Eckstein M, Suvehara D. Needle thoracostomy in the prehospital setting. *Prehosp Emerg Care.* 1998;2(2):132-135.
20. Cheskes S, Turner L, Thomson S, Aljerian N. The impact of prehospital continuous positive airway pressure on the rate of intubation and mortality from acute out-of-hospital respiratory emergencies. *Prehosp Emerg Care.* October-December 2013;17(4):435-441.
21. Aguilar SA, Lee J, Dunford JV, et al. Assessment of the addition of prehospital continuous positive airway pressure (CPAP) to an urban emergency medical services (EMS) system in persons with severe respiratory distress. *J Emerg Med.* August 2013;45(2):210-219.
22. Niederman MS. Challenges in the management of community-acquired pneumonia: the role of quinolones and moxifloxacin. *Clin Infect Dis.* 2005;41(S2):S158-S166.
23. Halm EA, Teirstein AS. Clinical practice. management of community-acquired pneumonia. *N Engl J Med.* 2002;347(25):2039-2045.

24. Tupper J, Visser S. Anaphylaxis: a review and update. *Can Fam Physician*. 2010;56(10):1009-1011.

25. Ring J, Grosber M, Mohrenschlager M, Brockow K. Anaphylaxis: acute treatment and management. *Chem Immunol Allergy*. 2010;95:201-210.

26. Chen SC, Markmann JF, Kauder Dr, Schwab CW. Hemopneumothorax missed by auscultation in penetrating chest injury. *J Trauma*. 1997;42(1):86-89.

27. Diggs LA, Yusuf JE, De Leo G. An update on out-of-hospital airway management practices in the United States. *Resuscitation*. July 2014;85(7):885-892.

28. New A. Oxygen: kill or cure? prehospital hyperoxia in the COPD patient. *Emerg Med J*. 2006;23(2):144-146.

29. Keenan SP, Sinuff T, Cook DJ, Hill NS. Does noninvasive positive pressure ventilation improve outcome in acute hypoxemic respiratory failure? a systematic review. *Crit Care Med*. 2004;32(12):2516-2523.

30. Bledsoe BE, Anderson E, Hodnick R, Johnson L, Johnson S, Dievendorf E. Low-fractional oxygen concentration continuous positive airway pressure is effective in the prehospital setting. *Prehosp Emerg Care*. April-June 2012;16(2):217-221.

31. Spijker EE, de Bont M, Bax M, Sandel M. Practical use, effects and complications of prehospital treatment of acute cardiogenic pulmonary edema using the Boussignac CPAP system. *Int J Emerg Med*. April 8, 2013;6(1):8.

32. Sullivan R. Prehospital use of CPAP: positive pressure = positive patient outcomes. *Emerg Med Serv*. 2005;34(8):120-126.

33. Kallio T, Kuisma M, Apaspaa A, Rosenberg PH. The use of prehospital continuous positive airway pressure treatment in presumed acute severe pulmonary edema. *Prehosp Emerg Care*. 2003;7(2):209-213.

34. Pang D, Keenan SP, Cook DJ, Sibbald WJ. The effect of positive pressure airway support on mortality and the need for intubation in cardiogenic pulmonary edema: a systematic review. *Chest*. 1998;114(4):1185-1192.

35. Vital FM, Saconato H, Ladeira MT, et al. Non-invasive positive pressure ventilation (CPAP or bilevel NPPV) for cardiogenic pulmonary edema. *Cochrane Database Syst Rev*. 2008;3:CD005351.

36. Frascone RJ, Wewerka SS, Burnett AM, Griffith KR, Salzman JG. Supraglottic airway device use as a primary airway during rapid sequence intubation. *Air Med J*. March-April 2013;32(2):93-97.

37. Frascone RJ, Russi C, Lick C, et al. Comparison of prehospital insertion success rates and time to insertion between standard endotracheal intubation and a supraglottic airway. *Resuscitation*. December 2011;82(12):1529-1536.

38. Gabrielli A, Layon AJ, Wenzel V, et al. Alternative ventilation strategies in cardiopulmonary resuscitation. *Curr Opin Crit Care*. 2002;8(3):199-211.

39. Hubble MW, Brown L, Wilfong DA, et al. A meta-analysis of prehospital airway control techniques part 1: orotracheal and nasotracheal intubation success rates. *Prehosp Emerg Care*. 2010;14(3):377-401.

40. Burnett AM, Frascone RJ, Wewerka SS, et al. Comparison of success rates between two video laryngoscope systems used in a prehospital clinical trial. *Prehosp Emerg Care*. April-June 2014; 18(2):231-238.

41. Bjoernsen LP, Lindsay B. Video laryngoscopy in the prehospital setting. *Prehosp Disaster Med*. 2009;24(3):265-270.

42. Kim YM, Kang HG, Kim JH, et al. Direct versus video laryngoscopic intubation by novice prehospital intubators with and without chest compressions: a pilot manikin study. *Prehosp Emerg Care*. 2011;15(1):98-103.

43. Walls RM. Management of the difficult airway in the trauma patient. *Emerg Med Clin North Am*. 1998;16(1):45-61.

44. Walls RM. Management of the difficult airway in the trauma patient. *Emerg Med Clin North Am*. 1998;16(1):45-61.

45. Walls RM, Murphy MF. *Manual of Emergency Airway Management*. 3rd ed. Philadelphia, PA: Lippincott Williams & Wilkins; 2008.

46. Granholm T, Farmer DL. The surgical airway. *Respir Care Clin N Am*. 2001;7(1):13-23.

47. Jabre P, Combes X, Leroux B, et al. Use of gum elastic bougie for prehospital difficult intubation. *Am J Emerg Med*. 2005;23(4):552-555.

48. Bioernsen LP, Lindsay B. Video laryngoscopy in the prehospital setting. *Prehosp Disaster Med*. 2009;24(3):265-270.

49. Angelotti T, Brock-Utne J. New methods for direct verification of correct endotracheal tube placement. *Anesth Analg*. 2007; 105(4):1168.

50. Ruetzler K, Roessler B, Potura L, et al. Performance and skill retention of intubation by paramedics using seven different airway devices—a manikin study. *Resuscitation*. 2011;82(5):593-597.

51. Steen PA, Kramer-Johansen J. Improving cardiopulmonary resuscitation quality to ensure survival. *Curr Opin Crit Care*. 2008;14(3):299-304.

52. Ristagno G, Gullo A, Tang W, Weil MH. New cardiopulmonary resuscitation guidelines 2005: importance of uninterrupted chest compression. *Crit Care Clin*. 2006;22(3):531-538.

53. Gatward JJ, Thomas MJ, Nolan JP, Cook TM. Effect of chest compressions on the time taken to insert airway devices in a manikin. *Br J Anaesth*. 2008;100(3):351-356.

54. Cockcroft DW. Management of acute severe asthma. *Ann Allergy Asthma Immunol*. 1995;75(2):83-89.

55. Kelly HW. Risk versus benefit considerations for the beta(2)-agonists. *Pharmacotherapy*. 2006;26(9):164S-174S.

56. Tashkin DP, Fabbri LM. Long-acting beta-agonists in the management of chronic obstructive pulmonary disease: current and future agents. *Respir Res*. 2010;11(1):149-162.

57. Cherry DK, Burt CW, Woodwell DA. National ambulatory medical care survey: 2001 summary. *Adv Data*. 2003;337:1-44.

58. Papiris S, Kotanidou A, Malagari K, Roussos C. Clinical review: severe asthma. *Crit Care*. 2002;6(1):30-44.

59. McLean-Tooke AP, Bethune CA, Fay AC, Spickett GP. Adrenaline in the treatment of anaphylaxis: what is the evidence? *BMJ*. 2003;327(7427):1332-1335.

60. Kane KE, Cone DC. Anaphylaxis in the prehospital setting. *J Emerg Med*. 2004;27(4):371-377.

61. Simons FE, Gu X, Simons KJ. Epinephrine absorption in adults: intramuscular versus subcutaneous injection. *J Allergy Clin Immunol*. 108(5):871-873.

62. Siafakas NM, Vermeire P, Pride NB, et al. Optimal assessment and management of chronic obstructive pulmonary disease (COPD). *Eur Respir J*. 1995;8:1398-1420.

63. Petty TL. The combination of ipratropium and albuterol is more effective than either agent alone. *Chest*. 107(5S):183-6S.

64. Weber EJ, Levitt MA, Covington JK, Gambrioli E. Effect of continuously nebulized ipratropium bromide plus albuterol on emergency department length of stay and hospital admission rates in patients with acute bronchospasm: a randomized, controlled trial. *Chest*. 1999;115:937-944.

65. Van Noord JA, Bantje T, Eland ME, Korducki L, Cornelissen PJ. A randomized controlled comparison of tiotropium and ipratropium in the treatment of chronic obstructive pulmonary disease. *Thorax*. 2000;55(4):289-294.

66. Bichara MD, Goldman RD. Magnesium for treatment of asthma in children. *Can Fam Physician*. 2009;55(9):887-889.

67. Rowe BH, Bretzlaff JA, Bourdon C, Bota GW, Camargo CA Jr. Magnesium sulfate for treating exacerbations of acute asthma in the emergency department. *Cochrane Database Syst Rev*. 2000;2: CD001490.

68. Jones LA, Goodacre S. Magnesium sulphate in the treatment of acute asthma: evaluation of current practice in adult emergency departments. *Emerg Med J*. 2009;26(11):783-785.

69. Rowe BH, Spooner CH, Ducharme FM, et al. Early emergency department treatment of acute asthma with systemic corticosteroids. *Cochrane Database Syst Rev*. 2001;1:CD 002178.

70. Knapp B, Wood C. The prehospital administration of intravenous methylprednisolone lowers hospital admission rates for moderate to severe asthma. *Prehosp Emerg Care*. 2003;7(4):423-426.

71. Singh JM, Palda VA, Stanbrook MB, Chapman KR. Corticosteroid therapy for patients with acute exacerbations of chronic obstructive pulmonary disease: a systemic review. *Arch Intern Med.* 2002;162(22):2527-2536.
72. Schweiger TA, Zdanowicz. Systemic corticosteroids in the treatment of acute exacerbations of chronic obstructive pulmonary disease. *Am J Health Syst Pharm.* 2010;67(13):1061-1069.
73. Choo KJ, Simons E, Sheikh A. Glucocorticoids for the treatment of anaphylaxis: Cochrane systematic review. *Allergy.* 2010;65(10):1205-1211.
74. Ignarro LJ. After 130 years, the molecular mechanism of action of nitroglycerin is revealed. *Proc Natl Acad Sci U S A.* 2002;99(12):7816-7817.
75. Mattu A, Lawner B. Prehospital management of congestive heart failure. *Heart Fail Clin.* 2009;5(1):19-24.
76. Mosesso VN, Dunford J, Blackwell T, Griswell JK. Prehospital therapy for acute congestive heart failure: state of the art. *Prehosp Emerg Care.* 2003;7(1):13-23.
77. Sacchett A, Ramoska E, Moakes ME, et al. Effect of ED management on ICU use in acute pulmonary edema. *Am J Emerg Med.* 1999;17(6):571-574.
78. Jarnoik J, Mikkelson P, Fales W, Overton DT. Evaluation of prehospital use of furosemide in patients with respiratory distress. *Prehosp Emerg Care.* 2006;10(2):194-197.
79. El-Orbany M, Connolly LA. Rapid sequence induction and intubation: current controversy. *Anesth Analg.* 2010;110(5):1318-1325.
80. Maslow AD, Regan MM, Israel E, et al. Inhaled albuterol, but not intravenous Lidocaine, protects against intubation-induced bronchoconstriction in asthma. *Anesthesiology.* 2000;93(5):1198-1204.
81. Robinson N, Clancy M. In patients with head injury undergoing rapid sequence intubation, does pretreatment with intravenous lignocaine/lidocaine lead to an improved neurological outcome? A review of the literature. *Emerg Med J.* 2001;18:453-457.
82. Butler J, Jackson R. Towards evidence based emergency medicine: best BETs from Manchester Royal Infirmary. Lignocaine premedication before rapid sequence intubations in head injuries. *Emerg Med J.* 2002;19(6):554.
83. Feng CK, Chan HK, Liu KN, et al. A comparison of lidocaine, fentanyl, and esmolol for attenuation of cardiovascular response to laryngoscopy and tracheal intubation. *Acta Anaesthesiol Sin.* 1996;34(2):61-67.
84. Helfman SM, Gold MI, DeLisser EA, Herrington CA. Which drug prevents tachycardia and hypertension associated with tracheal intubation: lidocaine, fentanyl, or esmolol? *Anesth Analg.* 1991;72(4):482-486.
85. Albanese J, Viviand X, Potie F, et al. Sufentanil, fentanyl, and alfentanil in head trauma patients: a study on cerebral hemodynamics. *Crit Care Med.* 1999;27(2):407-411.
86. Fastle RK, Roback MG. Pediatric rapid sequence intubation: incidence of reflex bradycardia and effects of pretreatment with atropine. *Pediatr Emerg Care.* 2004;20(10):651-655.
87. Yeung JK, Zed PJ. A review of etomidate for rapid sequence intubation in the emergency department. *CJEM.* 2002;4(3):194-198.
88. Bergen JM, Smith DC. A review of etomidate for rapid sequence intubation in the emergency department. *J Emerg Med.* 1997;15(2):221-230.
89. Schenarts CL, Burton JH, Riker RR. Adrenocortical dysfunction following etomidate induction in emergency department patients. *Acad Emerg Med.* 2001;8(1):1-7.
90. Hohl CM, Kelly-Smith CH, Yeung TC, et al. The effect of a bolus dose of etomidate on cortisol levels, mortality, and health services utilization: a systematic review. *Ann Emerg Med.* 2010;56(2):105-113.
91. Sagarin MJ, Barton ED, Sakles JC, et al. Underdosing of midazolam in emergency endotracheal intubation. *Acad Emerg Med.* 2003;10(4):329-338.
92. Davis DP, Kimbro TA, Vike GM. The use of midazolam for prehospital rapid-sequence intubation may be associated with a dose-related increase in hypotension. *Prehosp Emerg Care.* 2001;5(2):163-168.
93. Russo H, Bressolle F. Pharmacodynamics and pharmacokinetics of thiopental. *Clin Pharmacokinet.* 1998;35(2):95-134.
94. Diza-Guzman E, Mireles-Cabodevila E, Heresi GA, et al. A comparison of methohexital versus etomidate for endotracheal intubation of critically ill patients. *Am J Crit Care.* 2010;19(1):48-54.
95. Orser BA, Pennefather PS, MacDonald JF. Multiple mechanisms of ketamine blockade of N-methyl-D-aspartate receptors. *Anesthesiology.* 1997;86(4):903-917.
96. Filanovsky Y, Miller P, Kao J. Myth: ketamine should not be used as an induction agent for intubation in patients with head injury. *CJEM.* 2010;12(2):154-157.
97. Adembri C, Venturi L, Pellegrini-Giampietro DE. Neuroprotective effects of propofol in acute cerebral injury. *CNS Drug Rev.* 2007;13(3):333-351.
98. Schow AJ, Lubarsky DA, Olson RP, Gan TJ. Can succinylcholine be used safely in hyperkalemic patients? *Anesth Analg.* 2002;95(1):119-122.
99. Martyn JA, White DA, Gronert GA, et al. Up-and-down regulation of skeletal muscle acetylcholine receptors. Effects on neuromuscular blockers. *Anesthesiology.* 1992;76(5):822-843.
100. Martyn JA, Richtsfeld M. Succinylcholine-induced hyperkalemia in acquired pathologic states: etiologic factors and molecular mechanisms. *Anesthesiology.* 2006;104(1):158-169.
101. Vachon CA, Warnder DO, Bacon DR. Succinylcholine and the open globe: tracing the teaching. *Anesthesiology.* 2003;99(1):220-223.
102. Hunter JM. New neuromuscular blocking drugs. *N Engl J Med.* 1995;332(25):1691-1699.
103. Paton F, Paulden M, Chambers D, et al. Sugammadex compared with neostigmine/glycopyrrolate for routine reversal of neuromuscular block: a systematic review and economic evaluation. *Br J Anaesth.* 2010;105(5):558-567.
104. Patanwala AE, Stahle SA, Sakles JC, Erstad BL. Comparison of succinylcholine and rocuronium for first-attempt intubation success in the emergency department. *Acad Emerg Med.* 2011;18(1):10-14.

CHAPTER 35

Shock and Hemorrhage

Christopher J. Fullagar

INTRODUCTION

The evaluation and treatment of shock in the prehospital environment presents unique challenges to the EMS physician. Decisions regarding the balance between sophisticated field treatment and minimizing transport time to definitive care must continually be evaluated. The benefit of advanced care in the field has been questioned.[1-3] Some studies have demonstrated that the addition of the physician on the scene may increase scene time in certain scenarios, while other studies have not observed this effect.[3] This is likely related to the prehospital training and experience of the physician. Balancing physician intervention with scene time is an important part of the care of the patient in shock and must be explored during the EMS education of residents and fellows.

OBJECTIVES

- Describe the identification of shock in the field.
- Describe the initial management of shock in the field.
- Analyze the causes of shock.
- Examine how to treat specific causes of shock while in the prehospital setting.
- Present the use of advanced vascular access and pressors in the field.
- Discuss the use of tourniquets and hemostatic agents for severe hemorrhage.

CARE OF SHOCK IN THE FIELD

Physician participation in the field is routine in the Franco-German model of prehospital care and is becoming more common in the United States. Participation in the field also allows the physician to gain a first-hand perspective on how the system works. The physician is often in a position to have an effect on protocols, provider education, and operational matters that affect patient care. For those in training, participation in the field provides them with critical insight into the challenges and limitations of caring for patients in the out-of-hospital setting. Without an understanding of the differences inherent in the provision of prehospital emergency care, it is often less than productive to apply in-hospital evaluation and treatment techniques in the field environment. To treat a patient in shock effectively in the field environment requires a knowledge base specific to EMS.

Shock is a state of decreased perfusion resulting in inadequate delivery of oxygen to the tissue. Typically, the body has exhausted its ability to compensate for the stressors it is experiencing. The principles for management of shock include the maintenance of perfusion while supporting ventilation and oxygenation. The precise degree of resuscitation of the patient depends on a number of factors and has been the topic of significant discussion in the literature.[4] The prehospital environment presents unique challenges when treating a patient in shock. Equipment and supplies are typically limited in the field environment. Austere conditions such as temperature extremes, darkness, and precipitation may hamper care of the patient in shock. Temperature control is a significant factor. Initial studies indicated that therapeutic hypothermia may have beneficial effects on patients after return of spontaneous circulation (ROSC), although further evaluation of this is required.[5] Alternatively, trauma patients requiring massive transfusion with a core temperature less than 34°C is associated with a mortality rate >85%. Maintaining an adequate environment in the ambulance

may be challenging. Factors as simple as opening the doors to the back of the ambulance on a cold day may have a significant effect on the cabin temperature. Warmed saline may not be as readily available in the field. For hypothermic patients, interventions such as invasive warming may not be practical or even possible in the field environment. This is to say nothing of the patient who cannot be removed from the elements such as is the case with vehicle entrapment or patients in remote locations.

SHOCK RECOGNITION

Identification of the patient in shock may not be as apparent in the field environment as it may be in the hospital. Equipment is limited and environmental factors such as temperature and vibration may affect the accuracy of that equipment. Skin color and temperature that is consistent with shock may be difficult to differentiate from a normal response to outdoor environmental factors. Peripheral vasoconstriction in colder environments may render distal SaO_2 monitors useless. Other equipment such as $EtCO_2$ detectors and prehospital ultrasound, which can indicate poor ventilatory exchange and ventricular collapse respectively, may not be available to assist in the diagnosis of shock.

SHOCK TYPES

Shock is generally divided into four main categories: hypovolemic, cardiogenic, obstructive, and distributive. While the overarching goal of shock management is to support adequate perfusion, specific interventions tailored to each type of shock are important.

◼ HYPOVOLEMIC SHOCK

Hypovolemic shock results from decreased intravascular volume. Decreased preload leads to a compensatory increase in both cardiac output and systemic vascular resistance. Etiologies may include hemorrhage or other fluid losses such as gastrointestinal, insensible losses, burns, and third spacing.

◼ CARDIOGENIC SHOCK

Cardiogenic shock is secondary to a failure of the cardiac pump itself. Systemic vascular resistance increases to compensate for diminished cardiac output. Etiologies include arrhythmias, cardiomyopathies, and mechanical abnormalities such as valve dysfunction. In all of these cases the ability of the heart to maintain adequate cardiac output is overwhelmed, leading to inadequate systemic perfusion.

◼ OBSTRUCTIVE SHOCK

Obstructive shock is sometimes classified as a type of cardiogenic shock as the heart is unable to maintain output due to an extracardiac etiology. This type of shock is secondary to mechanical impedance of forward flow such as saddle pulmonary embolism (PE) or tension pneumothorax.

◼ DISTRIBUTIVE SHOCK

In distributive shock, systemic vascular resistance is compromised. Cardiac output is increased in an effort to compensate for the vasodilatory effects that cause distributive shock. Distributive shock includes septic shock, anaphylaxis, and other systemic inflammatory processes. Neurogenic shock may fall into this broader category.

◼ COMBINED SHOCK

In addition to the broad categories above, a particular process may produce different types of shock simultaneously. Sepsis is an excellent example of this. In addition to the vasodilatory effects of the inflammatory mediators (distributive shock), the septic patient may also have a component of hypovolemic shock secondary to decreased oral intake, insensible losses, and GI losses. Myocardial irritability may also result in cardiac arrhythmias inducing a component of cardiogenic shock.

GENERAL CONSIDERATIONS IN THE MANAGEMENT OF SHOCK

Initial management of the patient in shock follows the typical mantra of critical care patient management. Consideration of the primary survey with the establishment of high flow oxygen administration, cardiac monitoring, and establishment of IV access, typically two large bore IVs, is compulsory in the field as it is in the hospital. Limitations of equipment, space, or personnel may limit interventions to those that have the highest priority, but, in general, all of these are critical initial steps in the general field management of the patient in shock. While the necessity of establishing two large bore IVs has been challenged, it warrants consideration that in the chaotic scene environment one should anticipate that a single IV may become inadvertently dislodged by a combative patient or patient moving mishap.[6] With any advanced procedure the understanding of when not to perform an intervention is often as critical as knowing when to perform one. Any intervention must be weighed against scene time, provider safety, and issues of sterility.

BASIC LIFE SUPPORT

Initial interventions need not be advanced to have a significant beneficial effect on the patient in shock. It is important not to overlook or underestimate the effect of basic life support (BLS) intervention on a critical patient. Simple positioning of a patient in supine or slightly elevating the feet can be beneficial to maintaining perfusion. The importance of BLS care is amplified in an environment where advanced equipment is limited. Aggressive basic hemorrhage control with direct pressure and tourniquets, when needed, can have a profound effect on patient outcome. Other BLS maneuvers, such as proper basic stabilization of a pelvic fracture, are essential. Overlooking basic interventions such as these could prove fatal during transport if not properly implemented.

PARENTERAL FLUID HYDRATION

Normal saline solution is a satisfactory choice for initial resuscitation. Lactated Ringer's has also been suggested in the treatment of trauma-induced shock. Lactated Ringer's fails to show significant benefit over normal saline in the immediate phases of resuscitation and may not be available in the field.[4] Rapid administration of fluid must be tempered with the risks of volume overload which may result in pulmonary edema and hemodilution. In addition, the cooling effect of unwarmed saline administration may compound hypothermia in a patient in shock. According to the Hagen-Poiseuille equation of fluid dynamics flow is inversely proportional to length and exponentially proportional to diameter (**Figure 35-1**). Rapid instillation fluids are best administered via a short, large bore line. Hence, shorter peripheral IVs are preferable to longer central lines for rapid volume administration. The question whether to administer large quantities of fluid rapidly or to delay fluid administration continues to be unanswered. There is no definitive evidence for or against the use of rapid or high-volume administration of fluid in patients with uncontrolled hemorrhage in trauma.[4] Many practitioners will titrate fluid hydration in trauma to various end points such as maintenance of the patient's mental status or an arbitrary systolic blood pressure such as 90 mm Hg or mean arterial pressure of 60 mmHg.

VOLUME EXPANDERS

The determination of colloid versus crystalloid infusion in the treatment of shock has long been discussed. Albumin and hetastarch are two common examples of colloids. Initially, there were theoretical advantages of colloid infusion including less risk of pulmonary edema and faster volume expansion. A number of studies failed to demonstrate that colloids provided any significant benefit over crystalloid.[7] The use of colloid in trauma resuscitation has fallen out of favor due to poor efficacy and higher cost compared to crystalloid.

VASOPRESSORS

The decision regarding when and how to administer vasopressors in the field to a patient in shock depends, in part, on the cause of the shock itself (**Table 35-1**). Patients who are fluid overloaded, for example, may require vasopressors sooner than those who can tolerate volume resuscitation. Pressor choices are often limited in the field and relatively infrequently used. This coupled with cost and other factors such as shelf life or need for temperature control further contribute to limit the choices of pressors in most advanced life support (ALS) ambulances. There may be additional choices, however, in critical care transport units or in EMS physician vehicles. These units may handle a higher proportion of critical calls and cover a wider geographic area. Vasopressors are often recommended to be administered via a central line. This is mainly because of the sclerotic complication should extravasation of the pressor occur in the periphery. In the prehospital environment placement of a central line is often not practical for a number of reasons. Space is limited and, in an uncontrolled environment, it may be difficult to maintain sterility. This is not to mention the potential for injury to the providers from the sharps required to perform this procedure. In the field vasopressors are often started peripherally until after arrival to the hospital, when a central line can safely and more practically be placed. The choice of vasopressor agents used in EMS may vary. In most cases, the choice is often limited to one or perhaps two agents. While no individual agent has been determined to be superior to another, there are some differences among the available agents[8] (**Table 35-2**). In addition, certain agents may be associated in a greater number of adverse events such as increase incidence of arrhythmias with dopamine compared with norepinephrine.[9]

TABLE 35-1	**Common Vasopressors**
Drug	Dose
Dopamine	• Low dose: $<5\,\mu g/kg/min$ • Moderate dose: $5\text{-}10\,\mu g/kg/min$ • High dose: $>10\,\mu g/kg/min$
Dobutamine	$2.0\text{-}20\,\mu g/kg/min$
Epinephrine	• For refractory hypotension • Typical dosing is $1\text{-}4\,\mu g/min$ (1:10,000 solution) • For anaphylaxis, the dose and route change, based on the presence of shock: • *Without evidence of shock*: $0.3\text{-}0.5$ mg ($300\text{-}500\,\mu g$) IM q $5\text{-}10$ min (1:1000) • *With evidence of shock*: 0.1 mg ($100\,\mu g$) IV, which is 1.0 mL of 1:10,000 dilution IV given slowly over $3\text{-}5$ min or infused at $5\text{-}15\,\mu g/min$
Norepinephrine	$0.03\text{-}3.0\,\mu g/kg/min$
Vasopressin	• 0.04 U/min • Not titrated
Phenylephrine	• $0.5\text{-}8\,\mu g/kg/min$ • $100\text{-}180\,\mu g/min$ IV drip
Isoproterenol	$2\text{-}10\,\mu g/min$
Milrinone	$50\,\mu g/kg$ bolus, and then $0.25\text{-}1\,\mu g/kg/min$

Reproduced with permission from Marshall JP, Rollstin A, Chiu W, Chiu WC. Vasopressors and inotropes. In: Farcy DA, Chiu WC, Flaxman A, Marshall JP, eds. *Critical Care Emergency Medicine*. New York, NY: McGraw-Hill; 2012:chap 16.

$$\text{Flow} \propto \frac{\pi r^4}{8L}$$

FIGURE 35-1. Fluid catheter radius and length effect on flow. Adaptation of the Hagen-Poiseuille equation demonstrating the relationship among the catheter radius (r), catheter length (L), and rate of fluid flow.

TABLE 35-2 Physiological Effects of Vassopressors

Drug	MAP	SVR	HR	CO
Dopamine (moderate–high dose)	Increased	Increased	Increased	Increased
Dobutamine	Variable	Decreased		Increased
Epinephrine	Variable	Increased	Increased	Increased
Norepinephrine	Increased	Increased	0 → decreased	Increased
Vasopressin	Increased	Increased		Increased
Phenylephrine	Increased	Increased	0 → decreased[a]	0 → increased
Isoproterenol	Decreased	Decreased	Increased	Variable
Milrinone	Variable	Decreased		Increased

CO, cardiac output; HR, heart rate; MAP, mean arterial blood pressure; SVR, systemic vascular resistance

[a]Phenylephrine can produce reflex bradycardia as a side effect of hypertension. Reproduced with permission from Marshall JP, Rollstin A, Chiu W, Chiu WC. Vasopressors and inotropes. In: Farcy DA, Chiu WC, Flaxman A, Marshall JP. eds. *Critical Care Emergency Medicine*. New York, NY: McGraw-Hill; 2012:chap 16.

BLOOD

Carrying of blood in the field poses a number of challenges. Blood supply is limited and the lack of availability of type and crossmatch necessitates the use of O negative blood. Blood has a limited shelf life and must be kept within a narrow temperature range. This limits blood to some air and ground critical care transport units. In some areas, blood is carried in a designated physician response unit. This potentially allows a larger potential response area than placing the blood on a unit that covers a single jurisdiction.[10]

TRANEXAMIC ACID

Tranexamic acid (TXA), an antifibrinolytic agent, has garnered significant attention as studies have indicated a significant reduction in mortality when used in trauma patients. The use of TXA has been advocated in a wide spectrum of patients with traumatic bleeding, not simply those who are most severely injured.[11] TXA is classified as an antifibrinolytic agent, antihemophilic agent, hemostatic agent, and lysine analog. The exact mechanism of action responsible for the observed decrease in mortality among trauma patients is not known.[12] The recommended infusion of TXA is 1 g over 10 minutes followed by 1 g over 8 hours. It is suggested that TXA be started as soon as practical, making this an attractive adjunct for the prehospital phase of trauma resuscitation. In the CRASH-2 trial, TXA (or placebo) was started within 3 hours of the trauma.[8] As the use of TXA is becoming more widespread it will be interesting to see how the results compare with use on a larger scale.

BICARBONATE

There remain varying opinions regarding the use of bicarbonate for acidotic patients in shock. Studies have failed to show a benefit from bicarbonate administration in morbidity, mortality, or improved cellular function in the acidotic patient.[13] In the field it would be rare to have precise knowledge of a patient's pH. While there is no evidence that bicarbonate has a significant effect on the patient in septic shock, many practitioners will administer bicarbonate for a profoundly low pH. Generally, correction beyond a pH of 7.25 is not recommended, although some prefer lower values. While typically available in the prehospital setting, the use of bicarbonate in the field for this indication is further limited by lack of patient data and utility.

PNEUMATIC ANTISHOCK GARMENT

Recent literature regarding the use of pneumatic (PASG) and nonpneumatic antishock garments has centered on use in areas of the world with limited medical resources, particularly associated with the treatment of postpartum hemorrhage. In the United States, many EMS systems have reduced or eliminated the use of PASGs citing a number of drawbacks and lack of evidence showing definitive benefit for the patient in shock. Some of the issues include the amount of time required to properly deflate the garment once the patient arrives at the trauma center. There has also been discussion regarding increased mortality in patients with penetrating chest trauma with and general questions about the shunting of blood to uncontrolled internal injuries. Furthermore, inflation of the abdominal compartment may compromise ease of breathing. The position statement of the National Association of EMS physicians entitled "Use of the Pneumatic AntiShock Garment (PASG)" has been moved to the "historical" section of the page.

TRANSPORT DECISIONS

The transport of a patient in shock is in part determined by the etiology underlying the shock presentation. Decisions regarding hospital capabilities versus proximity must be considered. Since trauma outcomes revealed that bypassing a local hospital in favor of a trauma center improved outcomes, this concept has since been applied to other etiologies of shock. For example, a patient in cardiogenic shock secondary to ST-segment elevation myocardial infarction (STEMI) may be best served at a facility that can provide emergent percutaneous transluminal coronary angioplasty (PTCA) intervention. States may designate certain centers for particular presenting conditions such as strokes. Other presentations may be more difficult to triage in this way as the extent of the assessment of the patient may be limited in the ambulance. EMS physicians may be able to anticipate the needs of the patient and determine the best facility based on patient presentation and hospital specialty service availability.

TREATMENT OF SPECIFIC CAUSES OF SHOCK

HYPOVOLEMIC SHOCK

The mainstay of the treatment of hypovolemic shock is generally fluid repletion. Administering fluids in this instance is preferred over the use of vasopressors as the former helps correct the underlying problem. While specific end points are somewhat controversial, and will vary depending on the particular scenario such as trauma, objective signs can be used to determine the adequacy of treatment. Perhaps more important than a particular blood pressure number, signs such as mental status and skin color should facilitate in determining whether further fluid therapy is warranted. While not all trauma patients may warrant aggressive fluid resuscitation, those that are in severe shock require some volume repletion. Initial administration of isotonic saline is the typical starting point in prehospital emergency care. If more than 2 or 3 L are required, blood can be considered if it is available. In the absence of blood, TXA may be an alternative in the setting of severe hemorrhage if started in a trauma system that uses it. Colloids are generally not recommended. Surgical intervention is the definitive treatment for major trauma and rapid transport to an appropriate trauma center should not be delayed.

CARDIOGENIC SHOCK

The prehospital treatment of cardiogenic shock is best managed according to the underlying etiology. In some cases, such as STEMI, destination decisions may come into play. Although many hospitals can provide fibrinolytic medication, not all can provide PTCA capability. There is evidence to suggest that patients fare better when transported to a facility that can provide PTCA providing the transport is less than 90 minutes.[14] The EMS physician, either on scene or remotely, can influence destination and mode of transport decisions on a case-by-case basis. For patients in remote locations, air medical transport may be the only practical way to deliver the patient to the best-suited facility or, in some cases, the only advanced care available. While there are no uniform national utilization guidelines for air medical transport at this time, the EMS physician may assist in identifying which patients might be most appropriate for this intervention. Acute decompensated heart failure may also be treated effectively in the field. Medications to reduce preload and diurese, such as nitroglycerin and furosemide, are often carried on advanced life support units. Particular caution must be exercised in patients with aortic stenosis. The availability of prehospital noninvasive positive pressure ventilation (NPPV) has also expanded in many regions. Patients with acute pulmonary edema and dyspnea may benefit significantly from NPPV in the prehospital setting. Patients with hypercarbia appear to fare particularly well with NPPV. Mortality seems to be reduced more significantly in patients with acute decompensated heart failure secondary to acute myocardial ischemia or infarction.[15]

OBSTRUCTIVE SHOCK

Treatment of obstructive shock, such as pulmonary embolism, is somewhat limited in the prehospital setting. Initial treatment is centered on resuscitation and hemodynamic stabilization of the patient in shock. The mainstay of treatment is the prevention of recurrent embolism in the acute setting after the initial event. Anticoagulation is rarely available in the field. Fluids, vasopressors, and respiratory support are the mainstay of field treatment of PE.

DISTRIBUTIVE SHOCK

Anaphylactic reaction is a true medical emergency and prompt intervention in the prehospital setting is paramount to survival. Initial intervention is intramuscular (IM) epinephrine injected into the thigh.[16] Epinephrine administration for anaphylaxis should be instituted prior to second-line treatments such as antihistamines and corticosteroids. There are no absolute contraindications to epinephrine administration in the setting of anaphylaxis.[17] For patients who are refractory to repeated IM administration of epinephrine, some suggest the use of intravenous epinephrine. If this is considered, it must be done with the utmost caution in the prehospital setting, as it is not the ideal setting to administer IV epinephrine. Often the advanced provider is working alone and multitasking. The epinephrine dose must be carefully calculated and, in some cases, mixed. IV pumps are often not available. One recommendation is to draw up 0.1 mg (0.1 mL of the 1:1000 solution) into 10 cc of normal saline. This provides a concentration of 1:100,000 which may be administered over 10 minutes.[18] Ideally, this should be administered by IV pump and titrated to effect. Continuous cardiac monitoring is required and the infusion should be stopped if the patient develops arrhythmia or chest pain. Patients with anaphylaxis may have upper airway involvement as manifested by stridor, lower airway involvement/bronchospasm and/or hypotension. IV fluid bolus may be initiated after initial epinephrine administration if distributive hypotension is present. Allergic bronchospasm may benefit from bronchodilators. EMS physicians may also consider addition of inhaled anticholinergics or magnesium sulfate administration in refractory cases. Magnesium sulfate is often carried on the ambulance. For this indication, magnesium sulfate should be administered 2 g IV over 20 to 30 minutes in adults. Another consideration for physicians is the administration of glucagon for patients on β-blockers therapy in the setting of refractory anaphylactic hypotension. While glucagon supply may be limited in the ambulance, initial dose of 1 mg IV every 5 minutes is a reasonable starting point, although starting doses as high as 5 mg or more have been recommended, and may be considered as the situation and medication supply allows.

SEPTIC SHOCK

The choice for the best sedative agent to use in the field may still spur some controversy.[19] While a single dose of etomidate has been shown to suppress adrenal secretion of cortisol, there has been no evidence linking this with increased mortality.[20] Many still feel as though etomidate is

the best choice given the potential drawbacks of the alternatives. Others prefer ketamine as an alternative to etomidate in such instances.[21] One of the mainstays of the treatment of septic shock is the administration of IV fluid.[22] Some patients require 5 L of IV fluid in the first 6 hours of treatment. Patients will need to be monitored closely for the development of pulmonary edema particularly if there are underlying comorbidities that predispose them to this. Dividing the fluid administration into smaller boluses interspersed with clinical evaluation for pulmonary edema is possible without compromising the overall rapid infusion of needed fluids.

Vasopressors are the next line of intervention although they should be avoided until the patient's fluid deficit has been properly corrected. There are instances in the field, however, when vasopressors must be initiated before the fluid balance is completely corrected, particularly in the cases of profound hypotension or the development of pulmonary edema. While there is no definitive evidence to suggest a particular vasopressor in the setting of sepsis, there are some data to suggest that norepinephrine, if available, should be considered over dopamine. This is primarily because dopamine has been associated with an increased incidence of arrhythmias.[7]

ADVANCED VASCULAR ACCESS

INTRAOSSEOUS VASCULAR ACCESS

The availability of adult intraosseous (IO) access is now widely available in the prehospital setting. For rapid and safe vascular access in the field environment the IO may be the most practical method when intravenous (IV) access is difficult or impossible. Incidence of infection such as osteomyelitis is uncommon following IO access. Complications are generally considered minimal.[23] IO insertion techniques and locations may vary among the available devices. Removal may also be different based on the particular device used. Generally, the IO device should be left in place for no more than 24 hours. Although limited, this provides ample time to secure alternate vascular access in the hospital. Medications given via the IO route have been shown to have rapid systemic absorption.[24] Medications that can be given via the IV route may also be administered IO.

VENOUS CUTDOWN

With the increased availability of IO access in the field, venous cutdown is not often required for rapid access in the out-of-hospital environment. While saphenous vein cutdown may be of use in the pediatric population, IO access may be preferred in critical field situations.

CENTRAL VENOUS ACCESS

Central venous access has traditionally been practiced by some air medical and ground critical care transport agencies. Physicians with experience establishing these lines in the hospital may be inclined to initiate central lines in the field. Again, with the availability of adult IO access, central venous access has become less relied on in critical care scenarios in the field. Concerns regarding complications such as pneumothorax and sepsis may be more of a risk in the field setting. Ultrasound may not be available and difficulty may be encountered attempting to maintain strict sterility. The time it takes to perform the procedure may prolong delivery of the patient to definitive care. In addition, central venous access generally requires multiple sharps such as a scalpel, and needles for suture, lidocaine administration, and initial vascular access, all of which may pose a hazard to the providers in the austere field environment.

UMBILICAL VEIN CUTDOWN

The EMS physician faced with a critical premature or term newborn may consider performing an umbilical vein cutdown if peripheral or IO

TABLE 35-3	Complications of Umbilical Vein Cutdown

Thromboembolic events

Bacteremia/sepsis (particularly heart and liver)

Intracardiac placement or migration

- Arrhythmias
- Cardiac perforation
  - Pericardial effusion
  - Cardiac tamponade

Portal vein placement

- Thrombosis of hepatic vein
- Infusion of hypertonic or vasospastic solution
  - Hepatic necrosis
- Necrotizing enterocolitis
- Perforation of colon

access is unsuccessful or unavailable.[25] This decision is tempered by the complications that may occur (**Table 35-3**).[26] In addition, proper equipment, such as the appropriate catheter, may not be available. Generally a 5-French catheter for term infants and 3.5-French catheter for preterm infants are recommended. Typically, 4 to 5 cm of catheter length is required for emergency access. With any procedure done on a newborn it is important to consider hypothermia and maximize heat retention in the field environment.

SPECIAL ISSUES IN HEMORRHAGE CONTROL

■ TOURNIQUETS

The management of massive trauma in the field has developed from our experience with military and civilian tactical medical support. Not long ago tourniquets were a last resort for hemorrhage to be used only after all other methods of bleeding control failed. Now, in many areas, the use of tourniquets has been moved up on the algorithm as we have learned the importance of aggressive hemorrhage control and the relative safety of limited-time tourniquet application. The overstated concern of the complications of tourniquet use in the field expressed by previous EMS teaching contrasted with the experience in the operating room when tourniquet use occurs routinely for relatively extended periods. In this setting, it is not uncommon for a tourniquet to be on for 1 to 2 hours. The 2-hour upper limit for surgical patients is customary and likely derived from animal studies that show changes at the 2- to 3-hour mark. These changes, however, are typically temporary and there is no evidence to suggest that leaving a tourniquet up for greater than 2 hours should necessarily be contraindicated in the rare instances in which it is necessary.[27] Some EMS protocols recommend loosening the tourniquet periodically for brief intervals if prolonged use is required. On the other hand, if severe bleeding is not adequately controlled by the initial tourniquet, a second tourniquet may be added proximal to the first. Accurate documentation of the time of tourniquet application is recommended, and in prehospital settings, is often written on the patient's forehead or on the commercially available tourniquet on the provide tag (**Figure 35-2**).

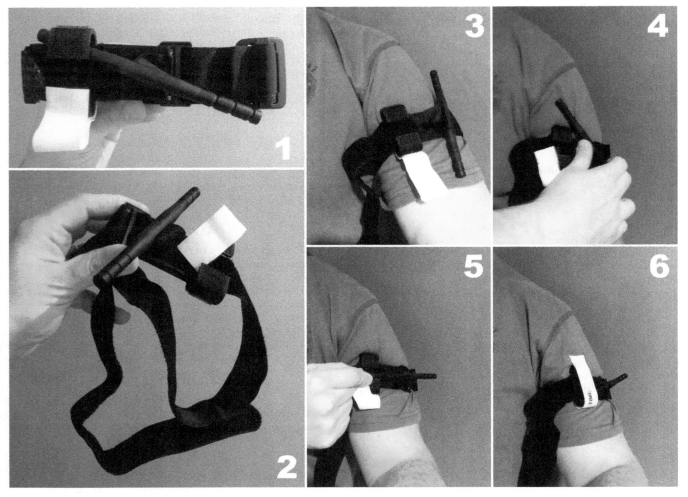

FIGURE 35-2. Combat application tourniquet (CAT).

HEMOSTATIC BANDAGES

The use of hemostatic bandages has been well demonstrated in the combat environment. EMS and combat medicine share many similarities. Operating in critical situations with limited resources in austere environments is reciprocally applicable. The drawbacks of hemostatic bandages have largely been addressed. Exothermic reactions, localized tissue necrosis, and difficulty corralling the loose granulations have been remedied by revised formulations packaged in self-contained bandages. Hemostatic bandages are particularly useful to control severe bleeding in areas where tourniquet use would not be possible such as the head, neck, and trunk. These bandages may also be used as adjunct to tourniquets in severe extremity bleeding and should be considered when assembling EMS physician field equipment (**Figure 35-3**).

PROTOCOL DEVELOPMENT

There has been a general push to standardize the care that EMS provides across systems. When developing protocols it is important to consider the national standards. There are, however, variations that may contribute to differences among protocols of different regions. Transport times, availability of resources (equipment and personnel), overall geography, and availability of other transport modalities, such as air medical services, may influence individual protocols. Considering the capabilities of the receiving hospitals in a system contributes to the optimization of care that is provided to the patient.

Physical space and financial resources are practical limitations that warrant consideration when developing protocols. Anything that is added to the EMS repertoire might be done at the expense of some other intervention, equipment, or procedure that might have a more beneficial impact for a greater number of patients. For example, it may not be practical to equip every ambulance in a particular system with TXA or blood for the few times that it will be used in massive hemorrhagic shock. An alternative may be to equip a special vehicle with expanded capacity to manage low-volume high-acuity patients which is available to augment a larger geographic area such as a supervisor's

vehicle, physician response unit, or air medical service. That would allow limited resources on the general EMS units to be dedicated to more practical and beneficial capabilities. Alternatively, it may not be practical for an EMS physician (or other specialized unit) to carry all of the medications that are available in the system particularly if the model is such that the physician will typically be meeting with an ALS ambulance. There should, however, be sufficient equipment with the physician vehicle to allow at least initial management of any medical emergency should the physician arrive on scene before the ambulance.

Capacity to maintain competency in rarely used procedures is another limited resource to consider when developing protocols. There may be instances in which it would not be practical to train an entire EMS system for certain, rarely used procedures but having an EMS physician available to perform that intervention may be reasonable. An EMS physician may draw on experience and training not available to many EMS providers. In addition, a single physician could potentially cover many smaller jurisdictions.

SUMMARY

The EMS physician has a number of roles in the field management of the patient in shock. Patient care, education, and administrative responsibilities such as protocol development and quality improvement measures are all part of those roles. Shock management in the prehospital environment necessitates an evaluation of the underlying etiology with limited diagnostic resources and effective initiation of a plan based on the inciting process. In the field, the EMS physician has the skills and equipment to perform many interventions. This must be tempered with the wisdom of knowing what must be done on scene, during transport or deferred until arrival at the hospital. Often, basic life support interventions will take precedence and have the most profound effect on the management of the patient in shock. Advanced interventions are secondary and should be employed at the right time, for the right patient, in the right setting. A properly educated, proficient EMS physician who works well as part of the EMS team can have a profound effect on many direct and indirect aspects of the out-of-hospital care of the patient in shock.

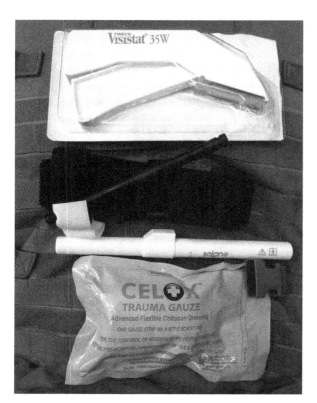

FIGURE 35-3. Some hemorrhage control devices. From top to bottom: wound stapler, CAT, disposable cautery, hemostatic gauze.

KEY POINTS

- There are four categories of shock: cardiogenic, hypovolemic, obstructive, and distributive.
- Normal saline is the preferred crystalloid for volume resuscitation.
- Blood products are preferred for hemorrhagic shock but technical challenges prevent widespread deployment of blood products in many EMS systems.
- Tourniquets, tranexamic acid (TXA), intraosseous (IO) access, and hemostatic dressings are being deployed more frequently in the civilian EMS environment.
- Medical antishock trousers (MAST) or pneumatic antishock garments (PASG) are infrequently utilized for resuscitation of hemorrhagic shock due to lack of proven benefit and presence of potential for harm in some circumstances. The NAEMSP has relegated its previous MAST/PASG position statement to historical interest only, and no longer recommends their use.

REFERENCES

1. Stiell IG, Nesbitt L P, Pickett W, et al. The OPALS Major Trauma Study: Impact of advanced life-support on survival and morbidity. *CMAJ*. 2008;178:1141-1152.
2. Stiell, IG, Wells GA, Spaite, DW, et al. The Ontario Prehospital Advanced Life Support (OPALS) study Part II: Rationale and methodology for trauma and respiratory distress patients. OPALS Study Group. *Ann Emerg Med*. 1999;34:256-262.

3. Stiell IG., Spaite DW, Field B, et al. Advanced life support for out-of-hospital respiratory distress. *N Engl J Med.* 2007;356:2156-2164.

4. Kwan I, Bunn F, Roberts I. Timing and volume of fluid administration for patients with bleeding. *Cochrane Database Syst Rev.* 2003;3:1-16.

5. Reynolds BR, Forsythe RM, Harbrecht BG, et al. Hypothermia in massive transfusion: have we been paying enough attention to it? *J Trauma Acute Care Surg.* 2012;73:486-491.

6. Merlin MA, Kaplan E, Schlogl J. Study of placing a second intravenous line in trauma. *Prehosp Emerg Care.* 2011;15:208-213.

7. Finfer S, Bellomo R, Boyce N, et al. A comparison of albumen and saline for fluid resuscitation in the intensive care unit. *N Engl J Med.* 2004;350:2247-2256.

8. Havel C, Arrich J, Losert H, et al. Vasopressors for hypotensive shock. *Cochrane Database Syst Rev.* 2011;5:1-81.

9. De Backer D, Biston P, Devriendt J, et al. Comparison of dopamine and norepinephrine in the treatment of shock. *N Engl J Med.* 2010;362:779-789.

10. Merlin MA, Grembowicz JJ, Cortacans HP, et al. Docs on demand. *EMS Magazine.* 2008;37:44-45.

11. Roberts I, Perel P, Prieto-Merino D, et al. Effect of tranexamic acid on mortality in patients with traumatic bleeding: prespecified analysis of data from randomized controlled trial. *BMJ.* 2012;345e5839.

12. Shakur H, Roberts I, Bautista R. Effects of tranexamic acid on death, vascular occlusive events, and blood pressure in trauma patients with significant haemorrhage (CRASH-2): a randomized, placebo= controlled trial. *Lancet.* 2010;376:23-32.

13. Kraut JA, Madias NE. Treatment of acute metabolic acidosis: a pathophysiological approach. *Nat Rev Nephrol.* 2012;8:589-601.

14. DeJaegere PP, Serruys PW, Simoons ML. Should all patients with an acute myocardial infarction be referred for direct PTCA? *Heart.* 2004;90:1352-1357.

15. Weng CL, Zhao YT, Liu QH. Meta-analysis: noninvasive ventilation in acute cardiogenic pulmonary edema. *Ann Intern Med.* 2010;152:590-600.

16. Simmons FER, Gu X, Simmons KJ. Epinephrine absorption in adults: intramuscular versus subcutaneous injection. *J Allergy Clinical Immunol.* 2001;108:871-873.

17. Kemp SF, Lockey RF, Simons FE. Epinephrine: the drug of choice for anaphylaxis. A statement of the World Allergy Organization. *Allergy.* 2008;63:1061-1070.

18. Brown SGA, Blackman KE, Stenlake V, et al. Insect sting anaphylaxis; prospective evaluation of treatment with intravenous adrenaline and volume resuscitation. *Emerg Med J.* 2004;21:149-154.

19. Schenarts CL, Burton JH, Riker RR. Adrenocortical dysfunction following etomidate injection in emergency department patients. *Acad Emerg Med.* 2001;8:1-7.

20. Hohl CM, Kelly-Smith CH, Yeung TC, et al. The effect of a bolus dose of etomidate on cortisol levels, mortality, and health service utilization: a systematic review. *Ann Emerg Med.* 2010;56:105-113.

21. Jabre P, Comber X, Lapostolle F, et al. Etomidate versus ketamine for rapid sequence intubation in acutely ill patients: a multicenter randomized controlled trial. *Lancet.* 2009;97:293-300.

22. Rivers E, Nguyen B, Havstad S, et al. Early goal-directed therapy in the treatment of severe sepsis and shock. *N Engl J Med.* 2001;345:1368-1377.

23. Voigt J, Waltzman M, Lottenberg L. Intraosseous vascular access for in-hospital emergency use: a systematic clinical review of the literature and analysis. *Pediatr Emerg Care.* 2012;185-199.

24. Tan BKK, Chong S, Koh ZX, et al. EZ-IO in the ED: an observational, prospective study comparing flow rates with proximal and distal tibia intraosseous access in adults. *Am J Emerg Med.* 2012;30:1602-1606.

25. Abe KK, Blum GT, Yamamoto LG. Intraosseous is faster and easier than umbilical venous catheterization in newborn emergency vascular access models. *Am J Emerg Med.* 2000;18:126-129.

26. Hermansen MC, Hermansen MG. Intravascular catheter complications in the neonatal intensive care unit. *Clin Perinatol.* 2005;32:141-156.

27. Fitzgibbons PG, DiGiovanni C, Hares S, et al. Safe tourniquet use: a review of the evidence. *J Am Acad Orthop Surg.* 2012;20(5):310-319.

CHAPTER 36

Decreased Consciousness and Severe Agitation

Noel Wagner

INTRODUCTION

It is common for an EMS physician to encounter patients experiencing an alteration in their level of consciousness. This can present as a decrease in the level of consciousness in which the patient will exhibit confusion or a more significant alteration to the point of coma. An individual may also present with acute agitation, confusion, and violent and uncontrollable behavior.

Traditionally decreased consciousness and acute agitation are often viewed as separate entities. In reality, both states are divergent points on a continuum. For example, a hypoglycemic patient may be simply confused, comatose, or combative and dangerous. The acutely agitated patient may require restraint and sedation prior to receiving care that may be very similar to that given to a patient with decreased consciousness.

The EMS physician is a tremendous asset in caring for a patient with an altered mental status. He or she brings a breadth and depth of knowledge that will provide a significant differential diagnosis list while having the ability to provide physician level care in the unusual circumstances that require such care.

The purpose of this chapter is to develop an understanding of these altered states, identify causes, and develop treatment plans that can be employed in the field whether a cause is identified or not. This chapter also gives particular attention to the acutely agitated state and the approach and treatment that is required to attempt to prevent a police or EMS provider–related death.

Although an overview of the approach and treatment of the altered state is provided, it must be emphasized that individual conditions may require different or modified treatment depending on the situation.

OBJECTIVES

- Identification of conditions causing altered level of consciousness.
- Discuss treatment priorities and plans.
- Discuss current understanding of excited delirium and treatment.
- Discuss restraint and takedown techniques.
- Overview chemical restraint and sedation.

PROVIDER SAFETY CONCERNS

When attempting treatment of an altered patient, provider safety is paramount. Not only must the EMS physician be aware of direct danger from a combative patient, or an unconscious patient who suddenly regains consciousness, he or she must also maintain vigilance to the surrounding scene. Dangerous factors that may have contributed to the patient's condition may still be present. Refer to Chapter 30 for a full discussion on this topic.

CAUSES

There are many potential causes of altered mental status. The classic mnemonic is AEIOU TIPS (see **Box 36-1**). This provides a concise overview of multiple entities that may lead to altered consciousness. This section will focus on specific conditions that may be identified and corrected in the field setting. This section will also discuss conditions that may

Box 36-1	
Altered Mental Status (AEIOU TIPS)	
A	Alcohol
E	Endocrine, Electrolytes, Encephalopathy
I	Insulin
O	O_2, Opiates
U	Uremia
T	Toxidromes, Trauma, Temperature
I	Infection
P	Psychiatric, Pharmacy
S	Space occupying CNS lesion, Subarachnoid hemorrhage, Stroke, Sepsis, Shock

require presumptive treatment based on suspicion alone in the absence of field diagnostics.

The ABCs are as applicable in the altered mental status patient as any other patient, if not more. Airway and breathing issues may readily account for alterations in mental status. Hypoxia, hypoventilation, hypercapnia, and carbon monoxide poisoning are high on the list of initial concerns. Pulse oximetry is now ubiquitous in the prehospital setting and readily assists in diagnosing hypoxia. Less common, but gaining in popularity, are end-tidal CO_2 detectors which are a tremendous asset in evaluating ventilatory status and impending respiratory failure. A more recent addition to the prehospital environment is the CO monitor. Its presence is still sporadic, but when available it is able to give a confirmation of suspected CO exposure as well as a quantifiable number by which the EMS physician can evaluate the level of poisoning and possibly affect the destination hospital if hyperbaric treatment facilities are available.

If circulation, measured as blood pressure of perfusion status, is altered, then this etiology must be addressed. These scenarios are beyond the scope of this chapter and are fully discussed in other chapters such as Chapter 35 or Chapter 39. Acute blood loss is addressed in the chapters on gastrointestinal emergencies (Chapter 41), blunt and penetrating trauma (Chapter 54), and wounds and hemorrhage (Chapter 57).

Blood glucose problems are rapidly detectable in the field and low levels are easily corrected. IV administration of D50 has long been the mainstay for correcting hypoglycemia in adults that is not amenable to more basic interventions such as oral intake of foods or liquids that are high in sugar content. Recently there has been investigation on the use of alternative IV dextrose solutions.[1] D10 administration in adults showed equal time to regain consciousness without the characteristic posttreatment hyperglycemia that is present with D50 administration. Currently, D50 remains the standard of care in this country, but more dilute solutions are apparently efficacious and may be administered to adults at the discretion of the EMS physician. D10 (<1 year old) and D25 (1-12 years old) are recommended for children.[2] Some EMS systems utilize D12.5 in place of D10[3] for ease of conversion which should hopefully increase safety. If IV access is unobtainable, IM/SQ glucagon may be administered. The dose is 1 mg IM/SQ for patients greater than 20 kg (44 lb). Patients below approximately 20 kg should receive 0.5 mg IM/SQ.

Electrolyte abnormalities are not easily identifiable in the field and usually require a significant level of presumption. Traditionally, a patient undergoing heavy exertion in a hot environment and who has been ingesting only free water would be suspected of hyponatremia, especially if a new onset seizure is observed. This should be expanded to any excessive fluid consumption during strenuous activity, regardless of fluid type.[4] Psychogenic polydipsia could result in hyponatremia in the setting of a psychiatric patient who has unrestricted water consumption. Treatment for uncomplicated hyponatremia would consist of 0.9% NS IV. Three percent NS could be considered if the patient is in extremis, is experiencing repetitive or protracted seizures unresponsive to benzodiazepines, or has lapsed into a comatose state. In such situations where cerebral edema and herniation is suspected, 50 to 100 mL of 3% saline may be bolused[5,6] followed by up to 200 mL over the next 4 to 6 hours. Three percent saline should be stopped once signs of cerebral edema and herniation have ceased.

Hypernatremia and severe dehydration are suspected by a history of decreased fluid intake and by clinical presentation. The treatment of both entities would be 0.9% NS IV. Dehydration to the point of mental status changes would require significant boluses of NS due to significant volume depletion. As long as the patient remains symptomatic from dehydration, there is no upper limit on NS administration, as long as pulmonary edema and other signs of fluid overload are monitored. Acute hypernatremia may also be corrected quickly. However, a slower correction should be employed, in the hospital setting, for sodium levels that are suspected to have been high for a longer time.

Hyperkalemia is most often suspected in a dialysis patient. Altered mental status is not the hallmark of hyperkalemia, but its presence could lead to arrhythmias which could induce an altered mental status prior to progression into cardiac arrest. The ECG may be beneficial in diagnosing peaked T waves or a sine wave, but it may be nondiagnostic if the patient has a sinus tachycardia or PSVT that precludes thorough examination of the morphology. Suspicion of hyperkalemia is enough to warrant treatment with IV calcium chloride with or without sodium bicarbonate.

Alcohol consumption is a common practice in this country and ethanol intoxication is always a high concern in a patient with an altered mental status. No specific antidote exists and support of the airway and respiratory status is warranted. This is the ideal patient to employ not only pulse oximetry, but end-tidal CO_2 monitoring as well to monitor for changes in the respiratory status that may not be appreciated by physical examination alone. This approach would also apply to other sedative medications. Blood glucose abnormalities should not be overlooked in someone who is intoxicated, or just appears intoxicated.

Opiates are a classic cause for altered mental status.[7,8] Pinpoint pupils and decreased consciousness are the hallmarks, although a person occasionally may present in an agitated state. The treatment is naloxone (Narcan) IV, IM, or IN. The usual starting dose is between 0.4 and 2 mg, but there is no upper limit on the amount of naloxone that may be administered and large doses may be required in large overdoses and in certain opiates.[9] Since narcotic overdose does not have a test in either the field or hospital, the EMS physician must have an index of suspicion, or a blanket treatment plan, to utilize Narcan (naloxone). Usage in patient with compromised respiratory status is unquestionable. Usage in patient with a lesser degree of alteration is less clear. The EMS physician must remain cognizant about the potential for mixed drug overdoses. Removal of the opiate effect and its sedative properties may result in unopposed effects of cocaine, methamphetamine, PCP, or something similar. It may also precipitate acute narcotic withdrawal which may create a combative and uncooperative patient. In these situations, the EMS physician is usually best served by weighing the patient's airway and ventilatory status along with the perceived safety of the patient and providers. If any of these are compromised, administration is warranted. If none are compromised, diagnostic trials of naloxone in the field are unwarranted and supportive care is recommended until this patient arrives at the hospital. However, it is important to consider that there is a growing availability of public access naloxone programs, and that the patient may have already received 2 mg of naloxone prior to arrival of EMS providers.[10-13]

On a related note, flumazenil (Romazicon) should not be utilized in the prehospital setting for suspected benzodiazepine overdoses or overdoses of unknown etiology. The safety of its usage in such situations is questionable[14-16] and should be avoided. Fatal, intractable seizures are possible and are a significant concern. Supportive airway and breathing management are safer options.

Other substances such as cocaine, methamphetamines, or PCP may also be encountered and usually present with agitation but may also include hallucinations, aggression, and violence. No specific antidote exists, but benzodiazepines are appropriate and large amounts may be necessary for effect in such patients. If the patient progresses into excited delirium, then more aggressive measures may be indicated and will be discussed later in this chapter.

CNS injury is often suggested by history provided by the patient or bystanders. Sometimes, the mechanism is less clear and requires a high index of suspicion. Stroke, both hemorrhagic and ischemic, may mimic CNS injury. No specific prehospital intervention is available to the EMS physician and supportive care and transport to the most appropriate facility is warranted.

Psychiatric conditions are widespread and more commonly lead to agitation rather than a depressed level of consciousness. An acute psychotic episode is characterized by abrupt disturbance of thought, behavior, and mood.[17] Anxiolysis and mild sedation may be required to provide comfort to the patient, provide safety, and prevent deterioration. When the acute psychotic episode includes agitation and violence, the patient has crossed into excited delirium, which will be discussed in more detail later in this chapter. Other specific psychiatric conditions are discussed in Chapter 51.

Temperature regulation issues and environmental exposure can lead to alterations in consciousness and can be addressed in the field. Thermometers may or may not be available so presumptive treatment may be required. Patient and environmental clues can be used to develop a suspicion of hyper- or hypothermia. Warming or cooling as needed is appropriate and can be accomplished in the prehospital environment and is discussed in Chapter 37.

While temperature abnormalities undeniably need treatment, acidosis treatment is less clear. An acidotic state is not reliably identified in the field setting so the EMS physician must be presumptive to suspect this state. Patients exhibiting hyperventilation may be showing a clinical sign of respiratory compensation, or the increased respiratory rate may be attributed to something entirely unrelated. Behavior such as vigorous fighting and physical exertion or history obtained from bystanders may lead the EMS physician to suspect an acidotic state. Some acidotic conditions such as DKA are usually best treated with ventilatory support, fluids, ensuring adequate volume status and transport. Infection and sepsis also benefit from similar care.

EXCITED DELIRIUM

Excited delirium has recently gained increased attention in the emergency medicine and EMS literature. The National Association of Medical Examiners has accepted excited delirium syndrome as a legitimate diagnosis for some time. Recently, the syndrome (ExDS) has been recognized by the American College of Emergency Physicians.[18] It is of interest that this condition is not universally acknowledged and there is continued debate as to the existence of such a condition. This disagreement occurs in the lay press[19] as well as in some fractions of the medical community. For example, the American Psychiatric Association does not list excited delirium as a diagnosis.[20]

Of those that do agree with its existence, some minor semantics are noted. Some state that excited delirium is the event that a patient experiences and the term excited delirium syndrome only applies when death is the outcome.[17] Others use the term excited delirium syndrome to refer to the premortem state as well as the postmortem diagnosis.[18] Regardless, certain characteristics of the condition are appreciated (see **Box 36-2**). Excited delirium syndrome results in a patient who is out of control, psychotic, untiring, and violent. This patient invariably has law enforcement contact and a resultant struggle. Control techniques such as chemicals (pepper spray or mace), conducted energy devices (CED), or restraint holds may be employed. Occasionally, the patient deteriorates and the result is death.

The exact causative etiology of excited delirium is unknown, but there is a strong prevalence of substance abuse and, to a lesser extent, mental illness. The main substances involved are cocaine, methamphetamine, PCP, and alcohol. Mental illness makes up a smaller proportion of those affected, often with concurrent substance abuse, but occasionally without. Most patients are male and young.

The actual cause of death is uncertain. It is postulated that death is due to severe acidosis, hyperthermia, and undefined cardiac arrhythmias.[18] Di Maio and Di Maio postulate that the cardiac abnormality is torsades de pointes (TdP) due to QT-interval prolongation.[17] They believe that the intense struggle resultants in massive catecholamine release. The struggle also produces significant hyperkalemia. The hyperadrenergic state protects against the effects of hyperkalemia but as the struggle stops the potassium level starts to fall. The patient then experiences a sudden and severe drop in potassium and may be suddenly significantly hypokalemic. This may trigger torsades de pointes and resultant cardiac arrest.

The best treatment for excited delirium is rapid and aggressive intervention.[17,18] Minimizing the amount of struggle through decisive physical control, rapid sedation, and chemical restraint may be lifesaving. Sodium bicarbonate use is tempting when faced with the marked acidosis that is invariably present, but a word of caution is in order. Simply treating the apparent acidosis cannot be supported as there is no specific literature in regard to this plan of action. Many conditions present with acidosis and sodium bicarbonate is not an appropriate treatment. Examples include diabetic ketoacidosis and traditional cardiac arrest. Also, Di Maio and Di Maio's theory of hypokalemic-induced TdP should give pause. The logic of giving medications traditionally used to counter the effects of potassium (sodium bicarbonate and calcium) must be questioned in the absence of any scientific literature to indicate their use.

The worst possible outcome of excited delirium syndrome is cardiac arrest. Since most excited delirium-induced cardiac arrests are asystolic arrests,[21-23] vasopressin should be the first-line therapy.[24,25] Additionally, the patient is already in a hyperadrenergic state and providing additional epinephrine has not proven successful in resuscitating prior ExDS cardiac arrests. Magnesium should be administered early in the arrest since torsades de pointes is strongly suspected as an etiology.

PATIENT EVALUATION/ AIRWAY MONITORING

As for all patients, those with decreased consciousness and severe agitation must be evaluated. The patient who is comatose or altered yet cooperative will not pose much of an evaluation dilemma. Traditional examination techniques and equipment (pulse oximetry, blood glucose monitor, cardiac monitor, stethoscope, etc) can be employed and information can be obtained.

Evaluation of a patient usually starts with an assessment of their mental status. This invariably is the first observation that is obtained since it is often accomplished while approaching the patient. Formal GCS testing is likely to be impractical in the agitated patient. It is not a first-line assessment in the patient with decreased consciousness as other evaluations and treatments must be considered first. The AVPU scale (see **Box 36-3**) has emerged as both a quick and accurate method to assess mental status. It can be assessed in a few seconds and often can occur in synchronization with the ABC assessment. It can be easily monitored and provides an easily interpreted piece of information for the prehospital team as well as the receiving facility.

Monitoring the patient's airway is simplified in a patient with decreased consciousness. Conventional methods of auscultation, pulse oximetry, CO_2 and visual observation are easily employed. Whether the patient is intubated or not, ongoing assessment is relatively simple and straightforward.

The traditional methods of examination and airway monitoring are not practical when the patient will not cooperate or even allow you to be safely in their presence. A much more rudimentary form of assessment must be employed. The EMS physician will have to visualize the respiratory status from afar. Effort and sounds will be appreciated from a distance without the aid if a stethoscope or pulse oximetry. Unfortunately, respiratory rate, effort, and sounds are often confusing information in the presence of acute agitation, physical activity, and fighting. A decrease in physical activity can signal a lessening desire to fight and resist or be an ominous sign of impending collapse. This distinction is not always readily apparent and the worst outcome must be anticipated and preparations made. Positioning may offer some clue to airway and breathing status if the patient is in an unusual position (ie, tripod). The ability to speak only in few word phrases could be due to severe respiratory compromise or a sign of a psychiatric condition or intoxicants. Skin color can potentially be appreciated and a bluish hue to the lips or extremities may be the only supportive piece of information that the EMS physician is afforded.

One of the most important observations for physical examination and airway monitoring is to note the respiratory status and its stability or change over time. While rate and effort may be deceiving due to the agitation, an acute change may signal deterioration and herald impending doom. Significantly increased or decreased rate or effort may signal that there is new airway and ventilation issue, a worsening of a preexisting one, or a worsening of the patients underlying medical condition. This change, if appreciable, should signal the EMS physician that immediate action is needed. Once an agitated patient is calmed or sedated, conventional measures for airway monitoring can be employed.

A complication of caring for such patients is that they may attempt to bite or spit at the care providers. Surgical masks and commercially available spit shields run the risk of becoming wet and impeding air exchange. A nonrebreather mask properly placed and attached to an oxygen source will provide some impedance to airborne saliva. Devices designed for oxygen administration such as nonrebreather masks should *always* be attached to an oxygen source. Any method used must be continually monitored as part of your ongoing airway assessment.

TREATMENT PRIORITIES

After scene safety is assessed and maximized, the ABCs are the next priority. Full details of these procedures are discussed in other chapters. Proper attention to adequate air exchange and control of serious hemorrhage is important. Decreased blood pressure requires treatment for shock (Chapter 35) in the absence of response to the rapidly correctable conditions discussed below.

Cervical spine immobilization has been a cornerstone of prehospital care in this country for decades. Recently debate has evolved regarding the appropriateness of cervical immobilization in certain subsets of patients (see Chapter 55). This debate will likely continue and develop over time. The current recommendation is to guard against a potential unstable cervical spine injury in a patient with decreased consciousness or a comatose state by utilizing a cervical collar and immobilization on a long backboard.[26] The agitated patient presents a different concern. The benefit of a cervical collar and immobilization on a backboard in a patient who is actively fighting and resisting spinal precautions is probably dubious at best. Additionally, agitated patients fighting against restraints may worsen their condition. A patient so combative and uncooperative that physical force is required for immobilization should probably have this modality deferred.

Rapidly correctable conditions should be the next focus. These include hypoxia, hypoglycemia, and narcotic overdose. In the absence of a functioning pulse oximeter, or the inability for a patient to cooperate with its usage, presumptive oxygen should be administered. Hypoglycemia is also easily detected in the prehospital environment and should be treated with IV dextrose or glucagon. A potential narcotic overdose can then be addressed with administration of naloxone (Narcan). Hypotension, fluid depletion, dehydration, and electrolyte abnormalities can then be addressed.

After rapidly correctable conditions are addressed, or if the patient's condition makes addressing these impossible, then focus shifts to restraint and control of an agitated patient. Physical and chemical restraints should be employed if safety is jeopardized and are discussed in more depth later in this chapter.

Core temperature abnormalities can then be addressed. If a thermometer is not available, the EMS physician will have to rely on environmental and historical clues as well as physical examination findings and consider presumptive treatment. Since the patient has an altered mental status it is advised that the physician be aggressive in treating even suspected temperature abnormalities.

At the end of the list of interventions, the EMS physician must decide if an acidotic state is suspected and whether presumptive treatment is in order.

PATIENT SAFETY ISSUES

Patient safety is both extremely important and difficult to ensure for the altered patient. Not only is the patient unable to communicate needs and concerns or cooperate with your care plan, they are often actively resisting attempts to help them and may be acting in a fashion that is dangerous to themselves as well as others.

Positional asphyxia has been a concern. This includes the prone position, hog tying, hobble tying, and pressure applied to a patient's upper torso. Some earlier observers and researchers discussed the dangers and condemned these practices.[27-30] More recent research has cast significant doubt on the theory that positional asphyxia is caused by routine practices utilized by police and other providers.[31-33]

Conducted energy devices, commonly referred to as tasers, have become a popular tool in law enforcement. They utilize electricity to incapacitate an uncooperative person.[34,35] They have been condemned in the lay press[36,37] and their use has resulted in lawsuits.[38] Proponents cite that taser use in itself is not dangerous and has proven innocuous in controlled laboratory trials.[39,40] The concern about arrhythmias seems dubious since it has been noted that time of collapse is remote from the application of the CED making an electricity-induced arrhythmia highly unlikely.[41,42] Additionally, the US Department of Justice recently concluded:

> Law enforcement need not refrain from using CEDs to place uncooperative or combative subjects in custody, provided the devices are used in accordance with accepted national guidelines and appropriate use-of-force policy. The current literature as a whole suggests that deployment of

a CED has a margin of safety as great as or greater than most alternatives. Because the physiologic effects of prolonged or repeated CED exposure are not fully understood, law enforcement officers should refrain, when possible, from continuous activations of greater than 15 seconds, as few studies have reported on longer time frames.[43]

The bottom line is that tasers are present in modern law enforcement and the will have to be factored into the care for the uncooperative patient. The EMS physician will often receive care of a patient who has been tased. This will factor into the plan of immediate care as well as continued care.

Once the patient is cooperative, in control and calm, there does not appear to be a delayed effect of the taser. A literature search by Vilke et al covering 22 years (1988-2010) showed that the routine performance of laboratory studies, electrocardiograms, or ongoing cardiac monitoring in asymptomatic, awake, and alert patients could not be supported.[44] The review does caution that this applies only to asymptomatic patients. Anyone experiencing symptoms, exposure >15 seconds, intoxication, or symptoms of excited delirium may require additional evaluation and treatment as warranted. The patient's condition leading up to the tasing, the events surrounding the tasing, and the patient's complaints and findings after the event are factors in determining the need for evaluation. The act of tasing in itself, viewed independently of any other information, does not mandate hospital evaluation. The EMS physician can provide this information to EMS providers or law enforcement if a question of disposition arises. If EMS or police policy dictates transport, this information may be used to utilize a BLS resource or even law enforcement transport.

Chemical sprays have also received some controversy. The most common of these is oleoresin capsicum, commonly known as pepper spray. As with other control modalities, they have been denounced.[45,46] Various studies have failed to show negative effects.[47,48]

RESTRAINT/TAKEDOWN

A patient who is merely upset or mildly agitated should not be treated with aggressive measures. Calming techniques and mild sedation are probably all that is required. This is all dependent on the patient not being dangerous or in danger. When a patient is severely agitated, uncontrollable, and violent, then restraint becomes necessary. The National Association of EMS Physicians states that patient restraint should be employed when a patient becomes dangerous to themselves or others.[49] This decision should be made with a thought to balancing a patient's dignity and liberty with a concern about their safety and the safety of others.[50]

The levels of restraint start with a progression that provides attempts at verbal calming, a show of force, physical take down and restraint, ending with chemical restraint. This restraint hierarchy does not need to proceed to the highest level if a lower level of restraint is effective in preventing patient and provider injury and provides safety to all. Likewise, just as physical and chemical restraint should be considered last resorts, they should not be shied away from in a patient in extremis and who is an immediate danger to themselves or others. A dire situation may require going to the last steps first if danger to the patient, providers, or others is evident.

Performing physical restraint in the field is a challenging task. A team will need to be assembled, usually in an expeditious fashion. The assembled ad hoc team may include not only the EMS physician, but also EMS, fire, and law enforcement personnel. Regardless of the composition of the restraint team, it is beneficial that all have previous training in patient restraint although this is not always possible. All members should perform a quick huddle to establish goals and roles of all members. Tactics and phrases can be communicated so that everyone understands the desired progression of the takedown and restraint. This can be brief lasting less than a minute or can be more detailed if time allows.

An adequate number of providers are important for a proper takedown. The traditional teaching is there should be a minimum of five providers

Restraint Checklist

Airway

- Difficulty
- Unusual sounds
- Vomitus/other obstructions

Breathing

- Adequate
- Color appropriate

Pressure remove

- Chest
- Neck
- Abdomen

Position

- Make sure patient is in the position that you intended

Appropriate limb restraints

- Monitor circulation

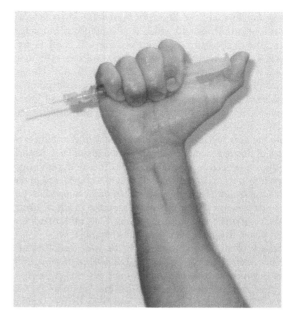

FIGURE 36-1. Suggested technique for medication administration in an acutely agitated and out-of-control patient. Grasping the syringe in this fashion will maximize both control of a sharp object as well as speed of administration.

for the restraint and takedown: one for each limb and one for the head. An additional team member would be ideal to safely apply restraints or administer medication. Two persons should approach from the front and two from the rear. This allows for some indecision on the part of the patient should they decide to attack. If they do attack in any direction, then there are two members of the team that will be behind the patient to restrain him or her. Extremities should be controlled at the joint.

This approach is under optimal circumstances and may need to be modified as the situation demands. A paucity of providers may result in a decision to wait for more persons to arrive or to attempt a modified take down. Also, a large or extremely active patient may require more than the traditional five providers. Each situation will be different and the EMS physician is in an ideal position to help with this decision.

The EMS physician is probably a more valuable resource if he or she is not part of the restraint team. This is contingent on the number of available bodies allowing this. The EMS physician is more beneficial in that they have airway and examination expertise and can serve as the safety person in watching for potential restraint complications (see **Box 36-4**). As the person on scene with the highest level of medical training, this keeps them in the position to continuously observe and monitor the patient and alter the treatment plan as needed. Additionally, the EMS physician is then in the position to administer medications to provide sedation and chemical restraint. If a rapidly acting sedative is selected (ie, ketamine),[51] then the patient may be safely immobilized by the restraint team until sedate and then safely transferred to physical restraints without a struggle. This enhances both patient and provider safety as there is no additional struggle to place the patient in restraints. It also allows for the patient to receive sedation as soon as possible and limits the time of struggle.

The proper position of restraint has had much controversy. As discussed earlier, the theory of positional asphyxia has waxed and waned. There is no unanimous consent on the proper position. One benefit of having EMS involved is that there is usually a stretcher available that can be utilized for patient restraint and treatment. It appears that sitting on the stretcher with the upper torso in an upright position is the most desirable position. This avoids the controversy of the prone and other positions and theoretically provides the least impediment to respiratory effort. Four-point restraints can then be employed. It is commonly suggested that one arm be restrained above the patients head to prevent the patient from either tipping the stretcher or moving and assuming a position other than what was intended.

Leather restraints are preferred to other devices in that they are secure and will offer the most protection to the patient and providers, but they are difficult to remove quickly in the event of clinical deterioration. Soft restraints are the next most desired. They are not as secure and patients have been known to rip through soft restraints in an acutely agitated state. They can be quickly cut in an emergency. Improvised gauze dressings and handcuffs or zip ties are a last resort. Gauze (or similar) restraints can tighten and compromise circulation or loosen and become ineffective. Handcuffs and zip ties are not designed for a patient who does not have the mental status to stop moving while they are inflicting damage to underlying structures. These may be better than no restraint when patient safety is at stake, but other restraint methods should be employed if available. They should be considered temporary restraints (at best) when there use in unavoidable.

Once restrained, monitoring is of the utmost importance. Priorities include airway preservation and guarding against impingement of the chest, abdomen, and neck (**Figure 36-1**).

SEDATIVES/CHEMICAL RESTRAINT

Sedation, or chemical restraint, is the final modality on the restraint hierarchy. A patient who continues to struggle while physically restrained is at risk of injuring themselves. This is particularly true if improvised restraints have been used. Also, the act of physical restraint does nothing to address the patients underlying medical or psychiatric condition. It has been shown that struggling against restraints is a detriment to normal physiology with pH levels as low as 6.25 being experienced.[52] It is unclear if sedation will prevent bad outcomes in cases of acute agitation, but excited delirium has an often fatal endpoint if left untreated. It is strongly encouraged that aggressive treatment be employed when the diagnosis of excited delirium is entertained. Such treatment may still be met with an undesirable outcome, but the lack of treatment is not appropriate as this does not offer any attempt to redirect a fatal cascade while it is in progress. Simply stated, the possibility of a bad outcome in spite of sedation and chemical restraint does not justify failure to utilize it in an attempt to correct metabolic worsening and potential cardiopulmonary collapse.

When sedation is administered, benzodiazepines have a long-standing tradition as first-line agents. They enjoy a considerable safety margin with virtually no medication or drug interactions that would preclude its use in an agitated patient. Additionally, benzodiazepines have a positive effect on the seizure threshold which is advantageous in many agitated conditions. The classic benzodiazepine is diazepam. It offers rapid onset IV. There is a considerable history of its use and safety. Its main drawback is that it is not a reliable intramuscular medication due to erratic absorption.[53] Lorazepam offers the same advantages of valium and provides consistent IM absorption. The major drawback of lorazepam is that it requires refrigerated storage, something not uniformly found in an ambulance or EMS physician vehicles.

Possibly the most versatile benzodiazepine is midazolam. It offers the advantages of diazepam and lorazepam when given IV, is absorbed well IM, and does not need refrigeration. It has the most rapid onset of all benzodiazepines. Its main drawback is that it is considered to have more respiratory depression (at high doses) than other benzodiazepines. The respiratory depression effect of benzodiazepines is felt to likely be due to the rapidity of onset and administration. With midazolam having the most rapid onset, this most likely accounts for this trait.

A drawback of all benzodiazepines is the wide variation in dosages required for effect. There can be a 10-fold difference or more in the effective doses between various patients. Sometimes massive doses may be required to achieve the desired effect. This may be up to 15 to 20 mg of lorazepam, 200 to 500 mg of diazepam, and 30 to 40 mg of midazolam.[54] Additionally, although they do not usually have direct hemodynamic effects, they may contribute to hemodynamic instability in large doses or in combination with previously ingested substances. This is particularly true with alcohol or narcotics. Finally, when administered IM midazolam and lorazepam still have and onset time of 10 minutes or greater. This can seem like an eternity in an acutely agitated patient.

Ketamine, a dissociative anesthetic, has emerged as a potent tool in the sedation of the acutely agitated patient. There is little literature to support its use in the acutely agitated patient,[55] but it does offer many theoretical and practical advantages. It provides rapid and consistent control without the wide variation in dosage seen with benzodiazepines. It is also rapidly effective IM which is a tremendous attribute when faced with an actively struggling and acutely agitated patient. Ketamine has no negative effects on blood pressure. It is also a bronchodilator and respiratory drive is preserved even at the height of its dissociative effect. Seizures are possible but infrequent.

Haloperidol has a long tradition of safe use in the acutely agitated patient. It provides sedation and control while preserving respiratory drive. It has recently come under scrutiny for cardiac side effects and the FDA has issued a warning for the use of haloperidol.[56] This is primarily due to documented cases of QT interval prolongation and torsades de pointes. It is of note that over 70% of deaths attributed to TdP after haloperidol administration were from IV administration which is an off label use and not FDA approved. Higher doses are also noted to have higher risk of QT prolongation and TdP. The FDA advises caution in patients who have other QT-prolonging conditions, including electrolyte imbalance (particularly hypokalemia and hypomagnesaemia), have underlying cardiac abnormalities, hypothyroidism, familial long QT syndrome, or are taking drugs known to prolong the QT interval. It is often impossible to definitively exclude many of these conditions in the prehospital setting especially in a patient who is acutely agitated and uncooperative. Some authors go as far as to say that haloperidol should never be used.[17] Others are strong supporters and note that its historical track record, lack of respiratory effects, and lack of hypotension are strong indications for its continued usage.[57] This author does not recommend the use of haloperidol for control of excited delirium. It makes little sense to use a medication with documented arrhythmia risks in a subset of patients already at risk for cardiac arrhythmias. Even if a bad outcome is unrelated to haloperidol, this fact may not be appreciated. If the EMS physician decides to use haloperidol it should be given IM and in recommended starting dosages (see **Table 36-1**).

The ultimate chemical restraint would be the use of paralytics. Their dose and administration are discussed in Chapter 34. The benefit of paralytics is that they offer definitive and predictable control of an agitated, combative patient when given IV. A potential downside is that they eliminate the respiratory drive in a severely acidotic patient who may be at the limits of respiratory compensation. The window for safe intubation is likely markedly narrowed and the need to support ventilation (not just oxygenation) during the procedure is paramount due to the likelihood of severe acidosis and the tenuous respiratory compensation that is occurring. Additionally, paralytics require IV administration for rapid, uniform onset. While IM administration is pharmacologically possible, the onset curve will be longer. How this affects a combative and uncooperative patient is unknown. There is potential to decrease respiratory function in a graduated fashion while the patient is still uncooperative with oxygenation, ventilation, or even airway monitoring. No information exists to guide the EMS physician as to whether this is problematic beyond the theoretical.

Etomidate deserves mention since the EMS physician may have access to this medication for airway control. It is a medication not traditionally utilized for rapid control of an agitated and potentially violent patient so extensive evaluation of its use in unavailable. It may provide immediate,

TABLE 36-1	Chemical Restraint Medications						
Medication	Class	Dose[a]	Route	Onset	Duration	Advantages	Disadvantages
Versed (midazolam)	Benzodiazepine	5 mg every 5 m	IM, IV, IN	1-2 m IV / 10-15 m IM	2 h IV / 4-6 h IM	IM absorption, most rapid benzodiazepine onset	Respiratory depression at higher doses[b]
Valium (diazepam)	Benzodiazepine	10-20 mg every 5 m	IV[c]	1-5 m	15-60 m	Classic, well-established track record	IV only
Ativan (lorazepam)	Benzodiazepine	2-4 mg every 5 m	IM, IV, IN	5-20 m IV / 20-30 m IM	6-8 h	IM absorption	Slowest benzodiazepine onset, refrigeration required
Ketalar (ketamine)	Dissociative anesthetic	1-2 mg/kg IV / 5 mg/kg IM/IN	IM, IV, IN	30 s IV / 3 m IM	5-10 m IV / 15-25 m IM	Rapid, reliable IM results	Seizure potential (low incidence)
Amidate (etomidate)	Anesthetic agent	0.3-0.6 mg/kg	IV	1 m	3-5 m	Very short acting, lowers ICP	IV only, uncommonly used in severe agitation
Haldol[d] (haloperidol)	Typical antipsychotic	5 mg	IM	20 m	hours	Long history of safe use, preserves respiratory drive	Arrhythmia concerns, lowers seizure threshold, long onset, rare hypotension

[a]Conventionally accepted starting doses. Some situations will require higher starting doses and total requirements may be significantly higher.

[b]Benzodiazepine-induced respiratory depression is possibly due to rapidity of onset. With midazolam having the most rapid onset of all benzodiazepines, this may explain the higher incidence of respiratory depression.

[c]Diazepam may be given IM, but erratic absorption precludes this as a viable and reliable route.

[d]The author of this chapter does not endorse haloperidol if excited delirium is suspected.

short duration sedation of a patient, allowing for proper restraint and treatment. Its main disadvantage is that it only works IV, and this is often problematic in the setting of acute agitation. Due to it being administered IV and its lack of track record in acute agitation, it is probably not preferred to other medications listed in this text, but it should not be eschewed for definitive patient control and protection if other agents are not available. At best, it is a segue medication for rapid control, but must be immediately followed by another medication. It may be useful for immediate control, advanced airway placement and then be followed by massive doses of benzodiazepines (since the airway is controlled) and consideration of paralytic medication.

Sedation and chemical restraint must be individualized based on the patient presentation. A patient who is only mildly to moderately agitated is best served with a benzodiazepine in moderate amounts. When the patient crosses into excited delirium, more aggressive control is indicated and ketamine is the desired medication. Massive doses of benzodiazepines may also be employed. Paralytics are a last resort when the patient is uncontrollable by other medications and their safety is still in peril. The discussed medications are summarized in Table 36-1.

PRACTICAL CONSIDERATIONS

A few practical notes regarding how to administer medications are in order. One question that arises is how to administer medication IM in a combative, struggling patient. Clothing is often in place and obstructs the safest and most convenient site of IM administration: the vastus lateralis muscle (the midanteriolateral thigh). Epinephrine is a medication that is recommended to be given IM through clothing as necessary in life-threatening situations.[58] Insulin has also received support in the literature for administration through clothing.[59] Consequentially, all of the medications in this chapter should be given through clothing if necessary, especially since they are being administered in critical, life-threatening situations.

Additionally, the standard 3- to 5-mL injection limit for IM medication administration should not apply to a patient who is agitated making medication administration dangerous. The purpose of the limit on injections is patient comfort and the prevention of fibrosis due to muscle damage from larger volume injections. Neither of these concerns are valid in a patient who is possibly about to deteriorate into cardiopulmonary arrest. IM medications should be given quickly and without regard to amount. Grasping the barrel of the syringe with the fingers and palm and using the thumb on the plunger (see Figure 36.1) will provide both maximum injection speed and control over the sharp object. Aspiration of the needle is not necessary as almost all medications administered IM can also be given IV (the exception being haloperidol). A needle that is slightly larger than what would be used for a typical injection can be used. Up to a 19-gauge needle can be employed if necessary to administer medication more quickly to help remove a sharp object from the vicinity of a combative patient. The needle length should be at least 1.5 in to ensure reaching the muscle belly. Longer needles may be needed for markedly obese patients.

Intranasal (IN) medication administration has been gaining popularity. Most of its usage has been for seizure control[60,61] or sedation in the hospital setting.[62] How this technique will fare in an acutely agitated, uncooperative patient is unclear. The clear advantage of not having to bring a sharp object near a fighting patient is a significant factor that makes this an attractive route to consider. This advantage may be offset by the EMS physician needing to put his or her hand in the vicinity of the combative patient's mouth. Medications of appropriate concentration will need to be selected that conform to the 2 mL maximum volume (1 mL per naris) of this administration method. Amounts that exceed this could run out and be lost or be swallowed and relegated to PO ingestion and the resultant delay in onset.

Intraosseous access is also an alternative route that may be considered. It is difficult to accomplish in a combative patient, but may prove easier than IV access in some situations. Medication needs as well as personnel resources available will dictate whether the EMS physician should attempt this route of access.

- Hypoxia, hypoglycemia, and narcotic overdose are rapidly correctable causes of altered mentation in the prehospital environment.
- Neither conducted energy devices such as tasers, nor chemical sprays ever been scientifically proven to be causative of patient mortality or severe morbidity.
- Physical and chemical restraints can be accomplished in a humane manner and can prevent injury or death.
- The EMS physician should be knowledgeable about and prepared to treat a broad differential of causes of mental status changes that range from decreased consciousness to severe agitation.
- The EMS physician should be aware of potential complications that can arise from different types of physical restraint and should allow for appropriate chemical restraint to mitigate the risk of these complications.
- Excited delirium is a medical emergency with potential for severe morbidity and mortality. It must be recognized and managed rapidly and appropriately with use of fast-acting sedatives followed by assessment and treatment of potential medical or toxic causes.

REFERENCES

1. Moore C, Woollard M. Dextrose 10% or 50% in the treatment of hypoglycaemia out of hospital? A randomized controlled trial. *Emerg Med J.* 2005;22(7):512-515.
2. Drugs for pediatric emergencies: Committee on Drugs. *Pediatrics.* 1998;101(e13):1-11.
3. Saginaw Valley Medical Control Authority. Pediatric altered mental status protocol. http://saginawvalleyems.org/protocols/approved/Sec_3PediatricTreatmentProtocols.pdf. Accessed August 22, 2011.
4. Almond CSD, Shin AY, Fortescue EB, et al. Hyponatremia among runners in the Boston Marathon. *N Eng J Med.* 2005;352:1550-1556.
5. Vaidya C, Warren H, Freda BJ. Management of hyponatremia: providing treatment and avoiding harm. *Cleve Clin J Med.* 77(10):715-726.
6. Ayus JC, Arieff A, Moritz ML. Editorial. *N Eng J Med.* 2005;353(4):427.
7. Seaman EL, Levy MJ, Lee Jenkins J, Godar CC, Seaman KG. Assessing pediatric and young adult substance use through analysis of prehospital data. *Prehosp Disaster Med.* October 2014;29(5):468-472.
8. Knowlton A, Weir BW, Hazzard F, et al. EMS runs for suspected opioid overdose: implications for surveillance and prevention. *Prehosp Emerg Care.* July-September 2013;17(3):317-329.
9. Drugs.com. Narcan informational sheet. http://www.drugs.com/pro/narcan.html. Accessed August 24, 2011.
10. Davis CS, Southwell JK, Niehaus VR, Walley AY, Dailey MW. Emergency medical services Naloxone access: a national systematic legal review. *Acad Emerg Med.* October 2014;21(10):1173-1177.
11. Goodloe JM. Not so fast on naloxone? There's growing support for non-paramedic use, but keep these cautions in mind. *EMS World.* May 2014;43(5):51-52.
12. Zuckerman M, Weisberg SN, Boyer EW. Pitfalls of intranasal naloxone. *Prehosp Emerg Care.* October-December 2014;18(4):550-554.
13. Weber JM, Tataris KL, Hoffman JD, Aks SE, Mycyk MB. Can nebulized naloxone be used safely and effectively by emergency medical services for suspected opioid overdose? *Prehosp Emerg Care.* April-June 2012;16(2):289-292.
14. Hoffman RS, Goldfrank LR. The poisoned patient with altered consciousness: controversies in the use of a "coma cocktail." *JAMA.* 1994;274:562.
15. Haverkos GP, DiSalvo RP, Imhoff TE. Fatal seizures after flumazenil administration in a patient with mixed overdose. *Ann Pharmacother.* 1994;28(12):1347-1349.
16. Weinbroum AA, Flaishon R, Sorkine P, et al. A risk-benefit assessment of flumazenil in the management of benzodiazepine overdose. *Drug Saf.* 1997;17(3):181-196.

17. Di Maio TG, Di Maio VJM. *Excited Delirium Syndrome: Cause of Death and Prevention.* Boca Raton, FL: Taylor & Francis Group; 2006.

18. White Paper Report on Excited Delirium Syndrome. ACEP Excited Delirium Task Force, September 10, 2009. http://www.fmhac.net/assets/documents/2012/presentations/krelsteinexciteddelirium.pdf. Accessed May 25, 2015.

19. NPR. Excite delirium: diagnosis or cover-up? http://www.npr.org/templates/story/story.php?storyId=7608386. Accessed August 3, 2011.

20. American Psychiatric Association. *Diagnostic and Statistical Manual of Mental Disorders.* 4th ed., text revision. Washington, DC: American Psychiatric Association; 2000.

21. Stratton SJ, Rogers C, Brickett K, et al. Factors associated with sudden death of individuals requiring restraint for excited delirium. *Am J Emerg Med.* 2001;19(3):187-191.

22. O'Halloran RL, Frank JG. Asphyxial death during prone restraint revisited: a report of 21 cases. *Am J Forensic Med Pathol.* 2000;21(1):39-52.

23. Stratton SJ, Rogers C, Green K. Sudden death in individuals in hobble restraints during paramedic transport. *Ann Emerg Med.* 1995;25(5):710-712.

24. McIntyre KM. Vasopressin in asystolic cardiac arrest. *N Eng J Med.* 2004;350(2):179-181.

25. Wenzel V, Krismer AC, Arntz HR, et al. European resuscitation council vasopressor during cardiopulmonary resuscitation study group. A comparison of vasopressin and epinephrine for out-of-hospital cardiopulmonary resuscitation. *N Eng J Med.* 2004;350(2):105-113.

26. EMS spinal precautions and the use of the long backboard. *Prehosp Emerg Care.* 2013 Jul-Sep;17(3):392-393. http://www.naemsp.org/Documents/Position%20Papers/POSITION%20EMS%20Spinal%20Precautions%20and%20the%20Use%20of%20the%20Long%20Backboard.pdf. Accessed May 25, 2015.

27. Reay DT, Howard JD, Fligner CL, Ward RJ. Effects of positional restraint on oxygen saturation and heart rate following exercise. *Am J Forensic Med Pathol.* 1988;9(1):16-18.

28. Roeggla M, Wagner A, Muellner M, et al. Cardiorespiratory consequences to hobble restraint. *Wien Klin Wochenschr.* 1997;109(10):359-361.

29. Pollanen MS, Chiasson DA, Cairns JT, Young JG. Unexpected death related to restraint for excited delirium: a retrospective study of deaths in police custody and in the community. *CMAJ.* 1998;158(12):1603-1607.

30. O'Halloran RL, Lewman LV. Restraint asphyxiation in excited delirium. *Am J Forensic Med Pathol.* 1993;14(4):289-295.

31. Chan TC, Vilke GM, Neuman T, Clausen JL. Restraint position and positional asphyxia. *Ann Emerg Med.* 1997;30(5):578-586.

32. Schmidt P, Snowden T. The effects of positional restraint on heart rate and oxygen saturation. *J Emerg Med.* 1999;17(5):777-782.

33. Ross DL. Factors associated with excited delirium deaths in police custody. *Mod Pathol.* 1998;11:1127-1137.

34. Taser International. www.taser.com. Accessed August 23, 2011.

35. Roberts JR. The medical effects of TASERs. *Emergency Medicine News.* February 2008:11-14.

36. NPR. Tasers implicated in excited delirium deaths. http://www.npr.org/templates/story/story.php?storyId=7622314. Accessed May 25, 2015.

37. The Christian Science Monitor. Three deaths in one weekend puts Taser use by cops in crosshairs. http://www.csmonitor.com/USA/Justice/2011/0808/Three-deaths-in-one-weekend-puts-Taser-use-by-cops-in-crosshairs. Accessed August 10, 2011.

38. The Bay City Times. Judge awards $1 million in Brett Elder wrongful death suit against Bay City, police. http://www.mlive.com/news/bay-city/index.ssf/2011/08/judge_awards_1_million_in_bret.html. Accessed August 22, 2011.

39. Ho JD. Rhetoric vs. reality. *Emergency Medicine News.* February 2008:4-6.

40. Sloane C, Vilke G. 'Death by tasercution' rare. *Emergency Medicine News.* February 2008:4-6.

41. Ideker R, Dosdall D. Can the direct cardiac effects of the electric pulses generated by the TASER X26 cause immediate or delayed sudden cardiac arrest in normal adults? *Am J Forensic Med Pathol.* 2007;28(3):195-201.

42. Vilke G, Sloane C, Bouton K, et al. Physiologic effects of a conducted electrical weapon on human subjects. *Ann Emerg Med.* 2007;50(5):569-575.

43. United States Department of Justice. NIJ Special Report: study of deaths following electromuscular disruption. May 2011. https://www.ncjrs.gov/pdffiles1/nij/233432.pdf. Accessed August 23, 2011.

44. Vilke GM, Bozeman WP, Chan TC. Emergency department evaluation after conducted energy weapon use: review of the literature for the clinician. *J Emerg Med.* 2011;40(5):598-604.

45. Van Derbeken J. Retired scientists cite pepper spray dangers. The San Francisco Gate. http://articles.sfgate.com/1997-11-07/news/17763125_1_pepper-spray-spray-s-active-ingredient-heart-rate. Accessed August 30, 2011.

46. ACLU of Southern California. Pepper spray update, June 1995. http://www.aclu-sc.org/attach/p/Pepper_Spray_New_Questions.pdf. Accessed August 30, 2011.

47. United States Department of Justice. NIJ Special Report: the effectiveness and safety of pepper spray. April 2003. https://www.ncjrs.gov/pdffiles1/nij/195739.pdf. Accessed August 30, 2011.

48. Chan TC, Vilke GM, Clausen J, et al. Impact of oleoresin capsicum spray on respiratory function in human subjects in the sitting and prone maximal restraint positions. US Department of Justice Report. May 18, 2000. Washington, DC. https://www.ncjrs.gov/pdffiles1/nij/grants/182433.pdf. Accessed May 25, 2015.

49. Kupas DF, Wydro GC. National Association of EMS Physicians Position Paper: patient restraint in emergency medical services systems. http://www.naemsp.org/Documents/Position%20Papers/POSITION%20PatientRestraintinEMSSystems.pdf. Accessed May 25, 2015.

50. Brice JH, Pirrallo RG, Racht E, et al. Management of the violent patient. *Prehosp Emerg Care.* 2003;7:48-55.

51. Ho JD, Smith SW, Nystrom PC, et al. Successful management of excited delirium syndrome with prehospital ketamine: two case examples. *Prehosp Emerg Care.* April-June 2013;17(2):274-279.

52. Hick JL, Smith SW, Lynch MT. Metabolic acidosis in restraint-associated cardiac arrest: a case series. *Acad Emerg Med.* 1999;6(3):239-243.

53. IPCS INCHEM. Diazepam. http://www.inchem.org/documents/pims/pharm/pim181.htm. Accessed August 22, 2011.

54. Roberts JR. Rapid tranquilization of violently agitated patients. *Emergency Medicine News.* November 2007:15-18.

55. Hick JL, Ho J. Ketamine chemical restraint to facilitate rescue of a combative "jumper." *Prehosp Emerg Care.* 2005;9:85.

56. United States Food and Drug Administration. Information for healthcare professionals: Haloperidol (marketed as Haldol, Haldol Deaconate and Haldol Lactate). http://www.fda.gov/Drugs/DrugSafety/PostmarketDrugSafetyInformationforPatientsandProviders/DrugSafetyInformationforHeathcareProfessionals/ucm085203.htm. Accessed August 3, 2011.

57. Roberts JR. Rapid tranquilization of violently agitated patients. *Emergency Medicine News.* December 2007:14-16.

58. EpiPen® autoinjector. http://files.epipen.gethifi.com/footer-pdfs/patient-packaging-insert-pdf/Prescribing-Information.pdf. Accessed August 15, 2011.

59. Fleming DR, Jacober SJ, Vandenberg MA, et al. The safety of injecting insulin through clothing. *Diabetes Care.* 1997;20(3):244-247.

60. Holsti M, Dudley N, Schunk J, et al. Intranasal midazolam vs rectal diazepam for the home treatment of seizures in pediatric patients with epilepsy. *Arch Pediatr Adolesc Med.* 2010;164(8):747-753.

61. McMullan J, Sasson C, Pancioli A, et al. Midazolam versus diazepam for the treatment of status epilepticus in children and young adults: a meta-analysis. *Acad Emerg Med.* 2010;17(6):575-582.

62. Klein EJ, Brown JC, Kobayashi A, Osincup D, Seidel K. A randomized clinical trial comparing oral, aerosolized intranasal, and aerosolized buccal midazolam. *Ann Emerg Med.* 2011;58(4):323-329. http://download.journals.elsevierhealth.com/pdfs/journals/0196-0644/PIIS0196064411005026.pdf. Accessed August 26, 2011.

CHAPTER 37

Drowning, Hypothermia, and Hyperthermia

Peter Tilney

INTRODUCTION

Environmental exposures lead to numerous emergency calls throughout the United States and beyond each year and result in potentially devastating conditions. Appropriate prehospital care may make the difference for patients experiencing these serious, and sometimes fatal, exposures. By knowing the risks and recognizing the signs, early detection and proper intervention can be instituted.

OBJECTIVES

1. Define and differentiate between the terms: drowning and near drowning.

2. Describe the signs and symptoms that occur during the drowning process and the prognosis of individuals who have undergone this process.

3. Describe the general management of drowning victims.

4. Comment on the inherent risks associated with water operations (covered in greater detail in Chapter 72).

5. Describe the cardiovascular and neurological findings of severe hypothermia.

6. Detail the initial management of life-threatening hypothermia and list deviations from usual ACLS during cardiac arrest or periarrest scenarios.

7. Describe the cardiovascular and neurological findings of severe hyperthermia.

8. Detail the management of life-threatening hyperthermia.

DROWNING

▓ EPIDEMIOLOGY AND DEFINITIONS

Although substantial efforts have been taken by health care advocates and public health providers to develop appropriate prevention strategies, drowning remains a significant cause of morbidity and mortality in not only the United States, but also worldwide. The global statistics vary widely on the annual number of deaths from submersion injuries, but depending on sources cited, annual death rates range from 150,000 to 500,000 deaths per year.[1,2,3-5] For each death that occurs, there are two to four other related water-related injuries that require hospitalization.[6]

In the United States, drowning is the second leading cause of death in children only surpassed by deaths from motor vehicle accidents.[2] Of those who survive the drowning episode, one-third will suffer from significant morbidity due to irreversible anoxic brain injuries.[7] The populations most at risk for submersion injuries are infants and toddlers aged 1 to 4 years. Children in this age bracket account for approximately 27% of all deaths due to submersion.[1] Of those patients, males are more apt to suffer from drowning injuries when compared to their female counterparts.[7]

Most submersion injuries occur in freshwater, even in states with large areas of coastal access. The sites of drowning also vary with age. In the young infant population (<1 year), 55% of drownings occur in the bathtub.[1] In older children, up to 50% occur in local swimming pools, followed by freshwater bodies of water (lakes, rivers, and streams).[1,2,6,7] It is important to note in older children and adults that greater than 50% of submersion injuries are associated with the concurrent use of alcohol and drugs.[1,6,7]

For many years, the specific definitions of the types of submersion injuries have been blurred. In 2002, the First World Congress on Drowning met in Amsterdam to delineate definitions based on the mechanism of injury and subsequent physiologic sequelae.[2] At the meeting, members defined drowning as the process of experiencing respiratory impairment from submersion or immersion. Patients who have had a mechanical obstruction due to a liquid medium regardless of outcome are said to have been involved in a drowning incident.

Since 2002, the definition of near drowning is slowly being phased out of use by medical professionals due to fact that it is imprecise and has a high level of interpretation by providers. However, it is worth defining due to fact that it is still common verbiage. Near drowning is defined as surviving, at least initially, after being submerged in a liquid medium. Since the decision in 2002 for a standard definition, further delineations have become increasingly irrelevant and for the sake of simplicity have not been included in the text.

As defined by the World Congress on Drowning in 2002[2]:

> Drowning is a process resulting in primary respiratory impairment from submersion/immersion in a liquid medium. Implicit in this definition is that a liquid/air interface is present at the entrance of the victim's airway, preventing the victim from breathing air. The victim may live or die after this process, but whatever the outcome, he or she has been involved in a drowning incident.

▓ PATHOPHYSIOLOGY

The process and subsequent continuum of drowning begins the moment the airway is obstructed by the noted liquid medium. Initially, victims are able to hold their breath briefly. This short period is immediately followed by laryngospasm due to the presence of liquid in the posterior oropharynx. This choking response represents the first anoxic insult that the patient experiences in the drowning process. If uncorrected, the patient will become even more hypoxic and hypercarbic due to the fact that gas exchange is inhibited. Depending on multiple physiologic factors and the mechanism of injury, 90% to 98% of cases, the laryngospasm will resolve resulting both swallowing and aspirating the liquid into the pulmonary tissues.[2]

In earlier literature, providers would describe those patients who had aspirated water, detritus, and vomitus to have suffered a "wet drowning." Those who had limited abnormal findings on examination or autopsy were to have suffered from a "dry drowning" due to persistent laryngospasm. However, given the fact that the amount of water that can be found in drowning victim's pulmonary tissues can vary widely with no definable pattern, the differentiation between dry and wet drownings has also been discarded. The reason for this is due to the fact that most victims have a degree of fluid in the pulmonary tissues if the mechanism of death is associated with a submersion injury. It is important to note, however, that if the victim has no fluid in the lungs or respiratory tissues, the cause of death is not due to drowning. Fluid will not infiltrate the lungs or associated tissues without active respiratory effort.[2,6]

The initial hypoxemia that the victim suffers secondary to the apnea of submersion is then exacerbated by a variety of factors including surfactant washout, pulmonary hypertension, and intrapulmonary shunting. As fluid is aspirated, profound alterations in arterial oxygenation occur. Left uncorrected, alveolar collapse, atelectasis, or mechanical obstruction leads to acute lung injury and acute respiratory distress syndrome (ARDS) or noncardiogenic pulmonary edema.

The debate concerning whether respiratory collapse is exacerbated depending on the fluid in which the patient is submerged, salt versus fresh water, continues. Multiple studies have been completed examining the effects of hyper- and hypotonic fluids on blood volume and electrolyte abnormalities in this population, and it has been found that only a small population of less than 15% of individuals has documented physiologic electrolyte changes from the aspiration of the surrounding liquid medium.[2] The end result, however, is the same. Whether it is due to mechanical obstruction, dilution of surfactant, loss of osmotic gradient, a ventilation and perfusion mismatch occurs, leading to profound hypoxemia.

Dysrhythmias and complete cardiovascular collapse can occur at the time of the initial hypoxic insult or several minutes after the noted laryngospasm has abated. If the victim is rescued prior to a prolonged period of submersion, the hypoxemia, acidosis, and subsequent electrolyte abnormalities will resolve with basic resuscitation. It is uncommon for drowning patients to suffer a primary ventricular fibrillation or ventricular tachycardic arrest giving the mechanism of injury. However, isolated events have been described anecdotally in lab models or in those patients who aspirate large volumes of fluid.

In the first several minutes of a drowning injury, cerebral ischemia occurs due to the cardiovascular compromise that occurs with submersion. The degree of injury to the brain and the remainder of the nervous system are dependent on the duration and severity of the initial hypoxic-ischemic injury. If the patient is extracted from the liquid medium and resuscitated appropriately, secondary ischemic injuries, including cerebral edema, can occur further exacerbating the initial insult. More than 10% of drowning survivors suffer permanent effects.[1,6]

Recovery of victims of drowning events vary widely based on duration of submersion injures, associated trauma, other medical conditions, and surrounding environmental factors. In young healthy patients, periods of submersion between 2 and 5 minutes are moderately well tolerated. However, submersions for greater than 25 minutes for all patients are associated with high morbidity and mortality rates.[6,7] Many drowning patients present with associated hypothermia due to the immersion in the surrounding environment. Hypothermia as a whole can be indicative of prolonged duration in the water and is associated generally with a much poorer prognosis. In some cases, the cold temperature can limit end-organ perfusion and is associated with some anecdotal cases of prolonged submersion with little to no long-term deficits.[6] Given the variability of factors, overall prognosis in victims of drowning incidents is difficult to predict.[7]

In patients who still have physiologic signs of spontaneous circulation at the time of rescue, the prognosis of recovery is variable. In those victims who are awake and oriented at the time of arrival in the emergency department, they typically survive without neurologic deficits if there is no respiratory compromise at the time of evaluation.[1,6,7] Those patients who arrive with altered mental status, but responsive to pain (ie, a GCS of 6 or greater) also typically survive without neurologic sequelae greater than 90% of the time.[6,7] However, those patients who arrived and were noted to be obtunded (with a GCS of 5 or less) tended to have poor outcomes.[2,6,7] Between 10% and 23% of those patients were neurologically affected and of those impaired patients, 39% died soon after their arrival and 17% had irreversible and incapacitating brain injuries.[2]

TREATMENT

Drowning emergencies can occur in a variety of environments. Proper initiation of prehospital care can heavily impact the overall morbidity and mortality in many cases. Bystander interventions, especially in children, are not uncommon. The role of the prehospital provider is to begin the initial resuscitation promptly to restore normal ventilation and circulation as quickly as possible. Concurrently, rescuers must not only begin basic cardiopulmonary resuscitative measures, but must also consider simultaneously the mechanism of injury and provide cervical spine precautions if applicable and prevent further heat loss if the patient is affected by the surrounding environment.

The initiation of the resuscitation will begin the assessment and establishment of an airway if indicated. If the patient is spontaneously breathing and there is no evidence of any traumatic injury, the patient should be placed in the left lateral decubitus position with supplemental oxygen. However, in most cases, the patient will be apneic and require clearing of the airway and subsequent positive pressure ventilation. As discussed previously, most patients will swallow large amounts of water during the drowning process, which can lead to significant gastric distention. Rescuers should be prepared for an abundance of vomiting and plan for immediate treatment to minimize further risk of an additional pneumonitis. In this early portion of the resuscitation, abdominal thrusts and the "Heimlich" maneuver are contraindicated. They have not shown to be

beneficial and can precipitate further vomiting and are associated with additional complications.[1,2,6] If the patient remains hypoxemic or continues to be obtunded, placement of a definitive airway (endotracheal intubation, Combitube, or King Airway) will prevent further aspiration and will continue to facilitate appropriate oxygenation and ventilation.

The resuscitation should continue with appropriate cardiac monitoring. As per advanced cardiac life support (ACLS) protocols, pulses should be routinely assessed, and if are not present, CPR should continue. Bystanders and prehospital providers have a variety of monitoring devices available. Automated external defibrillators are available at a variety of locations and have been used in many resuscitations successfully. Advanced Life Support EMS providers routinely use manual defibrillators and monitoring devices, thus demonstrating further benefits for activating a 9-1-1 response.

Once the patient arrives in an appropriate receiving facility, treatment is focused minimizing further hypoxia. If the patient remains obtunded, and a definitive airway has not been established, rapid sequence intubation is required. Patients who are able to protect their airway can be supported with supplemental oxygen or BiPAP. Positive pressure ventilation can aid in minimizing the respiratory effort of the patient until the respiratory status improves. FiO_2 and PEEP should be titrated appropriately to maintain oxygen saturations of greater than 96%.

Additional sequelae following a drowning episode are common. Pulmonary edema and subsequent ARDS is a routine finding due to variety of factors including surfactant washout. These patients benefit from elevated PEEP or BiPAP levels to increase alveolar recruitment and ventilation. Diuretics have been used with some success, but it is important to assess the patient's fluid status prior to their routine administration. Lastly, the use of antibiotics is indicated when there is concern for immersion in grossly contaminated fluids. Their routine use is not indicated unless signs and symptoms occur. Other complications including traumatic injuries, hypothermia, and underlying comorbidities need to be addressed during each individual resuscitation. Overall outcomes are dependent on the quality and efficiency of the initial resuscitation and subsequent restoration of optimal oxygenation and ventilation.

■ WATER RESCUE OPERATIONS

When a water rescue team is activated for deployment, operations must be conducted in a safe and efficient manner. These specialty-trained teams undergo vigorous training and preparation to not only rescue victims, but also to conduct the deployments in a safe and efficient manner. Members adequately prepare for missions by not only perfecting skills as individual members by taking swiftwater rescue technician (SRT) courses and education on prehospital emergency care, but they will continuously train as a team to establish clear pathways and effective methods of recovery to minimize risk to the team and maximize the beneficial outcome.

During the course of rescue operations, standard operating procedures (SOPs) are typically defined prior to deployment to minimize adverse outcomes and mission failure. These protocols follow similar guidelines utilized in other rescue situations and are based on the Incident Command System (ICS). Once the mission is activated, staff must make rapid decisions during the course of the initial scene evaluation:

1. What is the nature of the call?

2. Is the activation for a rescue of living individual(s) or recovery of deceased victims?

3. What are the hazards?

4. Is there a need for additional resources beyond the scope of the first responders?

Once the initial scene assessment is completed, rescue operations can commence. Despite its simplicity, the standard Talk-Reach-Throw-Row-Go is still the standard in water rescue operations.[8] Most scenarios requiring rescue personnel require the active intervention of providers, but all attempts should be made to minimize risk. There are clear examples when the standard operation procedures of water rescue cannot retrieve the victim without harming either the victim or placing the team at extreme risk. Helicopter utilization may be appropriate for patient extrication in these situations.

Once the patient is in a safe environment, trained personnel must complete rapid assessment for injuries and illnesses. In most cases, these patients are likely to have multiple complaints including traumatic injuries, hypothermia, and potentially, respiratory distress from inhalation of water. They will require aggressive management and transport to the nearest appropriate facility for evaluation and treatment.

HYPOTHERMIA

EPIDEMIOLOGY AND PATHOPHYSIOLOGY

The maintenance of the normal core body temperature is dependent on the body's inherent metabolism as well as the interaction with surrounding environmental conditions promoting heat loss. The human body functions optimally with a core temperature between 36.4°C and 37.5°C. Hypothermia is defined as an unintentional decrease in core temperature to less than 35°C (95°F) with severe hypothermia categorized as a body core temperature less than 28°C (82.4°F). At this temperature, body systems responsible for maintenance of homeostasis begin failing and further insult can occur easily.

Hypothermia occurs primarily due to three factors: decreased heat production, increased heat loss, and impaired thermoregulation. In order to maintain "normothermia," multiple body systems must be operating optimally to ensure homeostasis. To promote cellular respiration and metabolism, sufficient quantities of fuel (ie, food) must be available for consumption. Hypoglycemia can further exacerbate the inability of body temperature maintenance. Heat production can also be limited due to endocrinologic inadequacies including hypothyroidism and hypopituitarism. Other systemic failures can also further impair thermoregulation, including the inability to shiver, extremes of age, and inactivity.

The most common reason, however, for hypothermia is due to heat loss.[9,10] Each year, there are multiple cases of fatalities due to environmental exposure with greater than 50% of these fatalities occurring in elderly patients in urban areas.[9] It is important to identify the causative factors associated with primary hypothermia (accidental hypothermia) in order to treat patients effectively. Heat loss occurs as a result of the patient's interaction with surrounding environment through evaporation (cooling by conversion of fluid to vapor), conduction (transfer of heat by direct contact), convection (transmission of heat by moving particles), and radiation (nonparticulate heat emission). Heat loss can be further exacerbated through vasoactive medications, including illicit drugs, as well as damage to the skin seen in large-scale burns.

When treating patients with cold-related injuries, it is important to identify that there is a spectrum of illness seen with a decrease in body temperature. Mild and moderate hypothermia will be discussed in further detail in later chapters. Severe hypothermia is defined as a core temperature of less than 28°C (or 82.4°F). Patients with severe hypothermia have significant alterations in critical body systems. These patients typically will present obtunded and comatose with noted global loss of cerebral reflexes. EEG activity, if measured, will be minimal or completely silent with temperatures less than 26°C.[9,10] Ocular reflexes will not be present concurrently.

As with all other body systems in hypothermia, the cardiovascular system will be significantly affected. Cardiac output will be decreased significantly and is readily apparent in noted hypotension that may not be correctable with vasoactive medications. As the temperature continues to drop, the myocardium will also have noted sequelae. Bradycardia occurs initially and is followed by myocardial irritability, as evidenced by cardiac dysrhythmias. These include Osborn waves and prolongation of the PR, QRS, and QT intervals.[9-11] (**Figure 37-1**). The 12-lead tracing shows Osborn waves (J waves) in leads II, V5, and V6. With further decreases in temperature less than 28°C, the myocardium is susceptible to ventricular fibrillation and eventually asystole.

As patient's temperature decreases significantly, further organ system failures can occur. Similar to the effects categorized previously, patient's respiratory status deteriorates with additional cooling. Depression of the respiratory centers result in blunting of airway reflexes, bradypnea, and eventually, respiratory arrest occurs if the cooling is not corrected.[9-11] Pulmonary edema can occur with rewarming and reassessment is vital to

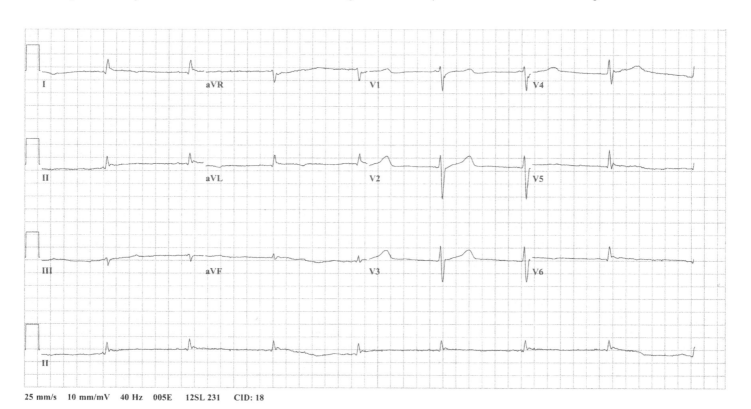

25 mm/s   10 mm/mV   40 Hz   005E   12SL 231   CID: 18

FIGURE 37-1. Noted Osborn or J waves in leads II, V5, and V6 in a 88-year-old male with hypothermia.

TABLE 37-1	Signs and Symptoms of Severe Hypothermia
Organ System	Clinical Manifestations in Severe Hypothermia
Nervous system	Altered mental status, confusion
	Obtundation, coma
	Loss of ocular reflexes, and dilated/fixed pupils
	Decrease in or loss of EEG activity
Cardiovascular system	Bradycardia, Osborn/J waves
	Hypotension, loss of peripheral pulses dysrhythmias
Respiratory system	Bradypnea, apnea
	Pulmonary edema
Renal system	Oliguria, loss of renal perfusion
Hematologic system	Thrombocytopenia, anemia, leucopenia, coagulopathy
Musculoskeletal system	Muscular rigidity, frostbite

maintain appropriate oxygenation and ventilation. Renal failure, hypoglycemia, frozen or poorly perfused extremities, coagulopathy are all additional sequelae seen in severe hypothermia (**Table 37-1**).

▓ TREATMENT

Management of the severely hypothermic patient requires an understanding of human pathophysiology combined with a rapid assessment of the insult that the patient has encountered. Initial actions focus on the removal of environmental stimulus, the prevention of further cooling, and evaluation of other associated conditions. Once placed in a safe environment, attention is then focused on aggressive rewarming. Similar to other types of resuscitations, initial assessment and treatment focuses on basic cardiopulmonary stabilization.

If the patient is obtunded at the time of initial patient contact, consideration must be made to ensure that the etiology of the patient's altered mental status is due to hypothermia. During the initial assessment, blood glucose and evaluation of pupils to assess the possibility of narcotic use may be completed while initiating other critical interventions. The determination of the patient's temperature should also occur early in the resuscitation. Esophageal probe placement or rectal temperatures are the most accurate means of assessing core temperature. Continuous temperature monitoring is required in patients with severe hypothermia during the rewarming process.

Immediate attention should be focused on determining whether patients have a patent airway and are oxygenating appropriately. If the patient is breathing on her or his own and is protecting the airway, warm humidified oxygen can be applied. In most cases of severe hypothermia, the patient will require endotracheal intubation for airway protection and establishment of a definitive airway. It is important to note that neuromuscular blockade used in rapid sequence intubation (ie, rocuronium and succinylcholine) will not work in patients with body temperatures less than 86°F and should be avoided.[9-11] If the jaw is clenched, nasotracheal intubation or other BLS maneuvers may be necessary to maintain the airway.

After the definitive airway is placed, an orogastric tube can be placed to relieve gastric distention. Lastly, a Foley catheter can be placed to monitor urine output during the course of the rewarming process. There are now several companies that manufacture catheters with temperature sensors to aid in monitoring body temperatures during the resuscitation.

Once the initial stabilization has occurred, aggressive active rewarming must then take place. Fluid resuscitation should immediately begin with intravenous fluids heated to 40°C - 42°C. These fluids will not actively rewarm the patient; rather they will prevent further heat loss.[9,10] In many cases, the crystalloid administered will treat associated hypotension. It has been recommended not to use lactated Ringer in these resuscitations due to liver's inability to metabolize lactate effectively when in a hypothermic state.[10]

Although the treatment for severe hypothermia is rewarming, there is little agreement in how to complete this task effectively without additional injury. In patients with severe hypothermia, there is little role for passive rewarming methods. As noted previously, initial treatment methods focus on arresting further hypothermic insult. Therefore, active rewarming methods are required to treat this subset of patients.

Active external rewarming utilizes a variety of methods to treat severe hypothermia.[12] Each method, however, has its controversies and side effects.[13-15] Devices used include hot water immersion, heated blankets, forced air rewarming, and heating pads. Immersion in hot water has been long utilized in patients with mild to moderate hypothermia. However, it is not typically used in severely affected patients due to the fact that appropriate monitoring and resuscitation cannot occur easily. Burns and thermal injuries can occur with the use of heating blankets, pads, and radiant heat sources. Forced air rewarming (ie, Bair Huggers) can be used appropriately, will prevent further heat loss, and provide radiant heat transfer. External rewarming techniques, however, can cause peripheral vasodilation, which can exacerbate noted hypotension. Further complications can occur due to the transport of cold blood to the core, resulting in a core temperature decrease (afterdrop) before results of treatment are seen.

Recent development in technology in the last several decades has focused on active core rewarming. These internal rewarming techniques began with the instillation of fluids into truncal cavities. Heated irrigation has been used in peritoneal dialysis as well as closed thoracic lavage.[10,11,16] Both methods instill large volumes of fluid into noted cavities; however, these require specialized training and knowledge of surgical techniques.

Additionally, there are other methods used in extracorporeal blood rewarming, including hemodialysis, arteriovenous rewarming, venovenous rewarming, and cardiopulmonary bypass. Dialysis has been used successfully in patients who not only require active core rewarming, but also concurrent treatment for severe renal dysfunction and the removal of certain ingested toxins. Cardiopulmonary bypass is the most efficient core rewarming technique and can raise temperatures 1°C to 2°C every 3 to 5 minutes, but is labor intensive and not available at all facilities.[10,11]

As the human body core temperature drops in severe hypothermia, the patient's myocardium becomes more irritable and is prone to significant cardiac dysrhythmias, resulting in compromised cardiac output. As with other critical systems, the primary treatment is to rapidly warm the patient. Most dysrhythmias will resolve spontaneously once the core body temperature is increased toward baseline. Initially, circulatory support by health care providers is dependent on identifying whether a pulse is present. Nonlethal rhythms including bradycardia and atrial fibrillation require basic supportive care and careful handling. At temperatures less than 32°C (86°F), the possibility of converting a patient from a nonlethal rhythm to ventricular fibrillation, ventricular tachycardia, or asystole is increased according to the irritability discussed previously.[10,11] These patients require gentle handling to minimize risks of spontaneous conversion.

Those hypothermic patients without a pulse require aggressive rewarming in addition to extensive resuscitation measures. If the patient is found to be in ventricular fibrillation or ventricular tachycardia, an initial defibrillation is warranted. Typically, attempts will be unsuccessful at temperatures less than 32°C; however, aggressive rewarming should occur with concurrent CPR and airway management.[11] As the temperature is increased 1-2 degree Celcius, additional attempts at defibrillation can occur. Once the body temperature achieves 30°C to 32°C (86°F to 89.6°F), antidysrhythmic and vasoactive medications can be utilized successfully.[10,11] Given that the body's metabolism is altered at low temperatures, the lowest indicated dose is indicated in hypothermia patients. Higher levels of these medications can lead to systemic toxicity.

Antidysrhythmic and vasoactive medications are useful adjuncts in patients with severe hypothermia. However, their efficacy remains largely unknown. Treatment should focus on aggressive rewarming rather than standard advanced cardiac life support protocols.

If the patient continues to remain hypotensive during the resuscitation, warm intravenous fluids are indicated for volume replacement. Vasopressor therapy has minimal effect on persistent hypotension and can result in worsening dysrhythmias.

Patients with severe hypothermia require an efficient and multifaceted approach during resuscitation. Aggressive rewarming must occur simultaneously with other resuscitative techniques. With this combination of therapies, effects seen after a significant drop in core body temperature, specifically a core afterdrop, will be minimized. Even though the effects of the initial insult can be mitigated with initial treatment, numerous other complications can occur after the patient is rewarmed including rhabdomyolysis, electrolyte imbalance, ARDS, and disseminated intravascular coagulation. Continued monitoring and reassessments will be required to ensure a successful outcome.

HYPERTHERMIA

Hyperthermia is the elevation of core body temperature due to an excess of heat production, and inability to decrease heat transfer to the ambient environment. Similar to the continuum of severity of illness seen in hypothermia, heat-related effects occur in a like fashion, based on the degrees above normal body temperature. The key difference, however, is that once the core temperature reaches 105.8°F (41°C), cellular apoptosis occurs and complex proteins begin to break down.[11] If uncorrected, significant physical impairment and noted sequelae can occur. There is a significant morbidity and mortality related to thermal illness with heat stroke, resulting in the death of greater than 12% of adult patients with body temperatures in excess of 41°C.[11] Thus, aggressive treatment to minimize these effects is essential to ensure appropriate outcomes.

There is a significant difference between heat-related illness and basic fevers. Febrile illness is normal physiologic response by the body that results in an elevation of core body temperature by pyrogenic stimuli (ie, infection). This elevation remains under the control of thermoregulatory centers in the hypothalamus and brainstem and rarely exceeds 41°C.[17] In heat-related illness, however, there is no thermoregulation and thus body temperatures increase unchecked, leading to significant physiologic injury. It is also critically important to differentiate between heat-related illness and that of malignant hyperthermia (MH) that occurs secondary to a triggering agent. These include such medications as volatile halogenated anaesthetic agents and depolarizing muscle relaxants. Malignant hyperthermia has also noted sequelae including rigidity, and hypercapnia which is not identified in patients with heat stroke. Lastly, MH can be corrected with the use of dantrolene, whereas heat stroke requires rapid cooling by traditional means.[17]

Heat-related illness occurs primarily in warm climates and is exacerbated by conditions affecting thermoregulatory control. These include mental illness, chronic medical conditions, occupational hazards, and insufficient acclimatization. Rapid increases in body temperature occur when heat production occurs unchecked, and heat dissipation is inhibited. Signs and symptoms occur at various degrees of severity ranging from the mild discomfort related to heat stress to the emergent sequelae of heat stroke. The mild to moderate conditions of heat-related illness are outlined in Chapter 47. The remainder of this section will focus on the identification and treatment of the emergent heat stroke.

Heat stroke is the third leading cause of death behind cardiac disorders and head/ neck trauma in athletes.[11,18] Between 350 and 400 deaths occur annually, of which almost 50% occur due to ambient weather conditions.[18] All humans are at risk for heat-related illness; however, the population of the young, elderly, and those with chronic conditions, which inhibit appropriate thermoregulations, can be particularly affected. Heat stroke is defined as an elevation of core body temperature to greater than or equal to 41°C with accompanying alterations in the central nervous system (CNS), including altered mental status, ataxia, and other neurologic sequelae.

Heat stroke has been further delineated into classic and exertional, based on the mechanism of injury. Classic heat stroke occurs primarily

in compromised patients over the course of several days, usually during environmental conditions which include elevated temperature and humidity. Typically, patients with classic heat stroke present with anhydrosis, but this is not a firm criterion. This population of patients will also present with CNS dysfunction that is manifested by altered mental status, seizures, or coma. In addition, patients can present with signs and symptoms consistent with systemic volume loss from earlier diaphoresis and other insensible losses. Tachycardia, hypotension, and respiratory alkalosis from hyperventilation can be seen in some of these patients.

Exertional heat stroke occurs primarily in poorly acclimatized young patients including athletes and military personnel who participate in strenuous activities and are not adequately prepared for the conditions. These patients present not only with elevated core body temperatures and CNS alteration, but they also demonstrate sequelae resulting from significant hypovolemia. Common manifestations include severe tachycardia, hypotension, and tachypnea. Gastrointestinal signs and symptoms make occur as well including nausea, vomiting, and diarrhea, thus exacerbating the noted dehydrated state even further.

As a result of these sequelae, patients with exertional heat stroke can develop significant lab abnormalities including acute renal failure (increased BUN and creatinine), rhabdomyolysis (elevated CPK), and in extreme cases disseminated intravascular coagulation (DIC). Alterations in electrolytes also occur as a result of the acute volume loss including hypokalemia, hypocalcemia, and hypoglycemia. Lactic acidosis and liver dysfunction can also occur.

When patients present with CNS dysfunction in a warm environment, it is critical that the provider differentiate between heat-related illness and acute hyponatremia. With serum sodium levels less than 130 mmol/L, alterations in sensorium, seizures, and obtundation can occur.[18] Health care providers must assess core temperatures in order to differentiate between the two diagnoses. Exertional hyponatremia can occur in similar environments. However, the hyponatremia is due to an excessive amount of water intake prior to, during, and after physical exercise without attention to simultaneous salt loss. If the sodium is not corrected, persistent seizures, coma, and even death may occur (**Table 37-2**).

Treatment of heat stroke requires prompt assessment of critical systems and prompt cooling. Airway, breathing, and circulation must be addressed immediately. With CNS alteration, airway management must be an initial consideration. Simultaneously, the patient must be removed from further exposure followed by rapid cooling. In cases where there is potential for rapid deterioration of the patient, survival from heat-related illness is significantly increased with cooling that brings core body temperature to within normal limits within 30 to 60 minutes of identification.[18,19]

There are a variety of techniques that can be used to cool patients rapidly. Each has a level of efficacy and can be applied based on the condition of the patient. As noted, the first interventions required are to remove the patient from the heat source, and to remove any clothing that is impeding heat dissipation. In the prehospital environment, air conditioning, and icepacks to critical areas including the groin, axilla and anterior portions of the neck are reasonable locations to initiate cooling.

TABLE 37-2	Signs and Symptoms of Heat Stroke
	Clinical Manifestations of Severe Hyperthermia: Heat Stroke
Organ System	Temperature Greater Than 41°C
Nervous system	Altered mental status: confusion, ataxia, obtundation
	Dizziness, vertigo, syncope
Cardiovascular system	Tachycardia, hypotension, hypovolemic shock
Respiratory system	Tachypnea
Renal system	Prerenal azotemia, electrolyte abnormalities
Hematologic system	Thrombocytopenia, anemia, coagulopathy
Skin	Anhydrosis, hot and flushed skin, diaphoresis

The most effective method of rapid cooling is to immerse patients in cold water baths.[11,17-19] If the patient is critically ill (requiring airway management and other invasive procedures), this may be impractical or impossible depending on the circumstances.

Techniques derived from desert warfare place hyperthermic patients on mesh stretchers and regularly douse them with cold water, while simultaneously operating large fans to drop temperatures through evaporative heat loss.[11,18] Although studies comparing the two above methods have not been completed, the two techniques may be useful for different patient populations.

Once cooling has been initiated and addressed, additional treatment of related complications can occur. Patients with CNS dysfunction including persistent seizures will require benzodiazepines. These will include lorazepam at doses between 2 to 4 mg IV with a maximum of 8 mg IV during a 12-hour period. The patient with volume depletion will require extensive rehydration. Intravenous access may be initially difficult to obtain, given patient's fluid status. However, newer options including intraosseous access may be useful. Vasopressor and inotropic support is rarely indicated given the etiology of the hypovolemia and these medications can cause further harm by releasing catecholamines that may further elevate core body temperature. Rhabdomyolysis can occur with severe cases of heat illness. Adequate fluid resuscitation and alkalinization of the urine can minimize the renal effects of muscle breakdown and subsequent myoglobin release. Cardiopulmonary effects including dysrhythmias typically resolve with normalization of core body temperatures.

Severe heat-related illness with body temperatures of greater than 41°C and concurrent CNS dysfunction is considered a life-threatening emergency.[17-19] Irreversible damage can occur at these temperatures in as little time as 45 minutes.[18] Immediate cooling and supportive care of critical systems are essential in minimizing the sequelae of hyperthermia.

CONCLUSION

When patients suffer from the effects of hyper- and hypothermia, a spectrum of complications can occur. In severe cases, it is imperative that the provider completing these critical resuscitations have a clear understanding of the underlying pathophysiology in order to best treat these populations of patients successfully. With aggressive and well-directed therapy, outcomes can be successful and adverse effects can be minimized.

KEY POINTS

- Patients who have had a mechanical obstruction due to a liquid medium regardless of outcome are said to have been involved in a drowning incident.
- The choking response is the first insult that occurs during the drowning process.
- If patients suffer from a "true" drowning, there will be fluid noted within the lungs.
- There has been no identifiable difference between overall outcomes of patients who suffer from drowning between fresh and saltwater.
- Overall prognosis in drowning incidents can be evaluated at the time of hospital arrival. Those who arrive awake, alert, and in no acute respiratory distress tend to survive without sequelae. However, those who arrive obtunded with a GCS less than 5 have poor survival outcomes.
- Resuscitation should focus on restoring baseline oxygenation and ventilation as quickly as possible to limit any anoxic brain injury.

- Swiftwater rescue requires proper training and preparation to ensure successful retrieval of victims. Basic ICS principles and protocols are typically used in combination with the "talk, reach, throw, row, go" mantra of swiftwater rescue.
- Severe hypothermia is defined as a body core temperature of less than 28°C (82.4°F).
- Hypothermia can occur due to heat loss or lack of heat production.
- In severe hypothermia, all critical systems are affected including nervous, cardiovascular, respiratory, and hematologic.
- Restoration of function is dependent on aggressive active core rewarming. Rewarming techniques include removal from cold environment, radiation heat therapy, warm IV fluids, and if available invasive core rewarming techniques (dialysis or cardiac bypass).
- Defibrillation and the use of ACLS and vasopressor medications are considered ineffective until body core temperatures reach 30°C-32°C. They should be avoided until body temperature reaches this temperature to avoid toxicity.
- In situations where return of spontaneous circulation is a possibility (ie, exclusion of lethal injuries including frozen chest, decapitation) cardiopulmonary resuscitation and rewarming should occur should continue until 30°C-32°C is achieved.
- In patients with severe hypothermic injuries, complications occur routinely and should be expected including rhabdomyolysis, ARDS, DIC, and renal abnormalities.
- Heat stroke is defined as an elevation of core body temperature to greater than or equal to 41°C with accompanying alterations in the central nervous system (CNS), including altered mental status ataxia and other neurologic sequelae.
- Classic heat stroke occurs primarily in compromised patients over the course of several days, usually during environmental conditions which include elevated temperature and humidity leading to elevated core temperatures and altered sensorium.
- Exertional heat stroke presents in patients who have been participating in rigorous physical activity in a hot environment leading to an elevation in body core temperature, CNS dysfunction, and concurrent hypovolemia.
- Severe heat-related illness can affect multiple critical organ systems, leading to CNS dysfunction, hypovolemic shock, electrolyte abnormalities, and renal failure.
- In severe heat stroke, treatment focuses on decreasing core body temperature as rapidly as possible to minimize the effects of the heat-related illness.
- Cooling techniques include cold water immersion, evaporative heat loss (cooling in front of a fan), ice packs to the groin and axilla, cool IV fluids.
- Additional treatment for complications includes benzodiazepines for seizures, airway management, IV hydration, and alkalinization of the urine for rhabdomyolysis.

REFERENCES

1. Salomez F, Vincent JL. Drowning: a review of epidemiology, pathophysiology, treatment and prevention. *Resuscitation*. December 2004;63(3):261-268.
2. Layon AJ, Modell JH. Drowning: update 2009. *Anesthesiology*. June 2009;110(6):1390-1401. PubMed PMID: 19417599.
3. Claesson A, Lindqvist J, Herlitz J. Cardiac arrest due to drowning—changes over time and factors of importance for survival. *Resuscitation*. May 2014;85(5):644-648.

4. Vähätalo R, Lunetta P, Olkkola KT, Suominen PK. Drowning in children: Utstein style reporting and outcome. *Acta Anaesthesiol Scand*. May 2014;58(5):604-610. doi: 10.1111/aas.12298. Epub 2014 March 3.

5. Dyson K, Morgans A, Bray J, Matthews B, Smith K. Drowning related out-of-hospital cardiac arrests: characteristics and outcomes. *Resuscitation*. August 2013;84(8):1114-1118.

6. Burford AE, Ryan LM, Stone BJ, Hirshon JM, Klein BL. Drowning and near-drowning in children and adolescents: a succinct review for emergency physicians and nurses. *Pediatr Emerg Care*. September 2005;21(9):610-616.

7. Zuckerman GB, Conway EE Jr. Drowning and near drowning: a pediatric epidemic. *Pediatr Ann*. June 2000;29(6):360-366.

8. Ray S. *Swiftwater Rescue: A Manual for the Rescue Professional*. Asheville, NC: CFS Press; 1997.

9. Kempainen RR, Brunette DD. The evaluation and management of accidental hypothermia. *Respir Care*. February 2004;49(2):192-205.

10. Hanania NA, Zimmerman JL. Accidental hypothermia. *Crit Care Clin*. April 1999;15(2):235-249.

11. Seto CK, Way D, O'Connor N. Environmental illness in athletes. *Clin Sports Med*. July 2005;24(3):695-718, x.

12. Nordberg P, Ivert T, Dalén M, Forsberg S, Hedman A. Surviving two hours of ventricular fibrillation in accidental hypothermia. *Prehosp Emerg Care*. July-September 2014;18(3):446-449.

13. Sran BJ, McDonald GK, Steinman AM, Gardiner PF, Giesbrecht GG. Comparison of heat donation through the head or torso on mild hypothermia rewarming. *Wilderness Environ Med*. March 2014;25(1):4-13.

14. Hu C, Spotila J. Mobile warming: lessons learned in hypothermia prevention under difficult field conditions. *JEMS*. October 2012; 37(10):46-48.

15. Lundgren JP, Henriksson O, Pretorius T, et al. Field torso-warming modalities: a comparative study using a human model. *Prehosp Emerg Care*. July-September 2009;13(3):371-378.

16. Van der Ploeg GJ, Goslings JC, Walpoth BH, Bierens JJ. Accidental hypothermia: rewarming treatments, complications and outcomes from one university medical centre. *Resuscitation*. November 2010;81(11):1550-1555.

17. Jardine DS. Heat illness and heat stroke. *Pediatr Rev*. July 2007;28(7): 249-258. Erratum in: *Pediatr Rev*. December 2007;28(12):469.

18. Howe AS, Boden BP. Heat-related illness in athletes. *Am J Sports Med*. August 2007;35(8):1384-1395. Epub 2007 Jul 3.

19. Lugo-Amador NM, Rothenhaus T, Moyer P. Heat-related illness. *Emerg Med Clin North Am*. May 2004;22(2):315-327, viii.

CHAPTER 38 Neurological Emergencies

Charles I. Beaudette
Jeremy Joslin

INTRODUCTION

Neurological problems represent a wide range of presentations. The complaint may be as vague as confusion or lethargy or as specific as hemiparesis or aphasia. The underlying pathologies are numerous and encompass primary neurologic disorders as well as sequelae of metabolic, infectious, and toxic causes. Psychiatric disorders are complex and may also masquerade as a neurological issue. In the prehospital setting, it is very challenging and can be very difficult to elicit the etiology of the neurologic presentation. Historical information from the patient if possible, family, and bystanders is important for the early differentiation and treatment of these patients (**Table 38-1**).

Neurological emergencies require transport to hospitals for definitive care. Depending on the region and hospital system in the area, undifferentiated neurologic presentations should ideally be sent to the hospital system with stroke care. Protocols and interfaculty agreements are important for efficient, quality transports. Delays in transport can be deleterious. In events where delays occur, medical control should be involved to assist with timely and appropriate patient care.

ISCHEMIA STROKE

The incidence of stroke in the United States is 178,000 strokes per year.[1] Stroke affects about 3% of adults[2] and is the third leading cause of death in the United States, accounting for 137,000 deaths annually.[3]

TABLE 38-1 Neurological Problems in EMS

Common complaints:

Altered mental status

Confusion

Unresponsiveness

Hemiparesis

Seizure

Dizziness

Underlying pathology:

Cerebrovascular accident and transient ischemic attack

Intracranial hemorrhage

Migraine

Todd paralysis

Seizure

Hypertensive encephalopathy

Pharmacology

Toxins

Metabolic derangements

TABLE 38-2 Stroke Chain of Survival

Detection recognition of stroke signs and symptoms

Dispatch call 9-1-1 and priority EMS dispatch

Delivery prompt transport and prehospital notification to hospital

Door immediate ED triage

Data ED evaluation, prompt laboratory studies, and CT imaging

Decision diagnosis and decision about appropriate therapy

Drug administration of appropriate drugs or other interventions

Approximately 29% to 65% of stroke patients utilize EMS systems,[4] and the EMS system is integral to care for stroke patients. The American Heart Association recognizes the chain of survival for stroke treatment (**Table 38-2**). In cases of alteration in mental status, the diagnosis may be difficult to make in the field. One study showed a correlation with elevated blood pressure in altered mental status patients in the field and an increased risk of stroke.[5]

In December 1995, The NINDS trial[6] was published in the *New England Journal of Medicine*. This study was a randomized, double-blind trial of intravenous recombinant tissue plasminogen activator (t-PA). This study suggested that t-PA was beneficial when given within 3 hours of onset of the ischemic stroke. This study established the commonly accepted protocol for administration of tape, and subsequent trials and analysis indicate the importance of adhering to the NINDS protocol. Significant controversy exists regarding the risks and benefits of systemic thrombolytic therapy for stroke. The International Stroke Trial 3 (IST-3) data seem to show lack of benefit and presence of harm; however, the conclusions support the use of thrombolytics in the appropriate setting.[7] Medical directors and EMS physicians must develop protocols and have CQI that enable this type of high acuity care. Several considerations must be addressed from having the appropriate critical care prehospital team, well-established protocols for patients on t-PA drips, and the plan of care in the event the patient decompensates. The appropriate receiving hospitals need to be identified. Criteria for consideration of t-PA therapy are listed in **Table 38-3**.

Prehospital considerations include accurate accounts of the historical events surrounding the neurologic event, an accurate patient medication list with knowledge of recent administrations and modifications in mediations, last time patient seen normal, recent surgeries, list with knowledge of recent , and whether there was presence of a seizure. An important differentiation between "last time seen normal" and onset of the symptoms must not be confused. Patients who suffer an ischemic stroke are often confused or aphasic. This type of information needs to be obtained from prehospital witnesses and family members. A detailed history of the patient's medications should be elicited with emphasis on antiplatelet and anticoagulant medications. Hypoglycemic medications and narcotic history should be obtained as patients with extremes of glucose and narcotic overdose may present with an initial neurologic complaint. In the event the patient is unable to communicate, witnesses or family members should either accompany the patient to the hospital or EMS must obtain names and phone numbers so the receiving physicians can contact them to clarify information. In consideration for t-PA there are several historical components, which will include or exclude the patient from t-PA. Hemorrhagic conversion of an ischemic stroke is

TABLE 38-3 Inclusion/Exclusion Criteria for tPA

Inclusion Criteria

- Onset of symptoms <3 hours before beginning treatment (Onset time is defined as either the witnessed onset of symptoms or the time last known normal if symptom onset was not witnessed.)
- Diagnosis of ischemic stroke causing measurable neurological deficit
- Aged ≥18 years
- Potential risks and benefits of IV tPA treatment discussed with the patient and/or family members and they have verbalized understanding (to be documented in the patient's record). If the patient unable to give verbal consent and no family available, IV tPA can be given under Emergency Doctrine. Written informed consent not required for IV tPA when given within 3 hours of symptom onset

Exclusion Criteria

- Significant head trauma or prior stroke in previous 3 months
- Symptoms suggest subarachnoid hemorrhage
- History of previous intracranial hemorrhage
- Intracranial neoplasm, arteriovenous malformation, or aneurysm
- Recent intracranial or intraspinal surgery
- Arterial puncture at noncompressible site in previous 7 days
- Elevated blood pressure (systolic >185 mm Hg or diastolic >110 mm Hg)
- Active internal bleeding
- Blood glucose concentration <50mg/dL (2.7mmol/L)
- Acute bleeding diathesis, including but not limited to: platelet count <100 000/mm³
- (In patients without history of thrombocytopenia, treatment with
- IV rtPA can be initiated before availability of platelet count but should be discontinued if platelet count is <100,000/mm³.)
- Heparin received within 48 hours, resulting in abnormally elevated aPTT greater than the upper limit of normal
- Current use of anticoagulant with INR >1.7 or PT >15 seconds (In patients without recent use of oral anticoagulants or heparin, treatment with IV rtPA can be initiated before availability of coagulation test results but should be discontinued if INR is >1.7 or PT is abnormally elevated by local laboratory standards.)
- Current use of direct thrombin inhibitors or direct factor Xa inhibitors with elevated sensitive laboratory tests (such as aPTT, INR, platelet count, and ECT; TT; or appropriate factor Xa activity assays)
- CT demonstrates multilobar infarction (hypodensity >1/3 cerebral hemisphere)

Relative Exclusion Criteria

Recent experience suggests that under some circumstances—with careful consideration and weighting of risk to benefit—patients may receive fibrinolytic therapy despite one or more relative contraindications. Consider risk to benefit of IV rtPA administration carefully if any of these relative contraindications are present:

- Only minor or rapidly improving stroke symptoms (clearing spontaneously)
- Seizure at onset with postictal residual neurological impairments
- Major surgery or serious trauma within previous 14 days
- Recent gastrointestinal or urinary tract hemorrhage (within previous 21 days)
- Pregnancy

To extend IV tPA to 4.5 hours from symptom onset/last known normal, the following additional criteria *must* be met:

- The patient is <80 years of age
- The patient does not have a history of both diabetes *and* stroke
- The patient is not taking warfarin (Coumadin) or any other anticoagulant regardless of INR/coagulation results
- NIHSS is <25
- Written informed consent obtained from the patient and/or family—required when IV tPA given within the 3- to 4.5-hour window

of significant concern when considering t-PA.[8] There is a very specific exclusion criterion for t-PA. Refer to Table 38-3.

Selection of receiving hospital: Several diagnostic studies are required for determination of patient's candidacy for thrombolytics. The patient requires a multitude of laboratory studies including platelet counts and coagulation studies. A CT scan must be performed. While most emergency departments have CT capabilities, there are considerations within local systems which should be addressed, such as the need to call in a CT technician from home, prompt access to radiologist interpretation. Occasionally a CT scanner must be taken out of service for hours or days for maintenance. When this occurs, the EMS system much adjust accordingly. These delays should be conveyed to the transport team and the decision should then be made to send the patient to the most appropriate facility, which may necessitate diversion from the initially intended hospital. Receiving facilities should have a system in place for handling possible CVAs (AHA stroke guidelines 2013).[9]

■ TRANSPORT CONSIDERATIONS

Supportive measures include supplemental oxygen in hypoxic patients, electrocardiographic monitoring, head of bed to 30% to prevent aspiration, and continuous monitoring for neurologic changes. A 12-lead ECG is recommended as part of the initial workup for ischemic CVA (Stroke guidelines 2007) and performance of this test en route to the hospital may be reasonable, though it should not result in delay of other treatments or transport. During disaster and limited resources, EMS physicians should assist with triage decisions regarding transportation and diagnostic studies. Patients who could receive t-PA may warrant transportation prior to those with less severe complaints. Conversely, utilization of resources should be in the context of facilitating treatment or actionable diagnostic studies. Patients known to be excluded from thrombolytic therapy may be given lower triage assignment.

Helicopter transport of stroke patients is utilized to expeditiously transport patients in appropriate settings.[10] One study suggests it is a cost-effective method of delivering stroke care.[11] Regardless of transport mode, prehospital stroke center activation is currently of significant area of focus.[12] Electrocardiogram should be performed on all patients with suspected ischemic stroke (AHA 2007). Many ambulances can provide this capability and may obviate the need for electrocardiogram and the associated delay at the hospital.

Medical directors must consider educating their providers on the recognition of stroke and stroke mimics. In addition to choosing a prehospital stroke evaluation strategy, it may be appropriate to educate providers on conditions such as Todd paralysis, Bell palsy, other unilateral facial nerve palsies, dystonic reactions with dysarthria, anticholinergic toxidrome, and demyelinating diseases.

Studies focusing on prehospital delivery of thrombolytics may show future benefits. One study of simulated stroke patients revealed the feasibility of utilizing prehospital telemedicine to evaluate stroke patients.[13] A German study showed a reduction in time to thrombolytics by using prehospital thrombolytics in a specialized ambulance equipped with a CT scanner.[14]

INTRACRANIAL HEMORRHAGE

The inciting event in intracranial hemorrhage may be trauma, berry aneurysm rupture, hypertension, or malignancy. In the prehospital setting, the type of bleed will likely not be known. During interfacility transport the type of bleed may have already been determined. In all ICH, neurologic deficit can occur with mass effect placing pressure on specific structures (cranial nerves, tonsils). Other signs are produced by globally increasing intracranial pressure, which results in decreased perfusion to the brain. For the stated reasons, continuous neurologic monitoring is essential.

Cerebral perfusion pressure is the common pathway for delivery of oxygen to and removal of waste from the brain. Cerebral perfusion pressure equals the difference of mean arterial pressure minus intracranial pressure. Thus management of blood pressure is critical to the patient with ICH. However, exact targets for reduction are based on expert opinion. In patients with SBP >200 mm Hg, aggressive BP reduction to 140 mm Hg is reasonable.[15]

Transport considerations for patients with ICH include airway protection, anticipation of deterioration en route, maintaining normal partial pressure of CO_2, and managing cerebral perfusion pressure. Early intubation should be considered in obtunded or moribund patients. It is reasonable and acceptable to intubate an otherwise intact and stable airway for transport, to ensure intubation en route is avoided. The most experienced provider under the most preferable circumstances should perform the procedure in an ideal situation. Intubation provides protection of airway from aspiration or collapse of surrounding structures, ensures passage of oxygen to the blood, and when combined with end tidal capnography provides control of CO_2 tension. Intubation requires sedation and there is risk of pharmacologic blood pressure derangement and transient hypoxia, both of which can be deleterious to patients with hemorrhagic stroke. Appropriate transport crews are necessary in these types of situations.

SEIZURE

Consider seizure as a contributing factor to other findings and complaints. Seizure may explain a syncopal episode, and a postictal state may explain one's altered mental status and confusion. Nonconvulsive status epilepticus may present as coma or prolonged confusion. Toxic and metabolic derangements can present as seizure. Consideration of hypoglycemia and hypoxia in the seizure patient is important to a full and comprehensive approach to one's patient

Description of the seizure and events surrounding the seizure can help determine the type of seizure and in some cases differentiate from nonepileptiform seizures. Seizures are classified as generalize or partial, with generalized seizures involving both hemispheres of the brain, and partial involving a focal portion of the brain. Generalized seizures require loss of cognition since the entire cortex is involved, and the postictal period may be brief or prolonged. During partial seizures cognition is preserved, and presentation may be motor or sensory derangements, and occasionally psychological changes occur. Partial seizures with secondary generalization begin at a specific cortical focus and spread to involve both hemispheres with accompanying loss of cognition.

Status epilepticus is a life-threatening seizure disorder, consisting of continuous seizure greater than 15 minutes, or two or more seizures without return to normal level of consciousness between them. Mortality is between 3% and 22%. While the time duration of status epilepticus is inconsistent across definitions, continuous seizures that last >5 minutes are atypically long in duration and warrant aggressive management with benzodiazepines. In addition to rectal diazepam and IM and IV midazolam, it may be appropriate to consider potential use of buccal or intranasal versed.[16-19] Holsti et al showed particular success with intranasal midazolam in the prehospital setting as compared to rectal diazepam.

KEY POINTS

- Hypoglycemia has a wide range of manifestations. Always check glucose on patients with neurologic findings, particularly in stroke, seizure, and altered level of consciousness.
- In ischemic stroke, time is brain and suspected strokes should be rapidly transported to appropriate facilities. The 3-hour window is an outer time limit, not an acceptable goal for treatment.
- Ischemic stroke treatment with thrombolytics requires specific historical information, including the last time seen normal. If this is not reliably obtained from the patient or witnesses, the patient will not be a candidate for thrombolytics.
- Maintaining normal blood pressure and oxygenation, as well as CO_2 tension, without extreme deviation from physiologic ranges, is important for both ischemic and hemorrhagic strokes.
- Recognize and aggressively manage status epilepticus.

REFERENCES

1. Rosamond W, Flegal K, Furie K, et al. American Heart Association Statistics Committee and Stroke Statistics Subcommittee. Heart disease and stroke statistics—2008 update: a report from the American Heart Association Statistics Committee and Stroke Statistics Subcommittee. *Circulation.* 2008;117(4): e25-146.
2. Pleis JR, Ward BW, Lucas JW. Summary health statistics for U.S. adults: National Health Interview Survey, 2009. *Vital Health Stat 10.* 2010;249:1-207.
3. Heron M, Hoyert DL, Murphy SL, Xu J, Kochanek KD, Tejada-Vera B. Deaths: final data for 2006. *Natl Vital Stat Rep.* 2009;57 (14):1-134.
4. Adams HP, del Zoppo G, Alberts MJ, et al. Guidelines for the early management for adults with ischemic stroke. *Circulation.* 2007;115:e478-e534.
5. Irisawa T, Iwami T, Kitamura T, et al. An association between systolic blood pressure and stroke among patients with impaired consciousness in out-of-hospital emergency settings. *BMC Emerg Med.* December 17, 2013;13:24.
6. Tissue plasminogen activator for acute ischemic stroke. The National Institute of Neurological Disorders and Stroke rt-PA Stroke Study Group. *N Engl J Med.* 1995;333(24):1581-1587.
7. Whiteley WN, Thompson D, Murray G, et al. Effect of alteplase within 6 hours of acute ischemic stroke on all-cause mortality (third International Stroke Trial). *Stroke.* 2014;45(12): 3612-3617.
8. Wang W, Li M, Chen Q, Wang J. Hemorrhagic Transformation after Tissue Plasminogen Activator Reperfusion Therapy for Ischemic Stroke: Mechanisms, Models, and Biomarkers. *Mol Neurobiol.* 2014.
9. Jauch EC, Saver JL, Adams HP Jr, et al. Guidelines for the early management of patients with acute ischemic stroke: a guideline for healthcare professionals from the American Heart Association/American Stroke Association. *Stroke.* 2013; Mar;44(3): 870-947.
10. Silliman SL, Quinn B, Huggett V, Merino JG. Use of a field-to-stroke center helicopter transport program to extend thrombolytic therapy to rural residents. *Stroke.* 2003; Mar;34(3):729-733.
11. Silbergleit R, Scott PA, Lowell MJ, Silbergleit R. Cost-effectiveness of helicopter transport of stroke patients for thrombolysis. *Acad Emerg Med.* 2003; Sep;10(9):966-972.
12. Sozener CB, Barsan WG. Impact of regional pre-hospital emergency medical services in treatment of patients with acute ischemic stroke. *Ann N Y Acad Sci.* September 2012;1268:51-56.
13. Wu TC, Nguyen C, Ankrom C, et al. Prehospital utility of rapid stroke evaluation using in-ambulance telemedicine: a pilot feasibility study. *Stroke.* August 2014;45(8):2342-2347.
14. Ebinger M, Winter B, Wendt M, et al. Effect of the use of ambulance-based thrombolysis on time to thrombolysis in acute ischemic stroke: a randomized clinical trial. *JAMA.* April 23-30, 2014;311(16): 1622-1631.
15. Morgenstern LB, Hemphill JC 3rd, Anderson C, et al. American Heart Association Stroke Council and Council on Cardiovascular Nursing. Guidelines for the management of spontaneous intracerebral hemorrhage: a guideline for healthcare professionals from the American Heart Association/American Stroke Association. *Stroke.* 2010;41(9):2108-2129.
16. Scott RC, Besag FM, Neville BG. Buccal midazolam and rectal diazepam for treatment of prolonged seizures in childhood and adolescence: a randomised trial. *Lancet.* 1999;353(9153):623-626.
17. Camfield PR. Buccal midazolam and rectal diazepam for treatment of prolonged seizures in childhood and adolescence: a randomised trial. *J Pediatr.* 1999;135(3):398-399.
18. Fişgin T, Gurer Y, Teziç T, et al. Effects of intranasal midazolam and rectal diazepam on acute convulsions in children: prospective randomized study. *J Child Neurol.* 2002;17(2):123-126.
19. Holsti M, Sill BL, Firth SD, Filloux FM, Joyce SM, Furnival RA. Prehospital intranasal midazolam for the treatment of pediatric seizures. *Pediatr Emerg Care.* 2007; Mar;23(3):148-153.

CHAPTER 39

Cardiovascular Emergencies

Stacy N. Weisberg

Joseph Tennyson

Marie King

Erryn Leinbaugh

INTRODUCTION

Heart disease has been the leading cause of death in America for over 80 years. An estimated 935,000 people in America suffer a myocardial infarction each year at an estimated annual cost of $151.6 billion.[1,2] Although the development of EMS is often ascribed as a response to America's shocking rates of morbidity and mortality from motor vehicle accidents, emergency cardiac care has also driven EMS development and in many ways has become the central mission of modern EMS. From some of the first work on prehospital cardiac care as published by Frank Pantridge et al in 1967[3] to large multisystem studies of cardiac arrest survival published in the past few years, it is clear that much progress has been made. Yet the basic tenets of prehospital cardiac care remain simple: identification of the patient with a cardiac emergency; stabilization; selection of an appropriate receiving facility; safe and timely transport to that facility.

OBJECTIVES

- Understand the goals of prehospital treatment for patients with acute coronary syndrome.
- Discuss destinations, including options for treatment as well as transfer.
- Learn about treatment options for patients diagnosed with arrhythmias.
- Consider high-risk patients and special cardiac situations and equipment.
- Discuss other etiologies of chest pain and approaches for these patients.

ACUTE CORONARY SYNDROME (ACS)

■ GENERAL APPROACH TO CHEST PAIN

The prehospital approach to the ACS patient begins with identification of potential patients. Emergency medical dispatch (EMD) has been designed to assist with this, but these programs tend to overtriage and, as they rely on data from the lay public, can also fail to identify ACS patients.[4] For this reason, any dispatched chief complaint suggestive of ACS should be considered as such until it can be properly verified.

Upon arrival, scene safety is always the first step after which a brief scene size-up should be conducted to ensure that adequate equipment and resources are either present or have been requested. After quickly assessing airway, breathing, and circulation, it is essential that a focused history and physical examination be obtained, even if the patient has classic complaints of left-sided chest pain and shortness of breath.

If a patient is complaining of atraumatic chest pain, he or she should be placed on a cardiac monitor and 12-lead ECG obtained. Prehospital ECG has been shown to improve outcomes in patients with STEMI and non-STEMI patients.[5] IV access should be attempted and appropriate medical therapy started. Package the patient for transport, and transport the patient to the most appropriate facility. The patient needs to be monitored throughout the call for signs of deterioration, with changes in patient status addressed promptly (Table 39-1).

TABLE 39-1	Standard Approach to the ACS Patient
Standard prehospital approach to the ACS patient:	
ABCs	
Focused history and physical examination	
Identification of potential ACS patient	
Cardiac monitor applied	
12-lead ECG obtained	
IV access	
Pharmacologic therapy, with early oxygen and aspirin	
Destination decision	
Notify destination of patient/activate cath lab	
Safe transportation of patient	

Multitasking with limited providers and resources is the overarching principle in the approach to a patient with chest pain. Therefore, the physician on scene needs to be proficient in starting IVs, properly administering a variety of medications (Table 39-2), and utilizing and troubleshooting all the equipment in the transporting vehicle. Transportation should begin as soon as feasible. The team's approach should be goal oriented, for example, reaching definitive care quickly and safely, rather than task oriented, for example, obtaining IV access before proceeding to the next step.

If a prehospital diagnosis of ACS is made, determining the most appropriate destination becomes one of the most essential components of patient care. Many EMS systems utilize point-of-entry plans; these should be followed whenever possible. As a general principle, the patient should be transported to the nearest facility capable of providing definitive cardiac care. In most locations, this is a facility that provides emergent interventional cardiac catheterization. In rural locations, the transport time to such a facility may be prohibitive. Therefore, an appropriate facility may be one capable of administering thrombolytic therapy. Many factors, including time of day and weather conditions, affect such a decision. Prehospital delivery of medications like ticagrelor[6] and glycoprotein IIb/IIIa inhibitors[7,8] does not appear to improve outcomes.

Mode of transportation can also be a critical element of patient care. ACLS-trained providers should transport ACS patients whenever available. However, in locations where transport time to definitive care is short and arrival of ACLS-trained providers will be significantly delayed, BLS transport may be a reasonable option. On the other end of the spectrum, helicopter or fixed-wing transport can rapidly provide skilled personnel to transport even the sickest ACS patient. Air medical transport should

TABLE 39-2	Prehospital ACS Medications
Prehospital ACS Medications	Notes
Aspirin	For all potential ACS patients; only absolute contraindication is allergy
Oxygen	Generally by nasal cannula; applied early in patient encounter
Nitroglycerin	Sublingual usually sufficient in the field; strongly consider IV access first. Caution in inferior MI
Morphine	Concern for increased mortality in UA/NSTEMI. Remains Class I intervention for STEMI
Fibrinolytics	Not commonly used; for special situations/systems only
Heparin	Rarely given in the field; common for ALS/critical care transports. Consider initial bolus without continuous infusion for transport
β-Blockers	May increase mortality early in MI; no longer routinely used

be reserved for patients who are time critical, meaning transport time will be reduced compared to that provided by ground-based ALS units with the time savings, providing benefit to the patient, or for patients who are care critical, meaning that the patient requires medical therapies or medications en route which cannot be provided by the ALS ground units.

PREHOSPITAL TREATMENT ACS

Treatment of the patient diagnosed with ACS begins with initial stabilization. This includes immediate assessment of airway, breathing, and circulation and addressing any problems identified. Supplemental oxygen should be provided (at least 2 L or more as indicated) and continuous cardiac monitoring implemented. Insert two IVs, preferably 20 g or larger. If the patient is ambulatory on arrival, he or she should be placed in a seated position and restricted from further ambulation.

The mainstay of pharmacologic therapy for ACS is aspirin; no other prehospital pharmacologic therapy approaches aspirin in reducing mortality.[9] Four 81-mg aspirin tablets constitute the most common dose, chewed, not swallowed, as this speeds absorption. The only absolute contraindication to aspirin is an aspirin allergy.

The patient with chest pain or pressure and adequate blood pressure should receive nitroglycerin sublingually (0.4 mg) repeated every 5 minutes typically up to three doses if discomfort persists; however, additional doses can be given if blood pressure remains stable and pain continues. Consider ensuring functional IV access prior to administering nitroglycerin due to possible hypotension. This is more common if the myocardial infarction (MI) involves the right ventricle. Therefore, if evidence of inferior MI is present on the initial 12 lead, right-sided leads should be performed. If the right ventricular is involved, the patient will be preload dependent, meaning his or her symptoms will respond better to intravenous fluids instead of nitroglycerin. Consider a continuous infusion of nitroglycerin if chest pain persists, blood pressure is adequate, and transport times are sufficiently long.

In a patient with a diagnosed ACS who continues to have chest pain after three doses of sublingual nitroglycerin, morphine may be administered for pain control. The role of morphine in patients with unstable angina or non-ST-elevation myocardial infarction (NSTEMI) is questionable due to concerns for increased mortality,[10] though it is still a class I intervention for patients experiencing an ST-elevation myocardial infarction (STEMI)[11] (**Figure 39-1**). Pain management with fentanyl may be a more acceptable alternative to morphine.

Additional pharmacologic therapies for ACS are not routinely given in the prehospital setting. Unfractionated heparin is used for anticoagulation in the hospital setting, but is not a practical option prehospitally due to difficulties with administration, laboratory testing, and unpredictable anticoagulation effects. It is slowly being replaced by low-molecular-weight heparins,[12] which again are typically administered in the hospital setting. β-Blockers have traditionally been used early in ACS, although they are no longer indicated in the prehospital and ED environments due to concerns for cardiogenic shock and studies that do not demonstrate benefit with early administration.[13]

Rural EMS systems with transport times to a PCI capable facility in excess of 90 minutes may be candidates for a prehospital fibrinolysis protocol. If fibrinolysis is considered, it needs to be done immediately after identification of an STEMI, and should be done with the use of a specific fibrinolytic checklist and in consultation with the receiving facility.[11]

The receiving facility needs to be notified of an incoming patient as soon as possible, in keeping with local protocols. Many EMS systems allow for transmission of prehospital ECGs, which can enable the receiving physician to review the ECG and facilitate activation of the catheterization team. Ideally, transmission of the ECG should not delay patient transport. Should the cardiogram demonstrate an STEMI, the catheterization team should be activated prior to patient arrival, in accordance with local and institutional protocols. Bypassing non-PCI centers has been shown to be safe[14] and is recommended if the time between first medical contact and balloon at the destination facility is less than 90 minutes and transport times are under approximately 30 minutes.[11]

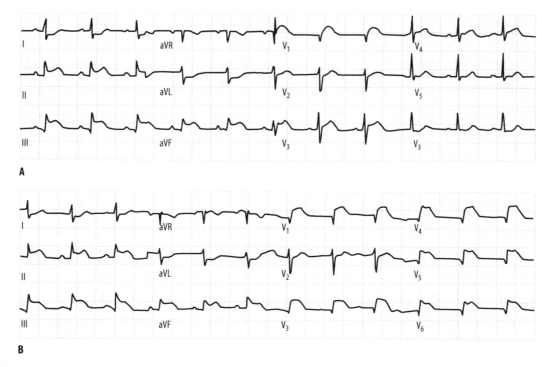

FIGURE 39-1. ST-elevation myocardial infarction. **A:** Inferior wall myocardial infarction with ST elevation in lead V₁. ECG showing inferior ST-segment elevation myocardial infarction, also with ST-segment elevation in lead V₁ suggestive of right ventricular infarction. **B:** Inferior wall myocardial infarction with right ventricular leads. Same patient with placement of right ventricular leads, showing ST-segment elevation in V₃R, V₄R, V₅R, and V₆R compatible with right ventricular infarction. (Courtesy of J. Stephan Stapczynski, Maricopa Medical Center. Reprinted with permission from Tintinalli JE, Stapczynski JS, Ma OJ, Cline DM, Cydulka RK, Meckler GD, eds. Tintinalli's Emergency Medicine: A Comprehensive Study Guide, 7th ed. New York, NY: McGraw-Hill; 2011.)

▣ CONSIDERATIONS FOR INTERFACILITY TRANSFER OF PATIENTS WITH ACS

Non-PCI capable hospitals with door-to-departure time of less than 30 minutes may consider rapid transfer as an acceptable option to fibrinolysis. ACS patients require the most rapid method of transfer that will safely deliver them to the destination hospital. In some systems ground transport via an ALS crew may be faster than air medical transport with a critical care crew. Regardless of the method chosen, transfer of ACS patients is a common occurrence, and transporting crews should be well practiced in efficiently moving the patient through the system from one hospital to the other as quickly and safely as possible.

One method of decreasing times for interfacility transfers is to use bolus dosing of medications in place of continuous intravenous infusions for medications such as nitroglycerin, heparin, and GP2B3A inhibitors.[15] Most interfacility transports are short enough that the duration of action of bolus medications is sufficient for the transport. This also serves to decrease the complexity of the patient encounter for the prehospital provider who no longer needs to focus on monitoring and troubleshooting pumps and can pay more attention to overall patient status and needs.

The prehospital provider transferring a patient with a diagnosed ACS should be prepared to treat complications associated with the patient's condition. Arrhythmias are the most commonly encountered condition. Cardiogenic shock is one of the most serious complications of MI, and requires vigilance to diagnose. Hypotension is the cardinal marker of cardiogenic shock in the out-of-hospital environment. Fluid boluses are the first line of treatment, remembering the patient with a right-ventricular infarct is preload dependent and so will improve hemodynamically with fluid boluses but the patient with left ventricular involvement will rapidly develop pulmonary edema. The most commonly available vasopressor in the prehospital setting is dopamine, and may be necessary to treat hypotension in the cardiogenic shock patient. Due to the arrhythmogenic potential of dopamine, careful monitoring of the patient's cardiac rhythm is necessary.

Intra-aortic balloon pumps (IABPs) are sometimes placed during cardiac catheterization for the management of cardiogenic shock. The prehospital provider may transfer a patient with an IABP in place. This is a specialized instrument requiring careful monitoring and an understanding of how to troubleshoot the device in case of malfunction or deterioration in patient condition. This understanding is outside the knowledge base of many physicians and most prehospital providers. Therefore, IABPs should only be transported by providers who have received specific training in their use or with the addition of a specialty team who routinely performs such transfers.

ARRHYTHMIAS

▣ APPROACH TO THE PATIENT

Similar to treatment in the emergency department, the approach to prehospital care of any patient with a cardiac arrhythmia focuses on identification of the dysrhythmia, assessing patient stability, and immediate treatment of any potentially life-threatening rhythms. When assessing the stability of the patient, one should evaluate for presence of chest pain, hypotension (SBP < 100), alteration of mental status, diaphoresis, and changes in skin color. The distinction between stable and unstable or borderline patients will help determine which of several possible treatments is most appropriate. For example, a 60-year-old male with a heart rate of 140 who is awake, alert, mentating well, and does not complain of chest pain may benefit from vagal maneuvers and intravenous fluids. If this same patient were complaining of dyspnea and chest pain, adenosine would be indicated. Similarly, if the patient has chest pain and a systolic blood pressure of 85, then electrical synchronized cardioversion would be indicated.

The goals of prehospital care versus definitive care in the emergency department should be clear. As a physician taking part in prehospital care, it may be appealing to attempt to identify and treat all medical conditions. It should be emphasized that the goals of prehospital care remain to stabilize the patient and transport them to an appropriate facility for definitive care.

▣ TACHYDYSRHYTHMIAS

The upper limit of normal rate for an adult heart is 100 beats per minute. Once the stability of the patient has been assessed and presence of a tachycardia has been established, the next step in management is to further classify the rhythm based on the width of the QRS complex. The normal QRS duration is 120 ms, which constitutes three small boxes on a standard 12-lead ECG. Thus any tachycardia with a QRS within this range is a narrow complex tachycardia whereas any tachycardia with a QRS complex wider than this is considered a wide complex tachycardia. The approach and treatment options for both are outlined below.

Narrow-Complex Tachycardia Once a narrow-complex tachycardia has been established, the distinction should be made between regular and irregular rhythms.

In a stable patient with minor symptoms (eg, palpitations) and a narrow-complex tachycardia with regular rhythm, consider sinus tachycardia or more broadly supraventricular tachycardia (SVT) as an etiology (**Figure 39-2**). In addition to intravenous fluids, if there is no evidence of volume overload, vagal maneuvers such as Valsalva maneuver should be attempted. Although there is evidence supporting the use of carotid massage, the concern for embolization of plaques prevents this from being recommended in the field, especially for patients over 50. Studies in the emergency department suggest that these maneuvers will convert up to 25 % of SVT,[16] although studies of prehospital effectiveness are limited.[17] In a symptomatic but stable patient in whom these maneuvers fail, pharmaceutical intervention should be considered.

Adenosine is considered by most to be the agent of choice for treating SVT.[18]

A 90% conversion rate has been reported when administered as an initial dose of 6 mg via rapid intravenous push, followed by 12 mg rapid intravenous push for up to two additional doses if needed.[19] This agent has the benefit of being extremely short-lived in the bloodstream and also being relatively safe if inadvertently administered to a ventricular-derived tachycardia. Verapamil and diltiazem are also options for the treatment

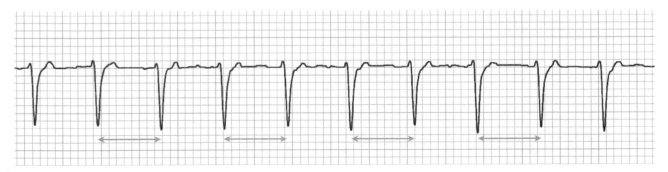

FIGURE 39-2. Supraventricular tachycardia. (Reprinted with permission from Knoop KJ. *The Atlas of Emergency Medicine.* 3rd ed. New York: McGraw-Hill; 2010.)

of SVT. Verapamil is initiated at a dose of 2.5 to 5 mg IV followed by 5 to 10 mg in 25 minutes if conversion is not achieved. Diltiazem is given at 0.25 mg/kg over 2 minutes for the first dose, followed by 0.35 mg/kg over 2 minutes in 15 minutes if needed. Both Verapamil and Diltiazem carry the risk of inducing hypotension and heart failure if inadvertently given to a patient with a wide-complex tachycardia.[20] As it has been estimated that as high as 20% of wide-complex tachycardias can be mistaken for SVT in the field, consider using adenosine as the first-line agent.

In an unstable patient, synchronized cardioversion starting at 50 J should be the first-line approach. If cardioversion is required and time allows, consider administering one or more of the following as needed to assist in patient comfort: diazepam 2.5 to 5 mg IV, midazolam 0.5 –to 2.5 mg IV, morphine sulfate 2 to 10 mg IV, or fentanyl 1 μg/kg IV.

In very rapid heart rates, it can be difficult to appreciate the regularity of the rhythm or the presence of p-waves. If an ECG obtained after adenosine administration does not demonstrate p-waves, consider atrial fibrillation or flutter as an etiology.

The most common narrow-complex irregular tachycardia is atrial fibrillation. Many patients presenting with atrial fibrillation will have minor symptoms, and no specific prehospital treatment is needed. In these cases, stabilization of other conditions and transport should be the goals of care. If the patient is unstable, synchronized cardioversion as outlined above remains the first-line treatment. There are several options for the symptomatic but stable patient, which should be considered in any patient with a heart rate above 140 to 150.

Diltiazem can be administered as described above. Although not frequently required prehospitally, after the initial bolus diltiazem may be continued as an infusion with a rate of 10 to 15 mg/h. This is often seen in interhospital transfers. Amiodarone (150 mg slow IV push over 10 minutes) is another treatment option that is useful in cases where a calcium channel blocker is contraindicated (Wolff-Parkinson-White syndrome, second- or third-degree heart block, severe hypotension, or cardiogenic shock) (**Figure 39-3**). After an initial IV bolus a continuous infusion is also possible at a rate of 1 mg/min. As with other drips, this will likely be more common in interhospital transfer.

In patients who are on β-blockers as part of their home medication regimen, consider metoprolol as an agent for rate control with an initial dose of 2.5 to 5 mg over 2 minutes followed by repeat doses of 5 mg at 5 minute intervals to a maximum of 15 mg. It is important that calcium channel blockers and β-blockers not be given to the same patient as this may have an additive effect on AV nodal blockade.

WIDE COMPLEX TACHYCARDIA

Patients with a heart rate over 100 and a QRS >−120 ms have a wide complex tachycardia (WCT) (**Figure 39-4**). Causes of a wide complex tachycardia range from ventricular in origin to SVT with aberrant conduction. It can be challenging to differentiate these etiologies in the prehospital setting. As such, it is prudent that treatment options be compatible with ventricular tachycardia.

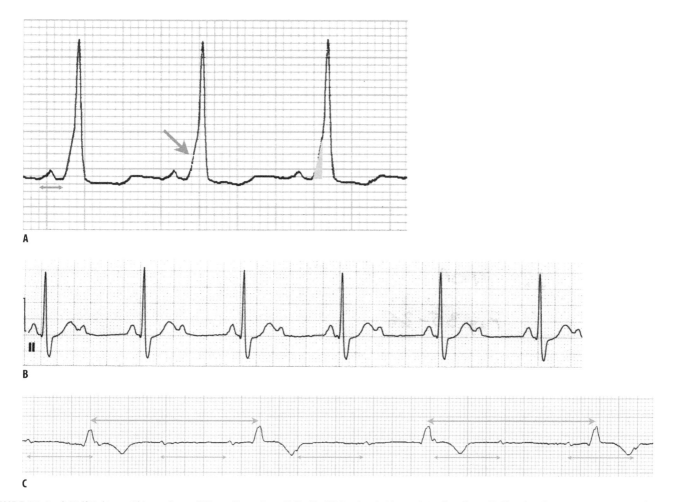

FIGURE 39-3. A: Wolf-Parkinson-White syndrome. (ECG contributor: James V. Ritchie, MD. Reprinted with permission from Knoop KJ. *The Atlas of Emergency Medicine*. 3rd ed. New York: McGraw-Hill; 2010.) **B:** Second-degree heart block (Mobitz II). (Reprinted with permission from Stone CK, Humphries RL. Current Diagnosis & Treatment: *Emergency Medicine*, 7th ed. New York: McGraw-Hill, 2011.) **C:** Third-degree heart block. (Reprinted with permission from Knoop KJ. *The Atlas of Emergency Medicine*. 3rd ed. New York: McGraw-Hill; 2010.)

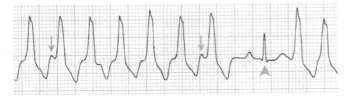

FIGURE 39-4. Ventricular tachycardia. (ECG contributor: James V. Ritchie, MD. Reprinted with permission from Knoop KJ. *The Atlas of Emergency Medicine*. 3rd ed. New York: McGraw-Hill; 2010.)

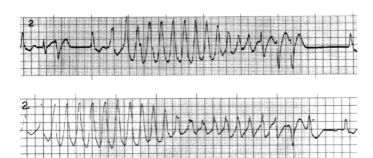

FIGURE 39-5. Torsades de pointe. (Reprinted with permission from Tintinalli JE, Stapczynski J, Ma O, Cline DM, Cydulka RK, Meckler GD, T, eds. *Tintinalli's Emergency Medicine: A Comprehensive Study Guide*. New York, NY: McGraw-Hill; 2011.)

Similar to other dysrhythmia, the unstable patient should undergo synchronized cardioversion, although the initial dose should be 100 J. Symptomatic but stable patients or borderline patients should be treated pharmacologically.

Medical treatment options for WCT include amiodarone dosed as described above. Alternatively, lidocaine 1 to 1.5 mg/kg IV with subsequent

dosing of 0.5 to 0.75 mg/kg IV every 3 to 5 minutes to a total dose of 3 mg/kg may be used. Lidocaine can be infused continuously at a rate of 2 to 4 mg/min IV if the boluses successfully convert the rhythm.

Torsades de point, or twisting of the points, is a rare etiology of polymorphic ventricular tachycardia (**Figure 39-5**). The prehospital treatment of choice is electrical cardioversion for unstable patients. Magnesium sulfate 1 to 2 g IV over 1 to 2 minutes and transcutaneous pacing (TCP) are recommended for patients who fail to convert.

■ BRADYDYSRHYTHMIAS

The prehospital approach to the bradycardic patient (HR under 60) begins with evaluating patient stability as outlined above (**Figure 39-6**). Administration of atropine sulfate 0.5 mg IV push every 3 to 5 minutes up to total dose 3 mg is indicated in symptomatic but stable patients. Additionally, transcutaneous pacer pads should be placed to prepare for the possibility of patient deterioration. In unstable patients, TCP is immediately indicated, although atropine may be given as above while preparing for TCP.

Options for continuous IV infusions to support heart rate in the hypotensive patient include dopamine 2 to 20 mg/kg per minute and epinephrine 2 mg to 10 mg/min IV. In the specific case where β-blocker or calcium channel blocker toxicity is the suspected cause for bradycardia, consider calcium chloride 10% 1 g IV and glucagon 1 to 5 mg IV.

■ HEART BLOCKS

Interruptions in the conduction system of the heart can cause various forms of heart block. There are two types of heart block that must be considered in the prehospital setting due to their inherent instability.

A Mobitz II second degree heart block (Figure 39-3B) is the result of a conduction block within the His-Purkinje system. The P-R intervals remain constant with intermittently dropped beats. This unstable rhythm has a high propensity for progressing to a complete heart block. Pharmacologic treatment is often ineffective and a low threshold for transcutaneous pacing should be observed.

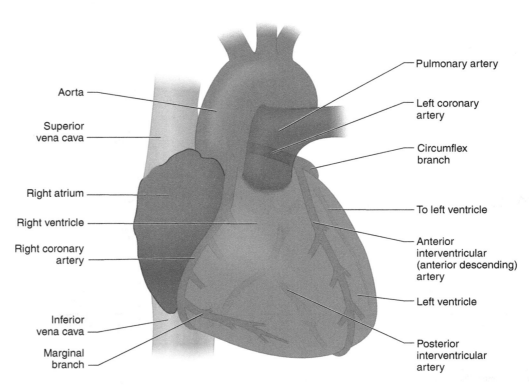

FIGURE 39-6. Left ventricular assist device. LVAD carries blood from the left ventricle to the aorta. (Reprinted with permission from Tintinalli JE, Stapczynski J, Ma O, Cline DM, Cydulka RK, Meckler GD, T. eds. *Tintinalli's Emergency Medicine: A Comprehensive Study Guide*. New York, NY: McGraw-Hill; 2011.)

A complete heart block or third degree block refers to a complete dissociation between the atrial and ventricular conduction system. The block may be nodal, in the His-Purkinje system or in the bundle branches of the conduction system. In this clinically unstable rhythm, transcutaneous pacing should be initiated as described above.

SPECIAL CONSIDERATIONS

PERIARREST FACTORS (Hs AND Ts)

There are many well-described causes of cardiac arrhythmias and cardiac arrest that are reversible. The American Heart Association refers to these conditions as the "Hs and Ts", which should be considered in all patients with cardiac emergencies. The Hs consists of *hypovolemia, hypoxia, hydrogen ions* (acidosis), *hyperkalemia* or *hypokalemia, hypothermia, hypoglycemia,* and *hyperglycemia.* The Ts are *toxins,* (cardiac) *tamponade, tension pneumothorax, thrombosis* (myocardial infarction), *thromboembolism* (pulmonary embolism), and *trauma.*[21] Based on this list, reasonable prehospital interventions include IV fluids, supplemental oxygen, glucose or (if available) insulin administration, needle decompression of the chest in unstable patients with signs of tension pneumothorax (hypotension, decreased breath sounds on one side, deviated trachea), aspirin, and morphine.

RENAL FAILURE PATIENTS

Because of a predisposition to electrolyte abnormalities, patients with advanced renal failure pose a particular difficulty in treating arrhythmias. In particular, hyperkalemia can cause a life-threatening bradycardia that can progress to a wide-complex arrhythmia if not corrected. Upon obtaining a history of renal failure, consider hyperkalemia as a cause of the arrhythmia and rapidly administer sodium bicarbonate 1 to 2 amps intravenously and calcium carbonate (10 mL of 10%) or calcium gluconate. After checking capillary blood glucose, dextrose −50% and insulin 10 units IV can also be given. Finally, nebulized albuterol will also help transiently low serum potassium levels. It is important to note that lidocaine is contraindicated in hyperkalemic patients.[22]

WOLF-PARKINSON-WHITE SYNDROME (WPW)

WPW is a preexcitation syndrome that occurs when an accessory conduction pathway exists from the atria to the ventricles (Figure 39-3A). This pathway predisposes affected individuals to a reentrant tachycardia and also atrial fibrillation. Agents that slow nodal conduction (β-blockers, calcium channel blockers, adenosine) should be avoided in these patients as these agents may actually increase the heart rate through the accessory pathway. Suggested interventions in stable but symptomatic patients have included procainamide (30 mg/min, maximal dose 17 mg/kg) and amiodarone administered as above (8 M). Procainamide, however, is difficult to administer in the field and requires 40 to 60 minutes to achieve therapeutic levels in the bloodstream.[23] Amiodarone has been listed by the AHA as the drug of choice for the treatment atrial fibrillation in the setting of WPW.[21] However, it should be used with caution as the potential for increased ventricular rate and deterioration to ventricular fibrillation does exist.[24]

AICDS

Automated implantable cardioverter-defibrillator devices (AICDs) have been utilized with increasing frequency to treat patients at risk for ventricular dysrhythmias, including patients with CHF. Although AICDs are designed to convert tachydysrhythmias, they may not achieve conversion, may fail to fire or may fire inappropriately. Patients experiencing arrhythmias despite the presence of an AICD should be treated the same as a patient without an AICD. Important distinctions are as follows: (1) If TCP is indicated, pacer pads should not be placed directly over the AICD. They should be placed anterior and posterior and 10 cm from the device. (2) If the AICD continues to fire inappropriately, a magnet placed over the device will cause it to revert to "factory" settings, thus

possibly preventing continued shocks. If there is any question regarding the appropriateness of the device firing, rapid transfer to an emergency department is a better option.

LVADS

Left ventricular assist devices are implanted pumps used to enhance LV function (Figure 39-6). These devices are becoming more common in the outpatient setting as a "bridge to transplant" for congestive heart failure patients.[24,25] Complications of these devices include failure of the power supply and mechanical malfunction.[26] If a power failure is suspected, some models can be powered by a hand pump that the patient is instructed to have available at all times. In the case of a malfunction, the patient will likely present with symptoms of hypovolemia, right-sided heart failure and pulmonary hypotension.[27] In this case, transport to the facility at which the device was implanted should be strongly considered. Finally, the presence of an LVAD complicates CPR by creating the potential of dislodging the tubing, resulting in massive hemorrhage. If applicable, the use of a hand pump in lieu of CPR should be considered.

MANAGEMENT OF THE CHF PATIENT

Prehospital management of the CHF patient has undergone major changes in the last decade, primarily due to the development of portable CPAP machines. This has greatly reduced the need for prehospital intubation and its associated complications for these patients.[28] Many of the challenges of managing CHF in the prehospital setting, however, remain unchanged.

Primary among these challenges is making the proper diagnosis of CHF. Dyspnea can be the presenting chief complaint for many medical conditions. Differentiating between CHF and pneumonia, especially prehospitally, can be exceptionally difficult. A focused history and careful physical examination are essential.

If CHF is the presumed cause of a patient's respiratory distress, initial management should include management of airway, breathing, and circulation, with supplemental oxygen and a 12-lead ECG obtained early in the patient encounter. The patient should be sitting upright with an IV in place. Nitroglycerin is often given for preload reduction, blood pressure permitting. Furosemide is commonly administered intravenously at twice the patient's daily dose, up to 80 mg. CPAP can be applied to the patient who maintains the ability to protect his or her airway, and titrated to effect. Potentially modifiable causes of CHF should be sought and treated if found. These include atrial fibrillation with a rapid response, cardiac tamponade, cardiogenic shock, and exposures to organophosphates.

Patients who are obtunded, whose mental status declines while on CPAP, or who present in flash pulmonary edema with pink frothy sputum coming from their nose or mouth should be considered for intubation or other placement of a supraglottic airway. The management of the airway will be dependent on protocols, available medications (sedatives, paralytics), and service practice.

OTHER CAUSES OF CHEST PAIN

There are many causes of chest pain in addition to ACS, CHF, and dysrhythmias. Some of these include aortic dissection, pulmonary embolism, infections, inflammatory conditions, and trauma.

Aortic dissection cannot reliably be differentiated from ACS in the prehospital setting, although a careful history and physical examination could bring it higher on the differential. No specific prehospital treatments exist aside from rapid transport to a facility with appropriate surgical capabilities. Blood pressure control is a mainstay of management, but would not be initiated in the prehospital setting. However, providers may be responsible for monitoring blood pressure during an interfacility transfer with a continuous infusion of antihypertensive medication.

Pulmonary embolism is a cause of chest pain that often goes unrecognized. Careful attention to airway, breathing, and circulation and transport to an appropriate facility are the only generally available pre-hospital interventions. The mainstay of treatment for most emboli is anticoagulation that is either given as a single injection prior to patient transfer or run as a continuous infusion during the transfer, requiring no intervention from the provider doing a patient transfer.

Pneumonia is another cause of prehospital chest pain and can be easily confused with CHF. Clues to lead the prehospital provider to consider a diagnosis of pneumonia include a dyspneic patient with fever, one-sided lung findings on auscultation, and hypotension. While antibiotics are not usually given in the prehospital setting, initial fluid boluses should be considered.

Pericarditis should be considered in any patient with compatible ECG findings (PR depression being the most distinctive) and a history of positional chest pain. In the patient in whom ACS cannot be excluded, treating for ACS en route to an appropriate receiving facility brings little risk.

Pneumothorax should be suspected in any patient with sudden onset of dyspnea and chest pain, recent trauma, or a tall, thin body habitus. It is treated in the prehospital setting with needle decompression on the affected side if the patient is in severe respiratory distress or becomes hemodynamically unstable.

Gastroesophageal reflux disease (GERD) and other esophageal disorders are common causes of chest pain that should never be diagnosed in the prehospital setting. Anxiety is another common prehospital presentation that can cause significant chest pain and dyspnea. Any presentation of chest pain or dyspnea diagnosed in the field as anxiety should be made with great care and be reevaluated frequently.

Trauma to the chest, abdomen, or back can present as chest pain. Because many prehospital encounters occur in public areas and most patients are fully clothed, the prehospital provider may not visualize the patient's chest or back on initial examination and so may miss a traumatic injury. For this reason, visual inspection of the chest and back, including both axillae, should be carried out as soon as possible in any patient presenting with chest pain.

CONCLUSION

Chest pain is a commonly encountered prehospital presentation. Diagnosing acute coronary syndrome prehospitally can have significant impact on patient management. The prehospital provider must be able to accurately diagnose the etiology of a patient's chest pain to the best of his or her ability, determine the stability of the patient, and transport that patient to the most appropriate destination. Many consequences of the patient's condition such as pain, arrhythmias, and shortness of breath can and should be managed during the transport for both patient comfort and patient safety. Providers well trained in the management of chest pain will be able to significantly enhance patient outcomes.

KEY POINTS

- All patients complaining of chest pain should be taken seriously with an immediate assessment, including vital signs, monitor, and obtaining a 12-lead ECG.
- Prehospital ECG has been shown to improve outcomes in patients with STEMI and non-STEMI patients.[5]
- Utilize point-of-entry plans for destination decisions when transporting a patient with a diagnosed ACS.
- Prehospital delivery of medications like ticagrelor and glycoprotein IIb/IIIa inhibitors does not appear to improve outcomes.
- Thrombolytics may be considered when a patient cannot be rapidly transported to a hospital capable of performing emergent cardiac catheterization.
- For patients with arrhythmias, first determine if the patient is stable or unstable, tachycardic or bradycardic. Then determine if

the rhythm is a wide complex, narrow, or a heart block and treat accordingly. For all unstable rhythms, consider cardioversion or pacing as the first line of therapy.

- Consider hyperkalemia as a cause of arrhythmia in a patient with renal failure.
- Treat patients with diagnosed Wolff-Parkinson-White syndrome and arrhythmias with amiodarone.
- Congestive heart failure can be difficult to diagnose. If one is confident with the diagnosis, consider treating with a diuretic. Respiratory distress can also be treated with CPAP.
- There are many causes of chest pain beyond ACS; however, always consider the life-threatening diagnoses first such as aortic dissection, pulmonary embolism, and tension pneumothorax and treat the patient accordingly.

REFERENCES

1. Centers for Disease Control and Prevention (CDC). Prevalence of heart disease–United States, 2005. *MMWR Morb Mortal Wkly Rep.* February 16, 2007;56(6):113-118.
2. Lloyd-Jones D, Adams R, Carnethon M, et al. Heart disease and stroke statistics–2009 update: a report from the American Heart Association Statistics Committee and Stroke Statistics Subcommittee. *Circulation.* January 27, 2009;119(3):e21-e181.
3. Pantridge JF, Geddes JS. A mobile intensive-care unit in the management of myocardial infarction. *Lancet.* August 5, 1967;2(7510): 271-273.
4. Reilly MJ. Accuracy of a priority medical dispatch system in dispatching cardiac emergencies in a suburban community. *Prehosp and Disaster Med.* March-April 2006;21(2):77-81.
5. Quinn T, Johnsen S, Gale CP, et al. Effects of prehospital 12-lead ECG on processes of care and mortality in acute coronary syndrome: a linked cohort study from the Myocardial Ischaemia National Audit Project. *Heart.* June 2014;100(12):944-950.
6. Montalescot G, van 't Hof AW, Lapostolle F, et al. Prehospital ticagrelor in ST-segment elevation myocardial infarction. *N Engl J Med.* September 11, 2014;371(11):1016-1027.
7. Auffret V, Oger E, Leurent G, et al. Efficacy of pre-hospital use of glycoprotein IIb/IIIa inhibitors in ST-segment elevation myocardial infarction before mechanical reperfusion in a rapid-transfer network (from the Acute Myocardial Infarction Registry of Brittany). *Am J Cardiol.* July 15, 2014;114(2):214-223.
8. Hermanides RS, Ottervanger JP, Dambrink JH, et al. Risk of bleeding after prehospital administration of high dose tirofiban for ST elevation myocardial infarction. *Int J Cardiol.* May 17, 2012;157(1):86-90.
9. Randomized trial of intravenous streptokinase, oral aspirin, both, or neither among 17,187 cases of suspected acute myocardial infarction: ISIS-2. ISIS-2 (Second International Study of Infarct Survival) Collaborative Group. *Lancet.* August 13, 1988;2(8607):349-360.
10. Meine TJ, Roe MT, Chen AY, et al. Association of intravenous morphine use and outcomes in acute coronary syndromes: results from the CRUSADE quality improvement initiative. *Am Heart J.* June 2005;149(6):1043-1049.
11. O'Connor RE, Brady W, Brooks SC, et al. Part 10: Acute coronary syndromes: 2010 American Heart Association guidelines for cardiopulmonary resuscitation and emergency cardiovascular care. *Circulation.* 2010;122:S787-S817.
12. Armstrong PW, Chang WC, Wallentin L, et al. Efficacy and safety of unfractionated heparin versus enoxaparin: a pooled analysis of ASSNET-3 and -3 PLUS data. *CMAJ.* May 2006 9;174(10)1421-1426.
13. Al-Reesi A, Al-Zadjali N, Perry J, et al. Do beta-blockers reduce short-term mortality following acute myocardial infarction? A systematic review and meta-analysis. *CJEM.* May 2008;10(3):215-223.

14. Le May MR, Davies RF, Dionne R, et al. Comparison of early mortality of paramedic-diagnosed ST-segment elevation myocardial infarction with immediate transport to a designated primary percutaneous coronary intervention center to that of similar patients transported to the nearest hospital. *Am J Cardiol*. November 15, 2006;98(10):1329-1333.

15. Weisberg S, Fitch J, Towner D, et al. Transporting without infusions: effect on door-to-needle time for acute coronary syndrome patients. *Prehosp Emerg Care*. April 6, 2010;14(2):159-163.

16. Lim SH, Anantharaman V, Teo WS, et al. Comparison of treatment of supraventricular tachycardia by Valsalva maneuver and carotid sinus massage. *Ann Emerg Med*. 1998;31(1):30.

17. Smith G, Morgans A, Boyle, M. Use of the Valsalva manoeuvre in the prehospital setting: a review of the literature. *Emerg Med J*. 2009;26:8.

18. Furlong R, Gerhardt RT, Farber P, et al. Intravenous adenosine as first-line prehospital management of narrow-complex tachycardias by EMS personnel without direct physician control. *Am J Emerg Med*. 1995;13(4):383.

19. McCabe JL, Adhar GC, Menegazzi JJ, et al. Intravenous Adenosine in the Prehospital Treatment of Paroxysmal Supraventricular Tachycardia. *Ann Emerg Med*. 1992;21(4):358-361.

20. DiMarco JP, Miles W, Akhtar M, et al. Adenosine for paroxysmal supraventricular tachycardia: Dose ranging and comparison with verapamil. Assessment in placebo-controlled, multicenter trials. *Ann Intern Med*. 1990;113:104.

21. AHA. Management of symptomatic bradycardia and tachycardia. *Circulation*. 2005;112:67.

22. McLean SA, Paul ID, Spector PS. Lidocaine-induced conduction disturbance in patients with systemic hyperkalemia. *Ann Emerg Med*. 2000;36(6):615.

23. Fengler BT, Brady WJ, Plautz CU. Atrial fibrillation in the Wolff–Parkinson–White syndrome: ECG recognition and treatment in the ED. *Am J Emerg Med*. 2007;25(5):576-583.

24. Boriani G, Biffi M, Frabetti L, et al. Ventricular fibrillation after intravenous in Wolff-Parkinson-White syndrome with atrial fibrillation. *Am Heart J*. 1996;131:1214-1216.

25. Delgado DH, Rao V, Ross HJ, Verma S, Smedira NG. Mechanical circulatory assistance: state of art. *Circulation*. 2002;106(16):2046.

26. Ranjit J, Kamdar F, Liao K, et al. Improved survival and decreasing incidence of adverse events with the Heartmate II left ventricular assist device as bridge-to-transplant therapy. *Ann Thorac Surg*. 2008; 1235(86):1227.

27. Riddle, WA. The high-tech heart: LVAD emergencies in pre-transplant patients. *JEMS*. 2007;32(8). http://www.jems.com/articles/2007/07/high-tech-heart-lvad-emergenci.html. Accessed August, 2011.

28. Hubble MW, Richards ME, Jarvis R, et al. Effectiveness of prehospital continuous positive airway pressure in the management of acute pulmonary edema. *Prehosp Emerg Care*. October-December 2006;10(4)430-439.

CHAPTER 40

Pulmonary Emergencies

Margaret Strecker-McGraw
Taylor Ratcliff

INTRODUCTION

There are inconsistent data on the percentage of EMS calls involving pulmonary emergencies. A search of the literature reveals respiratory calls make up approximately 11% to 15% of all EMS requests.[1,2] Few publications actually define the types of calls and concomitant demographics of those patients. After the terrorist attacks of 9/11, there was an increase in "syndrome surveillance" across the country primarily in an attempt to discover aberrant trends in the incidence of pulmonary disease. Despite attempts to classify the number of disease presentations, including using EMS/9-1-1 call records, the information remains scarce.[3]

Nevertheless a patient with a pulmonary emergency is an anxiety-provoking situation for both the patient and the prehospital provider.

OBJECTIVES

1. Discuss demographics of respiratory disease pertaining to EMS, including percent of EMS calls, the incidence and increase of acute and chronic lung disease, as well as fatality data from respiratory distress.

2. Understand and be able to integrate knowledge about normal respiratory physiology including normal versus positive pressure ventilation, mechanics of gas exchange, and the CNS control of respiratory drive.

3. Discuss and list common causes of respiratory illness including pathophysiology, presentation, and treatment for asthma, COPD, CHF, and lung malignancy.

4. Describe differences between acute and chronic respiratory conditions including chronic and acute phases of respiratory failure.

5. Discuss and list causes, presentation, and treatment for other acute medical causes of respiratory distress including PE, pneumonia, pulmonary edema, croup, and epiglottitis.

6. List and discuss other nonmedical causes of respiratory distress including asphyxiants, respiratory toxins, and foreign body airway obstruction.

7. Describe the indications for prehospital endotracheal intubation.

8. Discuss the use of supraglottic airway devices and their role in prehospital care.

9. Describe the physiology and indications for use of prehospital noninvasive positive pressure ventilation.

10. Discuss and understand the RSI process including indications and medications.

According to the CDC, in 2007 the number of visits to ambulatory cares sites in the United States, including physician offices, hospital outpatient, and emergency departments for chronic and unspecified bronchitis, as a primary diagnosis, was 11.7 million, and for other chronic obstructive pulmonary disease conditions, as a primary diagnosis, was 6.1 million.[4]

Health statistics provided by the CDC for US adults in 2009 reveal the number of noninstitutionalized adults diagnosed with chronic bronchitis as 9.9 million or 4.4% of the US population. The percent of noninstitutionalized adults who had been diagnosed with emphysema was 4.1 million (2.2%) of the population. The number of deaths in the United States from chronic/unspecified bronchitis per 100,000 population is 0.2. The number of deaths per 100,000 population from emphysema is 4.2 and for other chronic lower respiratory diseases excluding asthma per 100,000 population is 36.8.[5]

These statistics reveal that COPD is responsible for a significant economic burden on society and a significant medical burden on EMS responders.

RESPIRATORY PHYSIOLOGY

Two conical lungs, whose inferior borders overlie the diaphragm and have apices that extend above the first ribs, are covered with a visceral pleura. This pleura is in close proximity to the parietal pleura, which covers the inside of the pleural cavities. Only a thin layer of pleural fluid separates the parietal and visceral pleura. The parietal layer secretes 2400 mL of fluid daily, which is reabsorbed by the visceral layer. The pleura are a dynamic layer protecting the lung and pleural cavity from infection while transmitting the forces of respiration without damage to the underlying lung parenchyma.[6,7]

The trachea bifurcates at the carina, forming the right and left mainstem bronchi. Each side continues branching multiple times eventually down to a terminal bronchiole, which enters an acinus or the beginning of the respiratory zone. The acinus has several generations of branching and ultimately ends in the terminal alveolar sacs (**Figure 40-1**).

Pulmonary circulation consists of mixed venous blood from the pulmonary arteries whose origins are in the right ventricle. After passing through the pulmonary capillary beds, where carbon dioxide is discharged and oxygen gas is absorbed via diffusion, the blood returns via the bronchial veins to the pulmonary veins and ultimately the left atrium. Pulmonary circulation is a low-pressure system with typical pulmonary artery pressures of 20 mm Hg systolic and 12 mm Hg diastolic.[8,9]

The graph shown in **Figure 40-2** gives a visual conception of the common lung volumes and measurements used in pulmonary physiology. One can see from the graph that there is always a residual amount of volume in the lungs even after a forced expiration. A typical adult will have a tidal volume of approximately 0.5 L but volumes depend on height, weight, age, gender, and disease status. Females may have a decrease in vital capacity of up to 25% of a typical male. Children typically have much smaller volumes and any calculations for respiratory interventions should be based on weight (Figure 40-2).

■ GAS EXCHANGE IN THE LUNGS

In order to understand the basic respiratory physiology, in the following discussion, a few definitions need to be introduced:

Minute ventilation: the total amount of new air moved into the respiratory passages each minute. On average this is approximately 6 L/min.

Alveolar ventilation: the amount of air reaching the alveoli per minute.

Anatomic dead space: the amount of air in the respiratory anatomy that does not participate in gas exchange (trachea, bronchi, etc).

Tidal volume: the amount of air that moves into the lungs with each breath.

Ventilation: movement of air into lungs. When discussing gas exchange, it refers to the movement of CO_2 out of the lungs.

Perfusion: movement and distribution of blood through the pulmonary circulation.

Diffusion: movement of O_2 and CO_2 across the air-blood barrier or alveolar capillary membrane. O_2 and CO_2 are exchanged via simple diffusion and passively move down a partial pressure gradient. For most individuals, the arterial blood becomes fully saturated with oxygen early in inspiration, and the rate of uptake of oxygen depends on capillary blood flow.

The diffusion capacity depends on the thickness of the alveolar wall, the area available for gas exchange, and the partial pressure difference between the two sides. If the thickness of the wall increases (pulmonary edema), or the alveolar complex is destroyed (emphysema), the diffusion capacity is lower.

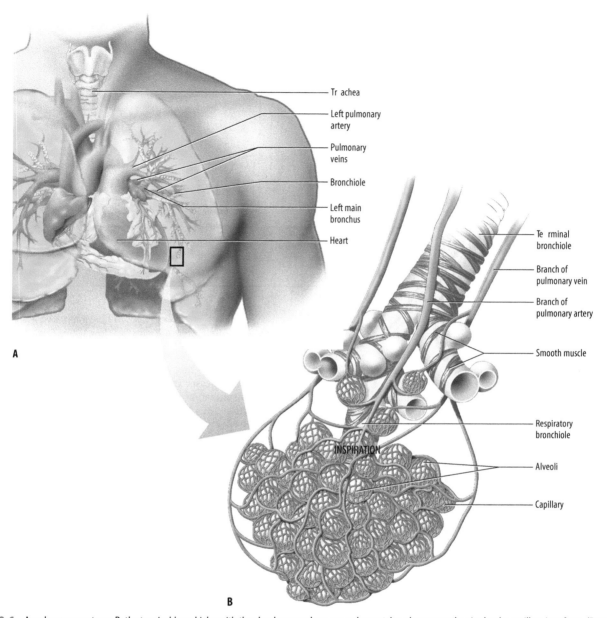

FIGURE 40-1. A: pulmonary anatomy. B: the terminal bronchioles with the alveolar sacs where gas exchange takes place across the air-alveolar capillary interfaces. (Reproduced with permission from Barrett KE, Barman SM, Boitano S, Brooks HL. Ganong's Review of Medical Physiology, 23rd ed. New York, NY: McGraw-Hill; 2010. Figure 35-1.)

CNS CONTROL OF RESPIRATORY DRIVE

The pacemaker activity for respiration is in the respiratory control centers of the brain. It is primarily an involuntary process influenced not only by neural control, but also by chemical control, some voluntary control, body temperature, drugs, pain, emotion, sleep, baroreceptors, and proprioceptors. Neural control of respiration includes factors responsible for alternating inspiration/expiration, rhythm, factors that regulate rate and depth of ventilation (vagal nerve input), and factors that modify respiratory activity, both voluntary (speech) and involuntary control (sneeze, cough).

The medullary rhythmicity area is the respiratory control center of the central nervous system located in the medulla. The medullary respiratory control center is the primary control center and provides output to the respiratory muscles.

The respiratory control center can be divided into the inspiratory center and the expiratory center. The inspiratory center spontaneously controls the diaphragm and intercostal muscles responsible for inspiration.

Two other centers in the pons, the apneustic center and the pneumotaxic center influence medullary respiratory output.

Molecules such as oxygen, carbon dioxide, and hydrogen influence respiration. Deviation from the normal concentrations of these molecules will change the rate, depth, or rhythm of respiration as sensed by chemoreceptors located in the medulla, carotid arteries, and the aortic arch (eg, elevated CO_2 or hypercapnia decreases blood pH and is sensed by chemoreceptors in the medulla). The medulla then increases the rate and depth of respiration (hyperventilation) to blow off CO_2 during expiration to return the pH to a normal or near normal range. Conversely, if CO_2 and hydrogen levels fall below the baseline level, hypocapnia may result. Hypocapnia results in slow, shallow breathing called hypoventilation. Likewise, when oxygen levels fall and carbon dioxide and pH remain normal, respiratory rate will increase until oxygen levels return to normal.

To some extent, respiration can be controlled voluntarily because of neural pathways between the cerebral cortex and the respiratory control center (eg, hyperventilation). Respiration may increase with

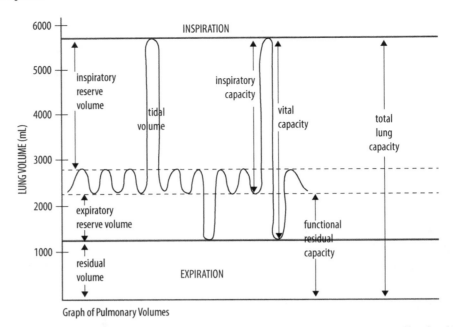

FIGURE 40-2. Lung volume is depicted in milliliters of air. Notice the sine wave of normal tidal volume as one breathing at rest interrupted by a forced inspiration, a forced expiration and then a combined maximum inspiration with forced expiration. (Reproduced with permission from Hall JE, ed. Guyton & Hall Textbook of Medical Physiology, 13th ed. Philadelphia: Elsevier; 2016. Figure 38-6. Copyright Elsevier.)

hyperthermia and decrease in response to hypothermia. Certain drugs and medications can affect respiration. For example, narcotics such as Demerol and morphine can reduce the rate and depth of breathing while adrenaline, amphetamine, and cocaine typically have the reverse effect.

Pain and emotions often increase respiration. Emotions such as crying are controlled by the hypothalamus and limbic system that, in turn, stimulate the respiratory center and increase respiration. When the pain or emotion subsides, respiration returns to normal. Baroreceptors are pressure receptors located in the carotid and aortic sinuses that sense changes in blood pressure. Changes in respiration are inversely proportional to changes in blood pressure. For example, when blood pressure increases, respiration decreases. Proprioceptors are receptors located in muscles, tendons, and joints that sense movement. During exercise, these receptors transmit signals to the respiratory center that increase the rate and depth of respiration.

COMMON CAUSES OF RESPIRATORY DISTRESS

In this section, common medical causes of respiratory distress will be presented. For each, this section will highlight the pathophysiology (causes) as well as the typical clinical presentation and general treatment.

■ COPD AND ASTHMA PATHOPHYSIOLOGY

The prevalence and incidence of asthma is very high in the Western world.[10] The number of people with asthma continues to grow. One in 12 people (about 25 million, or 8% of the population) had asthma in 2009, compared with 1 in 14 (about 20 million, or 7%) in 2001.[11]

Asthma is a disease that is reversible and episodic. It is characterized by a chronic inflammatory disorder of the airways coupled with airway hyper-responsiveness that leads to recurrent episodes of wheezing, shortness of breath, chest tightness, and coughing. Children will often be awakened from a sound sleep with an episode and it may consist primarily of coughing (cough variant asthma). These episodes are associated with reversible airflow obstruction and between acute attacks, the patient often returns to a normal respiratory pattern. Patients with persistent inflammation may have lung remodeling over time, which eventually leads to a loss of lung function. Asthma patients tend to be younger patients and are more likely to have an allergy trigger or a strong family history.

Obstructive lung disease can be classified into two categories: chronic bronchitis and emphysema. Patients with COPD have significant fixed airway obstruction that remains, even when the disease in under control. Both diseases cause chronic cough and shortness of breath. Chronic inflammation causes structural changes and irreversible airflow limitation. This can be caused by an increase in resistance of the conducting airways or an increase in compliance due to destruction of the airway walls or both. Destruction of the lung parenchyma, also by inflammatory processes, leads to the loss of alveolar attachments to the small airways and decreases lung elastic recoil; in turn, these changes diminish the ability of the airways to remain open during expiration. Often, COPD patients have right heart failure and chest remodeling. Cigarette smoking is a primary cause of COPD. Other environmental and genetic factors can cause COPD including exposure to air pollution, second-hand smoke, occupational chemicals, and a history of childhood respiratory infections.[12]

Chronic bronchitis is characterized by chronic cough and sputum production. A working definition of chronic bronchitis can be defined as a chronic, productive cough for 3 months during two successive years in which other causes for chronic cough have been excluded.[13]

Emphysema is destruction and irreversible enlargement of the air spaces distal to the terminal bronchioles. The destruction of the alveoli reduces expiratory flow by decreasing the elastic recoil present in healthy lung parenchyma. Destruction of the airspace walls is found upon histologic examination. Bullae, radiolucent areas larger than 1 cm in diameter that indicate severe local destruction, may be seen in macroscopic examination and on radiographs.

One must be cautious in diagnosing COPD in the field as other disease states may also present with breathlessness, wheezing, and sputum production. Remembering the adage, "All that wheezes is not asthma," may help keep a broadened differential.

Clinical Presentation Clinically, patients have chronic difficulty breathing that persists daily and is acutely exacerbated by an inflammatory stimulus such as an infection, allergens, or noncompliance with medications, etc. Differentiating asthma from COPD is sometimes difficult and the patient's age, medical and social history are typically helpful. Asthma patients may be younger at age of onset but that is variable. Most COPD patients will be older and may be thin, have pursed lip breathing (exhalation), as well as clubbed or stained fingertips from long-term smoking. However, many patients have both asthma and COPD. Both diseases will present with increased work of breathing, and variably cough and wheeze. Wheezing is the clinical hallmark of bronchospasm and a diagnostic sign in COPD and asthma that patients will benefit from bronchodilator therapy. However, be warned that in severe cases, patients may not be able to move enough air through the lungs to generate wheezing. Quiet lungs in the setting of respiratory distress is an ominous sign. Vital signs will commonly show an increased heart and respiratory rate as well as decreased oxygen saturations. Asthmatics can typically compensate and maintain near normal oxygenation until severe, whereas COPD patients are typically chronically hypoxic and may have low oxygen saturations at baseline.

Treatment Chronic treatment of both conditions involves inhaled bronchodilators and also the use of steroids to reduce chronic inflammation. Treatment in the acute setting is similar. The ABCs should be managed first and supplemental oxygen given. For patients at risk for immediate respiratory failure, assisting ventilations or intubation should be considered. In alert patients a trial of CPAP or BiPAP may be appropriate.[14,15] In asthma, high flow oxygen can be utilized liberally. However, in mixed disorders or COPD, oxygen should be titrated to keep pulse oximeter readings between 92% and 95%. Prolonged high flow oxygen in COPD can suppress the hypoxic respiratory drive and has been linked to worsened long-term outcomes.

Bronchodilators such as albuterol (Ventolin) and levalbuterol (Xopenex) are the mainstays of prehospital treatment and can be given in a range of dosing based on severity from a "unit dose," typically 2.5 mg of albuterol to continuous nebulizer treatments lasting 30 minutes or more and delivering 10 to 20 mg of albuterol in some cases. Providers should remember that in addition to bronchodilation, β-agonists have activity on the heart and can produce significant tachycardia and hypertension which can be harmful in some patients with cardiovascular disease. The patient should be monitored for high heart rate, significant hypertension, or signs of cardiac ischemia such as chest pain or ECG changes. Ipratropium bromide (Atrovent) is a nebulized medication adjunct that can be combined with. Atrovent works by reducing airway secretions and synergizing bronchodilatory medications. Atrovent is used primarily in the prehospital and ER setting and has been less effective in the inpatient chronic care setting.

Steroids and IV fluids are also a mainstay of treatment and can be given in a variety of doses and ranges. Chronic therapy is usually delivered via inhaled steroids. For acute treatment, methylprednisolone (Solu-Medrol) and dexamethasone (Decadron) are common choices. Whether administered orally, IV, or IM, these medications take around an hour or more for onset of action and do not offer immediate benefit. Additionally, IV volume replacement is an important consideration as most patients with respiratory distress are volume depleted from increased respiratory losses and reduced oral fluid intake.

Severe COPD and asthma that do not respond to conventional treatment may require other β-agents such as subcutaneous epinephrine, terbutaline, or in some cases an IV infusion of those medications. Again, this carries a risk of significant increases in cardiac demand.

Lastly, the patient with complete respiratory failure and severe alterations in mental status will require intubation. However, intubation should be considered the last resort for obstructive lung disease patients. Mechanical ventilation of COPD and asthma patients is difficult and perilous. Responders must remember that air trapping continues to occur and ventilation requires more time for exhalation. Normal intubated patients require approximately 1 second for inhalation and 2 seconds for exhalation, thus a 1:2 ratio. COPD and asthma patients may benefit from a ratio of 1:3 or more requiring slower ventilation rates and making oxygenation difficult. Continue aggressive treatment for bronchospasm even after intubation with in-line β-agonist nebulizer treatments and continued IV medications.[16]

▪ PULMONARY EDEMA AND CHF PATHOPHYSIOLOGY

Just as gases can diffuse across the thin alveolar membrane in the lungs, so can fluids. However, in the case of fluids this is typically due to hydrostatic or osmotic forces. Any fluid, excluding pus/blood, in the lungs can be termed "pulmonary edema" although the term is classically used to describe fluid that enters the alveoli from the capillary circulation. Pulmonary edema has many causes ranging from heart failure to alveolar injury (such as in ARDS, inhalation injury, burns, etc) or overly aggressive resuscitation with IV fluids. Congestive heart failure (CHF) is a common cause of pulmonary edema encountered by EMS. The right heart pumps blood into the pulmonary circulation and an impaired left heart is unable to "pump out" blood from the right heart. The high pressure in the pulmonary circulation causes fluid to shift into the alveoli. Left-sided heart failure produces pulmonary edema and symptoms whereas right heart failure produces the peripheral signs of heart failure, leg swelling, etc. Most patients have impairment of both sides of the heart and left-sided heart failure in the United States is most commonly due to ischemic heart disease (CAD).

Clinical Presentation EMS providers may encounter patients with new onset or existing CHF. Exacerbations may come on abruptly or gradually worsen over several days. Patients with CHF may give a worsening history of the disease as well as weight gain or increased peripheral edema in the time period preceding the trouble. Frequently, poor adherence to medications, diuretics, or excessive fluid or salt intake can cause CHF exacerbations. Patients will typically appear with increased work of breathing and distress. Coughing may be present and may produce classic "pink frothy" sputum, giving them a nickname of "pink puffer." Vital signs are highly variable depending on how poor the patient's cardiac function is. Heart rate and blood pressure can range from high to low. And oxygen saturations may be low or normal. The most complicated CHF patient is one who has significant respiratory distress paired with hypotension and bradycardia. This is a clear sign of a very sick heart and contraindicates many mainstays of treatment for CHF. The lung examination classically reveals coarse crackles in the lung bases, formally called rales. This sound is produced from fluid in the small airways.

Treatment The goal for CHF and pulmonary edema is fundamentally simple—get the fluid back into the circulation and out of the alveoli. The ABCs must be managed and if airway or breathing adequacy is questioned, CPAP, BiPAP, or intubation may be indicated.[17,18] For pulmonary edema from a non-CHF source, that is, IV fluids, altitude, irritants, etc, treatment involves stopping the offending agent and using positive pressure ventilation. Every CHF patients should have supplemental oxygen and positive pressure ventilation via NIPPV. For the "warm" CHF patient—those with adequate heart rate and blood pressure—the addition of nitrates is indicated. A common prehospital regimen is up to three sublingual nitroglycerin tablets followed by some nitroglycerin paste administration. For advanced providers, establishing a nitroglycerin IV infusion is also an option that allows rapid titration of treatment. Remember to ask all patients about use of erectile dysfunction drugs such as Viagra or Cialis. For the "cold" CHF patient—those with bradycardia or hypotension—treatment is far more difficult. Oxygen can still be used but nitrates must initially be avoided and CPAP is questionable based on its tendency to reduce venous return and lower blood pressure. Intubation should be performed if airway patency and breathing are not adequate and once done, hypotension may need to be treated initially with judicious IV fluid boluses if any suspicion of "intravascular" volume depletion is present (ie, recent hx of vomiting, diarrhea, etc). Vasopressors may be needed to support blood pressure. Dopamine is a good choice because of its positive effect on blood pressure, heart rate, and cardiac contractility as well. Once blood pressure and heart rate are corrected, CPAP and nitrates can carefully be administered to help mobilize pulmonary edema.[19]

▪ LUNG MALIGNANCY PATHOPHYSIOLOGY

Cancer remains the second most common cause of death in the United States and lung cancer remains in the top five malignancies.[20] At present, EMS providers render care to a large geriatric population with a significant incidence of lung malignancy. Lung malignancy is mentioned in this chapter because it presents with a variety of features that cause respiratory distress, ranging from acute to more chronic. Malignancy can cause bleeding, inflammation, physical obstruction, and mass effects that all reduce functional lung capacity or cause other problems such as pulmonary edema or pneumothorax.

Clinical Presentation For many patients, a nagging cough, worsening shortness of breath, or hemoptysis (coughing up blood) may be the first signs that lead to a diagnosis of lung cancer. For others, worsening disease may produce symptoms that mimic obstructive lung disease, CHF, or predispose the patient to recurrent infections like pneumonia. For patients with existing lung malignancy, the clinical presentation is highly variable. The above features may produce COPD or CHF type symptoms with wheezing, rales or rhonchi, and increased work of breathing. Decreased immune function in the lungs can lead to infection with a clinical picture of pneumonia with sputum, fever, and worsening shortness of breath. Also, unlike some other respiratory illness, the malignancy can erode structures within the lungs. Spontaneous pneumothorax or erosion into blood vessels producing massive bleeding or hemothorax is possible. Patients may have massive hemoptysis (bloody sputum) that cannot be controlled and compromises the airway.

Treatment Treatment of symptoms is the best approach. Supplemental oxygen provides a great deal of comfort for most patients with lung malignancy. Albuterol or other bronchodilatory medications should be used for wheezing and steroids may have some role in reducing inflammation. Pulmonary edema treatment is best accomplished with CPAP as other measures that would work on CHF-like nitrates and diuretics are less effective. IV fluids and pain medication should also be considerations but not in amounts that will depress or labor breathing further. Intubation is indicated for complete respiratory failure but the EMS provider should ensure that the patient does not have a DNR order or specific directive against mechanical ventilation. Intubation may also be required for massive hemoptysis if the airway cannot be kept clear. Evidence of pneumothorax should be treated with pleural decompression of the affected side. In lung cancer patients who request palliative treatment, oxygen, CPAP, and pain medication is the mainstay of treatment.

ACUTE AND CHRONIC RESPIRATORY CONDITIONS

A detailed list of causes of respiratory distress and the timeline associated with each is presented in Chapter 34. Related to this, the EMS responder must be able to differentiate between chronic stable disease and acute exacerbations. Asthma, COPD, and CHF patients all have baseline daily symptoms. This will include physiologic compensation mechanisms and routine medications for control of these disease processes. For all of these patients, the EMS provider must also differentiate between respiratory distress and respiratory failure in these patients.

Asthma patients with chronic disease may appear normal and have normal function outside of exacerbations. Asthma onset has a typical bimodal onset presenting either in early childhood or later in adult life. Most patients will develop symptoms such as coughing and wheezing, especially in response to allergens, infection, and exercise. Diagnosis is clinical with a history, physical examination, and pulmonary function testing (PFT) for confirmation if needed. Asthmatics may have a family history or also suffer from other common ailments such as allergies, eczema, or other inflammatory conditions such as arthritis and irritable bowel syndromes. Daily therapy with long-acting bronchodilators and inhaled steroids produce good symptom control for many patients.

COPD although similar to asthma in clinical presentation has a different pathophysiology and course. Most patients develop COPD from chronic lung irritants, most commonly cigarette smoking in the United States. Some are from direct use and others from heavy second-hand smoke in households with smokers, etc. Others may have injury from workplace environmental exposures or chronic infections. A small portion of the population may have a condition called α_1-antitrypsin (A1AT) deficiency where the elastic fibers surrounding the alveoli and bronchioles age and breakdown prematurely. This is genetic in nature and not related to exposure. Generally, COPD will present after the fifth to sixth decades of life and will continue to worsen if the person continues to smoke, etc. The exception is the A1AT patient who may have disease at a younger age. Chronic therapy involves the same as for asthma patients, but also with the addition of ipratropium bromide (Atrovent) inhalers and then typically requiring supplemental home oxygen at some point. Both asthma and COPD patients are extremely sensitive to any decreases in baseline lung function, with infection being one of the most common causes of deterioration and exacerbation from baseline.[21]

Congestive heart failure is also a slowly progressive and insidious disease that is typically encountered later in life. As a patient's left heart function declines either from heart disease, pulmonary disease, or other causes, pulmonary symptoms worsen. Depending on overall heart function and the ability to contract and eject blood, the ejection fraction (EF), patients will have variable needs and treatment. Mild CHF may produce minimal daily symptoms and may be controlled with oral diuretics and dietary fluid and salt restriction. Severe CHF may require numerous medications including aggressive diuretics, hormone modifying agents, and long-acting oral nitrates. Many patients will become oxygen dependent and have significant distress when trying to sleep, lying flat, etc. Many CHF patients may already use CPAP when sleeping, or in some severe cases, continually during the day. Acute CHF exacerbations may result from a variety of problems ranging from superimposed infection, worsening heart disease (such as silent MI, etc), or commonly medication and/or dietary noncompliance. Many EMS providers may answer calls for other complaints and find patients in CHF decompensated states.[22] The most severe CHF patients in end-stage heart failure may require portable IV infusions of medications to increase heart rate and contractile function like Milrinone and some may have implanted portable ventricular assist devices like the LVAD. Patients with an LVAD or similar device have an implanted impeller or other pumping device in the left heart that is surgically implanted and connected to an external battery/control pack that is connected to wires externalized through the chest. These are typically installed in patients who have failed all other therapy and are end stage. Recent research has shown that LVADs may provide up to another year of life for end-stage CHF patients and that number continues to increase.[23] Of note, patients with such devices may not have a palpable pulse due to the continuous flow of blood from the LVAD as opposed to the contractile flow normally produced by the heart. EMS responders should ask the patient or immediate family for help troubleshooting problems with the LVAD as they have been extensively trained by the manufacturer.

Remember that in cases of chronic disease, the human body can compensate for wide variations in disease and physiology given enough time. Acute illness finds the body unprepared to compensate and rapidly throws off body physiology, compensatory mechanisms, and defenses. When this happens, chronic respiratory conditions can turn into respiratory failure.

▓ ACUTE AND CHRONIC RESPIRATORY FAILURE

Respiratory failure is a syndrome rather than a single disease process and the overall frequency of respiratory failure is not well known.[24]

The mortality rate associated with respiratory failure depends on the etiology. For acute respiratory distress syndrome, the mortality rate is approximately 45% in most studies.[25] For an acute exacerbation of COPD, the mortality rate is approximately 30%.

Respiratory failure is situation whereby the system fails in oxygenation, ventilation, or both. In practice, respiratory failure is defined by a PaO_2 of less than 60 mm Hg or a $PaCO_2$ of more than 50 mm Hg. Respiratory failure may be acute or chronic. Acute respiratory failure may present with dramatic changes in acid-base status. It usually develops over minutes to hours and the pH is usually less than 7.3. Hypoventilation, V/Q mismatch, and shunt are the most common pathophysiologic causes of acute respiratory failure.

Chronic respiratory failure is found to have less dramatic acid-base changes. It usually develops over weeks or months and allows for renal compensation and an increase in bicarbonate retention with a less dramatic decrease in pH. Chronic respiratory failure may actually go undetected if careful observation is not included in your examination or review of previous health evaluations is not undertaken. The clinical presentation is important and chronic hypoxemia as manifested by polycythemia or cor pulmonale suggests a chronic nature.

Respiratory failure is classified as either hypoxemic or hypercapnic and may be acute or chronic. Type 1 respiratory failure, the most common form, is hypoxemic and is characterized by a PaO_2 of less than 60 mm Hg with a low or normal $PaCO_2$. Cardiogenic or noncardiogenic pulmonary edema, pneumonia, and pulmonary hemorrhage are examples of acute lung disease that causes type 1 respiratory failure.

A $PaCO_2$ of more than 50 mm Hg characterizes hypercapnic respiratory failure, or type 2 respiratory failure. Hypoxemia is common in these patients. The acid-base status depends on the level of bicarbonate which, in turn, is dependent on the duration of hypercapnia. Drug overdose, neuromuscular disease, COPD, asthma, and chest wall abnormalities are common etiologies of this particular type of respiratory failure.

OTHER ACUTE MEDICAL CAUSES OF RESPIRATORY DISTRESS

Acute medical causes of respiratory distress are those that arise within minutes to hours to days and can be single in presentation or superimposed on chronic existing disease.

RESPIRATORY INFECTIONS PHYSIOLOGY

Pulmonary infections are one of the major causes of acute respiratory distress and involve all age groups, but again are more prevalent in the young and the old. Children and adults suffer from all manner of pathogens that affect the lungs including viruses (likely the most common) as well as bacteria and less commonly fungal infections. All are capable of causing lung inflammation, causing edema and swelling of the airways and causing pulmonary edema or secretions that block air exchange in the alveoli.

Clinical Presentation For viral respiratory infections, usually the triad of "cough, coryza (runny nose, watery eyes), and fever" are present. Cough is a uniform feature of almost all lung infections as inflammation promotes coughing and expulsion of mucus and other infectious debris in the lungs. Cough in children can be classified as "brassy," "barky," or sometimes having a "seal bark" type quality. A barky or seal bark cough is commonly associated with upper respiratory infections that inflame the larynx such as croup and respiratory syncytial virus (RSV). Viral respiratory infections are volatile and may present rapidly with many patients becoming ill in as little as 24 hours.

Bacterial lung infections are commonly termed *pneumonia* and in contrast may take days to progress in severity. There are numerous pathogens that affect human lungs and the disease course ranges from mild with recovery within a week to those that are uniformly fatal like *Bacillus anthracis* (anthrax). Clinically cough is still a major feature, deep and "chesty" in nature, often with production of thick foul smelling sputum. Patients will develop progressive symptoms of fever, malaise, and chills.

Fungal and other atypical lung infections tend to be less common and are usually confined to immunocompromised patients, such as those with HIV or diabetes. Also patients who have structural lung disease like chronic bronchitis or cystic fibrosis are at increased risk. Symptoms in these patients may be vague with fevers, cough, and malaise existing for weeks to months. Tuberculosis is one such infection caused by the organism *Mycobacterium tuberculosis* that has features of both a bacteria and a fungal organism. The incidence of tuberculosis in the United States continues to be very low, 3.8 cases per 100,000 persons in 2009, thanks to advanced surveillance and monitoring of cases. Foreign born or visiting persons from other countries where tuberculosis is prevalent may bring the disease to the United States. Immunocompromised patients are also at increased risk. Clinical symptoms include chronic cough with symptoms for weeks to months, night sweats, weight loss, and bloody sputum are all hallmarks (although this can present in many pulmonary diseases).[26]

Epiglottitis is a bacterial upper airway infection that affects mainly the epiglottis and larynx, causing swelling of the upper airway, epiglottis, and glottic opening. Previously seen mainly in children, the Hib and other vaccines have reduced the incidence and shifted this disease toward adults. Children may present with high fevers, malaise, severe sore throat, and a minimum of cough. They also fail to swallow saliva and airway secretions producing drooling. Most will sit up in a "tripod" fashion. Adults may have a similar complaint with a hoarse voice and complaints of severe sore throat.

Respiratory Infection Treatment Treatment for patients with acute pulmonary infections remains the same regardless of the etiology. Protection of the rescuer is paramount. EMS providers should wear PPE that provides protection for contact/droplet and airborne pathogens such as a gown, gloves, and an N95 respirator mask. Every patient with a presumed infectious respiratory disease should be treated as hazardous until proven otherwise. Once the patient has been assessed, if their condition permits, it is simplest to place an N95 respirator mask on the patient as opposed to the entire crew. This also prevents droplet spread of infection to ambulance surfaces and at the receiving hospital.

Initial assessment should focus on ensuring that ABCs are intact. High flow oxygen can be provided and if assessment reveals impending respiratory failure, NIPPV or intubation should be considered. Low pulse oximetry readings should respond to high flow supplemental oxygen. Patients with hypoxia refractory to supplemental oxygen administration should be reassessed to ensure work of breathing and tidal volume is adequate, if not, again NIPPV or intubation should be considered. Breath sounds will frequently be coarse and reveal rhonchi or rales. In a patient with no history of CAD or heart failure, this frequently is due to secretions and mucus from the inflammatory process. If wheezing or stridor is present, an inhaled β_2 agonist such as albuterol should be considered; the use of Atrovent may have benefit as well. IV fluids should be administered in boluses as needed for dehydration and hypotension. The use of steroids in the EMS setting is controversial and may not be beneficial. Some patients may benefit from steroids but their impact is generally in the inhospital setting over the total course of treatment. Steroids may be more beneficial in patients with superimposed asthma or COPD.

Patients, specifically children, with suspected epiglottitis or other upper airway inflammation are at high risk of airway compromise and have different treatment priorities. Excessive agitation and crying on part of the patient can cause laryngospasm or complete obstruction of the airway. Measures should be taken to keep these patients calm and comfortable and any treatment causing agitation or distress should be avoided. In patients with suspected epiglottitis, it is acceptable to calmly transport them in the parent's arms in a position of comfort. Supplemental humidified oxygen or β_2- agonists can be provided via blow-by technique if this does not agitate the patient. However, in the background, the EMS provider should have an immediate plan in place for placement of a needle cricothyrotomy or a surgical airway in older patients should the airway become obstructed. The receiving hospital should be informed of the EMS provider's clinical suspicion so that personnel and equipment can be readied for any needed airway procedures. Adult treatment is similar to pneumonia as above.

PULMONARY EMBOLUS PHYSIOLOGY

A pulmonary embolus, commonly termed PE, is an obstruction that blocks blood flow to a portion of the lung's circulation ranging from severe to clinically insignificant. The blockage can be variable, most commonly being a "thrombus" or blood clot, but can also be an "embolus" such as dislodged cholesterol, air, or amniotic fluid. A PE can typically be found in the pulmonary arteries or the smaller pulmonary arterioles that carry deoxygenated blood to the heart. This obstruction, if large enough, causes a backup of blood flow into the right heart and prevents efficient oxygenation.

Clinical Presentation The patient's clinical symptoms are determined in large part by the size of the PE and the amount of blood flow that it obstructs. Patients may have tiny PEs that remain unnoticed whereas large PEs that obstruct the main pulmonary trunk frequently cause immediate death. Although PE is a great disease mimic with many presentations, patients classically present with sudden onset of shortness of breath and frequently chest pain, cough, and sometimes bloody sputum. PEs can also present with syncope, stroke-like symptoms, seizures, and other complaints that make PE diagnosis challenging. PE should always be on the EMS provider's differential for sudden onset shortness of breath. A good clinical history may reveal risk factors for increased blood clotting such as prolonged immobility or recent surgery, malignancy, smoking, use of birth control hormones, pregnancy, or a past history of blood clots or hypercoagulable state. Vital signs are typically abnormal with mild tachycardia being a major feature, often in addition to low oxygen saturations on pulse oximetry. Another feature is the 12-lead ECG. Although only present in up to 20% of patients, the "S1Q3T3" pattern may be noted with an S-wave in lead I, a pathologic Q-wave and an inverted or abnormal T wave in lead III. However, this is not sensitive or specific and the ECG is more valuable in ruling out other causes of symptoms such as acute MI or other arrhythmia. Lastly, patients with significant hypoxia will show a poor response to high flow oxygen with continued low oxygen saturations.

Treatment for Pulmonary Embolus Treatment for patients with suspected pulmonary embolus is supportive. ABCs should be ensured and breathing can initially be supported with high flow oxygen or NIPPV if desired although it is not clear whether this is highly effective. Intubation may be required. Circulation is frequently an issue and both tachycardia and hypotension may be encountered. In most cases, the tachycardia is sinus and is compensatory; efforts at slowing the heart rate may be detrimental. Blood pressure can be treated initially with crystalloid IV fluid boluses taking care not to precipitate pulmonary edema and after adequate volume is restored. Vasopressors such as dopamine or norepinephrine may be required to support blood pressure. Limited prehospital treatment options are available for patients with severe PE. Rapid transport to the hospital is required for unstable patients where blood thinning agents such as heparin may be used, and more aggressive treatments such as clot lysis with tPA or endovascular procedures to "retrieve" the clot. EMS providers with routine long transport times and a tPA procedure for STEMI patients may want to discuss tPA options with their medical director for PE.[27]

MEDICAL, NONPULMONARY CAUSES OF RESPIRATORY DISTRESS

Not all patients with a subjective complaint of "shortness of breath" or with visible increased work of breathing have a pulmonary problem. Any variation in oxygen delivery, mechanical air movement, or circulation of blood will cause symptoms.

MECHANICAL DYSFUNCTION

Any physical restriction on chest wall movement or cause that obstructs this process can cause shortness of breath and increased work of breathing. Commonly this can come from injury to the ribs with resultant pain and "splinting," injury to the diaphragm muscle (either trauma or nerve innervation), or increased abdominal pressure. Any increased abdominal pressure will be translated up to the diaphragm, from either hiatal hernias, abdominal fluid–like ascites, or masses/bowel obstruction, etc. In small children, excessive crying and "air swallowing" can produce enough pressure and displacement to cause respiratory distress.

CIRCULATORY AND METABOLIC DYSFUNCTION

Patients with high metabolic demands will commonly have what appears to be respiratory distress or tachypnea. High metabolic states create wastes such as CO_2 that must be eliminated. They body will increase the breathing rate to compensate. The best example of this is a patient with diabetic ketoacidosis (DKA). Fever is another cause, especially in children.

Abnormal pulmonary circulation can cause respiratory distress as well. Any factor that disrupts or shunts blood away from the pulmonary circulation will cause symptoms. Examples include pulmonary emboli that we have discussed already and other circulatory shunts where arterial and venous blood mixes together. An example of this is the dialysis patient who may form a large fistula allowing blood to mix and bypass the pulmonary circulation.

For most patients with nonrespiratory causes of shortness of breath, maximization of oxygenation is the main priority. Usually little can be done about things like shunts or hiatal hernias except to place the patient in a position of comfort and give high flow oxygen. If breathing and oxygenation are completely inadequate, mechanical ventilation should be considered.

FOREIGN BODY AIRWAY OBSTRUCTION

Foreign body airway obstruction affects all age groups but are most common in the small children and older adults. Small toys, pills, buttons, coins, and other small objects are frequently encountered by toddlers and small children and can readily turn into an acute airway obstruction. Elderly patients will commonly present with choking episodes during mealtime and may have a food bolus obstruction. Children may choke on food items as well and objects that fit snugly into the pediatric larynx and trachea may be difficult to remove. Examples are foods such as peanuts, grapes, and hot dogs. Parents should be cautioned to avoid these foods or cut them lengthwise to decrease the diameter. Dental appliances such as bridges and partial teeth are a common cause of choking in the elderly as well.

The clinical presentation typically usually involves a sudden onset of either complete airway obstruction, with apnea, cyanosis, and decompensation, or possibly the acute onset of coughing and stridor. Especially for children, the actual event may not be witnessed and the care provider may find the patient unresponsive or in extremis. In contrast, adult patients usually present with a history of eating or ingestion. Exceptions to these cases are intoxicated or impaired patients with disabilities who may not be able to summon help or give a history.

Management should follow the American Heart Association algorithm where the EMS provider must promptly analyze the situation and determine that a foreign body airway obstruction is likely to be present. For awake children and adults, age appropriate abdominal thrusts should be administered. The EMS provider should be prepared for the patient to decompensate and be ready to provide additional care. For the unresponsive patient, American Heart Association BLS CPR measures should be initiated. Advanced rescuers may try direct visualization of the foreign body under direct laryngoscopy with a laryngoscope and removal with Magill forceps. As a last resort, a surgical airway may be considered for obstructions that cannot be removed.[28]

TOXIC INHALATION AND ASPHYXIANTS

The EMS provider may encounter patients with respiratory distress due to toxic inhalations and either accidental or recreational exposure to asphyxiants. The complete range of toxic gases and inhalants is far too broad to be addressed in this book but can be classified into one of a few main categories. Simple asphyxiants cause harm by displacing oxygen but are relatively inert and pose no overall toxic role or cause physiologic damage. Good examples of these are the inert industrial gases such as helium, argon, nitrogen, and carbon dioxide. In high enough concentration, these all displace oxygen, causing respiratory distress, hypoxia, and eventually unresponsiveness and death.

Other gases are cellular asphyxiants that alter the way oxygen is used at the cellular level. Examples of this include the inhalation of products of combustion. Typically gases from a residential house fire contain both carbon monoxide and cyanide. Both of these agents prevent oxygen from being used by individual cells. Cell metabolism becomes anaerobic and generates large amounts of acidic waste, causing metabolic acidosis. Other gases react with the lining of the alveoli, damaging the surface for gas exchange. Examples of these gases are ammonia, chlorine, and phosgene. Many toxins affect multiple body systems and areas.

Regardless of the exposure, strict precautions must be observed and only trained rescuers should access and treat patients until proper decontamination has been done. Patients with toxic inhalations may continue to "off-gas" or exhale toxins even after being decontaminated externally. Adequate ventilation, in-line filters, or scrubbers should be used to deal with exhaled gases if indicated. Treatment for victims of simple asphyxiants involves immediate removal from the agent and supportive ventilation and oxygenation. The EMS provider must always suspect the presence of other gases or contaminants are involved until proven otherwise.

Patients exposed to cellular toxins such as cyanide may rapidly decline and become critically decompensated. Toxins may cause airway edema and swelling, necessitating early intubation. Aggressive ventilation, fluid, and blood pressure correction may be needed. If available, a toxin-specific antidote should be employed such as a cyanide kit or other tool to "reverse or block" the cellular effects of the toxin. The local HAZMAT authority or the Poison Control Center should be contacted in all of these cases for treatment information.

INDICATIONS AND STRATEGIES FOR AIRWAY MANAGEMENT

The decision to intervene on behalf of a patient and manage the airway is broad, ranging from clear indications for patients in cardiac arrest to other more difficult decisions for patients with a potential for deterioration. The actual techniques and considerations are discussed in Chapter 59; however, we will discuss the theory here of when to intervene and with what approach.

First and foremost, the decision to secure and manage a patient's airway is one that must be taken with great care and concern. Especially in the case of rapid sequence (RSI) or pharmaceutically assisted intubation (PAI), the EMS provider is making a decision to take away whatever spontaneous or self-initiated airway support and breathing the patient has and makes a commitment to replace that with what must be a secure, effective, and sufficient airway and ventilation strategy. This decision cannot be taken lightly.

NONINVASIVE POSITIVE PRESSURE VENTILATION

Noninvasive positive pressure ventilation (NIPPV), either bilevel positive airway pressure (BiPAP) or constant positive airway pressure (CPAP) has continued to revolutionize the treatment of respiratory distress. NIPPV is a very effective treatment adjunct for almost any patient with difficulty breathing provided that they are awake and alert, able to protect their own airway, and have a sufficient baseline level of spontaneous breathing.

Originally indicated for CHF, research about NIPPV has found it to be effective in patients with asthma, COPD, pneumonia, drowning, etc. CPAP or BiPAP fits over the patients' nose and/or mouth and provides a consistent level of airway pressure. Remember from the physiology section above, during end expiration and before active inhalation, airway pressures reach zero and then become negative. CPAP or BiPAP negates this pressure and keeps small airways and alveoli "propped" open, allowing more time for gas exchange and recruiting inactive or collapsed lung segments. Also, the pressure provides a positive gradient "pushing" fluid (water, serum, etc) back into the circulation.

It should be considered in any respiratory distress patient who continues to decline or worsen despite medical therapy and in most cases should be attempted before intubation as many times intubation can be delayed or avoided. NIPPV can be problematic in patients with hypotension as it worsens the venous return to the heart and may lower blood pressure but otherwise has few contraindications. Also, recall that any type of positive pressure ventilation will worsen pneumothorax.

Chapter 59 discusses the mechanical properties and techniques for the use of NIPPV.[29,30]

INDICATIONS FOR INTUBATION AND MECHANICAL VENTILATION

In general, patients require mechanical ventilation due to failure to ventilate, failure to oxygenate, or airway problems. The decision to intubate is sometimes difficult and clinical experience is invaluable for those situations that do not have an immediate yes or no decision tree. Most patients who need to be intubated have one or more of the following indications:

1. Inability to maintain the airway patency or airway obstruction (eg, acute laryngeal edema, anaphylaxis, airway trauma, and epiglottitis)
2. Inability to protect the airway against aspiration (loss of gag reflex)
3. Anticipated loss of control of the airway (eg, deteriorating mental status, laryngeal edema, neck trauma, circumferential neck or facial burns, acute stridor, etc)
4. Inability to ventilate (inability to blow off CO_2)
5. Inability to oxygenate

Inability to ventilate is characterized by reduced alveolar ventilation which manifests as an increase in the $PaCO_2$ >50 mm Hg. This may be due to neurological problems (including head injury, spinal cord injury, CVA, etc), myopathic disorders (including myasthenia gravis or an exacerbation of multiple sclerosis), structural or anatomical problems (flail chest, pleural effusions, pneumothorax or hemothorax, airway obstruction), or gas exchange problems (ARDS, pulmonary embolism, COPD exacerbation).

Inability to oxygenate, leading to hypoxemia, primarily occurs at the pulmonary capillary-alveolar interface. This can be due to diffusion defects, which interferes with gas exchange. This can be caused by thickening of the alveolar wall (pulmonary fibrosis) or increased extracellular fluid (pulmonary edema). Ventilation perfusion mismatch (V/Q mismatch or "shunting") can also lead to the inability to oxygenate. Both "dead-space ventilation" (alveoli are perfused but not ventilated) and "shunt" (alveoli are ventilated but not perfused) can be found in the same lung. Inability to oxygenate can also occur at the cellular level, due to poisoning by hazardous exposures such as cyanide.

In addition, there may be a problem with oxygen delivery and utilization: if the cardiac output is low, if the patient is edematous, or if a specific pathology interferes with the normal processes. For example, an acute MI with resulting poor cardiac output would interfere with delivery and poor oxygenation would result.

Patients are usually intubated for controlled mechanical ventilation as an endotracheal tube or tracheostomy will provide a good seal for controlled ventilation: inspired volumes and pressures are consistent, compared with noninvasive methods.

Additionally, for the EMS provider, the EMS medical director may have a specific set of qualifications and standards for proceeding with intubation. This may include a checklist or a requirement to contact online medical control prior to proceeding. In general, the whole patient picture must be considered to time intubation effectively, and the key is to identify early signs of respiratory failure and intervene before complete failure occurs and cardiopulmonary arrest ensues.

INTUBATION AND VENTILATION MODALITIES

Once the decision has been made to perform advanced airway management, the modality becomes based on the certification level and skills set of the EMS provider. For EMT or ECA providers who are limited to "assisting ventilation" with a BVM only, this technique is difficult but can be effective with patient cooperation. The prevalence of CPAP and BiPAP has nearly replaced this technique.

EMS responders trained in endotracheal intubation can proceed once the patient has become obtunded, losing protective airway reflexes, or once the decision has been made to proceed with RSI/PAI.

For all providers, the use of the supraglottic airway has been in practice in EMS for some time. Products such as the Combitube, King airway, and other supraglottic products have traditionally been used as rescue airways for failed intubation but are now effective enough to find a place in the toolbox of many EMS providers. Many EMS medical directors grant authorization to EMT providers for placement of supraglottic airways. Although not the "gold standard" for tracheal isolation and prevention of aspiration, today's supraglottic airways have a proven track record for ease and rapidity of use as well as high success rates for ventilation. Remember that even in cardiac arrest, current trends are moving toward rapid placement of a supraglottic airway.

■ PHARMACEUTICALLY ASSISTED OR RAPID SEQUENCE INTUBATION

Rapid sequence (RSI) or pharmaceutically assisted intubation (PAI) is another tool the EMS provider has for treating respiratory emergencies. The use of RSI and in some literature endotracheal intubation in the prehospital setting is a topic of great debate. Certain EMS medical directors do not grant this right and other health care professional organizations believe that RSI and/or intubation is too specialized and complicated for prehospital use.[31] In light of this, the EMS industry must be very judicious about when and how RSI is utilized. In well-trained hands, RSI is effective and may improve intubation rates.[32] One can compare RSI to a game of "Russian Roulette" where a bullet is loaded into the chamber of a gun and the revolver chamber is spun randomly. When the EMS provider sedates and paralyzes a patient, removing all of their protective airway reflexes and any ability to spontaneously breathe, the gun is loaded and cocked. If the EMS provider is then unable to either place an airway or ventilate the patient, the result is as deadly as the proverbial "bullet to the head." EMS providers with RSI privileges must be well trained, proficient, understand the mechanics and medications, and also know when not to use RSI techniques. If assessment of the airway and patient reveals a low probability for successful ventilation or intubation, it is best to consider another method.

■ RSI PHARMACOLOGY

RSI or PAI consists of one central theory—using pharmaceutical medications to remove consciousness, muscle tone, and in most cases, protective airway reflexes to allow the passage of an endotracheal tube on an otherwise awake patient. Usually a two-drug combination is used with the initial medication being the "induction" agent and the second being the "paralytic."

The induction agent is typically a strong sedative or dissociative drug that at the intended dose produces unconsciousness, amnesia, relaxation, and in some cases, analgesia. Different medications can produce these results and some common ones are etomidate (Amidate), midazolam (Versed), Propofol, ketamine, and in some cases, high-dose opiates such as fentanyl or morphine. All of these medications at the intended doses produce relaxation, amnesia, and unconsciousness. However, only some have pain modulating properties. They all have side effects including variable amounts of respiratory depression, hypotension, and some cardiovascular side effects ranging from tachycardia to bradycardia. The choice of induction drug varies and can be selected based on the desired side effects or lack thereof. Etomidate and midazolam are some of the most common used medications in the prehospital environment.

The second medication is the paralytic that creates a blockade between the muscle cells and the innervating nerve cell, called the neuromuscular junction (NMJ). Two major classes exist, being depolarizing and nondepolarizing paralytics. Only one major depolarizing paralytic is in widespread use today, succinylcholine. This medication works by firing or "depolarizing" all of the skeletal muscle cells in the body and keeping them in a "refractory" state where they will not fire again until the medication wears off. Succinylcholine is well adapted to RSI because the onset of action is very rapid (15-60 seconds) depending on the dose and normally wears off within 10 to 15 minutes. This allows the intubation to occur and then if complications arise, usually the patient can be ventilated until the

effects are gone. Succinylcholine, however, is complicated by a large side effect and contraindication profile; most of which relate to its tendency to elevate serum potassium. Thus it cannot be used in renal patients or other patients who might already have high serum potassium (hyperkalemia). The nondepolarizing paralytics also work by blocking the NMJ but do not cause the depolarization of the muscle cells. This eliminates the concerns about potassium release and does not raise the serum potassium level. There are many different types of nondepolarizing agents and selection is based mainly on the desired duration of action. The downside of many nondepolarizing agents is the slow onset of action (1-3 minutes) and the long duration of action (30 minutes-1/2 hours). Rocuronium (Zemuron) known quaintly as "rock" is a favored prehospital medication as at the proper dose, the onset of action is rapid and similar to succinylcholine. However, rocuronium does last two to three times longer than succinylcholine depending on the dose. It is important to know that there is no reversal agent for succinylcholine and few EMS services carry medications to reverse the nondepolarizing agents.

After intubation, the patient must be continued on an agent(s) that provide continued sedation and analgesia as the original RSI medications will wear off typically within 5 to 10 minutes. Favored regimens are a combination of versed/fentanyl or propofol. Patients should be secured to avoid inadvertent removal of the IV lines or the ET tube. In addition, judicious IV fluids should be continued as most RSI and sedation medications cause vasodilatation and hypotension.

KEY POINTS

- COPD and asthma levy a significant burden on the EMS system and the health care system in general
- COPD, which encompasses chronic bronchitis, emphysema, and asthma, is an obstructive pulmonary disease with an inflammatory component.
- Emphysema and chronic bronchitis are irreversible, progressive diseases; asthma is reversible unless lung remodeling takes place.
- The physiology of respiration is a complex process that has multiple structural, chemical, and neurologic controls.
- Respiratory failure is situation whereby the system fails in oxygenation, ventilation or both.
- The decision to intervene on behalf of a patient and manage the airway is broad, ranging from clear indications for patients in cardiac arrest to other more difficult decisions for patients with a potential for deterioration.
- Noninvasive positive pressure ventilation (NIPPV), either bilevel positive airway pressure (BiPAP) or constant positive airway pressure (CPAP), has continued to revolutionize the treatment of respiratory distress.
- NIPPV is a very effective treatment adjunct for almost any patient with difficulty breathing provided that they are awake and alert, able to protect their own airway, and have a sufficient baseline level of spontaneous breathing.
- Originally indicated for CHF, research about NIPPV has found it to be effective in patients with asthma, COPD, pneumonia, drowning, etc.
- Most patients who need to be intubated have one or more of the following indications:
  1. Inability to maintain the airway patency or airway obstruction (eg, acute laryngeal edema, anaphylaxis, airway trauma, and epiglottitis
  2. Inability to protect the airway against aspiration (loss of gag reflex)

3. Anticipated loss of control of the airway (eg, deteriorating mental status, laryngeal edema, neck trauma, circumferential neck or facial burns, acute stridor, etc)

4. Inability to ventilate (inability to blow off CO_2)

5. Inability to oxygenate

- EMS providers with RSI privileges must be well trained, proficient, understand the mechanics and medications, and also know when not to use RSI techniques.

REFERENCES

1. Sporer KA, Johnson NJ. Detailed analysis of prehospital interventions in medical priority dispatch system determinants. *West J Emerg Med.* February 2011;12(1):19-29.

2. Munjal KD, Silverman RA, Freese J, et al. Utilization of emergency services in a large urban area: description of call types and temporal trends. *Prehosp Emerg Care.* 2011;15:371-380.

3. Buehler JW, Sonricker A. Syndromic surveillance practice in the United States: findings from a survey of state, territorial, and selected local health departments. *Adv Dis Surveill.* 2008;6(3). http://faculty.washington.edu/lober/www.isdsjournal.org/htdocs/articles/2618.pdf.

4. Centers for Disease Control. Summary Health Statistics for U.S. Adults: National Health Interview Survey, 2009. Tables 3,4. http://www.cdc.gov/nchs/fastats/copd.htm.

5. American Lung Association. State of lung diseases in diverse communities 2010. www.lungusa.org.

6. Wang NS. Anatomy and physiology of the pleural space. *Clin Chest Med.* March 1985;6(1):3-16.

7. Finley DJ. Anatomy of the pleura. *Thorac Surg Clin.* May 2011;21(2):157-163, vii.

8. Grotberg JB. Respiratory mechanics and gas exchange. *Standard Handbook of Biomedical Engineering and Design.* New York: McGraw-Hill; 2004:chap 4.1. http://unhas.ac.id/tahir/BAHAN-KULIAH/BIO-MEDICAL/NEW/HANBOOK/0071449337_ar004-Respiratory_Mechanics_And_Gas_Exchange.pdf.

9. Grotberg JB. Respiratory mechanics and gas exchange. *Standard Handbook of Biomedical Engineering and Design.* New York: McGraw-Hill; 2004:chap 4.2. http://unhas.ac.id/tahir/BAHAN-KULIAH/BIO-MEDICAL/NEW/HANBOOK/0071449337_ar004-Respiratory_Mechanics_And_Gas_Exchange.pdf.

10. Eder W, Ege M, von Mutius E. The asthma epidemic. *N Engl J Med.* November 23, 2006;355:2226-2235.

11. CDCVitalSigns. Asthma in the U.S. May 2011. http://www.cdc.gov/VitalSigns/Asthma/index.html.

12. Global Strategy for the diagnosis, management and prevention of COPD. Global Initiative for Chronic Obstructive Lung Disease (GOLD). 2010. http://www.goldcopd.org.

13. Vestbo J, Hurd SS, Agustí AG, et al. Global strategy for the diagnosis, management, and prevention of chronicobstructive pulmonary disease: GOLD executive summary. *Am J Respir Crit Care Med.* February 15, 2013;187(4):347-65. http://www.goldcopd.org/uploads/users/files/GOLD_Report_2013_Feb20.pdf.

14. Cheskes S, Turner L, Thomson S, Aljerian N. The impact of prehospital continuous positive airway pressure on the rate of intubation and mortality from acute out-of-hospital respiratory emergencies. *Prehosp Emerg Care.* October-December 2013;17(4):435-441.

15. Aguilar SA, Lee J, Dunford JV, et al. Assessment of the addition of prehospital continuous positive airway pressure (CPAP) to an urban emergency medical services (EMS) system in persons with severe respiratory distress. *J Emerg Med.* August 2013;45(2):210-219.

16. NHLBI Consensus Report on Asthma Management 2007. NIH Publication Number 08-5846. http://www.nhlbi.nih.gov/guidelines/asthma/asthsumm.pdf.

17. Bledsoe BE, Anderson E, Hodnick R, Johnson L, Johnson S, Dievendorf E. Low-fractional oxygen concentration continuous positive airway pressure is effective in the prehospital setting. *Prehosp Emerg Care.* April-June 2012;16(2):217-221.

18. Spijker EE, de Bont M, Bax M, Sandel M. Practical use, effects and complications of prehospital treatment of acute cardiogenic pulmonary edema using the Boussignac CPAP system. *Int J Emerg Med.* April 8. 2013;6(1):8.

19. Heart Failure Society of America1, Lindenfeld J, Albert NM, et al. HFSA 2010 comprehensive heart failure practice guideline. *J Card Fail.* June 2010;16(6):e134-e156.

20. Kochanek KD, Xu J, Murphy SL, Miniño AM, Kung HC. Deaths: preliminary data for 2009. *Natl Vital Stat Rep.* March 16, 2011;59(4):1-51.

21. Kemp SV, Polkey MI, Shah PL. The epidemiology, etiology, clinical features, and natural history of emphysema. *Thorac Surg Clin.* May 2009;19(2):149-158.

22. Muzzarelli S, Leibundgut G, Maeder MT, et al. Predictors of early readmission or death in elderly patients with heart failure. *Am Heart J.* August 2010;160(2):308-314.

23. Sheikh FH, Russell SD. HeartMate® II continuous-flow left ventricular assist system. *Expert Rev Med Devices.* January 2011;8(1):11-21.

24. Kaynar AM. Respiratory failure. September 28, 2010. http://emedicine.medscape.com/article/167981-overview.

25. Phua J, Badia JR, Adhikari NK, et al. Has mortality from acute respiratory distress syndrome decreased overtime? A systematic review. *Am J Respir Crit Care Med.* February 1, 2009;179(3):220-227.

26. CDC. Tuberculosis (TB). Fact sheet. Trends in tuberculosis, 2013. http://www.cdc.gov/tb/publications/factsheets/statistics/TBTrends.htm.

27. Ouellette DR. Pulmonary embolism. http://emedicine.medscape.com/article/300901-overview.

28. Berg RA, Hemphill R, Abella BS, et al. Part 5: adult basic life support: 2010 American Heart Association Guidelines for Cardiopulmonary Resuscitation and Emergency Cardiovascular Care Science. 2010; 122(18 suppl 3):S685-S705.

29. Vital FM, Ladeira MT, Atallah AN. Non-invasive positive pressure ventilation (CPAP or bi-level NPPV) for cardiogenic pulmonary edema. *Cochrane Database Syst Rev.* July 6, 2008;(3):CD005351.

30. Ward NS, Dushay KM. Clinical concise review: Mechanical ventilation of patients with chronic obstructive pulmonary disease. *Crit Care Med.* May 2008;36(5):1614-1619.

31. Hubble MW, Brown L, Wilfong DA, Hertelendy A, Benner RW, Richards ME. A meta-analysis of prehospital airway control techniques part I: orotracheal and nasotracheal intubation success rates. *Prehosp Emerg Care.* July-September 2010;14(3):377-401.

32. Gangadharan L, Sreekanth C, Vasnaik MC. Prediction of difficult intubations using conventional indicators: Does rapid sequence intubation ease difficult intubations? A prospective randomised study in a tertiary care teaching hospital. *J Emerg Trauma Shock.* January 2011;4(1):42-47.

CHAPTER 41

Gastrointestinal Emergencies

Debra Lee

INTRODUCTION

Abdominal pain, vomiting, diarrhea, and constipation are exceedingly common symptoms. In 2007, 10.8 million cases presented to emergency departments with gastrointestinal complaints, representing 9.2% of ED visits.[1] Twenty-one to forty-one percent of these patients, despite a full complement of diagnostic testing, leave the ED without a clear diagnosis.[2] There is diagnostic complexity in differentiating benign self-limited disease versus serious life-threatening conditions when evaluating these common gastrointestinal complaints. Patients arriving via EMS transport are more likely to require hospital admission, suggesting that EMS providers will encounter a sicker subset of the overall ED population.[3] Evaluation of these patients is often a challenge as is the provision of education and medical oversight to the EMS provider and system.

Differentiating the seriousness of gastrointestinal complaints begins at the time of dispatch. Dispatch protocols often attempt to address severity of illness and consideration of pathology originating from an alternate organ system when determining the response to the "sick" or "abdominal pain" call types. It has been suggested that dispatch protocols relying on age and gender classification alone result in significant overtriage.[4] Potential overuse of advanced life support (ALS) must be weighed against the benefits of ALS response: early electrocardiogram (ECG) interpretation, intravenous fluids, and medication administration. The diagnostic complexity of gastrointestinal complaints requires providers to approach them with a high level of suspicion and thorough evaluation, especially in higher risk populations such as the elderly, immunocompromised, women of childbearing age, and individuals with chronic disease.

OBJECTIVES

- Discuss the assessment of gastrointestinal emergencies.
- Understand common causes of gastrointestinal symptoms.
- Identify life-threatening gastrointestinal conditions.
- Discuss appropriate out-of-hospital management.
- Identify life-threatening nongastrointestinal conditions that commonly present with gastrointestinal symptoms.
- Discuss the use of ultrasound and other point-of-care testing in the prehospital environment.
- Discuss the use of narcotics for abdominal pain in the prehospital environment.
- Discuss the use of antiemetics for nausea or vomiting in the prehospital environment.

EVALUATION

Patients often present with one or more complaints, typically abdominal pain with associated symptoms such as nausea, vomiting, anorexia, diarrhea, or constipation. Atypical presentations of gastrointestinal conditions such as alterations in mental status, syncope, or jaundice with or without abdominal pain are responsible for some of the diagnostic uncertainty. The key to the appropriate diagnosis comes with a history and physical examination that is as complete as possible. Consideration of past medical and surgical history can significantly impact the differential diagnosis. The provider should complete the history with full awareness of time of onset, duration of the pain, the quality of the pain, the region or radiation of the pain, factors that provoke or palliate, and the severity

of the symptoms. Utilization of a rapid assessment mnemonic such as OPQRST is helpful and should be encouraged (**Table 41-1**).

Symptoms with an acute onset are of great concern in the practice of emergency medicine but gastrointestinal disease associated with high morbidity and mortality may have a more indolent presentation. An acute onset of symptoms of abdominal pain may increase concern for perforated viscous or nongastrointestinal causes such as abdominal aortic aneurysm, aortic dissection, ruptured ectopic pregnancy, or testicular/ovarian torsion. A slower onset of symptoms may indicate an inflammatory or infectious process such as appendicitis or colitis. Understanding the quality of painful symptoms is helpful in determining visceral versus somatic types of pain. Visceral symptoms tending more toward dull, aching pains with somatic symptoms often described as sharp, well-localized pain. Visceral pain is often referred to other locations and difficult to pinpoint. The location where the patient feels referred visceral pain is determined during fetal development and therefore subject to some variation. Classically, referred pain to the right shoulder is attributed to gallbladder disease. Pancreatic, aortic and renal colic often refers to the back.

Provoking factors may include oral intake as in the case of biliary disease, gastric ulcers, or mesenteric ischemia; pain with sudden movements may indicate peritoneal irritation as with appendicitis or peritonitis. Palliating factors may alternatively include oral intake, rest, or medications. Severe symptoms would heighten concern though the presence of even mild symptoms especially in the elderly, young, immunocompromised, and chronically ill may indicate serious disease. These populations warrant special consideration in the assessment of gastrointestinal symptoms.

The past medical and surgical history will direct the development of the differential and are therefore important pieces of information to obtain. Knowledge of a previous history of peptic ulcer disease in the patient with sudden onset, severe abdominal pain would increase concern for a ruptured viscous. A history of abdominal surgery would raise the diagnosis of a bowel obstruction higher on the differential.

The physical examination is of the most benefit when a clear differential is in mind when performing the examination. The patient's general appearance will provide insight into the severity of illness. Identification of the "sick" patient is a vital skill for any clinician. Special attention should be paid to the level of discomfort, mental status, color, and respiratory pattern. The absence of severe pain is not unexpected in elderly or immunocompromised patients. An alteration in mental status may indicate a serious metabolic derangement such as acidosis, uremia, or hyperammonemia though it may also be a result of poor perfusion and shock. Jaundice or pallor would be of a concern in patients at risk for liver failure, hepatitis, or severe anemia. Kussmaul-type respiratory pattern may be an indicator of acidosis.

Inspection of the abdomen yields important information especially in patients who are unable to provide a reliable history. A distended abdomen from ascites or obstruction is notable. Chronic changes such as the caput medusa may indicate the presence of liver disease. Cullen or Grey Turner sign would raise concern for intraperitoneal bleeding. The presence or absence of surgical scars should be noted as this may have significant impact on the differential diagnosis.

Auscultation can be difficult in the prehospital environment and the presence or absence of bowel sounds is of limited clinical utility. The

TABLE 41-1	Rapid Assessment Mnemonic
O	Onset
P	Palliating and provoking factors
Q	Quality
R	Region, radiation, and referral
S	Severity
T	Timing—presence, progression previous episodes

TABLE 41-2 Differential Diagnosis of Abdominal Pain Based on Location

Diffuse Pain

Aortic aneurysm (leaking, ruptured)
Aortic dissection
Appendicitis (early)
Bowel obstruction
Diabetic gastric paresis
Familial Mediterranean fever
Gastroenteritis
Heavy metal poisoning
Hereditary angioedema
Malaria

Mesenteric ischemia
Metabolic disorder
 (Addisonian crisis, AKA,
 DKA, porphyria, uremia)
Narcotic withdrawal
Pancreatitis
Perforated bowel
Peritonitis (of any cause)
Sickle cell crisis
Volvulus

Right Upper Quadrant Pain

Appendicitis (retrocecal)
Biliary colic
Cholangitis
Cholecystitis
Fitz-Hugh-Curtis Syndrome
Hepatitis
Hepatic abscess
Hepatic congestion
Herpes zoster
Myocardial ischemia
Perforated duodenal ulcer
Pneumonia (RLL)
Pulmonary embolism

Left Upper Quadrant Pain

Gastric ulcer
Gastritis
Herpes zoster
Myocardial ischemia
Pancreatitis
Pneumonia (LLL)
Pulmonary embolism
Splenic rupture/distension

Right Lower Quadrant Pain

Aortic aneurysm (leaking, ruptured)
Appendicitis
Crohn disease (terminal ileitis)
Diverticulitis (cecal)
Ectopic pregnancy
Endometriosis
Epiploic appendagitis
Herpes zoster
Inguinal hernia
(incarcerated, strangulated)
Ischemic colitis
Meckel diverticulum
Mittelschmerz
Ovarian cyst (ruptured)
Ovarian torsion
Pelvic inflammatory disease
Psoas abscess
Regional enteritis
Testicular torsion
Ureteral calculi

Left Lower Quadrant Pain

Aortic aneurysm (leaking, ruptured)
Diverticulitis (sigmoid)
Ectopic pregnancy
Endometriosis
Epiploic appendagitis
Herpes zoster
Inguinal hernia
 (incarcerated, strangulated)
Ischemic colitis
Mittelschmerz
Ovarian cyst (ruptured)
Ovarian torsion
Pelvic inflammatory disease
Psoas abscess
Regional enteritis
Testicular torsion
Ureteral calculi

Reprinted with permission from Tintinalli JE, Stapczynski JS, Ma OJ, Cline DM, Cydulka RK, Meckler GD, eds. Tintinalli's Emergency Medicine: A Comprehensive Study Guide, 7th ed. New York, NY: McGraw-Hill; 2011.

presence of hyperactive bowel sounds may be noted in patients with bowel obstruction. The utility of percussion in the prehospital environment is also of limited clinical utility. Environmental factors will make it difficult to differentiate the tympany associated with bowel obstruction versus the shifting dullness associated with ascites.

Most of the information from the abdominal examination is yielded from palpation. Tenderness to palpation in specific locations or quadrants may focus the differential. Voluntary guarding is a protective mechanism that is often found with focal tenderness. Rebound tenderness is indicative of peritoneal inflammation with rigidity on physical examination indicating diffuse peritoneal inflammation and a potential "surgical abdomen" (**Table 41-2**).

DIAGNOSTIC TESTING

Point-of-care testing (POC) is possible in the prehospital arena but its use is generally limited to response with *urban search and rescue* (USAR) or *disaster medical assistance teams* (DMAT); however, some advanced POC

has been done in the standard prehospital setting.[5-16] Hemoglobin and hematocrit have utility in the assessment of gastrointestinal hemorrhage. The metabolic panel, blood gas, and lactate are useful tools to assess the patient's metabolic state and as part of the evaluation for mesenteric ischemia or in the evaluation of patients with extra abdominal causes of gastrointestinal complaints such as diabetic ketoacidosis, hypercalcemia, hyponatremia, or acute kidney injury.

The *12-lead electrocardiogram* should be utilized to assess patients with gastrointestinal complaints at risk for potential cardiac pathology such as an acute coronary syndrome or arrhythmia. Elderly patients, women, and diabetics are more likely to present with atypical symptoms of an acute coronary syndrome. The ECG may also be used to assess for metabolic derangements resulting from gastrointestinal illness or causing gastrointestinal symptoms such as hypokalemia or hypercalcemia.

There is no reported data regarding the utilization of *radiographs* in the prehospital setting but as with point-of-care testing the equipment may be available especially in the setting of an extended disaster response. While using these tools in the prehospital setting is a foreign concept

TABLE 41-3	Differential of Acute Abdominal Pain	
Diagnosis	Symptoms	Signs
Appendicitis	Classically vague periumbilical or epigastric pain that migrates to the RLQ Anorexia, nausea, vomiting Low-grade fever	Abdominal tenderness Fever Voluntary or involuntary guarding Rebound tenderness Rovsing, psoas, or obturator sign
Biliary colic, cholecystitis, cholangitis	Acute crampy, colicky RUQ, or epigastric pain May radiated to the subscapular area Nausea, vomiting Fever or chills with cholecystitis and cholangitis	RUQ tenderness Murphy sign Fever with cholecystitis/cholangitis
Bowel obstruction	Crampy diffuse abdominal pain Nausea, vomiting No flatus or stool passage Bloating History of previous surgery or bowel obstruction	Abdominal distention Abdominal tenderness Fever Abnormal bowel sounds Peritoneal signs may indicate strangulation
Mesenteric ischemia	Gradual to acute onset Poorly localized, unrelenting abdominal pain Nausea, vomiting, diarrhea	Classically, pain "out of proportion" to examination Physical examination varies depending on the duration of ischemia May develop hypovolemia and sepsis
Ectopic pregnancy	Abdominal or pelvic pain Vaginal bleeding Amenorrhea Nausea, vomiting Dizziness Referred pain to shoulder	Abdominal or pelvic tenderness Adnexal tenderness Adnexal mass
Ovarian torsion	Abrupt onset Severe unilateral abdominal or pelvic pain Nausea, vomiting	Unilateral abdominal or pelvic tenderness Tender adnexal mass
Testicular torsion	Abrupt onset Severe unilateral abdominal or testicular pain Nausea, vomiting	Unilateral testicular tenderness High riding testicle with a horizontal lie Loss of cremasteric reflex on the affected side
Diverticulitis	LLQ abdominal pain Nausea, vomiting Change in stool pattern (frequency or consistency) Constipation Diarrhea Rectal bleeding	LLQ tenderness, guarding, rebound Fever Heme-positive stools If perforation, potential for tachycardia, high fever, sepsis
Gastroenteritis	Intermittent, crampy abdominal pain Poorly localized Diarrhea Nausea, vomiting	Nonspecific abdominal examination Absence of peritoneal signs Fever

during normal working conditions, the EMS physician must be aware of their availability and utility. Radiographs are of limited utility but may be helpful in the evaluation for free air in the abdominal cavity, the presence of pleural effusion/infiltrate, or to evaluate for a bowel obstruction.[17]

The use of *ultrasound* has become the standard of practice in emergency medicine for a variety of applications.[18] Prehospital ultrasound in military, ground, and aeromedical applications has been shown to be of some utility in smaller studies focused primarily on the evaluation of trauma using the Focused Assessment Sonography in Trauma (FAST) examination.[19-22] The utility of prehospital ultrasound by paramedics is an area of significant interest.[23-30] In a majority of the studies on prehospital ultrasound, emergency physicians performed the scan or reviewed images remotely.[31-32] ALS providers have demonstrated the ability to perform and interpret FAST and abdominal aortic (AA) examinations in the field though further validation is necessary.[33] Larger studies to

determine whether prehospital ultrasound could affect clinical outcomes are needed (**Table 41-3**).

LIFE-THREATENING GASTROINTESTINAL CONDITIONS

■ PERFORATED VISCOUS

Perforated viscous typically presents with an acute onset of abdominal pain followed by severe diffuse abdominal pain as the patient develops a chemical and bacterial peritonitis. Perforated esophagus is heralded with the acute onset of epigastric or chest pain as gastric contents evacuate into the mediastinum, resulting in a chemical and bacterial mediastinitis. Penetrating trauma is the most common cause of perforated viscous though any condition resulting in a loss of integrity of the bowel wall may result in perforation. Peptic ulcer disease, appendicitis, diverticulitis, bowel obstruction, and ischemia are frequent causal factors. The examination typically includes diffuse tenderness with or without rebound; rigidity may result as the peritonitis develops. Free air on upright chest x-ray or abdominal x-ray is frequently missed with sensitivities described at less than 25%.[17] The prehospital treatment for both conditions is supportive and in virtually all cases surgical repair is needed. Mortality remains high especially in patients with multiorgan failure at just under 20%.[34,35]

GASTROINTESTINAL BLEEDING

The presentation of gastrointestinal bleeding may be subtle but the morbidity and mortality are significant. The mortality of gastrointestinal bleeding is 10% with a higher mortality associated with the more prevalent upper gastrointestinal bleeding versus lower gastrointestinal bleeding.[36-38] NSAIDs, aspirin, and glucocorticoids use contributes to the development of gastrointestinal bleeding and are important elements of the history to obtain. Increased mortality is seen in patients of increased age and in those using anticoagulant and antiplatelet agents.[39,40] Patients typically present with symptoms of hematemesis, hematochezia, or melena though there are more subtle presentations with symptoms of hypovolemia or anemia. Upper gastrointestinal bleeding is primarily the result of peptic ulcer disease followed by bleeding from esophageal varices. Lower gastrointestinal bleeding is most often caused by diverticular disease followed by the presence of vascular dysplasia. Prehospital care is supportive. Intravenous access with two large bore catheters should be established. An ECG and cardiac monitoring should be considered, especially in elderly patients at risk for an acute coronary syndrome.

ISCHEMIC BOWEL

Patients with ischemic bowel typically present with symptoms of abdominal pain, classically described as pain out of proportion to the clinical examination. The overall mortality is high at 60% to 80%.[41] It is imperative to be able to identify the conditions involving impaired flow to the mesenteric arteries or veins through either thrombosis, embolism, or another decreased flow state such as a closed loop bowel obstruction. Presentations will vary according to the cause of ischemia. Embolic disease will present acutely. Patients with thrombotic disease may describe symptoms of intestinal angina and weight loss. Ischemic colitis may present with bloody diarrhea, with or without pain. While some of these low flow states may be subclinical, the high mortality is a result of bowel necrosis. Patients will develop clinical signs of peritonitis, hypotension, and a metabolic gap acidosis. Prehospital care is supportive but prehospital care providers should be educated to maintain a high level of suspicion especially in elderly patients and those who have risk factors for embolic and thrombotic disease.

SERIOUS GASTROINTESTINAL CONDITIONS

BOWEL OBSTRUCTION

Bowel obstruction makes up 15% of ED admissions for abdominal pain and is a common entity with a majority of obstructions involving the small bowel.[42] Nearly all bowel obstructions are admitted to the hospital. Management is typically conservative in cases that do not exhibit signs of peritonitis or ischemia. The majority of small bowel obstructions are attributed to the presence of intra-abdominal adhesions. Large bowel obstruction is most commonly caused by malignancy followed by volvulus of the sigmoid or cecum. Management of large bowel obstructions typically involves surgical repair though the volvulus of the sigmoid colon can be decompressed through colonic endoscopy; the risk of recurrence warrants surgical repair at a later time. The mortality for small bowel obstruction is 4% while large bowel obstruction trends toward 10%. The higher mortality is thought to be in part due to the higher age at incidence of LBO versus SBO though factors such as delayed diagnosis, complications of ischemia, or bowel infarct will increase mortality.

APPENDICITIS

Appendicitis is a common disease with a lifetime risk for men and women of 8.6% and 6.7%, respectively. The overall mortality is low at 1% but increases to 4% with complications of perforation and abscess.[43] The difficulty in diagnosis is reflected in its frequent association to medical malpractice claims.[44] Atypical presentations complicate the diagnosis, in part due to the varied position of the appendix within the abdominal cavity. Patients may therefore describe left-sided, suprapubic, pelvic, testicular, or flank pain and associated symptoms may include dysuria, urinary frequency, constipation, or diarrhea. The classic presentation for appendicitis includes the poorly differentiated periumbilical pain which moves to the right lower quadrant with subsequent tenderness at McBurney point with guarding and rebound as peritonitis sets in. Additional physical examination findings that are identified with appendicitis include the Rovsing, obturator, and psoas signs. Fever, nausea, vomiting, and anorexia are also classically described. Appendicitis may be present in patients at any age and atypical presentation and diagnosis complicated by perforation is seen more often at the extremes of age.[45]

DIVERTICULOSIS/DIVERTICULITIS

Diverticulosis is an exceedingly common disease with increased incidence with every decade of life and an overall prevalence of 25%.[46,47] Diverticulitis will develop in 10% to 15% and diverticular bleeding will occur in 3% to 5%.[48] Ninety percent of diverticula are located in the descending or sigmoid colon though they can develop in any part of the colon. Patients will typically present with left lower quadrant pain which may be associated with nausea, vomiting, fever, constipation, or diarrhea. Some will report dysuria and frequency if the adjacent urinary bladder becomes inflamed, thus complicating the diagnosis. Patients will typically be tender over the inflamed diverticula. Potential complications include bleeding, perforation, abscess formation, and the development of colonic fistulas. The overall mortality is low though patients with recurrent symptoms may require surgical intervention.[48]

BILIARY DISEASE

Biliary disease is spectrum of conditions including cholelithiasis, cholecystitis, choledoclithiasis, and cholangitis. Cholelithiasis is a common diagnosis with an overall prevalence of 10% to 15% of the adult population. Risk factors for the development of gallstones include female gender, obesity, rapid weight loss, and a genetic predisposition seen especially in Hispanics and American Indians.[49] The term *biliary colic* refers to the pain produced by the contraction of the gallbladder against the gallstone blocking the cystic duct. Persistent obstruction will ultimately result in increased pressure within the gallbladder, resulting in inflammation and ischemia of the gallbladder wall. Mortality from cholelithiasis itself is rare but complications of biliary obstruction from gallstones can be significant. The classic presentation includes pain radiating to the right shoulder or scapula after a fatty meal. Murphy's sign is pain on palpation to the right upper quadrant with deep inspiration. Nausea, vomiting, steatorrhea, and fever may be present. Jaundice may be present but significant hyperbilirubinemia and diffuse jaundice would indicate prolonged biliary obstruction more likely seen with choledoclithiasis, cholangitis, or an obstructive malignancy. Charcot triad of fever, right upper quadrant pain, and jaundice is described in patients with cholangitis. Abdominal ultrasound to assess for gallbladder stones, gallbladder wall thickening, and common bile ductal dilatation is indicated in the ED though application in the prehospital environment has not been reported.

PANCREATITIS

Pancreatitis has an overall mortality of 5% though the mortality can increase dramatically to 47% for a subset of individuals who develop an extrapancreatic disease, systemic inflammatory response (SIRS), pancreatic necrosis, organ failure, and acute respiratory distress syndrome (ARDS).[50] The pathogenesis of pancreatitis is evenly split between gallstone pancreatitis and alcohol induced pancreatitis, which are the causative agents in

80% to 90% of cases. Other causes of pancreatitis include trauma, steroid use, mumps, autoimmune disease, scorpion bites, hypercalcemia, hypertriglyceridemia, post-ERCP, and idiopathic.[51] Patients typically report a dull epigastric pain often radiating to the back. Shortness of breath may be described in patients who have developed pulmonary effusions or if they are developing ARDS. Dizziness, lightheadedness, syncope, alteration in mental status, as well as hypotension may represent the development of SIRS. Close monitoring of vital signs including blood pressure and oxygen saturation is recommended as the development of organ failure is associated with a significant increase in mortality.[50]

COMMON GASTROINTESTINAL CONDITIONS

GASTROENTERITIS

Gastroenteritis is identified by symptoms of vomiting and diarrhea. The overall morbidity and mortality in the United States is low but patients often present for symptomatic relief. There is potential for significant dehydration especially in populations who are at the extremes of age. There are a variety of viral and bacterial causes of gastroenteritis. Identification of causal agents may be possible during periods of an outbreak of disease though confirmation of causal agents is not the norm and may lead to identification of a specific epidemic. Patients will typically present with a syndrome of vomiting and diarrhea often accompanied with abdominal cramping and fever. The history of recent travel, sick contacts, or recent ingestion of foods associated with bacterial contamination may help direct therapy. The goal of treatment is symptomatic relief and rehydration.

GASTRITIS AND PEPTIC ULCER DISEASE

The prevalence of peptic ulcer disease in the United States is high at 10% though hospitalizations and surgical interventions are on the decline. The overall mortality is low at 2.7% but raises significantly for complications of hemorrhage and perforation.[52] The classic presentation is of burning epigastric pain relieved by oral intake. Pain related to peptic ulcer disease is alternately described as sharp, dull, achy, or a "hungry" or "empty" type of pain. Episodic pain is often reported as these patients are prone to recurrence of symptoms. Complications of peptic ulcer disease include gastrointestinal hemorrhage and perforation.

SERIOUS NONGASTROINTESTINAL CONDITIONS PRESENTING WITH GI COMPLAINTS

ABDOMINAL AORTIC ANEURYSM

The symptomatic abdominal aneurysm typically presents with some element of abdominal or back pain. Syncope preceding severe abdominal or back pain should immediately raise concerns for a ruptured or leaking abdominal aortic aneurysm. Patients may describe abrupt onset of pain or a ripping or tearing sensation. This history may be difficult to obtain, especially in the setting of shock. Rapid identification of these lesions is paramount as the mortality of patients with rupture approaches 50%. Bedside ultrasound to identify an aneurysm or the presence of blood in the abdominal cavity is ideal.

ACUTE CORONARY SYNDROME

Acute coronary syndrome is the general classification for unstable angina, NSTEMI, and STEMI. Patients with advanced age, female gender, and diabetes are associated with atypical presentations of ACS. While a majority of patients with acute myocardial infarction present with symptoms of chest pain or dyspnea up to 18% present atypically.[53] The diagnosis of ACS should be considered in patients with significant cardiac risk factors and a benign physical examination. Patients may present with nausea, vomiting, or abdominal pain—typically with an abrupt onset—which may be associated with symptoms classically described with ACS such as diaphoresis, syncope, dizziness, shortness

of breath, or palpitations. A 12-lead ECG should be considered in these patients.

ECTOPIC PREGNANCY

The diagnosis of ectopic pregnancy should be considered for all women of childbearing age with abdominal pain. Young women with a history of amenorrhea or irregular periods, abdominal pain, and syncope should be treated as an ectopic pregnancy until proven otherwise. Sudden onset of abdominal or pelvic pain from tubal stretching or rupture is often accompanied with vaginal bleeding. Hypotension and shoulder pain from diaphragmatic irritation may result from ruptured ectopic pregnancy. Ultrasound may be helpful to determine the presence of intraperitoneal blood or to rule out an ectopic pregnancy.

OVARIAN TORSION

The presence of ovarian torsion should be considered in the female of childbearing age with a sudden onset of severe abdominal or pelvic pain. The classic presentation for torsion includes the sudden onset of severe pelvic or abdominal pain after exercise. The patient may have nausea or vomiting. The patient may have a history of previous ovarian cysts, current pregnancy with a large corpus luteal cyst, or ongoing treatment for infertility. Identification is key and typically performed with Doppler ultrasound. Rapid surgical intervention is required to maintain ovarian function.

TESTICULAR TORSION

The incidence of testicular torsion has a bimodal distribution, initially in the perinatal period and again during puberty. Patients will report a sudden onset of lower abdominal or testicular pain sometimes associated with nausea or vomiting. On physical examination a high-riding, firm, and tender testicle, often in a transverse lie, may be seen. The most sensitive physical finding is the loss of the cremasteric reflex on the affected side. Manual detorsion should be considered but if successful surgical repair will still be necessary.

DIABETIC KETOACIDOSIS

Diabetic ketoacidosis is the result of dehydration during a state of relative insulin deficit, resulting in elevated blood sugar and serum ketones. Abdominal pain, nausea, and vomiting are common symptoms of diabetic ketoacidosis. As the metabolic acidosis worsens, patients may present with Kussmaul respirations and alterations in mental status. Assessment of blood sugar is often helpful though further assessment and treatment rely on the basic metabolic panel and blood gas. A 12-lead ECG should be considered.

PREHOSPITAL MANAGEMENT

Prehospital management of gastrointestinal emergencies is primarily supportive. Diagnostic aids such as ECG and ultrasound are helpful in the assessment of gastrointestinal complaints and may help direct patient care. Airway management and control should be considered in any patient who presents with an alteration in mental status. Ventilation may be compromised in patients suffering with peritonitis or pancreatitis. Lung auscultation and pulse oximetry may reveal significant pathology associated with gastrointestinal complaints and should be treated with oxygen as needed. Hypotension may be present in patients with severe dehydration, sepsis, or anemia related to gastrointestinal bleeding and intravenous administration of saline or lactated Ringer is indicated.

Prehospital *analgesics* have been administered since the beginning of EMS though prehospital pain management remains an area for improvement.[54,55] Pain protocols using narcotic medications, typically morphine or fentanyl, have been effective in improving patient comfort and satisfaction with rare adverse effects. In review of 6212 patients, the major adverse effects of opioids were dizziness and itching, sedation was rare; two required naloxone but ventilatory support was not needed.[56] Arguments that analgesics diminish the diagnostic capability of receiving providers are unfounded but early administration of analgesics is shown to decrease pain.[57] The key to proper administration of prehospital analgesics is in protocol development with utilization of pain scale, close monitoring of the patient response, and a health quality improvement program.

Antiemetic medications are becoming more widely available to prehospital providers in the form of ondansetron. Previous studies demonstrated efficacy of droperidol though the subsequent black box warning has curtailed its use. Nausea and vomiting are common complaints potentially exacerbated by ambulance transport with motion sickness seen frequently in patients transported by ambulance.[58] Prevention of vomiting is desirable from the standpoint of patient comfort but also for the clinical benefits of decreasing risk of dehydration and aspiration. Ondansetron has been shown to be safe with minimal side effects and effective in alleviating symptoms of nausea and vomiting with oral dissolving tablet (ODT), intramuscular and intravenous administration.[59,60]

KEY POINTS

- Patients with gastrointestinal complaints present significant challenges to the EMS provider. A detailed history and physical is required though may yield nonspecific findings that do not point a definitive diagnosis.

- Providers must approach these patients mindful of potentially life-threatening conditions, extraabdominal sources of symptoms especially in populations who may present with atypical symptoms, or a more benign appearance such as the elderly or immunocompromised.

- Stabilization of ABCs is always the priority. Airway protection and intravenous fluid administration should be given when appropriate. Consideration of a comprehensive differential may significantly impact the ultimate disposition and treatment.

- Intervention with analgesic and antiemetic medications has not been shown to delay care or result in adverse outcomes. The integration of pain management and antiemetic protocols to facilitate treatment should be a consideration for every system.

REFERENCES

1. Niska R, Bhuiya F, Xu J. National Hospital Ambulatory Care Survey: 2007 emergency department summary. National health statistics report; no 26. Hyattsville, MD: National Center for Health Statistics; 2010.
2. Hastings RS, Powers RD. Abdominal Pain in the ED: a 35 year retrospective. *Am J Emerg Med.* 2011;29:711-716.
3. Hiestand B. The influence of emergency medical services transport on Emergency Severity Index triage level for patients with abdominal pain. *Acad Emerg Med.* 2011;18(3):261-266.
4. Kennedy JD, Sweeney TA, Roberts D, et al. Effectiveness of a medical priority dispatch protocol for abdominal pain. *Prehosp Emerg Care.* 2003;7(1):89-93.
5. Mullen M, Cerri G, Murray R, et al. Use of point-of-care lactate in the prehospital aeromedical environment. *Prehosp Disaster Med.* April 2014;29(2):200-203.
6. Tobias AZ, Guyette FX, Seymour CW, et al. Pre-resuscitation lactate and hospital mortality in prehospital patients. *Prehosp Emerg Care.* July-September 2014;18(3):321-327.
7. Shah A, Guyette F, Suffoletto B, et al. Diagnostic accuracy of a single point-of-care prehospital serum lactate for predicting outcomes in pediatric trauma patients. *Pediatr Emerg Care.* June 2013;29(6):715-719.
8. Guerra WF, Mayfield TR, Meyers MS, Clouatre AE, Riccio JC. Early detection and treatment of patients with severe sepsis by prehospital personnel. *J Emerg Med.* June 2013;44(6):1116-1125.
9. Schött U. Prehospital coagulation monitoring of resuscitation with point-of-care devices. *Shock.* May 2014;41(suppl 1):26-29.
10. Venturini JM, Stake CE, Cichon ME. Prehospital point-of-care testing for troponin: are the results reliable? *Prehosp Emerg Care.* January-March 2013;17(1):88-91.
11. Prosen G, Klemen P, Štrnad M, Grmec S. Combination of lung ultrasound (a comet-tail sign) and N-terminal pro-brain natriuretic peptide in differentiating acute heart failure from chronic obstructive pulmonary disease and asthma as cause of acute dyspnea in prehospital emergency setting. *Crit Care.* 2011;15(2):R114.
12. Sørensen JT, Terkelsen CJ, Steengaard C, et al. Prehospital troponin T testing in the diagnosis and triage of patients with suspected acute myocardial infarction. *Am J Cardiol.* May 15, 2011;107(10): 1436-1440.
13. Di Serio F, Petronelli MA, Sammartino E. Laboratory testing during critical care transport: point-of-care testing in air ambulances. *Clin Chem Lab Med.* July 2010;48(7):955-961.
14. Schuchert A, Hamm C, Scholz J, Klimmeck S, Goldmann B, Meinertz T. Prehospital testing for troponin T in patients with suspected acute myocardial infarction. *Am Heart J.* July 1999;138(1 pt 1):45-48.
15. Prause G, Ratzenhofer-Komenda B, Offner A, Lauda P, Voit H, Pojer H. Prehospital point of care testing of blood gases and electrolytes - an evaluation of IRMA. *Crit Care.* 1997;1(2):79-83.
16. Herr DM, Newton NC, Santrach PJ, Hankins DG, Burritt MF. Airborne and rescue point-of-care testing. *Am J Clin Pathol.* October 1995;104(4 suppl 1):S54-S58.
17. Van Randen A, Lameris W, Luitse J, et al. The role of plain radiographs in patients with acute abdominal pain at the ED. *Am J Emerg Med.* 2011;29:582-589.
18. American College of Emergency Physicians. Policy Statement: emergency ultrasound guidelines. *Ann Emerg Med.* 2009;53:550-570.
19. Lapostolle F, Petrovic T, Lenoir G, et al. Usefulness of hand-held ultrasound devices in out-of-hospital diagnosis performed by emergency physicians. *Am J Emerg Med.* 2006; 24(2):237-242.
20. Walcher F, Winlich M, Conrad G, et al. Prehospital ultrasound imaging improves management of abdominal trauma. *Br J Surg.* 2006;93:238-242.
21. Do JR, Mcmanus J, Harrison B. Use of ultrasonography to avoid an unnecessary procedure in the prehospital combat environment: a case report. *Prehosp Emerg Care.* 2006;10:502-506.
22. Ma OJ, Norvell JG, Subramanian S. Ultrasound applications in mass casualties and extreme environments. *Crit Care Med.* 2007;35(5 suppl):S275-S279.
23. Press GM, Miller SK, Hassan IA, et al. Prospective evaluation of prehospital trauma ultrasound during aeromedical transport. *J Emerg Med.* September 30, 2014;47(6):638-645.
24. Brun PM, Chenaitia H, Lablanche C, et al. 2-point ultrasonography to confirm correct position of the gastric tube in prehospital setting. *Mil Med.* 2014 Sep;179(9):959-963.
25. Jakobsen LK, Bøtker MT, Lawrence LP, Sloth E, Knudsen L. Systematic training in focused cardiopulmonary ultrasound affects decision-making in the prehospital setting - two case reports. *Scand J Trauma Resusc Emerg Med.* May 1, 2014;22:29.
26. Hu H, He Y, Zhang S, Cao Y. Streamlined focused assessment with sonography for mass casualty prehospital triage of blunt torso trauma patients. *Am J Emerg Med.* July 2014;32(7):803-806.
27. Widmeier K, Wesley K. Infection inspection: screening & managing sepsis in the prehospital setting, part 2 of 2. *JEMS.* March 2014;39(3):36-40.
28. Taylor J, McLaughlin K, McRae A, Lang E, Anton A. Use of prehospital ultrasound in North America: a survey of emergency medical services medical directors. *BMC Emerg Med.* March 1, 2014;14:6.
29. Herzberg M, Boy S, Hölscher T, et al. Prehospital stroke diagnostics based on neurological examination and transcranial ultrasound. *Crit Ultrasound J.* February 27, 2014;6(1):3.
30. Brun PM, Bessereau J, Levy D, Billeres X, Fournier N, Kerbaul F. Prehospital ultrasound thoracic examination to improve decision

making, triage, and care in blunt trauma. *Am J Emerg Med.* July 2014;32(7):817.e1-e2.

31. Boniface KS, Shokoohi H, Smith ER, et al. Tele-ultrasound and paramedics: real-time remote physician guidance of the Focused Assessment with Sonography for Trauma examination. *Am J Emerg Med.* 2011;29: 477-481.

32. Strode CA, Rubal BJ, Gerhardt RT, et al. Wireless and satellite transmission for prehospital focused abdominal sonography for trauma. *Prehosp Emerg Care.* 2003;7:375-379.

33. Heegaard W, Hildebrandt D, Spear D, et al. Prehospital ultrasound by paramedics: results of field trial. *Acad Emerg Med.* 2010;17: 624-630.

34. Kulkarni S, Niak A, Subramanian N. APACHE-II scoring system in perforative peritonitis. *Am J Surg.* 2007;194:549-552.

35. Ordonez CA, Puyana JC. Management of peritonitis in the critically ill patient. *Surg Clin North Am.* 2006;86:1323-1349.

36. Strate LL. Risk factors for mortality in lower intestinal bleeding. *Clin Gastroenterol Hepatol.* 2008;6(9):004-10.

37. Wilcox CM, Clark WS. Causes and outcome of upper and lower gastrointestinal bleeding: the Grady Hospital experience. *South Med J.* 1999;92:44.

38. Hussain H, Lapin S, Cappell MS. Clinical scoring systems for determining the prognosis of gastrointestinal bleeding. *Gastroenterol Clin North Am.* 2000;29(2): 445-464.

39. Loperfido S, Baldo V, Piovesana E, et al. Changing trends in acute upper-GI bleeding: a population-based study. *Gastrointest Endosc.* 2009;70:212-224.

40. Kumar R, Mills A. Gastrointestinal bleeding. *Emerg Med Clin N Am.* 2011;29:239-252.

41. Oldenburg W, Lau L, Rodenberg T, et al. Acute mesenteric ischemia. *Arch Intern Med.* 2004;164:1054-1062.

42. Hayden GE, Sprouse KL. Bowel obstruction and hernia. *Emerg Med Clin N Am.* 2011;29:319-345.

43. Vissers RJ, Lennarz WB. Pitfalls in appendicitis. *Emerg Med Clin N Am.* 2010;28: 103-118.

44. Brown TW. An epidemiologic study of closed emergency department malpractice claims in a national database of physician malpractice insurers. *Acad Emerg Med.* 2010;17(5):553-560.

45. Selbst SM, Friedman MJ, Singh SB. Epidemiology and etiology of malpractice lawsuits involving children in US emergency departments and urgent care centers. *Pediatr Emerg Care.* 2005;21:165-169.

46. Muers-Szojda MM. Diverticulosis and diverticulitis form no risk for polyps and colorectal neoplasia in 4241 colonoscopies. *Int J Colorectal Dis.* 2008;23(10):979-984.

47. Blachut K. Prevalence and distribution of the colonic diverticulosis. Review of 417 cases from Lower Silesia in Poland. *Rom J Gastroenterol.* 2004;13(4):281-285.

48. Parra-Blanco A. Colonic diverticular disease: pathophysiology and clinical picture. *Digestion.* 2006;73(suppl 1):47-57.

49. Stinton LM, Myers RB, Shaffer EA. Epidemiology of gallstones. *Gastroenterol Clin N Am.* 2010;39:157-169.

50. Tenner S, Baillie J; DeWitt J, Vege SS; American College of Gastroenterology. American College of Gastroenterology guideline: management of acute pancreatitis. *Am J Gastroenterol.* 2013; 108(9):1400-1416.

51. Privette TW, Carlisle MC, Palma JK. Emergencies of the liver gallbladder and pancreas. *Emerg Med Clin N Am.* 2011;29:293-317.

52. Wang YR. Trends and outcomes of hospitalizations for peptic ulcer disease in the United States, 1993 to 2006. *Ann Surg.* 2010;251(1): 51-58.

53. Saczynski JS, Yarzebski J, Lessard D, et al. Trends in prehospital delay in patients with acute myocardial infarction (from the Worcester Heart Attack Study). *Am J Cardiol.* 2008;102:1589-1594.

54. McManus, JG, Sallee DR. Pain management in the prehospital environment. *Emerg Med Clin N Am.* 2005;23:415-431.

55. Jennings PA, Cameron P, Bernard S. Epidemiology of prehospital pain: an opportunity for improvement. *Emerg Med J.* 2011;28(6):530-531.

56. Park CL, Roberts DE, Aldington DJ et al. Prehospital analgesia: systematic review of evidence. *J R Army Med Corps.* 2010;156(4 suppl 1): 295-300.

57. Manterola C, Astudiollo P, Losada H, et al. Analgesia in patients with acute abdominal pain. *Cochrane Database Syst Rev.* 2007;(3): CD005660.

58. Weichenthal L, Soliz T. The incidence and treatment of prehospital motion sickness. *Prehosp Emerg Care.* 2003;7:474-476.

59. Warden CR, Moreno R, Daya M. Prospective evaluation of ondansetron for undifferentiated nausea and vomiting in the prehospital setting. *Prehosp Emerg Care.* 2008;12(1):87-91.

60. Salvucci AA, Dquire B, Burdick M, et al. Ondansetron is safe and effective for prehospital treatment of nausea and vomiting by paramedics. *Prehosp Emerg Care.* 2011;15(1):34-38.

Endocrine and Immunologic Emergencies

David M. Landsberg

INTRODUCTION

While endocrine and immunologic emergencies may not hold the dramatic appeal of a multiple trauma they are no less fatal and often are definitively treated by medical intervention alone. The EMS physician stands to have a significant impact on the outcome of those diagnoses and management schema that fall outside the traditional ALS curriculum and yet are rapidly treated by appropriate medical intervention. In this chapter, we will review likely endocrine and immunologic emergencies that may be encountered in the field where there is opportunity for the EMS physician to provide diagnosis and intervention with those tools available in the prehospital environment.

OBJECTIVES

- Describe the initial prehospital evaluation and management of hyperglycemia, hyperglycemic hyperosmolar syndrome, and diabetic ketoacidosis.
- Describe the initial prehospital evaluation and management of hypoglycemia.
- Describe the initial prehospital evaluation and management of thyroid storm.
- Describe the initial prehospital evaluation and management of adrenal insufficiency.
- List causes of immune deficiency.
- List common autoimmune diseases in prehospital patients.
- Describe the initial prehospital evaluation and management of allergic reactions

THYROID EMERGENCIES

MYXEDEMA COMA

The initial approach to the patient with altered sensorium is covered in Chapter 36. Upon completion of the initial priorities and screening for the more common sources of altered sensorium the possibility of myxedema should always be considered. The clinical stigmata of generalized slowing across all organ systems are readily assessed without the need for advanced testing modalities. A careful history from family or friends as well as review of the patient's prescriptions, if available, may yield valuable clues to the diagnosis. Obviously specific history of thyroid disorder is pivotal and one should bear in mind that history of hypo- or hyperthyroidism suggests the diagnosis in the appropriate clinical context. A patient who is undergoing radioablative or pharmacologic therapy for hyperthyroidism is as much at risk as the patient who neglects to take their thyroid supplementation in the presence of diagnosed hypothyroidism. Further historical screening should focus on complaints of fatigue, cold intolerance, and especially somnolence.[1,2] The presence of an acute superimposed illness over baseline hypothyroidism can precipitate an acute crisis particularly when the diagnosis of hypothyroidism was previously undiscovered or underreplaced.[1,2] In addition to altered sensorium the expected physical examination findings include bradycardia and hypothermia along with hyporeflexia.[1,2] The classical skin and hair changes of the disease are further supportive as is any evidence of surgical thyroidectomy. A depressed $EtCO_2$ in the setting of normal minute ventilation may be a clue to the hypometabolic state.[3]

The management of myxedema focuses on the acute replacement of the deficient steroids. If practical, blood can be drawn and saved for later analysis of the TSH, free T4, and cortisol levels preceding treatment. The dose of T4 varies in the literature with no large-scale RCTs to convincingly support one dose over another but there is general agreement on a dose between 200 and 400 μg IV acutely.[4,5] It should also be remembered that the possibility of concomitant adrenal insufficiency exists and until that entity is excluded there must be concurrent supplementation of glucocorticoid.[4-6] A dose of 100 mg hydrocortisone IV or 4 mg dexamethasone IV is sufficient in this setting.[6,7] Apart from the aforementioned disease-specific therapy, standard treatment with large-volume isotonic crystalloid and vasopressors is appropriate for hemodynamic support.

THYROID STORM

The diagnosis of severe thyrotoxicosis is a clinical one and often requires the exclusion of many other more common entities. Thyroid storm may develop in a patient with long-standing hyperthyroidism or may be the initial presentation of the disease.[2,8] Consistent with other endocrine emergencies the presence of significant physiologic stressors can precipitate a storm.[9,10] Infection, trauma, iodine exposure, and thyroid surgery are all well described to have the potential to precipitate a crisis.[12] It should be noted that amiodarone exposure may be the inciting iodine source.[12] In general, it is the sympathomimetic properties of thyroid hormone excess that will be the most dramatic findings leading to the diagnosis. Tachycardia and hypertension leading later to hypotension as rate-related cardiomyopathy ensues is a typical progression.[8,9] Hyperpyrexia with warm and moist skin are often present.[10,11] Mental status changes favor agitation and psychosis but may conversely also present as coma.[10,11] The presence of hyperreflexia, tremor, goiter, and ophthalmopathy concurrently are strongly consistent with the diagnosis.[8-10,11]

Standard therapeutic regimens focus on controlling the adrenergic activity followed by disruption of hormone synthesis, release, and peripheral conversion. Not having the depth of pharmacologic options prehospitally that are present in the ED it would be reasonable to focus on β-blockade and glucocorticoid supplementation followed by thionamide and iodine treatment upon arrival at the receiving facility.[10,11] Propranolol 0.5 to 1 mg over 10 minutes and esmolol 250 to 500 μg/kg loading dose followed by an infusion at one-fifth that dose per minute are established protocols for this purpose.[8-10,11] The balance of the management is supportive.

ADRENAL EMERGENCIES

ADRENAL INSUFFICIENCY

Adrenal insufficiency may occur as a primary process or it may occur secondary to an initial illness or injury that precipitates the adrenal crisis. Secondary adrenal crisis may render treatment for the primary illness refractory to standard interventions. Adrenal insufficiency may arise from primary failure of the adrenal gland.[6,7] Alternatively it may arise secondary to failure at the level of the hypothalamus or pituitary.[6,7] While primary failure results in both glucocorticoid and mineralocorticoid deficiency and secondary failure generally results in isolated glucocorticoid deficiency, it is replacement of the glucocorticoid component that has the capacity to yield immediate results. Restoration of sodium, potassium, and water balance through correction of mineralocorticoid deficiency takes many days while vasodilatation and decreased cardiac inotropy will respond rapidly to glucocorticoid replacement. The most common cause of primary hypoadrenalism is autoimmune disease.[6,7] It is not clear whether this is entirely secondary to autoimmune disease alone or the steroid treatment so often obligated in management of the primary disorder. Given that the dose and duration of steroid therapy required to cause adrenal suppression is variable, the author recommends that adrenal insufficiency be considered in any patient who has received steroids in the last 30 days or who carries a chronic diagnosis that may reasonably have been treated with steroids when prescriptions are unknown. The clinical cue that should bring this diagnosis to mind is hypotension not responsive to standard therapy. The dosing regimen has been the subject of much study and debate over the last 30 years. Standard practice of

50 to 100 mg of hydrocortisone IV or 4 mg dexamethasone IV acutely can be expected to last at least 6 hours.[6,7,12] If practical a blood sample could ideally be drawn before treatment for later analysis of native cortisol level. If this is not possible, dexamethasone is the preferred agent as it will not interfere with the cortisol assay if an ACTH stimulation test is subsequently administered.[6,7]

PHEOCHROMOCYTOMA

This exceedingly rare diagnosis bears mentioning only to underscore that excessive hypertension or tachycardia should be managed in the usual manner with vasodilators and negative chronotropes as you would most similar presentations of other etiologies.

DIABETES MELLITUS

HYPOGLYCEMIA

The "diabetic wake-up" remains the prototype for definitive care delivered by ALS providers. It is the paramedic's version of "treat and release" and provides enormous job satisfaction and skill validation that should be appreciated by those supervising ALS providers. The EMS physician does not bring new medications or advanced treatments to the field to manage this diagnosis. The EMS physician does bring an exponentially broader armamentarium of differential diagnoses and understanding of pathogenic mechanisms that may potentially yield hypoglycemia outside of the straightforward scenario of insulin administration in the face of inadequate carbohydrate substrate.

Important sources of hypoglycemia not within the general scope of paramedic education include consideration of any process that may decrease the renal clearance of insulin or oral hypoglycemics. Signs of renal failure or any reason to have had decreased renal perfusion and/or injury in the setting of insulin administration may support this diagnosis. It is important to remember that sulfonylureas will present an analogous scenario. Hepatic failure and loss of is another potential source of hypoglycemia as is adrenal insufficiency previously discussed. Infection is generally a well-recognized cause of hyperglycemia but the metabolic load may also consume glucose and decrease insulin clearance, resulting in hypoglycemia as well. Analogous to this scenario is the metabolic load of rapidly progressive leukemia and lymphoma consuming the constituents of cellular metabolism.

HYPERGLYCEMIA

Isolated hyperglycemia is not life threatening in itself until the level rises high enough for hyperosmolarity to become the threat. The hyperosmolar state should be considered in the setting of a glucose reading that is immeasurably high on glucometry coupled with clinical signs of profound dehydration. The focus of treatment remains restoration of volume and euvolemia but only as much as is needed to support hemodynamics for transportation to definitive care. Attention should be given to the rate of correction of the hyperosmolarity as overly rapid correction can result in cerebral osmotic demyelination syndromes. As a practical matter even normal saline will be hypotonic to these patients and should be the only fluid administered prehospitally to any significant volume.

Diabetic ketoacidosis will be the other differential to consider in the setting of high glucometry and dehydration. Clinical clues to differentiating diabetic ketoacidosis (DKA) from hyperglycemic hyperosmolar syndrome (HHS) include the presence of large acetone by measurement or odor on examination. Abdominal pain is a very common presenting symptom of DKA and may help bolster this diagnosis.[13] It is felt to represent the splanchnic circulation's exquisite sensitivity to acidemia.[13] A clinical history of noncompliance and/or the presence of a known concomitant stressor help increase the diagnostic accuracy here. Standard treatment regimens for DKA focus on correcting the acidosis through facilitation of glucose transport by insulin and correction of the large intracellular dehydration that accompanies this diagnosis. It is reasonable to give parenteral insulin in this situation if there is confidence in the diagnosis. Isotonic fluids are also indicated and in large volumes can go a long way to correcting acidosis in the presence of relatively small doses of insulin.

IMMUNOLOGIC EMERGENCIES

Those immune emergencies that might frequently be encountered in the prehospital setting can be divided into immune mediated and autoimmune mediated. The former consisting of common allergic reactions from the indolent to the severe and the latter consisting of those reactions where the body attacks self-antigens.

IMMUNE MEDIATED

Anaphylaxis This disorder is a focus of ALS provider education and these providers are especially well prepared to recognize and treat such disorders. They are armed with both parenteral and inhaled β-agonists, antihistamines, and steroids for the management of these emergencies. As always, the EMS physician will add significantly to diagnosis in those cases where the presentation is atypical. The approach and management does not differ substantially from that which is provided in the ED for this primarily clinical diagnosis. The EMS physicians' latitude with dosing, however, may prove pivotal in severe cases.

Angioedema Angioedema presenting as a symptom of anaphylaxis is treated as anaphylaxis. Isolated angioedema such as is prototypically seen with ACE inhibitors is treated with steroids and antihistamines. Epinephrine is indicated if rapid airway closure is deemed to be occurring. In treating histamine-mediated angioedema, epinephrine is helpful but will not add to the management of bradykinin-mediated angioedema which is the mechanism when ACE inhibitors are causal. The EMS physician stands to add significantly to this management as isolated angioedema may not fit the ALS provider's protocol for anaphylaxis though can represent just as much of a threat.

AUTOIMMUNE MEDIATED

Presentations related to the underlying disease state will involve acute insults to targeted organs. Management will be supportive and directed at the presenting manifestations rather than the underlying disease in most cases. In the prehospital setting, hypertensive emergencies brought on by vasculitis will be treated as hypertensive emergency alone. Similarly, respiratory failure from a pulmonary-renal syndrome will be treated as respiratory failure with its usual cascade of supportive management. The EMS physician will bring a greater depth of understanding to these cases but as a practical consideration will not likely be considering immunomodulation with steroids in any but the most extreme cases. A scenario where outcome of the underlying disease may potentially be modulated prehospitally is in a patient presenting with pathognomonic temporal arteritis and visual changes. This is a potential pathology where the astute EMS physician may realize an opportunity based solely on history and clinical examination.[14] The initial dose of Solu Medrol in this instance is 1 g IV daily for 3 days.[14] If the full dose is not immediately available, a partial dose should be given on scene with the balance delivered on arrival at the ED.

KEY POINTS

- The EMS physician brings a broader scope and differential diagnosis to prehospital evaluation of potential endocrine and immunologic emergencies.

- Most endocrine and immunologic conditions are treated with symptomatic, supportive care in the prehospital environment.

- The EMS physician should be knowledgeable about the most common endocrine emergencies to present in the prehospital setting, including hypoglycemia, diabetic ketoacidosis, and adrenal crisis.

- Angioedema resulting from ACE inhibitors is not histamine related, and epinephrine is unlikely to have a beneficial effect as compared to epinephrine use in histamine-related angioedema resulting from an allergen exposure.

REFERENCES

1. Kwaku MP, Burman KD. Myxedema coma. *J Intensive Care Med.* July-August 2007;22(4):224-231. Review. PubMed PMID: 17712058.

2. Pimentel L, Hansen KN. Thyroid disease in the emergency department: a clinical and laboratory review. *J Emerg Med.* February 2005;28(2):201-209. Review. PubMed PMID: 15707817.

3. Ansarin K, Niroomand B, Najafipour F, et al. End-tidal CO(2) levels lower in subclinical and overt hypothyroidism than healthy controls; no relationship to thyroid function tests. *Int J Gen Med.* January 7, 2011;4:29-33. doi:10.2147/IJGM.S16252. PubMed PMID: 21403789; PubMed Central PMCID: PMC3056328.

4. Holvey DN, Goodner CJ, Nicoloff JT, Dowling JT. Treatment of myxedema coma with intravenous thyroxine. *Arch Intern Med.* January 1964;113:89-96. PubMed PMID: 14067598.

5. Arlot S, Debussche X, Lalau JD, et al. Myxoedema coma: response of thyroid hormones with oral and intravenous high-dose L-thyroxine treatment. *Intensive Care Med.* 1991;17(1):16-18. PubMed PMID: 2037720.

6. Koetz K, Kienitz T, Quinkler M. Management of steroid replacement in adrenal insufficiency. *Minerva Endocrinol.* June 2010;35(2):61-72. Review. PubMed PMID: 20595936.

7. Neary N, Nieman L. Adrenal insufficiency: etiology, diagnosis and treatment. *Curr Opin Endocrinol Diabetes Obes.* June 2010;17(3): 217-223. doi:10.1097/MED.0b013e328338f608. Review. PubMed PMID: 20375886; PubMed Central PMCID: PMC2928659.

8. Sarlis NJ, Gourgiotis L. Thyroid emergencies. *Rev Endocr Metab Disord.* May 2003;4(2):129-136. Review. PubMed PMID: 12766540.

9. Nayak B, Burman K. Thyrotoxicosis and thyroid storm. *Endocrinol Metab Clin North Am.* December 2006;35(4):663-686, vii. Review. PubMed PMID: 17127140.

10. Nayak B, Hodak SP. Hyperthyroidism. *Endocrinol Metab Clin North Am.* September 2007;36(3):617-656, v. Review. PubMed PMID: 17673122.

11. Franklyn JA, Boelaert K. Thyrotoxicosis. *Lancet.* March 24, 2012; 379(9821):1155-1166. doi:10.1016/S0140-6736(11)60782-4. Epub 2012 Mar 5. Review. PubMed PMID: 22394559.

12. Marik PE. Critical illness-related corticosteroid insufficiency. *Chest.* January 2009;135(1):181-193. doi:10.1378/chest.08-1149. Review. PubMed PMID: 19136406.

13. Umpierrez G, Freire AX. Abdominal pain in patients with hyperglycemic crises. *J Crit Care.* March 2002;17(1):63-67. PubMed PMID: 12040551.

14. Waldman CW, Waldman SD, Waldman RA. Giant cell arteritis. *Med Clin North Am.* March 2013;97(2):329-335. doi:10.1016/j.mcna. 2012.12.006. Epub 2012 Dec 22. Review. PubMed PMID: 23419630.

CHAPTER 43

Hematological and Oncological Emergencies

David M. Landsberg

INTRODUCTION

Hematological and oncological emergencies are sometimes overlooked in EMS planning and off-line medical direction and may seem less frequent than some trauma and medical conditions. However, these conditions are no less fatal and often seemingly complex when training and education in these areas are neglected. In some cases, the EMS physician stands to have a significant impact on the outcome of the patient with these conditions, and in other cases, may positively impact an important phase in the dying process for terminal patients. In this chapter, we will review likely hematological and oncological emergencies that may be encountered in the field where there is opportunity for the EMS physician to provide treatment in the field and improved medical direction to system providers on the proper management of these sometimes-complicated patient encounters.

OBJECTIVES

- List common causes of anemia in prehospital patients.
- Describe the initial prehospital evaluation and management of acute blood loss anemia.
- Describe the initial prehospital evaluation and management of hereditary anemias.
- Describe the initial prehospital evaluation and management of hereditary bleeding disorders.
- Describe the initial prehospital evaluation and management of disseminated intravascular coagulation.
- Discuss prehospital use of blood, blood products, and factors for acute nontraumatic anemia.
- Describe the initial prehospital evaluation and management of patients on chemotherapy.
- Briefly discuss care of terminal cancer patients in the prehospital environment.

ANEMIA

The focus of this section will be on anemia related to factors other than traumatic anemia which is covered in Chapter 57. The prehospital provider will often encounter symptomatic anemia which may be at the root of activating the 9-1-1 system though not as obvious as a 9-1-1 call for clinical bleeding. The chief complaint with symptomatic anemia is more likely to be related to the ramifications of decreased oxygen-carrying capacity than the knowledge that the RBC volume is compromised. The physical examination findings are well known to the reader as are the general principles of management. The question is what parts of the standard emergency department schema are applicable to the prehospital environment and how much of it is truly needed? We will divide the discussion into three sections. The first two sections will relate to insufficient RBC production or excessive RBC destruction with the third focusing on acute blood loss other than from traumatic causes.

■ INSUFFICIENT RBC PRODUCTION

Whether this reflects nutritional deficiency, bone marrow disorder, or dysregulation, there is little to do in the prehospital environment to diagnose the cause. Though history and physical may yield a working diagnosis this is of little practical importance as therapy will remain supportive with oxygen and maintenance of effective circulating volume.

While empiric treatment with folic acid or iron may seem reasonable if the diagnostic impression is strong enough, it is hard to argue that the effect of that treatment will be brisk enough that it is worth the trade of confounding the formal diagnostic evaluation to follow.

■ INCREASED RBC DESTRUCTION

Hemolysis is defined as RBC lifespan less than 100 days.[1] There are many conditions both acquired and inherited that may result in decreased RBC lifespan. Unlike the insufficient production algorithm above where we have little to offer prehospitally there are more opportunities within this population. The inherited hemolytic disorders offer the prehospital provider treatment opportunities related to the morphologic RBC changes that occur in these conditions.

Sickle Cell Anemia The acute presentations of sickle cell disease revolve around the vasoocclusive aspects of the disorder.[2] The most dramatic examples of these include the acute chest syndrome and CVA.[3-5] The prehospital physician, being able to recognize these states, can intervene with substantial but measured fluid therapy that might not otherwise fit standard prehospital protocols.[6] The EMS physician also has the opportunity to initiate early antibiotic therapy in those select patients who present with a sickle cell crisis with or without evidence of target organ embarrassment who have significant fever.[7] Given the functional asplenism of many of these patients, untreated bacteremia of encapsulated organisms can be rapidly fatal.[8,9] This is a true opportunity for the EMS physician to impact outcome to no lesser extent than securing an airway. Ideally the EMS physician who carries antibiotics would also carry blood culture vials to provide true ED standard of care within the prehospital setting. The national awareness of sepsis and its early treatment only underscore the impact that can be made in this population.[10]

Spherocytosis While the vasoocclusive complications of sickle cell disease are not typical of this disorder, there are significant issues of hypersplenism increasing the index of suspicion for splenic injury in these patients.[11] The other vulnerability here owes to the high proportion of these patients who eventually undergo splenectomy which places them at risk for the encapsulated organisms offering the EMS physician the same opportunities here as in sickle cell disease in the context of suspected sepsis.[11]

■ ACUTE BLOOD LOSS ANEMIA AND COAGULOPATHY

Gastrointestinal hemorrhage is the prototype for this disease state but retroperitoneal hemorrhage and spontaneous hemorrhage into muscle or viscera are also significant sources of morbidity and even occasional mortality.[12] The opportunity for the EMS physician here revolves around a deeper understanding of the multiple mechanisms in play including therapeutic or intrinsic coagulopathy. Rapid assessment of hemorrhage and the degree of circulatory compromise will fit standard prehospital practice but assessment of coagulopathy both clinically and through assessment of the patient's medication list may reveal opportunities not available to the ALS provider. Clinical signs of coagulopathy inclusive of purpura, hyphema, gingival bleeding, and/or inappropriate free bleeding from small hemostatic challenges such as IV punctures may be clues. Clinical tendency to bleed may also reflect platelet aggregation defects which are generally pharmaceutically induced.[13] In the setting of clinical coagulopathy and significant hemorrhage with evidence of anticoagulant administration or chronic liver disease the EMS physician is in a position to administer vitamin K empirically just as one would in the emergency department with laboratory confirmed elevated INR.[14] Acknowledging that the full normalization effect of this dose may not be seen for 24 hours, there is clinically important reversal within 6 hours and certainly earlier administration is better than later.[14] Immediate warfarin reversal may only be achieved with FFP or PCC discussed below.[14]

Tranexamic Acid (TXA) is an antifibrinolytic administered to control bleeding through its interruption of usual homeostatic fibrinolysis that is counterproductive in the setting of acute hemorrhage.[15-17] TXA has been studied in trauma populations with the 2010 CRASH-2 trial being the largest with over 20,000 randomized patients.[18] A significant mortality reduction from hemorrhage was seen along with an all-cause mortality reduction (5.7%-4.9% [$P = 0.0077$] and 16%-14.5% [$P = 0.0035$] respectively). Of note, administration of TXA more than 3 hours after injury was associated with significantly increased mortality (3.1%-4.4%, $P = 0.004$). In a US Military (MATTER trial) study of combat trauma in Afghanistan the positive effect was even more robust than seen in CRASH-2 with an all-cause mortality reduction from 23.9% to 17.4% ($P = 0.03$).[19] There is precedent for this intervention in the prehospital setting with London's Air Ambulance actively using TXA.[20]

Another avenue to consider is qualitative and/or quantitative platelet defects. A review of the patient's medication list and OTC medications may reveal ASA or NSAID use impairing platelet function. Platelet aggregation can be significantly improved through the administration of DDAVP 0.3 μg/kg over 30 minutes.[21] The clinical effect is rapid with platelet function assays returning to normal by 30 minutes and lasting up to 4 hours mediated through the liberation of stored vWF and Factor VIII.[21-23] This also makes this intervention ideal for acute bleeding in the setting of known von Willebrand disease or Factor VIII deficiency.[24]

DISSEMINATED INTRAVASCULAR COAGULATION

DIC and dilutional coagulopathy are indistinguishable without laboratory evaluation and even then can be difficult to discern unless dilutional coagulopathy can be excluded because massive hemorrhage is not present. In either event the transfusion of plasma is indicated and hypofibrinogenemia may be the most important piece of this coagulopathy.[25] Many will use cryoprecipitate in the setting of DIC due to its high fibrinogen content per unit volume. It is important to realize that plasma is also an appropriate choice and will just as surely raise your fibrinogen level though with higher overall transfusion volume to deliver the same dose of fibrinogen.[26] In the setting of massive hemorrhage this is likely of little clinical concern and may even be preferable as all plasma factors are being lost while the patient bleeds whole blood. It is important to remember that DIC is a secondary process.[26] Treatment of the primary process must at least be entertained while clotting factors are replaced. Control of hemorrhage as the inciting event is obvious but it is conceivable that occult sepsis might be missed as the primary insult among the drama of the DIC. This again presents a very real opportunity to initiate broad antibiotic therapy as soon as the patient enters the system rather than after the significant delay inherent to transport and standard ED evaluation. The treatment of DIC assumes access to blood products which is by no means ensured in the prehospital setting and discussed in the following section.

PREHOSPITAL TRANSFUSION OF BLOOD PRODUCTS

The presence of an EMS physician on scene simplifies many of the major clinical blockades to the use of blood products prehospitally but does little to ameliorate the administrative and regulatory obstacles inherent to this process.[27] Setting those aside for the moment and examining the clinical literature there is very little in the civilian EMS world to make a case for routine transfusion prehospitally. As physicians we well understand the need for blood transfusion to replace dramatic acute blood loss. We also understand that there is a growing literature about the role or acquired coagulopathy in the setting of hemorrhage and the role for coagulation factor administration to reverse it.[25] While this is standard validated practice in the ED, it is not yet clear that there is positive patient impact prehospitally though intuitively we would reason it should. There are EMS services both nationally and internationally that administer blood products prehospitally.[20,28] There are published descriptive studies notably from Australia, the United Kingdom, and the United States that demonstrate feasibility but no randomized trials to look at efficacy.[20,28] It is not known if studies done in the combat theater (which are largely descriptive and retrospective in nature as well) can be extrapolated to the civilian experience. For now it is simply not known whether prehospital transfusion improves patient outcome. It bears mentioning that a

very old product, freeze dried plasma (FDP), may have new life in this realm as French lyophilized plasma (FLYP).[29,30] FLYP is obtained from freeze-drying FFP and exposing it to ultraviolet light to inactive RNA and DNA pathogens.[30,31] The resultant compound is a dry powder with a 2-year shelf life that is ABO universally compatible and contains all clotting factors in physiologic ratios in almost identical doses to FFP.[30,31] Much of the complexity of storage and administration of standard blood products that complicates their use prehospitally is solved with this product. Though plasma will not carry oxygen it surely will reverse coagulopathy. It is not currently available in the United States. This will remain an area of controversy and avenue for further investigation in the immediate future. It will be up to each system to decide if the added complexity, cost, and potential transport delay associated with these interventions are justified in their particular patient population.

ONCOLOGICAL EMERGENCIES

More and more patients are living longer with malignancy with improved QOL and the prehospital provider can expect to see an increasing frequency of cancer-related calls for help.[32] Oncological emergencies are broadly divided into complications of disease and complications of therapy. We will explore both simultaneously and categorize by the organ system involved while discussing only those conditions so emergent that prehospital decisions can be expected to meaningfully impact outcome.

CENTRAL NERVOUS SYSTEM EMERGENCIES

The presence or absence of central nervous system (CNS) disease will often dramatically alter a patient's prognosis through its impact on functional status.[33,34] The more common CNS oncologic emergencies relate to the effects of local inflammation engendered by a growing focus of disease. Recognizing that acute changes in mental status or acute neurologic focality in this population may be attributable to this process offers an opportunity for early intervention that might otherwise be delayed. Emergent high-dose glucocorticoid in this scenario has the potential to avert permanent neurologic compromise.[35] The earliest finding in cord compression is often back pain.[35] A clinical history of back pain in a patient with active malignancy who now has a focal neurologic deficit ascribable to the spinal level at which the patient has had historical pain is a clear indication for immediate high-dose glucocorticoid.[35] There is little, if anything, to be lost and the aversion of a devastating neurologic injury to be gained. CNS metastases or primary CNS malignancy may similarly respond to steroids if local edema is felt to reasonably be the source of acute compromise. A CNS presentation may also be elicited by local ischemia similar to the presentation of CVA but with hyperviscosity or leukostasis as the source of vascular compromise.[36] Recognition of this possibility in the right clinical scenario such as acute leukemia or myeloma will give the astute EMS physician the opportunity to initiate dilutional therapy long prior to when it would otherwise have been initiated.[36,37]

CARDIOPULMONARY EMERGENCIES

Airway remains at the pinnacle of our treatment pyramid and any expanding lesion that compromises the patency of our airway draws our most urgent attention. As always, a patient who is able to maintain their airway and breathe for themselves should be supported in that endeavor.[38] The use of steroids, racemic epinephrine, and CPAP are all reasonable and often effective adjuncts to manage acute airway edema of various etiologies.[38,39] Even with an obstructing mass there is often a component of edema in the surrounding tissues that may offer opportunity for the prehospital provider. An isolated obstruction above the cords may be handled with cricothyrotomy if all else fails but the new complement of video laryngoscopes commercially available may offer the EMS physician an opportunity to safely visualize the obstruction and possibly even negotiate the airway successfully without resorting to surgical procedures.[40,41] These devices offer airway visualization without necessarily instrumenting the site of inflammation carrying the risks well understood by this reader. The author has had great success with these devices in such circumstances, and incidentally for this reader, also in fully immobilized patients with rigid collar intact.

More distal airway obstruction might be assessed and managed with a self-contained bronchoscope if the EMS physician is so trained and so equipped or might also be well visualized with a fiberoptic intubating stylette. This may yield just enough information to guide a narrow lumen endotracheal tube (ETT) correctly. Right or left mainstem obstructions might be well managed through the same process by directing the ETT into the open bronchus and excluding the compromised lung through inflation of the balloon within the patent mainstem. This maneuver may require a narrower than usual ETT. The same principle may be applied to unilateral pulmonary hemorrhage to prevent the hemorrhagic lung from inundating the good lung. Isolation of the good lung is usually enough to allow oxygenation but not until the hemorrhagic lung is tamponaded with a luminal balloon can the bleeding be controlled.

Cardiac tamponade is another source of acute or acute on chronic compromise.[35] Malignant effusions often grow very slowly over many months, steadily stretching the pericardium until the space may hold as much as a liter.[35,42] Despite the slow growth at some point this will compromise the patient enough that pericardiocentesis will be indicated. The EMS physician utilizing portable ultrasound will be able to prove this clinical suspicion in the field as well as assess the true degree of tamponade present.[43,44] The use of ultrasound will also give information about the echodensity of the collection and whether hemorrhage needs to be considered.[43,44] If hemorrhage is strongly suspected and clinical tamponade is present the EMS physician should consider leaving a drain at the time of pericardiocentesis which is elegantly handled through the use of a triple lumen catheter placed in the pericardial space via modified Seldinger technique.

The final cardiopulmonary differential to consider is those direct toxicities of certain chemotherapeutic regimens that may induce direct organ damage. A patient presenting with a picture of new parenchymal lung disease that does not seem to be infectious may, in fact, have been exposed to bleomycin or be suffering radiation or talc pneumonitis.[45,46] The pneumonitides are important to remember because they often respond to steroids and should receive them as soon as the diagnosis is strongly suspected.[45,46] New decompensated heart failure may come as a result of exposure to cyclophosphamide or doxorubicin.[47] Standard heart failure management approaches will apply.[47]

■ METABOLIC EMERGENCIES

Hypercalcemia Hypercalcemia may clinically resemble hypothyroidism with fatigue, constipation, apathy, and delirium being common manifestations.[35] The presence of underlying malignancy with known high rate of extensive bony metastases such as breast, lung, and myeloma are good clues to the diagnosis.[35] Prehospitally the management would focus on volume repletion with the provision of aggressive IVF. Steroids can be used as adjunctive therapy but are inferior to pamidronate or zoledronic acid which, due to cost, frequency of use and onset of action are impractical in the prehospital environment.[35]

Tumor Lysis Syndrome Tumor lysis syndrome (TLS) comes as a result of abrupt mass cellular death, often after initiation of chemotherapy most commonly in the setting of sensitive leukemias and lymphomas.[35] This can occur within 24 to 48 hours of initiating chemotherapy. There will be little to the clinical presentation to specifically make this diagnosis. In most cases, the chemistry panel will be needed to diagnose TLS. A clue for the EMS physician could be a prehospital diagnosis of likely hyperkalemia based on ECG changes. Placing that diagnosis in the context of a newly diagnosed leukemic who received chemotherapy 3 days ago and now has been oliguric for the last 24 hours could fairly strongly support a TLS diagnosis. The important thing for the EMS physician to remember is that these patients require aggressive hydration to avert renal injury and the more confidently the scenario suggests this diagnosis the more aggressive should be the fluid therapy.[35]

■ NEUTROPENIC FEVER

Most patients who have received a chemotherapeutic regimen that is likely to induce neutropenia will have been educated about the risks to their immune function. A patient who received such chemotherapy 1 to 2 weeks prior to prehospital presentation is assumed to be neutropenic in the context of a presentation that suggests infection until proven otherwise. It is never more true than it is in this situation that early antibiotics may make the difference between life and death.[48] The EMS physician presented with this situation is well advised to quickly draw cultures and initiate antibiotics. Even if the antibiotic you carry is less broad than you might otherwise choose in the ED it is still apt to cover the most likely pathogens and offers a significant opportunity in the care of this most fragile patient. Infection in an immunocompromised host can be rapidly fatal over hours.[48] As with lumbar puncture, do not delay life-saving treatment but do make every reasonable effort to get cultures.

TERMINAL PATIENTS

Death is entirely personal and is experienced uniquely by each individual and each family. Assumptions have no place here but well-worded questions that explore the patient's and family's understanding of the state of the disease as well as their preferences and their expectations will mark 2 to 3 minutes very well spent at the beginning of your encounter. The features unique to the prehospital environment where the EMS physician can substantially impact the plan are in the physician's clear understanding of what the hospital can and cannot do. The EMS physician is also equipped to explore if this patient had hoped to die at home and whether one more trip to the hospital runs a very real risk of that not happening. The EMS physician can meaningfully explore if transport is truly in the best interest of the patient and by virtue of physician skill set and authority may be able to facilitate meeting the patient's needs right in their own home, maximizing their quality and potentially even quantity of life. This may even extend to the provision of some social services depending on the resources of one's community.

Our ability as EMS physicians to bring hospital resources to the prehospital environment extends beyond the obvious treatment interventions of which this text is replete. The presence of the EMS physician on scene ensures that the right thing will always be done irrespective of any policy or protocol because we are the protocol and society has invested us with the breadth of experience and authority to always do the right thing. It is, after all, why we do what we do.

REFERENCES

1. Mohandas N, Schrier SL. Mechanisms of red cell destruction in hemolytic anemias. In: Mentzer WC, Wagner GM, eds. *The Hereditary Hemolytic Anemias.* New York: Churchill Livingstone; 1989:391.
2. Embury SH, Garcia JF, Mohandas N, Pennathur-Das R, Clark MR. Effects of oxygen inhalation on endogenous erythropoietin kinetics,

erythropoiesis, and properties of blood cells in sickle-cell anemia. *N Engl J Med.* 1984;311(5):291.

3. National Acute Chest Syndrome Study Group; Vichinsky EP, Neumayr LD, et al. Causes and outcomes of the acute chest syndrome in sickle cell disease. *N Engl J Med.* 2000;342(25):1855.

4. Gladwin MT, Vichinsky EN. Pulmonary complications of sickle cell disease. *Engl J Med.* 2008;359(21):2254.

5. Webb J, Kwiatkowski JL. Stroke in patients with sickle cell disease. *Expert Rev Hematol.* June 2013;6(3):301-316. doi:10.1586/ehm.13.25. PubMed PMID: 23782084.

6. Glassberg J. Evidence-based management of sickle cell disease in the emergency department. *Emerg Med Pract.* August 2011;13(8):1-20; quiz 20. Review. PubMed PMID: 22164362.

7. Bernard AW, Lindsell CJ, Venkat A. Derivation of a risk assessment tool for emergency department patients with sickle cell disease. *Emerg Med J.* October 2008;25(10):635-639. doi:10.1136/emj.2007.056689. PubMed PMID: 18843058.

8. Brousse V, Elie C, Benkerrou M, et al. Acute splenic sequestration crisis in sickle cell disease: cohort study of 190 paediatric patients. *Br J Haematol.* March 2012;156(5):643-648. doi:10.1111/j.1365-2141.2011.08999.x. Epub 2012 Jan 9. PubMed PMID: 22224796.

9. Morgan TL, Tomich EB. Overwhelming post-splenectomy infection (OPSI): a case report and review of the literature. *J Emerg Med.* October 2012;43(4):758-763. doi:10.1016/j.jemermed.2011.10.029. Epub 2012 Jun 21. Review. PubMed PMID: 22726665.

10. Dellinger RP, Levy MM, Rhodes A, et al. Surviving sepsis campaign: international guidelines for management of severe sepsis and septic shock: 2012. *Crit Care Med.* February 2013;41(2):580-637. doi:10.1097/CCM.0b013e31827e83af. PubMed PMID: 23353941.

11. Bolton-Maggs PH, Stevens RF, Dodd NJ, et al. Guidelines for the diagnosis and management of hereditary spherocytosis. *Br J Haematol.* August 2004;126(4):455-474. Review. PubMed PMID: 15287938.

12. Chan YC, Morales JP, Reidy JF, Taylor PR. Management of spontaneous and iatrogenic retroperitoneal haemorrhage: conservative management, endovascular intervention or open surgery? *Int J Clin Pract.* October 2008;62(10):1604-1613. Epub 2007 Oct 19. Review. PubMed PMID: 17949429.

13. Eikelboom JW, Hirsh J, Spencer FA, Baglin TP, Weitz JI. Antiplatelet drugs: Antithrombotic Therapy and Prevention of Thrombosis, 9th ed: American College of Chest Physicians Evidence-Based Clinical Practice Guidelines. *Chest.* February 2012;141(2 suppl):e89S-e119S. doi:10.1378/chest.11-2293. Review. PubMed PMID:22315278; PubMed Central PMCID: PMC3269069.

14. Holbrook A, Schulman S, Witt DM, et al. Evidence-based management of anticoagulant therapy: Antithrombotic Therapy and Prevention of Thrombosis, 9th ed: American College of Chest Physicians Evidence-Based Clinical Practice Guidelines. *Chest.* February 2012;141(2 suppl):e152S-e184S. doi:10.1378/chest.11-2295. Review. PubMed PMID: 22315259; PubMed Central PMCID: PMC3278055.

15. Napolitano LM, Cohen MJ, Cotton BA, Schreiber MA, Moore EE. Tranexamic acid in trauma: how should we use it? *J Trauma Acute Care Surg.* June 2013;74(6):1575-1586. doi:10.1097/TA.0b013e318292cc54. Review. PubMed PMID:23694890.

16. Perel P, Ker K, Morales Uribe CH, Roberts I. Tranexamic acid for reducing mortality in emergency and urgent surgery. *Cochrane Database Syst Rev.* January 31, 2013;1:CD010245. doi:10.1002/14651858. CD010245.pub2. Review. PubMed PMID: 23440847.

17. Rappold JF, Pusateri AE. Tranexamic acid in remote damage control resuscitation. *Transfusion.* January 2013;53(suppl 1):96S-99S. doi:10.1111/trf.12042. Review. PubMed PMID: 23301980.

18. CRASH-2 trial collaborators, Shakur H, Roberts I, et al. Effects of tranexamic acid on death, vascular occlusive events, and blood transfusion in trauma patients with significant haemorrhage (CRASH-2): a randomised, placebo-controlled trial. *Lancet.* July 3, 2010;376(9734):23-32. doi:10.1016/S0140-6736(10)60835-5. Epub 2010 Jun 14. PubMed PMID: 20554319.

19. Morrison JJ, Dubose JJ, Rasmussen TE, Midwinter MJ. Military Application of Tranexamic Acid in Trauma Emergency Resuscitation (MATTERs) Study. *Arch Surg.* February 2012;147(2):113-119. doi:10.1001/archsurg.2011.287. Epub 2011 Oct 17. PubMed PMID: 22006852.

20. Lockey DJ, Weaver AE, Davies GE. Practical translation of hemorrhage control techniques to the civilian trauma scene. *Transfusion.* January 2013;53(suppl 1):17S-22S. doi:10.1111/trf.12031. PubMed PMID: 23301967.

21. Franchini M. The use of desmopressin as a hemostatic agent: a concise review. *Am J Hematol.* 2007;82:731-735.

22. Flordal PA, Sahlin S. Use of desmopressin to prevent bleeding complications in patients treated with aspirin. *Br J Surg.* 1993;80:723-724.

23. Beck KH, Mohr P, Bleckmann U, Schweer H, Kretschmer V. Desmopressin effect on acetylsalicylic acid impaired platelet function. *Semin Thromb Hemost.* 1995;21:32-39.

24. Emma T, Emma L, Raza A. Treatment of patients with von Willebrand disease. *J Blood Med.* 2011;2:49-57. Published online 2011 April 20. doi: 10.2147/JBM.S9890Correction in: J Blood Med. 2013;4: 57-58. PMCID: PMC3262353.

25. Maegele M, Spinella PC, Schöchl H. The acute coagulopathy of trauma: mechanisms and tools for risk stratification. *Shock.* November 2012;38(5):450-458. doi:10.1097/SHK.0b013e31826dbd23. Review. PubMed PMID: 23042192.

26. Di Nisio M, Baudo F, Cosmi B, et al. Diagnosis and treatment of disseminated intravascular coagulation: guidelines of the Italian Society for Haemostasis and Thrombosis (SISET). *Thromb Res.* May 2012;129(5):e177-e1784. doi:10.1016/j.thromres.2011.08.028. Epub 2011 Sep 17.Review. PubMed PMID: 21930293.

27. Slapak C, Fredrich N, Wagner J. Transfusion safety: is this the business of blood centers? *Transfusion.* December 2011;51(12 pt 2):2767-2771. doi:10.1111/j.1537-2995.2011.03454.x. Review. PubMed PMID: 22150688.

28. Weiskopf RB, Ness PM. Transfusion for remote damage control resuscitation. *Transfusion.* January 2013;53(suppl 1):1S-5S. doi:10.1111/trf.12092. PubMed PMID: 23301968.

29. Statement on normal (whole, pooled) human plasma prepared by Committee on Plasma and Plasma Substitutes of the Division of Medical Sciences. National Research Council. *Transfusion.* March-April 1968;8(2):57-59. PubMed PMID: 5643632.

30. Sailliol A, Martinaud C, Cap AP, et al. The evolving role of lyophilized plasma in remote damage control resuscitation in the French Armed Forces Health Service. *Transfusion.* January 2013;53(suppl 1):65S-71S. doi:10.1111/trf.12038. PubMed PMID: 23301975.

31. Martinaud C, Civadier C, Ausset S, Verret C, Deshayes AV, Sailliol A. In vitro hemostatic properties of French lyophilized plasma. *Anesthesiology.* August 2012;117(2):339-346. doi:10.1097/ALN.0b013e3182608cdd. PubMed PMID: 22739764.

32. 61-year trends in US cancer death rates. Table 1.3. SEER Cancer Statistics Review. National Cancer Institute. 2010. http://seer.cancer.gov/archive/csr/1975_2010/results_merged/topic_historical_mort_trends.pdf.

33. Reck M, Thatcher N, Smit EF, et al. Baseline quality of life and performance status as prognostic factors in patients with extensive-stage disease small cell lung cancer treated with pemetrexed plus carboplatin vs. etoposide plus carboplatin. *Lung Cancer.* December 2012;78(3):276-281. doi:10.1016/j.lungcan.2012.09.002. Epub 2012 Oct 6. PubMed PMID: 23043970.

34. Rades D, Douglas S, Huttenlocher S, et al. Prognostic factors and a survival score for patients with metastatic spinal cord compression from colorectal cancer. *Strahlenther Onkol.* December 2012;188(12):1114-1118. doi:10.1007/s00066-012-0141-0. Epub 2012 Nov 1. PubMed PMID: 23111468.

35. McCurdy MT, Shanholtz CB. Oncologic emergencies. *Crit Care Med.* July 2012;40(7):2212-2222. doi:10.1097/CCM.0b013e31824e1865. Review. PubMed PMID: 22584756.

36. Stone MJ, Bogen SA. Evidence-based focused review of management of hyperviscosity syndrome. *Blood.* March 8,

2012;119(10):2205-2208. doi:10.1182/blood2011-04-347690. Epub 2011 Dec 6. Review. PubMed PMID: 22147890.

37. Ganzel C, Becker J, Mintz PD, Lazarus HM, Rowe JM. Hyperleukocytosis, leukostasis and leukapheresis: practice management. *Blood Rev.* May 2012;26(3):117-122. doi:10.1016/j.blre.2012.01.003. Epub 2012 Feb 23. Review. PubMed PMID: 22364832.

38. Sasidaran K, Bansal A, Singhi S. Acute upper airway obstruction. *Indian J Pediatr.* October 2011;78(10):1256-1261. doi:10.1007/s12098-011-0414-0. Epub 2011 May 11. Review. PubMed PMID: 21559808.

39. Williams B, Boyle M, Robertson N, Giddings C. When pressure is positive: a literature review of the prehospital use of continuous positive airway pressure. *Prehosp Disaster Med.* February 2013;28(1):52-60. doi:10.1017/S1049023X12001562. Epub 2012 Nov 9. Review. PubMed PMID: 23140660.

40. Struck MF, Wittrock M, Nowak A. Prehospital Glidescope video laryngoscopy for difficult airway management in a helicopter rescue program with anaesthetists. *Eur J Emerg Med.* October 2011;18(5):282-284. doi:10.1097/MEJ.0b013e328344e70f. PubMed PMID: 21430543.

41. Bjoernsen LP, Lindsay B. Video laryngoscopy in the prehospital setting. *Prehosp Disaster Med.* May-June 2009;24(3):265-270. Review. PubMed PMID: 19618365.

43. Labovitz AJ, Noble VE, Bierig M, et al. Focused cardiac ultrasound in the emergent setting: a consensus statement of the American Society of Echocardiography and American College of Emergency Physicians. *J Am Soc Echocardiogr.* December 2010;23(12):1225-1230. doi:10.1016/j.echo.2010.10.005. PubMed PMID: 21111923.

44. Arntfield RT, Millington SJ. Point of care cardiac ultrasound applications in the emergency department and intensive care unit—a review. *Curr Cardiol Rev.* May 2012;8(2):98-108. Review. PubMed PMID: 22894759; PubMed Central PMCID: PMC3406278.

42. Quint LE. Thoracic complications and emergencies in oncologic patients. *Cancer Imaging.* October 2, 2009;9(Spec No A):S75-S82. doi:10.1102/1470-7330.2009.9031. Review.PubMed PMID: 19965299; PubMed Central PMCID: PMC2797469.

45. Vasić L, Durdević P. [Radiation-induced lung damage—etiopathogenesis, clinical features, imaging findings and treatment]. *Med Pregl.* July-August 2012;65(7-8):319-325. Review. Serbian. PubMed PMID: 22924253.

46. Fyfe AJ, McKay P. Toxicities associated with bleomycin. *J R Coll Physicians Edinb.* September 2010;40(3):213-215. doi:10.4997/JRCPE.2010.306. Review. PubMed PMID: 21127762.

47. Volkova M, Russell R 3rd. Anthracycline cardiotoxicity: prevalence, pathogenesis and treatment. *Curr Cardiol Rev.* November 2011;7(4):214-220. Review. PubMed PMID: 22758622; PubMed Central PMCID: PMC3322439.

48. Maschmeyer G, Beinert T, Buchheidt D, et al. Diagnosis and antimicrobial therapy of lung infiltrates in febrile neutropenic patients: Guidelines of the infectious diseases working party of the German Society of Haematology and Oncology. *Eur J Cancer.* September 2009;45(14):2462-2472. doi:10.1016/j.ejca.2009.05.001. Epub 2009 May 23. Review. PubMed PMID: 19467584.

Renal and Urogenital Emergencies

Norma L. Cooney

INTRODUCTION

Urogenital complaints are common presentations to emergency departments and EMS providers. Although not the typical focus of prehospital education and planning, these clinical scenarios represent a potentially growing number of calls as more and more members of the public rely on EMS as their entry into the health care safety net. Despite the fact that these conditions are not the typical focus of EMS physicians and providers, appropriate care and attention can significantly impact the quality of care that these patients receive. In some cases, the prehospital patient encounter provides the needed clues to the diagnosis and proper management that would not otherwise be apparent. Even in cases where field care is not potentially definitive, attention to detail in the field and carefully relaying observations can speed diagnostic confirmation and intervention in the emergency department.

OBJECTIVES

- List common causes of hematuria in prehospital patients.
- Describe the initial prehospital evaluation and management of urogenital trauma.
- Describe the initial prehospital evaluation and management of priapism.
- Describe the initial prehospital evaluation and management of victims of sexual assault.
- Describe common complications of urological procedures affecting prehospital patient care (Foley/suprapubic catheters, nephrostomy tubes, kidney transplant, failure of dialysis catheters (ie, venous air embolism).
- Discuss flank pain.

The kidneys are the filter systems of the blood. They receive nearly 25% of the cardiac output, filtering 180 L per day though only approximately 1 L/day is excreted as urine. The bladder stores urine in a low-pressure system with a normal capacity of 400 to 500 cc. Injury or dysfunction of the mechanism of the filter or bladder can lead to significant illness.

HEMATURIA

Etiologies of hematuria are wide and varied. The most common causes are related to urogenital trauma, infection, nephritis, kidney stones, and tumors. It is important to note that medications may induce a red discoloration to the urine which may be mistaken for hematuria. These medications include but are not limited to sulfonamides, quinine, rifampin, and phenytoin. Posttraumatic hematuria may be secondary to renal or bladder injury. Infectious causes include hemorrhagic cystitis. Nephritis, kidney stones, and tumors are other causes. For the patient with flank pain that radiates into the groin (especially those with a history of renal colic) analgesia with narcotics and ketorolac may be appropriate in the prehospital setting. For older patients with no renal colic history the ketorolac should be omitted due to the potential for abdominal aortic aneurism to be masquerading as renal colic.

URINARY RETENTION

Patients with urinary retention typically present with acute lower abdominal pain and distention with an inability to urinate. In men older than 50 years of age, the most common cause is prostate hypertrophy. Other causes of urinary retention include obstructive, infectious and inflammatory, pharmacologic, neurologic, or other. Other common causes include prostatitis, cystitis, urethritis, and vulvovaginitis, and medication-induced urinary retention from anticholinergic and α-adrenergic agonist medications. Neurologic causes such as cortical, spinal, or peripheral nerve lesions may be the causation.

A history and a focused physical examination provide significant insight into the etiology of the patient's pain. The patient may have obvious distension of the lower abdomen and tenderness to palpation. Confirmation of a distended bladder is easily done with bedside ultrasound. One of the most common and easiest methods to measure bladder volume is the *prolate ellipsoid equation*: volume = length × width × height × 0.52. The diagnosis of urinary retention is defined as postvoid residual greater than 100 cc. This can be measured using a small ultrasound machine or passing a catheter into the bladder to collect the remaining urine.

Treatment is immediate decompression of the bladder with a straight catheter. Depending on the etiology of the urinary retention, a Foley catheter may need to be left in place until further diagnostic studies can be done. Pain medication should be strongly considered for treatment in the prehospital phase of care.

TESTICULAR TORSION

Torsion most commonly presents in puberty and occurs in 1 in 4000 per 25,000 males per year before the age of 25.[1-3] Torsion may be associated with trauma; however, this is not necessarily the case. Torsion of the testes is a urologic emergency. Patients typically have an acute onset of pain and nausea or vomiting secondary to pain. Patients may also complain of referred abdominal pain. The position of the testicle will be high and will lie in the transverse position of the affected testis. There will also be an abnormal cremasteric reflex.

Diagnosis is one made by clinical history and the physical examination. If a torsed testicle is suspected, an immediate detorsion of the testicle is necessary. If the testicle is not detorsed within 6 hours,[4,5] there is a high likelihood that the testicle may have irreversible ischemic. Manual detorsion using the "opening of a book" technique. Place the patient in the supine position or standing position. Manual detorsion of the testicle involves twisting outward and laterally. The testicle should be rotated outward 180° in a medial-to-lateral direction. Lateral rotation of the torsion has been described in up to a third of testicular torsions. Testicles may retorse after detorsion. In these cases surgical intervention is required.

Rotation of the testicle may need to be repeated two to three times for complete detorsion. Pain relief serves as a guide to successful detorsion. Resolution of the transverse lie of the testis to a longitudinal orientation, lower position of the testis in the scrotum, and return of normal arterial pulsations detected with a Doppler stethoscope are indicators of a successful detorsion.

PRIAPISM (BOX 44-1)

Priapism is defined as an erect penis for greater than 6 hours that has not returned to its natural flaccid state. There are two categories of priapism: low flow and high flow. In low-flow priapism, the blood cannot flow out of the penis. In high-flow priapism, the cause is typically secondary to a tear of an artery from penis or perineal injury.

Etiologies of priapism include sickle cell anemia, medications including Desyrel and Thorazine. Spinal cord injury, genitalia injury, black widow spider bites, carbon monoxide poisoning, and illicit drug use such as marijuana and cocaine may cause priapism.

Complications include ischemia, thrombosis, and impotence. Prehospital treatment begins with cold packs to the penis and perineum. Depending on the type of priapism, the patient may necessitate ligation of a vessel, intracavernous injection, surgical shunt, or aspiration. Interventions for ischemic priapism should begin within 4 to 6 hours

Box 44-1

Causes of Priapism[6]

Idiopathic

Drugs

Anticoagulants: **Heparin, Warfarin**

Antihypertensives: dihydralazine, guanethidine, labetalol, Nifedipine, phenoxybenzamine, prazosin

Antidepressants: phenelzine, trazodone, hypnotics, clozapine, diazepam

Blockers: tamsulosin, doxazosin, terazosin, prazosin

Recreational drugs: cocaine, ethanol, marijuana

Hematological disorders

Sickle cell anaemia

Leukemia

Multiple myeloma

Paroxysmal nocturnal hemoglobinuria

Thalassemia

Thrombocythemia

Henoch-Schönlein purpura

Metabolic disorders

Amyloidosis

Fabry disease

Gout

Diabetes

Nephrotic syndrome

Renal failure

Hemodialysis

Hyperlipidemic total parenteral nutrition

Trauma

Tumors (primary or metastatic)

Neurological disorders

(Modified from Box 1 from Cherian J, Rao AR, Thwaini A, Kapasi F, Shergill IS, Samman R. Medical and surgical management of priapism. *Postgrad Med J*. February 2006;82(964):89-94. With permission from BMJ Publishing Group, Ltd.)[6]

and include decompression of the corpora cavernosa by aspiration and intracavernous injection of sympathomimetic drugs. Prehospital care should include analgesia and if the patient is otherwise stable, transport to a hospital with on-call urological services.

SCROTAL ABSCESS/CELLULITIS

Scrotal abscesses are either superficial or intrascrotal. Superficial abscesses may be incised and drained without any significant complications. Intrascrotal abscesses must be surgically drained and require further investigation as to the etiology. Scrotal cellulitis typically presents with a swollen scrotum and pain. Patients may present with swelling and tenderness to the generalized area. There may be referred abdominal pain. If the infection has spread to more than a localized infection, the patient may have fevers, nausea, and vomiting.

An intrascrotal abscess may be secondary to epididymal infection, a testicular abscess that ruptures through the tunica albuginea, or drainage of appendicitis into scrotum through a patent processus vaginalis. Urethral stricture and neurogenic bladder with an alternate collecting device may be a source of a scrotal abscess.

Ultrasound is useful in detecting the location of the abscess. A superficial abscess to the scrotum can be treated with a simple incision and drainage procedure. Intrascrotal abscesses require surgical drainage. The cavity is typically left opened and packed. Typically the prehospital component of care is limited to analgesia and transport.

PHIMOSIS

Phimosis is defined as the inability to retract the foreskin over the glans penis. This is problematic if there is disruption of normal urinary function or if there is pain during sexual activities. Common treatments include steroid creams, manual stretching, changing masturbation habits, preputioplasty, and circumcision. No immediate prehospital intervention is required.

PARAPHIMOSIS

Paraphimosis occurs when the foreskin is retracted behind the glans penis and cannot return to the normal position. This stricture may cause reduced blood flow to the glans and the potential for an ischemic glans. This is a urologic emergency and can result in a gangrenous glans penis if not addressed in a timely fashion. In this retracted state, the glans tissues and penis may become swollen and subsequently more difficult to retract the foreskin back over the glans penis. Paraphimosis can typically be treated with compression of the glans penis and the return of the foreskin to its natural position. With analgesia an EMS physician may be able to reduce this in the prehospital setting; however, a penile block may be required to successful perform a reduction. In some cases a dorsal slit procedure may be needed. Only an initial attempt at manual (nonsurgical) reduction should be performed if attempted in the field.

SEXUAL ASSAULT

The sexually assaulted patient may present with varied complaints. The obvious genitourinary complaint may not be the primary complaint. Attention to details and the situation of the story are critical for appropriate evaluation and treatment of these patients. If the presenting symptom is *sexual assault* the police should be notified immediately especially if it is a minor. The adult patient must initiate their expressed wishes to file charges. In the case of an alleged sexual assault, one should make special considerations when dealing with the patient and handling articles of clothing. Collection of evidence (clothing or body fluids) is crucial to potential cases.

In the prehospital setting, one should not only be considerate of the particular handling of potential evidence, but must also remember that these patients may be the victim of significant trauma. A full screening evaluation should be done to determine if the patient has any life-threatening emergencies. After a complete medical evaluation, a sexual assault examination should be done at the hospital. This can be done by the emergency physician or by a designated regional sexual assault nurse examiner (SANE).

SANEs are specialists in one of the most well-known fields within the arena of forensic nursing.[7] SANEs have been most visible to sexual assault prosecutors, with programs in operation since the 1970s. SANEs are not available in every region. These nurses are specialists and experts in their field and a great resource to the patients and the medical community. They obtain a detailed history of the assault. If the patient is otherwise stable, transport to a hospital with a SANE program should be considered.

▪ HISTORICAL DETAILS

- Date and time of assault
- Location of assault
- Name of assailant and relationship of assailant to patient

- Mechanisms of injury
- Patient narrative of the assault (patient's history of the assault in her words)

The SANE specialist then conducts a forensic-oriented examination. Evidence is collected from all potential sources of the body including oral mucosa, finger nail beds, anus, vaginal wall, clothing, etc.

SOCIAL SERVICES

There are several types of abuse. They include *physical abuse, emotional abuse, neglect, isolation, financial or material exploitation, abandonment, sexual abuse, and self-neglect.* In an alleged assault case or suspect type of abuse, a social worker should always be involved to ensure the safety and well-being of the patient after the emergency department visit. A historical note, it was the passage of Title XX of the Social Security Act in 1974 that gave states permission to use Social Services Block Grant (SSBG) funds for the protection of adults as well as children.[8]

MANDATED REPORTERS

The circumstances under which a mandatory reporter must make a report vary from state to state. Typically, a report must be made when the reporter, in his or her official capacity, suspects or has reason to believe that a child has been abused or neglected. Another standard frequently used is in situations in which the reporter has knowledge of, or observes a child being subjected to, conditions that would reasonably result in harm to the child.[9]

Individuals designated as mandatory reporters typically have frequent contact with children. Such individuals may include:

- Social workers
- Teachers, principals, and other school personnel
- Physicians, nurses, and other health care workers
- Counselors, therapists, and other mental health professionals
- Child care providers
- Medical examiners or coroners
- Law enforcement officers

COMPLICATIONS OF RENAL/UROLOGICAL DEVICES

Several complications can occur with a *Foley* or *suprapubic* catheter. One of the most common is dislodgment of the catheter. Typically, the catheter is either pulled out accidentally when the patient is getting up out of bed or it is intentionally pulled out secondary to dementia or an altered mental status state. If there is a visible laceration, then pressure should be applied. However, typically there is no obvious tear. If this is the case, ensuring the patient is hemodynamically is most important in the prehospital medicine environment.

Nephrostomy tubes and *ureteral stents* are also common urological interventions that may prompt a call for EMS when there are complications. Pain or bleeding from stent migration or failure requires prehospital analgesia and transport to a hospital with urological services.

Dialysis catheter failure or bleeding from an *AV fistula* should prompt transport to a hospital with nephrology and a surgeon component in managing shunts. Patients who are suffering from decompensation due to missed dialysis should also be transported to a center with the same criteria. In cases where patients undergoing hemodialysis at an outpatient center experience acute chest pain and/or shortness of breath, or stroke-like symptoms, they should be transported in the left lateral decubitus position and preferentially taken to a hospital with emergency hyperbaric oxygen therapy services available because iatrogenic venous gas embolism can occur from faulty dialysis connections/catheters.[10] Stroke-like symptoms in this case would imply a pulmonary shunt or patent foramen ovale and a resulting arterial gas embolism to the brain.

UROGENITAL TRAUMA

STRADDLE INJURIES

A straddle injury is any injury to the genitalia, rectum, or perineum from a fall while straddling an object. This typically refers to blunt trauma; however, penetrating injury can also occur.[11] Straddle injuries can occur from falls in the home, falls at the swimming pool, playground equipment, skating, bicycle, and scooters accidents.[12] Some other causes include construction-related injuries, equestrian injuries, mechanical bull riding, and personal watercraft injuries. After direct trauma to the groin, the patient will develop pain, swelling, and bruising. Difficulty with urination may also occur. Associated injuries can include urethral injury, laceration of the perineum, and fracture of the pelvis. Prehospital management includes analgesia, cold packs, and precautions for pelvic fracture. A careful history should be obtained and caution should be taken in situations where trauma was not reported or when injury mechanism seems inconsistent. Ensuring a systematic approach to the evaluation and documentation of straddle injuries is an important component in the effort to avoid missing sexual abuse.[13] In cases of diabetics and other immune suppressed patients, consideration of cellulitis and Fournier gangrene is appropriate in the differential.

PENILE FRACTURE

Fracture of the penis is rupture of the tunica albuginea that also can result in injury to the corpora cavernosa and tearing of the urethra. This injury can lead to chronic issues including urethral stricture, impotence, and other related penile conditions. The mechanism of injury is typically related to sexual activity.[14] This condition typically presents with acute penile pain, detumescence, penile swelling and deviation, and inability or difficulty voiding. Because this condition has a high likelihood of urethral injury and is typically managed surgically, some effort should be made to transport otherwise stable patients to a hospital with on-call urological services. Pain control and avoiding manipulation are keys to prehospital care.

KEY POINTS

- The most commons causes of hematuria are urogenital trauma, infection, nephritis, kidney stones, and tumors.
- The diagnosis of urinary retention is defined as postvoid residual greater than 100 cc.
- Manual detorsion of the testicle involves twisting outward and laterally. The testicle should be rotated outward 180° in a medial-to-lateral direction.
- Prehospital treatment of priapism begins with cold packs to the penis and perineum.
- Paraphimosis can typically be treated with compression of the glans penis and the return of the foreskin to its natural position.
- In cases where sexual abuse is reported or suspected transport to a hospital with a SANE program should be considered.
- Straddle injuries can be associated with urethral injury, laceration of the perineum, and fracture of the pelvis. Prehospital management includes analgesia, cold packs, and precautions for pelvic fracture.

REFERENCES

1. Sharp VJ, Kieran K, Arlen AM. Testicular torsion: diagnosis, evaluation, and management. *Am Fam Physician.* December 15, 2013;88(12):835-840.
2. Wampler SM, Llanes M. Common scrotal and testicular problems. *Prim Care.* September 2010;37(3):613-626.

3. Ringdahl E, Teague L. Testicular torsion. *Am Fam Physician.* November 2006;74(10):1739-1743.

4. Mäkelä E, Lahdes-Vasama T, Rajakorpi H, Wikström S. A 19-year review of paediatric patients with acute scrotum. *Scand J Surg.* 2007;96(1):62-66.

5. Kiesling VJ Jr, Schroeder DE, Pauljev P, Hull J. Spermatic cord block and manual reduction: primary treatment for spermatic cord torsion. *J Urol.* November 1984;132(5):921-923.

6. Cherian J, Rao AR, Thwaini A, Kapasi F, Shergill IS, Samman R. Medical and surgical management of priapism. *Postgrad Med J.* February 2006;82(964):89-94.

7. American Prosecutor's Research Institute. The role of the sexual assault nurse examiner. National District Attorney's Association. 2007. http://www.ndaa.org/pdf/pub_role_sexual_assault_nurse_examiner.pdf. Accessed May, 2015.

8. Mixson PM, Public policy, elder abuse, and Adult Protective Services: the struggle for coherence. *J Elder Abuse Negl.* 2010 Jan;22(1–2):16-36.

9. Administration for Children and Families. Mandatory reporters of child abuse and neglect. U.S. Department of Health and Human Services. https://www.childwelfare.gov/systemwide/laws_policies/statutes/manda.pdf. Accessed May 2015.

10. Cooney DR, Kassem J, McCabe J. Electrocardiogram and X-ray findings associated with iatrogenic pulmonary venous gas embolism. *Undersea Hyperb Med.* March-April 2011;38(2):101-107.

11. Spitzer RF, Kives S, Caccia N, Ornstein M, Goia C, Allen LM. Retrospective review of unintentional female genital trauma at a pediatric referral center. *Pediatr Emerg Care.* December 2008;24(12): 831-835.

12. Saxena AK, Steiner M, Höllwarth ME. Straddle injuries in female children and adolescents: 10-year accident and management analysis. *Indian J Pediatr.* 2014;81(8):766-769.

13. Greaney H, Ryan J. Straddle injuries—is current practice safe? *Eur J Emerg Med.* December 1998;5(4):421-424.

14. Agarwal MM, Singh SK, Sharma DK, et al. Fracture of the penis: a radiological or clinical diagnosis? A case series and literature review. *Can J Urol.* April 2009;16(2):4568-4575.

Obstetric and Gynecologic Emergencies

Harry Wallus

Christian C. Knutsen

INTRODUCTION

Obstetric and gynecological issues are a common reason for patients to seek urgent and emergent care. The most significant of these for the prehospital provider involve some component of vaginal bleeding. When assessing the patient with vaginal bleeding, determining certain key factors are important such as duration of bleeding as well as quantity. Oftentimes, significant or brisk vaginal bleeding is defined by the patient changing one or more pads per hour. A family or personal history of a bleeding disorder may also provide key information as to the etiology of the bleed. Associated symptoms such as weakness, lightheadedness, and shortness of breath should be noted.

OBJECTIVES

- Describe the initial prehospital evaluation and management of vaginal bleeding.

- Describe the initial prehospital evaluation and management of patients in active labor (delivery procedure covered in Chapter 64).

- Describe the initial prehospital evaluation and management of pregnant patients with trauma.

- Discuss the indications for prehospital perimortem C-section (procedure covered in Chapter 64).

- Discuss the criteria for determining stability when evaluating for interfacility transport of an obstetrical patient (also discussed in Chapter 16).

VAGINAL BLEEDING

Physical examination of the patient with vaginal bleeding should initially focus on careful assessment of vital signs. Tachycardia and/or hypotension can indicate significant hypovolemia secondary to blood loss. Marked pallor or delayed capillary refill may indicate associated hypoperfusion. Signs and symptoms of shock must be recognized and addressed. An associated tender abdomen on examination may indicate a significant intra-abdominal hemorrhage and must be communicated to ED staff. Conversely, a patient who is normotensive without an elevated heart rate and a soft benign abdomen most likely has less significant pathology.

DYSFUNCTIONAL UTERINE BLEEDING

One of the more common reasons for vaginal bleeding or spotting in the nonpregnant patient is dysfunctional uterine bleeding (DUB). DUB is excessive noncyclic endometrial bleeding also described as anovulatory bleeding and most common in peri- and postmenopausal patients. DUB commonly presents as a slow persistent bleed, but excessive bleeding can occur.

ECTOPIC PREGNANCY

A more acute life-threatening cause of vaginal bleeding the prehospital provider must be familiar with is ectopic pregnancy. The incidence of ectopic pregnancy is as high as 19.7 per 1000 reported pregnancies.[1] Normally, implantation of a fertilized egg takes place within the endometrium of the uterus and is therefore referred to as an intrauterine pregnancy or IUP. Implantation in an ectopic pregnancy is inappropriately outside the uterus, most commonly within the fallopian tubes. Other possible locations for an ectopic pregnancy include the cervix, an ovary, and the abdomen. As the ectopic pregnancy progresses, the risk is organ rupture increases and can cause rapid, life-threatening interabdominal hemorrhage. Early consideration and recognition are imperative.

Ectopic pregnancy must be considered with a report of abdominal pain, missed or late menses, and vaginal spotting or bleeding. This history combined with signs of tachycardia, hypotension, or hypoperfusion can herald a potentially devastating intraabdominal bleed. Vagal stimulation from the abdominal bleeding may cause a relative bradycardia. IV access, preferably with two large bore IVs, should be established as soon as possible and fluid0esuscitation with normal saline begun. Supplemental oxygen should be provided. Rapid transport and notification of the patient's condition and possible diagnosis should be provided to the receiving facility to prepare the appropriate resources as soon as possible as this patient will most likely need an emergent obstetrics consultation and surgery.

MISCARRIAGE

A more common reason for a patient to present with abdominal pain, vaginal spotting or bleeding, and a missed or late period is a miscarriage or a spontaneous abortion (versus elective abortion through either pharmaceuticals or a planned procedure). The World Health Organization defines spontaneous abortion as loss of pregnancy before 20 weeks or loss of a fetus weighing less than 500 g. Different types of spontaneous abortion exist: threatened, inevitable, incomplete, complete, and missed. The particulars of each are not necessarily relevant in the prehospital setting and therefore do not need to be explored in detail. A thorough history includes determining last menstrual period, knowledge of pregnancy status, amount and duration of bleeding, passage of clots or potential fetal materials, and past obstetrics history (such as prior miscarriage). A detailed physical examination should take into account vital signs, signs and symptoms of hypoperfusion, and abdominal tenderness if present. Establishing an IV, providing supplemental O_2 and close monitoring of vital signs are prudent during transport. The prehospital provider should recognize this as a very emotional and upsetting time for the patient and take steps whenever possible to minimize her stress or discomfort.

COMPLICATIONS OF PREGNANCY

Prehospital care of the pregnant patient during the second half of pregnancy can be a challenging and anxiety provoking experience for the EMS physicians and providers. First and foremost, two patients are involved: the mother and the viable fetus. Secondly, this situation is not frequently encountered and therefore familiarity with the situation, potential complications, and treatment options may not be at the forefront of the provider's mind. The assessment and treatment of the pregnant patient should therefore be regularly reviewed. The goal of this section is to provide a review of the assessment and treatment of the most common issues of this unique patient population when they seek emergent care.

Prior to a discussion of the emergent conditions the gravid patient may face, an understanding of the basic physiological changes encountered in pregnancy is necessary. A number of changes involving the cardiovascular system take place in pregnancy. A pregnant woman can have 50% more blood volume than that of the nonpregnant women,[2] equating a volume of approximately 1500 mL. Also, heart rate and stroke volume increase, causing a physiologic tachycardia of pregnancy. The pregnant patient can have a heart rate 10 to 15 beats per minute above normal. While cardiac output increases, a decreased peripheral vascular resistance actually lowers the pregnant women's blood pressure. Lastly, venous return to heart in the supine position during the third trimester of pregnancy is compromised due to the gravid uterus resting on the inferior vena cava and decreasing cardiac preload, a phenomenon known as supine hypotensive syndrome. Pregnant patients must be placed on their left side to alleviate this syndrome. If immobilized after a trauma, the backboard should elevated on the right to allow the fetus to move to the left and improve venous return. All of these common physiological changes should be considered when assessing the pregnant patient.

Assessment of blood pressure, particularly hypertension, is of particular importance. Hypertension affects approximately 12% of pregnancies and contributes to approximately 18% of maternal deaths in the United States annually.[3] Hypertension during pregnancy is defined as a blood pressure of 140/90 mm Hg, a 20 mm Hg rise in systolic blood pressure or a 10 mm Hg rise in the diastolic pressure. Different categories of hypertension affect pregnancy. Patients with an established history of hypertension prior to the pregnancy have chronic hypertension. Hypertension that is mild develops in the third trimester and does not adversely affect the pregnancy is transient hypertension. Preeclampsia is the combination of hypertension and proteinuria with or without associated edema that occurs during the second half of pregnancy. Those with chronic hypertension may progress to preeclampsia or it may develop independently. Preeclampsia is a serious condition affecting 5% to 10% of pregnancies with signs and symptoms that include headache, visual disturbances, abdominal pain, confusion, and decreased urination. Patients with these signs and symptoms of preeclampsia or an elevated blood pressure require prompt ED evaluation. Notification prior to arrival to the receiving ED of the patient's diagnosis, signs and symptoms, or pertinent vital signs is extremely helpful.

▨ ECLAMPSIA

Eclampsia involves the signs and symptoms of preeclampsia along with seizures. The seizing pregnant patient in the second trimester of pregnancy requires immediate treatment with 4 to 6 mg of magnesium over 15 minutes. Prehospital providers should notify medical control immediately for assistance in managing this complicated patient in extremis. Communication to the medical control physician should include pertinent information such as age, pregnancy status (37 weeks, etc), vital signs if attainable, and any other pertinent diagnosis (for example, an established history of preeclampsia or hypertension). Prompt transport must take place as the definitive treatment for preeclampsia and eclampsia is delivery of the fetus. Early notification to the receiving facility is essential as obstetrical consultation and emergent deliver may be required. Seizure management and administration of magnesium are immediate concerns in the prehospital environment. Management of hypertension is a secondary concern in the prehospital setting.

▨ VAGINAL BLEEDING

Vaginal bleeding during the second half of pregnancy is particularly dangerous and is associated with fetal death in one-third of cases.[4] Two significant causes of late term bleeding include placenta previa and abruptio placentae.

Placenta Previa Placenta previa occurs when the placenta implants over the cervical os and is responsible for one-fifth of bleeding episodes during the second half of pregnancy (**Figure 45-1**). There are three categories of placenta previa: marginal (where the placenta implants next to but not over the cervix), partial (where the placenta covers a portion of the cervix), and complete (where the placenta covers the entire cervix). Placenta previa should be suspected with the onset of painless bright red bleeding during the late second and early third trimester.

Abruptio Placentae Abruptio placentae is the early or premature separation of the placentae from the uterine wall (**Figure 45-2**). The phenomenon occurs in approximately 1% of pregnancies and must be considered when the patient in her second half of pregnancy complains

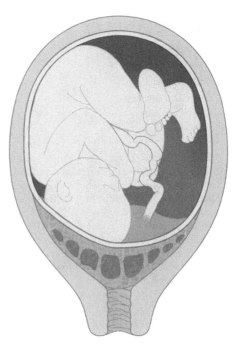

FIGURE 45-1. Complete placenta previa. (Reprinted with permission from Tintinalli JE, Stapczynski JS, Ma OJ, Cline DM, Cydulka RK, Meckler GD, eds. *Tintinalli's Emergency Medicine: A Comprehensive Study, 7th ed.* New York, NY: McGraw-Hill; 2011.)

of sudden onset of vaginal bleeding, abdominal pain, and a sense of constant contractions. Symptoms may also include dizziness, nausea, vomiting, or mild abdominal discomfort. On examination, the uterus is often firm and excessively tender. Abruptio placentae must be given significant consideration as it is one of the most serious complications of pregnancy and can be potentially devastating to mother and child.

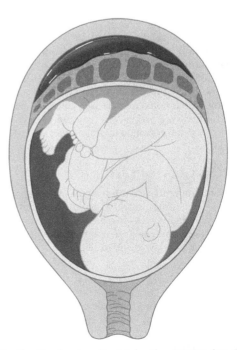

FIGURE 45-2. Abruptio placentae. (Reprinted with permission from Tintinalli JE, Stapczynski JS, Ma OJ, Cline DM, Cydulka RK, Meckler GD, eds. *Tintinalli's Emergency Medicine: A Comprehensive Study, 7th ed.* New York, NY: McGraw-Hill; 2011.)

Abruptio placentae may occur with trauma, stimulant abuse, or more commonly spontaneously with hypertension being a significant risk factor. Early consideration of the condition should be undertaken and steps to address potentially significant hemorrhage should be employed. Early notification of the receiving facility is again an important step to minimize any delay in mobilizing appropriate resources.

NORMAL DELIVERY

Precipitous delivery in the prehospital setting is a relatively uncommon event. Out-of-hospital births account for approximately 1 out of every 100 births annually in the United States.[5] Potential labor and delivery of the neonate should be considered in any pregnant patient with abdominal pain or cramping, back pain or pressure, or an urge to defecate without being able to do so. These potential signs of labor should be noted and steps taken to prepare for possible delivery in the prehospital setting. Providers should always locate and familiarize themselves with the sterile birthing kits in their vehicles. Typically, the primipara patient will have a more prolonged labor versus the multipara patient. While not always the case, however, providers must be aware that multipara patients may progress quickly to delivery.

There are essentially three stages of labor. *Stage one* is considered the time contractions begin and the cervix is fully dilated to 10 cm. Stage one is itself divided into three different periods. The latent phase consists mainly of thinning and effacement of the cervix. This stage typically takes 20 or more hours for first time mothers or closer to 10 hours for subsequent deliveries. The active phase begins when the cervix is thinned and effaced and dilated 3 to 4 cm. This is the most significant phase of cervical dilation and will take approximately 5 hours in primipara patients and 2 hours or less in multipara patients. The deceleration stage completes stage 1 when cervical dilation continues to the full 10 cm but at a slightly reduced pace. At this point the head is descending into the birth canal.

Stage two of labor is the time between full cervical dilation and delivery of the neonate. Delivery of the baby involves six cardinal movements of labor that include: (1) *engagement,* (2) *flexion,* (3) *descent,* (4) *internal rotation,* (5) *extension,* (6) *external rotation.* The delivery of the baby is most often in occiput anterior (OA) position or baby's head facing downward at delivery. As the baby crowns, or begins to emerge from the introitus, care should be taken to support the bottom of the perineum with the left hand while gentle counter pressure should be applied to the crown of the infant with the right to control delivery and decrease risk of perineal tear. As the infants head and chin emerge, the left hand supports the chin during the delivery. When the head fully emerges, both nares and the mouth should be suctioned to prevent aspiration. Care should be taken to depress the bulb syringe prior to insertion into any of these structures. At this stage, the infant's neck should be palpated for a nuchal cord present in approximately 25% of OA deliveries. If present, two fingers should be placed under the cord and it should be brought over the patient's head or reduced. If the cord is wound tightly, the cord may need to be clamped in the most accessible area with two clamps positioned closely together, cut taking care to cut away from the infant's neck and the cord removed. Delivery of the baby must occur quickly as the baby's oxygen delivery is stopped until spontaneous breathing begins.

Delivery of the infant's shoulders is next. Gentle traction in the downward direction will assist with delivery of the anterior shoulder and then gentle traction upward will assist in the delivery of the posterior shoulder. The delivery should be controlled by keeping the left hand in the area of the posterior axilla. Gloves, amniotic fluid, and blood can cause the infant to be quite slippery and care must be taken to ensure the infant is not inadvertently dropped. Keeping the infant close to your body decreases the risk of mishandling or dropping the infant. At this point, the baby is loosely wrapped in a blanket, sheet, or towel and gently stimulated and dried. If the child takes an initial vigorous breath and is crying, the mother may immediately hold the infant. The umbilical cord is cut 30 to 60 seconds after delivery after a clamp is placed 3 cm from the infant's body and a subsequent clamp just distal to it. The cord is then cut with sterile scissors. The third stage is delivery of the placenta. This should be allowed to progress naturally. Do not apply any retraction force to the umbilical cord as this can result in tearing of the cord or significant hemorrhage as the placenta prematurely separates from the uterus. This stage of labor typically takes 15 to 30 minutes and should be followed by gentle uterine massage to stimulate contraction of the uterus and thus decrease bleeding.

COMPLICATIONS OF DELIVERY

While thankfully uncommon, a number of complications during the delivery of the infant can occur. The three most common include cord prolapse, shoulder dystocia, and breech presentation.

CORD PROLAPSE

Cord prolapse occurs when the initial presenting part of the infant is the umbilical cord (**Figure 45-3**). With the umbilical cord in the vaginal canal, the descent of the baby's head blocks blood through the cord and threatens the baby's life. Gentle pressure should be placed on the presenting fetal part aside from the cord to reduce cord compression using two fingers in the vagina and elevating the presenting part. This position should be maintained and the patient should be transported to the ED immediately. Early notification should be made to the ED as emergency operative delivery of the baby is required. Attempts to reduce the cord should never be undertaken.

SHOULDER DYSTOCIA

Shoulder dystocia occurs when the anterior shoulder becomes stuck under the pubic bone after delivery of the head and the delivery of the infant arrests (**Figure 45-4**). Shoulder dystocia is often recognized by the turtle sign where the head repeatedly descends slightly with contractions and then retracts into the perineum.[6] If observed, several maneuvers

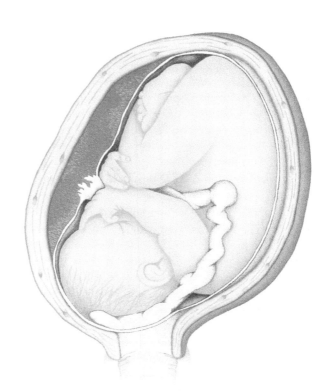

FIGURE 45-3. Cord prolapse. (Contributor: Judy Christensen. Reprinted with permission from Knoop KJ. *The Atlas of Emergency Medicine.* 3rd ed. New York: McGraw-Hill, 2010.)

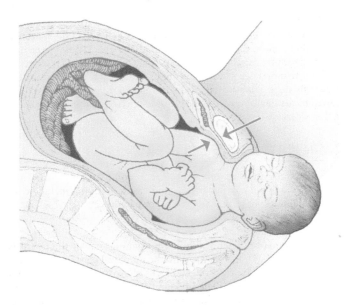

FIGURE 45-4. Shoulder dystocia. (Reprinted with permission from Reichman EF, ed. *Emergency Medicine Procedures*. 2nd ed. New York, NY: McGraw-Hill; 2013.)

must be attempted to deliver the baby. The first step is the extreme lithotomy position or McRoberts maneuver when the mother is on her back and her legs sharply flexed up to the abdomen and held in place by an assistant. This maneuver maximally opens the pelvic outlet. Next, firm suprapubic pressure can be applied to disimpact the anterior shoulder from the pubic symphysis. Never apply pressure to the fundus itself as this can further impact the shoulder. Next, a corkscrew maneuver, known as Wood maneuver, can be attempted where the provider presses on the posterior scapula of the infant with two fingers and attempts to rotate the shoulders 180° while simultaneously attempting to deliver the anterior shoulder. If unsuccessful, an attempt to deliver the posterior shoulder can be done where the posterior elbow is grasped and flexed, allowing the arm and then the posterior shoulder to be delivered with the anterior shoulder following. If all are unsuccessful, the mother can be moved onto her hands and knees and the maneuvers attempted again. The prehospital provider should be on the phone with medical control

getting instructions as to how to deal with these difficult scenarios and preparing for arrival.

■ BREECH PRESENTATION

The last delivery complication addressed in this chapter is breech presentation. There are several categories of breech presentation including frank, complete, incomplete, and footing (**Figure 45-5**). Frank and complete presentations usually deliver spontaneously without complication since they dilate the introitus nearly as well as a cephalad birth. The baby should be allowed to deliver spontaneously until the umbilicus is visible. At this point the provider should place their thumbs on the medial aspect of the thighs and deliver each leg one at time by pressing out laterally. The buttocks, or sacrum, should be facing anteriorly or up toward the provider. As the delivery progresses to the level of the shoulder blades, the infant should be grasped at the bony pelvis and rotated to 90° so the infant's right hip is now facing upward. The right arm should now be visible and a single digit should be placed and sweep the arm out and be delivered. The fetus should now be rotated 180° and the opposite arm should be delivered. Care must be taken to now deliver the flexed head. The provider should place an index and middle finger on the infant's maxilla (*not* oropharynx) and gently keep the head flexed to allow delivery. Never pull on the fetus as this may impact the head. Footling and incomplete breech presentations are fairly complicated and not considered safe for vaginal delivery. Therefore, when a single extremity is first seen, EMS providers should be educated on the need to contact medical control further instruction and EMS physicians should plan to be prepared to perform complicated deliveries when delay until C-section is not an option. If imminent delivery is apparent in this case, notification and a request for immediate obstetrical consultation on arrival are warranted and the potential need for neonatal resuscitation should be anticipated.

POSTPARTUM BLEEDING

Postpartum bleeding is categorized as either early (less than 24 hours) or late (greater than 24 hours and up to 6 weeks after delivery). The most common cause of early postpartum bleeding is uterine atony where the uterus fails to contract appropriately and continues to bleed. This can be addressed prehospitally with manually massage where a hand is placed over the abdomen and massages in a circular fashion in the area of the uterus. This technique should be attempted in all cases of early postpartum bleeding as it is noninvasive and will resolve the majority of cases.

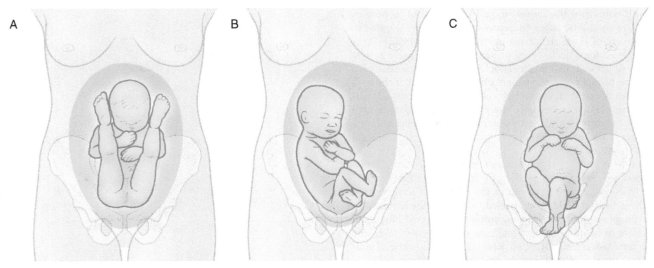

A   B   C

FIGURE 45-5. Breech presentation (A) frank breech (B) complete breech (C) footling breech. (Reprinted with permission from Reichman EF, ed. *Emergency Medicine Procedures*. 2nd ed. New York, NY: McGraw-Hill; 2013.)

moderate volume loss due to increased fluid state and then precipitously decompensate. Early recognition and treatment of compensated and decompensated shock are essential.

Assessment and management of the pregnant trauma patient should be rapid and aggressive. As with all trauma patients, the primary survey must address any airway issues as both the mother and the fetus have high oxygen demands. This is further complicated by a 25% residual capacity decrease in the mother due to a 3- to 4-cm elevation of the diaphragm during pregnancy. At minimum, high-flow O_2 through a nonrebreather mask should be applied. Circulatory issues should be addressed during the primary survey and any dangerous or life-threatening external hemorrhage controlled. During the secondary survey the provider should note fundal height. A fundus at the level of the umbilicus or higher may indicate a viable fetus. In the unfortunate event the mother decompensates, aggressive resuscitation may still lead to the delivery of a viable neonate. Careful note should be taken to illicit any abdominal pain as this could indicate placental abruption. During transport, the patient should be placed in the lateral decubitus position to avoid compression on the vena cava and the resultant supine hypotensive syndrome. If the patient is immobilized, the backboard may be slightly elevated (approximately 15%) with the patient adequately secured to accommodate this position. Lastly, a detailed history including past pregnancies, state of current pregnancy, any complications, comorbid conditions such as history of coagulopathy should be undertaken en route to the hospital anticipating the possibility of the patient decompensating rapidly for the reasons mentioned above.

CARDIAC ARREST

Cardiac arrest in the pregnant patient is an uncommon event that the prehospital provider must be prepared to address. There are several different factors that can lead to cardiopulmonary arrest in the pregnant patient including venous thromboembolism, severe pregnancy-induced hypertension, sepsis, amniotic fluid embolism, hemorrhage, and trauma. As with the trauma patient, early and aggressive airway management and oxygenation are essential. The pregnant patient is at increased risk of aspiration due to a lower esophageal sphincter tone as well as delayed gastric emptying; therefore, the airway should be secured with an ET tube when possible. Compressions should proceed as with the nonpregnant patient with one exception. The patient should again be placed in a lateral decubitus position to maximize venous return and resuscitative efforts. This may be accomplished by placing securing the patient to the backboard and elevating between 25° and 30° or by manually displacing the uterus to the left and upward during supine resuscitative efforts. ACLS protocols should be followed and appropriate medications administered as with the nonpregnant patient. Bicarbonate generally should be avoided as there is the possibility of increased fetal hypoxemia as the maternal acidosis resolves with administration (resulting in decreased hyperventilation and exhalation of pCO_2) while having no effect on the fetal circulation and its acidosis (as it is not thought to cross the placenta) and at the same time blunting the mother's natural compensatory mechanisms. Should the patient develop a pulseless ventricular tachycardia or ventricular fibrillation, defibrillation should proceed at the appropriate energy and intervals as with the nonpregnant patient. The prehospital provider should be aware that the EMS physician, emergency physician, or obstetrician can perform a perimortem cesarean section in an attempt to deliver a viable fetus and in turn improve the maternal hemodynamics (**Figure 45-7**). This procedure is ideally performed within 4 to 5 minutes (the "4-minute-rule") of the patient arresting although can be performed 15 minutes or greater from the event although the chances of delivering a neurologically intact viable fetus greatly diminishes the further out from the arrest one gets. Performing this procedure also carries some potential benefit to the mother in that it may improve the potential for ROSC; however, the EMS physician must ensure they are properly equipped and capable of performing the procedure in the field.[9]

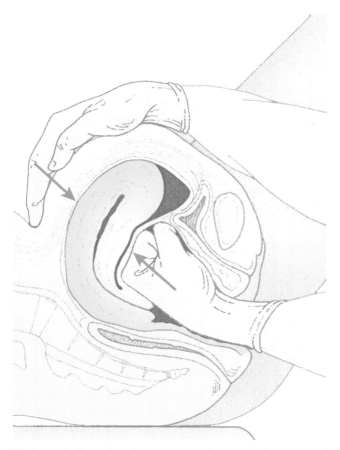

FIGURE 45-6. Bimanual uterine compression. (Reprinted with permission from Reichman EF, ed. *Emergency Medicine Procedures*. 2nd ed. New York, NY: McGraw-Hill; 2013.)

Should bleeding be brisk and potentially life threatening, after obtaining consent from the patient, one or more digits from the second hand may be placed intravaginally to attempt to compress the uterus upward and increased the effectiveness of the transabdominal massage (**Figure 45-6**). Adequate access with two large bore IVs should be established and fluid resuscitation should be begun anticipating significant volume loss and possibly shock. A second cause of early postpartum bleeding and common cause of late postpartum bleeding is retained products of conception. The most important role for the EMS physician and/or prehospital provider is to recognize the risk of significant bleeding and hence volume loss, anticipate and intervene appropriately with fluid resuscitation, monitor the patient closely and transport to an appropriate facility with obstetrical services, and provide early notification to the receiving facility.

TRAUMA IN PREGNANCY

According to trauma registry data significant trauma affects between 4.6% and 8.3% of pregnancies.[7] Maternal trauma is most commonly a result of motor vehicle accidents (55%), followed by falls (22%), assaults (22%), and burns (1%).[8] As discussed in previous sections the pregnant patient presents a unique challenge in that there are two patients being cared for, each with specific needs. The In these situations, the mother should be resuscitated aggressively as the well-being of the fetus is dependent on the stability of the mother.

Providers must again recognize the common physiological changes in pregnancy and how they may affect the presentation and assessment of the patient. Pregnant women may appear tachycardic and hypotensive, but may be simply demonstrating natural physiological changes of pregnancy. Conversely the patient may be able to tolerate mild to

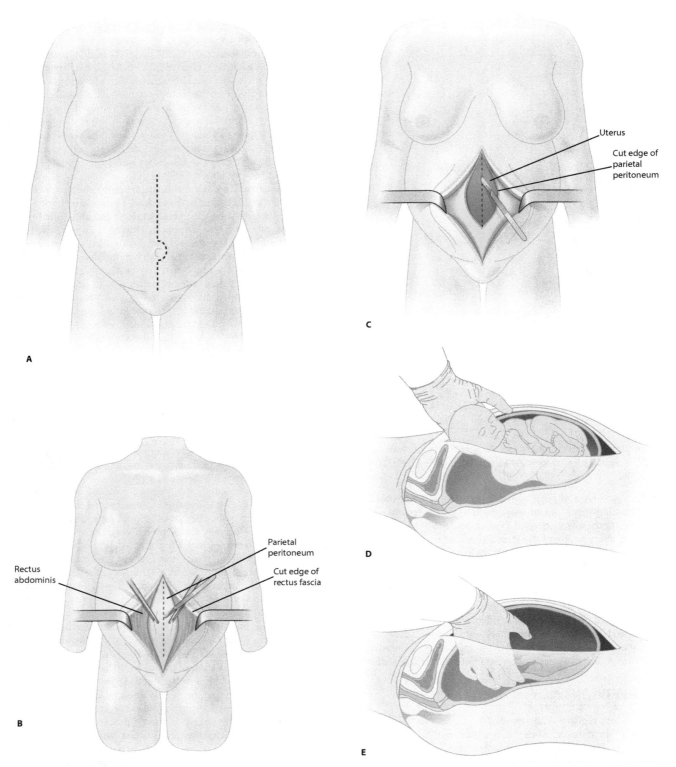

FIGURE 45-7. Procedure for perimortem cesarean section. (Reprinted with permission from Tintinalli JE, Stapczynski JS, Ma OJ, Cline DM, Cydulka RK, Meckler GD, eds. *Tintinalli's Emergency Medicine: A Comprehensive Study, 7th ed*. New York, NY: McGraw-Hill; 2011.)

3. Koonin LM, MacKay AP, Berg CJ, et al. Pregnancy-related mortality surveillance-United States, 1987-1990. *Morb Mortal Wkly Rep CDC Surveill Summ*. 1997;46:17-36.
4. Ajayi RA, Soothill PW, Campbell S, et al. Antenatal testing to predict outcomes in pregnancies with unexplained antpartum haemorrhage. *Br J Obstet Gynaecol*. 1992;99:122.
5. Curtin SC. Trends in the attendant, place, and timing of births, and in the use of obstetric interventions: United States, 1989-1997. *Natl Vital Stat Rep*. 1999;47:1-12.
6. Nocon JJ, McKenzie DK, Thomas LJ, Hansell RS. Shoulder dystocia: an analysis of risks and obstetric maneuvers. *Am J Obstet Gynecol*. 1993;168:1732.
7. Rosenfeld JA. Abdominal trauma in pregnancy: when is fetal monitoring necessary? *Postgrad Med*. 1990;88:89-91, 94.
8. Connolly AM, Katz VL, Bash KL, et al. Trauma in pregnancy. *Am J Perinatol*. 1997;14:331-336.
9. Katz VL. Perimortem cesarean delivery: its role in maternal mortality. *Semin Perinatol*. February 2012;36(1):68-72.

KEY POINTS

- EMS physicians should be knowledgeable and capable of managing obstetrical complications, and should ensure that their system EMS providers are well educated and trained in this area.
- Vaginal bleeding during pregnancy is by definition never normal and should be properly evaluated.
- Eclampsia should be initially managed with 4 to 6 g of IV magnesium.
- Even minor trauma in pregnancy can lead to significant complications and patients should be transported for evaluation and monitoring.
- Perimortem cesarian section should be performed in cases of maternal arrest within 4 to 5 minutes in order to improve maternal and fetal survival.

REFERENCES

1. Leads From the Mortality and Morbidity Weekly Report: ectopic pregnancy-United States, 1990-1992. *JAMA*. 1995;273:533.
2. Pritchard JA. Change in blood volume during pregnancy and delivery. *Anesthesiology*. 1965;26:393-399.

EMS Medicine: Poisoning and Envenomations

Jeremy Joslin

James Mangano

INTRODUCTION

The poisoned or envenomated patient represents a unique challenge to the EMS medicine practitioner. In many cases the offending medication, toxin, plant, or animal is unknown to the rescuer. Even when the offending agent is known, treatment can vary significantly based on severity of symptoms. Management of a patient with tricyclic antidepressant ingestion, for example, can range from benzodiazepines to bicarbonate to intravenous intralipid emulsion therapy. Proper education and training, coupled with robust, updated protocols, is needed to care for this group of patients effectively.

OBJECTIVES

- Describe important toxidromes for the evaluation of prehospital patients.
- Describe the initial prehospital evaluation and management of overdose on prescription medications.
- List common toxic ingestions and their antidotes (**Table 46-1**), including whether or not charcoal is indicated.
- Describe the initial prehospital evaluation and management of exposure to pesticides.

- Describe the initial prehospital evaluation and management of exposure to dangerous inhalants.
- Describe the initial prehospital evaluation and management of carbon monoxide poisoning.
- Describe the initial prehospital evaluation and management of insect envenomations.
- Describe the initial prehospital evaluation and management of reptile envenomations.
- Describe the initial prehospital evaluation and management of marine envenomations.

TOXIDROMES

Prehospital patients who are exposed to toxins or a drug overdose frequently display a set of signs and symptoms known as a toxidrome. **Table 46-2** describes the physiologic effects of several toxidromes. These effects are important clues to the exposure and can often guide management.

■ INITIAL PREHOSPITAL EVALUATION AND MANAGEMENT OF OVERDOSE ON PRESCRIPTION MEDICATIONS

Toxicological emergencies frequently present as a result of overdose on home prescription medications. Although it may appear obvious as to whether the overdose was accidental or intentional, the prehospital care provider should proceed with caution, and be very judicial with initial assumptions. In this sense, scene safety is a primary concern. A streetwise provider will enter the premises with caution, and law enforcement involvement should routinely be in place. While the patient who sustains accidental overdose on prescription medication may be of little threat, the patient who seeks to injure himself may be prepared to endanger

TABLE 46-1	Common Toxic Ingestions and Their Antidotes		
Ingestion	Common Antidotes	Other Therapies	Charcoal Indicated
Narcotics	Naloxone	Sodium bicarbonate (for wide complex dysrhythmias with propoxyphene)[1]	Not indicated
Benzodiazepines	Flumazenil		Not indicated
β-Adrenergic antagonists (beta blockers)	Glucagon	Phosphodiesterase inhibitors[2]	Indicated
	Calcium	Intravenous fat emulsion[3]	
	High-dose insulin maintaining euglycemia	Intra-aortic balloon pump	
	Inotropes and vasopressors	Extracorporeal circulation	
	Atropine	Cardiac pacing	
Calcium channel blockers	Atropine	Intravenous fat emulsion[4]	Indicated
	Calcium		
	Inotropes and vasopressors	Intra-aortic balloon pump	
	Glucagon	Extracorporeal circulation	
	High-dose insulin maintaining euglycemia	Cardiac pacing	
	Phosphodiesterase inhibitors		
Alkali substances	None available	Dilutional therapy[5,6]	Not indicated
Ethylene glycol	Ethanol	Pyridoxine[7]	Not indicated
	Fomepizole	Thiamine	
Iron	Deferoxamine	Continuous arteriovenous hemofiltration[8]	Not indicated
Tricyclic antidepressants	Sodium bicarbonate (for QRS prolongation)	Intravenous fat emulsion[9]	Indicated
	Benzodiazepines (for seizures)		
	Vasopressors and antidysrhythmics		
Acetaminophen	N-acetylcysteine		Indicated

TABLE 46-2	Toxidrome Drug Groups and Their Physiologic Characteristics
Anticholinergics	• Cause competitive inhibition of acetylcholinesterase receptors • Common offending agents include tricyclic antidepressants, antihistamines, and phenothiazines • Symptoms include "the anticholinergic flush," urinary retention, mydriasis, tachycardia, and dry mucous membranes
Cholinergics	• Cause overstimulation of cholinergic receptors by acetylcholine which is made overly abundant by inhibition of acetylcholinesterase • Common offending agents include organophosphates and carbamates (pesticides and insecticides), chemical warfare agents, toxic mushrooms • Symptoms include salivation, lacrimation, urination, diarrhea, emesis, bronchorrhea, paralysis, and fasciculations (SLUDGE)
Ethanol and other sedative-hypnotics	• Cause enhanced central nervous system inhibitory tone or alteration of normal glucose homeostasis • Common offending agents include ethanol and other alcohols, benzodiazepines, and barbiturates • Symptoms include ataxia, decreased mental status, decreased tone, nystagmus, and hyporeflexia
Opioids	• Cause overstimulation of opioid receptors • Common offending agents include heroin, morphine, hydrocodone, and oxycodone • Symptoms include altered mental status, respiratory depression, and hyporeflexia
Sympathomimetics	• Cause alterations in normal neurotransmitter production, release, or function • Common offending agents include cocaine and the amphetamine class of drugs such as khat, cocaine, methamphetamine, and MDMA • Symptoms include agitation, tremors, tachycardia, hypertension, hyperthermia, and seizures
Withdrawal from sedative-hypnotic	• Caused by alterations in neurotransmitter production, release, or function due to abrupt cessation of chronically used ethanol or a sedative-hypnotic agent • Symptoms include agitation, tremors, and seizures
Withdrawal from opioids	• Caused by alterations in neurotransmitter production, release, or function due to abrupt cessation of chronically used opioid agent • Symptoms include vomiting, rhinorrhea, piloerection, and diarrhea

Adapted from Wolfson AB et al (eds). Harwood-Nuss. *Clinical Practice of Emergency Medicine.* 5th ed. Philadelphia: Lippincott Williams & Wilkins, 2010; Ch 280, pg 1360.

the welfare of others. Finally, some patients who sustain an intentional overdose may have formulated a "backup" plan which may involve other means of self-harm. Beware the patient who has been medically resuscitated after an intentional overdose. They should not be left alone, and should be supervised so as to not ingest a secondary medication or produce another weapon of self-harm.

Medical priorities involve a rapid assessment of airway, breathing, circulation, and mental status. These elements will inform the building of a toxidrome, and guide further management. Any derangement of respiration or circulation should be managed accordingly. Further management should be in accordance with local and state protocols, and medical judgment. Refinement of any toxidromes should include integration of a full set of vital signs and 12-lead ECG with specific consideration of the QRS complex width and QTc interval length.

SPECIFIC INGESTIONS

ACETAMINOPHEN

Mostly nontoxic metabolites of acetaminophen are formed when it is taken in therapeutic doses since the drug can be conjugated with glucuronide or sulfate in the liver. However, acetaminophen can also be oxidized by cytochrome P-450 to N-acetyl-p-benzoquinoneimine (NAPQI) which is hepatotoxic. In acetaminophen overdose, a large amount of NAPQI is formed since the normal glucuronide and sulfate conjugation pathway is overwhelmed.

N-acetylcysteine (NAC) is the antidote in acetaminophen toxicity. NAC has three roles in overdose: preventing toxicity by preventing the formation of NAPQI, increasing the ability to detoxify by serving as a glutathione precursor and substitute, and treating the toxicity itself through nonspecific mechanisms.[10-12] NAC is very effective if given within the first 8 to 10 hours after an ingestion, but is still beneficial even if given late.[13] There is both an oral (Mucomyst) and intravenous (Acetadote) route of administration of NAC.

BENZODIAZEPINES

Benzodiazepines can be used as sedatives, as an induction agent of anesthesia, or as an anticonvulsant. Benzodiazepines work through

enhancement of the GABA receptors that lead to decreased neuronal firing. Decreased neuronal firing can lead to multiple CNS, respiratory, and cardiovascular issues, including lethargy, slurred speech, ataxia, coma, respiratory depression, and hypotension in overdose.

The treatment of a benzodiazepine overdose is supportive care; there is a reversal agent available, flumazenil, which may be used with extreme caution since acute GABA receptor antagonism in the setting of chronic GABA agonism can cause immediate withdrawal symptoms including seizure. Thus, the role of flumazenil is limited. In cases of mixed overdoses, flumazenil may lead to seizures or dysrhythmias since the benzodiazepine component may actually be protective of other agents' effects. In patients who are benzodiazepine dependent, flumazenil will induce withdrawal symptoms, including seizures. In patients who have had intravenous benzodiazepines, flumazenil may not reverse the respiratory depression. The most useful indication for flumazenil is in a benzodiazepine-naïve patient who has only taken a benzodiazepine, usually after procedural sedation.[14,15]

Initial Prehospital Evaluation and Management of Exposure to Pesticides When dealing with hazardous material incidents, scene safety and the safety of those around the incident are of upmost importance. When approaching the scene, approach cautiously, identify hazards, and secure the scene. When dealing with pesticide exposure, be aware that the exposure can be intentional self-harm (suicide attempt), accidental (farming incident), or an act of terrorism.

Part of securing the scene is the establishment of safety zones. In the hot or red (contamination) zone, contamination is actually present, personnel must wear the appropriate protective gear, limit the number of rescuers to those who are necessary, and bystanders are not allowed. In the warm or yellow (control) zone, life-saving emergency care and decontamination are performed and this is the area immediately surrounding the contamination zone. In the cold or green (safe) zone, normal triage, stabilization, and treatment are performed.

All patients in the hot zone are considered contaminated. As soon as the patient is contacted, and if conditions allow, airway, breathing, and circulatory support should begin. Cautious must be used if starting intravenous therapy as hazardous material may inadvertently be introduced into the patient. All clothing should be removed as soon as possible and skin should be washed with water and soap (triple wash: water, soap, water and rinsed again).

Organophosphates (OP) and nonorganophosphates (carbamates) are cholinesterase-inhibiting pesticides commonly used throughout the world. The toxicity is through the inhibition of cholinesterase, which increases the activity of all nicotinic and muscarinic receptors.[16] Carbamates bind cholinesterase transiently (due to rapid hydroxylation of the carbamate-AChE bond) and last minutes to hours. Aging, which is the irreversible binding of the pesticide to cholinesterase, can occur with organophosphates and makes these patients particularly challenging to manage.[17,18]

Symptoms of OP exposure can occur within 5 minutes, depending on the dose of the exposure. Symptoms can be variable because acetylcholine receptors are found in both the sympathetic and parasympathetic nervous systems.[19] There are several mnemonics associated with the cholinergic toxidrome, including SLUDGE (salivation, lacrimation, urination, miosis, defecation, GI distress, emesis) and DUMBBBELS (defecation, urination, miosis, bronchospasm, bronchorrhea, bradycardia, emesis, lacrimation, salivation).[20]

Death from OP is caused by respiratory failure and the subsequent hypoxemia. The antidotes for OP pesticide poisoning are atropine and pralidoxime. Atropine competitively antagonized acetylcholine at muscarinic receptors. Classically, atropine is given in doses high enough to cause "atropinization," which is where the patient's skin and mucous membranes are dry. These doses can be as 1 to 5 mg every 2 to 20 minutes.[21,22] Atropine does not reverse nicotinic effects, and therefore, the patient must be monitored for possible respiratory failure from delayed neuromuscular junction dysfunction.[23] There are several adverse effects of atropine; however, its benefit in pesticide poisoning usually outweighs the risks.[24]

Pralidoxime (2-PAM) is an oxime that can potentially reactivate inhibited cholinesterase.[25] Side effects are minimal and may only include emesis, hypertension, and possibly mild cholinergic effects with rapid infusion.[26] Due to the short activity of carbamates, the use of pralidoxime may not be indicated. If it is unknown which type of pesticide was used, giving pralidoxime will most likely not be detrimental if it was only a carbamate. Pralidoxime should not be given as the sole therapeutic agent and should be used only after a trial of atropine.

Diazepam may be considered an adjunctive therapy for OP poisonings as it may help with decreasing seizures and neuropathy. It is not recommended to be given routinely in all cases of exposure, but rather to be used with seizures and agitation as well as to aid intubation.[19,27,28] Activated charcoal should be considered if there is an ingestion of an insecticide.[29]

ABUSED INHALANTS

Dangerous inhalants are important source of exposure that prehospital providers must consider and be prepared to manage. Of utmost concern in responding these incidents is the scene safety outlined above. Numerous emergency responders have been subject to morbidity and mortality resulting from exposure to inhalants. Principles of management include the establishment of scene safety and proper HAZMAT response when indicated. Principles of patient decontamination are important even when dealing with inhalants. Once patient care is initiated, the basics of airway, breathing, and circulation must be rigorously assessed and managed.

Certain agents are purposefully inhaled in a recreational fashion, and their abuse may lead to significant illness or injury. Hydrocarbons (such as toluene, etc) may be "huffed" in an attempt to become intoxicated and euphoric. Some commonly abused products which have contained hydrocarbon propellants are brake cleaner, automotive degreasers, and spray paint. The hydrocarbons cause intoxication, but also sensitize the myocardium which is then susceptible to surges in adrenalin and other endogenous catecholamines. This stimulation can initiate ventricular tachycardia and lead to death. An unconscious patient found with a paper bag in hand and a ring of paint around the nose and mouth should raise concern of this "sudden sniffing death syndrome."[30]

Management of patients with exposure to these hydrocarbons requires calm response to avoid this excitation syndrome of ventricular tachycardia. Close cardiac monitoring should be initiated as soon as possible with the ability to manage any tachydysrhythmia utilizing intravenous medications or defibrillation/cardioversion. Although no specific antidotes are available, the use of benzodiazepines and β-blockers can be considered in the prehospital environment. Patients who have a history of chronic abuse should be evaluated for neurologic sequelae and impairment.

The alkyl nitrite inhalants are another recreationally abused inhalant and include the most common agent, amyl nitrite, which has a street name of "poppers." Amyl nitrites (and other impure street-derived nitrites such as butyl and isobutyl nitrites) are rapidly acting compounds used primarily to enhance sexual experiences and are commonly inhaled to produce a euphoric sensation perceived as a warm rush or high that is due to vasodilatation of cerebral and cutaneous blood vessels.[31-33] With high levels of exposure, nitrites can enter red blood cells and oxidize hemoglobin, forming methemoglobin, and ultimately methemoglobinemia. Headaches are a common side effect, but eye pain due to increases in intraocular pressure has also been described.[34]

Sutton et al describe an illustrative case where a 29-year-old man was brought to the emergency department exhibiting extreme lethargy and circumoral cyanosis. He reported inhaling amyl nitrite before the onset of symptoms. Vitals signs reported were a pulse of 112 beats/minute, blood pressure of 100/60 mm Hg, respiratory rate of 12 breaths/minutes, and pulse oximetry of 56% on 100% oxygen via nonrebreather mask. During intravenous access, the patient's blood was noted to appear chocolate brown. He was given the antidote for methemoglobinemia, methylene blue, and his mental status and pulse oximetry improved over the next several minutes.[35] Clinical pearls worth noting in the management of methemoglobinemia include

- Recognizing that methemoglobinemia can falsely increase pulse oximetry to 85% to 88%.
- Administration of methylene blue can falsely lower pulse oximetry readings.
- Utilizing pulse oximetry as a measurement of improvement is unreliable and not advised.

Nitrous oxide, also known as laughing gas, is a clear, odorless gas used in medicine and dentistry for its anesthetic effect. It can be obtained for recreational use in the form of whippets, which are small, pressurized tanks used to charge whip cream dispensers. Its effects include dissociative euphoria and intoxication. Delivery has been commonly been described to use balloons filled with the gas by a large tank, and then sold to users. A more dangerous method of administration is filling a large plastic bag with the gas, and then placing the bag over one's head in order to rebreathe the gas. As oxygen is consumed, however, simple asphyxiation may result. Resuscitative management includes keeping the patient safe from the resultant intoxication, administering oxygen when required, and considering administration of B_{12} once hospitalized for deficiencies caused by chronic use.

DANGEROUS INHALANTS

Emergency medical services should pay close attention to scene safety, especially when there is concern for leaked gases. Simplified, these dangerous inhalants can be considered noxious irritants or simple asphyxiants. A dangerous asphyxiant which has been implicated in first responder mortality is hydrogen sulfide. Hydrogen sulfide (H_2S) can be produced using ingredients found in household products, and has seen an increased use as a method of suicide. HS produces a smell of rotten eggs, but in higher concentrations may collapse and succumb before the foul odor can provide warning due to the swift olfactory fatigue HS can cause. Because it is heavier than air, it can present a challenge in rescue situations. First responders should always be wary of this "knockdown gas" when responding to a scene with a multiple unconscious patients.

Common irritating inhalants include chlorine gas, chloramines, and ethylene chloride. Because they are noxious, they frequently provide warning and allow for the victim to escape before morbidity can ensue. Chloramine gas, in particular, is a likely irritant to be encountered by EMS since it is most commonly produced by mixture of household bleach and ammonia products. First aid includes respiratory support with inhaled β-agonists and high flow oxygen. Invasive support is rarely required.

Because of the invisible dangers inherent with these dangerous inhalants, EMS and other first responders should be familiar with the scene heuristics that suggest the presence of these gases. The presence of gas tanks, industrial settings, drug paraphernalia, and multiple patients should all be considered elements of a possibly unsafe scene. Protocol development for EMS agencies should include scene considerations, but also management germane to the treatment and stabilization of these toxins as well.

PREHOSPITAL EVALUATION AND MANAGEMENT OF SMOKE INHALATION

There are several issues that arise when dealing with a patient who has experienced smoke inhalation. First and foremost, if the patient has been exposed to fire or a toxin rich atmosphere, they must be removed and placed in a safe area. With all hazardous situations, scene safety is of upmost importance. Airway, breathing, and circulation are key. There are three categories of toxic combustion products: simple asphyxiants, such as carbon dioxide, which displaces oxygen, irritant toxins, such as ammonia, sulfur dioxide, and hydrogen chloride, and chemical asphyxiants, which include carbon monoxide, hydrogen cyanide, hydrogen sulfide, and oxides of nitrogen (methemoglobinemia).[36-39]

Carbonaceous particulate matter, or soot, often adds to the challenge of managing a patient with smoke inhalation. Soot is not only dangerous because it contains acids, heavy metal, and other chemicals, but it also adheres to mucosal lining which extends the time that these materials can affect the body. In the prehospital evaluation of smoke inhalation patients, it is important to look for signs of soot and thermal injury in and around the airway to determine if a definitive airway is needed urgently. Respiratory compromise is the primary concern as a prehospital provider. The chemical irritants and heat can lead to airway edema and obstruction. Patients may complain of cough, chest tightness, and shortness of breath and quickly progress to stridor and respiratory arrest.[40-43]

Cyanide (CN), another combustion product, produces a functional hypoxia by blocking oxidative phosphorylation and formation of adenosine triphosphate (ATP). The initial symptoms of cyanide poisoning include headache, vertigo, agitation, confusion, coma, seizures, and death. A classic finding of CN poisoning is cherry red skin color which is the result of increased oxygen saturation of venous hemoglobin.[44,45] Hydroxycobalamin is simple to use, and has been studied in the prehospital environment with encouraging results.[46] A regional strategy commonly used for deployment utilizes supervisor vehicles or chief cars for ensuring its availability on fire scenes.

Carbon monoxide (CO), a major component in combustion products, causes hypoxemia, ischemia, and cellular asphyxia. The affinity to bind with hemoglobin is 250 times stronger than that of oxygen. The CO binding causes the oxygen-hemoglobin dissociation curve to shift to the left, lowering the amount of available oxygen to the cells. At low levels of carbon monoxide, the patient may experience headache, dizziness, and nausea/vomiting typical of a viral illness. At higher levels of CO, patients may experience seizure, coma, hypotension, dysrhythmias, and death.[47-50]

Providing high flow oxygen to patients with CO poisoning can decrease the half-life to 40 to 80 minutes and can further decrease the half-life of COHgb to less than 20 minutes if provided at pressures greater than 1 atm.[51,52] Amyl nitrate and sodium nitrite, which are commonly found in cyanide antidote kit, should be used with caution in victims of smoke inhalation because they form methemoglobinemia, which cannot carry oxygen, making oxygen-carrying capacity even worse in the patient

TABLE 46-3 Undersea and Hyperbaric Medical Society Patient Selection Criteria for Hyperbaric Oxygen Therapy

- Serious CO poisoning
  - Transient or prolonged unconsciousness
  - Neurological signs
  - Cardiovascular dysfunction
  - Severe acidosis
- Age greater than or equal to 36
- Exposure duration greater than 24 hours (even if intermittent)
- Initial COHb level greater than or equal to 25%

From Gesell LB. Hyperbaric oxygen therapy indications. The Hyperbaric Oxygen Therapy Committee Report, 12th ed. Undersea and Hyperbaric Medical Society; 2008.

poisoned with carboxyhemoglobin (carbon monoxide).[53] β-Agonist may be of some benefit since there may be a reversible component to the bronchoconstriction.[54] Nebulized heparin and N-acetylcysteine have been reported to limit pulmonary toxicity in children.[55]

The EMS physician should be keenly aware of the local resources and facilities available for treatment of these common illnesses and should incorporate this knowledge into local protocols. For example, symptomatic patients with known CO exposure who may benefit from hyperbaric oxygen therapy *might need transport* to a facility which is able to perform the therapy (**Table 46-3**).[56]

ENVENOMATIONS (TABLE 46-4)

PREHOSPITAL EVALUATION AND MANAGEMENT OF ENVENOMATIONS

Envenomations may be the result of an interaction with insects, arthropods, reptiles, amphibians, marine animals, and even mammals. The prehospital is most likely going to care for patients who have been envenomated by an arthropod, insect, snake, or marine animal. There are over 900,000 species of arthropods in the world. There is great variation in the venom produced by arthropods and they vary based on polypeptides, enzymes, histamines, serotonin, acetylcholine, and dopamine makeup.

Insect stings are likely to come from those of the order Hymenoptera ("membrane-winged"), and include Apidae (honeybees and bumblebees), Vespidae (yellow jackets, hornets, wasps), and Formicidae (ants). Anaphylaxis to Hymenoptera occurs in about 0.5% of the US population, accounting for approximately 40 deaths annually.

TABLE 46-4 Important Envenomations and Their Treatment

Common Name	Taxonomy	Antivenom Available	Local Therapy
Bark scorpion	*Centruroides sculpturatus*	Yes[57]	Lidocaine injection
Black widow	*Latrodectus* spp	Yes[58]	Cold compression
Brown recluse	*Loxosceles* spp	No	Cold compression
Rattlesnakes, Copperheads, Cottonmouths	*Crotalinae* family	Yes	Immobilization
Coral snakes	*Elapidae* family	No (discontinued)	Pressure immobilization
Portuguese man-of-war	*Physalia* spp	No	Vinegar or hot water[59,60]
Sea nettle	*Chrysaora* spp	No	Baking soda slurry[61]
Stingray	*Dasyatidae* family	No	Hot water immersion (122F)
Lionfish	*Pterois* spp	No	Hot water immersion (122F)

Anaphylaxis represents the most important condition that prehospital providers should be vigilant against.[62,63]

Treatment for Hymenoptera stings should focus on the standard anaphylaxis care which includes diphenhydramine, corticosteroids, and epinephrine.[64] Stingers should be removed by scraping or pinching out.[65] Some species' stingers detach from the insect's body and may continue to secret venom.

Fire ant venom inhibits sodium and potassium ATPase.[66] Anaphylaxis occurs in 0.6% to 6% of those stung. There can be local, large local, and systemic reactions. Local reactions only require cleansing and cold compresses and possibly vinegar or topical or locally injected lidocaine to decrease the pain of the sting. Large local reactions may be treated with corticosteroids, antihistamines, and pain medications. Systemic reactions are treated with either subcutaneous or intravenous epinephrine. For anaphylaxis, intramuscular administration of epinephrine is preferable to subcutaneous administration.[67]

A number of caterpillars can also cause envenomation. There are many differences in caterpillar venoms, which may cause symptoms that include pain and burning at the site of injection, to systemic effects, which include nausea, vomiting, fever, tachycardia, hypotension, and seizures. Some envenomation can even lead to DIC and intracerebral hemorrhage.[68,69] If caterpillar hair get into the eye, a myriad of symptoms may develop affecting the eye.[70] Treatment for caterpillar envenomations is symptomatic, and may include the use of analgesics, benzodiazepines, antihistamines, and corticosteroids. Ocular injuries are uncommon, and can be treated symptomatically by the EMS provider.[71] As with any condition requiring epinephrine use, close observation should be utilized in anticipation of any rebound phenomena.

REPTILE ENVENOMATIONS

A full description of the management of reptile envenomations is beyond the scope of this text. The EMS physician should be aware of the local epidemiology of venomous reptile bites, and should tailor the local EMS systems training and protocol development accordingly.

The prehospital management of venomous snakes benefits from identification of the offending snake at the taxonomic level of family/subfamily or lower. That is, knowing the difference between a Crotalidae and Elapidae can inform decisions on tourniquet use. In the United States, these two groups of snakes comprise all of the venomous snakes with an overwhelming majority of bites delivered by snakes in the Crotalidae subfamily. Prehospital management of snakebites by crotalids comprises of symptomatic care with limb splinting and transportation to a hospital where the use of antivenom can be considered. Tourniquets or compression bandages should not be used with crotalid envenomations despite recent guidelines published by the American Heart Association.[72-74]

Identification to the species level may be extremely difficult in the field. Although earnest in effort, attempts to capture or closely photograph a venomous snake can lead to additional envenomations and is generally not recommended. Several methods have been described to aid in identifying the species of snake responsible for a bite. These methods have included characterizations of the snake's head and eyes, as well as newer methods using characteristics of the scales and tail.[75] Snakes should never be transported to the emergency department alive. Dead snakes also pose a threat as fangs may still inadvertently deliver venom. A photograph of a dead snake is the safest method of communicating identifying information to hospital staff and consultants.

During evaluation of a patient who has been bitten, it is important to consider that "dry bites" make up a significant portion of crotalid bites. Whereas empiric treatment with antivenom for suspected Elapidae bites is usually considered, a wait-and-see approach to crotalid bites can be employed. Local and systemic symptom severity guide hospital treatment.

Venomous snakebite considerations:

- Juvenile crotalid snakes are not more poisonous than adult counterparts despite folklore that juvenile snakes have not learned how to conserve venom. On the contrary, data show that the larger the snake, the more severe the bite.[76]

- First aid should include marking the bite site and observing any local changes. Intravenous access, with crystalloid fluid administration, is recommended.

- Routine use of antihistamines or glucocorticoids is not supported.

- Suction devices, or other folk remedies, are not helpful and should be avoided.

- Prehospital use of crotalid antivenom is impractical, fraught with complications, and is not recommended.

MARINE ENVENOMATIONS

Marine animal envenomations are responsible for injury and illness both along the US coastal waterways and in home aquariums. It is important for EMS physicians practicing in coastal regions to have a familiarity with the local species which can cause morbidity and mortality. Animals found on the Pacific coasts can be considerably different from those found in Gulf Coast regions. Further, the composition of venom and stinging mechanisms can be significantly different from the venom of animals found in Asia and Australia. Little assumption should be made in management similarities amongst these regions.

In the United States, the three animals most likely to cause illness or injury from envenomation are the scorpion fish, rays, urchins, and Cnidaria. Although the scorpion fish are native to the Indo-Pacific, the *Pterois* (lionfish) have become an invasive species in US waters. Still, most envenomations are related to their high desirability in the home aquaria trade. Their long, venomous spines can inject a heat-labile toxin which can cause extreme pain and hyperemia. Prehospital care should focus on submersion of the affected body part, typically an aquarist's hand, into water made as hot as tolerable to the touch. Special attention should be paid to ensure the water is tested by someone other than the victim, and therefore not too hot to cause thermal injury. Patients who have been exposed to the *Pterois* toxin in the past may be immunogenically primed and may develop anaphylaxis.

Other common marine envenomations include stings by animals which protect themselves by large barbs. These include the rays and sea urchins. These animals invariably envenomate as a protective mechanism and are able to inflict significant pain on their victims. Prehospital first aid requires an assessment for clinically important trauma, assessment of any retained barbs or other foreign bodies, and application of pain management maneuvers. Pain management can be initiated by systemic analgesia, local wound anesthesia with agents such as lidocaine, or soaking an injured extremity in hot, nonscalding water using the same cautions described above. Formal evaluation for consideration of prophylactic antibiotics is recommended.

Perhaps the most common marine envenomations come from the stings of animals in the phylum Cnidaria which include corals, the scyphozoans which are the true jellyfish, the hydrozoans such as the Portuguese man-of-war (*Physalia physalis*), the cubozoans such as the box jellyfish (*Chironex fleckeri*), and anemones. These animals are alike in that they use stinging cells called nematocysts to cause painful envenomations. Envenomations can cause a variety of medical ailments besides pain including gastrointestinal distress, respiratory distress, neurologic dysfunction, allergic reaction, and death.

Despite their similar appearance and overlapping distribution, the true jellyfish, Portuguese man-of-war, and box jellyfish envenomations may benefit from slightly different first-aid treatments.[59] Since field identification may be difficult or impossible in many cases, a generic recommendation of vinegar, ammonia, hot water, or topical anesthetic are recommended as first-aid treatments.[59,60] Urine is not recommended. A gentle cleansing of the affected area with saltwater taking care to remove any remaining tentacles is important. The rescuer's hands should be gloved, and articles such as a credit card can be used to scrape off remaining tentacles and nematocysts.

REFERENCES

1. Sloth Madsen P, Strøm J, Reiz S, Bredgaard Sørensen M. Acute propoxyphene self-poisoning in 222 consecutive patients. *Acta Anaesthesiol Scand.* December 1984;28(6):661-665.
2. Travill CM, Pugh S, Noble MI. The inotropic and hemodynamic effects of intravenous milrinone when reflex adrenergic stimulation is suppressed by beta-adrenergic blockade. *Clin Ther.* October 1994;16(5):783-792.
3. Cave G, Harvey MG, Castle CD. The role of fat emulsion therapy in a rodent model of propranolol toxicity: a preliminary study. *J Med Toxicol Off J Am Coll Med Toxicol.* March 2006;2(1):4-7.
4. Bania TC, Chu J, Perez E, Su M, Hahn I-H. Hemodynamic effects of intravenous fat emulsion in an animal model of severe verapamil toxicity resuscitated with atropine, calcium, and saline. *Acad Emerg Med Off J Soc Acad Emerg Med.* February 2007;14(2):105-111.
5. Maull KI, Osmand AP, Maull CD. Liquid caustic ingestions: an in vitro study of the effects of buffer, neutralization, and dilution. *Ann Emerg Med.* December 1985;14(12):1160-1162.
6. Rumack BH, Burrington JD. Caustic ingestions: a rational look at diluents. *Clin Toxicol.* January 1977;11(1):27-34.
7. Nath R, Thind SK, Murthy MS, Farooqui S, Gupta R, Koul HK. Role of pyridoxine in oxalate metabolism. *Ann N Y Acad Sci.* 1990;585:274-284.
8. Banner W Jr, Vernon DD, Ward RM, Sweeley JC, Dean JM. Continuous arteriovenous hemofiltration in experimental iron intoxication. *Crit Care Med.* November 1989;17(11):1187-1190.
9. Harvey M, Cave G. Intralipid outperforms sodium bicarbonate in a rabbit model of clomipramine toxicity. *Ann Emerg Med.* February 2007;49(2):178-185, 185.e1-4.
10. Buckpitt AR, Rollins DE, Mitchell JR. Varying effects of sulfhydryl nucleophiles on acetaminophen oxidation and sulfhydryl adduct formation. *Biochem Pharmacol.* October 1, 1979;28(19):2941-2946.
11. Lauterburg BH, Corcoran GB, Mitchell JR. Mechanism of action of N-acetylcysteine in the protection against the hepatotoxicity of acetaminophen in rats in vivo. *J Clin Invest.* April 1983;71(4):980-991.
12. Slattery JT, Wilson JM, Kalhorn TF, Nelson SD. Dose-dependent pharmacokinetics of acetaminophen: evidence of glutathione depletion in humans. *Clin Pharmacol Ther.* April 1987;41(4):413-418.
13. Smilkstein MJ, Knapp GL, Kulig KW, Rumack BH. Efficacy of oral N-acetylcysteine in the treatment of acetaminophen overdose. Analysis of the national multicenter study (1976 to 1985). *N Engl J Med.* December 15, 1988;319(24):1557-1562.
14. Als-Nielsen B, Gluud LL, Gluud C. Benzodiazepine receptor antagonists for hepatic encephalopathy. *Cochrane Database Syst Rev.* 2004;(2):CD002798.
15. Flumazenil drug information, professional. Drugs.com. [cited 2013 Oct 23]. http://www.drugs.com/mmx/flumazenil.html.
16. Organic phosphorus pesticides. In: Hayes WJ, Laws ER, eds. Handbook of Pesticide Toxicology. 3rd ed. San Diego, CA: Academic Press; 2010.
17. Lotti M, Becker CE, Aminoff MJ. Organophosphate polyneuropathy: pathogenesis and prevention. *Neurology.* May 1984;34(5):658-662.
18. Wilson IB, Hatch MA, Ginsburg S. Carbamylation of acetylcholinesterase. *J Biol Chem.* August 1960;235:2312-2315.
19. Marrs TC. Organophosphate poisoning. *Pharmacol Ther.* 1993;58(1):51-66.
20. Tafuri J, Roberts J. Organophosphate poisoning. *Ann Emerg Med.* February 1987;16(2):193-202.
21. Eddleston M, Buckley NA, Checketts H, et al. Speed of initial atropinisation in significant organophosphorus pesticide poisoning—a systematic comparison of recommended regimens. *J Toxicol Clin Toxicol.* 2004;42(6):865-875.
22. Eddleston M, Dawson A, Karalliedde L, et al. Early management after self-poisoning with an organophosphorus or carbamate pesticide - a treatment protocol for junior doctors. *Crit Care Lond Engl.* December 2004;8(6):R391-R397.
23. Goldfranks on Organophosphates. p. 1640.
24. Robenshtok E, Luria S, Tashma Z, Hourvitz A. Adverse reaction to atropine and the treatment of organophosphate intoxication. *Isr Med Assoc J IMAJ.* July 2002;4(7):535-539.
25. Eyer P. Neuropsychopathological changes by organophosphorus compounds—a review. *Hum Exp Toxicol.* November 1995;14(11):57-864.
26. Quinby GE. Further therapeutic experience with pralidoximes in organic phosphorus poisoning. *JAMA J Am Med Assoc.* January 18, 1964;187:202-206.
27. Dickson EW, Bird SB, Gaspari RJ, Boyer EW, Ferris CF. Diazepam inhibits organophosphate-induced central respiratory depression. *Acad Emerg Med Off J Soc Acad Emerg Med.* December 2003;10(12):1303-1306.
28. Murphy MR, Blick DW, Dunn MA, Fanton JW, Hartgraves SL. Diazepam as a treatment for nerve agent poisoning in primates. *Aviat Space Environ Med.* February 1993;64(2):110-115.
29. Eddleston M, Juszczak E, Buckley NA, et al. Multiple-dose activated charcoal in acute self-poisoning: a randomised controlled trial. *Lancet.* February 16, 2008;371(9612):579-587.
30. Anderson CE, Loomis GA. Recognition and prevention of inhalant abuse. *Am Fam Physician.* September 1, 2003;68(5):869-874.
31. Newell GR, Adams SC, Mansell PW, Hersh EM. Toxicity, immunosuppressive effects and carcinogenic potential of volatile nitrites: possible relationship to Kaposi's sarcoma. *Pharmacotherapy.* October 1984;4(5):284-291.
32. Ridenour TA, Bray BC, Cottler LB. Reliability of use, abuse, and dependence of four types of inhalants in adolescents and young adults. *Drug Alcohol Depend.* November 2, 2007;91(1):40-49.
33. Romanelli F, Smith KM, Thornton AC, Pomeroy C. Poppers: epidemiology and clinical management of inhaled nitrite abuse. *Pharmacother J Hum Pharmacol Drug Ther.* 2004;24(1):69-78.
34. Newell GR, Mansell PW, Spitz MR, Reuben JM, Hersh EM. Volatile nitrites. Use and adverse effects related to the current epidemic of the acquired immune deficiency syndrome. *Am J Med.* May 1985;78(5):811-816.
35. Sutton M, Jeffrey B. Acquired methemoglobinemia from amyl nitrate inhalation. *J Emerg Nurs JEN Off Publ Emerg Dep Nurses Assoc.* February 1992;18(1):8-9.
36. Davies JW. Toxic chemicals versus lung tissue—an aspect of inhalation injury revisited. The Everett Idris Evans memorial lecture—1986. *J Burn Care Rehabil.* June 1986;7(3):213-222.
37. Dyer RF, Esch VH. Polyvinyl chloride toxicity in fires. Hydrogen chloride toxicity in fire fighters. *JAMA J Am Med Assoc.* January 26, 1976;235(4):393-397.
38. Stone J, Hazlett R, Johnson J, Carhart H. The transport of hydrogen chloride by soot from burning polyvinyl chloride. *J Fire Flammabl.* 1973;4:42-51.
39. Youn YK, Lalonde C, Demling R. Oxidants and the pathophysiology of burn and smoke inhalation injury. *Free Radic Biol Med.* 1992;12(5):409-415.
40. Edye LA, Richards GN. Analysis of condensates from wood smoke. Components derived from polysaccharides and lignins. *Environ Sci Technol.* 1991;25(6):1133-1137.
41. Hantson P, Butera R, Clemessy JL, Michel A, Baud FJ. Early complications and value of initial clinical and paraclinical observations in victims of smoke inhalation without burns. *Chest.* March 1997;111(3):671-675.
42. Morgan WK. The respiratory effects of particles, vapours, and fumes. *Am Ind Hyg Assoc J.* November 1986;47(11):670-673.
43. Herndon DN, Traber DL, Niehaus GD, Linares HA, Traber LD. The pathophysiology of smoke inhalation injury in a sheep model. *J Trauma.* December 1984;24(12):1044-1051.

44. Barillo DJ, Goode R, Esch V. Cyanide poisoning in victims of fire: analysis of 364 cases and review of the literature. *J Burn Care Rehabil.* February 1994;15(1):46-57.
45. Borron SW, Baud FJ. Acute cyanide poisoning: clinical spectrum, diagnosis, and treatment. *Arh Hig Rada Toksikol.* September 1996;47(3):307-322.
46. O'Brien DJ, Walsh DW, Terriff CM, Hall AH. Empiric management of cyanide toxicity associated with smoke inhalation. *Prehosp Disaster Med.* October 2011;26(5):374-382.
47. Ernst A, Zibrak JD. Carbon monoxide poisoning. *N Engl J Med.* November 1998 26;339(22):1603-1608.
48. Thom SR, Keim LW. Carbon monoxide poisoning: a review epidemiology, pathophysiology, clinical findings, and treatment options including hyperbaric oxygen therapy. *J Toxicol Clin Toxicol.* 1989;27(3):141-156.
49. Arturson G, Garby L, Robert M, Zaar B. The oxygen dissociation curve of normal human blood with special reference to the influence of physiological effector ligands. *Scand J Clin Lab Invest.* September 1974;34(1):9-13.
50. Weaver LK. Clinical practice. Carbon monoxide poisoning. *N Engl J Med.* March 2009 19;360(12):1217-1225.
51. Pace N, Strajman E, Walker EL. Acceleration of carbon monoxide elimination in man by high pressure oxygen. *Science.* June 16, 1950;111(2894):652-654.
52. Hardy KR, Thom SR. Pathophysiology and treatment of carbon monoxide poisoning. *J Toxicol Clin Toxicol.* 1994;32(6):613-629.
53. Curry S. Methemoglobinemia. *Ann Emerg Med.* April 1982;11(4):214-221.
54. Mellins RB. Respiratory complications of smoke inhalation in victims of fires. *J Pediatr.* July 1975;87(1):1-7.
55. Desai MH, Mlcak R, Richardson J, Nichols R, Herndon DN. Reduction in mortality in pediatric patients with inhalation injury with aerosolized heparin/N-acetylcystine [correction of acetylcystine] therapy. *J Burn Care Rehabil.* June 1998;19(3):210-212.
56. Gesell LB, ed. Hyperbaric oxygen therapy indications. The Hyperbaric Oxygen Therapy Committee report. Durham, NC: Undersea and Hyperbaric Medical Society; 2008.
57. Shelton CM, Chhim RF, Christensen ML. Recent new drug approvals. Part 1: drugs with pediatric indications. *J Pediatr Pharmacol Ther JPPT.* 2012;17(4):329-339.
58. Offerman SR, Daubert GP, Clark RF. The treatment of black widow spider envenomation with antivenin latrodectus mactans: a case series. *Perm J.* 2011;15(3):76-81.
59. Ward NT, Darracq MA, Tomaszewski C, Clark RF. Evidence-Based Treatment of Jellyfish Stings in North America and Hawaii. *Ann Emerg Med.* October 2012;60(4):399-414.
60. Auerbach PS. In reply to evidence-based treatment of jellyfish stings in North America and Hawaii. *Ann Emerg Med.* February 2013;61(2):253-254.
61. Burnett JW, Rubinstein H, Calton GJ. First aid for jellyfish envenomation. *South Med J.* July 1983;76(7):870-872.
62. Barnard JH. Studies of 400 Hymenoptera sting deaths in the United States. *J Allergy Clin Immunol.* November 1973;52(5):259-264.
63. Smoley BA. Oropharyngeal hymenoptera stings: a special concern for airway obstruction. *Mil Med.* February 2002;167(2):161-163.
64. Fisher M. Treating anaphylaxis with sympathomimetic drugs. *BMJ.* November 19927;305(6862):1107-1108.
65. Visscher PK, Vetter RS, Camazine S. Removing bee stings. *Lancet.* August 1996 3;348(9023):301-302.
66. Javors MA, Zhou W, Maas JW Jr, Han S, Keenan RW. Effects of fire ant venom alkaloids on platelet and neutrophil function. *Life Sci.* 1993;53(14):1105-1112.
67. Simons F, Gu X, Simons KJ. Epinephrine absorption in adults: intramuscular versus subcutaneous injection. *J Allergy Clin Immunol.* 2001;108(5):871-873.
68. Caovilla JJ, Barros EJG. Efficacy of two different doses of antilonomic serum in the resolution of hemorrhagic syndrome resulting from envenoming by Lonomia obliqua caterpillars: a randomized controlled trial. *Toxicon Off J Int Soc Toxinology.* June 1, 2004;43(7):811-818.
69. Arocha-Piñango CL, Guerrero B. [Hemorrhagic syndrome induced by caterpillars. Clinical and experimental studies. Review]. *Investig Clínica.* June 2003;44(2):155-163.
70. Cadera W, Pachtman MA, Fountain JA, Ellis FD, Wilson FM 2nd. Ocular lesions caused by caterpillar hairs (ophthalmia nodosa). *Can J Ophthalmol.* February 1984;19(1):40-44.
71. Pinson RT, Morgan JA. Envenomation by the puss caterpillar (Megalopyge opercularis). *Ann Emerg Med.* May 1991;20(5):562-564.
72. Seifert S, White J, Currie BJ. Pressure bandaging for North American snake bite? No! *Clin Toxicol.* December 2011;49(10):883-885.
73. Markenson D, Ferguson JD, Chameides L, et al. Part 13: First aid: 2010 American Heart Association and American Red Cross International Consensus on First Aid Science With Treatment Recommendations. *Circulation.* October 19, 2010;122(16 suppl 2):S582-S605.
74. American College of Medical Toxicology; American Academy of Clinical Toxicology; American Association of Poison Control Centers; European Association of Poison Control Centres and Clinical Toxicologists; International Society on Toxinology; Asia Pacific Association of Medical Toxicology. Pressure immobilization after North American Crotalinae snake envenomation. *Clin Toxicol.* December 2011;49(10):881-882.
75. Cardwell MD. Recognizing dangerous snakes in the United States and Canada: a novel 3-step identification method. *Wilderness Environ Med.* December 2011;22(4):304-308.
76. Janes Jr DN, Bush SP, Kolluru GR. Large snake size suggests increased snakebite severity in patients bitten by rattlesnakes in southern California. *Wilderness Environ Med.* 2010;21(2):120-126.

Environmental Injuries

CHAPTER 47

Marc-David Munk
Darryl J. Macias

INTRODUCTION

EMS providers often encounter patients who have become victims of environmental emergencies. Even in urban areas, patients may suffer from heat- or cold-related illnesses. In more remote areas, altitude illness, undersea illness, and decompression sickness may be encountered. Electrical injuries from both lightning and electrical sources may be seen. EMS workers need to understand how to stabilize these illnesses and injuries, while remaining safe.

OBJECTIVES

- Understand the pathophysiology, diagnosis, and management of hypothermia, frostbite, nonfreezing cold injury, and other cold-related injuries.
- Understand the pathophysiology, diagnosis, and management of heat stroke, heat exhaustion, and other heat-related injuries.
- Understand altitude-related illness, including AMS, HACE, HAPE.
- Understand the pathophysiology and treatment of undersea-related illnesses. Understand the diagnosis and management of electrical injuries.
- Understand the pathophysiology of electrical injuries.
- Understand that standard triage decisions may be reversed in the case of electrical injuries.
- Appreciate possible risks to the rescuer in electrical injuries.
- Understand the pathophysiology of decompression sickness.
- Understand barotrauma injuries
- Be familiar with treatment of diving and undersea injuries.

COLD-RELATED ILLNESS

MECHANISMS OF HEAT LOSS AND COMPENSATORY MECHANISMS

Heat transfer occurs through radiation, conduction, convection, and evaporation. Each of these mechanisms serves to transfer heat to and from the body. In homeostasis, these mechanisms of energy diffuse heat generated through the body's metabolic processes. Conduction is the transfer of heat between objects in direct contact. The amount of energy lost by a body in contact with another object depends on several factors, including the amount of the body in contact with the object, the conductivity of the objects, and the difference in temperature between the two objects. Conduction is a major cause of profound heat loss among victims who have fallen into cold water, for example. Convection is the transfer of heat caused by the movement of molecules of gas of liquid near the body. Convection explains why wind can exacerbate cold temperatures (the wind chill index). Radiation refers to the transfer of electromagnetic radiation between objects, in this case between humans and the environment. Evaporative heat loss takes place when water changes state, from liquid to gas. Heat loss increases with sweating.[1]

RISK/CONTRIBUTING FACTORS

Certain populations are more at risk for accidental hypothermia than others. Patients at either end of the human age spectrum are particularly at risk for hypothermia.

In the elderly, both metabolic and behavioral factors contribute to a propensity for rapid development of hypothermia in cold conditions.[2] In infants, increased surface area and absence of behavioral adaptations to cold exposure contribute to a high risk of hypothermia, even in ambient conditions.

Next, ingestion of certain medications places patients at risk for hypothermic illness. Medications can either interfere with thermogenesis or promote heat loss through various processes, including vasodilatation. Sedatives and psychotropic medications, including barbiturates, benzodiazepines, phenothiazines, lithium, and tricyclic antidepressants can all cause hypothermia.

Rescuers need to be vigilant for hypothermia in select populations: trauma patients, in particular, are vulnerable to hypothermia both as a consequence of their underlying injuries and hypovolemia. This is by virtue of the fact that they may have spent time in cold environments following their injuries, and as an iatrogenic consequence of standard trauma exposure and resuscitation practices.

HYPOTHERMIA

Hypothermia is generally defined as a core body temperature of 35°C or less, and is often categorized as being either primary or secondary in origin.[3] Primary hypothermia occurs when individuals are exposed to ambient conditions that exceed their ability to thermoregulate. This is distinct from secondary hypothermia, which occurs in patients with specific endocrine, neurologic, or metabolic conditions such as sepsis and cerebral lesions.[4] Primary (or accidental) hypothermia will be primarily discussed in this chapter.

Pathophysiology of Hypothermia Mammals maintain a careful equilibrium between heat loss and heat production. In humans, thermoregulation occurs via a complex sensory and transmission framework consisting of temperature sensitive sensors in the cutaneous tissues, the spinothalamic tract, the thalamus, and the hypothalamus.[5] The body can conserve and generate heat as a response using the autonomic, circulatory, and endocrine systems to stimulate thermogenesis. Hypothermia develops when cooling losses exceed the body's ability to maintain warmth.

Hypothermia has effects on all organ systems, but particularly the central nervous system, cardiac, renal, and hemostatic systems. Effects on the CNS are particularly pronounced: Cold depresses the central nervous system and amnesia, dysarthria, poor decision making, and delirium can be seen at even modestly decreased core body temperatures.[6] The cardiac system is similarly affected by cold. Cardiac output is affected by an impaired cardiac conduction system and by impaired myocardial contractility.[7] Dysrhythmias in moderate to severe hypothermia are common, and potentially lethal. Classically, tachycardia followed by bradycardia is described in cases of progressive hypothermia. Cold causes disruptions in the cardiac cycle, with prolongations of conduction time and electrocardiac intervals. These disruptions, combined with disruptions in transmembrane myocyte potentials, can incite multiple dysrhythmias, including reentrant tachycardias, atrial fibrillation, ventricular tachycardia, and ventricular fibrillation.[8] One ECG finding, the J (or Osborn) wave, is classically described in hypothermia.[9] This wave is classically seen on an ECG at the junction of the QRS complex and the ST segment.

The renal system responds to hypothermia by increasing diuresis, sometimes considerably. This "cold diuresis" effect is primarily caused by a relative central hypervolemia due to peripheral vasoconstriction, and leads to ongoing diuresis even in the face of relative dehydration.[10]

The hemostatic system is significantly affected by cold. Both coagulopathy and hypercoagulability can be seen in hypothermic patients. Coagulopathy can be caused by inhibitions in the coagulation cascade, thrombocytopenia, and platelet dysfunction.[11]

Clinical Presentation and Evaluation of Hypothermia Patients with hypothermia may be affected to varied degrees: Some, with severe hypothermia, may present in cardiac arrest. In these cases, determining whether hypothermia or some other medical/trauma etiology is responsible for the arrest may be difficult. Patients may be unconscious with pulses, and others may be conscious but have significantly diminished mentation. Patients with mild illness may present with or without shivering and may appear clinically intoxicated—confused, inattentive, and displaying slurred speech. Protective behaviors, such as heat-seeking efforts, may be ignored. It is important to be alert to the potential for hypothermic injury in patients otherwise suspected of being impaired by drugs of abuse.

Treatment of Hypothermia The decision to begin resuscitation can be difficult in patients found pulseless in cold conditions. In the absence of obviously lethal trauma, resuscitative attempts should as a rule be initiated, and continued until normothermia is achieved. There have been multiple case reports of patients successfully resuscitated even after prolonged periods of cardiac arrest.[12,13] Prehospital treatment for hypothermic patients not in cardiac arrest should be initiated as per **Box 47-1**.[14] Attention must be paid to ensuring that all traumatic injuries and medical comorbidities are assessed and managed, in addition to treatment of hypothermia. Aggressive attention should be paid to airway management: There is no reliable data to suggest that intubation induces lethal arrhythmias. Similarly, standard cardiac resuscitation efforts should be initiated.[15]

Rewarming Methods and Indications Prior to the initiation of rewarming, patients must have their temperatures measured accurately. The most accurate readings are taken from esophageal monitors (in the intubated patient) although rectal thermometers, while less accurate than esophageal probes, may be the best available option. Oral, external auditory, and bladder thermometers are unreliable instruments to measure true core body temperature.[16] The appropriate method of rewarming should be selected based on the severity of patient symptoms. Rewarming efforts can be divided into three categories: passive external, active external, and active internal methods.[17]

Passive external rewarming refers to efforts to protect and insulate patients from heat loss, in order to facilitate native thermogenesis. Such efforts are best reserved for cases of hypothermia in a selected population of younger, healthier patients.

In contrast, active rewarming refers to the transfer of heat from a source, to an affected patient. Active rewarming can be either external (heat applied to the external surface of the skin) or internal (invasive techniques designed to rewarm the blood and organs) as noted in **Box 47-2**. Active rewarming is required for patients with moderate to severe hypothermia and those with complicating comorbidities, such as age or metabolic complicating factors. Most active warming in the EMS environment will be active external warming, using heated bags of IV fluid, or water bottles placed in the groin and axilla. Other options include warm air convection devices modified for use with portable power systems. The decision to pursue invasive cooling should be made with consideration for the degree of hemodynamic instability as well as

---

Box 47-1

Prehospital Management of Hypothermia

1. Assess vital signs. Be aware that some patients may have significant bradycardia and present minimal cardiac output, adequate to support diminished metabolic demand. Endotracheal intubation and other airway maneuvers should be initiated as medically indicated.

2. Minimize further hypothermia by drying and insulating the patient: Remove wet clothing and wrap the patient in dry blankets.

3. Correct dehydration: Most patients with moderate to severe hypothermia benefit from a fluid challenge to correct dehydration. Warmed fluids should be used.

4. Initiate active rewarming to the torso. Hot water bottles or heated bags of IV fluid can be placed in the patient's axillae and groin. It is in practice difficult to provide a meaningful amount of rewarming to patients in the EMS setting.

5. Begin gentle transport to a receiving facility. Avoid rough handling of the patient, which may initiate cardiac arrhythmias.

Box 47-2

Active Rewarming Methods Commonly Used in EMS

Active external warming techniques

1. External heaters
2. Water bottles and warmed bags of IV fluids in groin/axilla
3. Circulated hot air
4. Immersion in warm water

Active internal methods (usually employed at receiving facilities)

1. IV infusions of warmed fluids
2. GI lavage via NG tube or rectal tube
3. Thoracic lavage via thoracostomy tube/peritoneal lavage via peritoneal incision
4. Hemodialysis
5. Extracorporeal blood rewarming
6. Cardiopulmonary bypass

---

the extent of hypothermia.[3] During all attempts at rewarming, attention should be paid to the possibility of afterdrop—the ongoing cooling of the core caused by relocation of cold peripheral blood into the relatively warmer core.[18] In dehydrated and significantly hypothermic patients, this translocation of cold can be life threatening. Afterdrop seems to be minimized by directing warming efforts to the torso, and by avoiding use of cold extremities until the core temperature is stabilized.

■ LOCALIZED COLD EMERGENCIES

Frostbite and Frostnip Frostbite refers to tissue injury and destruction caused by freezing. Frostnip, in contrast, is a mild temporary form of cold-induced injury and is also known as first-degree frostbite. These injuries are distinct from nonfreezing cold injuries such as trench foot, discussed separately. While frostbite remains a concern for outdoor enthusiasts, it is not uncommonly encountered in urban populations, particularly in the homeless. Second-degree frostbite refers to superficial frostbite where third- and fourth-degree refers to deeper injuries.

Pathophysiology of Frostbite Physiologic factors related to dermal circulation are the key to frostbite. Skin contains a complex system of capillaries with richly innervated arteriovenous connections. Cutaneous vascular tone is controlled by both direct local and systemic sympathetic vasoconstrictor fibers. In cold conditions, vasoconstriction occurs, predisposing subsequent local freezing injury. Frostbite injury begins with extracellular ice crystal formation, followed by intracellular ice formation, cellular dehydration, dysfunction, and subsequent death. Evidence has shown that frostbite and burn injuries share similar patterns of endothelial damage, edema, and inflammatory mediator release.

Clinical Presentation and Evaluation of Frostbite Frostbite has traditionally been categorized, like burns, by severity—although new classification schemes have more recently been proposed to better reflect prognosis. First-degree injury is typified by white or yellow skin accompanied by localized erythema and numbness. Superficial blisters are seen in second-degree injury, and deeper, blood filled blisters are seen in third-degree injury. Fourth-degree injury involves the deeper tissues, including muscle and bone. Regardless of the ultimate degree of severity, frostbite generally presents with a cold, initially numb, edematous affected area. Pain subsequently develops with rewarming. The extent of eventual tissue loss is poorly correlated to the affected area's clinical appearance. Several weeks are needed to determine the ultimate extent of any tissue loss.[19]

Treatment of Frostbite Field treatment of frostbite depends, to a great extent, on circumstances. The most important factor when making the decision to initiate the thawing of a frostbitten area is the likelihood of refreezing. Patients with short transport times should have wet clothing removed from the frostbitten area, but thawing efforts should generally be left for hospital staff to initiate. Patients with very long transport times, particularly in the aeromedical setting, may benefit from rewarming efforts so long as refreezing of the affected area can be prevented. Once in the ED, rapid rewarming, best done by immersing the affected area in a water bath at 104°F-108°F, is recommended. Analgesia and indicated tetanus prophylaxis are mandatory. Most literature promotes the use of inflammatory cascade inhibitors, such as aspirin and ibuprofen, to control thrombosis and tissue loss.[20]

Transport Decisions and Disposition Most small emergency departments can manage the initial treatment of severe frostbite. Once rewarming efforts have been initiated, subsequent management, including transfer for treatment and rehabilitation in specialized trauma units should be considered. Admission for all but the most trivial frostbite should be considered given the significant functional loss that can accompany this injury.

Mild hypothermia can be managed at most emergency departments. With severe hypothermia, transport to a center capable of initiating active internal warming should be considered. In such a case, the benefits of advanced-level ED care need to be weighed against the risks of prolonged ambulance transport.

Trench Foot Trench foot describes tissue damage caused by cold temperatures above freezing. Unlike frostbite, these injuries do not involve cellular freezing. Often an underdiagnosed injury, trench foot, like its cousin immersion foot, is caused by prolonged exposure to wet, cold conditions. Classically this condition has been described in soldiers who wear wet boots for prolonged periods, but has also been described in shipwreck survivors and in the homeless.[21] Trench foot is primarily caused by profound vasoconstriction and sympathetic response caused by prolonged cold exposure and decreased blood flow to the affected extremities. Endothelial damage and capillary leakage result. Eventual amputation is a possible outcome.

Clinical Presentation and Evaluation of Trench Foot Like frostbite, trench foot presents with pallor, edema, and loss of sensation. Because of the profound vasoconstrictive nature of this injury, decreased capillary refill, and severe pain remain hallmarks. Like frostbite, trench foot can result in significant tissue damage and long-term loss of function.[22]

Treatment of Trench Foot The primary goal of therapy for trench foot is the preservation of viable tissue. Rapid rewarming is thought to result in a sharp increase in tissue oxygen consumption. For this reason, rapid rewarming is avoided. Little recent data concerning optimum management of this condition are available: Best evidence suggests that affected extremities should be kept dry and slightly cooler than room temperature to reduce distal metabolic demand.[23,24]

HEAT-RELATED ILLNESS

When exposed to high temperatures, the body will attempt to dissipate excess heat through a range of thermoregulatory mechanisms. When the capacity of these mechanisms is overcome, heat-related illness occurs. Body heat is generated via basal metabolism, by exertion, and via exposure to the sun, hot objects, and warm ambient temperatures.[25] Excessive heat is toxic to cells and causes the release of inflammatory proteins. High temperatures denature proteins, interrupt cellular processes, and cause cell death.[26,27] The term heat-related illnesses refers to a range of conditions, including heat exhaustion, heat cramps, and both classic and exertional heat strokes.

■ PATHOPHYSIOLOGY OF HYPERTHERMIA

Mechanisms of Heat Regulation Humans are able to regulate their core temperatures via autonomic processes which modify the rates of heat production (shivering and changes to basal metabolism) and by heat loss (sweating and vasoconstriction/dilatation). Behavioral modification also serves a role in controlling temperature. When thermoregulatory mechanisms can no longer compensate for excessive heating, heat illness

develops. Depending on the degree and duration of heat exposure, illness along a continuum of severity may occur.

Mechanisms of Heat Dissipation Heat transfer, as in cases of hypothermia, can only occur via four processes: radiation, convection, evaporation, and conduction. At cool temperatures, radiation accounts for the bulk of heat loss. Evaporation is the second most important means of heat transfer. Conduction (the transfer of heat from the skin to the air) is relatively inefficient although convection, caused by the movement of air over the skin surface, improves this process.[28] At higher temperatures, the body can no longer radiate heat to the environment and evaporation becomes increasingly important for heat transfer. As humidity increases, evaporative heat loss decreases. For this reason, a combination of high temperature and high humidity can overcome the two main physiologic mechanisms that the body uses to dissipate heat.

■ RISK/CONTRIBUTING FACTORS

Age Age extremes are a well-appreciated risk factor for the development of heat-related illness. The elderly are more susceptible to heat stroke because of decreased sweating ability and decreased cardiovascular capacity to distribute blood flow to the skin.[29] In children, basal metabolic rate is higher than that of adults.

Medications Medications can contribute to the development of heat-related illness by either increasing the amount of basal heat production (thyroid hormone, amphetamines, tricyclics) or by decreasing the effectiveness of heat loss mechanisms (most anticholinergics and antihistamines).[30]

Environment Clearly, exposure to warm, humid climates places individuals at risk for heat-related illness. Certain populations, including professional and amateur athletes, military members, and outdoor enthusiasts are at risk for developing heat illness due to their exposure to the warm climates. Many members of these groups are often unwilling to modify their activities to suit warm ambient conditions.[31]

Preexisting Illness Patients with certain preexisting conditions are at risk for developing heat illness. Patients with endocrine abnormalities, illnesses causing dehydration, fatigue, sleep deprivation, and cardiovascular disease all have decreased abilities to respond to heat stress. The presence of obesity and lack of physical conditioning also contribute to the risk.

■ CLINICAL PRESENTATION AND EVALUATION OF HEAT ILLNESS

Heat Exhaustion Heat exhaustion occurs when salt, free water, or both is depleted through exposure to hot conditions. Patients with heat exhaustion may present with headache, nausea, malaise, and dizziness.[32] Their temperature may be normal or slightly elevated, but, unlike heat stroke, there are no central nervous system symptoms.

Heat Stroke Heat stroke represents the most severe manifestation of heat-related illness. It is a life-threatening emergency with high mortality if not promptly treated. Heat stroke can be divided into two categories, which differ by affected population and by presentation: These are classic and exertional heat strokes. Both forms present with hyperthermia (>40°C) and altered mental status and both are caused by heat leading to edema and destruction of tissue.[33,34]

Classic heat stroke is often seen in older adults and the chronically ill during heat waves. It often occurs in the form of epidemics. Compared to exertional heat stroke, classic heat stroke often occurs over days and is notable for its significant abnormalities in fluids and electrolytes.[34] In contrast, exertional heat stroke usually occurs when excess heat generated by muscular exercise exceeds the body's ability to disperse it. This form of heat stroke is commonly seen in athletes and in the young. Soldiers, particularly those at the beginning of training, are at high risk for this condition.

Both forms may present with prodromal dizziness, weakness, confusion. CNS symptoms seen in heat stroke include irritability, confusion, hallucinations, seizures, and coma.

▦ TREATMENT OF HEAT ILLNESS

Heat Exhaustion Heat exhaustion is treated with fluid and electrolyte replacement and rest in a cool environment. Patients with mild heat exhaustion may be treated with oral solutions. Parenteral fluids may be necessary in patients who appear to be hypovolemic. In the EMS setting, normal saline solution is the preferred IV solution although this may be modified in the ED once the patient's electrolyte status is determined.

Heat Stroke For patients with heat stroke, EMS providers should immediately initiate cooling. In the field, the best way to initiate cooling is by covering the victim with an ice and water bath. An IV should be initiated, and parenteral hydration initiated to correct underlying dehydration. The goal of therapy is to immediately lower core body temperature and correct dehydration.[35]

Immersion in ice water is the most effective means of rapidly lowering body temperature, but this may not be practical in the EMS setting. Immersion also limits the ability of rescuers to provide cardiac resuscitation is needed. Fanning and placing ice bags near the axillae and groin are other options. Cooling should be continued until core temperature reaches 38.5°C.[36]

It is understood that EMS services may not have the ability to perform rectal temperatures on patients, although many services do carry external auditory and forehead colorimetric thermometers. Without a measured temperature, the diagnosis of heat stroke may not be obvious. In the absence of a documented temperature, and in the highly suggestive clinical setting (such as a healthy individual who collapses after exercise in hot weather), cooling should be empirically begun; adverse outcomes from delays in cooling affected patients are severe.

In addition, it has been found that the temperature of patients arriving in the ED following EMS transport is often lower than the temperature on scene. This discrepancy, likely from cooling during transport, may lead the receiving physician to underdiagnose heat stroke.[37] An accurate thermometer should be considered essential equipment in any ambulance, given its ease of use, potential benefits, and lack of risk.

Transport Decisions and Disposition Patients with heat-related illness should be brought to the closest appropriate facility. Patients with heat stroke will likely merit ICU admission. Cooling for heat stroke must not be delayed, and should be initiated in the field, followed by rapid transport to the ED. Mass gatherings and community wide heat epidemics require further planning and EMS medical directors should coordinate planning for these events.[38,39]

ALTITUDE-RELATED ILLNESS

▦ MODERATE, HIGH, AND EXTREME ALTITUDES DEFINED

Moderate altitudes are above 1000 m, high altitude is between 2000 and 5500 m, and extreme altitude surpasses 5500 m.[40] This varies with barometric pressure and latitude as storms and increased latitude decrease barometric oxygen. Healthy individuals with an arterial oxygen saturation of 100% at sea level may saturate to 92% on arrival destinations at 2500 m,[41] and this can worsen in sick individuals.

▦ PHYSIOLOGY OF ACCLIMATIZATION[42-47]

See **Figure 47-1**.

▦ PRESENTATION, PATHOPHYSIOLOGY, AND TREATMENT OF HIGH-ALTITUDE ILLNESS

A. *Risk factors*: Travel to elevations above 2000 to 2500 m is associated with altitude illnesses.[40,48] The rate of acute mountain sickness (AMS) among conference delegates at 1920 to 2957 m in Colorado was 25%.[49] An important risk factor in high-altitude illness is referred to as ascending "too high too fast." Few studies give ideal ascent rates.[49,50] Sleeping at successive daily elevations of 500 m beyond 3000 m, or a previous history of altitude illness, increases risk.[49] Ascent rates of 300 to 500 m daily above 3000 m, with a complete rest day each third day, appears to be safe. "Climbing high and sleeping low" helps acclimatization,[51] which may not be applicable to those with preexisting medical illness.

B. Acute mountain sickness and high-altitude cerebral edema (HACE) is a continuum of improper acclimatization. AMS in its benign, self-limiting form is nonspecific. Headache (in 95%[40]), anorexia, lassitude, nausea/vomiting, dizziness, and insomnia from periodic breathing occurs beyond the first 4 hours above 2000 m.[44] The Lake Louise scoring system requires the presence of headache, and one other symptom.[44,52] Symptoms peak in 2 to 3 days, improving on day 5 at the same elevation. Dyspnea, peripheral edema, or tachycardia is not necessary for diagnosis.[40]

In its malignant form, AMS can lead to HACE, with ataxia on tandem gait walk testing,[53] and altered mentation is also seen. Focal neurologic findings are usually from other cerebrovascular causes,[54] still mandating rapid evacuation. Rule out carbon monoxide poisoning (from cooking inside a tent), hypothermia, hyperthermia, electrolyte

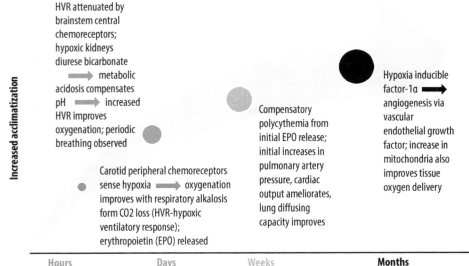

FIGURE 47-1. Physiology of acclimatization.

or glycemic disorders, cardiac disorders, migraine, infection, or drug/alcohol intoxication.

C. High-altitude pulmonary edema (HAPE) is a noncardiogenic pulmonary edema occurring beyond 3000 m[55] affecting 0.2% to 15% of travelers, depending on ascent rate and exercise intensity,[44] seen 36 hours upon altitude arrival.[51] A subtle nonproductive cough or inordinate dyspnea at moderate exercise, or at rest, may be seen,[44] while pink, frothy sputum occurs later. Patients fatigue more frequently than others.[51] Relative increases in tachycardia, tachypnea, hypoxia, and chest crackles on examination are seen.[44] Radiographs demonstrate right middle lobe patchy infiltrates, and ultrasound can aid the diagnosis.[56] Males, those with a history of HAPE, and increased pulmonary artery pressures (eg, pulmonary embolism, a unilateral pulmonary artery, or congenital cardiac disorders including a patent foramen ovale)[44,57] are at risk. Exaggerated increases of pulmonary artery pressures and increased capillary vascular permeability from inflammation at altitude are causative.[44] Rule out pneumonia, opiate overdose,[58] asthma, CHF from hypoxemia, and other causes of acute hypoxia.

D. *Other considerations*: High-altitude focal neurologic deficits responsive to descent or oxygen supplementation are frequent presentations of atypical migraines.[59] Apparent TIAs in those without cerebrovascular disease, with headache resolving with descent, are reported; these findings *without* headache in the elderly indicates cerebrovascular disease. Acute global amnesia and delirium without headache resolve with descent.[59] Cerebral venous thrombosis (headache with focal neurological findings not ameliorated with descent nor oxygen)[59] and lower extremity venous thrombosis can occur. Color blindness and high-altitude retinal hemorrhage (HARH) also exist.[51] Permanent altitude dwellers risk chronic mountain illness (CMS) with decreased HVR, increased pulmonary arterial pressures,[60] hypoxia, polycythemia, AMS symptoms, paresthesias, and CHF; living above 2500 m is a risk.[61] Reentrant pulmonary edema on return to high altitude ameliorates with continuous positive airway pressure (CPAP).[62] Stable coronary artery disease does not increase cardiac events below 3500 m.[63] COPD and asthma do not seem to increase risk of altitude illnesses below 3000 m.[64] COPD requiring supplemental oxygen during commercial airflight should apply the same precautions to altitude travel.

TREATMENT AND TRANSPORT CONSIDERATIONS

With the ABCs treat hypothermia, which aggravates high-altitude illness. Nonsteroidal anti-inflammatory agents benefit mild headaches. Use acetazolamide, 125 to 250 mg po bid (2.5 mg/kg po bid in children) for moderate symptoms, or insomnia at altitude which will accelerate acclimatization from diuresis a mild metabolic acidosis.[44,48] Paresthesias, appetite loss, sensitivity to sunlight, and a distaste for carbonated beverages are reported; allergies to sulfonamides contraindicate acetazolamide use.[44] Acetazolamide prophylaxis (125 mg po bid) is initiated 1 day before altitude arrival; consider this for those with previous AMS. Duration is useful for up to 5 days at a given altitude; increasing altitude warrants continuation of therapy.

Dexamethasone is used for acetazolamide contraindications, or for necessary rapid ascents, preventing AMS and HAPE. The drug masks symptoms without acclimatization; sudden discontinuation causes symptom recurrence. Prophylaxis with 2 to 4 mg po daily suffices; 8 to 10 mg po, IM or IV initially, then 4 mg every 6 hours until descent is achieved, treats severe AMS and HACE.[44] Supplemental oxygen is recommended; portable hyperbaric chambers is useful if descent is not possible. Individuals with CMS without HACE benefit from acetazolamide, supplemental oxygenation, and descent.[63]

Those without a HAPE history do not necessarily need prophylaxis. Clinicians often use nifedipine for prophylaxis and treatment of HAPE, 20 to 30 mg extended release tabs po bid daily. Prophylactic PDE 5 inhibitors relax pulmonary artery vasculature; sildenafil 50 mg po tid and tadalafil 10 mg po bid; yet treatment experience is limited.[44] Salmeterol may supplement nifedipine, but should not be used as HAPE monotherapy.[49]

Rest and supplemental oxygen without descent are useful in mild HAPE. Patients are given 4 to 6 L of oxygen, titrating SaO_2 to 92%. Mandatory reexamination in 24 hours with evidence of a room air SaO_2 >90% and crackle resolution allows patients to resume activities under supervision.[49] Portable hyperbaric chambers are useful if immediate descent or oxygen administration is not possible. CPAP ameliorates HAPE and reentrant pulmonary edema[49,63] in a hospital setting.

Dexamethasone may be added to HAPE patients with AMS or HACE, since HAPE and HACE may coincide.[49] Some recommend acetazolamide for HAPE, citing reductions in pulmonary arterial pressures.[44] The use of phosphodiesterase-5-inhibitors and nitroglycerin is contraindicated. Those with HACE, CNS findings, and unresolved HAPE should be hospitalized and should not reascend without medical clearance once symptoms resolve. Remote environments not accessible to vehicular travel may mandate air ambulance evacuation. A landing site may not be nearby, necessitating intermediate transport by other means. During inclement weather, it may be necessary to medically stabilize the patient on-site before transport.

ELECTRICAL AND LIGHTNING INJURIES

Electrical and lightning injuries may cause cardiopulmonary arrest and electrocution can cause deep insidious tissue burns leading to kidney failure and compartment syndromes. Lightning injuries can result in cardiopulmonary arrest with neurological injuries, with minor burns. Care for those in cardiac arrest first (reverse triage). Attention to rescuer safety takes precedence in both mechanisms of injury.

▨ ENVIRONMENTAL CONSIDERATIONS

Many *electrical injuries* are from occupational hazards; contact duration, AC or DC circuit, voltage, while current and pathway determine severity.[65] High amperages correlate with high mortality[66] and wet skin causes cardiac arrest without burns.[66] Victims cannot self-release from current in AC injury; DC current often catapults patients, inducing blunt trauma. Respiratory arrest or ventricular fibrillation can occur at 100 mA.[66]

Mortality from lightning injury is from ventricular fibrillation or asystole.[67] Injury occurs electrically, with heat production, and concussive forces as a result of discharge.[68] Exposure duration segregates lightning from electrical injury; lightning is a unidirectional massive current impulse unlike DC or AC, lasting milliseconds.[68] Lightning injury occur with direct strike, immediate contact with objects hit by lightning, side flash (energy down power cords into computers, television screens, or land telephones), ground current, and upward streamers; superficial burns are not often accompanied by internal injury from "flashover."[68]

▨ INJURY PRESENTATION

Electrical injury can lead to dysrhythmias, ischemic patterns, or ventricular fibrillation.[68,69] More "stable" rhythms resolve without sequelae; angina is a concern. Peripheral vessel damage causes compartment syndrome.[66] Injury severity is greater than expected from burn size alone; deep muscle injury leads to acute renal failure (ARF)[69]; correlated with fasciotomies and amputations.[70] Orthopedic injuries are reported.[71] The most common cause of death with *lightning* is ventricular fibrillation and asystole.[67,69] Asystole and respiratory standstill from injury to brainstem respiratory centers initially occurs; cardiac automaticity and contractions resume shortly, yet respiratory centers do not recover quickly. Without immediate ventilatory assistance, hypoxia causes secondary cardiac arrest.[69] Ventilation takes equal importance as perfusion in this biphasic arrest pattern.[68] ARF and compartment syndromes are uncommon in lightning injuries; both mechanisms of injury may cause secondary blunt traumatic injury.[69] CNS damage occurs 70% in both[66,71]; coma, seizures, visual loss, deafness, and aphasia may also occur. Dilated or unreactive pupils should not be initially used as criteria for brain death in lightning victims.[71] CNS disorders can occur short term, weeks to months after insult.[66]

Keraunoparalysis from lightning is a transient paresis with autonomic findings, affecting the lower limbs.[72] Tympanic membrane rupture, vertigo, cataracts, and Horner syndrome may occur.[71] Both mechanisms may cause CNS hemorrhage.[66,72] Late psychiatric sequelae has also been reported.[72,73] Electrical current tends to cause deep skin and tissue burns if the victim "freezes" to the circuit.[71] Skin findings from lightning include linear, punctate or feathering patterns, thermal burns, or combinations.[71] Linear burns are from steam burns due to flash vaporization of sweat or rainwater. Feathering burns (Lichtenberg figures), if present, are pathognomic, having fernlike patterns, and disappearing hours later without treatment as they are not true burns. Punctate burns are small, closely spaced circular burns rarely requiring grafting. Thermal burns from metal objects need standard burn care.[69] Cranial burns increase mortality fourfold; patients are twice as likely to suffer a cardiopulmonary arrest.[71]

PREHOSPITAL RESCUE AND TREATMENT

Electrocuted victims can transmit electricity, shocking rescuers. Cut off the current source first, or remove the patient from the source with nonconducting objects. Downed power lines pose danger. In lightning rescue, stay within traveling range of a grounded shelter. Lightening has been noted to cause potential MCI events.[74] Employ the following "30-30 Rule" for rescuers: If lightning is seen, count the time until thunder is heard. For 30 seconds or less, seek safe shelter immediately. Thunder without lightning means lightning may be within striking range. After the storm dissipates, wait 30 minutes after hearing the last thunder before leaving safety[75]; resuscitation is best in safe shelter.[67] "Reverse triage" is used to resuscitate pulseless apneic victims first; the "walking wounded" will probably not suffer cardiopulmonary decompensation,[69] and must seek safe shelter to avoid more strikes. With the ABCs, consider the possibility of blunt trauma and C-spine injury in all. Though uncommon in lightning, electric injury is associated with myoglobinuria; consider vigorous fluid therapy. Fluid resuscitation guidelines with burn formulas for insidious burns is difficult; use urine output to guide therapy. Mannitol or urinary alkalinization does not confer additional benefits to normal saline alone.[76] For transport, remember that helicopters are at high risk for lightning strike; limit rescuer exposure to aircraft.[68]

Definitive care should occur in cases of cardiopulmonary arrest, significant ECG abnormalities, CNS injury, burns, possible deep tissue injury, and women with viable pregnancies.[68] Victims of low-voltage electrical injury, uncomplicated lightning strikes, and histories of stable cardiac disease may be observed.[77] All children should go to the ED[71]; children with labial electric cord injury should be hospitalized.

DECOMPRESSION/UNDERSEAS ILLNESS

Decompression illness (DCI) is from intravascular/extravascular bubble formation due to sudden reductions in ambient pressure. It may have skin, musculoskeletal, pulmonary, cardiac, or CNS manifestations. DCI occurs in recreational or commercial scuba diving, and in aeronautical activities where sudden changes in air pressure could occur. Hyperbaric oxygen therapy (HBOT) is definitive.

SCUBA DIVING

Open scuba divers breathe pressurized air (21% oxygen) or oxygen enriched air (Nitrox with 28%-40% O_2) in single tanks capable of injury if mistreated. Closed scuba systems "recycle" air after scrubbing CO_2; additional gases supplement rebreathed gas. One can dive deeper; yet technical diving requires substantial training due to its complexity. See **Figure 47-2** for equipment differences.

DIVE PHYSICS AND PHYSIOLOGY

Sea level barometric pressure is 1 atmosphere (atm). For each 10 m (33 ft) of seawater (1 msw/33 ftsw) below surface, pressure increases by 1 atm; at 10 msw, the pressure is 2 atm, and so on. Gases and tissues compress at greater depths, expanding at lesser depths from pressure changes; thus, gas volume varies inversely to ambient pressure (Boyle law). More gas can be forced in or out of tissues, depending on pressure (Henry law); gas leaves rapidly if pressure is rapidly released. Inert nitrogen is 78% of air under pressure. Increasing pressure saturates more N_2 into tissues. Each gas (N_2, or O_2) acts as its own gas with its own effects under pressure (Dalton law). More unmetabolizable N_2 is loaded on deeper dives and released on ascent; N_2 is soporific; diving to 30 m (4 atm) loads more nitrogen into the CNS, inducing nitrogen narcosis; sport diving should not exceed 40 msw (**Figure 47-3**). Minimizing tissue N_2 saturation with dive computers/tables mitigate this, yet DCI can still occur. Slow recompression allows lung bubble elimination ("off-gassing"). On ascent, exhalation helps eliminate alveolar bubble buildup. Nitrox lessens N_2 load at the expense of diving at shallower depths: high-pressure brain

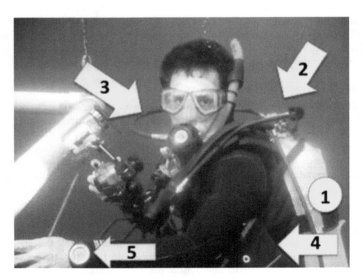
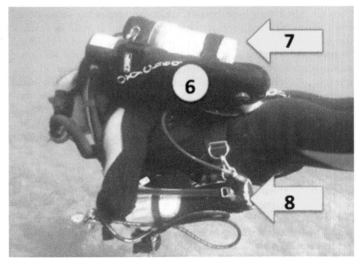

FIGURE 47-2. Open and closed circuit SCUBA systems. Limit for safe recreational open circuit scuba about 40 msw; closed technical systems allow deeper diving, especially when nitrogen replaced by helium, along with supplemental oxygen ("trimix"). **A**: open circuit SCUBA. (1) High-pressure air tank at 3000 psi. (2) First-stage regulator component reduces pressure at mouthpiece to ~150 psi. (3) Second-stage regulator one-way demand valve allows inspired air flow with ease at ambient pressure for proper lung expansion; exhaled air released into water via nonreturn exhaust valve in mouthpiece. (4) Buoyancy control vest controls depth; connected hose inflates or deflates device. (5) Pressure gauge/dive computer. **B**: Closed circuit SCUBA. (6) Mouthpiece connected to breathing bag system connected to high-pressure gas supply. (7) Carbon dioxide absorbing canister returns air devoid of carbon dioxide into rebreathing mix. (8) Additional tanks of gas (oxygen, helium). Problems: hypoxia from inadequate gas mix; greathing resistance with harder work, caustic gas when lime scrubbing agent and water mix; constant attentiveness to complex computers.

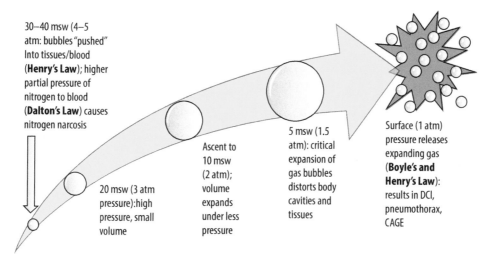

FIGURE 47-3. The deadly gas laws.

O_2 toxicity induces seizures at depths below 40 msw, depending on O_2 concentration. Adding helium (trimix) overcomes N_2 and O_2 limitations, increasing bottom time and depth. Such technical diving is hazardous: Breathing incorrectly calculated air mixes, and DCI from below 50 msw is deadly.[78] Dive times and profiles, and gas breathed help a physician determine gas uptake amounts.

DIVING DISORDERS

Descent contracts air volume (negative pressure) inside a mask, as well as in middle ear chambers and sinuses relative to outer pressure without equalization. Ocular and periorbital vessel engorgement occurs in mask squeeze, but this is prevented by exhaling air into the mask. Inability to equalize ears and sinuses can occur with rhinitis or masses, while eardrum perforation with water intrusion (middle ear barotrauma; MEB) results. Vertigo, vomiting, or panic from MEB may lead to uncontrolled ascent, which may result in DCI or even specifically arterial gas embolism (AGE). For MEB, keep the ear canal dry, avoid eardrops, and proscribe diving unless cleared by an ENT specialist. Topical nasal or systemic decongestants, analgesics, and benzodiazepines help. Inner ear barotrauma (deafness, tinnitus, vertigo, vomiting) mimics DCI, requiring rest, head elevation, antiemetics, and emergent referral for possible HBOT.[79] Unrelieved pressure ruptures lung tissue on ascent, resulting in pneumomediastinum, pneumothorax, or cerebral AGE as air goes into circulation.[80,81] Lung ultrasonography appears to be more sensitive than a chest radiograph for pneumothorax. A patient may require needle or tube thoracostomy, with hospital transfer for HBOT; cabin altitudes 150 m above departure must not be exceeded for air transport.[82] DCI comprises decompression sickness (DCS) and cerebral AGE. DCS pathology is bubble formation in blood/tissue from dissolved N_2. On ascent, bubbles distort and inflame tissues, causing microemboli and tissue ischemia. Lung microvasculature filters small bubbles; some bubbles may enter the arterial circulation[83] facilitated by a patent foramen ovale (PFO), causing "undeserved bends" (musculoskeletal DCS despite proper dive table practices).[84,85] Altitude exposure after diving adds to DCI risk.[86] DCS is organ specific, ranging from pruritus and malaise to cardiopulmonary arrest.[79] The "bends" (atraumatic musculoskeletal DCS) or skin findings (cutis marmorata) are Type 1 DCS; CNS findings (including and not limited to paresthesias, paresis, altered mentation, vertigo, incoordination, and loss of bowel or bladder function) characterize Type 2 DCS; both mandate urgent referral for HBOT.[87] Symptoms may take a day to present; suspect if a patient has unexplained findings plus DCS risk factors within the previous day.[88] The diagnosis is clinical; a careful examination (including a neurological examination) is necessary.[87] Cerebral AGE presents acutely, with unconsciousness or seizures quickly upon resurfacing; focal motor,

visual, or cognitive deficits may be seen.[80] Bubbles may occlude coronary arteries (causing dysrhythmias, ischemia, or cardiac arrest).[87] ACLS and transfer to the closest 24-hour emergency HBOT facility are mandatory.

INITIAL TREATMENT OF DCI

Supplemental 100% oxygen therapy beyond symptom resolution is recommended, allowing inert gas washout, ameliorating tissue hypoxia, and biochemical damage; those receiving oxygen have quicker symptom resolution.[89] In-water recompression is not recommended, especially in obtunded patients.[90] A head down position is proscribed, which may potentiate cerebral edema; a supine position is preferable.[87,91] Fluid rehydration ameliorates hemoconcentration. Supplemental glucose in normoglycemia, corticosteroids, or anticoagulants does not improve outcomes.[79] Lidocaine has been used for serious neurological cases at a dose of 1.5 mg/kg bolus, with an hourly infusion thereafter, however, should be done in consultation with a hyperbaric medicine physician and likely not appropriate for prehospital care.[87,84]

DISPOSITION AND TRANSPORT DECISIONS

Any suspicion of DCI warrants consideration for immediate transfer for HBOT, even after symptom resolution. HBOT is definitive therapy for DCI.[91] Mild symptoms (static or remitting limb pain, constitutional symptoms, rash, or stable nondermatomal sensory changes for 24 hours, with normal neurological examinations), should not worsen without HBOT; the risk-benefit ratio of a hazardous evacuation might preclude transfer. Contact the Diver's Alert Network at 1-919-684-9111 for the nearest hyperbaric chamber, or for other questions.

KEY POINTS

- Patients with mild hypothermia may present with or without shivering and may appear clinically intoxicated—confused, inattentive, and displaying slurred speech. It is important to be alert to the potential for hypothermic injury in patients otherwise suspected of being impaired by drugs of abuse.

- In the absence of obviously lethal trauma, resuscitative attempts in hypothermic patients should as a rule be initiated, and continued until normothermia is achieved.

- Most active warming in the EMS environment will be active external warming, using heated bags of IV fluid, or water bottles placed in the groin and axilla.

- Patients with short transport times should have wet clothing removed from the frostbitten area, but thawing efforts should generally be left for hospital staff to initiate. Patients with very long transport times, particularly in the aeromedical setting, may benefit from rewarming efforts so long as refreezing of the affected area can be reliably prevented.

- Heat stroke represents the most severe manifestation of heat-related illness. It is a life-threatening emergency with high mortality if not promptly treated.

- Without a measured temperature, the diagnosis of heat stroke may not be obvious. In the absence of a documented temperature, and in the highly suggestive clinical setting cooling should be empirically begun.

- High-altitude illnesses usually occur beyond 2000 m and that acclimatization is the physiological response to hypoxia at altitude.

- Inadequate acclimatization to hypoxia results in altitude-related illnesses, notably acute mountain sickness (AMS), high-altitude cerebral edema (HACE), and high-altitude pulmonary edema (HAPE). These potentially lethal disorders are treatable, and should be distinguished from diseases not related to ascent to high altitude. If in doubt, immediate descent to lower altitude is mandatory.

- Patients with HACE, CNS findings, and unresolved HAPE should be hospitalized and should not reascend without medical clearance.

- In electrical injuries, "reverse triage" is used to resuscitate pulseless apneic victims first; the "walking wounded" will probably not suffer cardiopulmonary decompensation.

- Any suspicion of DCI warrants consideration for immediate transfer for HBOT, even after symptom resolution.

REFERENCES

1. Webb P. The physiology of heat regulation. *Am J Physiol*. 1995;268 (4 pt 2):R838-R850.
2. Muszkat M, Durst RM, Ben-Yehuda A. Factors associated with mortality among elderly patients with hypothermia. *Am J Med*. 2002;113(3):234-237.
3. Hanania NA, Zimmerman JL. Accidental hypothermia. *Crit Care Clin*. 1999;15(2):235-249.
4. Larach MG. Accidental hypothermia. *Lancet*. 1995;345(8948):493-498.
5. Hardy JD. Physiology of temperature regulation. *Physiol Rev*. 1961;41:521-606.
6. Fischbeck KH, Simon RP. Neurological manifestations of accidental hypothermia. *Ann Neurol*. 1981;10(4):384-387.
7. Maaravi Y, Weiss AT. The effect of prolonged hypothermia on cardiac function in a young patient with accidental hypothermia. *Chest*. 1990;98(4):1019-1020.
8. Vassallo SU, et al. A prospective evaluation of the electrocardiographic manifestations of hypothermia. *Acad Emerg Med*. 1999;6(11):1121-1126.
9. Graham CA, McNaughton GW, Wyatt JP. The electrocardiogram in hypothermia. *Wilderness Environ Med*. 2001;12(4):232-235.
10. Granberg PO. Human physiology under cold exposure. *Arctic Med Res*. 1991;50(suppl 6):23-27.
11. Patt A, McCroskey BL, Moore EE. Hypothermia-induced coagulopathies in trauma. *Surg Clin North Am*. 1988;68(4):775-785.
12. Walpoth BH, et al. Accidental deep hypothermia with cardiopulmonary arrest: extracorporeal blood rewarming in 11 patients. *Eur J Cardiothorac Surg*. 1990;4(7):390-393.
13. Nordberg P, Ivert T, Dalén M, Forsberg S, Hedman A. Surviving two hours of ventricular fibrillation in accidental hypothermia. *Prehosp Emerg Care*. July-September 2014;18(3):446-449.
14. Lazar HL. The treatment of hypothermia. *N Engl J Med*. 1997;337(21):1545-1547.
15. Gilbert M, et al. Resuscitation from accidental hypothermia of 13.7 degrees C with circulatory arrest. *Lancet*. 2000;355(9201):375-376.
16. Hayward JS, Eckerson JD, Kemna D. Thermal and cardiovascular changes during three methods of resuscitation from mild hypothermia. *Resuscitation*. 1984;11(1-2):21-33.
17. van der Ploeg GJ, et al. Accidental hypothermia: rewarming treatments, complications and outcomes from one university medical centre. *Resuscitation*. 2010;81(11):1550-1555.
18. Grissom CK, et al. Spontaneous endogenous core temperature rewarming after cooling due to snow burial. *Wilderness Environ Med*. 2010;21(3):229-235.
19. McCauley RL, et al. Frostbite injuries: a rational approach based on the pathophysiology. *J Trauma*. 1983;23(2):143-147.
20. Heggers JP, et al. Experimental and clinical observations on frostbite. *Ann Emerg Med*. 1987;16(9):1056-1062.
21. Wrenn K. Immersion foot. A problem of the homeless in the 1990s. *Arch Intern Med*. 1991;151(4):785-788.
22. Golant A, et al. Cold exposure injuries to the extremities. *J Am Acad Orthop Surg*. 2008;16(12):704-715.
23. Edwards JC. The diagnosis and treatment of conditions of exposure; trench foot, immersion foot and frostbite. *Mo Med*. 1951;48(8):621-626.
24. Ramstead KD, Hughes RG, Webb AJ. Recent cases of trench foot. *Postgrad Med J*. 1980;56(662):879-883.
25. Roberts GT, et al. Microvascular injury, thrombosis, inflammation, and apoptosis in the pathogenesis of heatstroke: a study in baboon model. *Arterioscler Thromb Vasc Biol*. 2008;28(6):1130-1136.
26. Bouchama A, et al. Evidence for endothelial cell activation/injury in heatstroke. *Crit Care Med*. 1996;24(7):1173-1178.
27. Bouchama A, et al. Inflammatory, hemostatic, and clinical changes in a baboon experimental model for heatstroke. *J Appl Physiol*. 2005;98(2):697-705.
28. Hardy JD. *The physiology of temperature regulation. NADC MA United States Nav Air Dev Cen Johnsville Pa Aviat Med Accel Lab*. 1960;NADC-MA-6015:1-296.
29. Vandentorren S, et al. Mortality in 13 French cities during the August 2003 heat wave. *Am J Public Health*. 2004;94(9):1518-1520.
30. Olson KR, Benowitz NL. Environmental and drug-induced hyperthermia. Pathophysiology, recognition, and management. *Emerg Med Clin North Am*. 1984;2(3):459-474.
31. Epstein Y, et al. Exertional heat stroke: a case series. *Med Sci Sports Exerc*. 1999;31(2):224-228.
32. Ahmed A, Sadaniantz A. Metabolic and electrolyte abnormalities during heat exhaustion. *Postgrad Med J*. 1996;72(850):505-506.
33. Bouchama A, Knochel JP. Heat stroke. *N Engl J Med*. 2002;346(25):1978-1988.
34. Bouchama A. Features and outcomes of classic heat stroke. *Ann Intern Med*. 1999;130(7):613; author reply 614-5.
35. Smith JE. Cooling methods used in the treatment of exertional heat illness. *Br J Sports Med*. 2005;39(8):503-507; discussion 507.
36. Gaffin SL, Gardner JW, Flinn SD. Cooling methods for heatstroke victims. *Ann Intern Med*. 2000;132(8):678.
37. Sutton JR. Heatstroke from running. *JAMA*. 1980;243(19):1896.
38. Rrice K, Perron S, King N. Implementation of the Montreal heat response plan during the 2010 heat wave. *Can J Public Health*. February 11, 2013;104(2):e96-e100.
39. Lukins JL, Feldman MJ, Summers JA, Verbeek PR. A paramedic-staffed medical rehydration unit at a mass gathering. *Prehosp Emerg Care*. October-December 2004;8(4):411-416.
40. Richalet JP, Herry JP. *Medecine de l'alpinisme et des sports de montagne*. 4th ed. Paris, France: Masson; 2006:33-50.
41. Navitsky R, Macias D. Arterial oxygen saturation levels at moderate altitudes (abstract), Society of Academic Emergency Medicine Western Regional Conference; September 15, 1998; Newport Beach, CA.

42. Ward SA, Macias D, Whipp BJ. Is breath hold time an objective index of exertional dyspnea in humans? *Eur J Appl Physiol*. 2001;85:272-279.

43. Levine BD. VO2max: what do we need to know, and what do we still need to know? *J Physiol*. 2008;586:25-34.

44. Schoene RB. Illnesses at high altitude. *Chest*. 2008; 134:402-416.

45. Agostini P, Swenson ER, et al. High altitude exposure of three weeks duration increases lung diffusing capacity in humans. *J Appl Physiol*. 2011;110:1564-1571.

46. Semenza GL. HIF-1: mediator of physiological and pathophysiological responses to hypoxia. *J Appl Physiol*. 2000;88:1474-1480.

47. LaManna JC, Chavez JC, Pichiule P. Structural and functional adaptation to hypoxia in the rat brain. *J Exp Biol*. 2004;207:3163-3169.

48. Luks AM, McIntosh S, et al. Wilderness Medical Society consensus guidelines for the prevention and treatment of acute altitude illness. *Wilderness Environ Med*. 2010;21:146-155.

49. Basnyat B, Murdoch DR. High-altitude illness. *Lancet*. 2003;361: 1967-1974.

50. Bloch KE, Turk AJ, et al. Effect of ascent protocol on acute mountain sickness and success at Mustagh Ata, 7546m. *High Alt Med Biol*. 2009;10:25-32.

51. Macias DJ. Pathophysiology of high altitude illness. Lecture, University of New Mexico High Altitude Medicine Conference 2007; July 9, 2007; Chamonix, France.

52. Castellani JW, Muza SR, et al. Effect of hypohydration and altitude exposure on aerobic exercise performance and acute mountain sickness. *J Appl Physiol*. 2010;109:1792-1800.

53. Bird BA, Wright AD, et al. High altitude ataxia-its assessment and relevance. *Wilderness Environ Med*. 2011;22:172-176.

54. Basnyat B, Wu T, Gertsch JA. Neurological conditions at altitude that fall outside the usual definition of altitude sickness. *High Alt Med Biol*. 2004;5:171-179.

55. Gabry AL, Ledoux X, et al. High-altitude pulmonary edema at moderate altitude (< 2,400 m; 7,870 feet): a series of 52 patients. *Chest*. 2003;123;49-53.

56. Fagenholz PJ, Gutman JA, et al. Chest ultrasonography for the diagnosis and monitoring of high-altitude pulmonary edema. *Chest*. 2007; 131:1013-1018.

57. Allemann Y, Hutter D, Lipp E, et al. Patent foramen ovale and high-altitude pulmonary edema. *JAMA*. 2006;296:2954-2958.

58. Lawrence W. Raymond. Altitude pulmonary edema below 8,000 feet: what are we missing? *Chest*. 2003;123(1):5-7.

59. Basnyat B, Wu T, Gertsch JH. Neurological conditions at altitude that fall outside the usual definition of altitude sickness. *High Alt Med Biol*. 2004;5(2):171-179.

60. Leon-Velarde F, Villafuerte FC, Richalet JP. Chronic mountain sickness and the heart. *Prog Cardiovasc Dis*. 2010;52:540-549.

61. Penaloza D, Arias-Stella J. The heart and pulmonary circulation at high altitudes: healthy highlanders and chronic mountain sickness. *Circulation*. 2007;115:1132-1146.

62. Personal communication with Professor Osvaldo Paredes, Intensive Care Unit Director, Universidad Tecnologia Equinoccial, Quito, Ecuador. June 15, 2006.

63. Dehnert C, Bartsch P. Can patients with coronary heart disease go to high altitude? *High Alt Med Biol*. 2010;11:183-187.

64. Luks Am, Swenson ER. Travel to high altitudes with pre-existing lung disease. *Eur Respir J*. 2007;29:770-792.

65. Arnoldo BD, Purdue GF, Kowalske K, et al. Electrical injuries: a 20 year review. *J Burn Care Rehabil*. 2004;25:479-484.

66. Duff K, McCaffrey RJ. Electrical injury and lightning injury: a review of their mechanisms and neuropsychological, psychiatric and neurologic sequelae. *Neuropsychol Rev*. 2001;11:101-116.

67. Celik A, Ergun O, Ozok G. Pediatric electrical injuries; a review of 38 consecutive patients. *J Pediatr Surg*. 2004;39:1233-1237.

68. Maghsoudi H, Adyani Y, Ahmadian N. *J Burn Care Res*. 2007; 28:255-261.

69. Luz DP, Millan LS, Alessi MS, et al. Electrical burns: a retrospective analysis across a 5 year period. *Burns*. 2009;35:1015-1019.

70. Cancio LC, Jimenez-Reyna JF, Barillo D, et al. One hundred ninety five cases of high voltage electric injury. *J Burn Care Rehabil*. 2005: 331-340.

71. Koumbourlis AC. Electrical injuries. *Crit Care Med*. 2002;30: S424-S430.

72. Mofidi M, Kianmehr N, Farsi D, et al. An unusual case of bilateral anterior shoulder and mandible dislocations. *Am J Emerg Med*. 2010;28:745 e1-2.

73. Jain S, Bandi V. Electrical and lightning injuries. *Crit Care Clin*. 1999;15:319.

74. Schenk E, Wijetunge G, Mann NC, Lerner EB, Longthorne A, Dawson D. Epidemiology of mass casualty incidents in the United States. *Prehosp Emerg Care*. July-September 2014;18(3):408-416.

75. Zafren K, Durrer B, Herry JP, et al. Lightning injuries: prevention and on-site treatment in mountains and remote areas. Official guidelines of the International Commission for Mountain Emergency Medicine and the Medical Commission of the International Mountaineering and Climbing Federation (ICAR and UIAA MEDCOM). *Resuscitation*. 2005;65:369-372.

76. O'Keefe Gatewood M, Zane RD. Lightning Injuries. *Emerg Med Clin N Am*. 2004;22:369-403.

77. Cooper MA, Andrews CJ, Holle RJ, et al. Lightning injuries. In: Auerbach PS, ed. *Wilderness Medicine*. 5th ed. St Louis, MO: Mosby; 2007:67-108.

78. Rostain JC, Lavoute C, Risso JJ, et al. A review of recent neurochemical data on inert gas narcosis. *Undersea Hyperb Med*. 2011;38: 49-59.

79. Bennett PB, Marroni A, Cronje FJ, et al. Effect of varying deep stop times and shallow stop times on precordial bubbles after dives to 25 msw (82 fsw). *Undersea Hyperb Med*. 2007;34(6):399-406.

80. Diving and decompression. In: Brubakk AO, Neuman TS, eds. *Bennett and Elliott's Physiology and Medicine of Diving*. 5th ed. London: Saunders; 2003:17-600.

81. PADI. www.padi.com. Accessed August 20, 2011.

82. Parrish F, Pyle RL. Field comparison of open circuit scuba to closed circuit rebreathers for deep mixed gas diving operations. *Marine Tech Soc J*. 2002;36:13-20.

83. Personal communication with Peter Bennett, MD, St Lucia. October 3, 2004.

84. Wienke BR. Computer validation and statistical correlations of a modern decompression diving algorithm. *Comput Biol Med*. 2010;40: 252-260.

85. DeGorodo A, Vallejo-Manzur F, Chanin K, et al. Diving emergencies. *Resuscitation*. 2003;59:171-180.

86. Neuman TS, Jacoby I, Bove AA. Fatal pulmonary barotrauma due to obstruction of the central circulation with air. *J Emerg Med*. 1998;16:413-417.

87. Vann RD, Butler FK, Mitchell SJ, et al. Decompression illness. *Lancet*. 2010;377:153-164.

88. Blaivas M, Lyon M, Duggal S. A prospective comparison of supine chest radiography and bedside ultrasound for the diagnosis of traumatic pneumothorax. *Acad Emer Med*. 2005;12:844-849.

89. Nelson BP, Melnick ER, Li J. Portable ultrasound for remote environments part II: current indications. *J Emerg Med*. March 2011;40:313-321.

90. MacDonald RD, O'Donnel C, Allan GM, et al. Interfacility transport of patients with decompression illness: literature review and consensus statement. *Prehosp Emerg Care*. 2006;10:482-487.

91. Obad A, Marinovic J, Ljubkovic M, et al. Successive deep dives impair endothelial function and enhance oxidative stress in man. *Clin Physiol Funct Imaging*. 2010;30:432-438.

92. Ginsberg MD, et al. Temperature modulation of ischemic brain injury—a synthesis of recent advances. *Prog Brain Res*. 1993;96:13-22.

93. Melamed E, Glassberg E. [Non-freezing cold injury in soldiers]. *Harefuah*. 2002;141(12):1050-1054, 1090.

94. Cooper MA. A fifth mechanism of lightning injury. *Acad Emerg Med*. 2002;9:172-174.

95. Ritenour AE, Morton MJ, McManus JG, et al. Lightning injury: a review. *Burns.* 2008;34:585-594.

96. Cooper MA, Kotsos T, Gandhi MV, Neideen T. *Acute Autonomic and Cardiac Effects of Simulated Lightning Strike in Rodents.* Atlanta, GA: Society for Academic Emergency Medicine; 2001.

97. Soar J, Perkins GD, Abbas G, et al. European Resuscitation Council Guidelines for Resuscitation 2010 Section 8. Cardiac arrest in special circumstances: electrolyte abnormalities, poisoning, drowning, accidental hypothermia, hyperthermia, asthma, anaphylaxis, cardiac surgery, trauma, pregnancy, electrocution. *Resuscitation.* 2010;81:1400-1433.

98. Cherington M. Spectrum of neurologic complications of lightning injuries. *NeuroRehabilitation.* 2005;20:3-8.

99. Cohen MA. Clinical Pearls: struck by lightning. *Acad Emerg Med.* 2001;8:928-931.

100. Roeder WP, Cooper MA, Holle R, et al. Updated lightning recommendations for lightning safety—2002. *Bull Am Meteorological Soc.* 2003;84(2):261-266.

101. Thomas R. Towards evidence based emergency medicine: best BETs from the Manchester Royal Infirmary. Bet 1. Rhabdomyolysis and the use of sodium bicarbonate and/or mannitol. *Emerg Med J.* 2010;27:305-308.

102. Brown CV, Rhee P, Chan L, et al. Preventing renal failure in patients with rhabdomyolysis: do bicarbonate and mannitol make a difference? *J Trauma.* 2004;56:1191-1196.

103. Fish RM. Electrical injury: Part III: cardiac monitoring indications, the pregnant patient, and lightning. *J Emerg Med.* 2000;18:181-187.

104. Bailey B, Forget S, Gaudreault P. Prevalence of potential risk factors in victims of electrocution. *Forensic Sci Int.* 2001;123:58-62.

105. Carte AE, Anderson RB, Cooper MA. A large group of children struck by lightning. *Ann Emerg Med.* 2002;39:665-667.

106. Strauss M. Decompression illness. Lecture, Mountain and Marine Medicine Diving and Travel Medicine Series 2007; May 22, 2007; Bonaire, Netherlands Antilles.

107. Francis TJ, Mitchell SJ. Pathophysiology of decompression sickness. In: Bove A, ed. *Bove and Davis' Diving Medicine.* 4th ed. Philadelphia, PA: Saunders; 2004:165-174.

108. Answers to frequently asked questions. http://www.rebreather.com/RBFAQ.html. Accessed August 20, 2011.

109. NAUI Worldwide. www.naui.org. Accessed August 20, 2011.

110. Boyle R. A defence of the doctrine touching the spring and the weight of the air. In: *New Experiments Physio-Mechanical, Touching the Air.* Oxford, England: Oxford University Press; 1662:57.

111. Davies MJ, Fisher LH, Chegini S, et al. Asthma and the diver. *Clin Rev Allergy Imm.* 2005;29:131-138.

112. http://mostly-diving.co.uk/Diving/Info/NitroxCalc.htm. Accessed August 20, 2011.

113. Tetzlaff K, Shank ES, Muth CM. Evaluation and management of decompression illness-an intensivist's perspective. *Intensive Care Med.* 2003;29:2128-2136.

114. Saary MJ, Gray GW. A review of the relationship between patent foramen ovale and type II decompression sickness. *Aviat Space Environ Med.* 2001;72:1113-1120.

115. Germonpre P. Patent foramen ovale and diving. *Cardiol Clin.* 2005;23:97-104.

116. Freiburger JJ, Denoble PJ, Pieper CF, et al. The relative risk of decompression sickness during and after air travel following diving. *Aviat Space Environ Med.* 2002;73:980-984.

117. Allan GM, Kenny D. High altitude decompression illness: case report and discussion. *CMAJ.* 2003;169:803-807.

118. Navy Department. *Diving Medicine and Recompression Chamber Operations. NAVSEA 0910-LP-106-0957.* 6th rev ed. Washington, DC: Naval Sea SystemsCommand; 2008. *US Navy Diving Manual;* vol 5.

119. Shank ES, Muth CM. Case report on a diver with decompression injury, elevation of serum transaminases and rhabdomyolysis. *Ann Emerg Med.* 2001;37:533-536.

120. Longphre JM, Denoble PJ, Moon RE, et al. First aid normobaric oxygen for the treatment of recreational diving injuries. *Undersea Hyperb Med.* 2007;34:43-49.

121. Mitchell SJ, Pyle R, Moon RE. Therapy for decompression illness. In: Vann RD, Mitchell SJ, Denoble PJ, Anthony TG, eds. *Technical Diving Proceedings of the Diver's Alert Network 2008 January 18-19 Conference.* Durham, NC: Diver's Alert Network; 2009:178-203.

122. Blatteau JE, Pontier JM. Effect of in-water recompression with oxygen to 6 msw versus normobaric oxygen breathing on bubble formation in divers. *Eur J Appl Physiol.* 2009;106:691-695.

123. Mitchell SJ, Doolette DJ, Wachholz CJ, et al. *Management of Mild or Marginal Decompression Illness in Remote Locations.* Durham, NC: Diver's Alert Network; 2005

124. Weaver LK. Hyperbaric oxygen in the critically ill. *Crit Care Med.* 2011;39:1784-1791.

CHAPTER 48

Infectious Diseases and Bioterrorism

Russell D. MacDonald

INTRODUCTION

Prehospital personnel are usually the first health care personnel to encounter sudden illnesses or other health care emergencies in the community setting. Responding to these emergencies puts paramedic personnel at risk because the type, extent, and severity of this illness are not yet known. The Occupational Safety and Health Administration (OSHA) identifies there are more than 1.2 million community-based first-response personnel, including law enforcement, fire, and emergency medical service personnel, who are at risk for infectious exposure.[1] This large number highlights the need to protect these personnel against such exposures.

At one time, infectious disease and bioterrorism preparation were not a priority in some EMS agencies. Terrorism events such as the 1995 sarin gas attack on the Tokyo subway, the 2001 World Trade Center in New York City, the 2005 London Underground bombings, and the 2003 severe acute respiratory syndrome (SARS) outbreaks made preparedness a priority. This was especially true in Tokyo where first response personnel were not adequately prepared for acts of terrorism and were exposed to sarin gas,[2,3] and as emergency medical personnel responding to patients at the onset of the SARS outbreaks in Toronto[4] and Taipei[5] were exposed to or contracted SARS in significant numbers, and one paramedic died due to SARS. More importantly, in Toronto, the loss of paramedic availability for work due to exposure, illness, and quarantine impacted the ability to maintain staffing for many weeks during the outbreak.[6] These two examples highlight the need for EMS systems to adequately prepare and protect the workforce from potential exposure.

OBJECTIVES

- Describe the five types of infectious agents.
- Describe the seven modes of transmission of a contagious disease.
- Discuss the use of standard prehospital PPE and when additional PPE should be used (eg, respiratory).
- List common serious contagious and communicable diseases present in the prehospital environment.
- List appropriate immunizations for prehospital personnel.
- Describe how needlesticks and known exposures (HIV, hepatitis C, meningitis, TB) are managed.
- Discuss ways EMS agencies can help prevent, and respond to, certain epidemics (eg, influenza).
- List potential biological agents that may be released as an act of terrorism.
- Discuss how the approach to an MCI with a bioterrorism element changes the approach of EMS to the operations.
- Discuss stock-piling treatments for emergency responders and how to design a response plan to specific bioterrorism threats.

This chapter addresses communicable infectious disease and agents of terrorism in a manner relevant to EMS agencies and their personnel. The chapter is divided in three parts. The first is specific to infectious and communicable disease, describing the basics of communicable disease transmission and prevention, general approach to the patient with a suspected infectious or communicable disease, and specific disease conditions outlined by presenting complaint. The second is specific to agents of bioterrorism, and includes methods for detection and management of

those exposed. The second part also includes the fundamentals of decontamination. The third includes the EMS agency's role and planning for health care emergencies related to infectious disease, EMS interactions with public health agencies, and special considerations for EMS agencies in epidemics or pandemics.

Occupational health and safety is an important component of infection control and prevention of communicable disease in EMS. This includes aspects of routine EMS operations such as immunization of personnel, hand hygiene, personal protective equipment, sharps safety, and cleaning of equipment and disinfection. This is beyond the scope of this chapter and the reader should consult other resources dedicated to this subject.

INFECTIOUS AND COMMUNICABLE DISEASE

◾ TRANSMISSION AND PREVENTION

OSHA defines an occupational exposure as "a reasonably anticipated skin, eye, mucous membrane, or parenteral contact with blood or other potentially infectious material that may result from the performance of the employee's duties."[1] Infection control practices are designed to prevent exposure to blood or potentially infectious material, including cerebrospinal fluid, synovial fluid, pleural fluid, pericardial fluid, amniotic fluid, peritoneal fluid, and any other body fluid, secretion, or tissue.

Universal precautions is the term formerly used to describe aspects of the methods used to prevent exposure, but this term is no longer used by health care workers. The more favored terms are *routine practices* and *additional precautions*. These terms indicate the same basic, minimum level of precaution is taken for all patients.

The Association for Professionals in Infection Control and Epidemiology[7] defines *infection* as an invasion and multiplication of microorganisms in or on body tissue, causing cellular damage through the production of toxins, multiplication, or competition with host metabolism. Infectious agents capable of causing disease include bacteria, viruses, fungi and moulds, parasites, and prions. These five types of microorganisms can be differentiated by their appearance on microscopic examination, reproductive cycle, chemical structure, growth requirements and by other detailed criteria. While bacteria and viruses are the most common causes of illness in the developed world, parasites are more prevalent in other settings.

The ability of a microorganism to cause an infection is dependent on several factors. The *dose* is the amount if viable organism received during an exposure. Infection occurs when there is a large enough number to overwhelm the body's own defenses. *Virulence* refers to the ability of a microorganism to cause infection, and pathogenicity refers to the severity of infection. *Incubation* and *communicability period* are the intervals between when the organism enters the body and when symptoms appear, and the time during which the infected individual can spread the disease to others, respectively. The host status and resistance refer to the host's ability to fight infection, which can be influenced by immune function and immunization status, nutritional state, and presence of comorbid illness.

An *infectious* disease results from the invasion of a host by disease-producing organisms, such as bacteria, viruses, fungi, or parasites. A *communicable* (or contagious) disease is one that can be transmitted from one person to another. Not all infectious diseases are communicable. For example, malaria is a serious infectious disease transmitted to the human blood stream by a mosquito bite, but malaria is infectious, not communicable. On the other hand, chickenpox is an infectious disease which is also highly communicable because it can be easily transmitted from one person to another.

The mode of transmission is the mechanism by which an agent is transferred to the host. Modes of transmission include contact transmission (direct, indirect, droplet), airborne, vector-borne, or common vehicle (food, equipment). Contact transmission is the most common mode of transmission in the EMS setting, and can be effectively prevented using routine practices.

Direct contact transmission occurs when there is direct contact between infected or colonized individual and a susceptible host. Transmission may occur, for example, by biting, kissing, sexual contact. Indirect contact occurs by passive transfer of infectious agent to a susceptible host through a contaminated intermediate object such as contaminated hands, equipment, or surfaces are not washed between patient contacts. Examples of diseases transmitted by direct or indirect contact include human immunodeficiency virus (HIV), hepatitis, methicillin-resistant *Staphylococcus aureus* (MRSA), vancomycin-resistant enterococci (VRE), *Clostridium difficile*, and Norwalk virus.

Droplet transmission refers to large droplets generated from the respiratory tract of a patient when he/she coughs or sneezes, or during invasive airway procedures (intubation, suctioning). The droplets are propelled and can be deposited on the mucous membranes of the susceptible host. The droplets may also settle in the immediate environment and the infectious agents, remain viable for prolonged periods of time, and later transmitted by indirect contact. Examples of diseases transmitted by droplet transmission include meningitis, influenza, rhinovirus, respiratory syncytial virus (RSV), and SARS.

Airborne transmission is the spread of infectious agents to susceptible hosts by very small droplets containing the infectious agent. The droplets can remain suspended in the air for prolonged periods of time, disperse widely by air currents, and can be inhaled by susceptible host located at some distance from the source. Examples of diseases transmitted by airborne transmission include measles (rubeola), varicella (chicken pox), and tuberculosis.

Vector-borne transmission refers to the spread of infectious agents by an insect or animal (the "vector"). Examples of vector-borne illness include rabies, where the infected animal is the vector, and West Nile virus or malaria, where infected mosquitos are the vectors. Transmission or vector-borne illness does not occur between emergency personnel and their patients.

Common vehicle transmission refers to the spread of infectious agents by a single contaminated source to multiple hosts. This can result in large outbreaks of disease. Examples of this type of transmission include contaminated water sources (*E coli*), contaminated food (*Salmonella*), or contaminated medication, medical equipment, or IV solutions.

▓ IMMUNIZATIONS FOR EMS PROVIDERS

The Society of Healthcare Epidemiologists of America, Association for Professionals in Infection Control and Prevention, and the American Academy of Pediatrics support the mandatory vaccination of all health care workers and the routine screening for TB. Vaccinations commonly recommended include HBV (hepatitis B) vaccine, MMR, TDaP, chicken-pox vaccine, and the annual flu vaccine. The CDC published a *Morbidity and Mortality Weekly Report (MMWR)* on the topic on November 25, 2011, available on the Web site at http://www.cdc.gov/mmwr/preview/mmwrhtml/rr6007a1.htm.

▓ OCCUPATIONAL EXPOSURE OF PROVIDERS

Despite the use of reasonable practices it is possible to be exposed through various means to body fluids that may be sources for exposure to certain serious diseases. Adherence to OSHA standards requires development of an exposure control plan that contains the following elements: assessment of a provider exposure prone tasks and procedures, exposure control methods, HBV vaccination, postexposure evaluation and follow-up, hazard communication (including labeling, signs, bags, etc), information and training (initial and annual), record keeping, annual review of exposure plan and enforcement activities, maintenance of confidential provider medical records (for employment period plus 30 years), and training records. Providers have a right to immediate health care provider examination and management in cases of specific exposures and should be in compliance with the agency or employer policy. Providers should be trained on exposure prevention, as well as immediate postexposure self-care. Postexposure prophylaxis should be a component of the policy for providers with an exposure that warrants such care. Every agency should have an infection/exposure control officer and have a mechanism by which exposed providers are alerted to possible occult exposures (such as TB or meningitis) and provided with follow-up instructions.

GENERAL APPROACH AND PATIENT ASSESSMENT

The risk of communicable disease is not as apparent as other physical risks, such as road traffic, power lines, or firearms. Responding personnel must use the same level of suspicion and precaution when approaching a patient before the risk of communicable disease is known. The use of routine practices, as a minimum, is necessary for every patient encounter in order to mitigate this risk.

The risk assessment begins with information from an EMS dispatch or communication center, prior to making patient contact. Call-taking procedures must include basic screening information to identify potential communicable disease threats and provide this information to all responding personnel. The screening information can identify patients with symptoms of fever, chills, cough, shortness of breath, or diarrhea. The call taking can also identify if the patient location, such as nursing home, group home, or other institutional setting, poses a potential risk to the responding personnel. This information helps responding personnel determine what precautions are necessary before they make contact.

When patient contact is made, personnel can identify the patient at risk for a communicable disease. A rapid history and physical examination can raise suspicion for a communicable disease. The following screening questions help assess if the patient has a communicable disease:

- Do you have a new or worsening cough or shortness of breath?
- Do you have a fever?
- Have you had shakes or chills in the past 24 hours?
- Have you had an abnormal temperature (>38°C)?
- Have you taken medication for fever?

A screening physical examination will also identify obvious signs of a communicable disease. They may include any new symptom of infection (fever, headache, muscle ache, cough, sputum, weight loss, and exposure history), rash, diarrhea, skin lesions, or draining wounds.

All personnel must take appropriate precautions when a patient presents with any signs or symptoms suspected to be due to an infectious or communicable disease. All EMS and first responder agencies must provide appropriate training that enables personnel to identify at-risk patients and appropriate use of personal protective equipment (PPE).

SPECIFIC DISEASE CONDITIONS BY PRESENTING OR CHIEF COMPLAINT

This section will describe specific diseases grouped by common presenting complaints.

▓ RESPIRATORY INFECTIONS

Respiratory infections may be suspected when there are symptoms which classically include any combination of cough, sneeze, shortness of breath, fever, chills, or shakes. Infections above the epiglottis are classified as upper respiratory tract infections, while those below the epiglottis are classified as lower respiratory tract infections. Upper respiratory infections may be suspected when patients present with "cold" symptoms such as rhinorrhea, sneezing, lacrimation, or coryza. More localized and possibly more serious upper respiratory may present with symptoms such as throat pain, fever, odynophagia, dysphagia, drooling, stridor, or muffled voice. Lower respiratory infections typically present with any of fever, shortness of breath, pleural pain, cough, sputum, and generalized symptoms such as chills, rigors, myalgia, arthralgia, malaise, and headache. More atypical symptoms of respiratory infection may be found in children, the elderly, and the immunocompromised. Children with respiratory infection may present with gastrointestinal symptoms such as nausea, vomiting, abdominal pain, and diarrhea.[8,9] Elderly and the immunocompromised may not develop a fever in the presence of a respiratory infection.

Respiratory infections are spread when people cough or sneeze and the aerosolized respiratory secretions directly come in contact with the mouth, nose, or eyes of another person. As microorganisms in droplets can survive outside the body, indirect transmission can also occur when hands, objects, or surfaces become soiled with respiratory discharges. When respiratory infections are suspected in patients, EMS providers should use droplet precautions and apply them to a patient.

FEBRILE RESPIRATORY ILLNESS

Febrile respiratory illness should be suspected when a patient presents with any combination of fever, new or worse cough, and shortness of breath. It should be emphasized that the elderly and immunocompromised may not have a febrile response to a respiratory infection.

COUGH

PNEUMONIA

In addition to cough, shortness of breath, and fever, patients with pneumonia may also present with additional symptoms of tachypnea, increased work of breathing, chest or upper abdominal pain, cough productive of phlegm, sputum, or blood. Generalized systemic symptoms such as myalgia, arthralgia, malaise, and headache may also be present. Gastrointestinal symptoms such as nausea, vomiting, and diarrhea may be associated with pneumonia.[10]

The signs and symptoms traditionally associated with pneumonia are actually not predictive of pneumonia, whereas diarrhea, dry cough, and fever were more predictive of pneumonia. In elderly patients, the diagnosis of pneumonia is more difficult as both respiratory and nonrespiratory symptoms are less commonly reported by this patient group.[11]

Infectious agents that typically cause pneumonia include *Streptococcus pneumoniae, Mycoplasma pneumoniae, Chlamydia trachomatis, Chlamydia pneumoniae, Pneumocystis carinii, Haemophilus influenza.*[12] The incubation period from initial contact with the microorganism to development of symptoms is generally not well known for these organisms. For *Streptococcus pneumoniae,* it may be 1 to 3 days and *Mycoplasma pneumoniae* may range from 6 to 32 days. *Pneumocystis carinii* may appear 1 to 2 months after initial contact for those who are immunosuppressed. *Streptococcus pneumoniae* can be transmitted up to 48 hours after treatment is initiated. However, *Mycoplasma pneumoniae* can be transmissible for up to 20 days, and the organism may remain in the respiratory tract for up to 13 weeks posttreatment. The time period when transmissible is unknown for the other organisms listed.[13]

PERTUSSIS

Pertussis should be in the differential diagnosis of a patient presenting with chronic cough. Pertussis presents in three stages: first, a catarrhal stage lasting 1 to 2 weeks, followed by a paroxysmal stage lasting 1 to 6 weeks, and finally ending with a convalescent stage lasting 2 to 3 weeks. In the first stage, pertussis is virtually indistinguishable from any other respiratory illness, as it is characterized by runny nose, sneezing, low-grade fever, and a mild cough. The EMS provider may suspect pertussis in the second, paroxysmal, stage, when the patient has bursts of rapid coughs. The cough usually ends with a long high-pitched inspiratory effort described as a whoop, or it may end with vomiting. The third state is the period of recovery where the cough becomes less paroxysmal. In adolescents, adults, and the vaccinated, pertussis is milder and, hence, may be indistinguishable from other respiratory illnesses, even in the paroxysmal stage.

Pertussis is caused by the *Bordetella pertussis* bacterium and transmitted by the respiratory route with airborne droplets. Hence, respiratory and contact precautions should be undertaken with known or suspected

cases of pertussis. Unfortunately, routine precautions are not always sufficient because pertussis is most infectious during the nonspecific catarrhal period and the first 2 weeks of the paroxysmal phase. The time from infection to the development of symptoms is usually 7 to 10 days.[14]

Complications from pertussis most often occur in young infants. The major complication and most common cause of pertussis-related death is bacterial pneumonia. From 2001 to 2003, among the 56 pertussis-related deaths reported in the United States, 51 (96%) were among infants younger than 6 months of age.[15]

With the introduction of routine pertussis vaccination, pertussis had declined from about 140 cases per 100,000 population in the 1940s to about 1 per 100,000 population in the 1980s. However, since the 1980s pertussis rates have been steadily increasing. In 2002 in the United States, there were 3 cases per 100,000 population. The majority of cases were in children under 6 months of age, the age group most at risk of pertussis-related complications.[15]

Children in the United States are routinely vaccinated for pertussis in a four-dose schedule, starting at age 2 months. As these groups are often the source of infection in infants, an adolescent and adult vaccine was licensed in the United States in 2005. Pertussis is treated with macrolide antibiotics: erythromycin, clarithromycin, or azithromycin. Treatment ameliorates the illness and decreases the communicability period. Cases of pertussis treated with antibiotics should also be isolated for 5 days after antibiotic therapy has started to prevent further transmission. If exposed to a patient with pertussis, the contact should first assess their immunization status. In the event that the contact is nonimmunized, a 7-day course with macrolide antibiotics should be considered. Also, regardless of immunization status, if the contact is a child under age 1, a pregnant woman in the last 3 weeks of pregnancy, or if the person exposed has contact with infants or pregnant women in the last 3 weeks of pregnancy, macrolide antibiotic prophylaxis should be offered.[16]

INFLUENZA

Influenza classically presents with the abrupt onset of fever, usually 38 to 40°C, sore throat, nonproductive cough, myalgias, headache, and chills. Unfortunately, only about half of infected persons develop the "classic" symptoms of influenza infection.[17-19] Among those presenting with classic symptoms, studies have attempted to identify the signs and symptoms most predictive of influenza. Unfortunately, these clinical decision rules are no better than clinician judgment alone.[20]

Influenza is caused by a virus with three subtypes: influenza A, B, and C. Influenza A causes more severe disease and is mainly responsible for pandemics. Influenza A has different subtypes determined by surface antigens H (hemagglutinin) and N (neuraminidase). Influenza B causes more mild disease and mainly affects children. Influenza C rarely causes human illness and has not been associated with epidemics.[21]

Influenza transmission occurs primarily through airborne spread when a person coughs or sneezes, but may also occur through direct contact of surfaces contaminated with respiratory secretions. Hand-washing and shielding coughs and sneezes help prevent spread. Influenza is transmissible from 1 day before symptom onset to about 5 days after symptoms begin and may last up to 10 days in children. Time from infection to development of symptoms is 1 to 4 days.[22]

Influenza has been responsible for at least 31 pandemics in history. The most lethal "Spanish flu" pandemic of 1918 to 1919 is estimated to have caused 40 million deaths globally with 700,000 of those deaths occurring in the United States in a single year. In this pandemic, deaths occurred mainly in healthy 20 to 40 year olds, which differs from the usual young children and elderly pattern of mortality and morbidity in the seasonal outbreaks of influenza.

Individuals at high risk of influenza complications include young children, people over age 65, the immunosuppressed, and those suffering from chronic medical conditions. Complications of influenza include pneumonia, either the more common secondary bacterial pneumonia or rare primary influenza viral pneumonia; Reye syndrome in children taking aspirin; myocarditis, encephalitis, and death. Death occurs in about 1 per 1000 cases of influenza, mainly in persons older than age 65.

Studies estimate about 36,000 influenza-related deaths annually from 1990 to 1999 in the United States.[23]

Influenza vaccine is the principal means of preventing influenza morbidity and mortality. The vaccine changes yearly based on the antigenic and genetic composition of circulating strains of influenza A and B found in January to March, when influenza reaches its peak activity. When the vaccine strain is similar to the circulating strain, influenza vaccine is effective in protecting 70% to 90% of vaccinees younger than age 65 from illness. Among those aged 65 and older, the vaccine is 30% to 40% effective in preventing illness, 50% to 60% effective in preventing hospitalization, and up to 80% effective in preventing death. EMS providers should be immunized annually, typically in October.

Four antiviral drugs are available for preventing and treating influenza in the United States. Amantadine and rimantadine belong to a class of drugs adamantanes active against influenza A, and oseltamivir and zanamivir belong to the class of neuraminidase inhibitors active against influenza A and B. When used for prevention of influenza, they can be 70% to 90% effective in preventing influenza. When used for treatment, antivirals can reduce influenza illness duration by 1 day and attenuate the severity of illness. Antiviral agents should be used as an adjunct to vaccination, but should not replace vaccination. The CDC recommends influenza antivirals for individuals who have not as yet been vaccinated at the time of exposure, or who have a contraindication to vaccination, and are also at high risk of influenza complications. Also, if an influenza outbreak is caused by a variant strain of influenza not controlled by vaccination, chemoprophylaxis should be considered for health care providers caring for patients at high risk of influenza complications, regardless of their vaccination status. Since the 2005 to 2006 influenza season, a high proportion of influenza A viruses were resistant to the adamantanes. As a result, the CDC has recently recommended against the use of adamantanes for treatment and prophylaxis of influenza. The neuraminidase inhibitors continue to be recommended as a second line of defense against influenza. For prophylaxis, the neuraminidase inhibitors should be taken daily until the exposure exists or until immunity from vaccination develops, which can take about 2 weeks. For treatment, these antivirals should be started as soon as influenza symptoms develop, but no later than 48 hours after symptoms start, and treatment should continue for 5 days. In the setting of an influenza outbreak, EMS systems may opt to restrict duties for EMS providers who are not immunized or who have not yet received prophylactic antiviral therapy in attempt to prevent spread of the outbreak.[21]

AVIAN INFLUENZA H5N1

Influenza A virus infects humans and can also be found naturally in birds. Wild birds carry a type of influenza A virus, called avian influenza virus, in their intestines and usually do not get sick from them. However, avian influenza virus can make domesticated birds, including chickens, turkeys, and ducks, quite ill and lead to death. The avian influenza virus is chiefly found in birds, but infection in humans from contact with infected poultry has been reported since 1996. A particular subtype of avian influenza A virus, H5N1, is highly contagious and deadly among birds. In 1997 in Hong Kong, an outbreak of avian influenza H5N1 occurred not only in poultry, but also in 18 humans, 6 of whom died. In subsequent infections of avian influenza H5N1 in humans, more than half of those infected with the virus have died. In contrast to seasonal influenza, most cases of avian influenza H5N1 have occurred in young adults and healthy children that have come in contact with poultry infected, or surfaces contaminated with H5N1 virus. As of the end of 2007, there were 346 documented human infections with influenza H5N1 and 213 deaths (62%). Although transmission of avian influenza H5N1 from human to human is rare, inefficient, and unsustained, there is concern that the H5N1 virus could adapt and acquire the ability for sustained transmission in the human population. If the H5N1 virus could gain the ability to transmit easily from person to person, a global influenza pandemic could occur. No vaccine for H5N1 current exists, but vaccine development is underway. The H5N1 virus is resistant to the adamantanes, but likely sensitive to the neuraminidase inhibitors.[24]

SWINE INFLUENZA H1N1

In April 2009, the H1N1 influenza strain emerged and spread globally. It differed from prior influenza strains and the global population did not have a natural immunity to protect against this virus. While its overall burden of disease was not significantly higher than prior influenza strains, surveillance showed that it affected more young and healthy people than the regular seasonal flu. In June 2009, the World Health Organization (WHO) declared a pandemic, resulting in many national and subnational immunization programs directed targeting H1N1. In August 2011, WHO declared the pandemic over. Postpandemic strategies to limit impact of further outbreaks are focused on including the H1N1 strain in annual influenza vaccines, and careful monitoring and surveillance because the strain will likely continue to circulate in the population, along with other influenza strains, for several more years.

TUBERCULOSIS

Tuberculosis is caused by the *Mycobacterium tuberculosis* complex. The majority of active TB is pulmonary (70%), while the remainder is extrapulmonary (30%). Patients with active pulmonary TB will typically present with cough, scant amounts of nonpurulent sputum, and possibly hemoptysis. Systemic signs such as weight loss, loss of appetite, chills, night sweats, fever, and fatigue may also be present. Clinically, the EMS provider will be unable to distinguish pulmonary TB from other respiratory illness; however, certain risk factors may alert the EMS provider to the possibility of tuberculosis. These risk factors are immigration from a high-prevalence country, homelessness, exposure to active pulmonary TB, silicosis, HIV infection, chronic renal failure, cancer, transplantation, or any other immunosuppressed state.[25,26]

Active pulmonary TB is transmitted via droplet nuclei from people with pulmonary tuberculosis during coughing, sneezing, speaking, or singing. Procedures such as intubation or bronchoscopies are high risk for the transmission of TB. Respiratory secretions on a surface lose the potential for infection. About 21% to 23% of individuals in close contact with persons with infectious TB become infected through inhalation of aerosolized bacilli. The probability of infection is related to duration of exposure, distance from the case, concentration if bacilli in droplets, ventilation in the room, and the susceptibility of the host exposed. Effective medical therapy eliminates communicability within 2 to 4 weeks of starting treatment.[27]

If infected with TB, an individual may develop active TB with symptoms, or latent TB, which is asymptomatic. Time from infection to active symptoms or positive TB skin test is about 2 to 10 weeks. The risk of developing active TB is greatest in the first 2 years after infection. Latent TB may last a lifetime, with the risk that it may later progress to active TB. About 10% of patients with latent TB will progress to active TB in their lifetime.

If transporting a patient who is known or suspected of having TB, respiratory precautions should be undertaken by the EMS provider, in particular, a submicron mask. Patients should cover their mouth when coughing or sneezing, or wear a surgical mask. In the event of suspected exposure to a patient with active pulmonary tuberculosis, report the case and the exposure to the EMS system or public health authority. Close contacts should be monitored for the development of active TB symptoms. Two tuberculin skin tests should be performed, based on public health recommendations, on those closely exposed to patients with active TB.[28] Because the incubation period after contact ranges from 2 to 10 weeks, the first test is typically done as soon as possible after exposure, and the second test typically done 8 to 12 after the exposure. If the EMS provider or contact develops either active TB with symptoms or latent asymptomatic TB, as diagnosed with a new positive TB skin test, treatment should be sought.

Treatment for latent TB is typically isoniazid (INH) for 6 to 9 months.[28] This single-drug regimen is 65% to 80% effective. For active TB, a four-drug regimen is typically used for 2 months: isoniazid, rifampin, pyrazinamide, and ethambutol. This is followed by INH and rifampin for an additional 4 months. Several forms of multidrug-resistant (MDR)-TB and extensively drug-resistant (XDR)-TB have been identified.[29] These forms require aggressive, multidrug regimen for prolonged periods of time and are dependent on the organism's patterns of drug sensitivity and resistance. In all cases, a physician skilled in management of TB must initiate and monitor treatment and provide suitable follow-up. Public health officials must also be notified.[30]

SARS

It is difficult to distinguish SARS from other respiratory infections because patients present with symptoms similar to other febrile respiratory illnesses.[31] On initial presentation, reliance on respiratory symptoms alone is not sufficient to distinguish SARS from non-SARS respiratory illness.[32] Fever is the most common and earliest symptom of SARS often accompanied by headache, malaise, or myalgia.[33] In patients with SARS, high fever, diarrhea, and vomiting were more common as compared to other patients with other respiratory illnesses.[34] Cough occurred later in the course of disease and patients were less likely to have rhinorrhea or sore throat as compared to other lower respiratory tract illness.[35] Since clinical features alone cannot reliably distinguish SARS from other respiratory illnesses, knowledge of contacts is essential.[36] Contact with known SARS patients, contact with SARS-affected areas or linkage to a cluster of pneumonia cases should be obtained in the history.[37]

SARS was first recognized in 2003 after outbreaks occurred in Toronto (Canada),[38] Singapore, Vietnam, Taiwan, and China. The illness is caused by a coronavirus. The incubation period ranges from 3 to 10 days, averaging 4 to 5 days from contact to symptom onset. About 11% of those who develop SARS eventually die, usually due to respiratory failure. The risk of mortality is highly dependent on the patient's age and presence of comorbid illnesses. The case fatality is less than 1% for SARS patients less than age 24 and up to 50% for those age 65 and greater or those with comorbid illness.[39]

The coronavirus is found in respiratory secretions, urine, and fecal matter. Transmission is via droplet spread from respiratory secretions, with high risk transmission during intubation and procedures which aerosolize respiratory secretions. Transmission can also occur from fecal or urine contamination of surfaces. There have been no confirmed cases of transmission from asymptomatic cases. Preliminary studies show that transmission likely occurs after the development of symptoms with peak infectious period being 7 to 10 days after symptom onset, and declining to a low level after day 23 from onset of symptoms.[40]

If SARS is suspected, EMS providers must use all routine practices and additional precautions.[41] EMS systems may also elect to limit or avoid any procedures that may increase risk to EMS personnel. These include tracheal intubation, deep suctioning, use of noninvasive ventilatory support (CPAP, BiPAP), administration of nebulized medication, and any other procedure that may aerosolize respiratory secretions. During the SARS outbreaks in Toronto, EMS medical direction modified medical directives such that paramedics did not intubate patients or deliver nebulized therapy in the prehospital setting.[42] Finally, EMS personnel and systems must also notify the receiving facility of a patient suspected of SARS, permitting staff to have appropriate PPE in place and a suitable isolation room prepared for the patient.[43,44]

RASH

MRSA

Skin infections with onset in the community or hospital may be caused by *Staphylococcus aureus*. *Staphylococcus aureus* is a bacterium that normally secretes β-lactamases rendering them normally resistant to antibiotics such as ampicillin and amoxicillin. Methicillin, a type of β-lactam antibiotic, developed in 1959, was not broken down by these bacterial β-lactamase enzymes. However, in the 1960s, infections of Staphylococcus aureus were found to be resistant to methicillin and other β-lactam antibiotics, resulting in the emergence of methicillin-resistant *Staphylococcal aureus*.[45]

In addition to common skin and soft tissue infections, MRSA may less commonly cause severe and invasive infections such as necrotizing pneumonia, sepsis, and musculoskeletal infections such as osteomyelitis and necrotizing fasciitis. MRSA skin infections typically present as necrotic skin lesions, and are often confused with spider bites. The severity of MRSA skin infections may range from mild to severe. Unfortunately, there are no reliable clinical or risk factor criteria to distinguish MRSA skin and soft tissue infections from those caused by other infectious agents.[46]

Initially, MRSA infections were found in patients in health care facilities (health care–associated MRSA or HA-MRSA). However, community-acquired MRSA (CA-MRSA) infections are increasingly identified in people who did not have the traditional risk factors of those with HA-MRSA, specifically contact with health care facilities. These community-acquired strains are new MRSA strains, different from those which cause HA-MRSA. Regardless, both HA-MRSA and CA-MRSA can mimic infections caused by less-resistant bacteria, but are more difficult to treat.[47]

Transmission of MRSA is mainly through hand contact from infected skin lesions, such as abscesses or boils. About 1% of the healthy population is also colonized with MRSA, mainly in the anterior nares, but also in the pharynx, axilla, rectum, and perineum. Therefore, autoinfection may also be a route of infection. The transmissible period lasts as long as skin lesions continue to drain or as long as the carrier state remains. Newborns, the elderly, and the immunosuppressed are most susceptible.

Transmission of infection is prevented by routine precautions. Draining wounds should be covered with clean, dry, bandages. Contaminated surfaces should be cleaned with disinfectants effective against *Staphylococcus aureus*, such as a solution of dilute bleach or quaternary ammonium compounds. One study has showed that EMS ambulances may have significant degree of MRSA contamination, highlighting the need for proper cleaning and decontamination of all equipment and the vehicle itself after every patient transport.[48]

There are no data to support the routine use of decolonization of MRSA with antiseptic agents or nasal mupirocin. Decolonization may be considered in select circumstances, when a person has multiple recurrent infections of MRSA, or there is ongoing transmission in a well-defined group of close contacts. Little data are available on effective decolonization agents, but topical chlorhexidine gluconate or diluted bleach (3.4 g of bleach diluted in 3.8 L of water) is suggested.[49]

In those with skin or soft tissue infections, any drainage should be cultured. Abscesses should be incised and drained. Antibiotic therapy may be considered if there are signs of cellulitis, systemic illness, associated immunosuppression, extremes of age, facial infection, or failure of initial incision and drainage. The choice of therapy should be dictated by local susceptibility patterns. Clindamycin, doxycycline, and trimethoprim-sulfamethoxazole (TMP-SMX) are considerations for treatment of CA-MRSA skin and soft-tissue infections. HA-MRSA may be resistant to many more classes of antibiotics, and vancomycin or linezolid may be necessary.[50]

MEASLES

Measles is a viral disease which initially presents with a 2- to 4-day prodrome of fever, cough, runny nose, and possibly conjunctivitis. In the prodrome stage, the EMS provider will be unable to clinically distinguish measles from any other viral upper respiratory illness. A measles rash follows, beginning on the hairline, then involving the face and neck, and over 3 days, proceeding downward and outward to the hands and feet. The rash produces discrete red maculopapular (flat and raised) lesions initially, which may become confluent. Initially, the lesions blanch, and after 3 to 4 days become nonblanchable spots, which appear within 1 to 2 days before or after the maculopapular rash. Koplik spots, punctuate blue-white spots on the red buccal mucosa of the mouth, are pathognomonic for measles and would alert the EMS provider to the presence of measles.[51,52]

Measles has a 0.2% mortality rate, mainly due to pneumonia in children in developing countries. Cases of measles have declined dramatically since the introduction of live attenuated virus vaccine in 1963, with a record low of 34 cases in 2004. Sporadic outbreaks occur in populations that refuse vaccination. Children in the United States are routinely vaccinated with two doses of measles vaccine (MMR) at ages 12 to 15 months and ages 4 to 6 years.

Measles is transmitted by aerosol or droplet spread and is communicable from 4 days prior to appearance of the rash to 4 days after rash appearance. EMS providers will likely encounter the patient in the transmissible stage, and should use routine practices to prevent spread of disease.

The incubation period is approximately 10 days. Those who have not been immunized or have never acquired measles (born after 1957) are susceptible to infection if exposed. If susceptible and exposed, immunoglobulin should be given to children under age 1, pregnant women, and the immunocompromised within 6 days of exposure. For other susceptible persons, live measles vaccine may prevent disease if given within 72 hours of exposure. There is no treatment for measles, but vitamin A supplementation should be considered to prevent ocular complications.[53,54]

▓ RUBELLA

Rubella is a viral disease with a prodrome that precedes rash. Clinical diagnosis alone is unreliable. The prodrome, consisting of consists of fever, upper respiratory symptoms, and prominent lymphadenopathy, lasts 1 to 5 days and mostly present in older children and adults. During the prodrome, rubella is clinically indistinguishable from any other viral URTI. A maculopapular rash 14 to 17 days after exposure and lasting 3 days, typically follows the prodrome. Like measles, the rash starts on the face and progresses downward. In contrast to a measles rash, the rash due to rubella is fainter, does not coalesce, and is more prominent after a hot shower or bath. Associated symptoms may include arthralgias or conjunctivitis. Confirmation of rubella infection is by laboratory diagnosis of virus or antibody.[55]

Rubella is transmitted from respiratory secretions via airborne transmission or droplet spread, with an incubation period of 14 to 17 days. Even though rubella is most contagious when the rash is present, it may be transmitted by subclinical or asymptomatic cases of rubella, and 7 days before the onset of rash.

Life-threatening complications of rubella include encephalitis and hemorrhagic, but these are uncommon. The main objective of immunization is to prevent congenital rubella syndrome (CRS), the main complication of rubella. CRS occurs when a pregnant woman in early gestation, mainly in the first trimester, is exposed to rubella. CRS may lead to fetal death, premature delivery, and congenital defects including deafness, ocular, cardiac, and neurologic abnormalities.

There is no specific treatment of rubella, only preventative vaccination. Rubella immunization is part of the routine childhood vaccinations, administered as a live vaccine along with measles and mumps as "MMR." It is typically given at 12 months of age, and ages 4 to 6 years. Infants born to rubella immune mothers are protected for 6 to 9 months from transplacental maternal antibodies.[56]

If exposed to patients later diagnosed with rubella, immunity of the contact should be assessed. Subsequent immunization of the nonimmunized contact would not prevent infection or illness. In adults, rubella is generally a mild febrile disease, and control measures are aimed, preventing spread to nonimmunized pregnant women. In the case of spread, patients suspected of having rubella should be isolated with routine precautions in place. Pregnant women contacts should be investigated for immunity. In case of infection with rubella in nonimmune pregnant women in early pregnancy, counseling should be provided with consideration for abortion. Immunoglobulin in early pregnancy may also be given to modify or suppress symptoms, but there have been cases of CRS in spite of immunoglobulin therapy.[57-59]

▓ VARICELLA

Like measles and rubella, varicella starts with a prodrome which subsequently leads to a rash. In children, the prodrome of fever and malaise may be absent. Unlike measles and rubella, varicella infection, chickenpox, can be clinically diagnosed by the EMS provider based on a more pathognomonic rash. The pruritic rash progresses from macules to papules and then to vesicles which later crust over. The vesicles are unilocular and collapsible, in contrast to the multilocular and noncollapsible vesicles of smallpox. Lesions start on the scalp, progress to the trunk, and later move to the extremities.[60]

Varicella virus infection leading to chickenpox typically lasts 3 to 4 days, with an incubation period of 14 to 16 days. Transmission is by airborne droplets from the respiratory tract or by inhalation of aerosolized vesicular fluid from skin lesions. Chickenpox is transmissible 1 to 2 days before the onset of rash until all papules become crusted.[61]

Complications in children include secondary bacterial skin infections, pneumonia, and dehydration. Nonimmunized adults may have more severe complications, including encephalitis, transverse myelitis, hemorrhagic varicella, and even death. In the United States, only 5% of the reported cases of varicella are from adults, while 35% of the mortality occurs in adults. The case-fatality rate is 1 per 100,000 cases in children aged 1 to 14, but 25.2 per 100,000 cases in adults aged 30 to 49 years of age.

Maternal varicella 5 days before to 48 hours after delivery may result in neonatal infection and subsequent mortality as high as 30%. Varicella infection in the mother at 20 weeks of gestation can lead to congenital varicella syndrome, which includes skin scarring, extremity atrophy, and eye and neurologic abnormalities.

Since the licensure of varicella vaccine in 1995 in the United States, cases of chickenpox have declined from 83% to 94% by 2004. Varicella vaccine is recommended for all children without contraindication at 12 to 18 months of age, and is administered as one dose. Adults and adolescents age 13 years and older who do not have evidence of immunity should receive two doses of varicella vaccine.

Cases of chickenpox should be excluded from public places until the vesicles become dry. In the hospital, strict isolation measures should be undertaken to avoid contact with susceptible immunocompromised persons. Articles soiled by discharges from the nose and throat should be disinfected.

If exposed to chickenpox, contacts should assess their susceptibility based on their immune status. If previously infected or vaccinated, contacts are immune. Susceptible nonimmune contacts have three choices to prevent infection: vaccination, varicella zoster immunoglobulin, or antiviral drugs. Varicella vaccine can prevent illness or attenuate severity if used within 3 days of contact. Vaccine is recommended in susceptible individuals. Varicella zoster immunoglobulin (VZIG) is recommended for newborns, the immunocompromised, and pregnant women and can also modify severity or prevent illness if given within 96 hours of exposure. Antiviral drugs such as acyclovir, if used within 24 hours of onset of rash, can reduce the severity of disease. These are not recommended for routine postexposure prophylaxis, but can be considered in persons aged >13 years, and the immunocompromised.[62,63]

BITES

Bites require treatment for the physical injury itself, and treatment for the infectious disease exposure due to the bite. Infection rates from bites mainly depend on the animal which has caused the bite and the site of injury.[64] Cat bites can have an infection rate of up to 50%, while about 10% of dog bites become infected. Bites on the face, scalp, hand, wrist, foot, or joints have the highest rate of infection. Hands are the most common site of human, dog, and cat bites. Bite infections may cause cellulitis, osteomyelitis, abscess, septic arthritis, or even septicemia. In addition to antibiotic therapy, bites may also require treatment with rabies prophylaxis, tetanus prophylaxis, HIV, and hepatitis B prophylaxis. Prophylactic antibiotic treatment for bites depends on the specific infectious agents most commonly associated with the particular animal. Finally, EMS personnel should also be aware of the risk of transmission of hepatitis C due to human bites.[65]

▓ ANIMAL BITES

Bites by dogs and cats account for the vast majority of animal bites. In up to 75% of infected cat bites and 50% of infected dog bites, the causal infectious agent is *Pasteurella* species. This bacterium can produce an infection in as short as 12 hours. *Pasteurella canis* is most common organism in infected dog bites, while *Pasteurella multocida* is most common in cat bites. Other common organisms from infected cat and dog bites include *Streptococci, Staphylococci, Fusobacterium,* and *Bacterioides*.[64]

Preventing infection due to bites should begin with copious high-pressure irrigation with sterile saline solution. Prophylactic antibiotics are advised for hand bites from cats or dogs, and high-risk bites including any cat bite, deep dog bite punctures, and bites in immunocompromised individuals. Amoxicillin-clavulanic acid or cefuroxime, each for 5 days provides appropriate broad-spectrum activity. In penicillin-allergic patients, either azithromycin alone or clindamycin with levofloxacin can be given.[66,67]

HUMAN BITES

After dog and cat bites, humans are the next most common cause of bites. *Streptococci* species and *Eikenella corrodens* are the most common pathogens in infected human bites. Clenched-fist injuries, resulting from a flexed knuckle of a fist striking human teeth, are common and serious causes of human bite injuries. This type of injury often leads to serious deep infections because the patient usually offers an alternative mechanism for the hand injury, resulting in delayed antibiotic therapy. Human bites can also transmit HIV and hepatitis B and hepatitis C.[68]

Prophylactic antibiotics should be provided for all human bites that penetrate deeper than the epidermal layer, as well as bites to the hands, feet, or skin overlying joints or cartilaginous structures. Amoxicillin-clavulanic acid for 5 days is recommended as prophylactic therapy for human bites. In penicillin-allergic patients, a combination of clindamycin and a fluoroquinolone is a suggested regimen. Postexposure prophylaxis for HIV and hepatitis B should be considered for human bites according to a risk evaluation of the source. Patients should also be educated on the risk of transmission of hepatitis C.[69]

RABIES

Rabies is caused by rabies virus, a rhabdovirus of the genus *Lyssavirus* and may be transmitted by an animal bite. There is no treatment for rabies once it develops, and it has a mortality rate approaching 100%. The time from infection to development of disease is usually 3 to 8 weeks, and death is typically due to respiratory paralysis. To determine the risk of rabies transmission, knowledge is needed on the type of animal inflicting the bite, geographic location of the incident, the vaccination status of the animal and person, whether the bite was provoked or unprovoked, and whether the animal can be captured and tested.[70]

Patients receiving bites by animals suspected of having rabies should be given postexposure prophylaxis. For nonimmune individuals, prophylaxis consists of one dose of human rabies immunoglobulin, half given into the bite site, accompanied by a five-dose series of rabies vaccine on days 0, 3, 7, 14, and 28. Postexposure prophylaxis should always occur in consultation with local public health officials.[71]

In the United States in 2006, of all cases of rabies due to animal bites, 92% were related to wild animals and 8% to domestic animals. Among wild animals, rabies was most frequently found in raccoons, followed by bats, skunks, and foxes. Among domestic animals, cats were the most common cause of rabies, followed by dogs and cattle. Squirrels, guinea pigs, hamsters, chipmunks, gerbils, mice, rats, rabbits, and hares very rarely have rabies. In the United States, there have been two to three cases of human rabies each year for the last 10 years. Most were due to contact with bats, likely because bites from bats are superficial and not easily noticed. In the United States, Canada, and Western Europe, dogs account for less than 5% of animal rabies while in most developing countries, dogs account for more than 90% of cases of animal rabies.

Rabies immunization is not routinely recommended for the general population in North America, unless the person is engaged in activities that place them at high risk of acquiring rabies. These include rabies lab workers and veterinarians. Most agencies recommend that domestic dogs, cats, ferrets, and livestock be vaccinated against rabies. Routine rabies immunization for EMS personnel is not recommended.

Abnormal behavior in an animal or an unprovoked bite is more likely to indicate that a bite was from a rabid animal. This increases the risk of rabies transmission and postexposure prophylaxis should be offered. If a dog, cat, or ferret that caused a bite can be captured, it should be confined and observed for 10 days for the development of rabies symptoms. If rabies develops, the bitten individual should receive rabies postexposure prophylaxis. For any bites with bats, raccoons, skunks, or foxes, postexposure prophylaxis should be offered regardless of whether the animal is captured or not.[72,73]

TETANUS

Bites are at risk of being infected with *Clostridium tetani* because they are puncture wounds and/or contaminated with saliva. Live *Clostridium tetani* organisms are not present in the oral flora or humans or animals, but their resilient spores are ubiquitous and in the environment, soil, and feces. Crushed, devitalized tissue produced by bites favor the production of tetanus.[74,75]

Tetanus is an often fatal disease caused by the exotoxin of *Clostridium tetani*. The incubation period ranges from 3 to 21 days, during which time the spores transform into live bacteria which then produces an exotoxin. Clinically, the exotoxin leads to convulsive spasms of the skeletal muscles and generalized rigidity, mainly involving the jaw and neck. Patients with any form of bites should receive prophylaxis with 0.5 mL of tetanus toxoid intramuscularly if they have not received a booster immunization within the prior 5 years. Those who have not completed immunization series are not up to date with the immunization, or have an unknown immunization history should also receive tetanus immunoglobulin.[76]

ALTERED MENTAL STATUS, NECK STIFFNESS, HEADACHE

Meningitis refers to inflammation of the meninges covering the brain. It can be caused by infectious and noninfectious causes. Noninfectious causes include drugs, vaccines, systemic disease such as collagen vascular disorders, and malignancy. Infectious causes include viruses, bacteria, fungi, parasites, and rickettsiae.[77]

Meningitis is typically classified as bacterial meningitis versus aseptic meningitis. Aseptic meningitis refers to meningitis with cerebrospinal fluid absent of microorganisms on gram stain and/or routine culture. The most common cause of aseptic meningitis is viral agents.[78,79] Viral meningitis is generally more common, less severe, and requires supportive measures with no specific treatment. Bacterial meningitis, on the other hand, has a case-fatality rate of 13% to 37%, and as high as 80% in the elderly, despite appropriate antibiotic therapy. In addition, up to 20% of survivors of bacterial meningitis have permanent sequelae such as brain damage, hearing loss, or limb loss.[80,81]

Bacterial meningitis should be suspected when the patient presents with at least two of the four following symptoms: headache, fever, neck stiffness, or altered mental status. However, the EMS provider should be aware that only one of these symptoms may be present in the patient with bacterial meningitis.[82] Focal neurological symptoms such as extremity pain or temperature changes may be early signs. While a petechial rash is classically associated with bacterial meningitis, only 11% to 23% of patients with bacterial meningitis actually have a rash.[83] In the absence of diagnostic tests such as lumbar puncture, EMS personnel are unable to use clinical signs and symptoms alone to distinguish bacterial from aseptic meningitis.[84-86] Considering the rapid onset of symptoms and high morbidity and mortality with untreated bacterial meningitis, all patients with suspected meningitis should be treated as bacterial meningitis until proven otherwise.

Neisseria meningitidis and *Streptococcus pneumoniae* currently account for 80% to 85% of adult community-acquired meningitis. *Haemophilus influenzae* type b was formerly a leading cause of meningitis, but introduction of routine childhood vaccination is making this bacterium less prevalent. Less common causes include staphylococci, group B streptococci, and *Listeria*. *Streptococcus pneumoniae* is a more common cause of meningitis and mortality is also higher (30%) as compared to the mortality rate of (7%) meningitis caused by *Neisseria meningitides*. Since the introduction of routine childhood vaccination with *Haemophilus influenzae* type b, this is no longer a leading cause of meningitis.[87-89]

Transmission is by droplet spread from respiratory secretions. Therefore, respiratory and contact precautions should be undertaken when transporting patients suspected of meningitis. The time from transmission to the development of symptoms is about 2 to 10 days for *Neisseria meningitidis* and about 1 to 4 days for *Streptococcus pneumoniae*.

Empiric treatment of adult bacterial meningitis is vancomycin plus a third-generation cephalosporin, such as cefotaxime. In neonates, those over age 50, and those with altered immune status or alcoholism, ampicillin is added to cover *Listeria monocytogenes*. Treatment may last 14 -21 days depending on the infectious agent. In addition to treating the patient, EMS personnel exposed or in close contact to patients with meningitis may require prophylactic therapy. This is particularly important for personnel exposed to the patient's oral or respiratory secretions. Exposed personnel should contact their EMS agency or local public health agency immediately. Public health will likely provide prophylactic treatment with ciprofloxacin, ceftriaxone, or rifampin to prevent infection due to close contact.[90]

DIARRHEA

Diarrhea is practically defined by increased frequency, increased volume, and decreased consistency of stools. A strict definition is greater than three stools in a 24-hour period, with the stools being liquid enough to adopt the shape of the container in which they are placed. Acute diarrhea lasts 2 to 3 weeks, with chronic diarrhea lasting longer. Infectious diarrhea is commonly associated with nausea, vomiting, fever, abdominal cramps, and intestinal gas-related complaints. Diarrhea may be infectious or noninfectious in origin and the provider should attempt to rule out noninfectious causes, as most noninfectious causes are true diarrheal emergencies (mesenteric ischemia, GI bleed, bowel obstruction).

Infectious diarrhea may be caused by viruses, bacteria, protozoa, or helminthes. The diarrhea may be caused by the organisms themselves or the toxins they produce. Gastrointestinal infections are typically spread by contaminated water, contaminated food, contaminated environments, direct contact among humans, and hand-to-mouth transmission. The differential diagnosis can be narrowed by selectively testing stool specimens for bacterial culture, ova, parasites, *Clostridium difficile* toxin, and viral ELISA tests. These tests are not available in the prehospital setting, but history may identify prior testing results and the likely offending agent.[91,92]

To prevent spread of infection, EMS providers and systems must ensure routine practices and additional precautions are in place. In addition, equipment and transport vehicles must be thoroughly cleaned and decontaminated when transport involves a patient suspected of having infectious diarrhea.

Therapy that can be initiated by EMS providers includes isotonic fluid replacement and management of hypovolemia and sepsis. Antibiotic therapy and antimotility therapy should only be considered once a thorough assessment has been conducted in the hospital setting, as there are certain diarrheal conditions where such therapy may be inappropriate.

Acute infectious diarrhea may be bloody or watery, with bloody diarrhea signifying inflammatory destruction of the intestinal mucosa. Whether the diarrhea is watery or bloody provides clues as to the cause of the diarrhea, and the consequent sequelae: in watery diarrhea, the main concern is dehydration, while in bloody diarrhea, the main concern intestinal damage and sepsis.[91]

The most common causes of diarrhea are viruses, accounting for 50% to 75% of cases. As compared to bacterial diarrhea, viral diarrhea typically has less high fever, watery stools, whereas bacterial diarrhea typically has bloody stools with less severe abdominal pain. Among the viral causes of diarrhea, rotavirus[93] and the noroviruses[94] (Norwalk and Norwalk-like viruses) account for 50% of viral gastroenteritis. Adenoviruses are the second most common cause of acute viral gastroenteritis. Rotavirus diarrhea is most common cause of viral diarrhea in children and usually occurs in children between 6 and 24 months of age, as most individuals have antibodies by age 3. History and physical examination alone cannot clinically distinguish rotavirus from other enteric viral infections, as rotavirus infection presents with watery diarrhea, vomiting, fever, and abdominal pain. It usually diagnosed from rotavirus antigen in stools. In addition to transmission by the contact and the fecal-oral route, respiratory spread may also occur with rotavirus. The incubation period is 24 to 72 hours, with the period of communicability being up to 8 days from the start of the watery diarrhea. Two rotavirus vaccines are available for children, Rotarix and RotaTeq; RotaTeq is licensed for use in the United States. In 1999, RotaShield was withdrawn from the market after being associated with intussusception.

Diarrhea by norovirus causes signs and symptoms clinically indistinguishable from rotavirus: nausea, vomiting, diarrhea, and abdominal pain also occur with norovirus infection. In children, vomiting is more prevalent, whereas in adults, diarrhea is more common. Diagnosis is made by nucleic acid hybridization assays and RT-PCR. The incubation period is 12 to 48 hours and illness lasts for a shorter time than rotavirus diarrhea, 12 hours to 3 days. The period of communicability is unknown, lasting up to 7 days. Transmission routes are similar to rotavirus, including airborne transmission. There is currently no vaccine for norovirus infections.[95]

Bacterial diarrhea typically includes bloody diarrhea, as opposed to watery diarrhea; however, not all bacterial diarrhea is bloody. Bloody diarrhea is often referred to as dysentery. It is important to note that bloody diarrhea may not necessarily be due to infectious causes, and other causes of bloody diarrhea should be considered, such as mesenteric ischemia or a gastrointestinal bleeding. Common causes of bacterial diarrhea are *Salmonella, Shigella, Yersinia, E coli, Campylobacter*.[96,97]

E coli are classified by their O, H, and K antigens and also by their virulence properties.[98] *E coli* 0157:H7 is main serotype that causes bloody diarrhea through secretion of a potent Shiga-like cytotoxin. This serotype was responsible for a large outbreak of bloody diarrhea in the United States in 1982. This bloody diarrhea is notable for the absence of fever, and the subsequent 5% to 15% rate of development of hemolytic uremic syndrome (HUS), manifesting as pallor, jaundice, scleral icterus, dark urine, purpura, mucosal bleeding, dyspnea, and chest pain. The death rate of infections that lead to HUS is 3% to 5% even with ICU treatment. *E coli* 0157:H7 is found in healthy cattle and is spread to humans from undercooked beef, raw milk, and produce. The incubation period is typically 3 to 4 days and period of communicability can be up to 3 weeks in children. Antibiotics and antimotility agents are not recommended for this infection. Treatment is directed at HUS, which may require dialysis, steroids, or plasma therapy in the ICU setting.

Clostridium difficile is a bacterium that can cause a spectrum of mild watery diarrhea to severe colitis, which may progress to perforation of the colon and sepsis.[99-101] This infection is increasing in prevalence and frequently associated with health care settings.[100] More than 90% occur after or during antibiotic therapy. *C difficile* is also one of the most common cause of bacterial diarrhea in persons with HIV in the United States. The EMS provider may only suspect *C difficile*–associated diarrhea based on the risk factors, as it is clinically indistinguishable from any other watery diarrhea based on signs and symptoms. Diagnosis is confirmed by enzyme immunoassays of stool samples. EMS providers should notify transfer and receiving facilities that a patient has *C difficile*–associated disease, if known. Treatment is cessation of existing antibiotic therapy if possible, rehydration, avoidance of antimotility agents, and therapy with metronidazole or vancomycin, orally, for 10 days.[102]

JAUNDICE

■ HEPATITIS A

Hepatitis A can cause acute disease or asymptomatic infection, but not chronic infection.[103] Whereas more than 70% of older children and adults are symptomatic, in children younger than 6 years, 70% of infections are asymptomatic. Symptomatic illness is characterized by fever, jaundice, dark urine, in addition to malaise, anorexia, nausea . Jaundice is most common symptom. Unfortunately, the clinical signs and symptoms of hepatitis A are indistinguishable from other types of acute viral hepatitis. Diagnosis is usually by immunoglobulin (Ig) in blood, antihepatitis A immunoglobulin M in the acute phase, and antihepatitis A immunoglobulin G after 6 months.

Hepatitis A infection rarely progresses to fulminant hepatitis A, which can lead to death. In 2005, 0.6% of cases of hepatitis A progressed to fulminant hepatitis and died. Age and underlying chronic liver disease are risk factors for progression to fulminant hepatitis. Also, in 2005, the proportion of persons hospitalized with hepatitis A increased with age from 20% among children aged less than 5 years to 47% among persons aged greater than 60 years.

Hepatitis A is transmitted by the fecal-oral route from consumption of contaminated food or water. Rarely, hepatitis A can be transmitted by blood transfusion, particularly clotting factor concentrates. In the United States between 1990 and 2000, 45% of hepatitis A patients could not identify a risk factor for their infection. The time from infection to the presentation of symptoms, if any, is on average 28 days. Hepatitis A is most transmissible from feces 1 to 2 weeks before the onset of illness to about 1 week after the onset of jaundice.

If an EMS provider comes in contact with a patient suspected of having hepatitis A, routine practices and additional precautions can prevent spread of infection. Hepatitis A infection is prevented with vaccination administered in two doses 6 to 18 months apart. In 2005, ACIP recommended that all children aged 12 to 23 months of age receive the hepatitis A vaccination. International travelers, men who have sex with men, persons with clotting factor disorders and those with chronic liver disease should also be immunized. Hepatitis A vaccination is not routinely recommended for health care workers.

Unvaccinated persons who have been exposed to hepatitis A may be candidates for postexposure antihepatitis A immunoglobulin. This has been shown to be 85% effective in preventing hepatitis A infection if given within 2 weeks of exposure. Potential candidates include persons who have had household or sexual contact with a person with hepatitis A, persons who have shared illegal drugs with a person with hepatitis A, other food handlers working with another food handler diagnosed with hepatitis A, patrons of an infectious food handler if the food handler had diarrhea or poor hygiene, and staff and attendees at a child care center where a hepatitis A case has been diagnosed. Vaccination should supplement immunoglobulin administration in postexposure prophylaxis, but not replace it.[104-106]

HEPATITIS B

Hepatitis B infection can cause acute disease, chronic disease, or be asymptomatic.[107] Like hepatitis A, symptoms present more in adults than children, and symptoms are not specific for hepatitis B. Even about 50% of adults with acute infection are asymptomatic. When symptoms occur, they are divided into phases: prodromal, icteric phase, and convalescent phases. In the 3- to 10-day prodromal phase, nonspecific symptoms of malaise, weakness, and anorexia are the most common symptoms, but also low-grade fever, arthritis, rash, vague abdominal discomfort, nausea, and vomiting may occur. The icteric phase lasts 1 to 3 weeks and is characterized by jaundice, with dark urine and light stools starting 1 to 2 days before the onset of jaundice. In convalescence, jaundice disappears while malaise and fatigue may persist for weeks. Definitive diagnosis of hepatitis B is by serologic testing.

Most acute hepatitis B infection results in complete recovery, but in 1% to 2% of patients fulminant hepatitis infection occurs, with a 63% to 93% case-fatality rate. About 10% of acute infections progress to chronic infection, which leads to premature death from cirrhosis or liver cancer in 25% of cases. In the United States, an estimated 51,000 new hepatitis B infections occurred in 2005.

Hepatitis B is transmitted by percutaneous or mucosal exposure to infected blood or blood products. Transmission can also occur from

saliva, semen, vaginal secretions, cerebrospinal, pleural, peritoneal, pericardial, amniotic, or synovial fluid. Transmission to health care workers can occur not only from needlesticks or other sharp injuries, but also through cutaneous scratches or abrasions. The hepatitis B virus can exist for at least 7 days outside the body on inanimate surfaces, and infection can occur by touching skin lesions or mucous membranes with any contaminated equipment. This is particularly important in the EMS setting, and emphasizes the need for adherence to routine practices and additional precautions and proper cleaning and decontamination of equipment and vehicle surfaces. If the hepatitis B (HBs) antigen is present in the blood of a source, the source is communicable for hepatitis B. If infected, the incubation period is on average 60 to 90 days.

Hepatitis B vaccination is recommended for all infants at birth, age 1 to 2 months, and at 6 to 18 months. For unvaccinated adults, a three-dose schedule is recommended for those at increased risk of hepatitis B infection, which includes health care workers.

If percutaneous or mucous membrane exposure occurs to blood that may contain hepatitis B, postexposure prophylaxis with hepatitis B immune globulin (HBIG) may be considered. Before doing so, the vaccination status of the exposed person with hepatitis B should be assessed. If vaccinated, the exposed person should have an assessment of protective antibody levels to hepatitis B, as about 5% of vaccinees may not respond to the hepatitis B vaccine. If available, the source blood should also be assessed for the presence HBs antigen, which signifies infection with hepatitis B and communicability. If an individual is exposed to HBsAg positive fluid and is nonimmunized or lacks protective antibody levels, HBIG should be given within 24 hours, and hepatitis B vaccination also started.[108-110]

HEPATITIS C

About 60% to 80% of persons initially infected with hepatitis C are initially asymptomatic. Among the few 15% to 30% who become symptomatic, clinical signs and symptoms are similar to other acute viral hepatitis illnesses, and include jaundice, fatigue, dark urine, abdominal pain, anorexia, and nausea. Diagnosis of hepatitis C is by serologic testing.[111]

Unlike the other viral hepatitis infections, in up to 85% of hepatitis C infections, persistent infection develops. Among those with chronic infection, 70% develop chronic liver disease, and 1% to 5% of those died prematurely from their chronic liver disease. It is estimated that 20,000 new HCV infections occurred in the United States in 2005, and 3.2 million Americans are chronically infected with hepatitis C.

Hepatitis C is transmitted by mucosal or percutaneous exposure to infectious blood or blood-derived body fluids. Sexual contact can lead to transmission, but is a far less efficient route of transmission. The period of transmission may persist in infected persons indefinitely. If infected, the incubation period is on average 6 to 9 weeks, and it may take up to 20 years before the onset of liver disease.

There is currently no vaccine available to prevent hepatitis C, and postexposure prophylaxis with hepatitis C immunoglobulin has not been shown to be effective. EMS providers must rely on routine practices and additional precautions to prevent occupational and nosocomial transmissions. Disposable injection equipment should not be reused and properly disposed of, and reusable injection equipment should be appropriately sterilized.[112,113]

BIOLOGICAL WEAPONS

This section describes, in brief, the most common potential biologic agents that may be used in terrorist activities or weaponized and dispersed over large populations. This section also includes the fundamentals of decontamination in the event of a suspected biologic weapon exposure. This section is not intended to be all-inclusive or comprehensive, ant the reader should consult resources specific to biologic weapons for further details regarding each agent and decontamination methods specific to each weapon.

ANTHRAX

The symptoms of anthrax are determined by the route of transmission of the bacterium which causes anthrax, *Bacillus anthracis*. There are three forms of anthrax: cutaneous, gastrointestinal, and inhalational.[114,115]

Cutaneous anthrax presents as a small, painless, pruritic papule, which progresses to an enlarging vesicle in 1 to 2 days. The vesicle ruptures and erodes leaving a necrotic ulcer that later gets covered with a black, painless, eschar. Pathognomonic features of anthrax include the presence of an eschar, lack of pain, and edema out of proportion to the size of the lesion. Associated symptoms include swelling of adjacent lymph nodes, fever, malaise, and headache. Cutaneous anthrax is caused by B. anthracis entering a cut or abrasion in exposed areas of the body such as the face, neck arms, and hands. The incubation period of cutaneous anthrax is 1 to 12 days. The case-fatality rate can be as high as 20% without antibiotic therapy, but 1% with therapy.

Gastrointestinal anthrax presents with more nonspecific symptoms. There are two forms: oropharyngeal and intestinal. Oropharyngeal anthrax starts with edematous lesions at the base of the tongue or tonsils that progress to necrotic ulcers with a pseudomembrane. Sore throat, fever, cervical adenopathy, and profound oropharynx edema are associated symptoms. This form of anthrax initially presents with fever, nausea, vomiting, abdominal pain, and tenderness that may progress to hematemesis, bloody diarrhea, and abdominal swelling from hemorrhagic ascites. Gastrointestinal anthrax is caused by consumption of meat contaminated with anthrax. The incubation period for intestinal anthrax is believed to be 1 to 7 days. The case-fatality rate of gastrointestinal anthrax is estimated to be 25% to 60%.

Inhalational anthrax initially causes nonspecific symptoms that mimic influenza. These early symptoms are low-grade fever, nonproductive cough, malaise, and myalgias. Two to three days later, the patient rapidly progresses to severe dyspnea, profuse sweating, high fever, cyanosis, and shock. Hemorrhagic meningitis occurs in up to half of patients. It is critical that the EMS provider attempt to distinguish any influenza-like illness from anthrax, because of the narrow window opportunity for successful treatment. Nasal congestion and rhinorrhea are not common with inhalational anthrax, but more common with influenza-like illness. Further, shortness of breath is more common in inhalational anthrax and less common in influenza-like illness. While not typically available to EMS providers, the chest x-ray demonstrates mediastinal widening or pleural effusion. These findings are the most accurate predictors of inhalational anthrax. Inhalational anthrax can be caused by inhalation of anthrax spores, commonly seen following intentional release of aerosolized anthrax, or from the processing of materials from infected animals, such as goat hair. The incubation period for inhalational anthrax is usually 1 to 7 days, but can be as long as 43 days. Case-fatality rate of inhalational anthrax can be as high as 97% without antibiotics and up to 75% with antibiotics.

Human-to-human transmission of any form of anthrax is rare. A vaccine for anthrax is licensed in the United States and is administered in a six-dose schedule with annual boosters thereafter. Vaccination is not currently recommended for emergency first responders or medical personnel; however, it may be indicated for certain military personnel. In cases of deliberate use of anthrax as a biological weapon, first responders should wear a full face respirator with HEPA filters or a self-contained breathing apparatus, gloves, and splash protection. If clothing is contaminated, it should be removed and placed it plastic bags. Soap and copious amounts of water should be used to decontaminate skin, and bleach should be applied for 10 to 15 minutes in a 1:10 dilution if there is gross contamination. If exposure to aerosolized anthrax occurs, postexposure prophylaxis with ciprofloxacin or doxycycline should begin and continue for 60 days. Vaccination given in three doses for postexposure prophylaxis should also be administered because of the persistence of anthrax spores in the lungs. Quarantine is not appropriate for persons exposed to anthrax as they are not contagious. Patients suspected of being infected with anthrax and requiring hospitalization should be immediately started on IV antibiotics such as ciprofloxacin, and one other active drug.

Other active drugs include doxycycline, rifampin, vancomycin, penicillin, ampicillin, chloramphenicol, imipenem, clindamycin, and clindamycin. Treatment should continue for 60 days or longer.[116-118]

BOTULISM

Botulism is caused by a neurotoxin produced by *Clostridium botulinum*, which ultimately leads to a flaccid paralysis. There are four forms of botulism based on site of toxin production: foodborne, wound, intestinal, and inhalational.[119]

In foodborne botulism, early symptoms are nonspecific gastrointestinal symptoms, and include nausea, vomiting, and diarrhea. This may progress to blurred vision, double vision, dry mouth, and difficulty in swallowing, breathing, and speaking. Descending muscle paralysis occurs, starting with shoulders, and progressing to upper arms, lower arms, thighs, then calves. Respiratory muscle paralysis ultimately leads to death. Food-borne botulism is caused by the ingestion of *Clostridium botulinum* toxin present in contaminated food, or by deliberate contamination as a biologic weapon. The incubation period is usually 12 to 36 hours. The case fatality rate in the United States is 5% to 10%.

Intestinal botulism is rare and occurs mainly in infants. It causes a striking loss of head control, constipation, loss of appetite, weakness, and an altered cry. Intestinal botulism occurs with ingestion of botulism spores, rather than ingestion of toxin. Spores, which may come from honey, food, and dust, germinate in the colon. The incubation period is unknown. It is estimated to cause 5% of deaths of sudden infant death syndrome. The case-fatality rate of hospitalized cases is less than 1%.

Wound botulism causes the same symptoms as food-borne botulism. The incubation period is up to 2 weeks. This is also a rare disease, caused by spores entering an open wound from soil or gravel. Inhalational botulism would be the most common form in the case of use of botulinum toxin as a biologic weapon. Symptoms would the same as food-borne botulism, but the incubation period may be longer.

There are no reported cases of person-to-person transmission of botulism. Therefore, EMS providers do not require any special equipment to manage a patient with suspected or known botulism infection. Supportive care is advised in all cases, including volume replacement. In the case of consumption of food suspected of being contaminated with botulism, treatment may include gastric lavage or whole bowel irrigation. In the case of suspected aerosol exposure to the toxin, clothing should be removed and placed in plastic bags, and the exposed person should shower thoroughly.

Antitoxin use should be considered and administered within 1 to 2 days of exposure. Treatment for botulism is botulinum antitoxin, given after blood is collected to determine the specific antitoxin. Patients should be transported immediately to a center with an intensive care unit. In intestinal botulism in infants, equine botulinum antitoxin should not be used. In the United States, an investigational human-derived botulinal immune globulin is available for infant intestinal botulism from the California Department of Health Services.[120-122]

PLAGUE

Plague is caused by the bacterium *Yersinia pestis*. Initial signs and symptoms may be nonspecific and include fever, chills, sore throat, malaise, and headache. Tender, swollen, warm, and suppurative lymph nodes, mainly in the inguinal area, often follow. This swollen lymph node is called a bubo, hence the term bubonic plague. Patients infected with the plague may then progress to septicemia, meningitis, pneumonia, or shock. When plague progresses to the lungs leading to pneumonic plague, person-person transfer may occur from infective respiratory droplets that are expelled with coughing. The exposed contact subsequently develops primary plague pneumonia. Untreated plague has a case-fatality rate of 50% to 90%. If treated, the death rate is 15%.

Plague is transmitted to humans by bites, scratches, respiratory droplets, or by direct skin contact. Bites from infected rat fleas are the most frequent source of transmission, but bites or scratches from cats may also transmit plague. Airborne droplets from the respiratory tract of cats or humans infected with pneumonic plague are another source of transmission. In case of deliberate use as a biologic weapon, plague bacilli would be transmitted via the aerosolized airborne droplets. Direct contact with tissue or body fluids of a plague-infected sick or dead animal can lead to transmission to humans through a break in the skin. The incubation period is 2 to 6 days for bubonic plague. For primary pneumonic plague, incubation period is shorter, typically 1 to 4 days.[123,124]

Prevention of infection is by controlling exposure to infected fleas. In addition environmental flea and rodent control can be effective means to prevent prevalence and subsequent transmission. A vaccine for bubonic plague exists, but not a vaccine for pneumonic plague. It is administered in a three-dose schedule with booster doses every 6 months. Commercial plague vaccine is no longer available in the United States.

For patients with pneumonic plague, strict isolation is indicated with precautions against airborne spread until 48 hours after start of antibiotic therapy. Antibiotic therapy for bubonic or pneumonic plague is effective if started within 8 to 18 hours of onset of symptoms. First-line antibiotics are streptomycin or gentamycin. Chloramphenicol is used to treat plague meningitis.

Close contacts of patients infected with pneumonic plague should be provided with chemoprophylaxis with tetracycline or chloramphenicol for 1 week after exposure ends. Close contacts include EMS and other medical personnel, household contacts, and face-to-face contacts. Contacts should also be placed under surveillance for 7 days. If contacts refuse antibiotics, they should remain in strict isolation for 7 days. Articles soiled with sputum or purulent discharges should be disinfected.

Yersinia pestis could be used as a potential biologic weapon disseminated through aerosol spread, leading to pneumonic plague. Many patients presenting with fever, cough, particularly hemoptysis in a fulminant course with high case fatality should raise suspicions for deliberate use as a biological weapon.[125-127]

SMALLPOX

There are two clinical forms of smallpox: variola major and variola minor. Variola major is the more severe form of disease with a case fatality rate of greater than 30%, while variola minor is less severe form with a case fatality rate less than 1%. All smallpox begins with a prodrome that lasts 2 to 4 days. The prodrome starts abruptly and consists of fever, headache, nausea, vomiting, muscle pain, headache, and malaise.

Variola major has four principal clinical presentations: ordinary, modified, flat, and hemorrhagic. Ordinary is the most common occurring in 90% of cases. Modified is mild. Flat and hemorrhagic forms are uncommon, but usually severe and fatal.[128]

In ordinary smallpox, after the prodrome, mucous membrane lesions in the mouth begin, called an enanthem. This consists of red spots on the tongue, oral and pharyngeal mucosa which enlarges and ulcerate quickly. Subsequently, a skin rash or exanthem develops, beginning as macules on the face. The exanthem progresses from the proximal extremities to the distal extremities and trunk within 24 hours. The macules progress to papules, vesicles, pustules, crusts. Crusts later separate, leaving depigmented skin and pitted scars. Case fatality for ordinary smallpox is about 30%.

Modified smallpox occurs in previously vaccinated persons. During the prodrome, fever is absent, and the illness is less severe. The skin rash is more superficial and progresses quickly, and lesions are less numerous. This form is more easily confused with chickenpox.

Flat smallpox has a more severe prodrome with skin lesions (exanthem) that are more soft and flat, and contain little fluid. Most cases are fatal. The enanthem in the mouth is more extensive, and fever remains elevated throughout the course of illness rather than remaining restricted to the prodromal period.

Hemorrhagic smallpox consists of a more severe and prolonged prodrome along with extensive bleeding into the skin, mucous membranes, and gastrointestinal tract. The skin rash remains flat and does not progress beyond the vesicular stage. Hemorrhagic smallpox is usually abruptly fatal between the fifth and seventh days of illness. Case fatality for hemorrhagic and flat smallpox is greater than 90%.

Variola minor produced a rash like ordinary smallpox but experience much less severe systemic reactions.

Transmission of smallpox is via inhalation of the virus from airborne droplets or fine particle aerosols originating from the oral, pharyngeal, or nasal mucosa of an infected person. This usually occurs from direct face-to-face contact within a distance of 6 ft. Transmission could also occur from physical contact with an infected person or with contaminated articles through skin inoculation. Transmission from dried skin crusts is uncommon. Smallpox is not transmissible during the incubation period, but becomes infectious with the first appearance of rash until the disappearance of all scabs, which is about 3 weeks. The incubation period of smallpox is an average 12 days, ranging from 7 to 19 days.

EMS personnel should be able to identify the rash due to smallpox, and try to distinguish it from other less virulent diseases, particularly chicken pox. It is important to identify smallpox because its presence indicates a medical and public health emergency. Differentiation can be made through the prodrome and the rash. In smallpox, patients have a severe febrile prodrome, whereas in chickenpox there is a short, mild prodrome or no prodrome. In smallpox, the rash consists of deep, hard, well, circumscribed lesions at the same stage of development, while in chicken pox, the lesions are superficial, not well circumscribed, and at different stages of development. In addition to chickenpox, other conditions may be confused with smallpox, such as herpes, impetigo, contact dermatitis, erythema multiforme, and scabies. Further information to differentiate these illnesses from smallpox is available from the CDC at http://www.bt.cdc.gov/agent/smallpox/.

The last naturally occurring cases of smallpox were identified in 1977, and in 1980 the World Health Organization declared smallpox officially eradicated from the planet. However, there remain two sources of smallpox virus in storage and for research purposes: one in the United States and one in Russia. Any new suspected cases of smallpox are a medical and public health emergency. Therefore, strict respiratory and contact isolation of confirmed or suspected smallpox cases must be undertaken. No antiviral drug is approved for the treatment of smallpox, but cidofovir may be useful as a therapeutic agent and could be used off-label under an investigational new drug protocol.

Contacts with suspect or confirmed smallpox cases should be wearing N95 fit-tested masks, and use routine practices and additional precautions. All bedding and clothing should be autoclaved or laundered in hot water with bleach. Contacts include first responders, laundry handlers, housekeepers, and lab personnel.

Smallpox vaccine is administered as one dose and success of vaccination is determined by a major reaction at the inoculation site, but its use as a childhood immunization was discontinued in 1972. In nonemergency situations, vaccination is recommended for public health, hospital, and other personnel who may need to respond to a smallpox case or outbreak. In an emergency situation, such as the intentional release of variola virus in a bioterrorist event, vaccination would be recommended for those exposed to initial release, contacts of confirmed or suspected cases, and those involved in direct care or transportation of confirmed or suspected cases. There are a number of uncommon but serious adverse reactions, precautions, and contraindications to smallpox vaccine, which should be reviewed before administration, at http://www.bt.cdc.gov/agent/smallpox/. Vaccinia immune globulin intravenous is available for the treatment of adverse reactions to smallpox vaccine. Smallpox vaccine can be used for postexposure prophylaxis in exposed contacts. If administered less than 7 days after exposure, contacts generally experience the mild, modified type of smallpox.[129,130]

TULAREMIA

Tularemia, caused by the bacterium *Francisella tularensis*, has various clinical manifestations related to the route of introduction. All forms have a sudden onset of nonspecific influenza-like symptoms, including high fever, cough, sore throat, chills, headache, generalized body aches. Sometimes, nausea, vomiting, and diarrhea may also occur. All forms may lead to sepsis, pneumonia, and meningitis. The clinical forms include ulceroglandular, glandular, oculoglandular, septic, oropharyngeal, and pneumonic.[131]

Ulceroglandular tularemia is the most common form. It begins at the skin site of the bite of a tick or fly. A papule appears that becomes pustular, later ulcerates, and finally develops into an eschar. Regional lymph nodes become swollen, painful, and tender and rarely suppurate and discharge purulent material. Glandular tularemia has no skin involvement, only regional lymphadenopathy similar to that which occurs with ulceroglandular disease. Oculoglandular tularemia is caused by the bacillus entering the eye; conjunctival ulceration occurs followed by regional lymphadenopathy of the cervical and preauricular nodes. Septic tularemia begins with nonspecific symptoms of fever, nausea, vomiting, abdominal pain, eventually leading to confusion, coma, multisystem organ failure, and septic shock.

Oropharyngeal tularemia is caused by consumption of contaminated water or food, leading to exudative pharyngitis which may be accompanied by oral ulceration. Abdominal pain, diarrhea, and vomiting may accompany this type. Regional lymphadenopathy again occurs, affecting the cervical and retropharyngeal nodes.

Pneumonic tularemia may be caused by not only lung exposure to an infective aerosol from soil, grain, or hay, but also to deliberate use of an infective aerosol as a bioterrorist attack. The clinical presentation may be cough, pleuritic pain, and rarely dyspnea. Chest x-ray findings would show hilar lymphadenopathy, bronchopneumonia, and hilar lymphadenopathy. Despite the lungs as the primary route of entry, it is not uncommon for tularemic pneumonia to present as nonspecific systemic signs without respiratory symptoms, and often normal chest x-ray.

Tularemia is transmitted through the skin, mucous membranes, lungs, and gastrointestinal tract. The bacteria pass through the skin by bites, oropharyngeal mucosa, and conjunctiva by contaminated water, or by contaminated blood or tissue while handling carcasses of infected animals. Through the gastrointestinal tract, it is transmitted by ingestion of insufficiently cooked meat of infected animals or by consumption of contaminated water. Finally, tularemia can be transmitted through the lungs by contaminated soil, handling contaminated furs, or deliberate aerosolization of the bacterium as a biological weapon. The incubation period is usually 3 to 5 days but can range from 1 to 14 days.

There is no documented person-person transmission of tularemia, including pneumonic tularemia. Routine precautions are adequate when transporting and caring for patients. The vehicle and equipment, however, must be thoroughly cleaned and decontaminated after patient transport.

A vaccine for tularemia exists; however, there is no commercial production as yet and its availability is under review by the US Food and Drug Administration. Streptomycin is the drug of choice for treatment of tularemia, with ciprofloxacin as an excellent alternative. Gentamycin and tetracycline are alternatives but show high relapse rates. Treatment should last 14 to 21 days. In a mass casualty situation doxycycline or ciprofloxacin for 14 days are the preferred choices for treatment, started as soon as possible after exposure.[132,133]

■ VIRAL HEMORRHAGIC FEVERS

Viral hemorrhagic fevers are caused by different distinct families of viruses and lead to similar clinical syndromes. In the case of bioterrorist attack, it is essential that first responders be able to recognize the illness associated with the intentional release of the biologic agent.

In hemorrhagic fever, the initial signs and symptoms are nonspecific and include high fever, headache, muscle aches, and severe fatigue. There may be associated gastrointestinal symptoms of nausea, vomiting, diarrhea, and abdominal pain. Respiratory symptoms of cough and sore throat may also occur. About 5 days after the onset of illness, a truncal maculopapular rash develops in most patients. As the disease progresses, bleeding would occur from internal organs, the mouth, eyes, ears, and from under the skin, which would be demonstrated as skin petechiae and skin ecchymose. Shock, coma, seizures, and kidney failure may ensure in severe cases.

Viral hemorrhagic fevers are caused by viruses in four families: arenaviruses, bunyaviruses, flaviviruses, filoviruses, causing diseases such as Ebola hemorrhagic fever, Hantavirus pulmonary syndrome, Lassa fever, Marburg hemorrhagic fever, Hemorrhagic fever with renal syndrome, and Crimean-Congo hemorrhagic fever.[134] Transmission occurs when humans have direct contact with infected animals, mainly rodents, or are bitten by a mosquito or tick vector. Once a person has become infected, some viruses can be transmitted from person to person, mainly by close contact with infected people, but also indirectly by objects contaminated with infected body fluids.

Transmission of viral hemorrhagic fever mainly occurs in the latter stage of illness when the patient suffers vomiting, diarrhea, shock, and hemorrhage. In the case of Ebola virus, there are reports of transmission within a few days of the onset of fever. The incubation period ranges from 2 days to 3 weeks and no transmission has been documented during the incubation period.

There is no vaccine or established cure for viral hemorrhagic fevers, except for yellow fever and Argentine hemorrhagic fever. Ribavirin or plasma has been used for treatment with some success. Prevention is the best method of control. To prevent infection, contact with rodents, and bites from ticks and mosquitos should be prevented. Person-person transmission can be prevented by strict adherence to routine practices and additional precautions. In addition, patients with known or suspected viral hemorrhagic fever must be isolated. While this is not possible in the EMS setting, the transporting vehicle can serve to isolate the patient from the scene and while in transit.

If personnel are exposed to viral hemorrhagic fever, they should be placed under surveillance for fever. Surveillance should occur twice daily for at least 3 weeks after exposure. In case of development of temperature above 38.3°C, patients should be hospitalized immediately with strict isolation. The World Health Organization and CDC have prepared an infection control manual specific to viral hemorrhagic fever management and control, with detailed and comprehensive strategies to prevent spread and protect health care workers during an outbreak.[135-138]

EMS RESPONSE TO SUSPECTED RELEASE OF BIOLOGICAL WEAPONS

Prehospital personnel are often called up to respond to situations where patient decontamination is required due to a suspected chemical, biological, radionuclear (CBRN), or other potentially hazardous agent. The type and source of the agent are not known at the time of response, and in some cases, personnel are not even aware a potentially harmful agent is present. For this reason, personnel from all public service agencies must ensure the scene is safe to approach prior to performing their roles. **(Box 48-1)**

■ SYSTEM RESPONSE AND COORDINATION

Incidents range from relatively confined site-specific events to rapidly expanding accidents that endanger an entire community. Successful management of an incident requires preplanning and interagency

---

Box 48-1

The Goals of EMS Personnel at Potential CBRN Response

1. Protect themselves and other responding personnel from exposure.
2. Identify the potential hazard and obtain accurate information on its health effects to permit medical care of the victims.
3. Decontaminate victims to minimize ongoing exposure and secondary contamination of personnel prior to transport to hospital.
4. Provide emergency medical care within scope and certification.
5. Prevent unnecessary contamination of vehicles used to transport victims.

coordination. Managing the victims necessitates the coordinating of many resources and agencies. First arriving units may have obtained important information about the chemicals involved. Specialized teams may be available to provide additional guidance in identifying and managing the hazardous agent and perform decontamination of equipment, environment, victims, and personnel. EMS personnel will transport victims once thoroughly decontaminated and manage medical problems en route to the hospital. In the setting of a large-scale disaster, the regional office of emergency services (or similar) may be involved in coordination and resource acquisition. Finally, the local hospital emergency department(s) must be involved in planning and practicing for these incidents because they will eventually receive and care for the victims.

DECONTAMINATION PROTOCOL

The first step is determining the need for decontamination. Responding personnel can do this by consulting local expertise, the regional poison control center, or other public service agency involved in CBRN responses. While many response and decontamination protocols exist, they share the following similarities. EMS and other first response personnel must be familiar with the protocols present in their area. A general decontamination protocol is presented. Agent- or contaminant-specific protocols exist, but they are beyond the scope of this chapter.

Field decontamination should take place before any victim is removed from the scene. The decontamination facility should be set up upwind, uphill, and upstream of the contaminated area. There should be adequate security to prevent others from entering the area and victims from leaving the area prior to decontamination. A reception area must be established to screen victims and triage them for any necessary medical care. The names, addresses, telephone numbers, and e-mail addresses of all personnel and victims who have been or may have been exposed at the scene should be recorded for future notification if it is subsequently determined that medical evaluation or treatment is required.

Victims should be triaged in the following priorities, from highest to lowest priority: victims who require prompt medical attention due to agent exposure or illness / injury; victims exhibiting signs or symptoms of agent exposure; victims who are contaminated but not exhibiting signs or symptoms of agent exposure; victims suspected of contamination but showing no signs of toxicity; and animals that provide critical support (guide dogs, etc) to humans known or suspected to be contaminated.

If personnel are entering an area with a contaminant, whether known or unknown, they should wear a NIOSH-certified CBRN self-contained breathing apparatus with a level A protective suit to prevent personal contamination. Personnel must be properly trained in safe use of protective clothing and equipment prior to their use in a potentially hazardous setting.

Personnel who are not members of the specialized team and properly outfitted with protective gear should not enter any contaminated area. They must wait at the perimeter for decontaminated victims brought to them. The specialized team working in the contaminated and decontamination areas should be trained and capable of providing initial airway and spine stabilization, along with basic decontamination techniques.

In a properly functioning response, the contaminated area is referred to as a "red" or "hot" zone. The contaminated area includes all areas that victims have traversed prior to the determination of their contamination status. Once this area(s) is determined, all personnel, patients, and visitors should be evacuated, and the immediate area cordoned off and security posted to keep people out of the area. Personnel wearing appropriate personal protective equipment will decontaminate victims in a "decontamination area or corridor," often referred to as a "yellow" or "warm" zone. The "green" zone is contaminant free and used for recovery. Rescuers in level A suits are typically only able to drag victims onto a backboard and drag them out of the hot zone for decontamination. If victims are not breathing, and if able to do so, personnel can administer oxygen with a reservoir or manually triggered delivery device. Rescuers should direct ambulatory victims toward the decontamination area.

Once in the decontamination area, decontamination should take precedence over medical care unless an immediate threat to life is identified and can be managed safely while decontamination is underway. The purpose of decontamination is to make an individual and their equipment safe by physically removing toxic substances quickly and effectively. Care should be taken during decontamination, because absorbed agent can be released from clothing and skin as a gas. If clothing is contaminated, the victim should be stripped and clothes double-bagged for to prevent further spread of contaminant. Clothing contaminated with dust should be removed dry with care taken to minimize any dust becoming airborne. If circumstances permit, a dust mask or respirator should be placed over the victim's nose or mouth. Dust should be brushed off the face prior to fitting the mask or respirator.

Flush the entire body with plain water for 2 to 5 minutes. If the eyes are contaminated, eye irrigation should be continued for at least 10 to 15 minutes. Saline is preferred for eye irrigation. If the contaminant is oily or greasy, soap may be used followed by additional flushing with water. The areas under nails should be cleaned with a scrub brush or nail cleaner. If there is any doubt about the potential for secondary contamination, decontaminate the victim. If victims are properly decontaminated before they are brought to the EMS personnel, they will pose very little, if any, risk to personnel or their vehicle. All leather items, wool, or other highly absorbent materials that cannot be decontaminated should be removed prior to providing care.

Prehospital health care personnel may need to repeat or continue decontamination procedures after receiving the victim at the perimeter. This is particularly true in cases such as eye exposures to corrosives or skin exposure to oily pesticides. Although specialized protective gear should not be necessary, it is prudent to wear personal protective gear that would be used when caring for a patient with an infectious or communicable disease.

Victims with obvious significant illness or injury will need rapid transport and treatment after initial stabilization and basic decontamination is carried out. In virtually all cases, patients with serious trauma or medical illness can be quickly stripped and flushed with water prior to delivery to prehospital personnel outside the cold zone. This is true even in cold or inclement weather. If this cannot be performed because of life-threatening conditions or other circumstances, then the vehicle must be protected and those providing care during transport and driving the vehicle must be properly fitted and trained with the appropriate level of specialized protective gear. However, every effort should be made to decontaminate the victim at the scene if the means to do so are available. In those jurisdictions where a prehospital care provider might be placed in such a situation without assistance from a properly trained specialist, advance arrangements for additional training and protective equipment should be made.

Victims with few or minimal symptoms are not necessarily safe from progression of illness. Many toxic substances have delayed onset effects, which may appear several hours later, after the victim has returned home. If the toxic substance is known, obtain consultation from the Poison Control Center to determine if delayed effects might be seen and for guidance on triage of asymptomatic or mildly symptomatic exposure victims. Any persons suspected of being exposed should be seen and evaluated by emergency department staff.

Responding EMS personnel will not normally need personal decontamination. In the circumstances where they have been in the hot zone or have attended to a victim who was not properly decontaminated, they should consider themselves to be potentially contaminated, and undergo appropriate decontamination.

If the transport vehicle is inadvertently contaminated, advise from the local environmental health department, specialized response team, or local cleanup companies should be sought on how to determine the level and location of the contamination and on how to clean it up. Advice should also be sought on how to preserve evidence for law enforcement, and dispose of or clean contaminated clothing and personal items.

THE EMS SYSTEM AND ITS WORKFORCE

This section describes the role and planning for health care emergencies due to infectious disease, EMS interactions with public health agencies, and special considerations for EMS agencies in epidemics or pandemics. EMS agencies have a responsibility in the health care sector that exceeds merely emergency response. The report "EMS Agenda for the Future" identifies EMS at the intersection of the health care, public health, and public safety sectors. As a key stakeholder in community health and typically the public's first point of contact with the health care system during an emergency, EMS systems must be proactive in protecting not only their personnel against infectious and communicable disease. More importantly, the EMS systems must be able to maintain this essential service during an outbreak and act as the first barrier to disease spread within the health care system as a whole.

■ EMS PLANNING

Each and every EMS agency must explore their existing infectious disease outbreak or pandemic operational plans and procedures. The plans and procedures must be up to date, and include a number of essential elements in order to be useful and functional during a true outbreak or pandemic. The plans must include the EMS agency's role in preparing for, mitigating, and responding to a health care emergency. EMS agencies should consult with, develop, and coordinate their plans in conjunction with other local, regional, and national agencies and governments to ensure the EMS roles and responsibilities are well defined and understood by all stakeholders. The agency's leadership and authority must also be delineated within the plan, and be consistent with local, regional, and national plans in order to avoid conflict during the actual emergency. If not already in place, the EMS agency should adopt an incident command or other similar system used by other public service agencies. Finally, the EMS agency should also participate in and have access to large regional or national emergency stockpiles of drugs, supplies, and equipment in the event of a large-scale incident. These stockpiles can be colocated with existing EMS resources, permitting their rapid deployment during a large-scale emergency situation.

Each EMS agency should also develop and participate in training exercises that will prepare the agency and its personnel for their role in local, regional, and national infectious disease emergencies. These exercises allow each agency to exercise their plans and procedures, and determine how these function together with those from other public service and health care agencies. The exercises also allow individual EMS providers to better understand their respective roles during an emergency. Most importantly, exercises allow EMS leaders and personnel to develop a personal relationship with others within the public service and health care systems that can enhance communication during an actual emergency.

Effective communication and dissemination of information is typically a major obstacle during any health care emergency or disaster. In order to avoid ineffective or erroneous communication between stakeholders, plans must include a defined process to gather, update, and disseminate factual information to all relevant stakeholders. In the EMS setting, this must include clinical standards, treatment protocols, and any procedures specific to that emergency. The plan must also include just-in-time training methods to ensure all EMS leadership and providers receive this information and any requisite training in a timely manner. Finally, the EMS agency's plan must include methods to coordinate the release of factual, consistent information to public sources (media, public, etc) as required.

■ EMS SURVEILLANCE AND MITIGATION

EMS agencies and their providers are often the first point of contact between the public and the health care system during an emergency. This first contact is the first opportunity to identify a potential threat and mitigate that risk. During the SARS outbreaks in Toronto and Taipei,

EMS providers were among the first health care workers infected with the virus.[4,5] Interfacility patient transport by EMS agencies was also identified as a cause of further spread of SARS between hospitals.[4,38]

To mitigate the risk to providers and the health care system, EMS agencies must quickly adopt and implement a multitude of surveillance, screening, and mitigation strategies to prevent further disease spread. During the SARS outbreaks in Toronto, all EMS personnel were screened and a surveillance system monitored all potentially exposed personnel.[6] A series of work and home quarantine measures were also implemented to prevent depletion of the EMS workforce and ensure there were sufficient staff to maintain emergency response capabilities. In addition, call-taking procedures were modified to screen all calls to an EMS dispatch center for any sign of communicable or infectious disease. Responding personnel would be advised of any call that screened positive. Finally, a provincial government developed and deployed an innovative EMS command, control, and tracking system to mitigate the risk of iatrogenic spread of SARS among health care facilities, health care workers, and patients due to interfacility patient transfers.[139] All EMS agencies should have plans to provide provider- and agency-level strategies for surveillance, screening, and mitigation in order to protect its personnel and the public at large.

Local and regional EMS agencies should identify the role that EMS agencies play in ongoing disease surveillance in order to quickly identify and mitigate the risk of disease once it occurs. Potential roles for EMS include real-time monitoring and analysis of patterns in call volume, call type, presenting complaint, location, and any other disease-specific factors for which data are routinely available at EMS dispatch centers. This data, when used alone, or in conjunction with other health care data, can help identify variations from normal or expected patterns in community health-seeking behavior. These temporal and spatial fluctuations may be the first evidence of a potential threat to community health.

Real-time monitoring is ongoing in many regional, state, and national programs. There are over 100 million emergency department (ED) visits in the United States annually. Data regarding chief complaint and discharge diagnosis can be tracked and integrated with data from EMS agencies, laboratories, and pharmacies (prescriptions filled)[140,141] to provide public health officials with methods to detect changes in disease patterns and health-seeking behaviors. For example, New York City developed an electronic-based emergency department syndromic system that transfers ED triage chief complaint data and EMS data, among other things, each day to the New York City Department of Health. The subsequent analyses permit rapid detection of emerging threats to public health. This Web-based application sent alert e-mail messages when syndromic analysis revealed an increase in the number of patients in predefined symptoms groups and was the first indicator of an influenza outbreak[141,142] 2 to 3 weeks before traditional detection systems. EMS agencies play a collaborative role in multiagency, multijurisdictional efforts as assist public health and other authorities to identify and track patients at risk of exposure and prevent further spread of disease.

■ CONTINUITY OF EMS OPERATIONS

EMS agencies should include, in their preparedness plans, a contingency to allow EMS to maintain its ability to respond to routine emergencies while meeting the needs of a major infectious disease outbreak. EMS will likely experience both an increased demand for service while facing potential loss of trained personnel due to illness and absenteeism. In addition, the agency may face increased emergency department diversions or off-load delays, and a shortage of equipment and supplies. Both limit the agency's ability to maintain adequate resources to meet its existing service mandate. Finally, it is likely that a health care emergency due to infectious disease be ongoing and of many weeks duration.

EMS should take into account the prolonged nature of this potential emergency when planning. Local, regional, and national EMS organizations should have a plan to shift personnel between jurisdictions and augment any inadequate numbers in EMS workforce. There must also be an adequate supply of essential equipment, supplies, and services should the supply chain be interrupted during an emergency. Finally, there should be an effective, reliable, communication system and protocols between EMS, public service, and health care agencies to ensure all stakeholders receive timely information and are aware of diversion and capacities at local and regional levels.

LEGAL AUTHORITY

It is not typically possible for routine EMS policies and procedures to take into account any possible situation or scenario. This is particularly true in the setting of a health care emergency or disaster. The emergency plans developed by EMS agencies should include approved policies and procedures that enable agencies to deviate from routine procedures in order to respond to a disaster or similar situation.

The plans should identify the legislative authority, administrative rules and regulations, and liability protection to support the role of EMS providers during an infectious disease outbreak or other public health emergency. The legal authority should permit EMS agencies and their providers modify established treatment procedures to respond to the evolving role of EMS during the emergency, while ensuring appropriate medical direction, education, and quality assurance are in place. The plans should also include authority and ability to move and license EMS assets, such as vehicles and personnel, if restrictions in movement of the general public are in place.

CLINICAL STANDARDS AND PROTOCOLS

EMS standards and treatment protocols may require rapid and repeated modification during an infectious disease outbreak as more information on the outbreak becomes available. Each EMS agency must have physician medical direction to provide oversight and input regarding these modifications, and rapid dissemination and training methods to ensure providers are appropriate informed and prepared to deal with the outbreak.

Medical directors and EMS agencies should also have methods to communicate with other health care agencies to ensure new EMS standards and protocols are consistent with those in other health care sectors. The medical examiner or coroner's office should be contacted to identify any new protocols and processes to manage facilities, and outpatient facilities to determine the need for EMS-based treat-and-release protocols that do not require patient transport to a health care facility under certain circumstances.

PROTECTING EMS WORKFORCE WELL-BEING

EMS is a key component of any country critical infrastructure, and EMS personnel would experience additional workplace stress during an outbreak or other related health care emergency. The EMS agency must have in place strategies to protect the EMS workplace and their families in order to maintain EMS operations during an outbreak.

EMS agencies must ensure all EMS personnel utilize routine practices and additional precautions (where indicated), and ensure the necessary infrastructure is in place to promote safe working practices to mitigate the risk of disease. Finally, EMS agencies must make available, at all times, an adequate amount of appropriate protective equipment and related supplies designed to prevent disease.

Where risk mitigation programs exist, EMS agencies muse ensure that EMS personnel receive priority access to these programs. In the event of a vaccine- or medication-preventable outbreak, EMS agencies must have an established plan to provide vaccination or appropriate prophylactic medication to all EMS personnel in a timely manner. In the event of potential contact with an infectious disease, EMS agencies must have mechanisms in place to determine if isolation or quarantine are necessary and provide suitable resources for this. Finally, EMS personnel and their families must have available the necessary support services, including counseling and mental health, both during and after an infectious disease outbreak.

- Infectious agents capable of causing disease include bacteria, viruses, fungi and moulds, parasites, and prions.
- Modes of transmission include contact transmission (direct, indirect, droplet), airborne, vector-borne, or common vehicle (food, equipment).
- Agents spread by airborne route include pertussis, rubella, influenza.
- Agents spread by droplet route include tuberculosis, measles, rubella, varicella, *Haemophilus influenzae* type B, *Neisseria meningitidis*, *Streptococcus pneumoniae*, coronaviruses, and SARS.
- Individuals at high risk of influenza complications include young children, people over age 65, the immunosuppressed, and those suffering from chronic medical conditions. Influenza vaccine is the principal means of preventing influenza morbidity and mortality. EMS systems may restrict duties for unimmunized personnel in attempt to prevent outbreak spread.
- Human bites can transmit HIV and hepatitis B and hepatitis C, in addition to other bacteria. Those receiving bites by animals suspected of having rabies should be given rabies postexposure prophylaxis.
- Patients should receive tetanus toxoid if not immunized in the prior 5 years, and immunoglobulin if they have not completed a primary tetanus immunization series.
- EMS personnel exposed or in close contact to patients with meningitis may require prophylactic therapy.
- There is no specific postexposure prophylaxis for hepatitis C, and unlike the other viral hepatitis infections up to 85% of hepatitis C infections develop persistent infection.
- Anthrax is spread by cutaneous, gastrointestinal, and inhalation routes. The case-fatality rate is highest with the inhalation route.
- The goals of EMS personnel at potential CBRN responses are protect themselves, identify potential hazard(s), decontaminate victims, provide emergency care, and prevent unnecessary contamination of vehicles.
- EMS agencies must have infectious disease outbreak or pandemic operational plans and procedures, including adoption of an Incident Command System and access to emergency stockpiles in the event of a large-scale incident.
- EMS physicians must be familiar with how to prevent spread of infectious diseases by developing and encouraging practices that mitigate the various modes of disease transmission.

REFERENCES

1. US Department of Labor. Occupational exposure to blood-borne pathogens: precautions for emergency responders. OSHA 3130. Washington, DC; 1992.
2. Okudera H. Unexpected nerve gas exposure in the city of Matsumoto: report of rescue activity in the first sarin gas terrorism. *Am H Emerg Med.* 1997;15:527-528.
3. Okamura T. Report on 640 victims of the Tokyo subway sarin attack. *Ann Emerg Med.* 1996;28:129-135.
4. Varia M, Wilson S, Sarwal S, et al. Investigation of nosocomial outbreak of severe acute respiratory syndrome (SARS) in Toronto, Canada. *CMAJ.* 2003;169(4):285-292.
5. Ko PC, Chen WJ, Ma MH, et al. Emergency medical service utilization during an outbreak of severe acute respiratory syndrome (SARS) and the incidence of SARS-associated coronavirus infection among emergency medical technicians. *Acad Emerg Med.* 2004;11:903-911.

6. Verbeek PR, McLelland IW, Silverman AC, Burgess RJ. Loss of paramedic availability in an urban emergency medical services system during a severe acute respiratory syndrome outbreak. *Acad Emerg Med.* 2004:11:973-978.

7. Association for Professionals in Infection Control and Epidemiology. *APIC Text of Infection Control and Epidemiology.* Washington, DC: APIC; 2002.

8. March MF, Sant'Anna CC. Signs and symptoms indicative of community-acquired pneumonia in infants under six months. *Braz J Infect Dis.* 2005;9(2):150-155.

9. Juven T, Ruuskanen O, Mertsola J. Symptoms and signs of community-acquired pneumonia in children. *Scand J Prim Health Care.* 2003;21:52-56.

10. Periera JCR, Escuder MML. The importance of clinical symptoms and signs in the diagnosis of community-acquired pneumonia. *J Trop Pediatr.* February 1998;44:18-24.

11. Hopstaken RM, Muris JWM, Knottnerus JA, Kester ADM, Rinkens PELM, Dinant GJ. Contributions of symptoms, signs, erythrocyte sedimentation rate and C-reactive protein to a diagnosis of pneumonia in acute lower respiratory tract infection. *Br J Gen Pract.* May 2003;53:358-364.

12. Marrie TJ. Community-acquired pneumonia: epidemiology, etiology, treatment. *Infect Dis Clin North Am.* 1998;12(3):723-740.

13. Pneumonia. In: Heyman DL ed. *Control of Communicable Diseases Manual.* 18th ed. Washington, DC: American Public Health Association; 2004:413-424.

14. American Academy of Pediatrics. Pertussis. In: Pickering LK, ed. *Red Book: 2000 Report of the Committee on Infectious Diseases.* 25th ed. Elk Grove Village, IL: American Academy of Pediatrics; 2000:435-448.

15. Pertussis. In: Atkinson W, Hamborsky J, McIntyre L, Wolfe S, eds. *Epidemiology and Prevention of Vaccine-Preventable Diseases.* 9th ed. Washington, DC: Public Health Foundation; 2006:79-96.

16. Cortese MM, Bisgard KM. Pertussis. In: Wallace RB, ed. *Maxcy-Rosenau-Last Public Health and Preventive Medicine.* 15th ed. New York, NY: McGraw-Hill Medical; 2007:111-114.

17. Monto AS, Gravenstein S, Elliott M, Colopy M, Schweinle J. Clinical signs and symptoms predicting influenza infection. *Arch Intern Med.* 2000:160:3243-3247.

18. Hoeven AM v d, Scholing M, Wever PC, Fijnheer R, Hermans M, Schneeberger PM. Lack of discriminating signs and symptoms in clinical diagnosis of influenza of patients admitted to the hospital. *Infection.* 2007;35:65-68.

19. Zambon M, Hays J, Webster A, Newman R, Keene O. Diagnosis of influenza in the community: relationship of clinical diagnosis to confirmed virological, serologic, or molecular detection of influenza. *Arch Intern Med.* 2001;161(17):2116-2122.

20. Stein J, Louie J, Flanders S, et al. Performance characteristics of clinical diagnosis, a clinical decision rule, and a rapid influenza test in the detection of influenza infection in a community sample of adults. *Ann Emerg Med.* 2005;46(5):412-419.

21. Centers for Disease Control and Prevention. Seasonal flu. http://www.cdc.gov/flu/. Accessed April 30, 2011.

22. Fiore AE1, Shay DK, Broder K, et al. Prevention and control of influenza: recommendations of the Advisory Committee on Immunization Practices, 2008. *MMWR Recomm Rep.* August 8, 2008;57(RR-7):1-60.

23. Influenza. In: Atkinson W, Hamborsky J, McIntyre L, Wolfe S, eds. *Epidemiology and Prevention of Vaccine-Preventable Diseases.* 9th ed. Washington, DC: Public Health Foundation; 2006:233-253.

24. Centers for Disease Control. Avian influenza (bird flu). May 7, 2007. http://www.cdc.gov/flu/avian/. Accessed April 30, 2011.

25. Brandli O. The clinical presentation of tuberculosis. *Respiration.* 1998;65:97-105.

26. Cohen R, Muzaffar S, Capellan J, Azar H, Chinikamwala M. The validity of classic symptoms and chest radiographic configuration in predicting pulmonary tuberculosis. *Chest.* 1996;109:420-423.

27. American Thoracic Society; CDC; Infectious Diseases Society of America. Treatment of tuberculosis. *MMWR Recomm Rep.* 2003;52(RR-11):1-77.

28. Targeted tuberculin skin testing and treatment of latent tuberculosis infection. *MMWR Recomm Rep.* 2000;49(RR-6):1-77.

29. Centers for Disease Control and Prevention (CDC). Extensively drug-resistant tuberculosis—United States 1993-2006. *MMWR Morb Mortal Wkly Rep.* 2007;56(11):250-253.

30. Tuberculosis Committee, Canadian Thoracic Society. *Canadian Tuberculosis Standards.* 5th ed. Ottawa, Canada: Canadian Lung Association; 2000.

31. Liu CL, Lu YT, Peng MJ, et al. Clinical and laboratory features of SARS vis-à-vis onset of fever. *Chest.* 2004;126;509-517.

32. Chan PKS, Tang JW, Hui DSC. SARS: clinical presentation, transmission, pathogenesis and treatment options. *Clin Sci.* 2006;110:193-204.

33. Wong WN, Sek ACH, Lau RFL, et al. Early clinical predictors of SARS in the emergency department. *CJEM.* 2004;6(1):12-21.

34. Chen SY, Su CP, Ma MH, et al. Predictive model of diagnosing probable cases of SARS in febrile patients with exposure risk. *Ann Emerg Med.* 2004;43(1):1-5.

35. Su CP, Chiang WC, Ma MH, et al. Validation of a novel SARS scoring system. *Ann Emerg Med.* 2004;43:34-42.

36. Wang TL, Jang TN, Huang CH, et al. Establishing a clinical decision rule of SARS at the Emergency Department. *Ann Emerg Med.* 2004;43(1):17-22.

37. Booth CM, Matukas LM, Tomlinson GA, et al. Clinical features and short-term outcomes of 144 patients with SARS in the greater Toronto area. *JAMA.* 2003;289(21):2801-2809.

38. Dwosh H, Hong H, Austgarden D, Herman S, Schabas R. Identification and containment of an outbreak of SARS in a community hospital. *Can Med Assoc J.* 2003;168:1415-1420.

39. Poutanen SM, Low DE, Henry B, et al. Identification of SARS in Canada. *N Engl J Med.* 2003;348:1995-2005.

40. Severe acute respiratory distress syndrome. In: Heyman DL, ed. *Control of Communicable Diseases Manual.* 18th ed. Washington, DC: American Public Health Association; 2004:480-486.

41. Seto WH, Tsang D, Yung RW, et al. Effectiveness of precautions against droplets and contact in prevention of nosocomial transmission of severe acute respiratory syndrome (SARS). *Lancet.* 2003;361(9368):1519-1520.

42. Verbeek PR, Schwartz B, Burgess RJ. Should paramedics intubate patients with SARS-like symptoms? *CMAJ.* 2003;169(4):199-200.

43. Interdisciplinary Respiratory Protection Study Group. Protecting health care workers from SARS and other respiratory pathogens: a review of the infection control literature. *AJIC March.* 2005;33(2):114-121.

44. Chen MIC, Chow ALP, Earnest A, Leong HN, Leo YS. Clinical and epidemiological predictors of transmission in severe acute respiratory syndrome (SARS). *BMC Infect Dis.* 2006;6(151):1-10.

45. Daum RS. Skin and soft-tissue infections caused by methicillin-resistant Staphylococcus aureus. *N Engl J Med.* 2007;357(4):380-390.

46. Klevens RM, Morrison MA, Nadle J, et al. Invasive methicillin-resistant Staphylococcus aureus infections in the United States. *JAMA.* 2007;298(15):1763-1771.

47. Siegel JD, Rhinehart E, Jackson M, Chiarello L. Management of multidrug-resistant organisms in healthcare settings 2006. Centers for Disease Control and Prevention. http://www.cdc.gov/ncidod/dhqp/pdf/ar/mdroGuideline2006.pdf. Accessed April 30, 2011.

48. Roline CE, Crumpecker C, Dunn TM. Can methicillin-resistant Staphylococcus aureus be found in an ambulance fleet? *Prehosp Emerg Care.* 2007;11(2):241-244.

49. Coia JE, Duckworth GJ, Edwards DI, et al. Guidelines for the control and prevention of methicillin-resistant Staphylococcus aureus in healthcare facilities. *J Hosp Infect.* 2006;63S:S1-S44.

50. Gorwitz RJ, Jernigan DB, Powers JH. JA Jernigan and participants in the CDC-convened experts' meeting on management of MRSA in the community. Strategies for clinical management of MRSA in

the community: summary of an experts' meeting convened by the Centers for Disease Control and Prevention. 2006. http://www.cdc.gov/ncidod/dhqp/ar_mrsa_ca.html. Accessed April 30, 2011.

51. American Academy of Pediatrics. Measles. In: Pickering LK, ed. *Red Book: 2000 Report of the Committee on Infectious Diseases.* 25th ed. Elk Grove Village, IL: American Academy of Pediatrics; 2000:385-396.

52. Centers for Disease Control and Prevention. Measles. In: *Travelers' Health: Yellow Book.* 2008 ed. http://wwwn.cdc.gov/travel/yellow BookCh4-Measles.aspx. Accessed April 30, 2011.

53. Measles. In: Heyman DL, ed. *Control of Communicable Diseases Manual.* 18th ed. Washington, DC: American Public Health Association; 2004:347-354.

54. Measles. In: Atkinson W, Hamborsky J, McIntyre L, Wolfe S, eds. *Epidemiology and Prevention of Vaccine-Preventable Diseases.* 9th ed. Washington, DC: Public Health Foundation; 2006:125-144.

55. Centers for Disease Control and Prevention. Rubella. In: *Travelers' Health: Yellow Book.* 2008 ed. http://wwwn.cdc.gov/travel/yellow BookCh4-Rubella.aspx. Accessed April 2011.

56. Plotkin SA, Reef S. Rubella vaccine. In: Plotkin SA, Orenstein WA, eds. *Vaccines.* 4th ed. Philadelphia, PA: WB Saunders; 2004:707-743.

57. Rubella. In: Heyman DL, ed. *Control of Communicable Diseases Manual.* 18th ed. Washington, DC: American Public Health Association; 2004:464-468.

58. Rubella. In: Atkinson W, Hamborsky J, McIntyre L, Wolfe S, eds. *Epidemiology and Prevention of Vaccine-Preventable Diseases.* 9th ed. Washington, DC: Public Health Foundation; 2006:155-169.

59. Reef SE. Rubella. In: Wallace RB, ed. *Maxcy-Rosenau-Last Public Health and Preventive Medicine.* 15th ed. McGraw-Hill Medical; 2007:108-110.

60. Centers for Disease Control and Prevention. Varicella. In: *Travelers' Health: Yellow Book.* 2008 ed. http://wwwn.cdc.gov/travel/yellow BookCh4-Varicella.aspx. Accessed April 30, 2011.

61. American Academy of Pediatrics. Varicella-zoster infections. In: Pickering LK, ed. *Red Book: 2000 Report of the Committee on Infectious Diseases.* 25th ed. Elk Grove Village, IL: American Academy of Pediatrics; 2000:624-638.

62. Chickenpox/herpes zoster. In: Heyman DL, ed. *Control of Communicable Diseases Manual.* 18th ed. Washington, DC: American Public Health Association; 2004:94-99.

63. Varicella. In: Atkinson W, Hamborsky J, McIntyre L, Wolfe S, eds. *Epidemiology and Prevention of Vaccine-Preventable Diseases.* 9th ed. Washington, DC: Public Health Foundation; 2006:171-192.

64. Talan DA, Citron DM, Abrahamian FM, Moran GJ, Goldstein ED. Bacteriologic analysis of infected dog and cat bites. *N Engl J Med.* 1999;340:85-92.

65. American Academy of Pediatrics. Bite wounds. In: Pickering LK, ed. *Red Book: 2000 Report of the Committee on Infectious Diseases.* 25th ed. Elk Grove Village, IL: American Academy of Pediatrics; 2000:155-159.

66. Presutti RJ. Prevention and treatment of dog bites. *Am Fam Physician.* 2007;63(8):1567-1572.

67. Turner TWS. Do mammalian bites require antibiotic prophylaxis? *Ann Emerg Med.* 2004;44:274-276.

68. Talan DA, Abrahamian FM, Moran GJ, Citron DM, Tan JO, Goldstein EJC. Clinical presentation and bacteriologic analysis of infected human bites in patients presenting to emergency departments. *Clin Infect Dis.* 2003;37:1481-1489.

69. Rittner AV, Fitzpatrick K, Corfield A. Are antibiotics indicated following human bites? *Emerg Med J.* 2005;22:654-655.

70. Manning SE, Rupprecht CE, Fishbein D, et al. Human rabies prevention—United States 2008: recommendations of the Advisory Committee on Immunization Practices. *MMWR Recomm Rep.* May 2008 7;57(RR-3):1-26, 28.

71. Centers for Disease Control and Prevention. Rabies. In: *Travelers' Health: Yellow Book.* 2008 ed. http://wwwn.cdc.gov/travel/yellow BookCh4-Rabies.aspx. Accessed April 30, 2011.

72. Rupprecht CE. Viral zoonoses—rabies. In: Wallace RB, ed. *Maxcy-Rosenau-Last Public Health and Preventive Medicine.* 15th ed. McGraw-Hill Medical; 2007:419-423.

73. Rabies. In: Heyman DL, ed. *Control of Communicable Diseases Manual.* 18th ed. Washington, DC: American Public Health Association; 2004:438-447.

74. Centers for Disease Control and Prevention. Tetanus—technical information. http://www.cdc.gov/vaccines/pubs/pinkbook/down loads/tetanus.pdf. Accessed April 30, 2011.

75. Agrawal K, Ramachandrudu T, Hamide A, Dutta TK. Tetanus caused by human bite of the finger. *Ann Plast Surg.* 1995;34(2):201-202.

76. Tetanus. In: Atkinson W, Hamborsky J, McIntyre L, Wolfe S, eds. *Epidemiology and Prevention of Vaccine-Preventable Diseases.* 9th ed. Washington, DC: Public Health Foundation; 2006:69-78.

77. Kumar R. Aseptic meningitis: diagnosis and management. *Indian J Pediatr.* 2005;72:57-63.

78. Tapiainen T, Prevots R, Izurieta HS, et al. The Brighton Collaboration Aseptic Meningitis Working Group. Aseptic meningitis: case definition and guidelines for collection, analysis and presentation of immunization safety data. *Vaccine.* 2007;25:5793-5802.

79. Lee BE, Davies HD. Aseptic meningitis. *Curr Opin Infect Dis.* 2007;20:272-277.

80. Centers for Disease Control. Meningococcal disease. October 12, 2005. http://www.cdc.gov/meningococcal/. Accessed April 30, 2011.

81. Van de Beek D, de Gans J, Tunkel AR, Wijdicks EFM. Community-acquired bacterial meningitis in adults. *N Engl J Med.* 2006;354:44-53.

82. van de Beek D, de Gans J, Spanjaard L, Weisfelt M, Reitsma JB, Vermeulen M. Clinical features and prognostic factors in adults with bacterial meningitis. *N Engl J Med.* 2004;351(18):1849-1859.

83. Valmari P, Peltola H, Ruuskanen O, Korvenranta H. Childhood bacterial meningitis: initial symptoms and signs related to age, and reasons for consulting a physician. *Eur J Pediatrics.* 1987;146(5):515-518.

84. Brivet FG, Ducing S, Jacobs F, et al. Accuracy of clinical presentation for differentiating bacterial from viral meningitis in adults: a multivariate approach. *Intensive Care Medicine.* 2005;31:1654-1660.

85. Nigrovic L, Kuppermann N, Malley R. Development and validation of a multivariable predictive model to distinguish bacterial from aseptic meningitis in children in the post-Haemophilus influenzae era. *Pediatrics.* 2002;110;712-719.

86. Dubos F, Lamotte B, Bibi-Triki F, et al. Clinical decision rules to distinguish between bacterial and aseptic meningitis. *Arch Dis Child.* 2006;91:647-650.

87. Kirkpatrick B, Reeves DS, MacGowan AP. A review of the clinical presentation, laboratory features, antimicrobial therapy and outcome of 77 episodes of pneumococcal meningitis occurring in children and adults. *J Infect.* 1994;29:171-182.

88. Østergaard C, Konradsen HB, Samuelsson S. Clinical presentation and prognostic factors of Streptococcus pneumonia meningitis according to the focus of infection. *BMC Infect Dis.* 2005;5(93):1-11.

89. Stephens DS, Greenwood B, Brandtzaeg P. Epidemic meningitis, meningococcaemia, and Neisseria meningitidis. *Lancet.* 2007;369:2196-210.

90. Fitch MT, van de Beek D. Emergency diagnosis and treatment of adult meningitis. *Lancet Infect Dis.* 2007;7:191-200.

91. Diarrhea, Acute. In: Heyman DL, ed. *Control of Communicable Diseases Manual.* 18th ed. Washington, DC: American Public Health Association; 2004:159-171.

92. Dubberke ER, Carling P, Carrico R, et al. Strategies to prevent Clostridium difficile infections in acute care hospitals: 2014 update. *Infect Control Hosp Epidemiol.* 2014;35(suppl 2):S48-S65.

93. Centers for Disease Control and Prevention. About rotavirus. http://www.cdc.gov/rotavirus/. Accessed May, 2015.

94. Parashar U, Quiroz ES, Mounts AW, et al. Norwalk-like viruses. Public health consequences and outbreak management. *MMWR Recomm Rep.* June 1, 2001:50(RR-9):1-18.

95. Centers for Disease Control and Prevention. "Norwalk-like viruses:" public health consequences and outbreak management. *MMWR Recomm Rep.* 2001;50(no. RR-9):1-13.

96. Centers for Disease Control and Prevention. Travelers' diarrhea. In: *Travelers' Health: Yellow Book.* 2008 ed. http://wwwn.cdc.gov/travel/yellowBookCh4-Diarrhea.aspx. Accessed April 30, 2011.

97. Chalmers RM, Salmon RL. Primary care surveillance for acute bloody diarrhea, Wales. *Emerg Infect Dis.* July-August 2000;6(4):412-414.

98. Centers for Disease Control and Prevention. CDC technical fact sheet about Escherichia coli. http://www.cdc.gov/ecoli/. Accessed May, 2015.

99. Centers for Disease Control and Prevention. Clostridium difficile—information for healthcare providers. http://www.cdc.gov/ncidod/dhqp/id_CdiffFAQ_HCP.html. Accessed April 30, 2011.

100. Sunenshine RH, McDonald LC. Clostridium difficile-associated disease: new challenges from an established pathogen. *Cleveland Clinic J Med.* 2006;73(2):187-197.

101. Gerding DN, Johnson S, Peterson LR, Mulligan ME, Silva J. Clostridium difficile-associated diarrhea and colitis. *Infect Control Hosp Epidemiol.* 1995;16(8):459-477.

102. Ministry of Health and Long-Term Care/Public Health Division/Provincial Infectious Diseases Committee. *Best Practices Document for Management of Clostridium difficile in All Health Care Settings.* Toronto, Canada: Queen's Printer for Ontario; November 2007.

103. Centers for Disease Control and Prevention. Hepatitis A—FAQs for health professionals. http://www.cdc.gov/hepatitis/HAV/HAVfaq.htm#general. Accessed April 30, 2011.

104. Viral hepatitis A. In: Heyman DL, ed. *Control of Communicable Diseases Manual.* 18th ed. Washington, DC: American Public Health Association, 2004:247-253.

105. Hepatitis A. In: Atkinson W, Hamborsky J, McIntyre L, Wolfe S, eds. *Epidemiology and Prevention of Vaccine-Preventable Diseases.* 9th ed. Washington, DC: Public Health Foundation; 2006:193-205.

106. Buffington J, Mast E. Viral hepatitis In: Wallace RB, ed. *Maxcy-Rosenau-Last Public Health and Preventive Medicine.* 15th ed. McGraw-Hill Medical; 2007:212-215.

107. Centers for Disease Control and Prevention. Hepatitis B—FAQs for Health Professionals. http://www.cdc.gov/hepatitis/HBV/HBVfaq.htm#overview. Accessed April 30, 2011.

108. Viral Hepatitis B. In: Heyman DL, ed. *Control of Communicable Diseases Manual.* 18th ed. Washington, DC: American Public Health Association; 2004:253-261.

109. Hepatitis B. In: Atkinson W, Hamborsky J, McIntyre L, Wolfe S, eds. *Epidemiology and Prevention of Vaccine-Preventable Diseases.* 9th ed. Washington, DC: Public Health Foundation; 2006:207-230.

110. Buffington J, Mast E. Viral hepatitis In: Wallace RB, ed. *Maxcy-Rosenau-Last Public Health and Preventive Medicine.* 15th ed. McGraw-Hill Medical; 2007:216-220.

111. Centers for Disease Control and Prevention. Hepatitis C—FAQs for health professionals. http://www.cdc.gov/hepatitis/HCV/HCVfaq.htm#section1. Accessed April 30, 2011.

112. Viral hepatitis C. In: Heyman DL, ed. *Control of Communicable Diseases Manual.* 18th ed. Washington, DC: American Public Health Association; 2004:261-263.

113. Buffington J, Mast E. Viral hepatitis In: Wallace RB, ed. *Maxcy-Rosenau-Last Public Health and Preventive Medicine.* 15th ed. McGraw-Hill Medical; 2007:221-226.

114. Inglesby TV, O'Toole T, Henderson DA, et al. Anthrax as a biological weapon, 2002. Update recommendations for management. *JAMA.* 2002;287(11):2236-2252.

115. Bell DM, Kozarsky PE, Stephens DS. Clinical issues in the prophylaxis, diagnosis, and treatment of anthrax. *Emerg Infect Dis.* 2002;8(2):222-225.

116. Anthrax. In: Heyman DL, ed. *Control of Communicable Diseases Manual.* 18th ed. Washington, DC: American Public Health Association; 2004:20-25.

117. Shadomy SV, Rosenstein NE. Anthrax. In: Wallace RB, ed. *Maxcy-Rosenau-Last Public Health and Preventive Medicine.* 15th ed. McGraw-Hill Medical; 2007:427-431.

118. Anthrax. In: Atkinson W, Hamborsky J, McIntyre L, Wolfe S, eds. *Epidemiology and Prevention of Vaccine-Preventable Diseases.* 9th ed. Washington, DC: Public Health Foundation; 2006:307-321.

119. American Academy of Pediatrics. Botulism. In: Pickering LK, ed. *Red Book: 2000 Report of the Committee on Infectious Diseases.* 25th ed. Elk Grove Village, IL: American Academy of Pediatrics; 2000:212-214.

120. Centers for Disease Control. Botulism. May 21, 2008. http://emergency.cdc.gov/agent/botulism/. Accessed May, 2015.

121. Botulism. In: Heyman DL, ed. *Control of Communicable Diseases Manual.* 18th ed. Washington, DC: American Public Health Association; 2004:69-75.

122. Marshall DL, Dickson JS. Ensuring food safety. In: Wallace RB, ed. *Maxcy-Rosenau-Last Public Health and Preventive Medicine.* 15th ed. McGraw-Hill Medical; 2007:852-853.

123. Campbell GL, Dennis DT. Plague and other *Yersinia* infections. In: Kasper DL, et al. eds. *Harrison's Principles of Internal Medicine.* 14th ed. New York: McGraw Hill; 1998:975-983.

124. Dennis DT, Gage KL. Plague. In: Armstrong D, Cohen J, eds. *Infectious Diseases.* Vol 2. 2nd ed. London: Mosby, Ltd; 2003:1641-1648, Sec 6.

125. Plague (pestis). In: Heyman DL, ed. *Control of Communicable Diseases Manual.* 18th ed. Washington, DC: American Public Health Association; 2004:406-412.

126. Staples JE. Plague. In: Wallace RB, ed. *Maxcy-Rosenau-Last Public Health and Preventive Medicine.* 15th ed. McGraw-Hill Medical; 2007:370-373.

127. Centers for Disease Control. CDC Plague home page. December 11, 2007. http://www.cdc.gov/ncidod/dvbid/plague/. Accessed April 30, 2011.

128. Centers for Disease Control and Prevention. Overview of smallpox, clinical presentations, and medical care of smallpox patients. http://emergency.cdc.gov/agent/smallpox/response-plan/files/annex-1-part1of3.pdf. Accessed April 30, 2011.

129. Smallpox. In: Atkinson W, Hamborsky J, McIntyre L, Wolfe S, eds. *Epidemiology and Prevention of Vaccine-Preventable Diseases.* 9th ed. Washington, DC: Public Health Foundation; 2006:381-305.

130. Smallpox. In: Heyman DL, ed. *Control of Communicable Diseases Manual.* 18th ed. Washington, DC: American Public Health Association; 2004:491-495.

131. Dennis DT, Ingelsby TV, Henderson DA, et al. Tularemia as a biological weapon. Medical and public health management. *JAMA.* 2001;285(21):2763-773.

132. Mead PS. Tularemia. In: Wallace RB, ed. *Maxcy-Rosenau-Last Public Health and Preventive Medicine.* 15th ed. McGraw-Hill Medical; 2007:424-427.

133. Tularemia. In: Heyman DL, ed. *Control of Communicable Diseases Manual.* 18th ed. Washington, DC: American Public Health Association; 2004:573-576.

134. Centers for Disease Control and Prevention. Viral hemorrhagic fevers—fact sheet. http://www.cdc.gov/ncidod/dvrd/spb/mnpages/dispages/Fact_Sheets/Viral_Hemorrhagic_Fevers_Fact_Sheet.pdf. Accessed May 6, 2011.

135. Centers for Disease Control and Prevention and World Health Organization. Infection control for viral haemorrhagic fevers in the African health care setting. Atlanta: Centers for Disease Control and Prevention; 1998: 1-198. http://www.cdc.gov/vhf/abroad/pdf/african-healthcare-setting-vhf.pdf. Accessed May, 2015

136. Centers for Disease Control. Management of patients with suspected viral hemorrhagic fever. *MMWR Morb Mortal Wkly Rep.* 1988;37(S-3):1-15.

137. Lassa fever. In: Heyman DL, ed. *Control of Communicable Diseases Manual*. 18th ed. Washington, DC: American Public Health Association; 2004:289-292.

138. LeDuc JW. Epidemiology of viral hemorrhagic fevers. In: Wallace RB, ed. *Maxcy-Rosenau-Last Public Health and Preventive Medicine*. 15th ed. McGraw-Hill Medical; 2007:352-362.

139. MacDonald RD, Farr B, Neill M, et al. An emergency medical services transfer authorization center in response to the Toronto severe acute respiratory syndrome outbreak. *Prehosp Emerg Care*. 2004;8:223-231.

140. Pollock DA. Emergency medicine and public health: new steps in old directions. *Ann Emerg Med*. 2001;38(6):675-683.

141. Barthell EN, Aronsky D, Cochrane DG, Cable G, Stair T. The frontlines of medicine project: a proposal for the standardized communication of emergency department data for public health uses including syndromic surveillance for biological and chemical terrorism. *Ann Emerg Med*. 2002;39(4):422-429.

142. Pavlin JA. Investigation of disease outbreaks detected by "syndromic" surveillance systems. *J Urban Health*. 2003;80(suppl 1):I107-I114.

CHAPTER 49

Pediatric Patients

Ella K. Cameron
Richard M. Cantor

INTRODUCTION

"The test of the morality of a society is what it does for its children."

~Dietrich Bonhoeffer

Infants, children, adolescents, and young adults create a unique population for health care providers. The initial approach to the pediatric patient should include creating a rapport with the child and parent, performing a primary examination, and developing a plan for treatment. The examination of a fussy child or a child who has special needs is particularly challenging. Awareness for the specialized pediatric patient interaction will go far in helping to get a good history and physical examination. The developmental changes throughout childhood will also impact the examination findings and major milestones should be noted as part of a history and normal examination (**Table 49-1**). Distinct anatomical and physiological differences distinguish the pediatric patient from the adult patient, creating a challenging clinical situation if the provider is unprepared. Notable increases in pediatric morbidity and mortality from trauma and respiratory complaints in tertiary care centers in the

1980s were directly related to a lack of specialty trained pediatric emergency providers. Multiple studies have confirmed these findings and in the late 1980s and 1990s more focus was devoted to developing pediatric emergency care training, curriculum, and prevention efforts (need references). Over the last several years there has been an explosion of pediatric critical care and pediatric emergency medicine literature that supports the field and its development. Our goal for this chapter is to provide a resource for basic pediatric assessment and intervention that will enable stabilization of the patient until a higher level of care is available.

OBJECTIVES

- List normal ranges for vital signs in different pediatric age groups.
- Describe key physiological differences in pediatric patients relating to the prehospital care of medical emergencies.
- Describe key physiological differences in pediatric patients relating to the prehospital care of trauma-related emergencies.
- List appropriate resuscitation fluid types, amounts, and rates for different age groups and indications.
- List drug doses for drugs commonly used in the prehospital environment.
- Briefly discuss RSI and the drugs used for sedation and paralysis in children, with a focus on differences from standard adult care.

TABLE 49-1	Developmental Milestones			
Age	Gross Motor	Visual-Motor/Problem Solving	Language	Social/Adaptive
1 mo	Raises head from prone position	*Birth:* Visually fixes *1 mo:* Has tight grasp, follows to midline	Alerts to sound	Regards face
2 mo	Holds head in midline, lifts chest off table	No longer clenches fists tightly, follows object past midline	Smiles socially (after being stroked or talked to)	Recognizes parent
3 mo	Supports on forearms in prone position, holds head up steadily	Holds hands open at rest, follows in circular fashion, responds to visual threat	Coos (produces long vowel sounds in musical fashion)	Reaches for familiar people or objects, anticipates feeding
4 mo	Rolls over, supports on wrists, and shifts weight	Reaches with arms in unison, brings hands to midline	Laughs, orients to voice	Enjoys looking around
6 mo	Sits unsupported, puts feed in mouth in supine position	Unilateral reach, uses raking grasp, transfers objects	Babbles, ah-goo, razz, lateral orientation to bell	Recognizes that someone is a stranger
9 mo	Pivots when sitting, crawls well, pulls to stand, cruises	Uses immature pincer grasp, probes with forefinger, holds bottle, throws objects	Says "mama, dad" indiscriminately, gestures, waves bye-bye, understands "no"	Starts exploring environment, plays gesture games (eg, pat-a-cake)
12 mo	Walks alone	Uses mature pincer grasp, can make a crayon mark, releases voluntarily	Uses two words other than mama/dad or proper nouns, jargoning (runs several unintelligible words together with tone or inflection), one-step command with gesture	Imitates actions, comes when called, cooperates with dressing
15 mo	Creeps up stairs, walks backward independently	Scribbles in imitation, builds tower of two blocks in imitation	Uses four to six words, follows one-step command without gesture	15-18 mo: uses spoon and cup
18 mo	Runs, throws objects from standing without falling	Scribbles spontaneously, builds tower of three blocks, turns two to three pages at a time	Mature jargoning (includes intelligible words), 7-10 word vocabulary, knows five body parts	Copies parents in tasks (sweeping, dusting), plays in company of other children
24 mo	Walks up and down steps without help	Imitates stroke with pencil, builds tower of seven blocks, turns pages one at a time, removes shoes, pants, etc	Uses pronouns (I, you, me) inappropriately, follows two-step commands, has a 50-word vocabulary, uses two-word sentences	Parallel play
3 y	Can alternate feet when going up steps, pedals tricycle	Copies a circle, undresses completely, dresses partially, dries hands if reminded, unbuttons	Uses a minimum of 250 words, three-word sentences, uses plurals, knows all pronouns, repeats two digits	Group play, shares toys, takes turns, plays well with others, knows full name, age, gender
4 y	Hops, skips, alternates feet going down steps	Copies a square, buttons clothing, dresses self completely, catches ball	Knows colors, says song or poem from memory, asks questions	Tells "tall tales," plays cooperatively with a group of children
5 y	Skips alternating feet, jumps over low obstacles	Copies triangle, ties shoes, spreads with knife	Prints first name, asks what a word means	Plays competitive games, abides by rules, likes to help in household tasks

Modified with permission from Strange GR, Ahrens WR, Schafermeyer RW, Wiebe RA, eds. Pediatric Emergency Medicine, 3rd ed. New York: McGraw-Hill; 2009. Table 1-6.

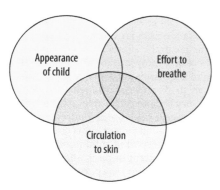

FIGURE 49-1. Three components of pediatric assessment. (Reproduced with permission from Strange GR, Ahrens WR, Schafermeyer RW, Wiebe RA, eds. Pediatric Emergency Medicine, 3rd ed. New York: McGraw-Hill; 2009. Figure 1-1.)

The unique differences between infants, children, and adults will guide the assessment and treatment of these patients. Three components of pediatric initial assessment include the **A**ppearance of the child, the child's **B**reathing, and an assessment of their **C**irculation by evaluating their skin (**Figure 49-1**). The combination of these ABCs allows for quick triage and emergent action if needed.

GENERAL CONCERNS

Pediatric care in the prehospital environment presents unique challenges for providers and medical directors.[10] The nature of the developing anatomy and physiology lends to complicated assessment considerations and the need for special equipment and skills. In order to address these issues Emergency Medical Services for Children Program was created under the Emergency Medical Services for Children (EMSC) Act of 1984.[11] The program brings together a multidisciplinary group of experts and under the management of the US DHHS's Health Resources and Services Administration (HRSA) and the US Department of Transportation National Highway Traffic Safety Administration (NHTSA).

TRANSPORTATION

The assessment and care of pediatric patients in the prehospital environment requires that providers have knowledge of age-specific physiology and stages of development, but also requires that EMS providers are properly equipped with the appropriate tools to safely and effectively evaluate, treat, and transport pediatric patients to appropriate destination facilities.

Because pediatric transports account for 4% to 13%[1] of transport volume in most EMS systems, and around 10.5%[2] of those transports involve care for seriously injured or ill pediatric patients, the care of pediatric patients could and should be considered to be a high risk but low volume event. As such, any tools that can assist the EMS provider in their accurate assessment of pediatric patients should be implemented by the EMS system. Such tools include pediatric weight or size-based drug dosage reference tables, as well as length-based pediatric assessment guides such as the Broselow Pediatric Emergency Tape.[3] Such assessment guides help providers rapidly identify or calculate weight-based doses of critical drugs or to identify which size-based pieces of equipment like endotracheal tubes, laryngoscope blades, or intravenous catheters are appropriate to use in the care of pediatric patients.[4-6]

Most states or jurisdictions have established minimal equipment standards that dictate the pediatric-specific equipment that is required to be carried by EMS vehicles in the jurisdiction. Additionally, several organizations, including NAEMSP, Emergency Medical Services for Children, ACEP, and the American College of Surgeons (ACS) have published recommended pediatric equipment guidelines for ambulances. In most EMS systems, it is probably not practical for EMS providers to carry a single "first-in bag" that contains all of the equipment and supplies

needed to care for both pediatric and adult patients. Such a bag would be prohibitively large and heavy due to the need to carry several sizes of endotracheal tubes, laryngoscope blades, and other size- or pediatric-specific items. Some systems may find it more practical and effective to equip their providers with specific pediatric equipment bags. Ideally, these bags would be similar to the standard adult "first-in bag" with regard to the cohorting and placement of certain pieces of equipment or supplies (airway, vascular access, etc). However, the pediatric bag should also be easily distinguished from the adult bag in order to avoid situations where inappropriate equipment is brought to a patient's side.

PACKAGING

In 2010 NHTSA released "Recommendations for the Safe Transportation of Children in Ground Ambulances." This document helped raise awareness that the sometimes common practice of transporting pediatric patients in the arms of caregivers who are secured to the ambulance stretcher is an unsafe practice. In a 2014 study by O'Neil et al, 14% of pediatric patients were transported in a parent's lap, 14% were unrestrained, and none of the children under the age of 3 were properly restrained.[7] Just as the civilian population must use a pediatric restraint device appropriate to a child's size when children are being transported in a private vehicle, EMS providers should follow a similar practice (**Figure 49-2**). Fortunately, several options for safe restraint exist. In many situations, the EMS provider can simply ask to use a family's own child restraint device while transporting the pediatric patient to a hospital. In situations where such a device is not available or practical to use, several manufacturers market devices specifically for use in the EMS environment to safely package pediatric patients of various sizes. Use of such devices reduces the need of EMS agencies to equip every transport

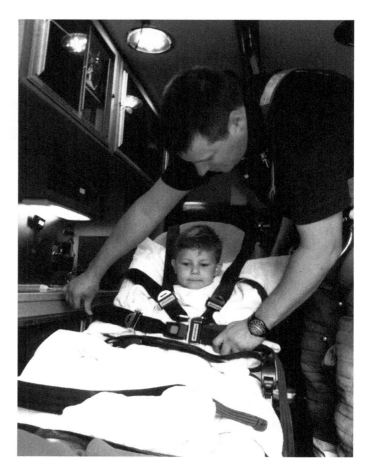

FIGURE 49-2. Children should be properly packaged. Providers may have difficulty using standard-size packaging techniques and equipment on young children.

vehicle with the wide variety of civilian child restraint devices that would be necessary to transport children of any size or age.

INTERFACILITY TRANSPORT

In addition to helping ensure that field providers are properly equipped, EMS physicians will also play an important role in developing pediatric care protocols, as well as developing guidelines to direct the dispatch of appropriately equipped and trained providers for execution of interfacility transport of pediatric patients. Depending on the EMS agency field provider and equipment resources, it may not be safe for a particular agency to perform interfacility transport of certain pediatric patients. Such circumstances are ideally defined in a prospective fashion and are detailed in a pediatric transport approval algorithm such as that depicted in **Figure 49-3**. In some cases, it may be beneficial or desirable to establish relationships with facilities that provide specific pediatric interfacility transport teams. In such circumstances, an EMS agency might provide the transport vehicle, but the receiving hospital would provide the equipment and pediatric critical care providers that are necessary to affect the safe and efficient transfer of critically ill neonatal or pediatric patients.[8]

TERMINATION OF RESUSCITATION

Just as pediatric patients require a different approach to assessment and treatment in the field due to age-related injury and illness patterns, there are some circumstances that occur in both the pediatric and adult population that will require a different operational approach by the EMS provider. Two examples include consent for treatment or refusal of care and withholding or termination of resuscitation in the field. The EMS physician should be familiar with the regulations in their specific operating jurisdiction regarding parental consent and refusal of care for pediatric patients. Chapter 24 provides more discussion of this topic.

Fortunately for patients, parents, and providers, EMS dispatches that result in the need to provide care for children in cardiopulmonary arrest are infrequent. However, unfortunately such circumstances do occur, and must be addressed prospectively with the development of appropriate protocols and guidelines. In these cases, protocols that have been developed to guide EMS providers in the decision to withhold or terminate resuscitative in the efforts for adult patients in cardiopulmonary arrest may not be appropriate to extrapolate to the pediatric population. Because of the significant social and psychological issues that caregivers are likely to experience during the critical illness or potential death of a child, it may be both reasonable and prudent for EMS systems to provide more aggressive field care and interventions than they would otherwise provide for an adult patient under similar circumstances. This care is likely to involve transport of children with no reasonable chance for survival to a hospital except in cases where there are obvious signs of prolonged death. Performing transport in these cases may allow for the engagement of specific social services and other support resources that will be necessary for family members or caregivers, and may provide more reassurance to both caregivers and EMS providers that "everything possible was done" to attempt to revive the child. In essence, EMS physicians and providers must recognize that in situations involving pediatric cardiopulmonary arrest with no chance for survival, provisions must be made for the care of the dying child as well for any family members or care givers who will almost certainly be affected by such a tragic event. It is necessary to note though that special care should be taken to both recognize and to not disturb evidence of potential child abuse or neglect in cases of out-of-hospital death of pediatric patients.

RESPIRATORY

Pediatric respiratory distress is a common presenting complaint in the emergency setting. If treated improperly, even mild respiratory distress can quickly develop into an acute respiratory emergency that has significant morbidity and mortality. The initial assessment of the child with a respiratory complaint includes airway evaluation for patency, work and quality of breathing, and an assessment of circulatory compromise from respiratory failure. Due to the immaturity of the central respiratory control younger infants and children are less likely to provide an adequate and sustained ventilatory response to a respiratory emergency. The

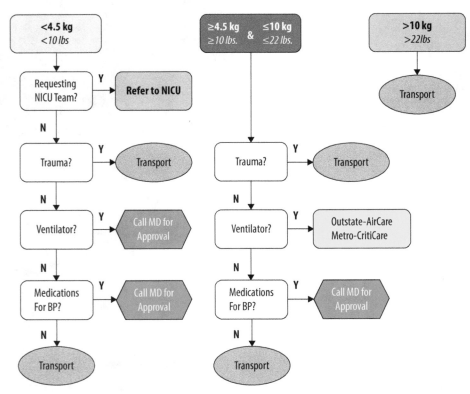

FIGURE 49-3. Pediatric transport approval algorithm.

patency of the airway must be established at the outset of evaluation. If there is a concern for obstruction, the examiner must evaluate for partial versus total occlusion of the airway. If a child has a *partial* airway obstruction, administer supplemental oxygen and maintain a position of comfort with all efforts directed to decrease worsening respiratory function. A *complete* airway obstruction will require back blows for a child less than 1 year old or repeat abdominal thrusts in a child after the first year of life. The method of blind finger sweep is no longer advocated but the use of Magill forceps under direct laryngoscopy remains an adjunct intervention for removal of an airway obstructed by a foreign body.

Assessment of work of breathing should include a general description of overall respiratory effort. The use of accessory muscles, retractions, nasal flaring, or abnormal breath sounds are hallmarks of respiratory distress. Differentiating between abnormal airway sounds such as stridor, wheezing, and grunting will often direct the choice of intervention. Stridor is an inspiratory, high-pitched sound produced by turbulent airflow at the level of obstruction which can develop in the upper airway from the nares to the subglottic region. Severe stridor can often be heard without the use of a stethoscope; mild stridor is best heard by auscultation at the level of the larynx. In a young infant causes of stridor may include congenital abnormalities; however, this hallmark of upper respiratory compromise is associated most commonly with croup, foreign body aspiration, or epiglottitis. Wheezing is a high-pitched continuous whistling musical sound that is produced by high-velocity turbulent airflow through a narrowed space. In mild distress, it often only noted during expiration. As obstruction worsens, however, both phases of respiration will be affected. The absence of wheezing may signal worsening respiratory effort as the patient becomes too fatigued to maintain the active process of respiration. Many etiologies can produce wheezing, including but not limited to asthma, bronchitis, bronchiolitis, foreign body, airway obstruction, severe allergic reaction, and many other inflammatory pathologies. An ominous sign in pediatric respiratory distress is grunting. It is a deep, low-pitched sound heard at the end of expiration that coincides with closure of the glottis. Grunting increases the positive end-expiratory pressure which prolongs the time for alveolar gas exchange and thereby will improve perfusion and ventilation. Grunting is a harbinger of impending respiratory collapse and the child should have immediate intervention. Patient positioning is also of great importance. Signs of impending respiratory collapse include tripoding, a patient who refuses to lie flat, or an infant who has head bobbing with each inspiration. Perhaps the most critical step in the assessment of respiratory complaints is the evaluation of perfusion as ventilatory collapse commonly precedes cardiopulmonary arrest. Pediatric patients have an enormous physiologic reserve and may maintain relatively normal vital signs until collapse is imminent. Tachycardia may present as an early indicator of compromise. Tachycardia has many contributing etiologies, including medications, pain, fear, and stress. Peripheral pulses, capillary refill, skin color, cold extremities, and decreased level of consciousness are all signs of dysfunctional perfusion and will provide an early warning of impending cardiopulmonary collapse.

Understanding and anticipating the differences in the pediatric airway is essential for successful airway management. Not only are there anatomical differences but physiological differences that will influence every aspect of airway evaluation and management. Anatomical differences illustrated in **Table 49-2** highlight the dynamic differences between the pediatric and adult airway. It is important to know these differences and plan accordingly. Placement of a towel or roll under child's shoulders creates a sniffing position which corrects for forward flexion of the head and allows the large occiput to be in line with shoulders, creating a better axis for inline airway anatomy and successful intubation. If tracheal intubation is indicated the best method is rapid sequence intubation (RSI). This method of airway management is a series of sequential steps that during the stress of an airway emergency are quickly recalled from training and when followed increase the likelihood of success. Prior to intubation the preparation of suction, oxygen by bag-valve-mask, equipment, as well as difficulty of intubation and the use of adjunct airway equipment should

TABLE 49-2	Comparison of Pediatric and Adult Airways	
	Pediatric	Adult
Tongue	Large relative to mouth	Relative to mandible
Epiglottis	Floppy and omega shaped	Flatter and firm
	Located at level of C3-C4	Located at level of C5-C6
Trachea	Smaller and shorter	
Larynx	Funnel shaped	Column shaped
	Angles posteriorly	Relatively straight
Narrowest point (upper airway)	Subglottic at cricoid ring	At vocal cords
Vocal cords	Short and concave	horizontal
Lung volume	~250 mL at birth	~6000 mL at adulthood

be considered. RSI steps include preparation, preoxygenation, pretreatment, sedation agent, paralyzing agent, intubation, and confirmation of endotracheal tube placement. Appropriate RSI medications, endotracheal tube sizes, and distance for placement are highlighted in **Table 49-3**. The majority of cardiopulmonary arrests in children are secondary to respiratory collapse; accordingly, it is a critical skill for emergency medicine providers to master the evaluation and management of pediatric airway and respiratory emergencies.

CARDIAC

Cardiac emergencies may range from a report of a self-limited apneic episode to an infant in full arrest. The important of a detailed history and physical cannot be overstated. Congenital heart disease (CHD) is present in approximately 0.96% of births.[9] Common cardiovascular presentations by age are seen in **Figure 49-4** and may guide differential diagnosis with respect to age of presentation. Cardiac lesions are most commonly described as cyanotic or noncyanotic in presentation.

Cyanotic cardiac lesions result from the infant's dependence on a patent ductus arteriosus that allows shunting of partially oxygenated blood. Common classification lists the "five Ts": truncus arteriosus, tetralogy of Fallot, transposition of the great vessels, tricuspid atresia, and total anomalous pulmonary venous return. Most of these cyanotic lesions will present within the first days of life. In contrast, left-sided outflow obstructive anomalies, such as hypoplastic left heart syndrome, coarctation of the aorta, and critical aortic stenosis, will present within the first few weeks of life as the ductus closes. They are therefore commonly referred to as "ductus-dependent" lesions. Their clinical presentation will include a shock-like syndrome with or without cyanosis. Immediate action to stabilize and resuscitate the infant is paramount. Initial interventions should include high flow oxygen, intravenous access (IO access if indicated), chest x-ray, ECG, bedside glucose, baseline labs, and blood gas analysis. The application of high flow oxygen will allow for differentiation between different etiologies for cyanosis. Analysis of an initial blood gas on room air comparing the PaO_2 values to a second blood gas taken while on high flow oxygen is referred to as the hyperoxia test and may be helpful in distinguishing between cardiac and pulmonary causes of cyanosis. A patient with respiratory etiology will improve on high flow oxygen. Fluid boluses should be considered in cases of shock with initial focus on airway, breathing, and circulation. The administration of prostaglandin E1 should be considered in these cases, as it will keep the ductus arteriosus patent and allow for continued right to left shunting of blood volume. The known side effects of prostaglandin E1 include apnea and elective intubation should be considered after its administration.

Noncyanotic cardiac lesions are most often the symptoms and signs of congestive heart failure (CHF). Clinical examination findings for CHF may include any of the following: failure to thrive, diaphoresis with

TABLE 49-3 RSI Drugs, Doses (mg/kg), Sizes, Distances

Age	2 mo	6 mo	1 y	3 y	5 y	7 y	9 y	11 y	12 y	14 y	16 y	Adult
Average weight (kg)	5	8	10	15	19	23	29	36	44	50	58	65
Preoxygenation												
Adjunctive agents (optional):												
Atropine (0.01-0.02 mg/kg): Use in all children or with ketamine	0.1	0.15	0.2	0.3	0.3	0.4	0.5	0.5	0.5	0.5	0.5	0.5
Lidocaine (1.5 mg/kg): Lowers ICP	8	12	15	22	28	35	44	54	66	75	90	100
Sellick maneuver												
Sedative												
Hypotension												
Etomidate (0.3 mg/kg):	1.5	2.4	3.0	4.5	6	7	9	11	13	15	17	20
Head trauma without hypotension												
Etomidate (see above) or Thiopental (3-5 mg/kg):	15-25	24-40	30-50	45-75	57-95	70-115	90-145	110-180	130-220	150-250	170-290	195-325
Status asthmaticus:												
Ketamine (1-2 mg/kg):	5-7	8-16	10-20	15-30	19-38	23-46	29-58	36-72	44-88	50-100	58-100	65-100
Paralyzing agent:												
Succinylcholine (1.0-1.5 mg/kg):	8	12	15	25	30	40	50	55	60	65	70	80
Rocuronium (0.6-1.0 mg/kg):	4	6	9	12	15	20	25	30	40	45	50	60
Intubate (tube size):	3.5	3.5	4.0	4.5	5.0	5.5	6.0	6.5	7.0	7.0 female, 8.0 male		
Tube depth at lip (cm):	11	12	13	14	15	16	18	19	20	22	22	22
Laryngoscope blade size:	1	1	1	2	2	2	2	2	3	3	3	3-4

Modified with permission from Strange GR, Ahrens WR, Schafermeyer RW, Wiebe RA, eds. Pediatric Emergency Medicine, 3rd ed. New York: McGraw-Hill; 2009. Table 23-2.

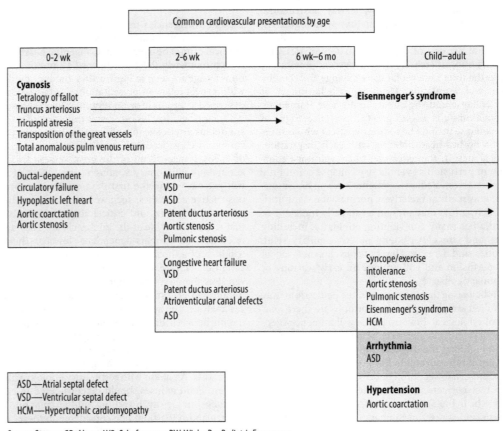

FIGURE 49-4. Common cardiovascular presentations by age. (Reproduced with permission from Strange GR, Ahrens WR, Schafermeyer RW, Wiebe RA, eds. Pediatric Emergency Medicine, 3rd ed. New York: McGraw-Hill; 2009. Figure 47-1.).

feeding, decreased activity, pulmonary edema, tachypnea, grunting, retractions, pallor, mottling, hepatomegaly, murmur, gallop, poor sleeping, and respiratory distress or shock. Again, immediate assessment of the ABCs is essential but after initial stabilization ECG, chest x-ray, labs, IV access, and echocardiography are indicated. The etiology of noncyanotic heart disease is differentiated by impact on pulmonary vascularity. Increase in pulmonary vascularity may be due to lesions such as atrial septal defect (ASD), ventricle septal defect (VSD), patent ductus arteriosus, (PDA), and atrioventricular septal defect. Lesions that do not cause pulmonary vascular increase include aortic stenosis, coarctation of the aorta, and pulmonary stenosis. Treatments appropriate for CHF include diuretics and inotropes.

TRAUMA

When assessing a pediatric trauma, classical ATLS protocols should be followed with the initial survey to include assessment of airway, breathing, circulation, disability, and exposure of patient followed closely by a secondary survey to identify immediate life-threatening injuries for which urgent intervention is indicated. Given the broad age range that composes this population an age-specific approach is warranted. Children respond differently than the adult trauma patient. Infants (less than 12 months old) are unable to communicate or verbalize their pain and injury and a high index of suspicion should exist for every organ system until it is proven to be uninvolved. In a toddler or young child their ability to localize pain or provide answers to direct questioning may be limited and a thorough examination is necessary. In the adolescent and young adult additional factors such as drugs and alcohol may complicate the history and physical.

There are age-specific injury patterns within the pediatric population (**Table 49**-4). Due to the relatively smaller size within the pediatric patient, the energy transmitted from basic traumatic forces is greatly magnified. Additionally, children have less adipose tissue, less connective tissue, and multiple organs in close proximity to one another, allowing for greater injury with even minimal force.

In younger children the head is disproportionately larger and as such more head injuries are noted in this population. Remember that the body will follow where the head leads and with many traumatic mechanisms the skull will often represent the first point of impact. Hypothermia is common in the injured pediatric patient. They are more prone to this

complication given their ratio of body surface area (BSA) to body size (highest at birth and decreasing as they reach adulthood). The skeletal structure of the child also changes with age and in younger children is often incompletely calcified. The absence of an overlying bony injury or fracture in no way rules out the possibility of a deeper insult. This is particularly important when evaluating a child for an injury to the lung (contusion) or the hepatosplenic axis. These unique anatomical differences result in well-recognized common mechanisms and associated patterns of disease (Table 49-4).

The goal of trauma assessment and management, no matter what age, remains the same: airway, breathing, and circulation. The anatomical and physiological differences as discussed in this chapter will prepare you to manage the emergency airway of a child as well as avoid the common pitfalls. It is important to remember that ventilatory abnormalities in children herald impending cardiac arrest unless managed aggressively and properly for age. The recognition of poor perfusion and shock is a critical step in stabilization. The patient should have two large bore IVs secured and if the provider is unable to do so after two failed attempts in an unstable patient an interosseous line should be placed. Capillary refill in a child may provide a better indication of perfusion since children possess extraordinary compensatory mechanisms. As such, measurable hypotension is a late finding. Fluid boluses are indicated and should be given rapidly by IV push 20 mL/kg (NS or LR) to be repeated once adequate perfusion is not restored. If the patient continues to have signs of shock a transfusion is indicated and should be given at 10 mL/kg bolus packed red blood cells. Reassessment of the patient after any and all interventions should be performed on an ongoing basis.

Nonaccidental trauma is a leading cause of death in infants (age <1 year). A high index of suspicion should be maintained when the history contains multiple traumatic emergency visits to multiple health centers, if there is a discrepancy in the history, late presentation of a child with injury, if the parents are perceived to be responding inappropriately, or if the history changes or does not match the severity of injury. There are some types of injury findings that should increase concern for nonaccidental trauma (**Box 49-1**).

It is important to note that the list is not inclusive of all indicators for child abuse and injury. If you suspect a child's injury is secondary tovnonaccidental trauma it is imperative to initiate further investigation by alerting the appropriate services in your area.

TABLE 49-4 Pediatric Injury Patterns	
Mechanism of Injury	Common Patterns of Injury
Motor vehicle collision (child passenger)	Unrestrained: multiple trauma, head and neck injuries, scalp and facial lacerations
	Restrained: chest and abdomen injuries, lower spine fractures (especially if improperly restrained)
Motor vehicle vs child pedestrian	Low speed: lower extremity fractures
	High speed: multiple trauma, head and neck injuries, scalp and facial lacerations
Fall from Height	Low height: upper extremity fractures
	Medium height: head and neck injuries, upper and lower extremity fractures
	High height: multiple trauma, head and neck injuries, upper and lower extremity fractures
Fall from bicycle	Without helmet: head and neck injury, scalp and facial injury, upper extremity fractures
	With helmet: upper extremity injury
	Striking handlebars: intra-abdominal injury

Modified from data in *ATLS: Advanced Trauma Life Support for Doctors (Student Course Manual)*, 8th ed. American College of Surgeons; 2008:245.

Box 49-1

Injury Findings That Should Increase Concern for Nonaccidental Trauma

Bruising in preambulatory children

—(or bruising in ambulatory children that is not explained by normal developmental milestones)

Injuries that do not match expected activity patterns

—(such as ears, inner arms or legs, buttocks, or trunk)

Injury or bruising to genitals or perianal area

Hematoma of the tragus of the ear

Scars or injuries in the shape of objects

Traumatic intracranial injuries in children under 2 years

—(for which there is no plausible explanation)

Rib or metaphyseal fractures in young children

Multiple fracture or fractures of varying age

Long bone or pelvic fractures in perambulatory children

—(or for which there is no plausible explanation)

Traumatic intra-abdominal injury

Concerning patterns of burns

NEUROLOGICAL

The challenging complaint of altered level of consciousness (ALOC) is often caused by serious pathology requiring aggressive investigation and treatment due to potential for significant irreversible damage. Given the considerable differential diagnoses that may lead to altered mental status (AMS) the primary assessment should be a rapid evaluation of airway, breathing, and circulation followed by a systematic, organized approach to history, and physical examination with particular attention to neurological examination and potential exposures to toxins. The primary evaluation of an altered child after initial ABCs will include exposure and disability. Important cutaneous findings include signs of infection (petechiae, purpura), shock (mottled appearance), organ failure (jaundice), and trauma are easily appreciated. The neurological examination (disability) is crucial. It should include evaluation of the respiratory pattern, any distinct breath odors, funduscopy, eye position, pupillary response, extraocular muscle movement, and the ability to follow both verbal and motor commands. A modified Glasgow coma scale is also used in the neurologic evaluation for children with ALOC (**Table 49-5**). Documentation of the initial physical examination is crucial as both administered medications and disease progression may change the examination findings. Potentially reversible causes for AMS such as hypoxia, opiate intoxication, and low blood glucose ought to be assessed quickly and as part of the initial resuscitation. The difficulty in assessing a patient with ALOC is not only due to the extensive differential but also to the limited ability to gather a detailed clear history. However, a detailed history should be attempted and should include questions about all medications or toxins in the house, potential exposure to trauma or ingestion, recent illness, past medical history of patient, prior history of similar episodes, vomiting or diarrheal episodes, and fever. A common mnemonic for remembering possible etiologies for AMS is listed in **Table 49-6**. The list is by no means exhaustive but merely a starting point for further diagnostic studies. After initial stabilization diagnostic

TABLE 49-5	Glasgow and Children's Coma Scale	
Glasgow	Children's	Score
Eye opening		
Spontaneous	Spontaneous	4
To command	To speech	3
To pain	To pain	2
None	None	1
Motor response		
Follows command	Spontaneous	6
Localizes pain	Withdraws to touch	5
Withdraws to pain	Withdraws to pain	4
Abnormal flexion (decorticate)	Abnormal flexion	3
Abnormal extension (decerebrate)	Abnormal extension	2
No response	No response	1
Verbal response		
Oriented	Coos, babbles, age-appropriate verbalizations	5
Confused	Irritable cry	4
Inappropriate words	Cries to pain	3
Incomprehensible	Moans, grunts	2
No response	No response	1 (Modified from Taylor, APLS)

Modified with permission from Strange GR, Ahrens WR, Schafermeyer RW, Wiebe RA, eds. Pediatric Emergency Medicine, 3rd ed. New York: McGraw-Hill; 2009. Table 6-1.

TABLE 49-6	Etiology of Altered Mental Status (Based on the Mnemonic "Tips From the Vowels")	
Mnemonic Device	Category	Cause
A	Abuse	Head trauma
		Shock
E	Epilepsy (and other causes of seizures)	Hypernatremia
		Hypocalcemia
		Hypoglycemia
		Hyponatremia
		Postictal state
		Status epilepticus
	Endocrine	Addison disease
		Hyperthyroidism
		Hypothyroidism
		Inborn errors of metabolism
	Electrolyte disorders	Hypercalcemia
		Hypernatremia
		Hyponatremia
I	Infection	Brain abscess
		Encephalitis
		Meningitis
		Sepsis
		Subdural empyema
	Intussusception	Neurologic presentation
O	Overdose	Alcohol
		Carbon monoxide
		Lead
		Opiates
		Salicylates
		Sedatives
U	Uremia (and other metabolic causes)	Hemolytic uremic syndrome
		Hepatic encephalopathy
		Hypoxia
		Renal failure
		Reye syndrome
T	Trauma	Child abuse
		Head trauma
		Hemorrhage
	Tumor	
I	Insulin-related problems	Diabetic ketoacidosis (DKA)
		Hyperglycemia
		Hypoglycemia
		Ketotic hypoglycemia
		Nonketotic hypoglycemia
P	Psychogenic	Diagnosis of exclusion
S	Shock	Anaphylactic
		Cardiogenic
		Hemorrhagic
		Hypovolemic
		Neurogenic
		Septic
	Stroke (and other CNS lesions)	Arteriovenous malformations
		Hemorrhage
	Shunt-related problems	Hydrocephalus
		Shunt dysfunction

Modified with permission from Strange GR, Ahrens WR, Schafermeyer RW, Wiebe RA, eds. Pediatric Emergency Medicine, 3rd ed. New York: McGraw-Hill; 2009. Table 6-1.

studies should be ordered and reviewed so that appropriate management is initiated in a timely fashion.

Hypoglycemia is a reversible cause of AMS and if not treated leads to coma, seizures, and irreversible brain injury. Presenting complaints for hypoglycemia often include focal neurological deficits and may be evaluated for other etiologies before lab values return with the correct diagnosis. Rapid blood glucose testing should be completed as part of the initial resuscitation and immediate treatment given to relieve symptoms. A blood glucose below 50 mg/dL is considered hypoglycemic and replacement may be given according to the "rule of 50," where the product of the concentration of glucose and volume (mL/kg) equal 50 (ie, 5 mg/kg of 10% dextrose). Further diagnostic evaluation of underlying causes for low blood glucose levels are indicated as multiple etiologies exist and possible rebound hyperglycemia may develop.

Syncope is a common presenting complaint to the emergency department. A thorough history and physical are essential as both intrinsic and extrinsic factors may trigger the event. Questions about drug use, supplement use, recent illness, vomiting, diarrhea, menses length and duration, activities just prior to event, or history of palpitations will help focus your investigation. Postural vital signs and an electrocardiogram are indicated as well as a pregnancy test in reproductive-aged females. Depending on the history, intravenous fluids, lab testing, radiological imaging, and urine testing may be indicated. It is important to understand the activity just prior to or at the time of syncope may indicate a significant cardiac pathology such as hypertrophic cardiomyopathy or arrhythmia. The majority of syncopal episodes in children, however, are due to non-life-threatening origins.

Seizures are a common presenting complaint in the pediatric emergency care setting. A myriad of etiologies, treatment modalities and diagnostic decisions result when a child presents with a shaking "spell." It is of upmost importance to gather a detailed history of the event and medical history: length of episode, description of episode, history of similar episodes, history of seizure disorder, antiseizure medications, age of child, and presence of fever. The return to baseline mental status is something that should be assessed and confirmed with caregiver to ensure that the patient does not have continued seizure activity.

Poisoning in children may have significant morbidity and mortality if toxins are not appropriately identified and treated. The history may provide a known toxin and quantity but often the ingestion is unknown and the clinical picture is one of altered mental status with no known toxin exposure. There are several known toxidromes that will assist in determining the type of exposure and therefore the choice of an appropriate antidote or supportive care (discussed in Chapter 46).

Management of suspected or known ingestions is variable depending on the toxin; however, there are several supportive measures that are universal. The initial assessment should include airway, breathing, and circulation evaluation and stabilization. Activated charcoal (1 g/kg in children under 6 years and 50-100 g in adolescent and adults) is most effective when administered within the first hour of ingestion and is noted to be effective in multiple doses with antimalarials, theophylline, barbiturates, carbamazepine, and dapsone. If the ingestion is known to be nontoxic the routine use of activated charcoal is not indicated. For caustic ingestions milk or water in small doses may be indicated. The induction of emesis and the use of cathartics are no longer recommended for management of suspected toxic exposures. Whole bowel irrigation decreases the time of absorption and should be considered in cases of iron, lead, lithium, delayed release calcium channel blockers, or in the case of drug packers. The dose is 100 to 200 mL/h (in small children 1-2 L/h) until the bowel contents are noted to be clear on defecation (roughly 4-6 hours). IV access should be secured and labs drawn. If an elevated anion gap metabolic acidosis is noted, an osmolar gap should be calculated to evaluate for toxic alcohol ingestion. Acetaminophen and salicylate levels should be included in a typical toxicologic workup as well as measurable levels of accessible or prescribed medications. The levels of various medications will dictate the need for antidote or, in some cases, dialysis. Disposition of the poisoned patient will depend on the substance ingested, the onset of action, level of toxicity, safety of discharge, education for accidental ingestion, and the need for continued monitoring.

TABLE 49-7 BLS Equipment and Supplies for Ambulances

Essential

Oropharyngeal airways: infant, child, adult (sizes 00-5)

Self-inflating resuscitation bag: child and adult sizes*

Masks for bag-valve-mask device: infant, child, and adult sizes

Oxygen masks: infant, child, and adult sizes

Nonrebreathing mask: pediatric and adult sizes

Stethoscope

Backboard

Cervical immobilization device‡

Blood pressure cuff infant, child, and adult sizes

Portable suction unit with a regulator

Suction catheters: tonsil-tip and 6-14 Fr

Extremity splints: pediatric sizes

Bulb syringe

Obstetric pack

Thermal blanket§

Water-soluble lubricant

Desirable

Infant car seat‖

Nasopharyngeal airways: sizes 18-34 Fr, or 4.5-8.5 mm¶

Glasgow coma scale reference

Pediatric Trauma Score reference

Small stuffed toy

Modified with permission from Strange GR, Ahrens WR, Schafermeyer RW, Wiebe RA, eds. Pediatric Emergency Medicine, 3rd ed. New York: McGraw-Hill; 2009. Table 48-2.

TABLE 49-8 ALS Equipment and Supplies for Ambulances

All ALS ambulances should carry everything on the BLS list, plus the following items:

Essential

Transport monitor

Defibrillator with adult and pediatric paddles

Monitoring electrodes: pediatric sizes

Laryngoscope with straight blades 0-2, curved blades 2-4

Endotracheal tube stylets: pediatric and adult sizes

Endotracheal tubes: uncuffed sizes 2.5-6.0, cuffed sizes

Magill forceps: pediatric and adult

Nasogastric tubes: 8-16 Fr

Nebulizer

IV catheters: 16-24 gauge

Intraosseous needles

Length/weight-based drug dose chart or tape

Needles: 20-25 gauge

Resuscitation drugs and IV fluids that meet the local standards of practice

Desirable

Blood glucose analysis system

Disposable CO_2 detection device

Modified with permission from Strange GR, Ahrens WR, Schafermeyer RW, Wiebe RA, eds. Pediatric Emergency Medicine, 3rd ed. New York: McGraw-Hill; 2009. Table 148-3.

The unique anatomical and physiological difference found in pediatric patients necessitates a specialized set of skills in both the initial history taking and examination. These variables also place this population of patients at risk for certain injury and exposure patterns. The physical and neurological development during these formative years is profoundly impacted by significant injury and disease, making the opportunity for successful intervention and treatment rewarding.

PREHOSPITAL EQUIPMENT

The Committee on Ambulance Equipment and Supplies and the National Emergency Medical Services for Children Resource Alliance has developed lists of BLS (**Table 49-7**) and ALS (**Table 49-8**) equipment to be carried on ambulances. This represents an expert consensus recommendation and not a regulatory determination.

KEY POINTS

- The EMS physician must have a thorough knowledge and understanding of pediatric anatomy, physiology, and the pathophysiology of common pediatric diseases states and injury.

- Airway compromise must be the first focus of pediatric assessment and resuscitation.

- The EMS physician should be familiar with the *pediatric assessment triangle* as well as other unique assessment skills and clinical skills that are necessary to provide care for the critically ill or injured children, especially since exposure to such cases is infrequent.

REFERENCES

1. Kannikeswaran N, Mahajan PV, Dunne RB, Compton S, Knazik SR. Epidemiology of pediatric transports and non-transports in an urban Emergency Medical Services system. *Prehosp Emerg Care*. October-December 2007;11(4):403-407.

2. Babl FE, Vinci RJ, Bauchner H, et al. Pediatric pre-hospital advanced life support care in an urban setting. *Pediatr Emerg Care*. 2001;17:5-9.

3. Hofer CK, Ganter M, Tucci M, Klaghofer R, Zollinger A. How reliable is length-based determination of body weight and tracheal tube size in the paediatric age group? The Broselow tape reconsidered. *Br J Anaesth*. February 2002;88(2):283-285.

4. Graves L, Chayen G, Peat J, O'Leary F. A comparison of actual to estimated weights in Australian children attending a tertiary children's' hospital, using the original and updated APLS, Luscombe and Owens, Best Guess formulae and the Broselow tape. *Resuscitation*. March 2014 ;85(3):392-396.

5. Abdel-Rahman SM, Ahlers N, Holmes A, et al. Validation of an improved pediatric weight estimation strategy. *J Pediatr Pharmacol Ther*. April 2013;18(2):112-121.

6. Abdel-Rahman SM, Paul IM, James LP, Lewandowski A; Best Pharmaceuticals for Children Act-Pediatric Trials Network. Evaluation of the Mercy TAPE: performance against the standard for pediatric weight estimation. *Ann Emerg Med*. October 2013;62(4):332-339.e6.

7. O'Neil J, Steele GK, Weinstein E, Collins R, Talty J, Bull MJ. Ambulance transport of noncritical children: emergency medical service providers' knowledge, opinions, and practice. *Clin Pediatr (Phila)*. March 2014;53(3):250-255.

8. Stroud MH, Trautman MS, Meyer K, et al. Pediatric and neonatal interfacility transport: results from a national consensus conference. *Pediatrics*. August 2013;132(2):359-366.

9. Jørgensen DE, Vejlstrup N, Jørgensen C, et al. Prenatal detection of congenital heart disease in a low risk population undergoing first and second trimester screening. *Prenat Diagn* 2015 Apr;35(4):325-330.

10. Gausche M, Seidel JS. Out-of-hospital care of pediatric patients. *Pediatr Clin North Am*. 1999;46:1305-1327.

11. Seidel JS, Henderson DP, Ward P, et al. Pediatric prehospital care in urban and rural areas. *Pediatrics*. 1991;88:681-690.

CHAPTER 50

Geriatric Patients

Teresita M. Hogan
Andrew Young
Jared Novack

INTRODUCTION

Adults aged 65 years and older are the foremost utilizers of EMS and are at excess risk for adverse events.[1] Studies overwhelmingly agree this high level of use by older adults is appropriate.[2-6] Elders have greater needs for emergency care than other age groups.[7] They are often acutely ill and nearly 30% of elder EMS patients require high intensity care. The potential exists for the elder population to overwhelm EMS networks due to their numbers and their complex interwoven needs that do not fit neatly into our systems design. EMS was designed for acute emergent action not for the multifaceted nuanced concerns experienced by our nation's elders. Understanding the full scope of this issue is essential to define opportunities for targeted improvements in practice and policy, thereby preparing EMS providers and systems for the oncoming geriatric tsunami.

OBJECTIVES

- Describe common physiological differences in geriatric patients.
- Describe common causes of altered mental status in geriatric patients.
- Describe key physiological differences in elderly patients relating to the prehospital care of trauma-related emergencies.
- Discuss blood thinning medications and the prehospital evaluation and management of geriatric patients.
- Describe common social and economic issues affecting overall health and well-being of geriatric patients.
- Describe the special features of the prehospital evaluation and management of nursing home and long-term care facility patients.
- Describe the initial prehospital evaluation and management of suspected elder abuse and neglect.

The aging demographic is well documented. In 2012, over 40 million people in the United States are aged 65 and older. This number is projected to more than double to 89 million in 2050. By 2050 fully one-fifth of the US population will be ages 65 and older.[8] Otherwise stated, from 2000 to 2050 the number of older adults is projected to increase by 135%, with those aged 85 years and older increasing by 350%.[9] This is particularly crucial since those over 85 have the highest rate of EMS transport.[10] The proportion of elder EMS use increases from 27% among those aged 65 to 84 years to 48% among those older than 85 years.[11] This could result in even greater proportions of the older and most complex EMS patients.[12]

Medicine's improving ability to treat disease has increased illness prevalence in elders,[13] augmenting demand for EMS beyond those of population numbers alone. Our health care workforce has a shortage of paraprofessional providers to meet this demographic need.[14] With age come illnesses not seen in younger persons, and atypical presentations of many diseases. Medical diagnosis and management of elders is complex and significantly different than in younger individuals. Symptoms are nonspecific and mask severe problems with high morbidity and mortality; comorbidities are common, and treatments vary. This requires existing providers to master geriatric issues.

The impact of the elder population on EMS can be anticipated and focuses on four main areas:

1. On the provider level, deficiencies in geriatric specific education have been acknowledged.[15] The need for paramedical personnel to train in geriatric topics prompted the American Geriatrics Society and the National Council of State EMS Training Coordinators to develop an optional course, "Geriatrics Education for EMS," which is now available to interested EMS providers.[16] As documented by the Institute of Medicine (IOM), geriatric specific competencies must be achieved and maintained: "Recommendation 4.2: All licensure, certification, and maintenance of certification for health care professionals should include demonstration of competence in the care of older adults as a criterion."[17] Reports such as this from the IOM may soon mandate compliance with geriatric specific education to maintain professional certification.

2. Since the 1990s, elders have required more time and resources, and had higher rates of admission to both the hospital and critical care units.[18-20] Older adults now compel a higher level of EMS to meet a greater proportion of severe illness, with life-threatening incidents occurring 5.2 times more frequently in this population.[21]

3. Current EMS are not set up for the needs of our aging population.[22-24] A true paradigm shift needs to occur from the current structure of emergency services delivery limited to acute interventions, to a broader model capable of managing complex subacute issues with acute decompensation. Providers will likely also face a change in focus from treatment of acute to more chronic illness.[14]

4. Finally, EMS must better manage transitions from long-term care, nursing homes, and elder day care facilities to optimize connections between patients using these entities and the modes of health care they require.[25]

ELDER PHYSIOLOGIC DIFFERENCES

Predictable physiologic changes occur as a function of aging, although the onset of these changes varies by many years among individuals. These can be general in nature or specific to an isolated organ system, thereby causing very specific failure of function. Some geriatric medical texts describe "the 1% rule" that most organ systems lose function at roughly 1% a year, beginning around age 30. Loss of function is undetected until a critical or threshold level is crossed. The higher the demand on an organ system, the less loss can be tolerated.

Table 50-1 lists major organ systems, the changes that occur with physiologic aging, and some of their clinical correlates.

ALTERED MENTAL STATUS IN THE GERIATRIC PATIENT

Altered mental status (AMS) is not a diagnosis but is a symptom heralding a wide array of medical, traumatic, and toxicologic syndromes.[26] AMS is found in only 4% to 10% of all ED patients[27] but exists in up to 30% of the elderly patient subset.[28] However, only 20% to 30% of these cases are recognized in the ED, resulting in increased mortality.[29] EMS workers can be pivotal in increasing recognition and improving treatment of this dangerous entity. AMS results from etiologies involving both a primary *central nervous system* (CNS) event as well as a secondary process affecting the CNS. Elderly patients are much more likely to have changes in mental status resulting from a secondary process. AMS has a bimodal distribution across age. Traumatic and toxicologic causes occur much more often in the younger adult, whereas in the elderly, neurologic etiologies and organ system dysfunctions are the most frequent causes of AMS.[30]

Accurate terminology for levels of cognitive impairment is essential for effective communication and treatment across health care settings. This can be seen in **Table 50-2**.

AMS is not a natural consequence of aging. In healthy individuals cognitive function is preserved even at extremes of age. AMS is a manifestation of disease states, toxins, medication interactions, metabolic abnormalities, or trauma. In order to care for geriatric patents any provider must take two important steps. First, eliminate age bias by understanding cognitive impairment is a disease state. Second, divide those with AMS into broad categories:

a. *Chronic alteration of mental status*: This category consists of the dementias, primarily Alzheimer disease. Alzheimer is overwhelmingly common, and it is predicted to attack up to 13.2 million in

TABLE 50-1	Major Organ Systems and Physiologic Aging	
Body Part	Change With Age	Importance in EMS
Brain	Atrophy Dementia	1. Intracranial hemorrhage with little trauma 2. Difficulty obtaining History/Physical, communication issues
Neurologic	Diminished reflexes Loss of proprioception Neuropathy	1. Loss of righting reflex causes falls 2. Loss of gag causes aspiration pneumonia
Teeth	Loss of dentition	1. Difficulty holding seal for bag ventilation
Ears	Hearing loss Vestibular dysfunction	1. Communication difficulty 2. Dizziness and fall risk
Eyes	Cataracts Arcus senilis Periorbital fat loss	1. Lens is cloudy, loss of visual acuity causes falls, and MVCs 2. White ring circling the cornea mistaken for trauma 3. Sunken eye mistaken for dehydration
Skin	Loss of collagen and elastin	1. Tenting at euvolemic levels mistaken for dehydration 2. Easy skin breakdown causing pressure ulceration with collar and backboard use or laying immobile on bed/floor
Neck	Decreased joint motion Increased spinal curvature	1. Propensity to fracture 2. Difficulty bagging and intubating 3. Need for special padding with immobilization
Chest wall	Loss of elasticity	1. Difficulty assessing breathing 2. More pulmonary injury with mild trauma 3. Easy rib fracture with CPR/hand placement important 4. Inability to see flail chest segments
Blood vessels	Atherosclerosis	1. Occult hypotension[a] 2. Delayed capillary refill without shock/vessel injury 3. Decreased distal pulses 4. Increased aortic dissections (medical and traumatic)
Heart	Decreased cardiac output Chronic Ischemic disease Conduction abnormalities	1. Loss of physiologic reserve 2. Congestive heart failure 3. Less response to medications 4. Edema to legs/feet 5. More frequent syncope 6. Ischemia and Infarction without pain 7. Stroke risk, dysrhythmias common
Lung	Diminished capacity	1. Loss of physiologic reserve 2. Easier fatigability and dyspnea 3. Use decreased tidal volumes when bagging
Abdomen	Decreased core muscle tone	1. Loss of guarding and rigidity with intraperitoneal bleeding or infection
Bones and Joints	Osteoporosis arthritis Increased spinal curvature at all levels	1. Chronic pain 2. Easy fractures 3. Easy falls 4. Decreased mobility 5. Need for special pads to immobilize
Extremities	Decreased muscle tone and mass Varicose veins Poor circulation	1. Loss of strength, increasing falls 2. Dependent edema, chronic skin changes 3. DVT risk 4. Ischemic risk

[a]Occult hypotension = state of shock or decreased perfusion not detected by routine vital sign measures

the United States by 2050.[31] Alzheimer is a chronic slowly progressive terminal disease and the sixth leading cause of death in elders.[32]

b. *Acute worsening of chronically altered mental status:* This is the second most common category encountered by EMS personnel and usually

results from a secondary process that affects the CNS. Overall, it should be understood that almost any disorder could cause AMS in elderly patients.[33]

c. *Acute alteration of baseline normal mental status:* This is the least common of all causes of AMS in elders encountered by EMS.

TABLE 50-2	Terminology in Altered Mental States
Term	Finding
Clouding of consciousness	Impaired capacity to think clearly and perceive
Confusion	Alteration in higher functions (memory, awareness)
Stupor	Less alert than usual, but not asleep
Obtundation	Appears asleep when not stimulated arouses easily
Coma	Unresponsive

Causes of AMS in the elderly population are distinct from those in younger patients. **Table 50-3** lists broad categories of AMS etiologies, more specific examples in each category, and percentages of elders who present with each category of AMS.

The key in assessment of AMS in elders is to *establish the new mental state in comparison to the baseline for that particular patient.* As the first health care provider on the scene, the paramedic has the opportunity to identify the acute problem as well as to establish the patient's baseline level of function. If the patient is stable, this baseline should be determined by whatever means possible. This may mean speaking to the patient, family members, or caregivers. In order to obtain this baseline level, ask about memory problems, ability to ambulate, communicate, and perform self-care. Second establish the timeframe over which this change has occurred. Did the change take months, days, or minutes? Does the change wax and wane? Query the caregivers about any possible precipitants. Was there a recent fall? Are there any medication changes? Also, simply ask what the caregiver thinks is going on. Finally, and perhaps more importantly, obtain contact information for the caregiver, so that future providers can quickly contact them.

EMS providers caring for elders must distinguish between two key situations:

1. *Delirium*: An abrupt disorientation for time and place, usually with illusions and hallucinations. The mind wanders, speech may be incoherent, and the patient is in a state of confusion. Additionally they can experience extremes of arousal and activity ranging from extreme excitement or agitation to acutely decreased consciousness and motor activity. This low slow activity is often unrecognized as delirium.

2. *Dementia*: A slow progressive loss of awareness for time and place, usually with inability to learn new things or remember recent events. The person may be lost in a time years prior to today. Remote memories may be intact. Total loss of function and regression to an infantile state may eventually result.[10]

The distinction between delirium and dementia is critical (**Table 50-4**). Delirium is an acute, reversible, potentially life-threatening problem that requires extreme emergency care. Acute change in mental status is a key feature of delirium. Delirium is a potentially life-threatening medical emergency.[34] Patients with delirium generally have underlying acute medical conditions that require rapid diagnosis and treatment.[35] It is usually important to describe delirium as a symptom secondary to some other disease process. This alerts the provider to discover the acute process underlying the delirium. Dementia, on the other hand, is very slowly progressive and requires support, but it is not an emergency treatment

TABLE 50-3	Causes of Acute AMS in Elder EMS Patients	
Category	Example	Percentage
Infection	UTI, pneumonia, meningitis, sepsis, acute abdomen	30-40
Medications/toxins	Anticholinergic, benzodiazepine, narcotics, alcohol	20-40
Neurologic	Stroke, seizure mass lesion	20-30
Metabolic	Electrolyte, endocrine, uremic, hepatic	15-25
Cardiovascular	AMI, hypertensive emergency, vasculitis	5-7

TABLE 50-4	Criteria Defining Delirium and Dementia	
Delirium		Dementia
Abrupt		Gradual
Reduced attention		Impaired recent memory
Disorganized thinking		Regression
At least two of the following:		
Reduced level of consciousness		Disjointed thinking
Perceptual disturbance -hallucinations, illusions		Poor judgment
Increased or decreased psychomotor activity		Loss of mental function

priority. Remember, comparing each patient to himself or herself in the recent past is the best clue to a critical problem. An acute or rapid deterioration signals delirium. Slow progression signals dementia.

GERIATRIC TRAUMA

Compared to younger people, elder patients frequently sustain injury as a direct result of their underlying medical conditions. Due to aging, the majority of these injuries are more severe and more difficult to diagnose and treat.[36] There are two key concepts to understanding geriatric trauma.

1. Physiologic changes make trauma increasingly more serious with advancing age:

   a. Identical mechanisms can cause more severe immediate injury in older adults as well as greater delayed or internal injuries.

   b. Vital signs may be normal in elders even in states of severe shock.[37]

   c. Physical examination can underrepresent extent of injury in older adults.

   d. Lower physiologic reserve can decrease ability to recover.

2. Trauma is often the direct result of underlying medical conditions. These conditions must often be addressed simultaneously with the treatment of injuries to stabilize the patient.

The older patient will likely require more interventions than the younger patient with identical injuries. This includes EMS evaluation and treatment, ED evaluation and treatment, surgical care, intensive care unit services, and all care up to and including rehabilitation. However, even obviously severely injured elders are less likely than younger patients to receive care in a trauma center.[37] The selective undertriage of elder patients with severe injury to level one trauma centers by EMS providers is well documented.[38-40]

The usually accepted physiologic triage variables of blood pressure and heart rate are not useful predictors of level one trauma interventions or mortality in older adults.[38] In fact, in trauma, the mortality of older adults increases at systolic blood pressure readings <110 mm Hg.[41] So vital signs considered normal in younger populations may represent shock in patients aged over 65 years. The finding of decreased end organ perfusion in the face of normal blood pressure and heart rate readings is termed *occult hypotension* and has been noted in over 40% of injured older adults.[42] The failure of trauma center diversion based on occult hypotension is high.

Low impact mechanisms such as ground level falls are known to cause severe traumatic injury and result in high mortality in older adults.[43] Simple ground level falls are reported to result in 34.6% of all deaths in elder patients.[44] The failure of trauma center diversion based on low-level mechanisms is high.

The Guidelines for the Field Triage of Injured Patients 2012[45] are the newest guiding principles from the American College of Surgeons, the Centers for Disease Control (CDC), and the National Highway Traffic Safety Administration (**Box 50-1**). These guidelines are intended to help prehospital providers select the most appropriate destination hospital for an individual patient. The new guidelines recognize that physiologic, anatomic, and mechanism of injury criteria all fail to identify older adults in need of level one trauma center care. They now propose a fourth level criteria or "Special Considerations" to correct this high rate of undertriage to level one centers for older adults.

SPINAL IMMOBILIZATION IN GERIATRIC TRAUMA INCLUDING GROUND LEVEL FALLS

Spinal immobilization is one of the most frequently performed EMS procedures. The topic of whether or not EMS providers can safely avoid immobilization is pertinent especially in elder patients who are at high risk of low mechanism fracture. A desire to avoid immobilization stems from elders who may not tolerate these devices and who are in jeopardy for skin breakdown and pressure ulceration. Fragile elder skin can breakdown in as little as 90 minutes on a backboard. Protocols to decrease immobilization performed variably well with respect to identification of patients with fracture; however, all were in agreement that they should be used with caution at extremes of age".[46] Immobilize the older adult spine earlier and for lesser indications than in the young. Fractures occur even in patients who are ambulatory posttrauma. Older patients especially those with arthritis sustain spinal injury with a lesser mechanism than younger more flexible patients.

Proper immobilization of elders requires the use of support pads as well as cushion pads. Support pads support areas of curvature above the plane of the backboard. EMS directors should consider specialized removable pads for older patients to support the areas behind the head, neck, and low back. Support pads serve to maintain comfort and ensure full immobilization. Additionally, because older patients have thin skin that can quickly be damaged simply by the weight of their body on a hard surface, cushion pads under pressure point areas of the sacrum, back, shoulders, and occiput should be used to minimize pressure ulcers. Cervical collars should be carefully fit to avoid pressure on the chin and sternum additionally cushion pads may need to be placed at these points. TCommercial backboards with support padding and cushion padding are now available from various manufacturers. If numbers of elder trauma transports are high systems should consider investing in this equipment.

GERIATRIC FALLS

Falls are a significant health risk in the older population and frequently have multiple causes. The scope of this problem is truly enormous with one-third of all people above age 65 and one-half of all people above age 85 sustaining at least one fall annually. Most falls occur at home, thus the EMS provider has the only opportunity to assess the fall where it occurs. Recognition and treatment of any acute illness that has contributed to the fall are as critical as is acquiring information about the patient and environment that can be useful in preventing future falls. To help gather this diverse information the FALLS mnemonic below may be helpful (**Box 50-2**).

Two actions are required from any prehospital care provider responding to a patient who sustained a fall:

1. Evaluate injuries suffered as a result of the fall itself.

2. Evaluate for a medical cause of the fall.

Falls in the elderly are a sentinel event. The fall itself is often the presenting symptom of a person's underlying medical deterioration. Every fallen elder should be evaluated for the underlying cause of the fall.

THE ANTICOAGULATED PATIENT

The use of oral anticoagulation in older adults is quite prevalent as anticoagulation is beneficial for the treatment of:

- Nonvalvular atrial fibrillation
- Congestive heart failure
- Cardioembolic CVA
- Valvular heart disease and prosthetic heart valves
- Ischemic heart disease
- Left ventricular dysfunction
- Venous thromboembolic disease, including pulmonary embolism and deep vein
- Peripheral vascular disease.

Approximately 26% of all patients with *intracranial hemorrhage* (ICH) are on anticoagulation therapy and have a doubling in the rate ICH mortality in a dose-dependent manner.[47] About 20% of elders on warfarin therapy also take daily antiplatelet agents.[48] This combined therapy expectedly increases the risk of ICH.[49] Poorly controlled blood pressure while on anticoagulation or antiplatelet therapy is also associated with high rates of ICH.[50] Even modest decreases in blood pressure can decrease ICH by 50%.

The complex topics of anticoagulation risk-benefit assessment, that is, fall risk, compliance, monitoring, and polypharmacy are beyond the scope of this chapter. Our focus is to understand that even mild trauma can have devastating consequences for patients who receive anticoagulation. Risk of traumatic intracranial hemorrhage (TICH) in anticoagulated patients has been underrecognized. Anticoagulated patients with simple ground level falls show a mortality of up to 30%.[51] We now know that with even mild head trauma and a normal Glasgow coma scale as many as 29% of these apparently benign patients sustain TICH. The type of anticoagulation (warfarin, aspirin, or clopidogrel) did not matter.[52]

It is important to note that antiplatelet agent use has increased fivefold since 1999 and is associated with increased incidence of ICH.[53] Recently the pharmacologic industry has developed new anticoagulants such as enoxaparin, prasugrel, fondaparinux, dalteparin, and dabigatran. As with their predecessors, these new agents carry increased risk of complicated bleeding. Some were specifically developed for ease of use, can be taken orally, and do not require serial monitoring.

The most important aspect relating to EMS and anticoagulation is quick identification of anticoagulant use. This may require not only history from patient and caregivers, but also a survey of the household including the refrigerator, as some of these agents require refrigeration. The identification and communication of anticoagulation is very important because there are no simple lab tests to detect or quantify the presence of these newer agents.

The EMS principles of basic care for an acutely bleeding patient remain the same regardless of the presence of anticoagulation. Lacerations should be wrapped and direct pressure applied, or proximal pressure in nonresponsive cases. Deep penetrating wounds may be packed. Large bore IV access should be obtained, and fluid resuscitation should be initiated for those with unstable vital signs, remembering that tachycardia may be masked in elders by altered physiology, as well as medications such as β-blockers or digoxin.

Anticoagulation-associated intracranial hemorrhage (AAICH) causes four distinct subtypes.

1. Spontaneous bleed without antecedent trauma.

2. Immediate TICH.

3. Delayed TICH.

4. Expanding TICH—In 50% of patients these strokes can continue to enlarge for 12 to 24 hours.[54]

These entities are responsible for 90% of anticoagulation-associated deaths.[55] Delayed TICH is reported in 1% of anticoagulated elders with head injury.[56] Expansion of existing ICH is also well known. In all cases anticoagulation-associated ICH is a medical emergency as even small hematomas can enlarge and cause damage or death.[57] In an elder with acute AMS look for the use of anticoagulation. If found, consider rapid transport to a high-level center.

Reversal of anticoagulation is essential in TICH. Time to reversal can be excessive even in the best settings. In some neuro-ICUs median reversal time was 30 hours during which hematoma expansion may occur.[58] Treatment options are expanding with introduction of both new anticoagulant agents and new reversal options. Treatment schemes are quite complex and include intravenous vitamin K, fresh frozen plasma, cryoprecipitate, unactivated prothrombin-complex concentrates, and recombinant factor VIIa. Some hospitals may not stock these drugs or use them in a routine manner. These reversal agents also have a high incidence of complications such as anaphylactic reactions,[59] and increased arterial thrombosis causing myocardial and cerebral infarctions.[60] Finally surgical intervention may be necessary in these patients after reversal of the anticoagulation. Thus the CDC guidelines state anticoagulated head injured patients should be preferentially transported to level one trauma centers.[46]

SOCIAL AND ECONOMIC ISSUES IN GERIATRIC PATIENTS

Elderly patients are especially vulnerable to multiple social and economic issues that affect their health and well-being. These contribute to elder use of emergency services. Of foremost impact is the issue of functional decline (FD). FD is the loss of certain abilities due to aging or age-related problems and ranges from high-level functional loss such as the ability to maintain employment or driving. FD is common affecting 12% of elders over 75. Self-care problems result in falls, dehydration, poor nutrition, and poor hygiene. Living alone has also been described as contributing to elder EMS use.

The term *instrumental activities of daily living* (IADL) refers to shopping, housekeeping, finances, cooking, transportation, and telephone use. The term activities of daily living refers to bathing, dressing, toileting, and ability to transfer. These terms define loss of function that most significantly increase need for specific elder services.

Examining elders with recent decline in IADLs or ADLs showed that 65% and 75%, respectively, reported decline directly contributed to need for emergency service.[61] Another study found that immobility or difficulty leaving the house was the primary for elders to call on emergency services.[62]

Access to health care and PCP directly relates to EMS use.[63] Elders without a PCP are 45% more likely to visit the ED than those with better health access. They account for a disproportionate share of ED visits across all levels of illness. This utilization is not explained by other sociodemographic factors. Twenty percent of ED visits by older community dwelling adults could potentially be prevented through primary care.[64]

Medication use, drug-drug interactions and drug-disease interactions cause significant adverse health effects for elders. Elders consume more than 30% of all prescription drugs.[65] Elder adverse drug events contribute to 7% to 11% of all ED visits[66] and 12% of hospital admissions.[67] EMS providers can be key in the identification of medication use, misuse, or drug reaction as the cause of elder patient problems. Obtaining medication history is a priority in the older population; this skill needs to be elevated to the level of acute assessment and not viewed as a tedious requirement.

THE NURSING HOME PATIENT

Nearly 25% of nursing home residents (NHRs) are transported at least once annually to an ED.[68] These patients account for more than 2.2 million ED visits annually in the United States.[69] The vast majority are transferred by ambulance.[70] The numbers are staggering with approximately 1.6 ED visits each year for every NHR in the United States.[71,72] Approximately 8% of all US NHR have one visit to an ED within a given 90 day period.[73] In ineffective transitions of care from NH to the ED and patient safety is quite vulnerable.[74]

NHRs, as a group, present to the ED with medical and surgical problems that differ from community-dwelling older adults.[75] Two-thirds of NHRs who present to the ED have cognitive impairment,[76] making the collection of historical data challenging, and increasing the importance of transfer documentation. However, 10% of NHR are transported to the ED without any written documentation, while important patient information is often missing in the 90% who arrive with paperwork.[76,77] NH personnel similarly report that NHR often return from the ED without notification, written documentation, or recommendations for care.

These facts highlight national challenges on appropriate delivery of health care to the NH population. As a point of frequent contact with NH patients EMS providers are in a unique position to affect positive changes and drive more appropriate health care utilization by this demographic. Clearly many of the most common chief complaints of nursing home patients including chest pain, shortness of breath, AMS, and fever require immediate ED evaluation. Need for ED care is highlighted by the fact that more than 90% of NHR received diagnostic tests, more than 70% received imaging tests, more than 70% underwent procedures, and approximately 70% received medications in the ED. Ultimately about 50% of NHR transported to the ED required hospital admission. As many as 67% of those transferred to an ED are classified as urgent or emergent prior to a physician evaluating the patient.[78]

Data show that it is difficult for EMS providers to serve as the instrument reducing NH to ED transfers due to the complexity of NHR presentations of acute illness. A study of 313 patients concluded that paramedics were not able to accurately determine which patients required ambulance transport or ED care.[79] Another study of 1180 patients showed paramedics with written guidelines have poor accuracy in determining the need for ALS or BLS ED transport, MD evaluation in 24 hours, or no MD care required.[80] This illustrates the difficulty of provider evaluations in reducing transports to the ED from nursing homes. NHRs are medically complex and even the most benign complaint can be masking serious medical emergencies. Although up to 40% of ED visits from nursing homes may be preventable most of these reductions result from the installation of midlevel providers at the NH or by improving patient safety measures and falls prevention.[81]

Numerous unnecessary ED transfers are due to lack of NH staff education and awareness of other viable care options. Many of these transfers are for specialty services such as interventional radiology for g-tube replacement or teams for procedures such as PICC line placement. Such procedures are only available during daytime business hours. Also, many of these services are not emergent so the patient can have the procedure routinely scheduled. Educating prehospital providers on what procedures need to be performed emergently and what can be deferred can lead to reduce transfers.[82]

Questions to address before ED transport:

- Do advanced directives obviate the need for further evaluation or treatment?
- Does the chief complaint require evaluation for emergent threat to life or limb?
- Is there any change from a patient's baseline level of function?
- Are the vital signs normal?
- Is the intervention for which the transfer is made something that the ED can provide at the time?

Another problem unique to nursing home to ED transfers is lack of communication between the referring facility and the ED. Two-thirds of NH to ED transfers present with some cognitive impairment, making obtaining an adequate history from the patient difficult.[83] NH forms become critical in these cases. However, there is poor documentation between NH and EDs.[84] Patients often arrive lacking critical data points including chief complaint, vital signs at the NH, baseline mental status, and advanced directives information.[85,86] Similarly, EDs fail to provide NHs adequate information detailing what care was provided while in the ED. This can result in ED reevaluation.[87] Implementation of a standardized transfer form that requires the referring facility to document certain data points decreases confusion for ED providers and reduces admission rates and length of admissions for nursing home patients. EMS directors should establish a standardized transport form that includes the information shown in **Table 50-5**.

Forms such as these have been shown to increase documentation rates of the listed data points.[88,89] These forms are recommended as an intervention to reduce hospitalizations.[90,91] Studies show that EMS monitoring of appropriate transfer forms completion and reporting results to the NHs director greatly increased full transfer form use.[92] EMS directors should consider implementing a similar feedback system with their regional nursing homes.[93]

TABLE 50-5	Essential Standardized NH Transport Form Content
Nursing home name	
NH contact information	
Name of NH charge nurse	
Patient name	
Patient date of birth	
Patient Social Security number	
Baseline cognitive statue	
Patient DNR status	
Reason for transfer	
NH vital signs	
Name of patient's PCP	

DNR, do not resuscitate; NH, nursing home; PCP, primary care provider.

ELDER ABUSE AND NEGLECT

Elder abuse is a particularly alarming area of elder care. Estimates of the frequency of elder abuse range from 2% to 10%.[94] Many patients who are victims of elder abuse, whether due to dependence of care, dementia, or other chronic diseases are afraid or unable to communicate the circumstances of their abusive situation. Since this issue is hidden, the EMS provider often has the most important role, that of recognition.[95]

Elder mistreatment is broadly defined as actions inflicting unnecessary suffering, injury, pain, loss, or violation of human rights upon a senior. There is an increase in morbidity in identified victims of elder abuse and neglect.[96] And although 95% of hospital care providers and prehospital care providers report believing that abuse is not a rare event, less than 50% have come in contact with what they thought was a case of else abuse.[96] Due to this discrepancy paramedical personnel are likely underreporting events of elder abuse. Therefore, they should be aware of the patient risk factors increasing the likelihood of abuse:

- Poverty
- Ethnic minority status
- Functional disability
- Decreased cognitive status
- History of recent worsening of cognitive status[97]

Currently, there is no federal law concerning elder mistreatment. Many state laws list abuse and neglect concurrently. Also, most state laws define a "mandated reporter" which often includes paramedics or EMTs, who must report suspected elder mistreatment to the appropriate agency.[98] In these states the mandate for prehospital providers to report is no different than that of hospital care providers. EMS directors should be aware of their individual state's laws regarding reporting mistreatment and set their practice guidelines accordingly.

Prehospital care providers should be aware of warning signs for elder mistreatment:

Bruises, cuts that are old or not consistent with current injury

Pattern of injury inconsistent with history

Cigarette/rope burns

Blood on person or clothes

Painful body movements not related to injury

Unaddressed pressure sores

Underweight, frail, or dehydrated appearing

Unclean appearance

Unsafe or unclean environment[6]

Discrimination between mistreatment and findings related to current or past accidental injury is difficult. If there is suspicion of abuse or neglect, findings should be documented objectively in the prehospital assessment note and report should be made to the agency responsible for further investigation. Even if a patient refuses transport, reporting is required. Cases show a social work referral made by EMS is helpful in identifying cases of neglect.[99] Providers need to remember that it would be much better to overreport suspect mistreatment than to underreport.

Overall, EMS detection and intervention in cases of elder abuse requires skilled observations either in repeated calls, findings on history or physical assessment, evaluation of living conditions, and good communication to hospital staff, or social services. This important contribution by EMS providers could drastically improve the patient's quality of life.

THE GERIATRIC EMERGENCY DEPARTMENT

Hospitals across the United States are developing geriatric emergency departments (GEDs). EMS directors are familiar with the concept of "centers of excellence" for given diseases and populations such as trauma center, stroke center, and pediatric ED. These all have specific requirements mandated and certified by external agencies that signify a higher level of care. As yet no external agency reviews GEDs, they are self-designated by each hospital's ownership. So current GEDs range from simple marketing tools with little to distinguish them from an undifferentiated ED, to areas that have only isolated physical plant changes, to departments where unique personnel with geriatric training offer specialized services. To offer better service and outcomes for elder patients takes more than better lighting and nonskid flooring. The American College of Emergency Physicians Geriatric Section and the Society for Academic Emergency Medicine Academy of Geriatric Emergency Medicine are defining domains for systems design to enhance emergency elder care delivery. Once these designs are studied and determined to improve outcomes then we will have standards that can be used to determine the components of geriatric centers of excellence. For now we believe that these components will likely require education of staff in geriatric topics, specific equipment to ensure patient safety, separate policies and protocols written for geriatric issues, and additional personnel to aid with social issues and transitions of care.

SUMMARY

This focus on geriatric patients as a special population is similar to the attention we have applied to other populations such as trauma or pediatric patients. The demographics of our aging population will soon make elder care a large part of what we do. Similar to these special populations, planning for the optimal care of geriatric patients will require changes in training, protocols, policies, and procedures. Let us reeducate, refocus, and retool our systems to best serve these vulnerable patients.

KEY POINTS

- The EMS physician should be familiar with the unique anatomical, physiologic, psychiatric, pathophysiologic, pharmacologic, and sociologic characteristics of the elderly population in order to fully understand how their unique needs must be met in the prehospital environment.
- Altered mental status is usually due to a secondary process and requires an approach with a broad differential diagnosis.
- Physiologic changes with age may mask serious injury or illness.
- "Normal" vital signs for the younger population may actually represent shock state for older patients.
- Anticoagulation with aspirin, Coumadin, clopidogrel, dabigatran (Pradaxa), or other anticoagulants results in a significant increase in the risk for traumatic intracranial hemorrhage even with ground level falls and a GCS of 15.
- New guidelines for field triage of injured patients include special age-related criteria to guide EMS disposition of injured elderly patients to Level I trauma centers.
- Falls should be considered a sentinel event and should be evaluated for traumatic injuries resulting from the fall, as well as potential medical causes for the fall.
- The EMS Physician should encourage EMS providers under their purview to embrace the critical role of serving as a communication liaison between nursing homes and emergency departments.

REFERENCES

1. Wolinsky FD, Liu L, Miller TR, et al. Emergency department utilization patterns among older adults. *J Gerontol A Biol Sci Med Sci.* 2008;63:204-209.
2. Ettinger WH, Casani JA, Coon PJ, Muller DC, Piazza-Appel K. Patterns of use of the emergency department by elderly patients. *J Gerontol.* November 1987;42(6):638-642.
3. Lowenstein SR, Crescenzi CA, Kern DC, Steel K. Care of the elderly in the emergency department. *Ann Emerg Med.* May 1986;15(5):528-535.
4. Nawar EW, Niska RW, Xu J. National Hospital Ambulatory Medical Care Survey: 2005 emergency department summary. *Adv Data.* June 29, 2007;(386):1-32.
5. Roberts DC, McKay MP, Shaffer A. Increasing rates of emergency department visits for elderly patients in the United States 1993 to 2003. *Ann Emerg Med.* June 2008;51(6):769-774. Epub 2007 Dec 11.
6. George G, Jell C, Todd BS. Effect of population ageing on emergency department speed and efficiency: a historical perspective from a district general hospital in the UK. *Emerg Med J.* May 2006;23(5):379-383.
7. Grueneir A, Silver MJ, Rochon PA. Review: emergency department use by older adults: a literature review on trends, appropriateness, and consequences of unmet health care needs. *Med Care Res Rev.* 2011;68:131.
8. Jacobsen LA, Kent M, Lee M, Mather M. America's aging population. *Popul Bull.* 2011;66(1):1-16. http://www.prb.org/pdf11/aging-in-america.pdf.
9. Wiener JM, Tilly J. Population ageing in the United States of America: implications for public programmes. *Int J Epidemiol.* 2002;31(4):776-781.
10. Svenson J. Patterns of use of emergency medical transport: a population-based study. *Amer J of Emerg Med.* 2000;18(2):130-134.
11. Shah MN, Glushak C, Mulliken R, et al. Prediction of emergency medical service utilization by elders. *Acad Emerg Med.* 2003;10:52-58.
12. McCaig LF, Burt CW. National Hospital Ambulatory Medical Care Survey: 2003 emergency department summary. *Adv Data.* 2005;(358):1-38.
13. Crimmins EM. Trends in the health of the elderly. *Annu Rev Public Health.* 2004;25:79-98.
14. Pawlson LG. Chronic illness: implications of a new paradigm for health care. Jt Comm J Qual Improv . 1994;20:33-39.
15. Peterson LN, Fairbanks RJ, Hettimger AZ, Shah MN. Emergency medical service attitudes toward geriatric prehospital care and continuing medical education in geriatrics. *JAGS.* 2009;57:530-535.
16. American Geriatrics Society. National Council of State EMS Training Coordinators, and Jones and Bartlett Publishers. About GEMS: history of GEMS. http://www.gemssite.com/about_history.cfm. Accessed February 13, 2012.
17. Institute of Medicine Committee on the Future Health Care Workforce for Older Americans, Institute of Medicine Report. *Retooling for an Aging America: Building the Health Care Workforce.* 2008. http://www.nap.edu/catalog/12089.html. Accessed February 12, 2012.
18. Strange GR, Chen EH, Sanders AB. Use of emergency departments by elderly patients: projections from a multicenter data base. *Ann Emerg Med.* 1992;21:819-824.
19. Strange GR, Chen EH. Use of emergency departments by elder patients: a five-year follow-up study. *Acad Emerg Med.* 1998;5: 1157-1162.
20. Singal BM, Hedges JR, Rousseau EW, Hogan TM. Geriatric patient emergency visits. Part I: Comparison of visits by geriatric and younger patients. *Ann Emerg Med.* 1992;21:802-807.
21. McConnel CE, Wilson RW. The demand for prehospital emergency services in an aging society. *Soc Sci Med.* 1998;46:1027-1031.
22. Adams JG, Gerson LW. A new model for emergency care of geriatric patients. *Acad Emerg Med.* 2003;10:271-274.
23. Schumacher JG. Emergency medicine and older adults: continuing challenges and opportunities. *Amer J of Emerg Med.* 2005;23:556-560.
24. Aminzadeh F, Dalziel WB. Older adults in the ED: a systematic review of patterns of use, adverse outcomes, and effectiveness of interventions. *Ann Emerg Med.* 2002;39(3):238-247.
25. Wiener JM, Skaggs J. *Current Approaches to Integrating Acute and Long-term Care Financing and Services. Public Policy Institute #9516.* Washington, DC: American Association of Retired Persons; 1995.

26. American College of Emergency Physicians. Clinical policy for the initial approach to patients presenting with altered mental status. *Ann Emerg Med.* 1999;33:251-280.

27. Cooke J. Depressed consciousness and coma. In: Marx JA, Hockberger RS, Walls RM, et al. eds. *Rosen's Emergency Medicine: Concepts and Clinical Practice.* 7th ed. Philadelphia, PA: Mosby Elsevier; 2010:106-112.

28. Wofford J, Loehr L, Schwartz E. Acute cognitive impairment in elderly ED patients: etiologies and outcomes. *Am J Emerg Med.* 1996;14:649-653.

29. Hustey FM, Meldon SW. The prevalence and documentation of impaired mental status in elderly emergency department patients. *Ann Emerg Med.* 2002;39(3):248-253.

30. Kanich W, Brady WJ, Huff JS, et al. Altered mental status: evaluation and etiology in the ED. *Am J Emerg Med.* 2002;20(7):613-617.

31. Hebert L, Scherr PA, Bienias JL, Bennett DA, Evans DA. Alzheimer disease in the US Population. *Arch Neurol.* 2003;60:1119-1122.

32. Heron MP, Hoyert DL, Murphy SL, et al. Deaths: final data for 2006. *Natl Vital Stat Rep.* 2009;57(14):1-34.

33. Singal BM, Hedges JR, Rousseau EW, et al. Geriatric patient emergency visits. Part 1: comparison of visits by geriatric patients and younger patients. *Ann Emerg Med.* 1992;21:802-807.

34. Inouye SK. Delirium in older persons. *N Engl J Med.* 2006;354:1157-1165.

35. Sanders AB. Missed delirium in older emergency department patients: a quality-of-care problem. *Ann Emerg Med.* 2002;39:338-341.

36. Lane P, Sorondo B, Kelly J. Geriatric Trauma Patients—are they receiving trauma center care? *Acad Emerg Med.* 2003;10(3):244-250.

37. Lehmann R, Beekley A, Casey L, et al. The impact of advanced age on trauma triage decisions and outcomes: a statewide analysis. *Am J Surg.* 2009;197:571-574.

38. Ma MH, MacKenzie EJ, Alcorta R, Kelen GD. Compliance with prehospital triage protocols for major trauma patients. *J Trauma.* 1999;46:168-175.

39. Phillips S, Rond PC 3rd, Kelly SM, Swartz PD. The failure of triage criteria to identify geriatric patients with trauma: results from the Florida Trauma Triage Study. *J Trauma.* 1996;40:278-283.

40. Chang DC, Bass RR, Cornwell EE, Mackenzie EJ. Undertriage of elderly trauma patients to state-designated trauma centers. *Arch Surg.* 2008;143:776-781.

41. Heffernan DS, Thakkar RK, Monaghan SF, et al. Normal presenting vital signs are unreliable in geriatric blunt trauma victims. *J Trauma.* 2010;69:813-820.

42. Martin JT, Alkhoury F, O'Connor JA, et al. 'Normal' vital signs belie occult hypoperfusion in geriatric trauma patients. *Am Surg.* 2010;76:65-69.

43. Spaniolas K, Cheng JD, Gestring ML, et al. Ground level falls are associated with significant mortality in elderly patients. *J Trauma.* 2010;69:821-825.

44. Chisholm KM, Harruff RC. Elderly deaths due to ground-level falls. *Am J Forensic Med Pathol.* 2010;31:350-354.

45. Sasser SM, Hunt RC, Faul M, et al. Centers for Disease Control and Prevention (CDC). Guidelines for field triage of injured patients: recommendation of the National Expert Panel on Field Triage. *MMWR Recomm Rep.* 2012;13(61):1-20.

46. Stroh G, Braude D. Can. An out-of-hospital cervical spine clearance protocol identify all patients with injuries? An argument for selective immobilization. *Ann Emerg Med.* 2001;37(6):609-615.

47. Rosand J, Eckman MH, Knudsen KA, et al. The effect of warfarin and intensity of anticoagulation on outcome of intracerebral hemorrhage. *Arch Intern Med.* 2004;164(8):880.

48. Shireman TI, Howard PA, Kresowik TF, Ellerbeck EF Combined anticoagulant-antiplatelet use and major bleeding events in elderly atrial fibrillation patients. *Stroke.* 2004;35(10):2362.

49. Dentali F, Douketis JD, Lim W, Crowther M. Combined aspirin-oral anticoagulant therapy compared with oral anticoagulant therapy alone among patients at risk for cardiovascular disease: a meta-analysis of randomized trials. *Arch Intern Med.* 2007;167(2):117-124.

50. Hart RG, Tonarelli SB, Pearce LA. Avoiding central nervous system bleeding during antithrombotic therapy: recent data and ideas. *Stroke.* 2005;36(7):1588.

51. Chisholm KM, Harruff RC. Elderly deaths due to ground-level falls. *Am J Forensic Med Pathol.* 2010;31:350-354.

52. Brewer ES, Reznikov B, Liberma RF, et al. Incidence and predictors of intracranial hemorrhage after minor head trauma in patients taking anticoagulant and antiplatelet medication. *J Trauma.* 2011;70(1):E1-E5.

53. Siracuse JJ, Robich MP, Gautam S, et al. Antiplatelet agents, warfarin, and epidemic intracranial hemorrhage. *Surgery.* 2010;148(4):724-730.

54. Sjöblom L, Hårdemark HG, Lindgren A, et al. Management and prognostic features of intracerebral hemorrhage during anticoagulant therapy: a Swedish multicenter study. *Stroke.* 2001;32(11):2567.

55. Fang MC, Go AS, Chang Y, et al. Death and disability from warfarin-associated intracranial and extracranial hemorrhages. *Am J Med.* 2007;120(8):700.

56. Peck, KA, Sise CB, Shackford SR, et al. Delayed intracranial hemorrhage after blunt trauma: are patients on preinjury anticoagulants and Prescription antiplatelet agents at risk? *J Trauma.* 2011;71(6):1600-1604.

57. Flibotte JJ, Hagan N, O'Donnell J, Greenberg SM, Rosand J. Warfarin, hematoma expansion, and outcome of intracerebral hemorrhage. *Neurology.* 2004;63(6):1059.

58. Lee SB, Manno EM, Layton KF, Wijdicks EF. Progression of warfarin-associated intracerebral hemorrhage after INR normalization with FFP. *Neurology.* 2006;67(7):1272.

59. Yasaka M, Sakata T, Minematsu K, Naritomi H. Correction of INR by prothrombin complex concentrate and vitamin K in patients with warfarin related hemorrhagic complication. *Thromb Res.* 2002;108(1):25.

60. Mayer SA, Brun NC, Begtrup K, et al. Efficacy and safety of recombinant activated factor VII for acute intracerebral hemorrhage. *N Engl J Med.* 2008;358(20):2127.

61. Wilber ST, Blanda M, Gerson LW. Does functional decline prompt emergency department visits and admission in older patients? *Acad Emerg Med.* 2006;13:680-682.

62. Shah MN, Glushak C, Karrison TG, et al. Predictors of emergency medical services utilization by elders. *Acad Emerg Med.* 2003;10(1):52-58.

63. Rosenblatt RA, Wright GE, Baldwin LM, et al. The effect of the doctor-patient relationship on emergency department use among the elderly. *Am J Public Health.* 2000;90(1):97-102.

64. Carter MW, Datti B, Winters JM. ED visits by older adults for ambulatory care sensitive and supply-sensitive conditions. *Am J Emerg Med.* 2006;24(4):428-434.

65. Knight EL, Avorn J. Quality indicators for appropriate medication use in vulnerable elders. *Ann Intern Med.* 2001;135(8 pt 2):703-710.

66. Hohl CM, Dankoff J, Colacone A, Afilalo M. Polypharmacy, adverse drug-related events, and potential adverse drug interactions in elderly patients presenting to an emergency department. *Ann Emerg Med.* 2001;38(6):666-671.

67. Mannesse CK, Derkx FH, de Ridder MA, et al. Contribution of adverse drug reactions to hospital admission of older patients. *Age Ageing.* 2000;29(1):35-39.

68. Bergman H, Clarfield AM. Appropriateness of patient transfer from a nursing home to an acute-care hospital: a study of emergency room visits and hospital admissions. *J Am Geriatr Soc.* 1991;39(12):1164-1168.

69. Wang HE, Shah MN, Allman RM, Kilgore M. Emergency department visits by nursing home residents in the United States. *J Am Geriatr Soc.* 2011;59(10):1864-1872.

70. Wang HE, Shah MN, Allman RM, et al. Emergency department visits by nursing home residents in the United States. *J Am Geriatr Soc.* 2011;59(10):1864-1872.

71. The Kaiser Family Foundation. United States: Total number of residents in certified nursing facilities; 2008-2011. State Health Facts.

http://www.statehealthfacts.org/profileind.jsp?ind=408&cat=8&rgn=1. Accessed May, 2015.

72. Harrington C, Carrillo H, Dowdell M, Tang PP, Blank BW. Nursing facilities, staffing, residents and facility deficiencies, 2005 through 2010. University of California, San Francisco, CA, October 2011. http://thenewsoutlet.org/media/documents/Nursing-Homes/Funding/Harrington-nursing-home-staffing-report.pdf. Accessed May, 2015.

73. Ouslander JG, Lamb G, Perloe M, et al. Potentially avoidable hospitalizations of nursing home residents: frequency, causes, and costs: [see editorial comments by Drs. Jean F. Wyman and William R. Hazzard, pp 760-761]. *J Am Geriatr Soc.* 2010;58(4):627-635.

74. IOM. *Crossing the Quality Chasm: A New Health System for the 21st Century.* Washington, DC: National Academy Press; 2001.

75. Gillick M, Steel K. Referral of patients from long-term to acute-care facilities. *J Am Geriatr Soc.* 1983;31(2): 74-78.

76. Jones JS, Dwyer PR, White LJ, Firman R. Patient transfer from nursing home to emergency department: outcomes and policy implications. *Acad Emerg Med.* 1997;4(9):908-915.

77. Stier PA, Giles BK, Olinger ML, Brizendine EJ, Cordell WH. Do transfer records for extended care–facility patients sent to the emergency department contain essential information? [abstract]. *Ann Emerg Med.* 2001;38(4 suppl):S102.

78. Jensen PM, Fraser F, Shankardass K, et al. Are long-term care residents referred appropriately to hospital emergency departments? *Can Fam Physician.* 2009;55(5):500-505.

79. Hauswald M. Can paramedics safely decide which patients do not need ambulance transport or emergency department care? *Prehosp Emerg Care.* 2002;6(4):383-386.

80. Pointer JE, Levitt MA, Young JC, Promes SB, Messana BJ, Adèr ME. Can paramedics using guidelines accurately triage patients? *Ann Emerg Med.* September 2001;38(3):268-277.

81. Caffrey C. Potentially preventable emergency department visits by nursing home residents: United States, 2004. *NCHS Data Brief.* 2010;(33):1-8.

82. Mercer S, Robinson S. Educating nursing home nurses on efficient use of the emergency department. *J Emerg Nurs.* 2008;34(1):74-76.

83. Wilber ST, Gerson LW, Terrell KM, et al. Geriatric emergency medicine and the 2006 Institute of Medicine reports from the Committee on the Future of Emergency Care in the U.S. health system. *Acad Emerg Med.* 2006;13(12):1345-1351.

84. Gillespie SM, Gleason LJ, Karuza J, et al. Health care providers' opinions on communication between nursing homes and emergency departments. *J Am Med Dir Assoc.* 2010;11(3):204-210.

85. Cwinn MA, Forster AJ, Cwinn AA, et al. Prevalence of information gaps for seniors transferred from nursing homes to the emergency department. *CJEM.* 2009;11(5):462-471.

86. Jones JS, Dwyer PR, White LJ, et al. Patient transfer from nursing home to emergency department: outcomes and policy implications. *Acad Emerg Med.* 1997;4(9):908-915.

87. Terrell KM, Miller DK. Challenges in transitional care between nursing homes and emergency departments. *J Am Med Dir Assoc.* 2006;7(8):499-505.

88. Terrell KM, Brizendine EJ, Bean WF, et al. An extended care facility-to-emergency department transfer form improves communication. *Acad Emerg Med.* 2005;12(2):114-118.

89. LaMantia MA, Scheunemann LP, Viera AJ, Busby-Whitehead J, Hanson LC. Interventions to improve transitional care between nursing homes and hospitals: a systematic review. *JAGS.* 2010;58(4):777-782.

90. Ouslander JG, Lamb G, Tappen R, et al. Interventions to reduce hospitalizations from nursing homes: evaluation of the INTERACT II collaborative quality improvement project. *J Am Geriatr Soc.* 2011;59(4):745-753.

91. Ouslander JG, Perloe M, Givens JH, et al. Reducing potentially avoidable hospitalizations of nursing home residents: Results of a pilot quality improvement project. *J Am Med Dir Assoc.* 2009;10(9):644-652.

92. Davis MN, Brumfield VC, Smith ST, et al. A one-page nursing home to emergency room transfer form: What a difference it can make during an emergency! *Ann Longterm Care.* 2005;13(11):34-38.

93. Ouslander JG, Lamb G, Perloe M, et al. Potentially avoidable hospitalizations of nursing home residents: frequency, causes, and costs: [see editorial comments by Drs. Jean F. Wyman and William R. Hazzard, pp 760-761]. *J Am Geriatr Soc.* 2010;58(4):627-635.

94. Lachs, MS, Pillemer K. Elder abuse. *Lancet.* October 2004;364(9441):1263-1272.

95. Rinker AG Jr. Recognition and perception of elder abuse by prehospital and hospital-based care providers. *Arch Gerontol Geriatr.* 2009;48(1):110-115.

96. Lachs MS, Williams CS, O'Brien S, et al. The mortality of elder mistreatment. *JAMA.* 1998;280(5):428-432.

97. Lachs MS, Williams C, O'Brien S, et al. Risk factors for reported elder abuse and neglect: a nine-year observational cohort study. *Gerontologist.* 1997;37(4):469-474.

98. Adult Protective Services. Institutional Abuse and Long Term Care Ombudsman Program laws. http://www.ncea.aoa.gov/NCEAroot/Main_Site/Library/Laws/APS_IA_LTCOP_Citations_Chart_08-08.aspx. Accessed March 15, 2012.

99. Kue R. Evaluation of an emergency medical services-based social services referral program for elderly patients. *Prehosp Emerg Care.* 2009;13(3):273-279.

CHAPTER 51

Mental Illness and Substance Abuse

Michael P. Wilson

Gary M. Vilke

INTRODUCTION

EMS providers are often called to evaluate patients who are behaving oddly or who are having an emotional or mental crisis. Although these conditions are not necessarily all from diagnosable psychiatric disorders, all involve—to some extent—disorders of thinking. These patients are therefore often labeled as "psychiatric," even if the cause of the patient's symptoms is from another medical condition.

OBJECTIVES

- Discuss the initial prehospital evaluation and management of the acutely psychotic patient.
- Discuss common psychiatric conditions in prehospital patients.
- Discuss the initial prehospital evaluation and management of the suicidal patient.
- Discuss the initial prehospital evaluation and management of the homicidal patient.
- Discuss commonly encountered drugs of abuse and their toxidromes.
- Discuss the involvement of law enforcement in prehospital psychiatric patients.
- Discuss some pitfalls associated with these conditions in the prehospital environment.

BACKGROUND

There are three key points to understanding behaviorally disordered patients. First, patients with odd behavior or who are having a mental or emotional crisis are "real patients." These patients need capable, caring EMS providers just as much as other patients who are suffering from medical conditions that can be treated with a paramedic drug kit. Providers who dismiss many of these patients as "just another psych patient" not only do not appreciate the varied causes of odd behavior, but may also miss an early opportunity to intervene in a potentially life-threatening condition. Second, these patients often present unique challenges to EMS providers. Since these patients often have impaired reasoning about their situation, they may have difficulty giving a history or answering questions like other patients. This can sometimes be frustrating to providers, especially those who are not used to utilizing creativity in order to obtain information. Finally, patients with impaired reasoning skills in chaotic environments may respond unpredictably. More so than with other types of patients, providers must always be mindful of their own safety as well as for others at the scene.

There are very few studies in the literature that specifically investigate prehospital management of behavior-disordered patients. Many of the recommendations in this chapter, therefore, are taken from the much larger literature on emergency department management of these patients. Nonetheless, prehospital providers are the "eyes and ears" of the clinicians who will eventually be treating these patients in the emergency department and will be the ones offering early intervention, which is key in the management of these patients.

COMMONLY ENCOUNTERED BEHAVIORAL CONDITIONS

Behaviorally disordered patients are common in the prehospital setting, although not all conditions have a definable psychiatric diagnosis. Such conditions include agitation and acute psychosis, suicidal patients, and homicidal patients. These conditions are often called *presentations* or *syndromes*, as each is only a label for symptoms which are produced by a variety of medical conditions. Each of these syndromes is discussed in turn.

■ AGITATION AND ACUTE PSYCHOSIS

Agitation and acute psychosis are challenging to specifically define. Most definitions include a disturbance or disorder in thinking with resulting excitement or restlessness on the part of the patient. Most providers "know agitation when they see it." Remarkably, however, most have difficulty defining agitation precisely. Likely this is because individual providers often have different comfort levels with restless or excited patients; an agitated patient to one provider may simply be an irritable or ornery patient to another.

Agitation experts, on the other hand, have defined agitation not as a diagnosis but rather as a collection of poorly defined symptoms. These symptoms usually involve some actions by the patient which cause some temporary disruption in the ability to care for that patient.[1] This can result from a primary psychiatric disorder, a medical condition such as low glucose or low blood oxygen, a metabolic disturbance or infection, thyroid disorder, substance use, head injury, or any other condition which impacts the function of the brain. Importantly, however, agitation also involves violence or the potential of violence, not just simply disregarding or resisting the following of instructions in the field.

Since agitation is difficult to define, it is also somewhat difficult to measure. Overseas, broadly defined psychiatric emergencies account for 12% of all EMS calls.[2] Inside the emergency department, providers diagnosed "mental disorders" more than 4 million times in 2006.[3] Based on these numbers, EMS providers do and will likely to encounter agitation or psychosis-related calls quite frequently. With challenges in funding of the public mental health system, these encounters are likely to grow in number.

Safety is the primary concern in the approach to the agitated patient. Agitated patients who attract police and EMS attention are usually already fairly excited or restless. In these patients, approaching lights and sirens or loud voices may escalate an unstable situation into a chaotic one. Providers should always be mindful of their own safety, as well as that of their partners and others at scene, when approaching these patients. In general, the safest initial method of approach to a behaviorally-disordered patient is verbal, as this can be done from a safe distance.[4] Ideally, one person should establish verbal contact with the patient so as to keep extra noise to a minimum.[5] Remember, most people—including patients—do not like it when multiple people are talking to them loudly at once, so try to avoid this if at all possible. Start the conversation by stating your name and asking the patient's name. Attempt to find out why the patient is agitated. The answer you get to this question can reveal a surprising amount of information. "I'm in pain," "I just broke up with my partner," or "There are Martians chasing me" all involve different issues that need to be addressed. They also usually have different treatments.

While conversing with the patient, personal safety is still paramount. Care should be given to respecting the patient's personal space and to remaining at least 2 arm lengths of distance from the patient. If the encounter is at night, responders should leave even more space so that sudden moves in the darkness to do not lead to compromised safety. Shining the flashlight directly in the eyes of the patient should be avoided as it may cause increased agitation/anxiety. The patient's behavior may be motivated by fear and calming their fears if possible is preferable to escalating them. These verbal techniques will often be so effective that patients can be willingly led to the quieter environment of the ambulance.

Sometimes, patients are so agitated that verbal communication is difficult if not impossible. In these instances, patients may need to be forcefully restrained. These events are high-risk, anxiety-provoking patient encounters, with a risk of injury to the patient as well as the provider. Given this, forceful takedowns are a last resort option after verbal de-escalation has failed. In general, these forceful takedowns are ideally performed primarily by law enforcement. EMS providers should avoid utilizing force without proper specialized training in takedown techniques or without the advantage of enough manpower (ie, overwhelming force).

Once the patient is calmed or subdued, assessment is the next step. If the patient continues to struggle against maximal restraint, medication can be used to further calm the patient (see **Table 51-1**). In most prehospital situations, the cause of the agitation is typically not known for certain, and so benzodiazepines are usually the first-line medications. Unless you are certain that the patient will need a long-acting medication, the shortest-acting benzodiazepine possible should be administered and will be based on local protocols and practice. See Table 51-1. The dose should be enough to calm the patient, not put them to sleep, as it will be difficult to assess a nontalking, overly sedated patient in the emergency department and oversedation often leads to additional unnecessary studies, like CT scans, to evaluate why the patient is so sedate and nonconversant.

The differential diagnosis of agitation is wide, including substance intoxication, substance withdrawal, electrolyte disturbances, thyroid dysfunction, brain injury, dementia, or psychiatric disorders such as schizophrenia. Clues from the scene and the patient's vital signs are therefore particularly important. Are there any injuries on the patient that might be causing agitation, particularly around the head? Are there any signs at the scene, such as needles or alcohol bottles that might provide clues?

Although it is often tempting to blame the patient's symptoms on "just psych," this should be the last diagnosis that EMS providers should consider. Always check both an oxygen saturation and a finger-stick glucose level, as these are easily correctable causes of agitation. Beyond this, there are a few considerations which can help further distinguish between psychiatric and medical causes of agitation (Table 51-1).

If the answer to any of these questions is yes, there is an especially strong likelihood that the patient may have a medical cause for their condition. Remember, however, that even patients with psychiatric disorders can get medical illnesses. It is probably safest to assume, therefore, that all patients with agitation have another cause for their symptoms until proven otherwise.

EXCITED DELIRIUM SYNDROME

Agitation that is so severe that it can cause sudden death is termed *excited delirium syndrome* (ExDS). ExDS, also known as agitated delirium, is a combination of altered mental status and combativeness.[6] Experts have debated the precise definition of ExDS in the literature, but there is general agreement that symptoms include tolerance to significant pain, rapid

TABLE 51-1 Distinguishing Psychiatric Illness From Medical Illness

- Does the patient not have a previous psychiatric history?
- Are there any features that point to some other diagnosis besides a psychiatric one?
  (Psychotic patients, for instance, are almost always alert and oriented. Lethargy and confusion are usually from a medical cause.)
- Are vital signs abnormal?
  (Although agitated patients can have elevated heart rates, this should resolve as the agitation resolves. There should never be a fever or low blood pressure.)
- Do the symptoms get better or worse over time (ie, waxing and waning)?
  (This is usually from a medical cause instead of a psychiatric one.)
- Did the symptoms have a sudden onset?
- Are there visual hallucinations?
  (These are usually from a medical cause.)
- Does the patient have a heavy drinking history?
- Has the patient recently started any new medications that might explain the symptoms?

TABLE 51-2 Useful Medications for Prehospital Agitation

Drug Name	Usual Dosage	Duration of Action
Midazolam (Versed)	2-5 mg IM/IV	Short acting
Lorazepam (Ativan)	1-2 mg IM/IV	Intermediate acting
Ketamine (Ketalar)	0.5-4 mg/kg IM/IV	Short acting
Diazepam (Valium)	5-10 mg IM/IV	Long acting

breathing, sweating, severe agitation, elevated temperature, poor awareness of police presence, lack of fatiguing, unusual or superhuman strength, and inappropriate clothing for the current environment. Not all of these signs or symptoms need to be present to diagnose ExDS. ExDS represents a true medical not psychiatric emergency. The diagnosis is often challenging, because the clinical signs and symptoms of ExDS can be produced by a wide variety of disease. Agitation, combativeness, and altered mental status, for example, can be produced by hypoglycemia, thyroid storm, certain kinds of seizures, cocaine, or methamphetamine use.

Prehospital personnel will not generally be able to differentiate between the multiple possible causes of ExDS. Instead, EMS personnel should simply recognize that the patient has a more severe agitation than is typical and symptoms consistent with ExDS. Especially if this agitation is unresponsive to agitation medications (see **Table 51-2**), these patients have a real medical emergency. High doses of sedating medications are often ultimately required, and initiation of therapy should begin in the field. All such patients will require transfer to an emergency department (ED) for further management and evaluation.

ExDS is not always fatal, but a significant proportion of these patients will have sudden death in the field, with estimates up to 11%.[7] The reasons for this are not fully understood. While many deaths from ExDS may not be preventable, there is a subset of patients who can be saved with early and proper intervention. This intervention includes early sedation, IV fluid if access can be safely obtained, and rapid transport. These should be started by EMS personnel en route to the hospital.

Agitated patients in the prehospital setting sometimes require restraint. Although verbal de-escalation should always be attempted first, patients with ExDS by definition are altered and so do not respond to verbal commands. Physical restraint for these patients is almost always required, and should be accomplished in such a way as to minimize the patient's exertional activity. These patients are typically aggressive and violent, and law enforcement should be the ones making tactical decisions on how to best restrain. Use of an electronic conduction device, such as a Taser, may be more preferable to fighting the patient physically, since heavy exertion can potentially worsen acidosis.[8]

Education about ExDS among medical and law enforcement personnel will hopefully lead to better awareness of this condition. Cooperative protocols between EMS and law enforcement should be created so as to more quickly identify and get EMS to scene prior to trying to restrain these patients. This will enable EMS to initiate treatment more quickly after restraint, and therefore optimize positive outcomes.

THE SUICIDAL PATIENT

Suicide was the 11th leading cause of death for all ages in 2007, and the Centers for Disease Control and Prevention (CDC) estimates that there are 100 to 200 attempts for every successful suicide.[9] Most patients who eventually suicide have visited a physician within the past month, even if they do not have a formal diagnosis of depression from a psychiatrist.[10] These statistics mean that it is likely that EMS providers will encounter a suicidal patient at some point, even if this patient does not have a formal diagnosis of a mood disorder, depression or is not on antidepressants.

In general, approaching a suicidal patient is no different than approaching an agitated patient. Providers should always keep in mind both the safety of the scene and their personal safety. Unless the patient is holding a weapon, however, risk to the provider is not usually as high. Providers should be much more mindful of patient safety. Ambulances are generally stocked with many sharp objects, and care should be taken to keep potential weapons away from the patient in case they decide to carry out their threat of self-injury.

Unless a patient is actively psychotic and agitated, and so poses a threat to the provider, restraints are not usually necessary. One exception is the air medical transport of a suicidal patient. Most experts recommend restraints during flight in case the patient acts out in order to avoid the patient taking down the aircraft. If the patient contacted help themselves, this is usually a positive sign that the individual wishes medical attention rather than to harm themselves. If the call was initiated by a third party, however, the patient should be kept under a close watchful eye. Patients who have already injured themselves in a suicide attempt should be treated exactly as any other patient. Providers should know not judge the patient for their actions, lecture them, or attempt to solve their psychosocial problems in a short ambulance ride.

Although practice patterns for evaluation and treatment of suicidal ideation in emergency departments vary widely across the country, EMS providers should treat all such patients the same. Patients who voice thoughts about harming themselves, especially if this is the reason that they called EMS in the first place, should be assumed to be at high risk for self-harm. This means that they should be transported to the closest most appropriate emergency department able to meet their needs for further treatment and evaluation. They should be monitored carefully during transport for self-harm.

THE HOMICIDAL PATIENT

In 2009, there were 15,241 murders in the United States, meaning that it likely that EMS providers will encounter either an individual who has just perpetrated a violent crime or one who is voicing violent thoughts.[11] These types of patients can prove especially challenging to providers.

In general, the strongest predictor of future violence is a history of violence.[12] These patients should therefore be approached with considerable caution, with attention to both the safety of the scene and the provider's personal safety. Restraint of these patients is not usually appropriate by EMS, as these patients will typically already be restrained by police with an accompanying police escort to the hospital. Ambulances are generally stocked with medical equipment that can be used as potential weapons, and this should always be considered when caring for a patient who may not have much to lose by escaping from police custody or who is not in control of his or her own actions.

Injuries should be cared for exactly as with any other patient. Although in police custody, homicidal patients still retain the right to refuse medical care. This should be honored if at all possible, if the patient has a capacity to make a reasonable informed decision and if the injuries are not life threatening.

THE INTOXICATED PATIENT

Drugs of abuse are commonly encountered by EMS providers, and it is important to understand what patients look like who are intoxicated with these substances. Prehospital treatments of each substance are also discussed.

ALCOHOL

Alcohol is by far the most widely abused drug that EMS providers are likely to encounter. Approximately 80% of men and 60% of women in developed countries have ever consumed alcohol, and 30% to 50% of these individuals have suffered some consequence, usually headache or interpersonal problem, for doing so.[13] According to the Centers for Disease Control and Prevention, nearly 42% of high school students have consumed alcohol in the last 30 days.[14] The consequences of children consuming alcohol can be especially severe, including school problems, social problems, and legal problems, usually for arrest while driving intoxicated or hurting someone while under the influence.[14]

The appearance of individuals who are acutely intoxicated with alcohol is fairly familiar to most EMS providers, and includes lowered inhibitions, incoordination, slurred speech, and nausea and vomiting in high doses. Withdrawal can be more difficult to recognize. At the severe end,

withdrawal from alcohol usually involves tremors, tachycardia, diaphoresis, and sometimes visual hallucinations and seizures. Mild to moderate withdrawal, on the other hand, may be notable only for restlessness and agitation with tachycardia being an early objective finding. Patients themselves may not wish to reveal a drinking history, and will often deny or minimize their daily alcohol use.

If recognized properly, withdrawal is usually not difficult to distinguish from active intoxication. For patients who are withdrawing from alcohol, national guidelines have called for treatment with benzodiazepines.[15] Although there are options for oral medication in the emergency department setting, intravenous treatment with an intermediate-acting or long-acting benzodiazepine as with agitation is usually appropriate in the prehospital setting (see Table 51-2). Other pharmacological options could include intranasal midazolam or use of ketamine.[16-18]

STIMULANTS

The most commonly encountered stimulants by prehospital providers are usually cocaine, often called "blow," "coke," or "candy," or methamphetamines, often called "bennies," "uppers," or "speed".[19] These drugs cause release of catecholamines, usually epinephrine and—to a lesser extent—norepinephrine, which create a state of excitement in users. Intoxicated patients are usually tachycardic, diaphoretic (unless dehydrated), hypertensive, and have piloerection (goose bumps). Occasionally, more severe complications of stimulant use can occur, including myocardial infarction or aortic dissection. These events, while rare, can be life threatening.[20]

Treatment of stimulant intoxication involves managing the symptoms. Benzodiazepines are the initial treatment of choice. Complications from substance abuse may be more severe in patients who are older or who already have coronary artery disease. However, all patients regardless of age should be placed on a cardiac monitor. Any patient who complains of chest pain associated with drug use, whether young or old, should receive an ECG if available and be placed on oxygen during transport, and follow local protocols for chest pain.

Withdrawal from stimulants produces the opposite clinical scenario, as these patients are usually lethargic and sleepy.[19] Although the diagnosis of stimulant withdrawal may be clear from the outset, these patients should always have a glucose and oxygen saturation checked in order to exclude other causes for their altered mental status.

SEDATIVE/HYPNOTICS

Barbiturates such as phenobarbital or pentobarbital (Nembutal), and benzodiazepines such as diazepam (Valium), lorazepam (Ativan), and alprazolam (Xanax) are commonly encountered sedative/hypnotics. These agents cause sedation, and intoxicated patients are therefore usually sleepy and lethargic.[19] Treatment is symptom based. Although the drug flumazenil (Romazicon) can be used to reverse benzodiazepine intoxication, many experts believe that this drug also lowers the seizure threshold. This makes its use more risky, especially in situations where the patient may have ingested more than one drug or if they have been chronically using benzodiazepines. The use of flumazenil should be limited, therefore, to situations in which the individual has ingested life-threatening doses of benzodiazepines, and are unable to protect their airway.

Withdrawal from benzodiazepines often causes anxiety, irritability, or seizures. Treatment of seizures in benzodiazepine withdrawal is often managed by giving more benzodiazepines, but of intermediate or long-acting type so that the person does not withdraw further from these agents.

OPIATES/OPIOIDS

Opiates are any derivatives of the opium poppy plant such as heroin or morphine.[19] The term opioids, on the other hand, describes any synthetic or semisynthetic chemical with actions similar to opiates, such as oxycodone (OxyContin), hydromorphone (Dilaudid), fentanyl (Sublimaze), or methadone (Methadose). In practice, this distinction makes little difference, as intoxication with opiates and opioids are managed identically.

Patients intoxicated with these substances are sleepy. In higher doses, patients become unresponsive and have respiratory depression. In addition, some opiates such as morphine can cause hypotension. Most opioids, with the notable exception of meperidine (Demerol), cause pupillary constriction. This pupillary constriction, along with slow respirations and altered mental status, may be the only clue to opioid intoxication.

The treatment of opioid intoxication is naloxone (Narcan). This medication can be given virtually by any route, including subcutaneously, intramuscularly, intravenously, or intranasally. Narcan has very few side effects.[21-23] Any patient with the combination of lethargy, hypopnea, and pupillary constriction should therefore be administered this medication.

Withdrawal from opioid medications causes diarrhea, piloerection (goose bumps), abdominal cramping, nausea and vomiting, general malaise, and yawning. The management of opioid withdrawal is generally outside the scope of practice for the prehospital provider, but generally involves treatment of symptoms through additional medications.

SYNTHETIC CANNABIS

A number of variants of synthetic cannabis are present in the community and typically go by the street names K2 or Spice. Intoxication may cause CNS depression or at times, altered mental status and agitation. Hallucinations and even seizures may occur.[24,25] Supportive care is appropriate for most, however, acutely agitated patients may require benzodiazepines.

HALLUCINOGENS

LSD and mescaline are commonly encountered hallucinogens.[19] While generally well tolerated in low doses, these substances may cause altered mental status, hyperthermia, sweating, and nausea in large doses. Treatment of hallucinogenic intoxication is symptomatic. Benzodiazepines can also be used if the patient is especially agitated.

Withdrawal from hallucinogenic substances, especially LSD, can be associated with flashbacks (ie, "bad trips"). Treatment of these withdrawal symptoms is generally outside the scope of practice for the EMS provider. However, benzodiazepines may be used if the patient is especially agitated.

CLUB DRUGS

"Club drugs" is a newer term for substances often used at dance parties. Commonly encountered club drugs include GHB or "Georgia home boy," ketamine or "special K," flunitrazepam (Rohypnol) or "roofies," and MDMA or "ecstasy".[19] Each of these drugs has a unique pharmacology, and shares the term "club drugs" only because of where they are most often administered.

MDMA is a type of amphetamine that shares many similarities with the stimulants discussed above. GHB and ketamine, on the other hand, are drugs that cause a dissociative state. At lower doses, these substances cause pleasurable sensations. At higher doses, intoxicated individuals may be catatonic or wide awake, but generally have no memory of the event. The hallmark of GHB intoxication is a catatonic individual who is bagged or ends up intubated for airway protection but then very rapidly becomes wide awake with few after effects of their mental state. Significant bradycardia can be associated with GHB as well. Ketamine, on the other hand, causes a longer-lasting feeling of dissociation (also called the "K hole"). Users may report out-of-body experiences.

BATH SALTS

The synthetic cathinones are widely abused, although it is thought that illegalization will decrease availability. The physiological and psychological effects of these drugs are unpredictable and users may be taking different substances with each ingestion.[26] Typically users suffer from a stimulant toxidrome and the effects may be indistinguishable from methamphetamine, MDMA, or cocaine.[27] Benzodiazepines and other sedative medications may be required for treatment of acute agitation. Homicidal and paranoid behavior is possible and self-abuse can also manifest.[28]

INVOLVING LAW ENFORCEMENT

As most EMS providers are not well trained in physical techniques used to subdue and the tactical use of force, involvement of law enforcement is critical. Law enforcement should accompany EMS providers any time the scene is unsafe, if a patient is agitated, if a patient is expressing violent thoughts or tendencies, or if a patient has committed a crime. If a patient is taken to a hospital against their will, the decision about restraint and transport should be made by law enforcement officials. EMS physicians and providers should always strive to be therapeutic in their interactions with patients.[29] Restraining patients, punishing them, or taking defensive actions "for safety's sake" should typically be left to law enforcement. EMS providers who cross the line into police work by restraining patients unnecessarily not only lose professional credibility, but open themselves to legal liability as well.

COMMON PITFALLS

There are several common pitfalls in managing behaviorally disordered patients in the prehospital setting:

- Failure to suspect medical etiology

    EMS providers should never blame the patient's symptoms on "just psych," unless other medical problems have been excluded first.

- Failure to check glucose or an oxygen saturation

    EMS providers should always check complete vital signs on all behaviorally disordered patients. Low blood glucose and low blood oxygen may cause agitation in many patients.

- Failure to recognize impaired level of decision making.

    An assessment of mental status is important in all behaviorally disordered patients. These patients, either by virtue of substance use, a medical condition, injury, or psychiatric disorder, have impaired reasoning about their condition. These patients are therefore often poor medical historians. This may be frustrating to providers who are not used to being creative, such as searching the scene carefully or talking to bystanders, in order to get information.

- Overuse of force

    EMS providers should only use the minimum of force to accomplish the primary objective of caring for the patient. Overuse of force is never appropriate, nor is using force in a way to punish or humiliate the patient.

- Failure to use appropriate amount of benzodiazepines.

    Patients may need to repeat dosing of medication in order to calm them. The dose of medication should be enough to calm the patient without putting them to sleep.

KEY POINTS

- EMS Physicians should be aware of three cardinal rules when addressing patients with behavior issues: assess for threats to provider safety, assess for threats to patient safety, and make attempts to calm the patient.

- Prehospital providers should assess for and report potential clues from the environment that may explain the patient's condition.

- Patients with behavior issues may be frustrating to EMS providers. Assessment for medical causes should be first priority after assessing for potential or existing threats to provider and patient safety.

- Few available studies guide the prehospital assessment and care of patients with behavioral issues.

- Suicidal patients, homicidal patients, and intoxicated patients present unique assessment and management challenges to the

EMS physician and provider, and providers should maintain a broad differential for medical, traumatic, toxic, and psychiatric causes for the patient's condition.

- Excited delirium is a relatively newly recognized, life-threatening condition that requires rapid recognition and appropriate intervention with physical restraint followed quickly by rapid acting pharmacologic restraint in order to minimize the risk for life-threatening electrolyte imbalance, lactic acidosis, rhabdomyolysis, hyperthermia, and cardiac arrhythmia/arrest.

REFERENCES

1. Allen MH, Currier GW, Hughes DH, Reyes-Harde M, Docherty JP. The Expert Consensus Guideline Series: treatment of behavioral emergencies. *Postgrad Med.* 2001;(Spec No):1-88.
2. Pajonk F-G, Schmitt P, Bideler A, et al. Psychiatric emergencies in prehospital emergency medical systems: a prospective comparison of two urban settings. *Gen Hosp Psychiatry.* 2008;30:360-366.
3. Pitts SR, Niska RW, Xu J, Burt CW. National Hospital Ambulatory Medical Care Survey: 2006 emergency department summary. *Natl Health Stat Report.* 2008;(7):1-38.
4. Vilke GM, Wilson MP. Agitation: what every emergency physician should know. *Emerg Med Rep.* 2009;30(19):233-244.
5. Richmond JS, Berlin JS, Fishkind A, et al. Verbal de-escalation of the agitated patient: consensus statement of the American Association for Emergency Psychiatry Project BETA De-escalation Workgroup. *West J Emerg Med.* 2012;13(1):17-25.
6. Vilke GM, DeBard ML, Chan TC, et al. Excited delirium syndrome (ExDS): defining based on a review of the literature. *J Emerg Med.* 2012;43(5):897-905.
7. Stratton SJ, Rogers C, Brickett K, Gruzinski G. Factors associated with sudden death of individuals requiring restraint for excited delirium. *Am J Emerg Med.* 2001;19:187-191.
8. Ho JD, Dawes DM, Nelson RS, et al. Acidosis and catecholamine evaluation following simulated law enforcement "Use of Force" encounters. *Acad Emerg Med.* 2010;17:E60-E68.
9. Ronquillo L, Minassian A, Vilke GM, Wilson MP. Literature-based recommendations for suicide assessment in the emergency department: a review. *J Emerg Med.* 2012;43(5):836-842.
10. Murphy GE. The physician's responsibility for suicide. II: errors of omission. *Ann Intern Med.* 1975;82:305-309.
11. The Disaster Center. http://www.disastercenter.com/crime/uscrime. htm. Accessed August 29, 2011.
12. Elbogen EB, Johnson SC. The intricate link between violence and mental disorder. *Arch Gen Psychiatry.* 2009;66(2):152-161.
13. Schuckit MA. Alcohol-use disorders. *Lancet.* 2009;373:492-501.
14. Fact sheets: underage drinking. Centers for Disease Control and Prevention. http://www.cdc.gov/alcohol/fact-sheets/underage-drinking.htm. Accessed August 28, 2011.
15. Wilson MP, Pepper D, Currier GW, Holloman GH, Feifel D. The psychopharmacology of agitation: consensus statement of the American Association for Emergency Psychiatry Project BETA Psychopharmacology Workgroup. *West J Emerg Med.* 2012; 13(1):26-34.
16. Keseg D, Cortez E, Rund D, Caterino J. The use of prehospital ketamine for control of agitation in a metropolitan firefighter-based EMS system. *Prehosp Emerg Care.* 2015;19(1):110-115.
17. Ho JD, Smith SW, Nystrom PC, et al. Successful management of excited delirium syndrome with prehospital ketamine: two case examples. *Prehosp Emerg Care.* April-June 2013;17(2):274-279.
18. Burnett AM, Salzman JG, Griffith KR, Kroeger B, Frascone RJ. The emergency department experience with prehospital ketamine: a case series of 13 patients. *Prehosp Emerg Care.* October-December 2012;16(4):553-559.
19. Commonly abused drugs. National Institutes of Drug Abuse. http://www.drugabuse.gov/DrugPages/DrugsofAbuse.html. Accessed August 28, 2011.
20. Alfonso L, Mohammad T, Thatai D. Crack whips the heart: a review of the cardiovascular toxicity of cocaine. *Am J Cardiol.* 2007; 100:1040-1043.
21. Davis CS, Southwell JK, Niehaus VR, Walley AY, Dailey MW. Emergency Medical Services Naloxone Access: a National Systematic Legal Review. *Acad Emerg Med.* October 2014;21(10):1173-1177.
22. Zuckerman M, Weisberg SN, Boyer EW. Pitfalls of intranasal naloxone. *Prehosp Emerg Care.* October-December 2014;18(4):550-554.
23. Knowlton A, Weir BW, Hazzard F, et al. EMS runs for suspected opioid overdose: implications for surveillance and prevention. *Prehosp Emerg Care.* July-September 2013;17(3):317-329.
24. Celofiga A, Koprivsek J, Klavz J. Use of synthetic cannabinoids in patients with psychotic disorders: case series. *J Dual Diagn.* July-September 2014;10(3):168-173.
25. Lisi DM. Designer drugs. Patients may be using synthetic cannabinoids more than you think. *JEMS.* September 2014;39(9):56-59.
26. Hall C, Heyd C, Butler C, Yarema M. "Bath salts" intoxication: a new recreational drug that presents with a familiar toxidrome. *CJEM.* March 1, 2014;16(2):171-176.
27. Glennon RA. Bath salts, mephedrone, and methylenedioxypyrovalerone as emerging illicit drugs that will need targeted therapeutic intervention. *Adv Pharmacol.* 2014;69:581-620.
28. John ME, Thomas-Rozea C, Hahn D. Bath salts abuse leading to new onset psychosis and potential for violence. *Clin Schizophr Relat Psychoses.* June 20, 2014:1-14.
29. Wilson MP, Sloane CM. Chemical Restraints, Physical Restraints, and Other Demonstrations of Force. In Jesus J, Grossman SA, Derse AR, Adams JG, Wolfe R, Rosen P) Ethical Problems in Emergency Medicine: A Discussion-Based Review, John Wiley & Sons, Ltd, Chichester, UK, 2012.

Trauma-Related Emergencies

Care of an Entrapped or Entangled Victim

Darren Braude

Ryan Lewis

INTRODUCTION

The most common source of entrapment and entanglement in most locales is the motor vehicle collision. Other potential sources include industrial accidents and agricultural incidents. It is imperative that medical providers have a standardized approach to these situations, have basic familiarity with safety issues and extrication concepts, and understand that the medical approach to these situations is unique.

OBJECTIVES

- Describe motor vehicle, industrial, and agricultural-related causes of entrapment and entanglement.
- List key nonmedical personnel and bystanders who are present on the scene, and may serve as a vital asset during these operations.
- Describe the initial approach to the entrapped and/or entangled victim.
- Provide a basic description of tools utilized by fire/rescue personnel during extrication operations.
- Describe the dangers associated with medical operations within a motor vehicle during extrication operations.
- Discuss unique challenges to airway management in a motor vehicle.
- Discuss management of hypotension and hemorrhage in the entrapped and/or entangled victim.
- Discuss the criteria associated with the consideration of field amputation.
- List other resources and personnel that may be helpful during this unique type of call.

INITIAL APPROACH TO THE ENTRAPPED OR ENTANGLED PATIENT

The initial approach to any scene should always be the same but special attention is necessary when arriving first. Scene safety begins with the call going out/dispatch notification. Activate all possible resources early; it is always better to turn away resources when they are not needed than to need them and be delayed because they are not on scene. Access point and direction should be considered for any potential hazardous materials involvement. Likewise, flow of traffic and positioning of vehicles should be considered during the initial approach. Medical vehicles should generally be close to the patient without jeopardizing contamination or damage to the ambulance. Positioning of medical vehicles should be in such a way as to be protected by larger vehicles such as fire apparatus. The path to and from the vehicle should be out of traffic—in many extended operations there will be multiple trips to and from

the vehicle for equipment or supplies; the more trips through or close to passing traffic, the more likely there is to be a secondary incident. Vehicles should be parked so as not to impede the loading of a patient into the ambulance and so as not to block the ambulance in at the scene. Upon arrival, there should be a visual scan for any downed lines or electrocution hazard.

If you are the first rescuer on scene an appropriate size-up should be made and conveyed to the communication center and other responders via radio in most cases. Basic information includes number and general acuity of patients and whether additional or fewer resources are needed and the response mode required on other incoming providers. Advise other responders of hazards to expect. In the common situation of an MVC with reported entrapment an appropriate size-up might be: "Fire Control, MD-1 arriving on scene. We have a single midsize vehicle into the center divider on the westbound side of the interstate, east of the Main Street on-ramp. There is major front-end damage with two victims apparently trapped. No fire or other hazards noted. Please continue all responders Code 3, start Heavy Rescue and launch the closest available helicopter. We will also need additional law enforcement for traffic control. I will be initiating care."

The proper protective equipment should be put on before exiting the vehicle and worn at all times. Physicians should never be on scene of an active rescue wearing scrubs without any proper protective equipment. Extrication gear with proper reflective/identification markings, helmet, eye protection, gloves, and heavy boots should be worn during the extrication.[1]

Many additional resources should be considered when on scene of an entrapped or entangled patient, particularly when they occur in the industrial or agricultural setting. On scene safety personnel from the industry are often intimately familiar with the operating systems and potential hazards of industrial machinery. Foremen, superintendents, or supervisors may also prove helpful in the direction of how to deactivate or cut power to machinery or devices posing dangers to the rescuers or patient (or causing the entrapment). Likewise, heavy equipment and machinery operators are beneficial in assisting with rescues that may involve the use of cranes, tractors, or heavy machinery. Engineers, linesman, electricians, and gas company personnel may also prove invaluable at the scene of an entrapped or entangled patient. Finally, coworkers of the trapped patient may be of assistance in determining the mechanism of entrapment and thus how to free the patient. Furthermore, coworkers often have emergency contact information for family, which in some rare cases may be needed if the patient is not expected to survive removal from the entrapment. In these thankfully rare cases, every effort should be made to safely allow for the family and patient to speak and be with one and other as the patient passes.

Medical responders must remember to balance extrication with patient care. Do no delay extrication for unneeded medical procedures or treatment—sometimes simpler is better. Medical responders should not delay active extrication in order to perform unnecessary procedures in the field. The need for monitoring equipment versus space and safety considerations should also be considered. Monitors utilized in confined space should be considered inert and proven to pose no threat of fire or explosion in highly volatile environments. Establish early incident command on scene and follow the structure. Prehospital scenes become much more chaotic when extended operations, extrications, and rescues are involved. Make every attempt to control the chaos and follow standard incident command guidelines and practices.

COMMON TYPES OF EXTRICATION MANEUVERS AND TOOLS

Some of the most common maneuvers in extrication from vehicles include simple door pops, roof flaps, roof removals, dash rolls, pedal pulls, airbag lifts, and the combination of any of these techniques. Many departments train with various techniques to accomplish each of these, but most have the same general technique or principles. Many of the principles such as spreading, pushing, cutting, rolling, or lifting utilized in vehicle extrication can be translated into other types of extrications; however, many more variables often exist independent of the extrication itself. This may include a broad approach to securing the scene, stabilizing debris/structures (structural collapse/disaster response), or multiple rescue types such as high-angle, confined space, and technical rescue in disaster, industrial, or agricultural incidents. Furthermore, in events of man-made disaster or incidents such as bombings or acts of terror there are often evidence preservation and law enforcement concerns to take into account as well.

Many different types of tools or brands of rescue tools are available for extrication, but most incorporate the same general principles and mechanisms of action. Some of the tools used to accomplish extrication are hydraulic spreaders, hydraulic cutters, winches, RAMS, airbags, gas cutters, power cutters/saws, and manual tools such as axes, rams, bolt cutters, and Halligan/Hooligan tools (**Box 52-1**; **Figure 52-1**).

MEDICAL ASSESSMENT

The medical evaluation of a prehospital trauma patient on scene is much different than that of the medical evaluation of that same patient in a trauma center. The same basic principles should exist; however, one must remember that at times, good medicine can lead to bad outcomes. In other words, sometimes simpler is better. Scene times should be minimized as much as possible to properly and safely treat the patient. Furthermore, safety concerns should be taken into consideration when attempting or planning complicated medical procedures that put rescuers at risk in an unstable scene.[2]

One major difference in prehospital medicine that is emerging from the battlefield is now the transition from the ABC mnemonic to the

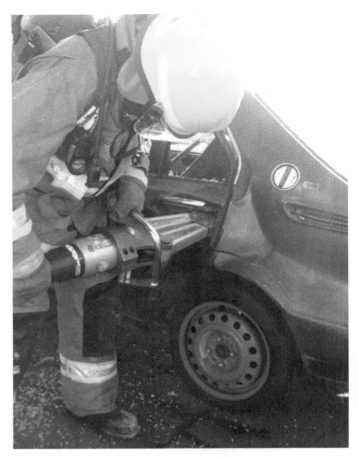

FIGURE 52-1. Hydraulic spreader. Fire personnel using a hydraulic spreader during an extrication exercise.

MARCH mnemonic. Prehospital data show that in most traumatic injuries, particularly battlefield injuries, massive hemorrhage is considerably more fatal than airway compromise. Therefore, the mnemonic MARCH was established for the order of assessment for prehospital patients in the tactical field. This can be translated to severely wounded patients entrapped or entangled on any scene (**Box 52-2**).

An additional approach to assessing patients in a prehospital setting may involve a remote assessment. This may be necessary if rescuers cannot safely approach a trapped patient and a quick assessment is needed to determine the risk versus benefit of immediate or delayed rescue. For example, if a patient is in an MVC involving a hazardous material and downed power lines, a remote assessment should be performed while an incident plan is being put together. If the patient has obvious injuries incompatible with life, then putting more lives at risk during an emergent and hasty rescue would not be prudent. Likewise, if the patient has only minor injuries and is trapped in a vehicle with a powerline lying over the top of it, one would not want to immediately rush in and risk

---

Box 52-1
Common Rescue/Extrication Tools
Hydraulic rescue tools
Hydraulic spreaders
Hydraulic cutters
RAMS
Powered equipment
Winches
Airbags
Gas cutters
Power cutters/saws
Manual tools
Glass break/seatbelt cutter
Windshield cutter
Axe
Sledge
Bolt cutters
Halligan/Hooligan tools

Box 52-2
Order of Assessment for Major Trauma (MARCH)
M = massive hemorrhage. Rapidly identify and stop any massive hemorrhage.
A = airway. Establish an airway.
R = respirations and respiratory system. Assist ventilation and decompress tension pneumothorax/place occlusive dressing over sucking chest wound.
C = circulation. Check pulse and perform CPR/ACLS if indicated.
H = hypothermia. Take active precautions to avoid hypothermia.

electrocution for an injury that is not life threatening to begin with. All rescuers must remember that injured rescuers only complicate the rescue and will almost guarantee assets being diverted from the patient to the injured rescuer, thus making the initial rescue even more complicated and prolonged.

PATIENT CARE DURING EXTRICATION

AIRWAY CONTROL

Challenges in airway management of the entrapped patient include, but are not limited to: limited patient access, the patient can rarely be optimally positioned, usual techniques may be impractical, the patients may have little reserve, and maintaining the airway during extrication may be as difficult as securing it in the first place.

For practical purposes patients may be divided into two groups: (1) those without a gag reflex and (2) those with a gag reflex who are maintaining their airway (conscious or unconscious) but need respiratory support. Patients who are entrapped in a vehicle without a gag reflex have a very poor prognosis from the outset. Airway interventions should be as rapid as possible without endangering the rescuer. Immediate placement of an extraglottic airway with gastric decompression capacity makes the most sense in the majority of cases though some providers may opt for endotracheal intubation when it can be done rapidly. Alternatives to traditional laryngoscopy techniques include face-to-face positioning (aka the Tomahawk), standing above the patient and video laryngoscopy.

Managing patients who are still maintaining their own airways but appear to be deteriorating, or no longer able to maintain critical oxygenation, is much more complicated. While many of these patients would be obvious candidates for rapid sequence intubation (RSI) in other situations, the risk to benefit ratio is clearly different when the patient is entrapped. RSI is particularly risky in this setting because the intubation itself is usually more difficult due to positioning, rescue techniques such as bag-valve-mask ventilation and surgical airways may also be more difficult, and the patient may not tolerate the hemodynamic effects of RSI medications and positive-pressure ventilation well. It is usually best for the patient to delay the procedure until after extrication, if at all possible. If the EMS physician decides that airway control cannot or should not be delayed, and there is sufficient safe access to the patient to perform the procedure, it is prudent to take as much time as possible to be confident of preparations. Rushing into an airway procedure on an entrapped patient without all equipment available and well-developed first attempt and backup plans can be disastrous. Rapid sequence airway (RSA) should also be considered an alternative to RSI in this setting. RSA combines the airway pharmacology of RSI with immediate placement of a newer generation extraglottic airway (EGA) with gastric decompression capability.[3] These devises are much faster and easier to insert in atypical positions and easier to reposition if they should become dislodged. Airway protection is not quite as good as with an endotracheal tube—but better than most providers realize—and this is clearly a unique circumstance where unconventional approaches should be considered.

Whether the airway is managed with an endotracheal tube or EGA, continuous capnography is imperative to monitor for device dislodgement during extrication. The patient should also be placed on a portable ventilator rather than managed with BVMV as soon as possible; this will maintain much more consistent ventilation and keep one additional person out of the way of those performing the extrication.

HEMORRHAGE CONTROL

Hemorrhage control of the entrapped patient depends on patient acuity, access, and rescuer safety. In general, the threshold for tourniquet use, much like in tactical medicine, should be lower.[4,5] Having a provider apply continuous direct pressure may be difficult for extended periods, may place that provider in an unsafe position, and may create an obstacle for those working on the extraction.

CERVICAL IMMOBILIZATION

While the spine should not be compromised, cervical immobilization adds another complication and delay to extrication. Spinal immobilization is also very uncomfortable for the patient over an extended period and can impact airway maintenance and respirations. The EMS physician may have the opportunity to impact care positively by making, or empowering other experienced providers to make, case-by-case exceptions to usual cervical immobilization guidelines for entrapped patients. For example, some system protocols may require cervical immobilization for all trauma patients with altered mental status yet the EMS physician may recognize that a particular patient that is entrapped in machinery below the shoulders and altered due to hemorrhagic shock may not have had sufficient force applied to the neck to cause a significant risk for injury. Similarly, a patient trapped in a vehicle with pelvic fractures after a high-force MVC would typically require immobilization on the basis of mechanism and distracting injury. The EMS physician on scene may, after personally examining the patient, feel comfortable discontinuing cervical precautions if they believe the patient examination is reliable despite potential distraction and there is no posterior neck pain or tenderness. A great deal of experience is necessary to make these decisions safely and even experienced providers are likely to disagree about the best management.

CHEMICAL EXTRICATION

Chemical extrication refers to the administration of analgesia, and possibly sedation, to the entrapped patient with the goal of minimizing discomfort and distress during the extrication process. The complicating factors include that these patients are often medically fragile as a result of the trauma incurred and may have an exaggerated response resulting in hypotension and oversedation at the same time that access to the patient to treat these complications may be limited. Despite these limitations chemical extrication, when performed cautiously, can be very humane.

The choice of medications and dose is critical to safety and must be tailored to the patient and circumstance. A patient with isolated injury to an extremity that requires major extrication and good airway access and vascular access is usually a candidate for aggressive chemical extrication. An unstable multisystem trauma patient with poor airway and vascular access is usually only a candidate for cautious analgesia, if anything at all.

Fentanyl is the usual choice for analgesia in these circumstances due to its rapid onset and excellent side effect profile; however, caution must be exercised in the sympathetic-dependent patient due to fentanyl's sympatholytic effect; it is prudent to start with smaller than usual doses in such patients. The addition of a sedative such as midazolam must be done very cautiously, especially if access to the patient's airway is limited, as response to benzodiazepines is often unpredictable and the combination of a narcotic and benzodiazepine is well known to cause potentiation. One small case series reported on the use of etomidate for chemical extrication.[6] *Etomidate* is hemodynamically stable though it can be associated with myoclonus and adrenal suppression; it also does not provide any analgesia. Another alternative is *ketamine*, which provides excellent analgesia at lower doses and analgesia with dissociative sedation at higher doses, while maintaining airway reflexes and blood pressure.[7,8] One retrospective study reported the use of ketamine for chemical extrication in 265 patients without complications. The precautions against ketamine in the setting of head injury have been recently relaxed though it is still wise to avoid if the patient is hypertensive.[9,10]

HYPOTENSION

Management of hypotension should always begin with a rapid assessment of likely causes. Before the provider becomes focused on hemorrhagic shock they must consider neurogenic and obstructive causes. While there is clearly controversy around aggressive control of blood pressure in the prehospital management of trauma, none of the existing literature applies to the blunt trauma patient with a prolonged prehospital course and/or potential crush injury.[11]

Control of hemodynamics should ideally begin prior to extrication as release of compression, pain and anxiety may result in further drops in blood pressure. Management of hemorrhagic shock should emphasize intravenous fluids and blood products may be administered on scene if available. The role of colloids and hypertonic saline is controversial but cannot be widely recommended.[12,13] While vasopressor agents are generally not recommended for management of hemorrhagic shock or the initial treatment of neurogenic shock they must be available and considered as a temporizing agent during the extrication process, especially when chemical extrication has been employed. Small bolus doses of phenylephrine are generally easy to administer and safe as long as the patient is not bradycardic, though it has not been evaluated in this setting.

CRUSH SYNDROME

Crush syndrome reflects the systemic complications of releasing muscle compression after a long enough period to have buildup of lactic acid, myoglobin, potassium, and other potential toxins, usually at least 1 hour, but potentially less.[14] The key to management is the initiation of intravenous hydration with isotonic saline at 1 to 1.5 L/h prior to release of the constriction.[15] Administration of sodium bicarbonate for alkalization may be considered as well. Use of diuretics is not generally advisable prior to extrication due to other potential complications and the inability for the patient to void easily or have a catheter placed. Providers should also be prepared to immediately treat the cardiac complications of hyperkalemia.

Rescuers managing the extrication procedure are often focused on freeing the patient as rapidly as possible without realizing the implications of crush syndrome. In cases where entrapment has been long enough for possible crush syndrome to develop, EMS physicians should communicate these concerns to the incident commander and advocate for reasonable delays to begin appropriate hydration, if it can be done safely, prior to patient release.

FIELD AMPUTATION

Field amputation is a high-profile though rarely applied prehospital procedure. Literature is primarily restricted to case reports and cases series, the largest involving a field amputation team in Dallas that has performed nine field amputation over 25 years of the team's existence.[16] EMS physicians may be called to evaluate appropriateness of the procedure, provide sedation and analgesia for the procedure performed by other physicians, or perform the procedure themselves (**Figure 52-2**) The decision to amputate may be complex and considerations related to this are discussed in Chapter 64 in more detail. If the EMS physician is not a surgeon, this may fall outside their usual scope of practice and comfort. EMS physicians who may potentially be called to such scenes should maintain a procedure for accessing the appropriate surgical personnel or should have the appropriate training, credentialing, and malpractice coverage to perform the procedure themselves.[17] If a surgical "go team" is utilized, all physicians and health care providers responding to a prehospital scene will require awareness training and must be familiar with the equipment available in the field.[18]

MOTOR VEHICLE CRASH (MVC)

By far, the most common causes of entrapment and/or entanglement are motor vehicle crashes. With vehicles being made of various composite materials designed to absorb impact by buckling, higher rates of driving speed, and the sheer number of people that drive vehicles, the likelihood of responding to an entrapped patien1t in an MVC at some point is nearly a guarantee. Kinetics and physics of a crash play a large part in the way a vehicle will deform upon impact and the injuries which may be seen secondary to the type of impact[19] Injuries are also highly dependent upon internal safety mechanisms and way a vehicle is manufactured (ie, the way a vehicle should come apart upon impact at certain control points). Some of the most common types of motor vehicle entrapments are caused by a deformity of the passenger compartment of some type, partial ejection of the occupant with impingement between the vehicle and another object, or penetration of the passenger compartment by an outside object.

Many types of passenger compartment deformity may occur. The most common type of structural deformity simply leads to the inability of access through the door secondary to lateral impacts or shifting of the alignment of the doors themselves. These extrications may be as simple as a door pop with a Halligan or crowbar, or as complicated as creating pinch points with hydraulic tools to get better bites and remove the door from the vehicle. Another type of deformity that may be encountered

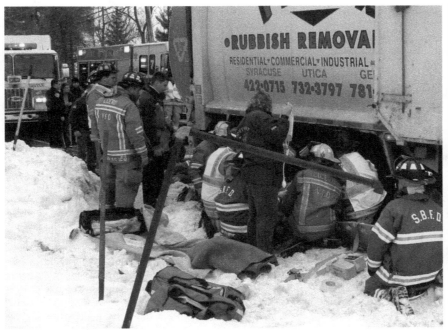
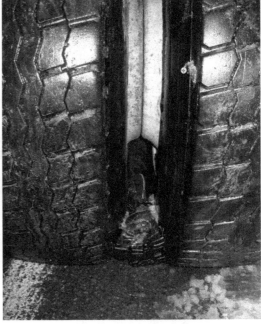

FIGURE 52-2. Evaluation for field amputation. **A:** An EMS physician (blue coat standing on the left with rescuers) equipped with an EMS vehicle, surgical supplies, and Gigli saw is on the scene of an auto versus pedestrian where a man has been run over by a garbage truck while backing. Crews work to lift the truck with airbags while the patient is stabilized. **B:** The patient's leg is shown protruding from between the tires of the truck.

is collapse of the steering column or movement of the patient underneath the steering column, causing entrapment between the seat and/or floor and the steering column. This may be overcome by using a winch mechanism to pull the column toward the front, hydraulic cutters to cut the steering wheel itself, or rams to roll the dash forward thus moving the steering column up and away, or some combination of these techniques. Additional types of structural collapse may include seat assembly breakdown, entrapment of body parts behind the accelerator or brake pedal, and the collapse of the roof of the vehicle. Some of the most difficult extrications to gain access to the patient and provide any advanced treatment include collapse of the roof or rollovers in which the vehicle is laying on its roof with collapse of the passenger compartment. This type of extrication may be lengthy and consists of several stages of removal/cutting of pieces of the vehicle to safely rollback or remove a roof. Keep in mind that these types of passenger compartment deformity may be caused by impacts with other vehicles or immovable objects such as barriers, poles, trees, buildings, or even the road itself as in rollovers.

DANGERS ASSOCIATED WITH EXTRICATION IN MVC

Many dangers are associated with response to a motor vehicle crash. The first thing any provider is taught in a prehospital course is always scene safety. Unfortunately, no scene will ever be completely 100% safe—that is simply not the world we live in. However, responders must be familiar with specific types of threats to themselves, their partners/crew, and any other individual on scene. Some specific dangers to pay specific attention to when responding to or on scene of an MVC are flow of traffic/passing vehicles, power lines, sharp debris, airbags and vehicle safety systems, unstable vehicles, hazardous materials, and fire hazards.[20]

The single biggest concern in working an MVC should always be the safe positioning and protection of vehicles and apparatus to divert flow of traffic safely away from rescuers. This often causes concern and may even cause tension with law enforcement on scene as it can create traffic nightmares; however, the safety of the rescuers and patients is the first priority and should never be put in jeopardy secondary to concerns over flow of traffic. Likewise, responders should make every attempt to position their vehicles out of the flow of traffic if not needed to protect the working scene, thus decreasing the chance of another MVC or the responders being struck by a passing vehicle while getting in or out of their vehicles. One should never assume that anyone sees your emergency lights and vehicle and that they will yield and give you the assumed safe area of operation. Always check your surroundings and be aware of approaching or passing vehicles while on scene.

Perhaps the most unexpected or hidden danger in an MVC is the vehicle's safety mechanisms themselves. With the advent of airbags and airbag systems, the patients have been much more protected; however, it has added an additional layer of concern for rescuers. One must remember that airbags do not always deploy as intended or they are set only to deploy with certain types of impacts. When working in and around the patient compartment, responders must determine if an airbag has deployed, and if it has not, they should make every attempt to render it safe prior to extrication (cut or remove battery cables from terminals). If it is not reasonable to make the airbag safe prior to assessment or extrication, rescuers should be aware of the potential unexpected deployment of a high pressure airbag, which may lead to serious injury to the rescuer or patient if struck by the bag or debris. Rescuers should make every attempt to avoid positioning themselves in the direct line of fire of airbags, should they deploy unexpectedly.

When approaching the scene, responders should be very aware of potential hazardous materials and/or downed power lines and make absolutely certain to clear the area visually prior to stepping out of your vehicle.[21] Unfortunately, there have been many preventable deaths of emergency responders when they are electrocuted on approach to the accident scene. Perhaps the most common and widespread danger to rescuers at the scene of an MVC is the threat of being cut or stabbed by broken glass, debris, or jagged metal. Finally, there is a threat of fire at the scene of any MVC. Although fires associated with extrication and fires that begin after arrival of rescue crews are exceedingly rare, rescuers must always assume there is a threat of fire and make every reasonable effort to protect the scene further (standby extinguishers, lines, sand/dirt on gas spills, etc).[22]

Despite the common system of medical responders not being actively involved with the operation of rescue tools themselves unless their primary duty on scene is rescue/fire, the medical responder should make every attempt to remain within the patient compartment or as close as possible to the patient in order to maintain the safety/protection of the patient and begin/continue emergent treatment. One must always be aware of the potential pinch points, direction of metal/debris being moved by extrication tools, broken glass, or glass which may break when extrication begins.[23]

INDUSTRIAL INCIDENTS/ENTRAPMENTS

Many different industries utilize complicated and dangerous machinery for the production, distribution, or manufacture of products. Some of the most difficult and dangerous entrapments/entanglements may be seen in this area. These include entanglement with machinery such as robotic or heavy machinery on assembly lines, entrapment in conveyor belts, or entrapment in, under, or between heavy machinery. Likewise, heavy equipment on construction sites or industrial sites always pose the threat of crush injury/entrapment between equipment and a solid object or other parts of the machine (ie, train cars), entrapment from loads being carried from the equipment, or structural collapse of equipment (ie, crane collapse). Rescues in these environments may include additional elements such as electrocutions, prolonged severe crush injury, thermal or chemical burns, traumatic amputation, or large mass casualty incidents with urban technical and heavy rescue assets required (eg,, construction site accidents with crane collapse or scaffolding collapse). One should always maintain a high index of suspicion for severe, complicated injury and extrication when responding to incidents at industrial or construction sites.

AGRICULTURAL INCIDENTS

Some of the most impressive and debilitating injuries may be seen with agricultural industry occurrences.[24] These types of events may include auger injuries, grain elevator injuries (explosions or entrapment in the grain itself), cotton gin accidents, processing plant incidents, or heavy machinery incidents. This is a specialized area and many classes in extrication techniques specific to agricultural equipment are offered. These may include topics such as how to remove a patient with severely entangled body parts from an auger and/or how to perform multifaceted rescues from grain elevators that often include confined space, high-angle, technical, and hazardous material techniques all rolled into one incident. As with industrial injuries, responders should always maintain a high index of suspicion for severe injury and/or entrapment when responding to an incident at an agricultural plant or business.

IMPALEMENTS

Impalements may occur in a variety of settings including construction, industrial, agricultural, and even motor vehicle accidents from impacts with trees or shrubbery or intrusions of pipe, rebar, steel, lumber, debris, or pieces of loads being hauled. This may include semitrucks that are in a frontal collision causing a shift of the load forward into the passenger compartment, especially dangerous for truckers carrying pipe, lumber, or steel, with nothing to really stop forward progression of loads except the passenger compartment itself.

Since is virtually never recommended to remove the impaled object from the patient in the field, impalements may be divided into those cases in which the patient and object may be easily and quickly transported and those in which substantial work must be undertaken to cut the object to a manageable size for transport. A wonderful but unfortunate example was the case of a patient impaled through the groin by the fork of an industrial forklift. In this case, the entire fork was removed from the vehicle and the patient transported with the impaled object in an open vehicle rather than ambulance! It is more common to be able to stabilize and cut an impaled piece of wood and metal close to the patient.

If the impaled object appears close to vital structures it is imperative that the object be well stabilized. It is also important to avoid injury to the patient during extrication from whatever tools are used and from the inadvertent heating of the impaled object. The patient will usually benefit from procedural sedation and analgesia if they can tolerate it hemodynamically. Caution must be used if access to the airway is limited.

KEY POINTS

- Encountering entrapment and entanglement circumstances is not uncommon in field care of patients.

- EMS physicians must have familiarity with the techniques and hazards associated with these events and should come equipped with proper personal protective equipment.

- EMS physicians must have operational experience, familiarity with field providers and rescuers, and possess advanced skills and equipment in order to provide maximal care during a response.

- Pharmacologic agents (sedatives, anxiolytics, and analgesics) may be as equally important tools as the hand and power tools used during extrication and disentanglement of entrapped patients.

REFERENCES

1. Siegel JH, Smith JA, Tenenbaum N, et al. Deceleration energy and change in velocity on impact: key factors in fatal versus potentially survivable motor vehicle crash (mvc) aortic injuries (AI): the role of associated injuries as determinants of outcome. *Annu Proc Assoc Adv Automot Med*. 2002;46:315-338.

2. Siegel JH, Smith JA, Siddiqi SQ. Change in velocity and energy dissipation on impact in motor vehicle crashes as a function of the direction of crash: key factors in the production of thoracic aortic injuries, their pattern of associated injuries and patient survival. A Crash Injury Research Engineering Network (CIREN) study. *J Trauma*. October 2004;57(4):760-777; discussion 777-8.

3. Braude D, Richards M. Rapid sequence airway (RSA)—a novel approach to prehospital airway management. *Prehosp Emerg Care*. 2007;11;1-3.

4. Bulger EM, Snyder D, Schoelles K, et al. An evidence-based prehospital guideline for external hemorrhage control: American College of Surgeons Committee on Trauma. *Prehosp Emerg Care*. April-June 2014;18(2):163-173.

5. Risk GC, Augustine J. Extreme bleeds: recommendations for tourniquets in civilian EMS. *JEMS*. March 2012;37(3):76-81.

6. Worf N, White S, High K. Chemical extrication of entrapped motor vehicle crash victims (abstract). *Air Med J*. 2005;24(5):206.

7. Keseg D, Cortez E, Rund D, Caterino J. The use of prehospital ketamine for control of agitation in a metropolitan firefighter-based EMS system. *Prehosp Emerg Care*. January-March 2015;19(1):110-115.

8. Burnett AM, Salzman JG, Griffith KR, Kroeger B, Frascone RJ. The emergency department experience with prehospital ketamine: a case series of 13 patients. *Prehosp Emerg Care*. October-December 2012;16(4):553-559.

9. Bredmose PP, et al. Prehospital use of ketamine for analgesia and procedural sedation. *Emerg Med J*. 2009;26:62-64.

10. Chesters A, Webb T, Ketamine for procedural sedation by a doctor-paramedic prehospital care team: a 4-year description of practice. *Eur J Emerg Med*. 2015 Jan 30 [Epub ahead of print].

11. Green SM, Roback MG, Kennedy RM, Krauss B. Clinical practice guideline for Emergency Department Ketamine Dissociative Sedation: 2011 Update. *Annals Emerg Med*. 2011;57:449-461.

12. Perel P, Roberts I, Ker K. Colloids versus crystalloids for fluid resuscitation in critically ill patients. *Cochrane Database Syst Rev*. 2013 Feb 28;2:CD000567.

13. Patanwala AE, Amini A, Erstad BL. Use of hypertonic saline injection in trauma. *Am J Health Syst Pharm*. 2010;67(22):1920-1928.

14. Gonzalez D. Crush syndrome. *Crit Care Med*. 2005;33(1 suppl):s34-s41.

15. Sever MS, Vanholder, R, Lameire N. Management of crush-related injuries after disasters. *New Engl J Med*. 2006;354:1052-1063.

16. Sharp CF, Mangram AJ, Lorenzo M, Dunn EL. A major metropolitan "field amputation" team: a call to arms … and legs. *J Trauma*. 2009;67(6):1158-1161.

17. Raines A, Lees J, Fry W, Parks A, Tuggle D. Field amputation: response planning and legal considerations inspired by three separate amputations. *Am J Disaster Med*. Winter 2014;9(1):53-58.

18. Zils SW, Codner PA, Pirrallo RG. Field extremity amputation: a brief curriculum and protocol. *Acad Emerg Med*. 2011;18(9):e84.

19. Methner P. Extrication scene tips for EMS personnel: EMS considerations to enhance scene operations and personal safety. *JEMS*. April 2004;29(4):28-30, 32,34-35.

20. Calland V. A brief overview of personal safety at incident sites. *Emerg Med J*. November 2006;23(11):878-882.

21. Krzanicki DA, Porter KM. Personal protective equipment provision in prehospital care: a national survey. *Emerg Med J*. December 2009;26(12):892-895.

22. Funk DL, Politis JF, McErlean M, Dickinson ET. Necessity of fire department response to the scene of motor vehicle crashes. *Am J Emerg Med*. November 2002;20(7):580-582.

23. Politis J, Dailey M. Extrication fundamentals. Proper care of the entrapped patient. *JEMS*. April 2010;35(4):41-47.

24. Augustine JJ. Man vs. machine. A farm accident leads to devastating injuries and a tough extrication. *EMS Mag*. June 2010;39(6):18, 20-21.

Field Triage and Transport Decision Making

John W. Lyng

INTRODUCTION

The daily operations of EMS systems focus on providing care and transport to individual patients with (usually) unlimited resources. This approach allows prehospital providers to attempt to maximize the chances of an individual's survival and reduce the morbidity they may experience from their injury or illness. In situations involving multiple/mass casualties incidents and disasters, the principles of "routine" field triage and transport decisions can change significantly, as the goals of patient care shift from doing the most good for a singular patient, to doing the most good for the most patients. Recognizing the regional variability inherent in prehospital emergency care, it is imperative for EMS physicians to understand the concepts in this chapter globally, but also to apply and understand them in the context of their local/regional EMS system(s). Specific aspects of daily operations are discussed elsewhere in the text.

OBJECTIVES

- Describe the theory behind the need for trauma triage in mass casualty incidents.
- Describe the major field triage methods, and detail their use.
- Describe the medical triage, transport, and treatment areas setup during an MCI.
- Discuss the role of the EMS physician in assisting the triage officer(s) and transport officer(s) in their duties.
- Discuss the pros and cons of the EMS physician limiting their role to aiding in the treatment area during an MCI.
- Discuss field triage and retriage in prolonged events, or during times of limited hospital/transportation resources.

TRIAGE: A BRIEF HISTORY

Triage, from the French *trier* meaning to sort, is a term initially ascribed to the process of sorting coffee beans. The transition from an agrarian process to a part of the medical evaluation process began with the efforts of Baron Dominique-Jean Larrey, Chief Surgeon of Napoleon's Army. Baron Larrey is credited with devising a system to identify and sort casualties of war on the battlefield and evacuate them via *ambulances volantes* to field hospitals.[1] In this first use of medical triage, the goal was to identify soldiers with injuries that were survivable, with focus placed on providing the care needed to return the soldier to the battlefield as quickly as possible in order to maintain a sufficient fighting force. Following the Napoleonic wars, the battlefields of subsequent military engagements saw further refinement of the triage processes as the technology of health care and warfare developed. The development of antibiotics and advanced surgical techniques, recognition and treatment of shock, utilization of helicopters, and institution of "buddy care" to initiate immediately lifesaving interventions all had a significant role in the reduction of combat fatalities from a rate as high as 30% during World War II to a rate of less than 10% in the Afghan and Iraqi wars.[1]

As with much of our present-day trauma care practices, civilian triage methods were subsequently derived from wartime practices that have been adapted to peacetime needs stemming from natural, industrial, and criminal/terror-related disasters and multiple/mass casualty incidents. Now, the medical literature is plentiful with acronyms such as START, JumpSTART, SAVE, SALT, and TSS, and products such as

triage kits containing color-coded tags, flags, tarps, vests, and other items are common in the consumer retail markets. For the end user, it can be challenging to determine which of several protocols and products are best chosen and implemented to maximize survival rates while maintaining a triage method that is cost-effective. One of these challenges is the lack of a universally accepted triage standard.

Several challenges exist behind the development and utilization of current triage methods, not the least of which is a paucity of evidence-based information on which to critically assess the accuracy and effectiveness of these schemes.

DEFINING THE NEED FOR TRIAGE

According to the World Health Organization, a disaster occurs when "normal conditions of existence are disrupted and the level of suffering exceeds the capacity of the hazard-affected community to respond to it."[2] The World Medical Association goes on to explain "from the medical standpoint, disaster situations are characterized by an acute and unforeseen imbalance between the capacity and resources of the medical profession and the needs of survivors who are injured or whose health is threatened, over a given period of time."[3]

Disasters are usually on a very large scale and involve a large geographic area, with examples including the 2010 Haiti earthquake, Hurricanes Katrina and Rita in the US Gulf Coast in 2005, and the 2004 Indian Ocean Tsunami. More common are mass casualty incidents (MCIs), defined as "a situation that places a significant demand on medical resources and personnel but in which local response capabilities are not overwhelmed despite a large number of patients requiring triage and medical treatment."[4]

In our daily prehospital and inhospital medical care, we expend significant resources with the goal of providing the greatest chance of survival for individual patients, that is, providing the "greatest good for the individual." In the vast majority of events, scarcity of resources during disasters and MCIs necessitates a paradigm shift toward rationing and equitable utilization of resources so we may provide the "greatest good for the greatest number."[5] In very limited circumstances, an exception to this premise exists. The concept of *reverse triage* deserves special mention with regard to the overall concept of utilization of resources. Two applicable definitions of this term apply. In the civilian setting, reverse triage refers to focusing care resources on the most critically injured or "expectant" patients. In this form, reverse triage is specifically applicable to the allocation of resources for multiple victims of a lightning strike, where there is a high potential for survivability of patients in cardiac arrest if they receive prompt CPR and defibrillation. For further discussion of care of the lighting-strike victim, the reader is referred to Chapter 47. In the military or tactical setting, reverse triage refers to prioritization of resources to the least injured personnel in order to return them to duty as quickly as possible in order to maintain strength of defending forces or control of the tactical environment. After an appropriate fighting or defensive/protective force is preserved, care can be provided to more critically injured personnel who are deemed salvageable by applicable triage and treatment schemata based on the combat or tactical environment and available treatment and evacuation resources.

TRIAGE AS PART OF A COORDINATED RESPONSE SYSTEM

Triage exists as part of a larger, comprehensive and integrated response to an MCI or disaster. As such, it must be recognized that triage operations do not exist in a silo, as they are affected by and affect the actions of other responding entities. Bostick et al discuss a concept of *systemic triage* and define four orders of triage that occur in the recognition, response, and recovery stages of a disaster.[6]

In systemic triage, first-order triage is established in the general community that may be or has been affected by the incident. First-order triage is used by public health to help disseminate information that may help prevent injury, decrease exposure to a threat, and help resources from becoming overwhelmed by providing risk-specific information to the community about appropriate self-protection practices, indications for seeking medical care, and appropriate venues to seek shelter or care. Examples of steps taken in first-order triage may be shelter in place, community evacuation, or specific disease call centers such as the Canadian SARs Hotline. Second-order triage occurs in the prehospital setting and involves the identification, sorting, treatment, and evacuation of casualties to appropriate locations for definitive care. Third-order triage occurs at sites of secondary or definitive care and involves assessment of the medical needs of arriving patients, stabilization and transfer to definitive care, or provision of definitive care. Use of treatment protocols and redistribution of patients are actions taken in this order of triage. Finally, Fourth-order triage occurs at the regional level and involves monitoring of the disaster and appropriate resource allocation, including actions like activating the strategic national (pharmaceutical) stockpile or redistributing human, supply, and equipment resources within the affected area.[6] Such a systemic approach allows for integration of the disaster response entities and maximizes the potential for increased casualty survival at each point of contact with victims and those at risk for disaster-related injury or illness. The coordination of response that is established by systemic triage is needed in order to provide victims of an MCI or disaster *equal opportunity of survival*, meaning all affected individuals are afforded equity in triage and the receipt of medical care that is consistent with their injuries and projected survivability, as well as prevailing resource constraints. This notion of equal opportunity in triage does not, however, guarantee either treatment or survival for all patients potentially affected by a catastrophic event.[6]

This chapter will focus second-order triage, the operations of triage in the identification of patients, their categorization, and prioritization for treatment and evacuation from an MCI/disaster scene. For more discussion regarding the role of EMS in disaster response, please see Section 12.

INJURY PATTERNS IN DISASTERS AND MCIs

With the exception of chemical, biologic, radiation, and nuclear (CBRN)-related events, an important concept to recognize about patients injured in disasters and MCIs is that their injuries tend to be similar to those that medical providers encounter in their regular daily trauma care.[5] Thus, most prehospital providers already possess the skills needed to evaluate and care for these patients. Although fortunately, as Frykberg discusses, "the great majority of initial survivors are *not* critically injured," the often large number of noncritical patients who must be assessed may make it more difficult to identify and provide immediate treatment to the 10% to 25% of patients who are critically injured.[5] Additional challenge exists in determining which patients may or may not be salvageable, and one of the most difficult principles for triage providers to adapt to is that circumstances may require them to abandon casualties that would normally (in day-to-day operations) undergo heroic measures regardless of their chances of survival.

CBRN events may add an additional level of complexity to the assessment of disaster and MCI victims. This is especially true because most EMS providers do not usually encounter patients injured by CBRN mechanisms during their daily operations and thus have less experience and potentially less knowledge and understanding of disease and toxicology mechanisms on which to base their assessment and categorization of CBRN injured patients. The issues of EMS provider safety, when, which type, and how to use personal protective equipment, and when, where, and how to perform patient decontamination increase the complexity of triage decisions.

Victims of chemical exposure may experience immediate or delayed injuries in the absence of physical trauma. Patients may initially be well-appearing casualties that later deteriorate and experience life-threatening conditions such as cholinergic toxicity. Thus frequent

retriage is a necessity. Providers also face challenges in the provision of immediately lifesaving treatment of chemically injured victims due to the availability, efficacy, and difficulty in administration of antidotes (ie, atropine and 2-PAM autoinjectors, the number of doses needed for effective treatment, etc). Furthermore, chemically exposed patients may pose an exposure risk to rescuers and require decontamination, which can slow the progress of moving patients from an incident scene to primary treatment and evacuation areas. Chemical-related events may occur in a discrete area or may be dispersed over a large geographic area depending on prevailing weather conditions and the nature of the chemical agent (a gas, vapor, or liquid).

Unlike chemical exposures, biologic exposures are unlikely to cause immediate injury and may have a latency period typically on the order of days. Although the initial exposure may have occurred at a discrete location, when patients begin to exhibit symptoms of their exposure they are unlikely to be confined to a discrete scene (ie, distributed over a larger geographic area). Therefore, the utilization of most primary triage methods is less likely to be effective during a biologic event.

The threat of a radiation exposure must be considered when developing a triage method that can be applied to "all hazards." Although capable of inflicting a significant psychological impact on a large population, radiation dispersion devices (RDD) or *dirty bombs* are more likely to inflict life-threatening traumatic injury that is a direct result of the explosion/blast forces rather than immediately life-threatening injury from the radiation exposure itself. Unless a patient is contaminated with radioactive material, the radiation-exposed patient poses no radiation risk to the rescuer (ie, a patient who gets an x-ray is exposed to radiation, but is not a risk to other people). Although the number of physically injured victims may be small, the psychological impact of RDDs may result in a large number of "worried well." While these patients are not likely to consume physical medical resources (medications, wound care supplies, etc) they do consume a significant number of personnel resources as they seek assessment and medical care. When considering the primary causes of injury in a dirty bomb event, it has been suggested that "no substantial revisions need to be made to MCI triage methods to account for radiation exposure."[7]

In difference to an RDD event, victims from a nuclear event are likely to suffer life-threatening injuries resulting from blast, thermal, and ionizing radiation mechanisms. The type of radiation exposure (α and β particles, and γ-rays), intensity of exposure, degree of contamination, and duration of exposure are likely to be higher in a nuclear event compared to an RDD detonation. Because sources of ionizing radiation are dispersed in the environment, ongoing exposure can occur for both victims and rescuers who remain in the primary contamination zone. Patients close enough to the source of the nuclear incident to receive enough radiation exposure to result in acute radiation sickness are also likely to be within the primary lethal blast zone (blast area roughly double the area where "survival possible" exposure of 2 to 4.5 Gy.[8]

ASSESSMENT OF THE EFFICACY OF A TRIAGE METHOD

A common theme among many of the literature resources reviewed for the development of this chapter is discussion regarding the lack of sufficient data on which to base evaluation of the efficacy of existing triage methods. Of the few articles that have attempted to validate existing triage methods, because there is little existing data available regarding outcomes from real-life utilization of triage methods to actual MCIs and disasters, most studies are based on data surrogates such as retrospective application of protocol assessment criteria to patients in trauma registries. Considering that prospective assessment of a particular triage method is likely impossible due to barriers in predicting disasters, lead time in training providers, and certain ethical challenges, the use of these surrogates for data and efficacy assessment are necessary.

In addition to the lack of adequate data, many articles also cited the lack of a universally accepted gold standard or outcome measure with which to compare various triage methods. However, several different concepts have been identified as critical variables that must be considered when evaluating or developing a triage method.

Frykberg discusses the concept of the *critical mortality rate*, the percentage of deaths only among the critically injured, suggesting that "the outcome of critically injured casualties is the best indication of the success of medical care in an MCI." By using this measure, triage methods would be compared based on their ability to identify and correctly categorize the critically injured patients, and would be judged on this specific survival score rather than on the overall disaster mortality rate (which would include the on-scene/immediate deaths as part of the entire fatality census).[5]

Several factors may influence the critical mortality rate achieved by a particular triage method. Ideally a triage method would correctly categorize each patient 100% of the time. However, certain rates of *undertriage*, inappropriate assignment of critically injured victims with life-threatening problems to a delayed category, and *overtriage*, assignment of noncritical casualties to immediate care, often occur. Undertriage places critical patients at risk of not receiving appropriate priority for treatment and transport. This may occur when victims have somewhat innocuous appearing injury patterns externally, but have significant internal injury (ie, small penetrating trauma from shrapnel). Conversely, casualties that have severe external injuries but have a low likelihood of survival may be overtriaged to the immediate category, rather than an "expectant" category. In either case, overtriage will lead to the consumption of resources that would best be utilized to care for the true "immediate" patients. Of the two, studies of MCI bombing events indicate that overtriage has been shown to have a greater negative impact, illustrating "a direct linear relationship between the rate of overtriage and the critical mortality rate of survivors".[9]

Both over- and undertriage can be an effect of the triage method or of the rescuer who is using the method. *Intrarater reliability* occurs when an instrument results in identical triage categorization if the same evaluator rates the same patient twice within a short time period.[10] *Interrater reliability* occurs when an instrument results in identical triage categorization of the same patient when evaluated by two different raters.[10] In a well-developed triage method, rates of intra- and interrater reliability would be high.

When authors discuss the "testing" of a triage method, it is important to understand exactly what is being tested. Is one testing whether the scheme can predict patient outcomes, whether providers use the scheme

accurately, or whether use of the scheme improves outcomes? In other words, when looking at the patient outcomes when a particular triage method has been utilized, it may be difficult to separate whether there was a success or failure of the tool itself, or success or failure in the ability of the providers to accurately/correctly use the tool.

The concept of *construct validity*, the ability of a test or process to assess what it is intended to assess, can be applied both to the validity of the triage method and in the tools used to assess the effectiveness of the method.[11] The construct validity of several primary triage methods (START, SMART, CareFlight) has been assessed in a few studies, but no such assessment has been applied to secondary triage methods.[10]

In the initial chaos of an MCI or disaster, a certain amount of inaccuracy of triage must be expected and accepted. This inaccuracy can be mitigated, however, by utilizing secondary and tertiary triage at each point in the patient evacuation process (ie, arrival at a treatment zone, just prior to departure from a treatment zone, upon arrival at a destination hospital, etc). Such serial reassessments can help increase the accuracy of their diagnosis, can increase triage accuracy, and decrease the rates of under- and overtriage.

MAJOR FIELD TRIAGE METHODS AND THEIR USE

Several triage methods have been proposed, and they are utilized to various degrees across the United States and internationally. In 2008, a consortium of specialists was convened in the United States to develop and propose a national standard triage guideline. In their review of existing literature and products, they identified nine existing triage methods. Several commonalities were identified between these systems, although it was found that there is a lack of uniformity in aspects such as patient assessment principles and commonality of language (ie, Priority I, II, III; Immediate, Delayed, Minimal; Emergent, Urgent, Nonurgent, etc) that may result in confusion, especially if neighboring jurisdictions use differing triage methods. This panel focused their efforts on reviewing primary triage methods, including *START, JumpSTART, Homebush, Triage Sieve, Pediatric Triage Tape, CareFlight, Sacco Triage Method, Military Triage,* and *CESIRA*. **Table 53-1** provides a summary comparison of these primary triage methods.

TABLE 53-1 Comparison of Existing Triage Systems

System	Coding	Status Assigned Based on	Interventions Allowed Before Categorizing as "Dead"	Comments
Simple Triage and Rapid Transport Treatment (START)	Immediate: red Delayed: yellow Walking wounded: green Deceased: black	Immediate: Resp. rate >30, slow capillary refill, or cannot follow commands Walking wounded: able to walk Deceased: not breathing after one attempt to open airway Delayed: all others	Open airway	• Modified version replaces capillary refill with radial pulse
JumpSTART	Immediate: red Delayed: yellow Minor: green Deceased: black	Immediate: respiratory rate <15 or >45 or irregular, or no palpable peripheral pulse, or inappropriate posturing or unresponsive (P or U on AVPU scale) Delayed: unable to walk, respiratory rate 15-45; and palpable peripheral pulse, and A or V on AVPU	Open airway, if not breathing and palpable radial pulse give five rescue breaths	• Developed for children ages 1-8 • Parallel to structure of START • Children carried to an ambulatory area should be assessed first • Modification for nonambulatory children
Homebush	Immediate: red Urgent: yellow Not Urgent: green Dying: white Dead: black	Immediate: not walking, breathing, but not able to follow commands, or no radial pulse, or resp. rate >30 Urgent: nonambulatory, do not meet other criteria	Open airway	• Based on START and SAVE triage • Category for Dying created so they can receive comfort care • Uses geographic triage with flags rather than individual tags

(continued)

TABLE 53-1   Comparison of Existing Triage Systems (*continued*)

System	Coding	Status Assigned Based on	Interventions Allowed Before Categorizing as "Dead"	Comments
	Also assigns radio phonetic categories: Immediate: Alpha Urgent: Bravo Not Urgent: Charlie Dying: Delta Dead: Echo	Not urgent: anyone who can walk Dead: not breathing Dying: patients determined to be beyond help		
Triage Sieve	Priority 1 (immediate): red Priority 2 (urgent): yellow Priority 3 (delayed): green Priority 4 (expectant): blue Dead white or black	Priority 1: not walking with respiratory rate <10 or >29, or capillary refill >2 s Priority 2: not walking with a respiratory rate 10-29 and cap refill <2 sec Dead: no airway	Open airway	• Heart rate of >120 bpm substituted for capillary refill in cold conditions or poor light • Does not use mental status
Pediatric Triage Tape (PTT)	Immediate: red Urgent: yellow Delayed: green Dead	Immediate: abnormally slow or fast respiratory rate, or abnormally slow or fast pulse rate Urgent: not walking with a capillary refill of <2 s Delayed: child who is walking, or an infant who is alert and moving all limbs Dead: not breathing	Open airway	• Requires a tape that uses height of patient to provide age-appropriate vital sign parameters (four sizes of the patient: 50-80 cm, 80-100 cm, 100-140 cm, and >140 cm) • Adaptation of Triage Sieve
CareFlight	Immediate: red Urgent: yellow Delayed: green Unsalvageable: black	Immediate: does not follow commands or no radial pulse Urgent: does not walk but obeys commands and has a radial pulse Delayed: walks Unsalvageable: not breathing with an open airway	Open airway	• No respiratory considerations • Can be used for pediatric patients
Sacco Triage Method	Group 1: high rate of deterioration Group 2: moderate Group 3: slow	Assigns an RPM score based on respiratory rate, pulse rate, and motor response	Open airway, decompress pneumothorax, stop exsanguination	• Provides a score for each patient; grouping of patients changes with available resources • Transport order by score, not group
Military Triage	Immediate Delayed Minor Expectant	Immediate: those who should be treated first, with a list of possible injuries Delayed: those who can have a delay of 6-8 hours before treatment Minor: those who will not have significant mortality if no further care is provided Expectant: those with signs of impending death who require vast resources for treatment	Open airway	• Based on NATO triage • Secondary Triage includes system for patient evacuation • Colors are often used to mark casualties when they have been triaged but colors can vary from unit to unit and are not universal
CESIRA	Red Yellow Green	Red: Unconscious, hemorrhaging, in a state of shock, insufficient respirations Yellow: none of the above with broken bones and other injuries Green: able to walk	Not applicable: prehospital providers in Italy may not determine death in the field	• No dead category, only physicians can declare death in Italy • Based on presenting problem • Name is based on order in which conditions are evaluated

AVPU, alert, voice, pain, unresponsive; NATO, North Atlantic Treaty Organization; RPM, respiratory rate, pulse rate, and motor response; SAVE, Secondary Assessment of Victim Endpoint.

Adapted with permission from Table 1: Comparison of Existing Mass Triage Systems in Lerner EB, Schwartz RB, Coule PL: Mass casualty triage: an evaluation of the data and development of a proposed national guideline. *Disaster Med Public Health Prep.* 2008;2 (suppl 1):S25-S34. Copyright © Society for Disaster Medicine and Public Health, Inc. 2008.

TRIAGE MEASURES

First, we will discuss some of the various measures that existing triage methods utilize in the categorization of patients. Then we will discuss the major triage methods that are in use in the United States, with mention of some valuable points illustrated by other systems.

Again, the goal of an effective triage method is to reduce both under- and overtriage. By using effective measures of injury, such as physiologic and anatomic criteria, rather than using mechanism of injury criteria to categorize patients, studies have shown that we can reduce rates of overtriage without increasing rates of undertriage.[5] Such physiologic and anatomic criteria include a Glasgow coma score

<14, a systolic blood pressure <90 mm Hg, and a respiratory rate <10 or >29 breaths per minute.

It is generally considered impractical to obtain a blood pressure reading using a sphygmomanometer in the initial triage phase of an event. This is because noisy and dark environments may make it difficult to hear and see well enough to use a blood pressure cuff, and because it is difficult to rapidly obtain such a measure on multiple patients. Therefore, certain surrogate measures of adequate perfusion, including assessment of a radial pulse or capillary refill, are utilized by most existing triage methods. Assessment of radial pulse likely carries the most utility, because it does not require special equipment to measure, and, unlike capillary refill, a radial pulse can be assessed in dark and cold environments.[12]

Even in normal day-to-day EMS and trauma operations, the calculation of an accurate Glasgow coma score (GCS) may be difficult.[12] However, there is good evidence to support the simplification of the GCS in the MCI setting. Dark environments may make it difficult for rescuers to assess a patient's eye response. Barriers to verbal communication, including language barriers, hearing impairment and hearing-related injuries, ambient noise, altered mental status, and endotracheally intubated patients may make it difficult to reasonably assess a patient's verbal response. Fortunately, several studies have shown that the motor score of GCS has highest predictive value for patient outcome.[7,13-17] Specifically, removal of the eye score from the total GCS did not lower predictive performance of the GCS. Additionally, although removal of the verbal score did result in statistically significant but mathematically minimal lowering of the performance of the GCS, the authors of the study advocated for the removal of the verbal score because of the aforementioned barriers to achieving a reliable verbal score. Finally, it was noted that the motor score held a near-linear relationship with mortality and was predictive of the need for intubation, admission to the ICU, and disability.[7,14] Based on several of these studies, it appears the motor component of the GCS has predictive validity, is easier to use on an MCI/disaster scene, and sufficiently identifies patients in need of immediate intervention or transport to a medical facility.[12,16,17]

START AND JUMPSTART

Simple Triage and Rapid Treatment (START) and JumpSTART (a variation of START that accounts for physiologic differences between pediatric and adult patients) are triage methods utilized by several jurisdictions in the United States and abroad. START was developed in 1983 by Newport Beach Fire and Marine Department and Hoag Hospital, Newport Beach, CA, and was updated in 1994. JumpSTART was developed in 1995 by the Miami, FL Children's Hospital and was modified in 2001. These methods are similar in that they first identify all walking wounded and categorize them as "minor" and direct them to a secondary triage area. Next is an assessment of apnea and respiratory rate, followed by assessment of perfusion using either the radial pulse or the capillary refill. Finally is an evaluation of mental status assessed by the ability of the patient to follow commands. **Figure 53-1** illustrates a combined START/JumpSTART triage algorithm. Incidents where START was utilized have been retrospectively reviewed for the rate of under- and overtriage. Additionally, the ability of providers to apply the START and JumpSTART methods using paper-based tests has also been assessed, although it is not known how well performance on a paper-based scenario predicts performance in the field.[12] With the exception of opening the airway (and providing five rescue breaths for apneic pediatric patients), neither START nor JumpSTART includes any other immediately lifesaving interventions in the protocols. One criticism of the START method is that it appears to undertriage elderly patients.[18]

TRIAGE SIEVE AND PEDIATRIC TRIAGE TAPE

The Triage Sieve is a method used widely in the United Kingdom and parts of Australia and was developed in 1995 by Hodgetts and Mackway-Jones.[19,35] Similar to START, this method assigns priority based on ability to walk, airway patency, respiratory rate, and pulse rate. This method first identifies the walking wounded and categorizes them as Priority 3/Delayed. Then the provider assesses for apnea and rate of breathing,

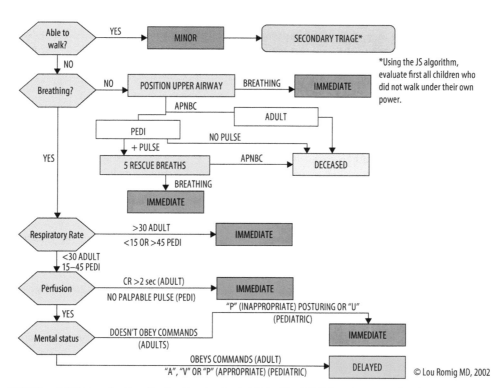

FIGURE 53-1 Combined START/JumpSTART triage algorithm. (Reprinted from Lou Romig, MD, Combined START/JumpStart Triage Algorithm. Miami, FL. 2002. http://www.jumpstarttriage.com/uploads/COMBINED_S-JS_ALGORITHM.gif.)

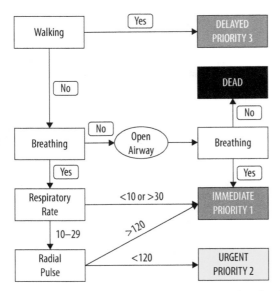

FIGURE 53-2 Triage Sieve algorithm. (Modified with permission from Crisis Medicine Training Network. Triage Sieve. Valhalla, South Africa, 2009. http://www.crisismedicine.co.za/registration.html.)

followed by assessment of perfusion by measuring the radial pulse. In difference to START's definition of abnormal breathing as >30 bpm, the Triage Sieve defines abnormal breathing as <10 or >29 breaths per minute. Triage Sieve also defines an abnormal pulse as >120/minute. There is no assessment of mental status or motor function (beyond ability to walk) in this method. Also, except for basic airway opening maneuvers, the protocol does not include other interventions for immediate life threats. **Figure 53-2** illustrates the Triage Sieve algorithm.

Similar to JumpSTART being a pediatric adaptation of START, the Pediatric Triage Tape (PTT) is a pediatric adaptation of Triage Sieve. The PTT is "a waterproof, nontear tape that relates the child's height/length to normal physiological variables so that their physiologic status can be assessed using age-appropriate norms."[20,35]

Malik et al documented the use of Triage Sieve at a train wreck in Pakistan.[21] There is no documentation of the use of the PTT in a real-world situation, although a few papers have assessed its utility using paper-based testing.[22] Additionally, attempts were made to validate the PTT using a surrogate data source. Wallis et al assessed the PTT's ability to retrospectively correctly identify pediatric trauma patients presenting to a South African trauma unit that had an Injury Severity Score of >15. They identified that with this population, the PTT had a sensitivity of 38% and specificity of 99%, and if it had been used in a similar real-life situation, rates of overtriage and undertriage would be 39% and 4%, respectively.[23]

HOMEBUSH (AUSTRALIA)

The Homebush Triage Standard was developed in Australia and utilizes START and SAVE. Unlike many response plans in the United States, the Homebush method does not utilize triage tags during the initial categorization of patients, but rather directs them to geographic areas on the disaster scene that have been marked with colored flags representing the different triage/treatment priorities. In addition to the Homebush method classifying patients into Immediate, Urgent, Non Urgent, Dying, and Dead, the method also assigns both a phonetic alphabet priority code (Alpha, Bravo, Charlie, Delta, Echo) and color code (Red, Yellow, Green, White, Black) in order to ensure clear radio communications and easy visual recognition. Like the US National Guideline for Mass Casualty Triage (SALT), the Homebush Triage Standard was suggested in order to establish a uniform method and familiar, common language of triage that all hospitals and ambulance services would utilize and allow for effective and efficient communication.[24]

MASS TRIAGE METHOD

The National Disaster Life Support (American Medical Association curriculum) suite of courses teaches a sorting method called MASS (Move, Assess, Sort, Send). This sorting method is adaptable to any of the major triage categorization systems and provides guidance on the process of on-scene evaluation and rapid sorting of patients. Utilizing the principle that patients who can walk and follow a command are likely to be less critically injured, patients who cannot walk but can otherwise move and follow a simple command are more severely injured, and those who cannot move and cannot follow a command are the most severely injured or dead, the MASS method employs a global sorting of patients in order to facilitate the identification of those patients who need to have a triage category of "immediate" ascertained as quickly as possible in order to effect maximal patient survivability.[25]

SALT

Recognizing that several triage methods were being utilized by various jurisdictions within the United States, and the problems inherent with the lack of a uniform standard practice (ie, lack of interoperability, lack of common language, different treatment and transport prioritization, etc) a panel of experts from the private and public sectors was convened in the United States in 2008. The consensus panel identified and reviewed existing triage methods in order to propose a National Guideline for Mass Casualty Triage. As part of their evaluation process, the panel identified "Model Uniform Core Criteria for Mass Casualty Triage."[26] These criteria earned the endorsement of the American Academy of Pediatrics (AAP), American College of Emergency Physicians (ACEP), American College of Surgeons—Committee on Trauma (ACSOT), National Association of Emergency Medical Technicians (NAEMT), National Association of EMS Physicians (NAEMSP), among several others.

In developing these core criteria, they established general criteria thought to be needed for a triage method to be effective (**Table 53-2**). Additionally, they recognized the need for a method of *global sorting*, guidelines for the provision of *lifesaving interventions*, and an algorithm for *individual assessment of triage category*.

In addition to these considerations, other authors have suggested that the ideal triage method will also be applicable by rescuers with a variety of backgrounds and levels of experience.[7] Key performance characteristics by which triage instruments should be examined to determine a standard guideline for triage that were identified by Armstrong et al include:

- Simplicity, for execution in chaos
- Time efficiency, when time equals lives

TABLE 53-2	General Considerations for an Effective Mass Casualty Triage Method

Triage methods and all their components must apply to all ages and populations of patients.

Triage methods must be applicable across the broad range of mass casualty incidents where there is a single location with multiple patients.

Triage methods must be simple, easy to remember, and amenable to quick memory aids.

Triage methods must be rapid to apply and practical for use in an austere environment.

Triage methods are resource dependent and the system must allow for dynamic triage decisions based on changes in available resources and patient conditions.

Triage methods must require that the assigned triage category for each patient be visibly identifiable (triage tags, tarps, markers).

Triage is dynamic and reflects patient condition and available resources at the time of assessment. Assessments must be repeated whenever possible and categories adjusted to reflect changes.

Adapted with permission from Table 1. General Considerations in Model uniform core criteria for mass casualty triage. *Disaster Med Public Health Prep.* 2011;5(2):125-128. Copyright © Society for Disaster Medicine and Public Health, Inc. 2011.

- Predictive validity, so that the assessment relates to the intended outcome, namely, the identification of the critically injured from the mass of walking wounded

- Reliability, in that it is reproducible (with both the same rater and between raters) across all hazards

- Accuracy, to minimize over- and undertriage

After reviewing the various existing triage methods, the consensus panel determined that although several of the triage methods reviewed met some of the Core Criteria, no single method existed that best fit all of the criteria. The panel then chose to design a new triage method: Sort, Assess, Lifesaving intervention, Treatment/Transport (SALT), which incorporates what were identified as the best characteristics of existing triage methods into a singular method that better meets the Core Criteria. It is recognized by the panel that SALT encounters the same limitations that existing methods do, the fact that it is based on Level V (expert opinion) evidence and needs to be validated through various possible methods. **Figure 53-3** illustrates the SALT triage method and **Table 53-3** defines the SALT triage categories.

In their invited commentary regarding SALT, Armstrong et al help clarify what SALT does that previous triage methods did not[27]:

- Focuses first on the mass of casualties by voice command sorting. Hearing loss and self-transport of the walking wounded may limit controlled casualty distribution from the scene.

- Assesses casualties briefly for explicitly defined lifesaving interventions with applicability in chemical and radiation hazards. Controlling hemorrhage, opening airway, decompressing the chest (for tension pneumothorax), and autoinjection for chemical injury are actions triggered by brief sensory observations.

- Separates expectant from dead with a new color, gray. SALT emphasizes the relative nature of the expectant category based on available

TABLE 53-3 SALT Triage Categories

Treatment/Transport Priority	Color	Treatments provided
Immediate	Red	Lifesaving interventions
Delayed	Yellow	Analgesics, splinting, basic burn, and laceration care
Minimal	Green	Basic first aid
Expectant	Gray	Comfort care, lifesaving interventions if resources become available (*recategorized as "immediate" in this instance*)
Dead	Black	

resources and the need for comfort care. Those casualties who are absolutely unsalvageable are unlikely to move out of the expectant category.

- Includes all ages; this instrument applies to adults and children, adding simplicity.

Although SALT has not been evaluated in an actual real-world event, two studies have assessed the ability of paramedics to accurately use the SALT method using paper-based and virtual reality–based examination techniques following an initial training session.[28,29]

SECONDARY TRIAGE METHODS

As previously mentioned, secondary and tertiary triage points can help increase the discrimination between critical and noncritical casualties. The Sacco Triage Method, Secondary Assessment of Victim Endpoint (SAVE), and Triage Sort are three methods of secondary triage that have

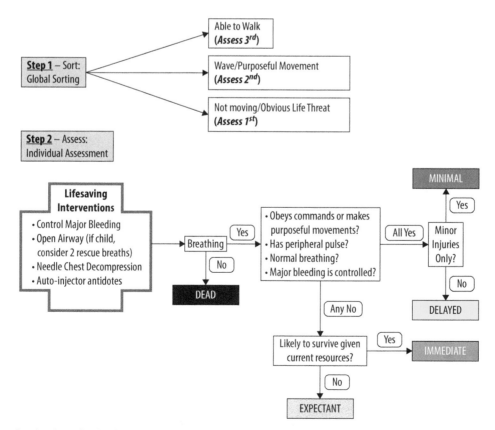

FIGURE 53-3 SALT triage algorithm. (Reproduced with permission from SALT Mass Casualty Triage. *Disaster Med Public Health Prep.* 2008;2(4):245-246. Copyright © Society for Disaster Medicine and Public Health, Inc. 2008).

been developed. Converse to the primary triage methods, the secondary triage methods, except for the Sacco Triage Method, have not been investigated for their validity.[10]

SACCO TRIAGE METHOD

The Sacco Triage Method is a proprietary software–based mathematical model that orders the treatment of patients based on their probability of survival, potential for deterioration, and available resources. This model was based on a set of physiologic scores including respiratory rate, pulse rate, and best motor response. This system is not a triage algorithm and it requires proprietary software, hardware, data entry personnel, communication with incident command or central dispatch, and resource availability reports. It is not designed as a primary triage algorithm, but may be useful when transport/evacuation resources are scarce and on-scene medical care must be prolonged. Additionally, because the method requires the use of proprietary software, it may be difficult for economically challenged jurisdictions to procure and implement. The Sacco Triage Method's use seems to be limited to a few jurisdictions in the United States.[10] When compared to other methodology for disaster triage, this method performed well.[30] When tested retrospectively this method performed well in pediatric patients.[31]

SAVE

Secondary Assessment of Victim Endpoint (SAVE) was developed for use at a casualty receiving area or on a primary scene where significant delays in evacuation to definitive care exist. It is designed to reassess patients and sort them based on survivability within a certain triage category when primary scene operations may be prolonged due to delays in transportation/evacuation of patients.[7] SAVE assumes that patients should be classified into one of three categories: (1) those who will die regardless of how much care they receive; (2) those who will survive whether or not they receive care; and 3) those who will benefit significantly from austere field interventions.[32] It is to the third subgroup that rescuers should direct limited resources, as they are expected to benefit most from their use.[32] The prioritization of patients into a subgroup using the SAVE concept is based on field outcome expectations "derived from existing survival and morbidity statistics."[32] Patients categorized as Immediate (Red) by the START method are assessed using SAVE first, followed by the Delayed (Yellow) and Minimal (Green) groups. Patients subsequently are moved to a treatment area if "1) morbidity or mortality may be reduced with treatment given the estimated time until there is access to definitive care; and 2) Treatment will not consume an inordinate amount of the limited resources and personnel available."[32] Although the remaining patients are initially excluded from receiving treatment, they should be frequently reassessed and moved to a treatment area should their condition change. Patients who are determined to most likely benefit from the earliest available evacuation to definitive care should receive first priority for transport. **Table 53-4** outlines the SAVE guidelines.

TRIAGE SORT

Similar to SAVE, Triage Sort was developed as a secondary triage tool to help establish treatment and transport priorities for patients who have been already categorized by a primary triage method. While SAVE is aimed at on-scene operations where there are limited medical resources and evacuation to definitive care will be delayed, Triage Sort was developed for use on scenes where resources have not been overwhelmed and categorizes patients based on a weighted score that combines the GCS, respiratory rate, and systolic blood pressure.[10] **Table 53-5** outlines the Triage Sort scoring and prioritization system.

TRIAGE TAGS

The utilization of triage tags is variable among the existing triage methods. Although they may allow for rapid visual identification of patients who have already been triaged, there are some disadvantages to their use. Unless deployed with the responding units, triage tags may be unavailable on scene when they are needed. Additionally, most tags are designed with

TABLE 53-4	Secondary Assessment of Victim Endpoint (SAVE) Guidelines

- Mangled Extremity Severity Score (MESS) to assess crush injury to extremities
- Glasgow coma score <8 in adults with significant head injury
- Abdominal trauma with refractory hypotension
- Chest trauma with abnormal vital signs
- Spinal trauma
- Burns with <50% probability of survival or adults >60 years old with an inhalational injury
- Adults with preexisting diseases
- Nontraumatic emergencies
- Special triage categories such as health care workers with minor injuries who with simple treatment may be able to assist in the medical response

Reproduced with permission from Table 4. Secondary Assessment of Victim Endpoint (SAVE) Guidelines in Nocera A, Garner A: An Australian mass casualty incident triage system for the future based upon triage mistakes of the past: The Homebush Triage Standard. *Aust NZ J Surg*. 1999;69:603-608.

TABLE 53-5	Triage Sort Scoring System					

			Scoring Parameters			
GCS	Points	Respiratory Rate	Points	Systolic Blood Pressure	Points
13-15	4	10-29	4	>89	4
9-12	3	>29	3	76-89	3
6-8	2	6-9	2	50-75	2
4-5	1	1-5	1	1-49	1
3	0	0	0	0	0
Total score		1-10	11	12	0
Treatment/transport priority		Immediate	Urgent	Delayed	Dead

tear-off sections. As patients are retriaged, the design of these tags allow for additional sections to be torn off if their condition deteriorates, but if the patient's condition improves they will require placement of a new triage tag. The SMART tag, made by TSG Associates, works around this problem by providing a tag that can be folded to display a patient's initial triage category, and refolded as the category changes based on the patient's improving or deteriorating condition.[33] In addition to issues with recategorization, some tags may be difficult to write on in inclement weather. If on-scene operations must be extended, a single tag may not provide sufficient space to record important care-related information. Advantages to the use of triage tags include the potential for improved patient tracking, especially with tags that incorporate a unique barcode identifier (as long as the facilities that will be caring for the patient have the correct software and hardware to read the barcode). Alternatives to use of triage tags is to sort patients by sending them to physically different areas marked by appropriately colored flags, tarps, or tents on the disaster scene corresponding to their triage category. The Homebush method used in Australia advocates for such geographical sorting over the use of tags.[24]

ON-SCENE OPERATIONS

In an MCI that occurs on a discrete scene, there may be a need to establish on-scene triage and treatment facilities. Larger-scale MCIs or disasters may occur over a larger geographic area, making a single triage location almost impossible to establish. Such circumstances may necessitate the creation of casualty collection points that can receive patients who "self-triage" as well as from EMS. In many large-scale events, many patients who seek treatment at a hospital do so via *self-triage*, meaning they arrive at the hospital by such means as private vehicles or public transportation rather than via EMS. If too many patients self-triage to a particular static resource (ie, a hospital or alternative treatment site), the site may become overwhelmed, thus further diluting the pool of available patient care resources, which can unnecessarily result in poorer patient outcomes including higher critical mortality rates. By creating casualty collection points, the emergency response system may help mitigate the effect of self-triage and can at least attempt to maintain control of the assessment, evacuation, and distribution of patients.

SCENE SETUP

Whether establishing operations at the scene of an MCI or at a casualty collection point, similar principles can guide the planning of how the base of operations is set up. Two common factors, regardless of the scene, are the need for an incident command post to be established, and the need to follow the principles of the incident command structure (ICS) outlined in the National Incident Management System (see **Figure 53-4**).[34] For further information regarding NIMS, please see Chapter 74. An Incident Command Post must be established, ideally in an area where access can be controlled but can still maintain a line of sight over critical operating areas such as the Immediate treatment zone and supply depot.

Suitable *ingress* and *egress* routes must be secured for the arrival and departure of patients and transport vehicles. Treatment zones should be created for each category of the patient: Immediate, Delayed, and Minimal. If resources allow, an Expectant treatment zone may also be established. Deceased patients should be left where they are found at the incident scene in order to avoid disturbing possible criminal evidence and to avoid utilizing resources that are needed to care for and transport salvageable patients.

■ PRIMARY SCENE/"GROUND ZERO"

If operations are established at the primary incident site (also known as "ground zero"), initial triage of patients is likely to occur where and when patients are found. As soon as a patient is categorized, they should be directed or assisted toward an appropriate treatment zone. If necessary, patients may be passed through a decontamination point as they are being distributed to their respective treatment zones (see **Figure 53-5**).

■ SECONDARY SCENE/CASUALTY COLLECTION POINTS

In some operations, it may be prudent or necessary to set up medical response operations at a location that is remote from the primary incident. Such sites are referred to as casualty collection points, are located in a secured location, and are often in between a primary scene and the locations of static facilities that will provide definitive care. At a casualty collection point, a specific point of triage should be established through which to funnel the flow of patients as they arrive by various means. Again, after a

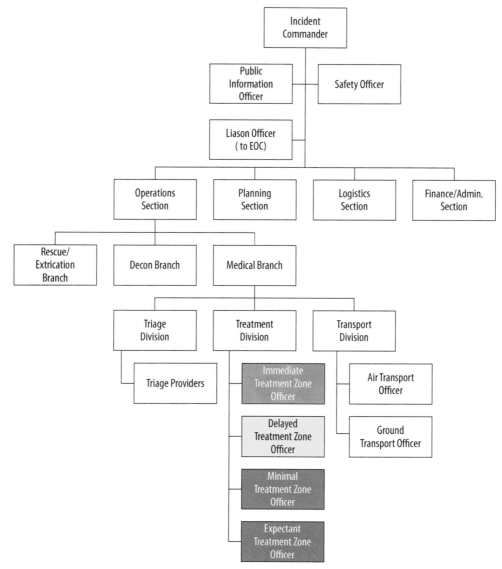

FIGURE 53-4 Command structure for various relevant ICS positions utilized during on-scene disaster operations.

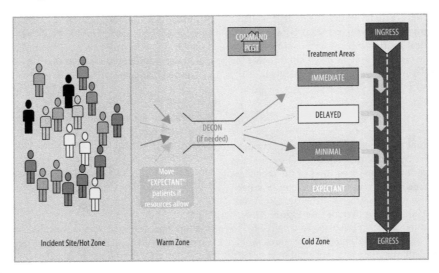

FIGURE 53-5 "Ground zero" triage.

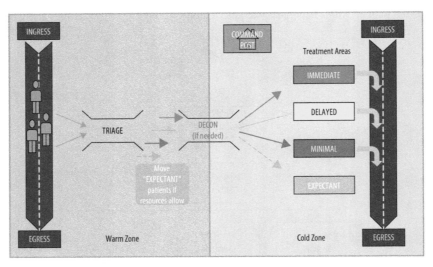

FIGURE 53-6 Casualty collection point triage.

patient has been categorized in triage, they should be directed or assisted toward an appropriate treatment zone. In order to maintain a unidirectional control of flow, points of ingress and egress should be separately established for both arriving and departing vehicles and patients (see **Figure 53-6**).

EVACUATION AND PATIENT DESTINATION CONSIDERATIONS

It should be understood that patients should be evacuated from the treatment zones as quickly as possible. If transport resources are readily available, only immediately lifesaving procedures should be performed on scene. Other interventions can and should be deferred to the destination facility or may be performed in transit. Cotransporting less severely injured patients with those who have more severe injuries (ie, a delayed patient with an immediate patient) may be an effective way to expedite evacuation of patients from the treatment zones, as long as cotransporting patients does not overwhelm the ability of the transporting providers to care for either patient. The goal of the triage, treatment, and transport process should be to evacuate all living casualties from the disaster scene or casualty collection point in a rapid manner. Utilization of alternative sources of transportation, such as public transportation or school buses, may be useful to evacuate and transport a large number of "minimal" patients in an environmentally controlled and secure vehicle, helping prevent added morbidity from prolonged environmental exposure. When possible, efforts should be made

to cotransport members of a family, especially when the family consists of young children, elderly adults, or those with special needs who may need a family member to serve as a guardian and representative.

The evacuation of patients from a scene or a casualty collection point must be done with knowledge of how the static care centers and hospitals are functioning based on their ability to operate following the event. This is true both with regard to the operational status of the hospitals' physical plants, but also with regard to the patient volumes they are receiving both from "organized" response systems and those patients who have self-triaged to the hospital.

The *geographic effect* refers to the premise that the hospital closest to the scene is often inundated with patients, which impairs their ability to effectively manage the number of casualties they are receiving.[5] By instituting a process called *leap frogging*, patients are diverted past the nearest treatment facility to other nearby hospitals, thus helping provide a more orderly and equitable distribution of patients among the available health care centers.[5]

THE EMS PHYSICIAN AND MCI/DISASTER OPERATIONS

In most circumstances, EMS providers who are active in the field at the time of the incident response will establish initial on-scene operations. However, as the nature of the incident is better understood and operational needs are defined, the presence of additional medical providers and supervisory personnel may be requested to the scene. The EMS physician(s) may be one of the resources that are called upon to provide on-scene assistance, although their exact on-scene role may differ depending on the situational needs. Potential EMS physician roles may include aspects of secondary triage, direct treatment, or to serve as an oversight/expert consultant.

We use caution here, to carefully define this physician role as one that should be filled by an EMS physician, that is, a doctor who has special training and knowledge in EMS and disaster field operations. Other physicians may be useful as on-scene medical providers, but only if they are capable of following specific instructions from the command structure.

Where and how the EMS physician is deployed may depend on the immediate needs of the scene, and as such, the deployment role may need to adapt as on-scene circumstances change.

THE EMS PHYSICIAN AS A SECONDARY TRIAGE OFFICER

In some cases, the EMS physician may best serve in a role as the triage officer. In the French disaster management response system, the *Red and White Plans*, a specially trained prehospital physician is dispatched to serve as the triage officer at a casualty collection point. The difference in the French Triage Method that makes a physician valuable in this role is that the system categorizes patients as absolute emergencies and relative emergencies, with a subsequent stratification of extreme emergency (EE), or first emergency (U1), second emergency (U2), and third emergency (U3). Each category is defined by a list of specific diagnosis such as cardiopulmonary failure (an EE), hemorrhagic gluteoperineal injuries (U1), compensated chest injuries, and head injures with a GCS >12 (U2), among others. This diagnosis-based stratification requires a sophistication of knowledge and experience that most EMS providers would not have, but that an EMS physician likely would.[7]

In a modification of the French approach, the EMS physician may serve well as a secondary triage officer in the "Immediate" and possibly the "Delayed" treatment zones. In this circumstance, the EMS physician(s) can utilize their more in-depth understanding of pathophysiology and injury management to help establish treatment and evacuation priorities for patients within each treatment zone. In this role, the EMS physician may serve as the secondary triage/treatment zone officer, or may serve a consultatory role to the EMS provider who is acting as the secondary triage/treatment zone officer.

THE EMS PHYSICIAN AS A TREATMENT PROVIDER

An alternative deployment of the EMS physician may be to serve as a *treatment provider* in the "Immediate" or "Delayed" treatment zones and become directly involved with patient care (**Figure 53-7**). In this role, the physician can perform simple lifesaving or life-maintaining interventions such as tube thoracostomy or hemorrhage control via vascular ligation. Obviously these interventions should be performed based on the availability of supplies and resources, and unless needed as an immediate lifesaving intervention, should not be performed if they will delay the patient's evacuation to definitive care. Other non-EMS physicians who self-respond to a scene or are uninjured/minimally injured casualties may also be useful as treatment providers in the Immediate and Delayed treatment zones. The caveat with utilizing any physician to provide or direct treatment for patients in a treatment zone is that they must recognize the limitations for immediate and ongoing care that exist in the given scene. It may be difficult for non-EMS physicians to recognize that a patient is not salvageable, and that other patients may benefit from the resources that could be expended trying to save an unsalvageable patient.

THE EMS PHYSICIAN IN AN OVERSIGHT ROLE OR EXPERT CONSULTANT

The advanced training, knowledge, and experience possessed by an EMS physician may make them most useful to serve a role in the Command Post to assist with scene oversight and/or as an expert consultant to the incident commander. As previously mentioned, the EMS physician may also be useful in a treatment zone by serving as an expert consultant,

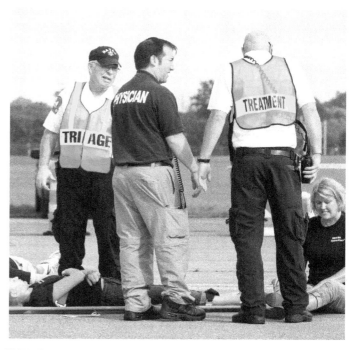

FIGURE 53-7 EMS physicians may augment triage and/or treatment roles. (Photo courtesy of Upstate Medical University Hospital, Syracuse, NY. Photographer: Robert Mescavage.)

directing the care being provided by other treatment providers (such as non-EMS physicians), but not becoming involved in directly providing patient care themselves.

Regardless of the role of the EMS physician on scene, care should be taken for their role to be clearly defined and maintained. Although the role may evolve over time, switching frequently between different roles will likely decrease the effectiveness of the EMS physician on scene and overwhelm the physician's capabilities. The EMS physician's role should be task oriented and follow the tenets of ICS/NIMS, especially with regard to maintaining span of control.

The World Medical Association provides excellent summary statements regarding the role of any physician in disaster response[3]:

- It is ethical for a physician not to persist, at all costs, in treating individuals "beyond emergency care," thereby wasting scarce resources needed elsewhere. The decision not to treat an injured person on account of priorities dictated by the disaster situation cannot be considered a failure to come to the assistance of a person in mortal danger. It is justified when it is intended to save the maximum number of individuals. However, the physician must show such patients compassion and respect for their dignity, for example, by separating them from others and administering appropriate pain relief and sedatives.

- The physician must act according to the needs of patients and the resources available. He/she should attempt to set an order of priorities for treatment that will save the greatest number of lives and restrict morbidity to a minimum.

CONCLUSION

Triage has been an evolving process that has developed over centuries into a dynamic system that has adapted to advances in the technology of war, the understanding of disease and injury, and in medical science and technology. We recognize that our current triage strategies are based mostly on "expert opinion," and as such existing methods have inherent flaws and shortcomings. The effort put forth by the panel that developed the US National Guideline for Mass Casualty Triage has been an excellent step toward establishing an evidence-based approach to triage methods and practices. Ongoing research, including postevent analysis of triage decisions and casualty outcome analysis, as well as evaluation of provider training techniques and provider knowledge retention must be pursued. Such efforts will further guide us in the development and refinement of a comprehensive all hazards triage standard that is interoperable, universal, validated, and maximizes patient survival. The EMS physician plays a key role in ongoing response planning, integration of EMS with other disaster response entities, and the advancement of the science of triage through research. As the science of triage progresses, we recognize that MCIs and disasters will continue to occur. We must remain flexible in our ability to "improvise, adapt, and overcome" as we rise to meet the challenges encountered during future disaster responses.

KEY POINTS

- Triage is a dynamic process, not a finite moment in time or a static process. It must occur at several steps between the onset of the incident to the final disposition of the patient.

- The EMS physician should advocate for the adoption of uniform standards of triage to ensure interoperability between agencies and jurisdictions on the local, regional, state, federal, and international levels.

- The EMS physician may play several important roles in the triage process including response planning and resource integration, as an active participant in on-scene response, and in postincident recovery.

- Resource availability and capability are limiting factors in the care provided during multiple casualty, mass casualty, and disaster incidents.

- EMS physicians should embrace their important role in the advancement of the body of knowledge related to triage practices. Using this knowledge, processes can be developed to validate triage methods so we can optimize our ability to provide the most benefit to the most patients.

REFERENCES

1. Mitchell GW. A brief history of triage. *Disaster Med and Public Health Prep.* 2008;2(suppl 1):S4-S7.
2. World Health Organization Regional Office for the Western Pacific: disasters. Manila, Philippines. 2011. World Health Organization. Emergency and humanitarian action: fact sheet. January 2005. http://www.wpro.who.int/mediacentre/factsheets/fs_20050104/en/. Accessed May, 2015.
3. World Medical Association. WMA statement on medical ethics in the event of disasters. Ferney-Voltaire, France. 2006. http://www.wma.net/en/30publications/10policies/d7/. Accessed May, 2015.
4. Lee CH. Clinical pearl—disaster and mass casualty triage. *Am Med Assoc J of Ethics.* 2010;12(6):466-470.
5. Frykberg ER. Triage: principles and practice. *Scand J Surg.* 2005;(94):272-278.
6. Bostick NA, Subbarao I, Burkle FM Jr. Disaster triage for large-scale catastrophic events. *Disaster Med and Public Health Prep.* 2008;2(suppl 1): S35-S39.
7. Cone DC, Koenig KL. Mass casualty triage in the chemical, biological, radiological, or nuclear environment. *Eur J Emerg Med.* 2005;12:287-302.
8. Kumar P, Jagetia GC. A review of triage and management of burn victims following a nuclear disaster. *Burns.* 1994;20:397-402.
9. Frykberg ER. Medical management of disasters and mass casualties from terrorist bombings: how can we cope? *J Trauma.* 2002;53:201-212.
10. Jenkins JL, McCarthy ML, Sauer LM. Mass casualty triage: time for an evidence-based approach. *Prehospital and Disast Med.* 2008;23(1):3-8.
11. Jewel N. *Statistics for Epidemiology.* Boca Raton, FL: CRC Press; 2004.
12. Lerner EB, Schwartz RB, Coule PL. Mass casualty triage: an evaluation of the data and development of a proposed national guideline. *Disaster Med and Public Health Prep.* 2008;2(suppl 1):S25-S34.
13. Jagger J, Jan JA, Rimel R. The Glasgow coma scale: to sum or not to sum? *Lancet.* 1983;2:97.
14. Healy C, Osler TM, Rogers FB, et al. Improving the Glasgow coma scale score: motor score alone is a better predictor. *J Trauma.* 2003;54:671-678.
15. Al-Salamah MA, McDowell I, Stiell IG, et al. Initial emergency department trauma scores from the OPALS Study: the case for the motor score in blunt trauma. *Acad Emerg Med.* 2004;11:834-842.
16. Garner A, Lee A, Harrison K, et al. Comparative analysis of multiple casualty incident triage algorithms. *Ann Emerg Med.* 2001;38:541-548.
17. Meredith W, Rutledge R, Hansen AR, et al. Field triage of trauma patients based upon ability to follow commands: a study in 29,573 injured patients. *J Trauma.* 2001;38:129-135.
18. Cross KP, Petry MJ, Cicero MX. A better START for low-acuity victims: data-driven refinement of mass casualty triage. *Prehosp Emerg Care.* 2014;19(2):272-278.
19. Hodgetts TJ, Mackway-Jones K. *Major Incident Management and Support: The Practical Approach.* London: BMJ Publishing; 1995.
20. Hodgetts TJ, Hall J, Maconochi I, et al. Pediatric triage tape. *Prehosp Immediate Care.* 1998;2:155-159.
21. Malik ZU, Pervez M, Safdar A, et al. Triage and management of mass casualties in a train accident. *J Coll Physicians Surg Pak.* 2004;14(2):108-111.
22. Kilner TM, Brace SJ, Cooke MW, et al. In 'big bang' major incidents do triage tools accurately predict clinical priority?: a systematic review of the literature. *Injury.* 2011;42(5):460-468.
23. Wallis LA, Carley S. Validation of the paediatric triage tape. *Emerg Med J.* 2006;23:47-50.
24. Nocera A, Garner A. An Australian mass casualty incident triage system for the future based upon triage mistakes of the past: the Homebush Triage Standard. *Aust NZ J Surg.* 1999;69:603-608.
25. National Disaster Life Support Foundation. Basic disaster life support (BDLS). Augusta, GA. 2007. http://www.ndlsf.org/index.php/courses/bdls. Accessed May, 2015.
26. Lerner EB, Schwartz RB, Coule PL. Model uniform core criteria for mass casualty triage. *Disaster Med and Public Health Prep.* 2011;5:125-128.
27. Armstrong JH, Frykberg ER, Burris DG. Toward a national standard in primary mass casualty triage. *Disaster Med and Public Health Prep.* 2(suppl 1):S8-S10.
28. Deluhery MR, Lerner EB, Pirrallo RG, et al. Paramedic accuracy using SALT triage after a brief initial training. *Prehosp Emerg Care.* 2011;15(4):526-532.
29. Cone DC, Serra J, Kurland L. Comparison of the SALT and SMART triage systems using a virtual reality simulator with paramedic students. *Eur J Emerg Med.* 2011;18(6):314-321.
30. Cross KP, Cicero MX. Head-to-head comparison of disaster triage methods in pediatric, adult, and geriatric patients. *Ann Emerg Med.* June 2013;61(6):668-676.e7.
31. Cross KP, Cicero MX. Independent application of the Sacco Disaster Triage Method to pediatric trauma patients. *Prehosp Disaster Med.* August 2012;27(4):306-311.
32. Benson M, Koenig KL, Schultz CH. Disaster triage: START, then SAVE—a new method of dynamic triage for victims of a catastrophic earthquake. *Prehosp Disas Med.* 1996;11(2):117-124.
33. TSG Associates. SMART tag: for triage that works. Halifax, UK. 2009. http://www.smartmci.com/products/triage/smart_tag.php. Accessed May, 2015.
34. Federal Emergency Management Agency. National Incident Management System (NIMS)—Incident Command. Washington, DC. 2011. https://www.fema.gov/incident-command-system-resources. Accessed May, 2015.
35. Crisis Medicine Training Network. Triage Sieve. Valhalla, South Africa. 2009. http://www.crisismedicine.co.za/pdfs/Triage%20SIEVE.pdf. Accessed May, 2015

Blunt and Penetrating Trauma

Doug Isaacs

Pam Lai

INTRODUCTION

Trauma and injury account for 182, 479 deaths in 2007, with approximately 31,224 due to penetrating injuries, that is, firearms, and 65,474 secondary to blunt mechanisms, such as motor vehicle collisions and falls.[1] These statistics do not include the numerous morbidities that may also be associated with these injuries. It is difficult to address the world of trauma and acute care medicine without discussing "the golden hour;" and the "platinum ten minutes" referring to the fact that any trauma resuscitation is divided into either success or failure within the first hour of medical attention, and the initial minutes where critical interventions take place. While numerous debates have raged since the inception of this concept, the underlying idea of prompt and effective medical care starting from the point of patient contact in the field, and therefore the importance of prehospital management of the trauma patient, is indisputable.

OBJECTIVES

- Understand the initial prehospital management of the trauma patient, including triage and transport criteria.
- Understand the prehospital management of specific injuries to the chest and abdomen and the surrounding controversies of their care.

MANAGEMENT OF THE TRAUMA PATIENT

The overall management of the trauma patient has not deviated as much as the care of other medical emergencies. This may be taken in the perspective of patients undergoing an acute myocardial infarction and the use of the defibrillator, various drugs, and transport destination centers. Alternatively, if a patient has undergone penetrating abdominal trauma, the response is similar to that performed in years past, with stabilization of the patient in the field and transportation of the patient to the nearest trauma center where the patient would receive definitive treatment in the operating room. Thus, this chapter, instead of going through the laborious task of delineating the relatively static role of prehospital trauma management, will instead explore some of the recent controversies along with the techniques and technologies that are being used in the prehospital field.

TRAUMA TRIAGE

Triage of the trauma patient in the field is oftentimes a complex, challenging, and much debated issue among prehospital providers. The American College of Surgeons' Committee on Trauma has defined an acceptable undertriage rate (seriously injured patient not taken to a trauma center) as 5%, whereas overtriage rates may be acceptably as high as 25% to 50%.[2] The relatively high allowance for the overtriage rate is tolerated so as to allow for an acceptable level of patients who may be undertriaged. Many studies have in fact reported overtriage rates to be as high as 90%.[3,4]

The importance of successful triage by prehospital providers is further emphasized with the development of regionalized trauma systems. It has been shown that the regionalization of receiving facilities, that is, the designation of hospitals to care for certain conditions such as trauma, burn, hyperbaric, or poisons (venomization) has significantly reduced mortality and morbidity.[5] Thus the decision of transport to one of these

specialized facilities may be critical for both definitive patient care as well as the appropriate utilization of resources both at the hospital level as well as in the prehospital field: Indeed, not every patient involved in a "trauma" may require the use of a level 1 trauma center.

While it may not be as appreciated in large urban EMS systems with multiple trauma centers, effective trauma triage becomes particularly important in rural systems where in many instances, a critical decision must be made in choosing between ground and aeromedical transport to the most appropriate facility. For best outcomes, the prehospital triage criteria should be optimized such that patients may be classified as (1) serious injury requiring transport to a trauma center or (2) noncritical injury that may be treated at a local nontrauma receiving hospital.

Prehospital triage criteria typically include various combinations of physiologic, anatomic, and mechanistic criteria. Initial studies have shown that while mechanistic indicators are useful in identifying and subsequently transporting severely injured patients to trauma centers, the results trend toward overtriage.[6] On the other hand, anatomic and physiologic criteria have generally added to the improvement of triage accuracy.[4,7] This, however, is not the case in blunt trauma where the reliable clinical assessment of internal organ damage may be severely limited.[4]

Various studies have shown mixed results in the reliability of EMTs and paramedics to effectively predict patients' injury severity. One widely used triage criteria is the Prehospital Index (PHI) which consists of five field criteria: systolic blood pressure, heart rate, respiratory status, level of consciousness, and the presence of penetrating truncal injury. In a 2010 study, the combination of EMT judgment, PHI, and a mechanistic scale involving the quantity of damaging energy transfer to the patient (high velocity impact or HVI) identified patients who would benefit from care at a level 1 trauma center, albeit with low sensitivities (74.2%) and high rates of overtriage (85.1%).[8] Another study showed that prehospital personnel with a similarly established triage scoring system (MAP, mechanism, anatomy, and physiology) used over a 10-year period were able to adequately distinguish patients in a rural environment that required helicopter transport to a trauma center with relatively high sensitivities, 93.8%, and an adequate rate of overtriage such that only a small increase in the rate of helicopter transports were recorded (7%-10%).[9] When patient triage was subdivided to include the assessment of the severity of injury to individual body regions, it was not shown to improve accuracy.[10] However, it has been shown that paramedics are best able to differentiate severe head injury, which is commonly based on a neurologic examination and determination of prehospital GCS score. A prehospital GCS <14 has been shown to be associated with severe head injuries with a sensitivity of 62% and specificity of 89%.[10,11] In contrast, paramedics were least able to identify severe blunt abdominal injuries.[10] A 2014 study revealed that 36% of helicopter transported trauma victims had only minor injuries and that apparent risks for overtriage included falls, penetrating injury, and being uninsured.[12]

ALS VERSUS BLS TRANSPORT

It has been reported that as much as 50% of injuries that eventually result in death occur at the scene with another 25% of these eventual deaths occurring within the first 24 hours of hospitalization.[13,14] Of the potentially survivable patients, one could surmise, that according to the dogma of trauma care, they would receive the most benefit by expeditious evaluation and care by prehospital personnel. Herein lies the question of how the patient would receive the most benefit: expeditious transport to an appropriate care center or thorough examination and potentially lifesaving interventions to be performed on the scene, such as basic airway management and hemorrhage control, and then transport for definitive care.

A major controversy in the prehospital care of trauma is the necessity of ALS (advanced life support) transport versus BLS (basic life support) transport. While the definitions of the levels of care may differ from system to system, in general the term ALS refers to a more sophisticated level of care potentially involving more invasive methods, including intravenous fluids, intubation, and the use of medications whereas BLS care typically involves patient assessment and temporizing measures for more definitive care at a hospital.

When dealing with trauma in the prehospital care setting, two strategies have typically been discussed: "scoop and run" versus "stay and play." The former deals with expedited transport to a high acuity trauma center with minimal prehospital treatments and the later refers to stabilization of the patient on the scene before transport. The terminology is not strictly related to ALS versus BLS transport but rather it seems to reflect global differences between prehospital care: United States and Canada favor the more expedited "scoop-and-run" dogma as opposed to Europe, which trends toward the "stay–and-play" approach.

And while prehospital ALS, whether with an on-scene physician or not, has theoretical advantages, the evidence supporting its effectiveness for treating trauma is limited. This may be attributed to the fact that all ALS providers, including paramedics and physicians, are ultimately limited in the type of interventions they may perform in the prehospital setting (due to historical nonavailability of sophisticated imaging or operative maneuvers). In addition, some studies have suggested that prolonged prehospital interventions may even cause more harm than benefit as the time to perform these interventions delays definitive care.[15] These findings have been shown to be dependent on the severity and location of the injury. For example, for patients with severe blunt head injury or who have sustained multiple injuries, these patients have been shown to have improved survivability with ALS care. However, it should be noted that these studies utilized air-medical transportation to definitive care.[16-18] In cases of multiple blunt trauma there has not been shown to be a difference between ALS and BLS care,[19-22] with some studies even suggesting improved care by BLS.[23,24] Of studies concerning penetrating or undetermined trauma, no difference in outcomes were observed among the relatively mildly injured patients, with 10% to 15% of those with an Injury Severity Score (ISS) greater than 15[22,25-28] with some studies showing improved outcomes for those treated by BLS.[29-33]

In 2007, it was seen that of patients who suffered penetrating thoracic trauma, seven of 88 (8.0%) EMS-transported patients via ALS survived until hospital discharge, whereas 16 of 92 (17.4%) survived after police or private transportation. After identifying that prehospital procedures occurred in 88.6% of patients treated by ALS, Seamon et al showed that for each procedure, patients were 2.63 times more likely to die before hospital discharge.[33] This phenomenon of increased patient survivability with layperson transportation following severe injury (ISS greater than 15) was also seen in an earlier study as well.[34]

On the other hand, smaller studies have shown the benefit of providing ALS care in cases of trauma. Small, uncontrolled studies have shown decreases in mortality in selective cases of falls and penetrating injuries.[35,36] Other studies have attempted to validate ALS prehospital care by comparing EMS systems among countries; however, comparison is oftentimes difficult[37] in that the term ALS is an ill-defined and heterogenous term that can be defined as care by two paramedics or on-scene physicians and can also differ in the method of transportation and may or may not include air-medical systems. The differences between paramedic driven and physician run ALS systems showed an overall improved intermediate survivability among those with physicians at the scene. However, when comparing between systems with the same provider type, significant variability was seen in overall patient outcomes by as much as a four-fold difference in overall death rates.[38] This heterogeneity highlights the fact that it is oftentimes difficult to make comparisons between ALS systems. A 2013 study by Seamon et al,[39] failed to show a benefit in outcomes when compared to BLS care of trauma patients. A 2014 Cochrane review study by Jayaraman et al, which included three studies meeting the study criteria, similarly concluded that there is currently no evidence that ALS training for ambulance crews improves outcome in trauma patients.[40]

CHEST TRAUMA

Thoracic injury accounts for as much as 25% of deaths from trauma or approximately 16,000 deaths annually in the United States (**Figure 54-1**). Many of the resulting injuries causing early death, including tension

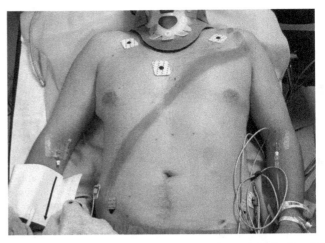

FIGURE 54-1. Blunt chest trauma—"seatbelt sign." (Photo contributor: Brad Russell, MD. Reprinted with permission from Knoop KJ. *The Atlas of Emergency Medicine.* 3rd ed. New York, NY: McGraw-Hill; 2010.)

pneumothorax, cardiac tamponade, or excessive hemorrhage can be treated and oftentimes the resulting death can be prevented in the prehospital setting.

Procedures such as needle decompression and chest tube thoracostomy have been used in the prehospital setting, to varying degrees of success.[41] Currently, the American College of Surgeons Advanced Trauma Life Support (ATLS) and Prehospital Trauma Life Support (PHTLS) courses both recommend the use of needle thoracostomy (NT) in the setting of tension pneumothorax as a bridging measure until definitive treatment with tube thoracostomy is established.[42,43]

Needle thoracostomy converts the life-threatening tension pneumothorax into a smaller simple, open pneumothorax. As a result, the compromise in respiratory effort is relieved at the cost of a small, open pneumothorax. In addition, since the diameter of the needle is insignificant compared to the human airway, respirations are not negatively affected.[18] While this is widely considered to be an easy, less invasive procedure that can be done in the prehospital setting, it is not without risks.[44-47] Complications have been shown to stem from delay of transport to a hospital for definitive care, misdiagnosis and misplacement of the needle thoracostomy, and inappropriate patient selection.[48,49]

Often the reported complications stem from insufficient cannula length that is used to decompress the pneumothorax in relation to chest wall thickness.[48-50] Current ATLS guidelines recommend a 5-cm needle catheter with the needle placed in the anterior chest wall at the second intercostal space in the midclavicular line. This is in spite of the fact that most commercially available needle angiocatheters used in the United States are 4.4 cm. A recent study looked at the predictability of failure rates of needle thoracostomy based on mean chest wall depth and found that the standard 4.4 cm angiocatheter would be unsuccessful in 50% of cases.[51]

Other studies have shown that the use of needle decompression is a relatively safe procedure when performed by paramedics in urban as well as aeromedical settings[47,49,52] (**Figure 54-2**). Studies have revealed that for patients with severe thoracic injury (AIS >4), needle thoracentesis use varied from 0% to 22%.[44] Patients were seen to sustain gunshot wounds, stab wounds, motor vehicle collisions, or other forms of blunt trauma. These large studies showed that among paramedics based in urban settings, little to no vascular injury, infection, or other complications were seen due to needle decompression.[43,44]

When dealing with tension pneumothoraces in the field, among the common signs and symptoms paramedics are taught to evaluate is tracheal deviation. It has been suggested to de-emphasize this physical finding from paramedic training in light of the fact that 0% to 1% of patients were reported to have this physical finding at the time of patient evaluation.[49,53] The frequency of inappropriate and inadequate needle decompression has been recently evaluated with the use of CT and

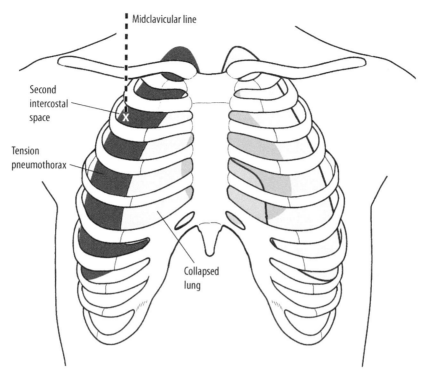

FIGURE 54-2. Needle thoracostomy. (Reprinted with permission from Tintinalli JE, Stapczynski JS, Ma OJ, Cline DM, Cydulka RK, Meckler GD, eds. *Tintinalli's Emergency Medicine: A Comprehensive Study Guide.* 7th ed. New York, NY: McGraw-Hill; 2011.)

ultrasound techniques. Blaivas has shown that out of 57 patients who had at least one needle thoracostomy attempted in the prehospital setting, 15 patients (26%) were reported to have no evidence of a pneumothorax on ultrasound examination or on CT.[54]

In contrast, tube thoracostomy is less accepted in the prehospital setting for the treatment and management of a pneumothorax, hemopneumothorax, or hemothorax. In general, chest tubes are not inserted in the prehospital setting due to concerns of on-scene time, sterility and infection, and the increased training that is involved with performing a more complicated procedure. These, in combination with appropriate patient selection, correct technique, and tube placement, reported complications of uncontrolled hemorrhage, iatrogenic damage to the heart or lungs make this a controversial prehospital procedure when performed by nonphysician prehospital providers.[55,56] Some systems utilize formal tube thoracostomy performance only by a critical care level provider with advanced training or an adequately trained and equipped EMS physician.

Some studies comparing the use of needle and tube thoracostomy in the same EMS system have shown that while tube thoracostomy had longer on-scene times, fewer patients were pronounced dead on arrival at the hospital, all while taking into account similar ISS, length of hospital stay, and overall mortality.[49] Incidences of lung damage or infection have been reported to be similar to ED tube thoracostomies and/or were seen to not be a significant complication in the prehospital setting.[49,57]

Another, perhaps more controversial, procedure is the role of the prehospital thoracotomy. While the emergency department thoracotomy is well established as the standard of care for certain instances of penetrating and blunt traumatic cardiac arrest, recent studies have continued to evaluate its efficacy with reported survival rates ranging from 1.8% to 27.5%.[58] Outcomes are drastically variable, with several reported mortalities as high as 100%, but it has been shown that survival improves with a decreased time lapse between arrest and definitive treatment in the operating room.[59-62] One of the first reported successful prehospital thoracotomies concluded that while its reported case study was successful, the practice itself should not be adopted as the prehospital standard of care.[63] US guidelines for the treatment of traumatic cardiac arrests report similar recommendations, stating that thoracotomies are "outside the remit

of prehospital care."[64] This is in stark contrast to many European EMS systems where physicians routinely are a part of prehospital care and are able to perform more invasive procedures than their US counterparts. In such cases, field thoracotomy may be reserved for single entry penetrating thoracic trauma with a witnessed arrest.

Much of the research and information on prehospital thoracotomies has been performed in Europe, and more recently in parts of Asia, where this has been the standard of care for many years. A recent study from Europe showed that out of 71 on-scene thoracotomies performed by physicians, 18% survived to hospital discharge.[65] Conclusions from the study suggested that survival was concurrent in patients with penetrating stab wounds and cardiac arrest secondary to pericardial tamponade, with better neurological outcome when thoracotomy was performed soon after the arrest.

Outcomes are more disparate when it comes to prehospital thoracotomies performed in the setting of blunt trauma, much as what has been reported for those performed in the emergency department.[66] In the United States, the overall survival rate after emergency thoracotomy in blunt trauma patients is reported to be 1.4%.[67] A recent study from Japan looked at survivability of prehospital thoracotomy in the setting of blunt trauma and found no survivors in a group of 34 patients.[68]

ABDOMINAL TRAUMA

Abdominal injuries are one of the more common types of trauma encountered in the prehospital field. Unrecognized abdominal injuries can have catastrophic results if not transported to an appropriate receiving facility for prompt definitive care. Traditionally, limitations as to what can be evaluated in the prehospital field precluded anything else but rapid transport. However, with the advent of newer technologies, such as portable ultrasound, and improved training to utilize these devices, there may be some additional information that may help triage and treat these patients.

Injuries from exsanguination from highly vascular organs, such as the liver, spleen, colon, small intestines, stomach, or pancreas may not be readily detected and are oftentimes missed until evaluation in the emergency department. The idea of point-of-care ultrasound has increased in use, extending its scope of practice into the prehospital setting.[69-71] Many of the initial studies concentrated on the use of ultrasound for the evaluation of trauma, utilizing the focused assessment sonography for trauma (FAST) or an extended FAST (eFAST) examination (**Figure 54-3**). However, the majority of these studies used physicians, nurses, or physician assistants and did not involve paramedics.[72-74]

A pilot study involving 104 patients showed that paramedics were able to adequately obtain and interpret prehospital FAST and abdominal aorta (AA) images with 100% confirmation of interpretation by a physician overreader.[75] The number of inadequate imaging was similar to a large prehospital study that involved prehospital physicians (approximately 7.7%).[71] Prehospital military studies have shown that early diagnostic ultrasound was one of the main factors that could decrease overall trauma mortality.[76] One study utilizing prehospital physicians showed that utilizing ultrasonography improved the accuracy of their physical examination such that their management of the trauma patient was altered in one-third of cases.[71]

Prehospital ultrasound is not isolated to the evaluation of abdominal trauma. Rather, it has some potentially far-reaching applications to evaluate cardiac resuscitation, pregnant patients (in the settings of breech positioning and fetal distress), as well as handling mass casualty incidents.[77-79]

Nonphysician aeromedical personnel were able to perform a cardiac ultrasound to evaluate for cardiac activity and pericardial effusion, with sensitivities and specificities of 100%.[80] One case study described the diagnosis of pericardial tamponade in the setting of penetrating trauma, with the return of spontaneous circulation after pericardiocentesis was performed en route to the hospital where an ED thoracotomy was performed shortly after patient arrival.[77]

In the setting of recent world events, the emphasis of mass casualty incident preparedness, from both natural or man-made causes, has been heightened to a new level. During the Second Lebanon War in 2006, a retrospective study performed at a level 1 trauma center showed that the emergency department and prehospital personnel were better able to screen which patients would be dispositioned to the operating room, CT scan, or observation unit.[78]

However, when ultrasound was used as an adjunct to Simple Triage and Rapid Treatment (START) mass casualty triage system,[81] it showed both an overtriage of 22.2% of yellow patients to the red category as well as an undertriage of 12.9%. Thus, solely relying on ultrasound as a triage tool or attempting to utilize it as an adjunct to triage may be of equivocal benefit.

The regionalization of medicine with its specialized centers for trauma, cardiac and invasive radiologic interventions, makes the potential role for prehospital ultrasound promising as it allows for more accurate EMS delivery of patients to the appropriate hospital for acute emergencies.

HEMORRHAGE CONTROL

Uncontrolled hemorrhage accounts for 50% of combat fatalities and 80% of civilian trauma fatalities in the United States.[82,83] Significant research and attention has therefore been paid to this phenomenon in the past few years, looking at some new and some revisited techniques for hemorrhage control, two of which will be discussed in this chapter.

HEMOSTATIC DRESSINGS

Up until the last 10 years, little advancement has been made in the control of external hemorrhage, as evidenced by much of our current techniques of gauze and pressure controlled bandages. Many of these products utilize naturally occurring substances, ranging from zeolites to plant-based chitin derivatives. Their efficacy has been tested in many studies in both the military and civilian literature with varying results.[84-88] with some studies even suggesting that these advanced hemostatic dressings are not superior to traditional gauze dressings.

The use of these products are ideally used for uncontrolled hemorrhage from wounds in areas that are not amenable to tourniquet application but are still accessible for compression, such as the trunk, groin, neck, and axilla. Many of the early versions of these products produced an exothermic reaction that resulted in local tissue damage and distal thromboli.[89] Newer housing for the active agents as well as the use of different active materials have negated this effect. Some current manufacturer compression times range from 2 to 5 minutes, which in many instances is similar if not longer than that compared to traditional gauze.[83-86,90,91]

TOURNIQUETS

Much controversy and debate has been made over tourniquets since its first use in 1674. Concerns are due to tourniquet-related tissue ischemic or neurologic injuries that result in extremity amputation.[92,93] Most complications are caused by improvised tourniquets, inappropriate use, and inadequate compression. A narrow, constricting tourniquet can cause irreversible injury to underlying tissue, including contractures, rhabdomyolysis and compartment syndrome, skin necrosis, and nerve injury.[91,92] A common mistake is inadequate compression that fails to occlude the artery and only occlude the venous return, which results in an increased rate of blood loss. When applying a tourniquet it should be fully applied with high enough pressure to completely impede both arterial inflow and venous outflow.

Anecdotal reports of benefit from tourniquet use have been seen in modern warfare from both the Korean and Vietnam conflicts as well as in Afghanistan and Iraq. Retrospective reviews of prehospital tourniquet use by the Israeli Defense Forces (IDF), which allows liberal use of tourniquets, revealed improvement in extremity hemorrhage control with very few adverse limb outcomes when tourniquet use was less than 5 hours. The 4-year analysis looked at the application of tourniquets to 91 patients and saw that 88% of the cases had no complications. Of the complications, all were neurologic with total tourniquet times ranging from 109 to 187 minutes.[94]

During the Iraq and Afghanistan conflicts, tourniquets were provided to each soldier. In a study performed at a combat support hospital, 232 patients were observed to have had an application of a tourniquet. Ninety percent survival was reported when the tourniquet was applied prior to the presence of shock, whereas only a 10% survival was observed after shock ensued. Transient nerve palsy was reported in 1.7% of patients and zero amputations were shown to have been caused by tourniquets.[95]

Of the possible complications from tourniquet use, nerve injury is the most common and can range from mild transient loss of function to

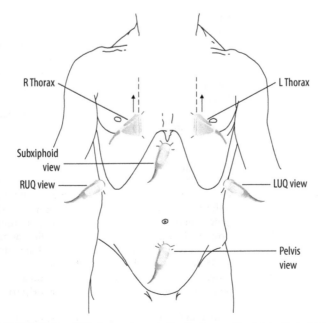

FIGURE 54-3. eFAST ultrasound examination for trauma. (Reprinted with permission from Knoop KJ. *The Atlas of Emergency Medicine.* 3rd ed. New York, NY: McGraw-Hill; 2010.)

permanent, irreversible damage. When all the motor nerves distal to the tourniquet are damaged, this results in limb paralysis that is oftentimes referred to as tourniquet paralysis syndrome.

Other complications may arise after the tourniquet is removed. Posttourniquet syndrome describes prolonged limb edema, weakness, dysesthesia, or pain after tourniquet removal. The hyperemia is a result of two factors: the mechanical flow of blood from a high pressure system to a lower pressure system, and from postischemic reactive hyperemia which reflects the increase in blood flow to restore neutral pH as well as to remove other metabolites. Nerve damage from posttourniquet syndrome is a resultant of prolonged ischemia, rather than from the mechanical stressors that result in tourniquet paralysis syndrome.

Recently civilian cases of successful use of tourniquets have led to recommendations for widespread deployment and training for use in appropriate circumstances.[96-102] Tourniquets should not be removed in the prehospital setting. Doing so may result in recurring hemorrhage and complications similar to crush syndrome, including rhabdomyolysis. When applying a tourniquet in the prehospital setting, care givers should be instructed when possible, to apply the tourniquet over bare skin, leaving the affected extremity and tourniquet exposed, document the time applied, and also note the neurovascular status of the distal limb.

INTRAVENOUS FLUIDS IN THE PREHOSPITAL SETTING

In the prehospital setting, it had been the standard of care in trauma patients to insert two large-bore IV catheters and infuse up to 2 to 3 L of crystalloid fluid even if the patient was not hypotensive. Research at the time did not demonstrate improved survival of those patients, and in some cases showed an in mortality with fluid administration.[103]

The drawback of administering large volumes of intravenous fluids is that it may worsen bleeding through injured vessels by dislodging already formed clots, increased blood pressure, or dilution of various clotting facors.[94]

The current concept employed by the military and trauma centers is that of permissive hypotension, where the systolic blood pressure is raised without reaching normotension. Blood pressures are typically raised to reach a mean arterial pressure of 60 to 70 mm Hg. A large study conducted compared the mortality rate of two groups of patients who sustained penetrating abdominal or thoracic injuries: one group who presented with a SBP < 90 mm Hg and a second group that was resuscitated to normotension.[104] A significant reduction in the mortality of the fluid-restricted group was found. Another study showed that while the overall mortality rate was identical between the two groups of patients, fewer complications and earlier hemostasis were observed in the fluid-restricted group.[105] In addition to avoiding dislodging clots and diluting clotting factors and platelets, it is also possible that reperfusion injury may be exaggerated if patients in hemorrhagic shock are resuscitated to normotensive status with crystalloid.

It should be emphasized that these studies were applied to patients with uncontrolled bleeding. A hypotensive trauma patient with an isolated extremity injury should be provided with hemostatic control as early as possible with use of direct compression, tourniquets, and/or hemostatic agents when appropriate.

Patient groups in which permissive hypotension may be detrimental include severe head trauma, pregnancy, elderly patients with cardiovascular disease, and entrapped patients with crush injury. More research to identify the best resuscitative strategies is currently ongoing, and will likely be most applicable when targeted at the prehospital setting.

TRANEXAMIC ACID

Massive transfusion protocols, fixed-ratio transfusion, and recombinant coagulation factors have all played, and some continue to play, a role in the resuscitation of hemorrhaging trauma patients. Disruption of the coagulation system has been well documented in numerous studies, with one reporting approximately 25% of seriously wounded trauma patients

presenting with abnormalities of the INRs that is directly associated with increased morbidity, mortality, and blood product use.[106] This "acute coagulopathy of trauma" has been speculated to involve the activation of protein C in conjunction with the inactivation of factors V and VIII and plasminogen activator inhibitor-1.[107]

TXA is an antifibrinolytic that inhibits both plasminogen activation and plasmin activity, thus resulting in the prevention of clot breakdown. TXA reduces the activity of plasminogen by occupying the lysine-binding sites on plasminogen, and hence preventing its binding to its lysine counterparts on fibrin. TXA has been historically used to control menstrual bleeding, hemorrhage after various surgeries, and the treatment of ruptured intracranial aneurysms, upper gastrointestinal hemorrhage, and traumatic hyphema, as well as hemophilia and von Willebrand disease.[108-110]

Two large studies have been conducted studying the efficacy of TXA in adult trauma patients at risk for significant bleeding. The authors of the CRASH-2 trial reported that TXA use resulted in a statistically significant reduction in the relative risk of all-cause mortality by 9%, with an even greater reduction in death as a result of hemorrhage on the day of the incident by 20%.[111] Another study (MATTERs) showed similar results with a lower unadjusted mortality with the patients who received TXA (17.4%) than those without treatment (23.9%).[112]

The widespread adoption of TXA is still debated in the setting of hemorrhaging trauma patients; however, the use of this antifibrinolytic seems a promising adjunct in the arsenal of resuscitating hemorrhaging trauma patients in the prehospital setting.

CONCLUSION

The prehospital treatment of trauma holds much promise with evolving technologies, training, and medical treatments. While the dogma of beneficial trauma resuscitation may still lie within "the golden hour," we have more weapons in our arsenal to treat our patients in the prehospital setting, making the most of our opportunities for the best patient care.

KEY POINTS

- Mechanism of injury criteria tends to overtriage injured patients to trauma centers.
- Addition of anatomic and physiologic criteria improves triage accuracy.
- Severe intraabdominal injures remain difficult to detect in the prehospital setting.
- Tourniquets are an important tool in prehospital hemorrhage management and are associated with infrequent complications.
- Overuse of crystalloid intravenous fluid may worsen patient outcome due to hemodilution, dislodgement of formed clot, and increases in blood pressure.
- Permissive hypotension is gaining acceptance as a traumatic injury management process across both civilian and military prehospital environments.
- The EMS physician should maintain an understanding of evolving tools in the management of hemorrhage and traumatic injury including tranexamic acid (TXA), hemostatic dressings, tourniquets, permissive hypotension, and developing triage processes to direct patient disposition.

REFERENCES

1. Xu J, Kochanek KD, Murphy SA, Tejada-Vera B. Deaths: final data for 2007. *Natl Vital Stat Rep*. 2010;58(19):1-135.
2. American College of Surgeons Committee on Trauma. Prehospital trauma care. In: *Resources for Optimal Care of the Injured Patient 2006*. Chicago, IL: American College of Surgeons; 2006:21-25.

3. Esposito T, Offner P, Jurkovich G, Griffith J, Maier R. Do prehospital trauma center triage criteria identify major trauma victims. *Arch Surg.* 1995;130:171-176

4. Cottington E, Young J, Shufflebarger C, Kyes F, Peterson F, Diamond D. The utility of physiologic status, injury site, and injury mechanism in identifying patients with major trauma. *J Trauma.* 1988;28:305-311.

5. Celso B, Tepas, J, Langland-Orban B, et al. A systematic review and meta-analysis comparing outcome of severely injured patients treated in trauma centers following the establishment of trauma systems. *J Trauma.* 2006;60:371-378.

6. Cooper M, Yarbrough D, Zone-Smith L, Byrne T, Norcross E. Application of field triage guidelines by prehospital personnel: is mechanism of injury a valid guideline for patient triage? *Am Surg.* 1995;61:363-367.

7. Cales, R. Injury severity determination: requirements, approaches, and applications. *Ann Emerg Med.* 1986;15:1427-1433.

8. Lavoie A, Emond M, Moore L, Camden S, Liberman M. Evaluation of the Prehospital Index, presence of high-velocity impact and judgment of emergency medical technicians as criteria for trauma triage. *CJEM.* 2010;12(2): 111-118.

9. Purtill M, Benedict K, Hernandez-Boussard T, et al. Validation of a prehospital trauma triage tool: a 10-year perspective. *J Trauma.* 2008;65:1253-1257.

10. Mulholland SA, Cameron PA, Gabbe BJ, et al. Prehospital prediction of the severity of blunt anatomic injury. *J Trauma.* 2008;64: 754-760.

11. Ross S, Leipold C, Terrigino C, et al. Efficacy of the motor component of the Glasgow Coma Scale in trauma triage. *J Trauma.* 1998;45:42-44.

12. Cheung BH, Delgado MK, Staudenmayer KL. Patient and trauma center characteristics associated with helicopter emergency medical services transport for patients with minor injuries in the United States. *Acad Emerg Med.* November 2014;21(11):1232-1239.

13. Demetriades D, Kimbrell B, Salim A, et al. Trauma deaths in a mature urban trauma system: is trimodal distribution a valid concept? *J Am Coll Surg.* 2005;201:343-348.

14. Trunkey DD. Trauma. Accidental and intentional injuries account for more years of life lost in the U.S. than cancer and heart disease. Among the prescribed remedies are improved preventive efforts, speedier surgery and further research. *Sci Am.* 1983;249:28-35.

15. Berlot G, Bacer B, Gullo A. Controversial aspects of the prehospital trauma care. *Crit Care Clin.* 2006;22:457-468.

16. Abbott D, Brauer K, Hutton K, Rosen P. Aggressive out-of-hospital treatment regimen for severe closed head injury in patients undergoing air medical transport. *Air Med J.* 1998;17:94-100.

17. Garner AA. The role of the physician staffing of helicopter emergency medical services in prehospital trauma response. *Emerg Med Australas.* 2004;16:318-323.

18. Davis DP, Peay J, Serrano JA, et al. The impact of aeromedical response to patients with moderate to severe traumatic brain injury. *Ann Emerg Med.* 2005;46:115-122.

19. Di Bartolomeo S, Sanson G, Nardi G, et al. HEMS vs. Ground-BLS care in traumatic cardiac arrest. *Prehosp Emerg Care.* 2005;9:79-84.

20. Iirola TT, Laaksonen MI, Vahlber TJ, et al. Effect of physician-staffed helicopter emergency medical service on blunt trauma patient survival and prehospital care. *Eur J Emerg Med.* 2006;13:335-339.

21. Klemen P, Grmec S. Effect of pre-hospital advanced life support with rapid sequence intubation on outcome of severe traumatic brain injury. *Acta Anaesthesiol Scand.* 2006;50:1250-1254.

22. Stiell IG, Nesbitt LP, Pickett W, et al. The OPALS major trauma study: impact of advanced life-support on survival and morbidity. *CMAJ.* 2008;178:1141-1152.

23. Thomas SH, et al. Helicopter transport and blunt trauma mortality: a mulitcenter trial. *J Trauma.* 2002;52:136-145.

24. Lee A, Garner A, Fearnside M, Harrison K. Level of prehospital care and risk of mortality in patients with and without severe blunt head injury. *Injury.* 2003;34:815-819.

25. Rainer TH, Houlihan KP, Robertson CE, et al. An evaluation of paramedic activities in prehospital trauma care. *Injury.* 1997; 28(9-10):623-627.

26. Suoimen P, Baillie C, Kivioja A, et al. Prehospital care and survival of pediatric patients with blunt trauma. *J Pediat Surg.* 1998;33: 1388-1392.

27. Owen JL, Phillips RT Conaway C, Mullarkey D. One year' trauma mortality experience at Brooke Army Medical Center: is aeromedical transportation of patients necessary? *Military Medicine.* 1999;164:361-365.

28. Sukumaran S, Henry JM, Beard D, et al. Prehospital trauma management: a national study of paramedic activities. *Emerg Med J.* 2005;22:60-63.

29. Adams J, Aldag G, Wolford R. Does the level of prehospital care influence the outcome of patients with altered levels of consciousness? *Prehosp Disaster Med.* 1996;11:101-104.

30. Nicholl JP, Brazier JE, Snooks HA. Effects of London helicopter emergency medical service on survival after trauma. *BMJ.* 1995;311:217-222.

31. Eckstein M, Chan L, Schneir A, Palmer R. Effect of prehospital advanced life support on outcomes of major trauma patients. *J Trauma.* 2000;48:643-648.

32. Liberman M, Mulder D, Lavoie A, et al. Multicenter Canadian study of prehospital trauma care. *Ann Surg.* 2003;237:153-160.

33. Seamon MJ, Fisher CA, Gaughan J, et al. Prehospital procedures before emergency department thoracotomy: 'scoop and run' saves lives. *J Trauma.* 2007;63:113-120.

34. Demetriades D, Chan L, Cornwell E, et al. Paramedic vs private transportation of trauma patients. *Arch Surg.* 1996;131:133-138.

35. Aprahamian C, Thompson BM, Towne JB. The effect of a paramedic system on mortality of major open intra-abdominal vascular trauma. *J Trauma.* 1983;23:687-690

36. Fortner GS, Oreskovich MR, Copass MK, Carrico CJ. The effects of prehospital trauma care on survival from a 50-meter fall. *J trauma.* 1983;23:976-981

37. Messick WJ, Rutledge R, Meyer AA. The association of advanced life support training and decreased per capita trauma death rates: an analysis of 12417 trauma deaths. *J Trauma.* 1992;33:850-855

38. Roudsari BS, Nathens AB, Cameron P, et al. International comparison of prehospital trauma care systems. *Injury.* 2007;38:993-1000.

39. Seamon MJ, Doane SM, Gaughan JP, et al. Prehospital interventions for penetrating trauma victims: a prospective comparison between Advanced Life Support and Basic Life Support. *Injury.* May 2013;44(5):634-638.

40. Jayaraman S, Sethi D, Wong R. Advanced training in trauma life support for ambulance crews. *Cochrane Database Syst Rev.* August 21, 2014;8:CD003109.

41. Warner KJ, Copass MK, Bulger EM. Paramedic use of needle thoracostomy in the prehospital environment. *Prehosp Emerg Care.* 2008;12:162-168.

42. Trauma Co. *Advanced Trauma Life Support.* 7th ed. Chicago, IL: American College of Surgeons; 2004.

43. National Association of Emergency Medical Technicians. *PHTLS: Prehospital Trauma Life Support.* 8th ed. Burlington, MA: Jones & Bartlett Learning, 2014.

44. Bulger EM, Nathens AB, Rivara FP, MacKenzie E, Sabath DR, Jurkovich GJ. National variability in out-of-hospital treatment after traumatic injury. *Ann Emerg Med.* 2007;49(3):293-301.

45. Heng K, Bystrzycki A, Fitzgerald M, et al. Complications of intercostal catheter insertion using EMST techniques for chest trauma. *ANZ J Surg.* 2004;74(6):420-423.

46. Spanjersberg WR, Ringburg AN, Bergs EA, Krijen P, Schipper IB. Prehospital chest tube thoracostomy: effective treatment or additional trauma? *J Trauma.* 2005;59(1):96-101.

47. Davis DP, Pettit K, Rom CD, et al. The safety and efficacy of prehospital needle and tube thoracostomy by aeromedical personnel. *Prehosp Emerg Care.* 2005;9(2):191-197.

48. Britten S, Palmer SH, Snow TM. Needle thoracentesis in tension pneumothorax: insufficient cannula length and potential failure. *Injury.* 1996;27(5):321-322.

49. Barton ED, Epperson M, Hoyt DB, et al. Prehospital needle aspiration and tube thoracostomy in trauma victims: a six-year experience with aeromedical crews. *J Emerg Med.* 1995;13(2):155-163.

50. Cullinane DC, Morris JA, Bass JG, Rutherford EJ. Needle thoracostomy may not be indicated in the trauma patient. *Injury.* 2001;32:749-752.

51. Stevens RL, Rochester AA, Busko J, et al. Needle thoracostomy for tension pneumothorax: failure predicted by chest computed tomography. *Prehosp Emerg Care.* 2009;13:14-17.

52. Warner KJ, Copass MK, Bulger EM. Paramedic use of needle thoracostomy in the prehospital environment. *Prehosp Emerg Care.* 2008;12:162-168.

53. Eckstein M, Suyehara D. Needle thoracostomy in the prehospital setting. *Prehosp Emerg Care.* 1998;2:132-135.

54. Blavias M. Inadequate needle thoracostomy rate in the prehospital setting for presumed pneumothorax: an ultrasound study. *J Ultrasound Med.* 2010;29:1285-1289.

55. Etoch SW, Bar-Natan MF, Miller FB, et al. Tube thoracostomy: factors related to complications. *Arch Surg.* 1995;130:521.

56. Newman PG, Feliciano DV. Blunt cardiac injury. *New Horizons.* 1999;7(1):26.

57. Spanjersberg W, Ringburg A, Bergs B, et al. Prehospital chest tube thoracostomy: effective treatment or additional trauma? *J Trauma.* 2005;59:96-101.

58. Rhee RM, Acosta J, Bridgeman A, et al. Survival after emergency department thoracotomy: review of published data from the past 25 years. *J Am Coll Surg.* 2000;190:288-298.

59. Tyburski JG, Astra L, Wilson RF, et al. Factors affecting prognosis with penetrating wounds of the heart. *J Trauma.* 2000;48:587-590.

60. Espositio TJ, Jurkovich GJ, Rice CL, et al. Reappraisal of emergency room thoracotomy in a changing environment. *J Trauma.* 1991;31:881-885.

61. Mazzorana V, Smith SR, Morabito DJ. Limited utility of emergency department thoracotomy. *Am Surg.* 1994;60:516-520.

62. Brown SE, Gomez GA, Jocobson LE. Penetrating chest trauma: should indications for emergency room thoracotomy be limited? *Am Surg.* 1996;62:530-533.

63. Wall MJ, Jnr Pepe PE, Mattox KL. Successful roadside resuscitative thoracotomy: case report and literature review. *J Trauma.* 1994;36:131-134.

64. Hopson LR, Hirsh E, Delgado J, et al. Guidelines for withholding or termination of resuscitation in prehospital traumatic cardiopulmonary arrest. *J Am Coll Surg.* 2003;196:106-112.

65. Davies GE, Lockey DJ. Thirteen survivors of prehospital thoracotomy for penetrating trauma: a prehospital physician-performed resuscitation procedure that can yield good results. *J Trauma.* 2011;70:E75-E78.

66. Corral E, Silva J, Suarez RM, et al. A successful emergency thoracotomy performed in the field. *Resuscitation.* 2007;75:530-533.

67. Rhee PM, Acosta J, Bridgeman, et al. Survival after emergency department thoracotomy: review of published data from the past 25 years. *J Am Coll Surg.* 2000;190:288-299.

68. Matsumoto H, Mashiko K, Hara Y. Role of resuscitative emergency field thoracotomy in the Japanese helicopter emergency medical service system. *Resuscitation.* 2009;80:1270-1274.

69. American College of Emergency Physicians. Policy statement: emergency ultrasound guidelines. *Ann Emerg Med.* 2009;53:550-557.

70. Mayron R, Gaudio FE, Plummer D, et al. Echocardiography performed by emergency physicians: impact on diagnosis and therapy. *Ann Emerg Med.* 1998;17:150-154.

71. Melniker LA, Leibner E, McKenney MG, et al. Randomized controlled clinical trial of point-of-care, limited ultrasonography for trauma in the emergency department: the first sonography outcomes assessment program trial. *Ann Emerg Med.* 2006;48:227-235.

72. Walcher F, Weinlich M, Conrad G, et al. Prehospital ultrasound imaging improves management of abdominal trauma. *Br J Surg.* 2006;93:238-242.

73. WalcherF, Petrovic T, Heegaard W, et al. *Prehospital ultrasound: perspectives from four Countries. Emergency Ultrasound.* New York, NY: McGraw Hill; 2008.

74. Nelson BP, Chason K. Use of ultrasound by emergency medical services: a review. *Int J Emerg Med.* 2008;1:253-259.

75. Heegaard W, Hildebrandt D, Spear D. Prehospital ultrasound by paramedics: results of field trial. *Acad Emerg Med.* 2010;17:624-630.

76. Blood CG, Puyana JC, Pitlyk PJ, et al. An assessment of the potential for reducing future combat deaths through medical technologies and training. *J Trauma.* 2002;53(6):1160-1165.

77. Polk JD, Merlino JL, Kovach BL, et al. Fetal evaluation for transport by ultrasound performed by air medical teams: a case series. *Air Med J.* 2004;23(4):32-34.

78. Byhahn C, Bingold TB, Twissler B, et al. Prehospital ultrasound detects pericardial tamponade in a pregnant victim of stabbing assault. *Resuscitation.* 2008;76:146-148.

79. Beck-Razi N, Fischer D, Michaelson M, et al. The utility of focused assessment with sonography for trauma as a triage tool in multiple-casualty incidents during the second Lebanon war. *J Ultrasound Med.* 2007;26:1149-1156.

80. Heegard W, Plummer D, Dries D, et al. Ultrasound for the air medical clinician. *Air Med J.* 2004;23(2):20-23.

81. Sztanjnkrycer MD, Baez AA, Luke A. FAST ultrasound as an adjunct to triage using the START mass casualty triage system: a preliminary descriptive system. *Prehosp Emerg Care.* 2006;10:96-102.

82. Sauaia A, Moore FA, Moore EE, et al. Epidemiology of trauma deaths: a reassessment. *J Trauma.* 1995;38:185-193.

83. Carey ME. Analysis of wounds incurred by U.S. Army Seventh Corps personnel treated in Corps hospitals during Operation Desert Storm, February 20 to March 10, 1991. *J Trauma.* 1996;40:S166-S169.

84. Wedmore I, McManus JG, Pusateri AE, Holcomb JB. A special report on the chitosan-based hemostatic dressing: experience in current combat operations. *J Trauma.* 2006;60:655-658.

85. Watters JM, Van PY, Hamilton GJ, et al. Advanced hemostatic dressings are not superior to gauze for care under fire scenarios. *J Trauma.* 2011;70:1413-1419.

86. Brown MA, Daya MR, Worley JA. Experience with chitosan dressings in a civilian EMS system. *J Emerg Med.* 2009. 37(1):1-7.

87. Pusateri AE, Holcomb JB, Bijan SK, et al. Making sense of the preclinical literature on advanced hemostatic products. *J Trauma.* 2006;60:674-682.

88. Arnaud F, Parreno-Sadalan D, Tomori T, et al. Comparison of 10 hemostatic dressings in a groin transaction model in swine. *J Trauma.* 2009;67:848-855.

89. Kheirabadi BS, Mace JE, Terrazas IB, et al. Safety evaluation of new hemostatic agents, smectite granules, and kaolin-coated gauze in a vascular injury wound model in swine. *J Trauma.* 2010;68: 269-278.

90. Achneck HE, Sileshi B, Jamiolkowski RM. A comprehensive review of topical hemostatic agents: efficacy and recommendations for use. *Ann Surg.* 2010;251:217-228.

91. Valeri CR, Vournakis JN. mRDH bandage for surgery and trauma: data summary and comparative review. *J Trauma.* 2010;71: S162-S166.

92. Navein J, Coupland R Dunn R. The tourniquet controversy. *J Trauma.* 2003;54(suppl):S219-S220.

93. Welling DR, Burris DG, Hutten JE, et al. A balanced approach to tourniquet use: lessons learned and relearned. *J Am Coll Surg.* 2006;203:106-115.

94. Lakstein D, Blumenfeld A, Sokolov T, et al. Tourniquets for hemorrhage control on the battlefield: a 4-year accumulated experience. *J Trauma.* 2003;54:S221-S225.

95. Kraugh JF, Walters TJ, Baer DG. Survival with emergency tourniquet use to stop bleeding in major limb trauma. *Ann Surg.* 2009;249:1-7.

96. Gates JD, Arabian S, Biddinger P, et al. The initial response to the Boston marathon bombing: lessons learned to prepare for the next disaster. *Ann Surg.* December 2014;260(6):960-966.

97. Callaway DW, Robertson J, Sztajnkrycer MD. Law enforcement-applied tourniquets: a case series of life-saving interventions. *Prehosp Emerg Care.* 2015;19(2):320-327.

98. Robertson J, McCahill P, Riddle A, Callaway D. Another civilian life saved by law enforcement-applied tourniquets. *J Spec Oper Med.* Fall 2014;14(3):7-11.

99. Jacobs L, Burns KJ. The Hartford Consensus to improve survivability in mass casualty events: process to policy. *Am J Disaster Med.* Winter 2014;9(1):67-71.

100. Bulger EM, Snyder D, Schoelles K, et al. An evidence-based prehospital guideline for external hemorrhage control: American College of Surgeons Committee on Trauma. *Prehosp Emerg Care.* April-June 2014;18(2):163-173.

101. Bobko J, Lai TT, Smith ER, Shapiro GL, Baldridge RT, Callaway DW. Tactical emergency casualty care? pediatric appendix: novel guidelines for the care of the pediatric casualty in the high-threat, prehospital environment. *J Spec Oper Med.* Winter 2013;13(4):94-107.

102. Galante JM, Smith CA, Sena MJ, Scherer LA, Tharratt RS. Identification of barriers to adaptation of battlefield technologies into civilian trauma in California. *Mil Med.* 2013;178(11):1227-1230.

103. Bickell WH, Wall MJ, Pepe PE, et al. Immediate versus delayed resuscitation for hypotensive patients with penetrating torso injuries. *N Engl J Med.* 1994;331:1105-1109.

104. Burris D, Rhee P, Kaufmann C, et al. Controlled resuscitation for uncontrolled hemorrhagic shock. *J Trauma.* 1999;46:216-233.

105. Yaghoubian A, Lewis RJ, Putnam B. Reanalysis of prehospital intravenous fluid administration in patients with penetrating truncal injury and field hypotension. *Am Surg.* 2007;73:1027-1030.

106. Gando S, Saitoh D, Ogura H, et al. Japanese Association for Acute Medicine Disseminated Intravascular Coagulation (JAAM DIC) Study Group. Disseminated intravascular coagulation (DIC) diagnosed based on the Japanese Association for Acute Medicine criteria is a dependent continuum to overt DIC in patients with sepsis. *Thromb Res.* 2009;123:715-718.

107. Brhoi K, Cohen MJ, Ganter MT, et al. Acute coagulopathy of trauma: hypoperfusion induces systemic anticoagulation and hyperfibrinolysis. *J Trauma.* 2008;64:1211-1217.

108. Lethaby A, Farquhar C, Cooke I. Antifibrinolytics for heavy menstrual bleeding. *Cochrane Database Syst Rev.* 2000:CD000249.

109. Cormack F, Chakrabarti RR, Jouhar AJ, et al. Tranexamic acid in upper gastrointestinal haemorrhage. *Lancet.* 1973;1:1207-1208.

110. Ro JS, Knutrud O, Stormorken H. Antifibrinolytic treatment with tranexamic acid (AMCA) in pediatric urinary tract surgery. *J Pediatr Surg.* 1970;5:315-320.

111. CRASH-2 trial collaborators. Effects of tranexamic acid death, vascular occlusive events, and blood transfusion in trauma patients with significant haemorrhage (CRASH-2): a randomized, placebo-controlled trial. *Lancet.* 2010;376:23-32.

112. Morrison JJ, Dubose JJ, Rasmussen TE, Midwinter MJ. Military Application of Tranexamic Acid in Trauma Emergency Resuscitation (MATTERs) Study. *Arch Surg.* 2012 Feb;147(2):113-119.

Head Injury and Spinal Cord Injury

Robert D. Greenberg

Clifford J. Buckley II

INTRODUCTION

Head and spinal cord injuries require special care and consideration. Rapid assessment, stabilization, extrication, and transportation to definitive care are the primary EMS objectives to facilitate the best opportunity for a functional outcome. Often, injuries to the head and spinal cord are not immediately obvious; therefore, reasonable precautions should be taken to prevent further injury. Detailed in this chapter are pieces of information pertinent to the physiology of brain and spinal cord injuries and the key ways to evaluate, manage, and stabilize patients suffering from these injuries.

OBJECTIVES

1. Describe the initial prehospital evaluation and management of head injury.

2. Describe the common causes and mechanisms involved in head trauma.

3. Discuss the role of EMS in the treatment of concussion, and in prevention of secondary brain injury.

4. Describe the initial prehospital evaluation and management of spinal trauma.

5. Discuss potential challenges in airway management in spinal trauma.

6. Discuss water-related spinal trauma.

7. Detail the criteria for the use of selective spinal immobilization.

8. Describe the potential harm to patients from spinal immobilization practices.

9. Discuss the debate concerning the use of spinal immobilization in penetrating trauma.

HEAD INJURY

The initial step in head injury management is the evaluation of mechanism of injury, history of present illness, and possible comorbidities, while maintaining situational awareness of the scene. Evaluation of a patient's mental status can be quickly attained through the use of the Glasgow coma scale (GCS) (**Table 55-1**). The GCS aims to give a reliable, reproducible, objective way of recording the conscious state of a patient for initial and subsequent assessments. It is commonly accepted and utilized in trauma care. Some experts advocate using the motor assessment only, but that is not the current care standard.[1]

A normal, awake patient should have a GCS of 15. Historically, patients with a GCS of 8 or lower have been considered for intubation as it is thought that their ability to protect their airway may be compromised. The lowest possible score is 3 and represents a patient with a complete lack of neurological response to stimuli and generally indicates a severe brain injury with an accompanying poor prognosis. The GCS is sometimes amended with an "I" for a patient that is intubated to indicate that the scale may be different due to sedation, chemical paralysis, or the noxious stimulus from the endotracheal tube. A 2014 study by Reisner et al revealed an association between poor outcomes from traumatic brain injury when GCS was abnormal and heart rate and blood pressure were also abnormal.[2]

In addition to the GCS, evaluation of physical findings includes bruising behind the ears (Battle sign) or around the eyes (raccoon eyes) as indicators of basilar skull fracture. If the patient is able to answer questions, evaluate for recall of the events that just transpired checking for loss of consciousness and orientation to person, place, and time. Also inquire about associated symptoms of dizziness, headache, nausea, vomiting, tinnitus, and/or vision disturbances. If the patient is ambulatory and/or cooperative, evaluation for signs of balance and motor disturbance can indicate more subtle signs of injury or intoxication. Examine the eyes for changes in pupil shape and reactivity. Fixed, dilated, and nonreactive pupils are ominous signs of serious brain injury.

MANAGEMENT/STABILIZATION

A common thread in the prehospital management of brain and spinal cord injury is hemodynamic stabilization. It is well accepted that hypotension and hypoxia are associated with poorer outcomes in head injured patients.[3] Just as with all trauma patients, the ABCs, (airway, breathing, and circulation) are the first priority in the management of brain and spinal cord injury. Blood pressure should not be lowered as part of a prehospital guideline.

Blood pressure should be monitored closely and consideration of cerebral blood flow must be a top priority for patient with presumed space-occupying bleeds. The main driving force behind CBF is cerebral perfusion pressure (CPP). CPP may be compromised in patients with large intracranial bleeds as the cerebral spinal fluid is forced from the intracranial space and the intracranial pressure rises in response to the loss of compensatory mechanisms. Cerebral perfusion pressure, which is responsible for allowing for proper oxygenation of the brain, is the sum of the mean arterial pressure (MAP), less the intracranial pressure. Normal intracranial pressure (ICP) is considered to be 5 to 15, but if a large intracranial bleed is suspected clinically, an ICP of >25 may be anticipated. CCP should be maintained at 70 mm Hg. When there is a presumed increase in ICP the equation yields a needed MAP of around 90 in order to maintain CCP.

$$CCP = MAP - ICP$$

$$CCP \text{ (goal of } 70 - 90 \text{ mm Hg)} = MAP \text{ (goal of } >90 \text{ mm Hg)} - ICP$$
$$(>25 \text{ mm Hg in severe head bleed})$$

Therefore, if the ICP was hypothetically 35 mm Hg, the MAP would need to be around 105 in order to ensure the proper CCP. This can be expressed as an algebraic formula, solving for MAP, expressed as x:

$$CCP = MAP - ICP$$

$$70 \text{ mmHg} = x \text{ mmHg} - 35 \text{ mmHg}$$

$$70 \text{ mmHg} + 35 \text{ mmHg} = x \text{ mmHg}$$

Therefore, the MAP required to maintain the CCP = 105 mm Hg

This is why hyperventilation, which is known to transiently decrease MAP (and therefore CPP), and mannitol should both be reserved for patients with signs of impending herniation. It is known that mortality increases approximately 20% for each 10 mm Hg loss of CPP. In ideal

Glasgow Coma Score	1	2	3	4	5	6
Eye	No response	Opens to pain	Opens to voice	Spontaneously open	N/A	N/A
Voice	No sound	Incomprehensible	Inappropriate words	Confused	Oriented	N/A
Motor	No movement	Extension to stimuli	Flexion to stimuli	Withdrawal from pain	Localized to pain	Obeys commands

TABLE 55-1 Glasgow Coma Scale

circumstances, CPP is maintained at 70 mm Hg and recommendations are to ensure maintenance of MAP >90 mm Hg. There is evidence that early hypotension (systolic blood pressure <90 mm Hg) is associated with an increase in morbidity and mortality. Unfortunately, there is not a reasonable way for the ICP to be monitored in the prehospital setting; however, during interfacility transports of patients who have had neurosurgical intervention, particular attention should be paid to ICP and calculations of CCP made at key points of the transport to ensure proper critical care of these severely injured patients.

◼ MECHANISMS OF INJURY

The mechanisms of head injury are complex, but follow the basic laws of energy. All mass in motion has inertia and thus a tendency to continue in motion. Often, head injuries result from rapid deceleration or direct blow and the brain is injured by colliding with the wall of the inner skull.[4] The brain can also be injured by disruption of cerebral vasculature. Rupture of arteries and/or veins inside the skull causes bleeding with resultant compression of the brain and is a life-threatening emergency.

The history and mechanism of injury may help identify potential secondary injuries. Prehospital personnel may be the only ones that have access to information at the scene to assist in the identification of life-threatening injuries once the patient has arrived at the hospiital.

◼ CONCUSSION AND SECONDARY INJURY

Rapid transport to definitive care is the priority once the ABCs and cervical spine are secured. Immediate extrication and evacuation may be necessary before beginning hemodynamic stabilization and the secondary survey if the scene is not secured. Often, and importantly for severely or multiple injured patients, the secondary survey can take place during transportation. After initial stabilization, it is prudent to survey for signs of concussion and secondary injury.

Concussions are common in closed head injury and should be taken seriously. Even though the patient may not be in critical condition, signs and symptoms of concussion can indicate significant brain injury. Loss of consciousness is a common historical feature that elevates the level of concern for brain injury. Amnesia is a common component of concussion and perseveration of questioning by the patient is frequent. Other signs of concussion include inappropriate somnolence, nausea, vomiting, clouding of thoughts, and headache.

Reassessment through serial GCS scoring can be utilized as a monitor of worsening brain injury. Changes in GCS can represent intracranial bleeding, brain herniation, or poor cerebral perfusion. Caution should be taken regarding the implications of administering medications that can alter the mental status or neurologic examination. Coordination and communication of prehospital medication protocols with receiving facilities should be maintained to avoid confusing clinical encounters.

◼ PENETRATING HEAD INJURY

Penetrating injuries to the head are particularly devastating. Penetrating trauma, particularly gunshot wounds, causes direct insult to the brain and often damages the cerebral vasculature. Penetrating head trauma may not always be obvious and, in the case of patients working around high-speed equipment, small materials can penetrate into the skull without evidence of an obvious entrance wound but may still cause devastating injury to the brain and related structures. Open skull fractures from penetrating trauma have poor morbidity and mortality numbers with 73% dead at the scene and 19% died at the hospital, with an overall mortality rate of 92%.[5] Transtentorial injuries are typically mortal. High velocity missiles cause cavitation and low velocity missiles (like small caliber bullets) tend to ricochet and tumble in the skull.

SPINAL TRAUMA

Spinal trauma can result in life-threatening injury and serious long-term morbidities for those involved. The immediate stabilization and management of spinal trauma may improve prognosis and therefore result in better outcomes with less neurological sequelae. The history surrounding the traumatic event can provide key information regarding the likelihood of spinal trauma. High-speed injuries, extreme flexion/extension injuries, direct blow, and diving injuries should all raise suspicion for spinal trauma. It should also be acknowledged that a high cervical spinal cord injury could mimic a significant closed head injury with complete paralysis appearing as unresponsiveness.

Patients complaining of neck or back pain, numbness, tingling, motor deficit, or weakness should be considered spinal trauma and possible cord injury until proven otherwise. Specific criteria for spinal motion restriction (SMR) will be discussed later in the chapter.

◼ ASSESSMENT

Much like brain injury, the same rules apply for the assessment of spinal trauma. Airway, breathing, and circulation are the priority. A patient without a patent airway, or who is not properly breathing or perfusing their organs will succumb regardless of the presence of spinal injury. Having a preventable death due to attempts at stabilizing a potential injury is not prudent. As previously discussed, the initial GCS will establish a baseline and help determine if there is a component of decreased mental status.

Patients with spinal trauma can have evidence of abnormal neurological function. Once stabilization and extrication are performed, a head to toe survey may be performed but should not delay transportation. Vertebral tenderness may represent spinal trauma, but may also be absent as the injury may not be superficial or palpable. A neurological examination checking mental status, motor function, sensation, and abnormal posturing is helpful as a baseline.[6,7] The higher the level of spinal cord trauma, the more devastating the neurological dysfunction. Very high spinal trauma can lead to respiratory failure and death so reassessment and monitoring are essential.

◼ MANAGEMENT/STABILIZATION

Cervical spine precautions have been the standard of care for patients with significant head injury and for patients with potential spinal injuries. For over 30 years, cervical spine precautions were considered standard measures taken to minimize further insult to the spinal cord or destabilization of the cervical vertebra. This is performed through spinal motion restriction with a variety of devices and the use of cervical collars and head blocks in conjunction with immobilization to a long spine board. However, recent studies and reviews have concluded that the variation in experimental results and the lack of proven benefit may indicate that cervical collars may not be the best practice in these patients. A recent systematic review summarized these points[8] (**Box 55-1**).

Classic cervical spine precautions with spinal motion restriction (SMR) have been recommended for patients with evidence or suspicion

---

Box 55-1

Summary Points on Routine Use of Cervical Collars From Recent Literature

- The existing evidence for using collars is inconsistent and not compelling.
- Current practice is mainly a result of the historical influence of poor evidence.
- There is a documentation number of harmful effects from collars.
- A practice change seems warranted based on a critical evaluation of the pros and cons of prehospital collar use in trauma patients.
- Temporary use of a rigid collar is an option during extrication procedures.
- Patients should be transported in a modified lateral recovery position in or to maintain (near) neutral spine alignment and airway patency.
- Prehospital management should not delay transportation of critically injured patients.

Data from Sundstrøm T, Asbjørnsen H, Habiba S, Sunde GA, Wester K. Prehospital Use of Cervical Collars in Trauma Patients: A Critical Review. *J Neurotrauma*. 2014; 31:531-540.

of spinal trauma. There are many techniques and numerous apparatus available to provide SMR. The historical rationale for keeping the patient's spine in alignment that there will be less chance that an injury to the bony spine will result in cord injury. Spinal trauma can be present without the injured patient having subjective knowledge of the injury.

As with brain injuries, frequent reassessment is important when caring for people with spinal injury. Always ensure that the ABCs are secured. Patients with spinal cord injury are prone to neurogenic shock. Neurogenic shock results from the loss of sympathetic tone, causing peripheral vasculature to be less responsive. The resulting circulatory collapse will present with hypotension and poor pulses on examination. Fluid resuscitation is always the first line of treatment, but additional pressor agents may also be required. Periodic neurological examinations can also be helpful in assessing developing neurological deficits.

AIRWAY MANAGEMENT

Airway management in the face of spinal trauma presents a precarious situation. People with spinal trauma who are unable to protect their airway require intubation or the use of other airway adjuncts. While securing an airway is obviously a priority, it is also essential that reasonable efforts be made to maintain cervical spine precautions throughout the intubation process. If possible, keep the cervical collar on when securing the airway, but if this is not possible, remove the cervical collar and manually secure the cervical spine. Prehospital intubation in patients with severe head injury is controversial.[9,10] A 2014 study by Karamanos et al revealed significantly higher mortality and worse oxygenation in a case-matched cohort of the patient when intubation was performed.[11]

WATER-RELATED SPINAL TRAUMA

As mentioned earlier, diving injuries are one of the common mechanisms of spinal trauma. Frequently, this results from diving into shallow bodies of water. The most common cause of spinal trauma from diving into pools happens from people diving into the upslope of the pool bottom. Some studies have suggested that diving-related injuries account for up to 14% of spinal cord injuries.[12] Young males are the group affected most by diving injuries. Not all water-related spinal trauma results from diving injuries. Boating accidents and other high-speed traumas must also be considered.

The mechanism of injury in diving injuries is typically a hyperextension injury resulting in spinal cord injury. Because the portion of the spine injured in water-related spinal trauma tends to be the cervical spine, the extent of the neurological damage can be catastrophic. Further complicating the spinal trauma is the presence of water and the risk for aspiration, drowning, and near-drowning, which greatly increase the morbidity and mortality in these traumas. Always ensure early appropriate airway management.

CRITERIA FOR THE USE OF SELECTIVE SPINAL MOTION RESTRICTION

Not every trauma patient requires SMR and it could potentially be harmful to do so unnecessarily. When arriving to a scene, a decision must be made on whether or not SMR is indicated or necessary. The National Emergency X-Radiography Utilization Study (NEXUS) developed a set of criteria to guide this decision[13,14] (**Box 55-2**). SMR should be implemented with

Box 55-2	
NEXUS Criteria	
1. Midline cervical tenderness	
2. Focal neurologic deficits	
3. Altered level of consciousness	
4. Evidence of intoxication	
5. Painful distracting injury	

TABLE 55-2	Clinical Clearance Protocol for Spinal Motion Restriction (SMR)
Level	Basic, Intermediate, Paramedic
Indication	Cervical Spine Clearance Cervical spine clearance may be appropriate for individuals that meet all of the criteria of the following algorithm. **Abnormal Mental Status? If No then continue;** **Intoxicated? If No then continue;** **Focal neurologic deficit? If No then continue;** **Neck pain? If No then continue;** **Midline neck tenderness? If No then continue;** **Painful or distracting injury? If No then may elect not to spinal restrict.** If the answer to any of the above questions is Yes, then the patient is not clinically cleared and the patient should have spinal motion restrictions applied. Documentation in the official record must be completed any time this procedure is performed.

Technique	• SMR decision
	  • If patient has *no* positive findings on above examination, may omit SMR
	  • If patient has *any* positive findings on above examination, or if unable to complete examination, SMR should be performed

Documentation	• Who made the decision to implement or not implement SMR and a justification for that decision with pertinent examination findings • Note any first responders who assisted in SMR prior to or during treatment • Any changes in patient's condition postprocedure

distracting injuries (ie, extremity fractures, lacerations, etc), neurological symptoms, intoxication, altered level of consciousness, and midline cervical tenderness.

It can be difficult to immediately identify distracting injuries. These injuries are extremely painful and cause the injured patient to be unaware that they may have neurological symptoms or midline cervical tenderness. There is not uniform agreement on exactly what a distracting injury is, but most sources do cite long bone injuries.[15] As a result, use discretion and, when in doubt, employ SMR. **Table 55-2** is an example of a field clearance tool used successfully in multiple EMS services.

HARM TO PATIENTS FROM SPINAL MOTION RESTRICTION PRACTICES

While SMR has been the classic teaching for over 40 years, there are potential risks to employing or overusing it. There is no significant valid research data to support that the routine use of spinal immobilization on a long spine board (backboard) prevents spinal cord injury, and there have been studies that do show it is markedly uncomfortable and may cause harm. The rigid cervical collar and backboard prevent movement, create pressure points, and are moderately painful. Prolonged SMR on a rigid backboard is associated with skin breakdown and pressure sores. This is especially true in the elderly when skin breakdown can be seen earlier when compared to a younger population.

SMR takes time to properly apply; it increases time on scene and may distract for other more emergent needs as well as diverting care from other patients. This can increase the amount of time before a patient receives definitive care and potentially increases exposure the perils of a scene. Upon arrival to the hospital, patients who have had SMR are more likely to be subjected to unnecessary tests and procedures. This may be in part to the discomfort caused by the procedure itself. Because the patient is restricted from being able to move their head, aspiration risk is increased should the patient need to vomit or cough up sputum. Lastly, the restricted patients are more difficult to secure an airway in and perform other potentially lifesaving procedures and testing on. The National Association of EMS Physicians (NAEMSP) and the American College of Surgeons Committee on Trauma (ACSCOT) have published a joint position statement that downplays the use of spine boards after initial extrication has been completed.[16] There is a growing body of literature that does not seem to support this time honored practice as the risks appear to be potentially greater than the benefits in this particular patient population. One paper showed that backboard times can be nearly an hour on average, with about half in the field and half in the ED.[17]

USE OF SPINAL MOTION RESTRICTION IN PENETRATING TRAUMA

Those suffering from penetrating trauma present a specific dilemma for prehospital providers as far as SMR is concerned. The evidence for using SMR in penetrating trauma, specifically gunshot wounds to the head, contradicts this as necessary.[18,19] In fact the joint position paper from NAEMSP and ACSCOM states: *"Patients with penetrating trauma to the head, neck, or torso and no evidence of spinal injury should not be immobilized on a backboard."*[16]

Some have speculated that the increased time on scene associated with SMR is detrimental to those with penetrating trauma and thus could be associated with increased mortality and morbidity. In fact, some studies have shown an associated increase in mortality in patients with SMR and penetrating trauma compared to those with penetrating trauma and no SMR. Overall the use of SMR in penetrating trauma does not appear to be beneficial.[20] Despite this fact, prehospital providers may still be inclined to utilize immobilization in these cases.[21]

CONCLUSION

Brain and spinal injuries represent a significant portion of traumatic injuries. For both brain and spinal injuries, the ABCs are the priority in management. As mentioned earlier, a patient without a patent airway, adequate breathing, nor satisfactory perfusion is going to die regardless of their other injuries. Efforts must be made to address the ABCs before moving on to the secondary survey. A head to toe approach to the secondary survey helps ensure that you do not miss subtle brain and spine injuries and other associated injuries. The Glasgow coma scale is a helpful tool for assessing mental status and can serve as a way to detect a deteriorating situation.

Having an understanding of the mechanisms of injury of various brain and spinal injuries can provide insight into the situation and guide further evaluation. Brain and spine injuries commonly compel spinal motion restriction (cervical spine precautions). Any patient with distracting injuries (perhaps excluding penetrating trauma), neurological symptoms, intoxication, altered level of consciousness, and midline cervical tenderness may still receive spinal motion restriction by convention; however, EMS physicians should be aware of this controversy and review current literature to guide practice and protocol changes. Spinal motion restriction can create some challenges when caring for the patient and prolonged backboard times may lead to real harm.

KEY POINTS

- Closed head injury can have a subtle presentation and consideration of concussion should be made.
- In severe head injury consideration of blood pressure support should be aimed at maintaining cerebral perfusion pressure based on a presumed elevation in ICP.
- Hyperventilation and the use of Mannitol should be discouraged up to the point of signs of early herniation.
- Penetrating head injury is almost always fatal (92%).

- Cervical spine immobilization with a rigid collar may be more harmful than beneficial based on recent evidence and persistent review of the literature is warranted.
- Spine immobilization with a long spine board may be more harmful than beneficial when used for more than initial extrication based on recent evidence and removal to simple spinal precautions as early as possible is likely prudent.
- Routine spinal immobilization for patients with penetrating trauma is not indicated.

REFERENCES

1. Cameron KL, Yunker CA, Austin MC. A Standardized Protocol for the Initial Evaluation and Documentation of Mild Brain Injury. *J Athl Train.* January-March 1999;34(1):34-42.
2. Reisner A, Chen X, Kumar K, Reifman J. Prehospital heart rate and blood pressure increase the positive predictive value of the Glasgow Coma Scale for high-mortality traumatic brain injury. *J Neurotrauma.* May 15, 2014;31(10):906-913.
3. Saul TG. Management of head injury. American College of Surgery Committee on Trauma. April 1998. https://www.facs.org/~/media/files/quality%20programs/trauma/publications/headinjury.ashx.
4. Barth JT, Freeman JR, Broshek DK, Varney RN. Acceleration-deceleration sport-related concussion: the gravity of it all. *J Athl Train.* July-September 2001;36(3):253-256.
5. Vinas F, Wyler A. Penetrating head trauma. *eMedicine. Medscape Reference.* June 2, 2011. http://emedicine.medscape.com/article/247664-overview. Accessed June 14, 2011.
6. Domeier RM, Evans RW, Swor RA, et al. The reliability of prehospital clinical evaluation for potential spinal injury is not affected by the mechanism of injury. *Prehosp Emerg Care.* 1999;3(4):332-337.
7. Meldon SW, Brant TA, Cydulka RK et al. Out-of-hospital cervical spine clearance: agreement between emergency medical technicians and emergency physicians. *J Trauma.* 1998;45:1058-1061.
8. Sundstrøm T, Asbjørnsen H, Habiba S, Sunde GA, Wester K. Prehospital use of cervical collars in trauma patients: a critical review. *J Neurotrauma.* 2014;31(6):531-540.
9. Sobuwa S, Hartzenberg HB, Geduld H, Uys C. Outcomes following prehospital airway management in severe traumatic brain injury. *S Afr Med J.* July 29, 2013;103(9):644-646.
10. Boer C, Franschman G, Loer SA. Prehospital management of severe traumatic brain injury: concepts and ongoing controversies. *Curr Opin Anaesthesiol.* October 2012;25(5):556-562.
11. Karamanos E, Talving P, Skiada D, et al. Is prehospital endotracheal intubation associated with improved outcomes in isolated severe head injury? A matched cohort analysis. *Prehosp Disaster Med.* February 2014;29(1):32-36.
12. World Health Organization. Water-related diseases: spinal injury. Geneva. 2001. http://www.who.int/water_sanitation_health/diseases/spinal/en/. Accessed June 14, 2011.
13. Hoffman JR, Wolfson AB, Todd K, Mower WR. Selective cervical spine radiography in blunt trauma: methodology of the National Emergency X-Radiography Utilization Study (NEXUS). *Ann Emerg Med.* October 1998;32(4):461-946. PubMed PMID: 9774931.
14. Hoffman JR, Mower WR, Wolfson AB, Todd KH, Zucker MI. Validity of a set of clinical criteria to rule out injury to the cervical spine in patients with blunt trauma. National Emergency X-Radiography Utilization Study Group. *N Engl J Med.* July 13, 2000;343(2):94-99. Erratum in: *N Engl J Med.* February 8, 2001;344(6):464. PubMed PMID: 10891516.
15. Wesley K. Selective spinal immobilization. *EMS World.* May 2004; 33(5):99-102, 104-106.

16. EMS spinal precautions and the use of the long backboard. *Prehosp Emerg Care*. July-September 2013;17(3):392-393.

17. Cooney DR, Wallus H, Asaly M, Wojcik S. Backboard time for patients receiving spinal immobilization by emergency medical services. *Int J Emerg Med*. June 20, 2013;6(1):17.

18. Haut ER, Kalish BT, Efron DT, et al. Spine immobilization in penetrating trauma: more harm than good? *J Trauma*. January 2010;68(1):115-120.

19. Connell RA, Graham CA, Munro PT. Is spinal immobilization necessary for all patients sustaining isolated penetrating trauma? *Injury*. December 2003;34(12):912-914.

20. Garcia A, Liu TH, Victorino GP. Cost-utility analysis of prehospital spine immobilization recommendations for penetrating trauma. *J Trauma Acute Care Surg*. February 2014;76(2):534-541.

21. Bouland AJ, Jenkins JL, Levy MJ. Assessing attitudes toward spinal immobilization. *J Emerg Med*. October 2013;45(4):e117-e125.

CHAPTER 56

Extremity Injuries

Joseph Tennyson
Stacy N. Weisberg
Mark Quale

INTRODUCTION

Musculoskeletal trauma is frequently encountered in the prehospital setting. In 2007, extremity injuries accounted for over 14 million emergency department visits within the United States.[1] Injuries from falls, motor vehicle accidents, sports activities, and pedestrian versus vehicle accidents are commonly encountered. It is imperative that EMS physicians know how to appropriately stabilize and manage these injuries as many result in limb or life-threatening conditions.

OBJECTIVES

- Understand the epidemiology of musculoskeletal extremity injuries in the prehospital environment.
- Recognize common injury patterns and their mechanisms.
- Be familiar with common immobilization techniques and equipment.
- Be familiar with common reduction techniques.
- Select appropriate destination facilities based on patients' injuries.

PREHOSPITAL EVALUATION OF MUSCULOSKELETAL TRAUMA

▒ PRIMARY SURVEY OF MUSCULOSKELETAL INJURIES

After ensuring the scene of the injury is safe, it is reasonable to consider adhering to the methodology described by courses such as ATLS and PHTLS (prehospital trauma life support) for performance of the primary and secondary survey. Management of airway compromise, respiratory failure, and life-threatening hemorrhage will be addressed elsewhere in this text.

▒ SECONDARY SURVEY OF MUSCULOSKELETAL INJURIES

The secondary survey identifies limb-threatening extremity injuries within its later portion as injuries to the head and thorax take early precedence. ATLS guidelines recommend the "ask, look, and feel" approach to evaluation. "Ask:" Awake and alert patients will help identify painful injuries, bleeding, or deficits. "Look:" Expose the patient's extremities and look for evidence of injury such as bleeding, swelling, deformity, discoloration, or cyanosis. Swelling, especially over large muscle groups, may be indicative of underlying fractures, hematoma formation, or crush injuries. Discoloration and cyanosis of distal extremities suggests ischemia of the affected limb. "Feel:" Palpate extremities to assess for tenderness, loss of sensation, deformity, crepitus, and distal pulses plus perfusion.[2]

Prior to manipulating any injured extremities, a distal neurovascular examination should be performed. Assess for key extremity pulses, such as radial artery pulses in the upper extremities and dorsalis pedis and posterior tibial artery pulses in the lower extremity. Compare pulses to the contralateral extremity. Also observe and compare capillary refill in distal nail beds. Capillary refill exceeding 2 seconds is generally abnormal. Evaluation of key sensory and motor groups will also provide important information and should be done during this assessment.

Extremities with grossly contaminated open fractures should have dirt and debris removed by saline irrigation or wiping followed by sterile dressing application. Vaseline dressings may be utilized as an initial layer over an open fracture with soft bulky dressings overlying.

Extremities with suspected fractures should be immobilized, preferably with a padded splint.

In general, prehospital reduction of fractures is discouraged. Fracture reduction is a painful process which is best accomplished with the assistance of procedural sedation in the emergency department setting. There are, however, situations where prehospital fracture reduction should be considered. These situations include fractures such as midshaft femur and unstable pelvic fractures, as well as fractures with associated neurovascular compromise or major hemorrhage. If distal pulses are absent in an extremity, immediate field assessment for reduction of a related fracture or dislocation by a trained provider should be considered.

Field reduction is controversial. The National Association of EMS Physicians condones fracture reduction by nonphysicians only if a prolonged transport to the hospital exists, while PHTLS recognizes that one to two attempts at prehospital reduction may be attempted if there is evidence of reduced circulation distal to the deformed extremity.[3] Generally, fracture reduction is done by recreating the forces which created the fracture followed by continuous axial traction at the distal portion of the extremity until it can be placed back into an anatomically neutral position. Should new neurologic deficit or worsened vascular examination occur after an attempted reduction, return the extremity to its initial position, immobilize it, and transport the patient immediately to a higher level of care.[4] Fracture and dislocation management of several selected fractures are reviewed later in this chapter.

PREHOSPITAL EXTREMITY IMMOBILIZATION

Any extremity with obvious or suspected injury following trauma should be immobilized. Without radiographs, it can be difficult to diagnose all but the most obvious fractures. Pain, deformity, open wounds, hematoma formation, or crepitus on palpation along an extremity is suggestive of an underlying fracture.

Splinting offers the benefit of reducing pain and preventing further vascular, muscle, and nerve damage to an injured extremity. It also prevents transforming closed fractures into open fractures.[3] On-scene extremity immobilization should not be conducted if it will delay transport of a patient with life-threatening injuries or prevent successful hemorrhage control in major bleeding. Often extremity immobilization can be conducted en route to the hospital, thus not delaying transport time.

Many types of commercially available splints now exist and it is important that each provider be experienced with the appropriate use of the various splinting and immobilization devices they intend to utilize. Splints can be divided into three major types: rigid, soft, and traction splints. The use of lower extremity traction splints is discussed within this chapter's section on femur fractures.

Rigid splints are manufactured out of plastic, malleable metals, wood, wire, or other materials. They tend to be less flexible and more supportive than soft splints and are usually padded. Rigid splints are usually secured to patients via circumferentially applied tape, bandages, or straps. The joints above and below the injury should be immobilized. In transporting, it is recommended, when possible, to leave the distal portion of the extremity (toes or fingers) outside of the splint so distal perfusion can be reassessed en route.

Vacuum splints are another type of splint used in the prehospital environment. Vacuum splints are very flexible and can be applied in a multitude of different positions. To apply this splint, one provider supports the injured extremity in the position desired for splinting, while the other provider wraps the splint along the length of the extremity and then secures it with a series of straps. Once applied longitudinally and strapped, a hand pump is attached to a small valve stem on the splint and is used to evacuate air from the splint. As air is evacuated, the splint forms to the shape of the injured extremity and becomes rigid. Vacuum splints have the advantage of being able to be applied to injured extremities found in a multitude of positions; this allows for minimal pain to the patient as movement of the extremity is minimized during the splinting process.

Soft splints include slings, bulky immobilizers, and air splints. Slings are used to immobilize suspected clavicle or shoulder injuries, as well as to support the weight of upper extremity splints for patient comfort. They are easy to apply and provide moderate immobilization of the upper extremity.

Bulky splints, such as a sheet of foam, pillow, or towel, can be wrapped around an injured extremity and secured with tape or ties when needed. Most often bulky splints are used to support an injured hand, wrist, or forearm injury.

Air splints come in a variety of shapes and sizes to fit different extremities. They are initially deflated and placed around the injured extremity and then inflated with air to provide support. It is important to note that air splints apply circumferential pressure to wounded extremities. This may exacerbate pain and may further distal ischemia. These splints should not be applied over open fractures. When transportation involves atmospheric pressures changes, as with aeromedical or mountain transport, expansion or decompression of the splint may occur and the pressure should be monitored. Due to some of the concern over these complications air splints may not be the best option for standard prehospital care.

MANAGEMENT OF SPECIFIC INJURIES

The majority of extremity injuries can be treated with a general approach involving hemorrhage control, gross decontamination, immobilization, and pain control. However, unique approaches to immobilization and reduction techniques are required for some injuries. Several specific injuries that may require specific immobilization or reduction are discussed within this section.

UPPER EXTREMITY INJURIES

SHOULDER DISLOCATIONS

Dislocated shoulders are frequently encountered in the prehospital setting and account for half of all dislocations seen in emergency department. Prehospital reduction of dislocations should be avoided by nonphysician providers unless there is a compelling neurovascular deficit associated, such as loss of distal pulses with an anticipated prolonged transport time. Traumatic injuries which need immobilization, such as a proximal humerus fracture, may appear similar on physical examination to a shoulder dislocation.

The three main subtypes of shoulder dislocations are anterior, posterior, and inferior. The most common dislocation is anterior (90%) and patients usually present with the arm supported on their effected side with a large defect inferior to the acromion (**Figure 56-1**). The injury usually occurs when a force is transmitted through an externally rotated and abducted arm. The axillary nerve can be injured in up to 15% to 55% of shoulder dislocations and should be assessed by checking sensation over the lateral deltoid.[5] Vascular injury is uncommon with shoulder dislocations, but radial pulses should always be assessed. Sling and swath immobilization is appropriate for transport of patient's with suspected shoulder dislocations.

If reduction is required due to the presence of distal ischemia and anticipated prolonged transport, one or two attempts at shoulder reduction may be attempted. There are a number of commonly used techniques for shoulder reduction including external rotation (modified Kocher), scapular manipulation, Milch, traction and counter traction, Stimson, FARES, Cunningham, and Hippocratic.

The external rotation technique is recommended for reduction in the field as this approach has few complications, can be easily employed in the prehospital setting, and often requires little analgesia if performed early. The scapular manipulation, Milch, traction and counter traction, Stimson, and FARES methods are impractical in most prehospital settings. The Cunningham technique is an excellent option, but does require a calm, cooperative patient and is best performed in a controlled and

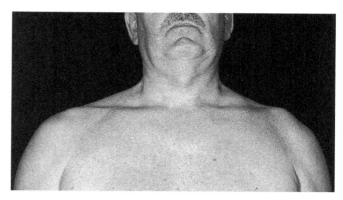

FIGURE 56-1. A patient whose right shoulder is anteriorly dislocated. There is a large defect inferior to the acromion on visual examination. (Photo contributor: Frank Birinyi, MD; Reprinted with permission from Knoop KJ, Stack LB, Storrow AB, Thurman RJ. *The Atlas of Emergency Medicine*. 3rd ed. McGraw-Hill; 2010. Figure 11.1.)

settling environment. The Hippocratic method should never be used, as it is associated with the significant threat of axillary nerve injury. To perform a shoulder reduction with the external rotation technique, the patient should be seated upright or at a 45° angle with arm adducted at their side. The practitioner supports the affected arm at the elbow with one hand and holds the patient's wrist with the other hand. Slow and steady force is applied to bring the patient's arm into 90° of external rotation. The shoulder may reduce (generally a "clunk" is felt or shoulder deformity disappears) at this point. If not reduced, the patient's arm should slowly be raised vertically until either resistance is met or the humerus is elevated to approximately 20° above the horizontal plane (**Figure 56-2**).

Posterior shoulder dislocations are frequently missed and commonly occur after generalized seizures and electrical injuries. Patients generally note severe shoulder pain and there is often posterior prominence of the shoulder with limited external rotation of the arm on examination. Neurovascular compromise is rare with posterior dislocations.

Inferior shoulder dislocations also known as Luxatio Erecta are very rare and result from hyperextension injury. The patient's arm will be positioned in roughly 180° of abduction. The head of the humerus is prominent and often palpable within the axilla. Vascular complications are highest among inferior dislocations most often affecting flow within the axillary artery. Reduction of inferior shoulder dislocations is often complicated with a frequent need for general anesthesia or surgical intervention for open reduction.

ELBOW DISLOCATIONS

Elbow dislocations present with severe pain, swelling, and elbow deformity. Posterior elbow dislocations are the most common (90%) and often result from falls onto an extended arm (**Figure 56-3**). Brachial artery injury and ulnar nerve injury may occur in up to 12% of elbow dislocations.[6] Reduction of a suspected elbow dislocation is not recommended in the prehospital environment unless critical limb ischemia is present with an associated prolonged transport time. Differentiating elbow dislocations from fractures requires radiographs as up to 60% of patients with elbow dislocations have an associated fracture.[7] Attempted reduction of a dislocation when a fracture exists can worsen injury. Fracture dislocations of the elbow generally require surgical management. Padded board or vacuum splints are well suited for immobilization of suspected elbow dislocations or fractures in the field. Attempts at elbow reduction are not recommended in the field.

CLAVICLE FRACTURES

Clavicle fractures are very common. They are often seen with sports injuries or seat belt injuries when force is applied directly over the clavicle or when the shoulder is forced into the chest. Clavicle injuries present with

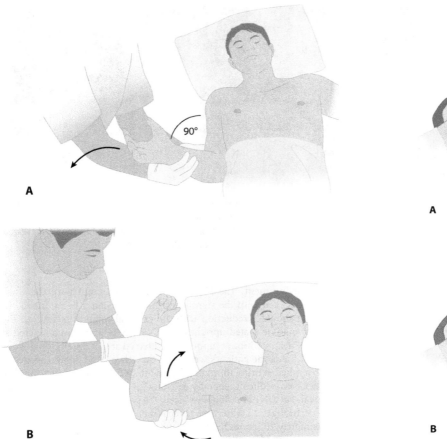

A

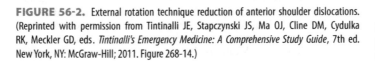

B

FIGURE 56-2. External rotation technique reduction of anterior shoulder dislocations. (Reprinted with permission from Tintinalli JE, Stapczynski JS, Ma OJ, Cline DM, Cydulka RK, Meckler GD, eds. *Tintinalli's Emergency Medicine: A Comprehensive Study Guide*, 7th ed. New York, NY: McGraw-Hill; 2011. Figure 268-14.)

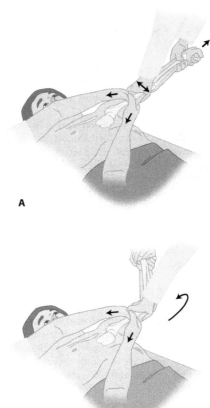

A

B

FIGURE 56-3. Reduction technique for posterior elbow dislocations. (Reprinted with permission from Tintinalli JE, Stapczynski JS, Ma OJ, Cline DM, Cydulka RK, Meckler GD, eds. *Tintinalli's Emergency Medicine: A Comprehensive Study Guide*, 7th ed. New York, NY: McGraw-Hill; 2011. Figure 267-7.)

pain, swelling, and possible skin tenting at the site of injury. Roughly 80% of fractures occur midclavicle, 15% distal, and 5% proximal.[8] Mid and distal clavicle fractures rarely have an associated neurovascular injury. Proximal clavicle fractures require large forces to the chest to fracture and have a higher incidence of thoracic vascular injuries, brachial plexus injury, and pneumothorax. Suspected clavicle fractures are stabilized in the field by immobilization of the affected upper extremity with a sling and swath.

■ HUMERUS FRACTURES

Humerus fractures result from direct blows to the upper arm or via axial loading. Proximal humerus fractures make up nearly 6% of all fractures and humeral diaphyseal fractures less than 2%.[9] Falls and motor vehicle injuries account for a large percentage of humerus fractures in the youth. Pathologic fractures can result from relatively minimal injuries in the elderly population. Proximal humerus fractures present with pain, swelling, and limited range of motion at the shoulder, making them difficult to differentiate from shoulder dislocations. Diaphyseal fractures often present with midshaft deformity. A low incidence of neurovascular injury is reported with humerus fractures. The radial nerve is most often injured, although median and ulnar nerve injuries can occur, while brachial artery involvement is rare.[10] Proximal humerus fractures are difficult to fully immobilize, but are well suited to immobilization with a sling and swath in the prehospital setting. Diaphyseal fractures should have a rigid splint applied for immobilization. Should neurovascular compromise exist with a prolonged transport, reduction

using longitudinal traction may be attempted and followed by application of a padded board splint.

Distal humerus fractures cause pain and swelling, often with associated deformity and instability of the elbow joint. These include supracondylar, intercondylar, and epicondylar fractures. Radial nerve injury is present in about 18% of distal humerus fractures as the radial nerve emerges from the spiral groove of the humerus and is tethered within the intramuscular septum.[11,12] Appropriate field management includes splinting with a padded board splint.

■ WRIST AND FOREARM FRACTURES

Wrist and forearm fractures are frequently encountered after falls onto an outstretched hand. Distal radius fractures are the most common. Patients present with pain and often deformity. Fractures such as Colles fractures are recognized for their classical "dinner fork" appearance where the wrist and hand are notably angulated dorsally. In other instances, the mechanism of injury, such as a direct blow perpendicular to the forearm to defend against an attack, will suggest an ulnar midshaft fracture (night-stick fracture). However, field examination is limited in discriminating many other wrist and forearm fractures plus proximal forearm fractures are often associated with dislocations at the elbow. Neurovascular examination should test function of the median, ulnar, and radial nerves plus assess radial and ulnar pulses. Field immobilization of simple wrist injuries suspicious for carpal involvement may only be splinted with a volar splint. Forearm injuries may be immobilized with a padded board splint.

RADIAL HEAD SUBLUXATION

Radial head subluxation, also referred to as nursemaid's elbow, is an injury often seen in young children. Subluxation is thought to occur when traction is placed on the extended arm of a child, such as by swinging a child by an arm or grabbing their arm to keep them from falling. The annular ligament of the radial head slips upward, allowing for subluxation at the radiocapitellar joint. It often presents acutely as inability of the child to use the affected arm.[11,12] Distressing pain is not associated, but the child will often support their arm at the side with the elbow pronated and have mild tenderness at the radial head. Basic field examination includes palpation of the injured extremity and distal neurovascular examination. In the prehospital environment, reduction is not recommended; rather the injured extremity should be splinted and treated with the presumption that a fracture or other injury exists.

HAND INJURIES

Prehospital care of hand injuries involves four main fundamentals: splinting and prevention of further injury, hemorrhage control, pain control, and care for amputed digits.[12] Examination of the hand should assess for gross injury, perfusion, and function initially. Radial and ulnar pulses should be palpated and evidence of distal perfusion to each digit of the affected hand should be assessed by observing capillary refill.

Neurological evaluation of the hand should assess the sensory and motor function of the median, ulnar, and radial nerves. Test the median nerve's motor function by thumb abduction and flexion of the first three digits. Sensory testing may be done at the palmar surface of the hand at the base of the index finger. Radial nerve motor function is checked by having the patient extend their fingers, wrist, and thumb. The radial nerve sensory function may be tested on the dorsal surface at the base of the thumb. The ulnar nerve is assessed by having the patient abduct and adduct their fingers against resistance; its sensory function is tested on the ulnar aspect of the hand.

Appropriate splinting of the injured hand may include a variety of splinting techniques including immobilization with a resting volar splint, finger splint, or gutter splint depending on the extent of injury.

It is often necessary to control hemorrhage associated with hand trauma. This is best addressed with direct pressure and elevation. Rarely do hand injuries require more aggressive hemostatic measures.

Finger and fingertip amputations occur frequently and when appropriately cared for can carry upward of a 75% replantation success rate.[13] Thus, it is important to obtain any amputated digit and store it appropriately. Amputation management is discussed later in this chapter.[12]

Limb-threatening injuries of the hand include crush injuries, high-pressure injections, compartment syndrome, amputations, and vascular injuries. Patients with limb-threatening injuries to the hand should be transported to a destination facility with hand specialty services available unless patient stability dictates otherwise.

LOWER EXTREMITY INJURIES

PELVIC FRACTURES

The pelvis is an extremely well-supported structure that generally requires a severe traumatic force to disrupt. High energy injuries resulting in complex fractures within the pelvic ring signify major trauma and carry an estimated 21% associated mortality.[14] Blunt trauma from falls, side impact motor vehicle accidents, motorcycle crashes, and pedestrian versus vehicle injuries are common causes of pelvic instability.[15]

The strong posterior attachments of the sacroiliac, sacrospinous, and sacrotuberous ligaments provide stability between the bones of the pelvic ring (**Figure 56-4**).[16] The pelvis protects the iliac arteries and its branches, pelvic venous plexus, and lumbar and sacral nerve roots which

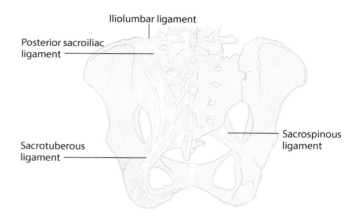

FIGURE 56-4. Major stabilizing ligaments of the pelvic ring. (Reprinted with permission from Tintinalli JE, Stapczynski JS, Ma OJ, Cline DM, Cydulka RK, Meckler GD, eds. *Tintinalli's Emergency Medicine: A Comprehensive Study Guide*, 7th ed. New York, NY: McGraw-Hill; 2011. Figure 269-1.)

course through the posterior pelvis. It also houses the genitourinary system plus the descending colon, sigmoid, and rectum. Hemorrhagic shock from pelvic injury occurs via three main mechanisms: arterial or venous plexus injury, fractures, and injury to other intrapelvic organs. Hemorrhage from the pelvic venous plexus accounts for 90% of cases of pelvic hemorrhage.[17]

Traumatic injuries to the pelvis are suspected in any patient after a high-energy injury or in any trauma patient presenting with hemodynamic compromise. There are four well-described patterns of pelvic injury based on the Young and Burgess classification system: lateral compression, anterior-posterior (AP) compression, vertical shear, and complex. Lateral compression injuries result when force applied laterally on the pelvis causes the sacroiliac joint to fracture and become disrupted with a corresponding lateral pubic ramus fracture. The hemipelvis affected rotates internally decreasing pelvic volume which may aid by tamponading bleeding, but injures pelvic vasculature and the genitourinary tract. Lateral compression fractures are the most frequent unstable pelvic fracture and are associated with side impact motor vehicle crashes, motor cycle accidents, or falls from a height onto the patient's flank. AP compression injury results from high-energy force transmitted anterior to posterior or vice versa through a patient. This pattern is often seen with pedestrian versus motor vehicle or head-on motorcycle collisions. The pubic symphysis disrupts and widens and the sacroiliac joints disrupt resulting in the "open book" injury. This pattern increases pelvic volume, allowing for large amounts of hemorrhage to occur. Vertical shear injuries often result after falls from height or motor vehicle crashes where large axial loading forces are transmitted through the femur into the pelvis. The affected hemipelvis disrupts at the sacroiliac joint and displaces vertically. Complex fractures represent a combination of any of the fracture patterns described.

Field examination for pelvic instability is conducted as part of the secondary survey after securing the ABCs and controlling major hemorrhage. Pelvic stability is assessed via a combination of approaches. In the unresponsive patient, physical examination is difficult and unreliable.

Visual examination should be conducted of the flank, perineum, and urethral meatus looking for ecchymosis, bleeding, or open fractures (**Figure 56-5**). Inspect and palpate the bony prominences of the iliac crests, pubic symphysis, and hips for step-offs, hematomas, or other deformities. The compression distraction maneuver is performed to assess for pelvic instability by applying gentle anterior to posterior pressure (compression) over the iliac crests as well as by applying a light outward force (distraction) assessing for any movement of the iliac crests or report of pain from the patient. Care should be used to ensure no worsening of an open-book-type injury. Indicators of sacroiliac joint disruption or an unstable compression or shearing injury to the pelvis may manifest as a rotational deformity of a leg, usually externally rotated,

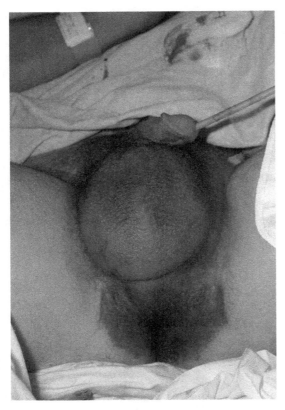

FIGURE 56-5. A vertical shear pelvic fracture presenting with scrotal edema plus perianal ecchymosis. (Photo contributor: Lawrence B. Stack, MD; Reprinted with permission from Knoop KJ, Stack LB, Storrow AB, Thurman RJ. *The Atlas of Emergency Medicine*. 3rd ed. McGraw-Hill; 2010. Figure 7.26.)

or as a discrepancy in leg length. Should any signs of pelvic injury be detected on physical examination, prehospital pelvic stabilization is recommended.

Examination of the pelvis alone has a poor sensitivity for the detection of pelvic fractures. A 2009 study of over 1500 patients demonstrated that the sensitivity of physical examination in detecting unstable pelvic fractures was only 8% in patients with a GCS of 13 or less.[18] In contrast, a study on alert patients with a GCS of 14 or greater noted that 67% of patients with a pelvic fracture complained of pain in the pelvis or low abdomen, while only 32% and 37% had pain with pelvic compression distraction maneuvers and palpation of the pubic symphysis, respectively.[19] In patients with altered mental status and hemodynamic instability, detection of unstable pelvic injuries can be very difficult to detect. Foremost, if the mechanism of injury suggests a high risk of pelvic fracture, pelvic stabilization should be considered.

Prehospital stabilization of pelvic fractures is most frequently accomplished by using a pelvic circumferential compression device (PCCD) or simple tied sheet. The use of MAST (military anti-shock trouser) trousers has fallen out of favor due to concerns of decreased venous return and difficulty obtaining access to the patients lower extremities once applied. PCCDs are generally defined as wraps or slings circumferentially placed and tightened around the pelvis, generally at the level of the femoral trochanters. A 2009 meta-analysis of 17 articles studying the effectiveness of PCCDs demonstrated their ability to reduce pelvic fractures and decrease pelvic volume, in turn leading to decreased hemorrhage.[20] There is little literature available to show clear mortality improvements by use of PCCDs; however, a small trial in 2010 utilizing PCCDs did demonstrate improved mean arterial pressures and decreased heart rates after placement in a small series of patients with pelvic fractures.[21]

If a PCCD is unavailable, a sheet may be wrapped around the iliac crests and femoral trochanters and tied in place. In general, approximately 40 lb of force is required to reduce the adult pelvis.[22] Do not overtighten such as to compromise blood flow to the lower extremities. Few complications have been reported from the use of PCCDs in the prehospital setting.

▨ HIP FRACTURES AND DISLOCATIONS

Hip fractures encompass three subtypes of proximal femur fractures: femoral head and neck, intertrochanteric, and subtrochanteric fractures. Although important to recognize the different anatomical classifications of hip fracture, they are managed identically in the prehospital environment. Over 250,000 hip fractures occur in the United States annually with 90% occurring in a population of over 50 years of age.[23] Unfortunately, there is a large amount of mortality from hip fractures. It is estimated that 14% to 36% of elderly will die within 1 year of their hip fracture.[24] Most hip injuries among the elderly result from falls and may have contributing conditions such as osteoporosis, malnutrition, and muscular weakness predisposing them to this injury.[25] Head-on motor vehicle collisions where axial load is transmitted up the femur are recognized for causing hip injuries and dislocations in the younger population.

Hip fractures generally present with severe pain causing inability to bear weight on the affected extremity. Patients will often localize this pain to the hip, groin, or low buttock. Classical examination findings are of a shortened and externally rotated leg. Pain is elicited at the hip by palpation at the level of the trochanter or by internal or external rotation or axial loading of the hip joint. Deformity, swelling, and ecchymosis may be present at the hip as well. Neurovascular examination should be assessed, although neurovascular complications of hip fractures are rarely reported.

Transport and immobilization of patients with suspected hip fractures focuses on patient comfort. Often, an injured patient will already have their injured extremity in a position of comfort. Transferring the patient with a scoop stretcher should be considered as logrolling onto a stretcher can be painful. Once on a stretcher, extremity immobilization with towels or pillows to support the patient in a position of comfort is recommended. Hip fractures are generally not immobilized with rigid splints and never with traction.

Hip dislocations as well as fracture dislocations require emergent evaluation. High speed motor vehicle accidents account for the majority of native hip dislocations, especially in the younger population.[25] Often multiple traumatic injuries are present simultaneously with a native hip dislocation. Prosthetic hips in elderly patients may dislocate with seeming little force or trauma, even occurring with actions as simple as sitting down. There are three main types of hip dislocations: anterior, posterior, and central. Ninety percent of hip dislocations are posterior dislocations which are frequently caused when large force is applied axially through the femur, dislodging (and often fracturing) the femoral head within the pelvic acetabulum.

Patients with posterior hip dislocations classically present with severe pain at the hip with the leg shortened, internally rotated, flexed at the hip, and adducted. Deformity and bony prominence may be palpated posterior to the hip joint. A thorough neurovascular examination is essential checking specifically for sciatic nerve function. The sciatic nerve courses just posterior to the hip joint capsule and can be easily injured with posterior dislocations. Anterior dislocations frequently occur when the hip is abducted and is suddenly struck and are at high risk for vascular compromise.

Attempted hip reduction in the prehospital setting is discouraged. Radiographs should be obtained to confirm dislocation and assess for concomitant fractures prior to any attempt at reduction.

▨ FEMUR FRACTURES

The strongest bone within the body, the femur requires high amounts of force to fracture. High-energy injuries such as head-on MVCs, pedestrian versus vehicle, and falls from greater than 20 ft are typical mechanisms.[26] Pathologic fractures from low impact falls are also commonly reported in the elderly. The incidence of femur fractures is about 1:10,000 in the general population; however, a threefold increase is observed in males less than 30 years and elderly over 80 years.[27] A 1986 study of MVCs demonstrated head-on collisions with an average velocity change of greater than 26 mph to have the highest incidence of femur injuries, followed by side-impact collisions with greater than 16 inches of intrusion, while rear-end collisions had no reported femur fractures.[28]

Femur fractures have a high incidence of reported hemodynamic compromise from associated blood loss. Examination noting pain, swelling, visible deformity, limb shortening, or a rotated extremity is common.

Large, expanding thigh hematomas may result from injury to the metaphyseal arteries which arise from various branches of the deep femoral artery and from the femur's vascular marrow supply. Weak or absent distal dorsalis pedis or posterior tibial artery pulses may identify vascular injuries early. Profuse bleeding causing upward of three units of blood loss into the thigh can result with up to 40% of isolated femur fractures requiring blood transfusions.[29]

Neurologic examination focuses on function of the sciatic nerve, although neurologic injuries associated with femur fractures are extremely rare.[30] Additionally, a thorough examination to rule out associated injury should be conducted. Hip fractures and ligamentous knee injuries commonly are observed in association with femoral injuries.[12]

Two primary approaches are available for the field stabilization of femur fractures: traction splinting and rigid splinting. Traction splinting was first attributed to decreasing mortality among soldiers in World War I by Sir Robert Jones using the Thomas Splint developed in the late 1800s.[31] No large trials exist to demonstrate benefit of traction splints over rigid splinting, thus benefit is based on small series and case reports. Most recently, traction splinting was attributed to decreasing morbidity among a small group of soldiers and civilians in the Gulf War.[32]

The primary roles of traction splints are to immobilize the extremity and prevent further soft tissue and vascular injury during transport. Secondary benefits of fracture reduction are alleviating pain, decreasing hemorrhage, lessening muscle spasm, and reducing risk of fat embolism. Decreased hemorrhage occurs with fracture reduction by minimizing the amount of elliptical free space surrounding the distracted bone fragments within the thigh.[3]

Important contraindications to traction splint application include nerve injury or suspected ipsilateral pelvic, hip, knee, tibia, or ankle factures. Should a contraindication for traction splinting exist, a commercially available rigid or soft splint should be used to maintain the extremity in its position of presentation. The use of traction splints for open femur fractures is in debate. There is concern that reduction of an open fracture could further contaminate the wound. If an open femur fracture is reduced with traction splinting, it is important to inform the receiving physician.

Several brands of commercial traction splints exist which can be placed within 2 to 5 minutes by two skilled providers. Examples include the Hare Splint (**Figure 56-6**), Sager Splint, and Kendrick Traction Device. We recommend reviewing and following the manufacturer's application instructions for each type.

KNEE INJURIES

The knee joint is prone to many injuries including fractures, dislocations, ligamentous, and meniscal injuries. Historical information about the mechanism of injury and any associated pain, inability to ambulate, locking, or popping is often helpful in identifying injuries of the knee. Examination with pain on palpation, deformity, ecchymosis, crepitus, or decreased range of motion should be suspicious for fracture or soft tissue injury. Assess neurovascular status of the distal extremity. Physical examination should also include assessment of all joints of the affected extremity as hip and ankle injuries may commonly occur with knee injuries. Should concern for fracture exist, splint or support the patient in a position of comfort.

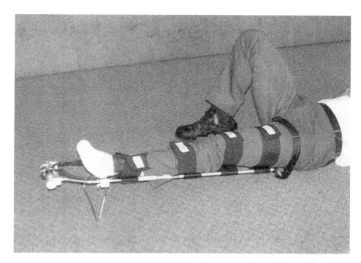

FIGURE 56-6. Example of a Hare traction splint. (Reprinted with permission from Tintinalli JE, Stapczynski JS, Ma OJ, Cline DM, Cydulka RK, Meckler GD, eds. *Tintinalli's Emergency Medicine: A Comprehensive Study Guide,* 7th ed. New York, NY: McGraw-Hill; 2011. Figure 2-7.)

KNEE DISLOCATIONS

Knee dislocations are rare, but represent orthopedic emergencies. Dislocation is defined as complete loss of tibiofemoral articulation. There are five types of knee dislocations: anterior, posterior, lateral, medial, and rotary. Tremendous energy is usually required to dislocate the knee joint. Motor vehicle accidents are a common cause; however, low impact forces are also reported to cause knee dislocations. Vascular injury, including arterial transection, thrombus, or other disruption may occur in upward of 22% of knee dislocations.[33]

Physical examination to identify a knee dislocation may be challenging secondary to pain, swelling, and limited range of motion. In severe cases, there is often a very noticeable visual defect from the dislocation.

Optimally, knee reductions should be performed in hospital. Field reduction may be considered if there is a loss of distal extremity perfusion in the setting of a prolonged transport time. Reduction of knee dislocations is successfully performed using longitudinal traction the majority of the time; however, operative reduction is sometimes necessary. Once reduced, the lower extremity should be splinted in 20° of flexion.[34] Serial vascular examinations of the lower extremity are required after knee reduction.

PATELLAR DISLOCATION

Patellar dislocation is common, representing about 2% of knee injuries, with an incidence as high as 5.8 per 100,000 and even higher among adolescents.[35,36] It occurs most commonly in adolescents and young adults as a result of rapid quadriceps flexion, hyperextension injury, or direct trauma to the knee. Rapidly pivoting on the sports field is often reported as the inciting mechanism. When dislocated, the patella has been derailed from the knee's intercondylar groove, its normal sliding tract. In the majority of dislocations the patella dislocates laterally and will present with anterior knee pain and the knee in flexion with the patella often palpable lateral to the intercondylar groove.

Reduction of the patella often occurs spontaneously in the field with passive knee extension. As with all dislocations, emergency department evaluation prior to attempted reduction may be preferred; however, when seen acutely by a properly trained provider or EMS physician, an attempt at field reduction may result in acute reduction and rapid pain control. If reduction is to be attempted, the procedure for lateral patellar dislocation reduction is simple. Slowly assist the patient's knee through passive extension while simultaneously applying a lifting force over the lateral edge of the patella until it slips back into the intercondylar groove. This procedure should be relatively well tolerated, although analgesia, and sometimes mild sedation, is commonly employed. If severe pain or resistance is encountered stop as this may signify a more serious injury or underlying fracture. Once reduced, reassess neurovascular status and splint the patient's leg in extension.[37]

TIBIAL PLATEAU FRACTURE

Although there are a multitude of different fracture patterns that may affect the knee, tibial plateau fractures are of particular significance for their high rate of associated neurovascular injuries. Tibial plateau fractures may occur from any combination of axial loading or varus-valgus forces. Common mechanisms include falls onto an extended leg and motor vehicle collisions. Lateral fractures of the plateau are most common and approximately 50% involve associated ligamentous or meniscal injury.[38] Physical examination with pain, swelling, or deformity over the proximal tibia is suggestive of this fracture. Decreased perfusion is an orthopedic emergency. For transport, the injured extremity should be splinted with the leg in extension; however, if pain is severe, supporting the patient with soft pillows or towels in a position of comfort is also appropriate.

LOWER LEG FRACTURES

Lower leg fractures include injuries of the tibia and fibula. Pedestrians struck by motor vehicles, falls, and sporting injuries are common causes of trauma to the lower leg. Physical examination of the lower extremity may show evidence of fracture by eliciting pain with palpation or noting visual deformity, ecchymosis, or swelling. Particular note should be made of any lacerations or puncture wounds over the tibia and fibula as these may signify open fractures. Distal vascular assessment should include palpation of both dorsalis pedis and posterior tibial arteries. Tibia and fibula injures should be splinted to immobilize both the knee above and ankle below.

Compartment syndrome is of particular concern with lower leg fractures, although it can occur within any extremity. The calf contains four fascial compartments, all of which have limited ability to stretch to accommodate pressure. An injury such as fracture, severe contusion, or vascular injury can cause pressure to build within a compartment. Once pressure builds to a level that prevents venous return, a rapid increase in compartment pressure occurs. This will eventually impede arterial flow and cause critical muscle ischemia. Should limb threatening ischemia occur within the thigh due to compartment syndrome, the leg will need emergent operative fasciotomy. Loss of distal pulses is a very late finding in compartment syndrome and therefore presence of distal pulses is not reliable to exclude compartment syndrome. Other findings of compartment syndrome include severe pain in an extremity out of proportion to injury, significant soft tissue tightness or swelling at the injury, pain with passive motion of involved muscle groups, and distal paresthesias or weakness.[39] Should a patient present with any concerns

for a compartment syndrome, emergent transport to the nearest emergency facility is indicated.

FOOT AND ANKLE FRACTURES

Foot and ankle injuries are among the most prevalent orthopedic injuries that present to emergency departments.[40] The majority of injuries represent ankle sprains; however, fractures and dislocations that are more serious may occur and may present similar to a sprain. Fractures of the lateral malleolus of the fibula are the most common and require less force to fracture than the medial malleolus. Patients with ankle fractures or dislocations will denote pain at the ankle joint and are generally nonambulatory. Deformity, swelling, and ecchymosis are all signs consistent with injury. Patient presentations concerning for ankle fracture should be immobilized to prevent movement at the ankle. Short leg posterior or sugar tong splints are ideal for field immobilization about the ankle.

EMS physicians should be aware of the Ottawa ankle and foot rules (**Figure 56-7**). The rules identify patients with ankle and midfoot injuries who are at high risk of fracture, and should have radiographs to evaluate for fracture. Sensitivity of the rules is demonstrated to be between 96.4% and 99.6% in repeated trials. Specificity is far lower, near 26.3% to 47.9%.[41] The rules help reduce the need for radiographic evaluation of ankle injuries through their high sensitivity.

The Ottawa ankle and foot rules identify patients at high risk for fracture if they have any of the following: (1) Are unable to bear weight immediately after the injury or for four steps in the emergency room. (2) Have bony tenderness along the distal 6 cm of the posterior tibia or medial malleolus. (3) Have bony tenderness at the distal 6 cm of the posterior fibula or lateral malleolus. 4) Have bony tenderness at the base of the fifth metatarsal or over the navicular. Of note, the Ottawa rules are not fully validated in patients less than 6 years of age or in patients who may have altered mental status or poor recall of the injuring event.

ANKLE DISLOCATIONS

A large amount of force is required to dislocate the ankle. This leads to significant soft tissue injury of the tendons and ligaments about the ankle and often involves a concomitant ankle fracture. Should neurovascular compromise exist in the setting of prolonged transport, reduction may be considered. Medial and lateral dislocations, with or without fracture, can typically be reduced and splinted if necessary in the field by a properly trained EMS physician. Reduction typically requires an assistant. Plantar flexion is applied to recreate the position of the initial injury followed by axial traction to the ankle. While the assistant maintains the axial traction the EMS physician grasps the distal tibia with one hand and applies lateral or medial traction (depending on the direction of dislocation), thus relocating the ankle. Neurovascular examination of the extremity must be repeated after reduction is accomplished. The ankle may be

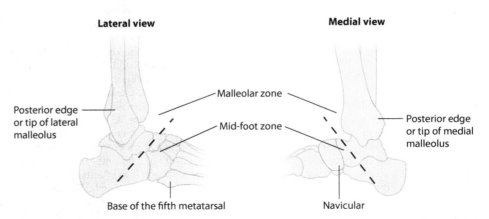

FIGURE 56-7. Ottawa ankle rules: Radiographs are required for any injuries of the midfoot and ankle if bony tenderness is elicited in the regions denoted in the figure. (Reprinted with permission from Tintinalli JE, Stapczynski JS, Ma OJ, Cline DM, Cydulka RK, Meckler GD, eds. *Tintinalli's Emergency Medicine: A Comprehensive Study Guide*, 7th ed. New York, NY: McGraw-Hill; 2011. Figure 273-4)

unstable and should be splinted and repeat examination for neurovascular status performed to ensure continued function after splinting.

FOOT FRACTURES

Foot fractures can be categorized into midfoot and forefoot injuries. The midfoot comprises the cuboid, navicular, and cuneiforms, while the forefoot includes the metatarsals and phalanges. Fractures of the foot usually present with pain, swelling, ecchymosis, or deformity at the site of injury. Examination should focus on palpation and visual inspection plus assess for neurovascular compromise. Dorsalis pedis pulses should always be assessed. If any concern for foot fracture exists, immobilization is appropriate for transport.

SOFT TISSUE INJURY

Sprains and strains are among the most commonly encountered soft tissue injuries evaluated by prehospital providers. Joint sprains commonly occur in the ankle, knee, wrist, fingers, and toes. Most frequent are ankle sprains, accounting for an estimated 85% of all soft tissue sprains.[42] Patients with sprains often present after sports-related injuries or low-energy falls. Obtaining a history of "rolling an ankle" or "twisting a knee" is a common low-energy mechanism. Ninety percent of ankle sprains occur after inversion injury. Injury after a high-energy injury, such as fall from height or motor vehicle collision, should be presumed to be a high at risk for fracture.

Differentiating sprains from fractures can be challenging without radiographs as many high-grade sprains can appear similar to fractures by examination. The Ottawa ankle rules (discussed prior) can help identify patients at highest risk for ankle and midfoot fractures. Pain, swelling, ecchymosis, and limited joint function are common examination findings.[43] As a rule, any extremity that is notable for deformity or neurovascular compromise is presumed to be fractured.

Prehospital treatment of sprains should focus on minimizing further ligamentous injury and decreasing pain and swelling. The PRICE (protect, rest, ice, compression, elevation) strategy is recommended for most sprain management. Protect: If a patient has a suspected ankle sprain, a strategy of temporary immobilization by applying an air brace or splint should be used. A Cochrane review demonstrated temporary immobilization for high-grade sprains with soft or semirigid functional supports has shown modest benefit over full immobilization or use of elastic bandaging.[44,45] Rest: The injured extremity should be supported and the patient should be discouraged from attempts at ambulation prior to physician evaluation. Moderate and severe sprains are often rested for a period of 1 to 3 days postinjury to allow for pain and swelling to decrease. Ice: Cold therapy is recommended by the American Academy of Orthopedic Surgeons for early management of ankle sprains.[43] Cold packs or an ice bag may be applied to injured areas to decrease pain and swelling. Compression: A temporary air brace or elastic wrap can serve a dual purpose of protecting and immobilizing the sprain as well as providing mild compressive force to help reduce further swelling. Elevation: Elevating the injured extremity on towels or pillows can aid to decrease swelling. Appropriate pain control should be administered to maximize patient comfort.

ACUTE LOW BACK STRAIN

Lumbosacral spine sprains and strains are very common within the United States and are estimated to be the fifth most common cause for physician visits.[46] When a patient presents with low back pain, identifying the exact etiology can be very difficult without laboratory or radiographic testing. The EMS physician must recognize signs and symptoms of emergent and urgent causes of low back pain to help identify high-risk patients. The differential for low back pain is extremely broad but includes lumbosacral sprain and strain, acute disc herniation, spinal stenosis, cauda equina syndrome, traumatic or compression fracture, infection, malignancy, and aortic aneurysm. Abnormal vital signs or patient history involving systemic symptoms, trauma, fevers, weakness, sensory changes, or difficulty with bladder or bowel function

is concerning for etiologies of low back pain other than lumbosacral sprain or strain.[47] Acute traumatic injury resulting in back pain should be handled with the possibility of fracture and involves stabilizing the low back with a long backboard should the patient have midline lumbar tenderness. Physical examination should assess distal neurovascular.

Prehospital treatment of lumbosacral sprains and strains involves identifying and treating patient pain. Allow patients to be in a position of comfort (unless immobilization is indicated) and identifying any items on history or examination consistent with more concerning etiologies. Opioid analgesia should be administered as indicated. External warming (chemical heat packs, etc) have also been demonstrated to alleviate acute low back pain during prehospital transports.[48]

AMPUTATION MANAGEMENT

Traumatic limb amputations often result from severe machine and industrial accidents. Oftentimes, proximal limb amputation results in a nonviable limb due to extreme tissue destruction and deformity of the extremity.[49] However, finger and fingertip amputations occur frequently and when appropriately cared for can carry upward of a 75% replantation success rate.[50] Thus, it is important to obtain any amputated tissue and store it appropriately.

The prehospital provider must focus on the safety of the patient and rapid transport to an appropriate facility. If life-threatening hemorrhage from the amputated limb is not controlled with direct pressure or other means, use of a tourniquet may be indicated.

When possible, obtain any amputated limb or digit and store it appropriately. To cool the amputated tissue, wrap it in saline soaked gauze and then place it within a sealed plastic bag to protect it from direct contact with any ice. Then place the bag containing the tissue within a second bag filled with ice or cool water and seal within a cooler for transport.[12]

CONCLUSION

Traumatic musculoskeletal injuries are encountered with great frequency in the prehospital environment. Ranging from severe life- and limb-threatening traumatic amputations and open fractures to minor soft tissue injuries, it is important that EMS physicians be proficient at managing musculoskeletal trauma. Understanding the mechanism of trauma and extent of injuries on examination will assist to focus on patient care priorities and determine appropriate selection of destination facilities.

KEY POINTS

- Major pelvic disruption with hemorrhage, major arterial hemorrhage, and crush syndrome as life-threatening injuries require immediate stabilization once identified during the trauma survey.
- The majority of extremity injuries are treated with a general approach involving hemorrhage control, gross decontamination, immobilization, and pain control.
- Except in the setting of certain fractures, such as midshaft femur and unstable pelvic fractures, or fractures with associated neurovascular compromise or life-threatening hemorrhage, prehospital fracture reduction is not recommended.
- In patients with suspected pelvic fractures and hemodynamic compromise pelvic stabilization should be considered.
- Traction splinting is indicated for the reduction of isolated midshaft femur fractures. Important contraindications to traction splint application include nerve injury or suspected ipsilateral pelvic, hip, knee, tibia, or ankle factures.
- Compartment syndrome is a particular concern in lower leg fractures. Loss of distal pulses is a very late finding and is not be relied on to "rule out" compartment syndrome

- EMS physicians should be aware of the Ottawa ankle and foot rules as they have a high sensitivity for identifying patients at high risk of fracture.
- Understand the indications for prioritizing transportation to trauma centers and other facilities with appropriate services for specific mechanisms and types of injuries.
- Patients with injuries that require specialty evaluation and management should be triaged to appropriate destination facilities.

REFERENCES

1. National Center for Health Statistics. Health US, National Hospital Ambulatory Medical Care Survey: 2008 emergency department summary. 2010. http://www.cdc.gov/nchs/data/ahcd/nhamcs_emergency/2008_ed_web_tables.pdf. Accessed May, 2015.
2. American College of Surgeons: Committee on Trauma. Musculoskeletal trauma. *Advanced Trauma Life Support Program for Doctors.* Chicago, IL: American College of Surgeons; 2004:208-209.
3. Melmed E, Blumenfeld A, Kalmovich B, et al. Prehospital care of orthopedic injuries. *Prehosp Disaster Med.* 2007;22:22.
4. Lee C, Porter KM. Prehospital management of lower limb fractures. *Emerg Med* 2005;22:660.
5. Serra J. Fractures and related injuries. In: Wilkerson JA, Moore EE, Zafren K, eds. *Medicine for Mountaineering and Other Wilderness Activities.* 6th ed. Seattle, WA: Mountaineers Books, 2010.
6. Visser CP, Coene LN, Brand R, et al. The incidence of nerve injury in anterior dislocation of the shoulder and its influence on functional recovery. A prospective clinical and EMG study. *J Bone Joint Surg Br.* 1999;81.
7. Hobgood ER, Khan SO, Field LD. Acute dislocations of the adult elbow. *Hand Clin.* 2008;24:1-7.
8. Perron A. Elbow injuries. In: Wolfson AB, Harwood-Nuss, A. eds. *Harwood-Nuss' Clinical Practice of Emergency Medicine.* Philadelphia, PA: Lippincott Williams & Wilkins; 2005:1046.
9. Post M. Current concepts in the treatment of fractures of the clavicle. *Clin Orthop Relat Res.* 1989;(245):89-101.
10. Court-Brown CM, Caesar B. Epidemiology of adult fractures: a review. *Injury.* 2006;37:691.
11. Shao YC, Harwood P, Grotz MR, Limb D, Giannoudis PV. Radial nerve palsy associated with fractures of the shaft of the humerus: a systematic review. *J Bone Joint Surgery Br.* 2005;87:1647.
12. Alho A. Concurrent ipsilateral fractures of the hip and shaft of the femur. A systematic review of 722 cases. *Ann Chir Gynaecol.* 1997;86.
13. Andrade A, Hern HG. Traumatic hand injuries: the emergency clinician's evidence-based approach. *Emerg Med Pract.* 2011;13:1.
14. Kim W, Lim JH, Han SK. Fingertip replantations: clinical evaluation of 135 digits. *Plast Reconstr Surg.* 1996;98:470.
15. Smith W. Early predictors of mortality in hemodynamically unstable pelvic fractures. *J Orthop Trauma.* 2007;21:31.
16. Williams-Johnson J, Williams E, Watson H. Management and treatment of pelvic and hip injuries. *Emerg Med Clin North Am.* 2010;28:841-859.
17. Standring, S. *Gray's Anatomy: The Anatomical Basis of Clinical Practice.* 40th ed. Edinburgh: Churchill Livingstone/Elsevier 2008.
18. Rice PL Jr, Rudolph M. Pelvic fractures. *Emerg Med Clin North Am.* 2007;25:795.
19. Shlamovitz G, Mower WR, Bergman J, et al. How (un)useful is the pelvic ring stability examination in diagnosing mechanically unstable pelvic fractures in blunt trauma patients? *J Trauma.* 2009;66:815-820.
20. Gonzalez RP, Fried PQ, Bukhalo M. The utility of clinical examination in screening for pelvic fractures in blunt trauma. *J Am Coll Surg.* 2002;195:740.
21. Spanjersberg WR, Knops SP, Schep NW, van Lieshout EM, Patka P, Schipper IB. Effectiveness and complications of pelvic circumferential compression devises in patients with unstable pelvic fractures: a systematic review of literature. *Injury.* 2009;40:1031.
22. Tan E, van Stigt SF, van Vugt AB. Effect of new pelvic stabilizer (t-pod) on reduction of pelvic volume and haemodynamic stability in unstable pelvic fractures. *Injury.* 2010;41:1239.
23. Bottlang M, Krieg JC, Mohr M, Simpson TS, Madey SM. Emergent management of pelvic ring fractures with use of circumferential compression. *J Bone Joint Surg Am.* 2002;84:43.
24. Cummings SR, Rubin SM, Black D. The future of hip fractures in the united states: numbers, costs, and potential effects of postmenopausal estrogen. *Clin Orthop Relat Res.* 1990;252:163.
25. Zuckerman JD. Hip fracture. *N Engl J Med.* 1996;334: 1519-1525.
26. Rudman N, McIlmail D. Emergency department evaluation and treatment of hip and thigh injuries. *Emerg Med Clin North Am.* 2000;18:29-66.
27. Browner BD. *Skeletal Trauma: Fractures, Dislocations, Ligamentous Injuries.* 2nd ed. WB Saunders; 1998.
28. Singer BR, McLauchlan GJ, Robinson CM, Christie J. Epidemiology of fractures in 15,000 adults: the influence of age and gender. *J Bone Joint Surg Br.* 1998;80:243-248.
29. Rastogi S, Wild BR, Duthie RB. Biomechanical aspects of femoral fractures in automobile accidents. *J Bone Joint Surg Br.* 1986;68:760-766.
30. Lieurance R, Benjamin JB, Rappaport WD. Blood loss and transfusion in patients with isolated femur fractures. *J Orthop Trauma.* 1992;6:175-179.
31. Spiegel PG, Johnston MJ, Harvey JP Jr. Complete sciatic nerve laceration in a closed femoral shaft fracture. *J Trauma.* 1974;14: 617-621.
32. Gray H. *The Early Treatment of War Wounds.* London: Frowde and Hodder and Stoughton; 1919.
33. Rowlands TK, Clasper J. The Thomas splint-a necessary tool in the management of battlefield injuries. *J R Army Med Corps.* 2003;149:291-293.
34. Wascher D, Dvirnak PC, DeCoster TA. Knee dislocation: initial assessment and implications for treatment. *J Orthop Trauma.* 1997;11:525.
35. Kelleher B. Knee dislocation in emergency medicine. 2011. http://emedicine.medscape.com/article/823589-overview.
36. Stefancin J, Parker RD. First-time traumatic patellar dislocation: a systematic review. *Clin Orthop Relat Res.* 2007;455:93.
37. Colvin AC, West RV. Patellar instability. *J Bone Joint Surg Am.* 2008;90:2751-2762.
38. Lu DW, Wang EE, Self WH, et al. Patellar dislocation reduction. *Acad Emerg Med.* 2010;17:226.
39. Scuderi GR, Tria AJ. *The Knee: A Comprehensive Review.* New Jersey: World Scientific 2010. http://search.ebscohost.com/login.aspx?direct=true&scope=site&db=nlebk&db=nlabk&an=340732. Accessed May, 2015.
40. Semer N. Fractures of the tibia and fibula. In: Lincoln, NE. ed. *Practical Plastic Surgery for Nonsurgeons.* Authors Choice Press; New York, 2007:205-219.
41. Title CI, Katchis SD. Traumatic foot and ankle injuries in the athlete. *Orthop Clin North Am.* 2002;33:587-598.
42. Bachmann LM, Kolb E, Koller MT, Steurer J, ter Riet G. Accuracy of Ottawa ankle rules to exclude fractures of the ankle and mid-foot: systematic review. *BMJ.* 2003;326:417.
43. O'Connor G, Martin AJ. Acute ankle sprain: is there a best support? *Eur J Emerg Med.* 2011;18:225.
44. Ivins D. Acute ankle sprain. *Am Fam Physician.* 2006;74:1714.
45. Kerkhoffs GM, Struijs PA, Marti RK, Assendelft WJ, Blankevoort L, van Dijk CN. Different functional treatment strategies for acute lateral ankle ligament injuries in adults. *Cochrane Database Syst Rev.* 2002;(3):CD002938.

46. Seah R, Mani-Babu S. Managing ankle sprains in primary care: what is best practice? A systematic review of the last 10 years of evidence. *Br Med Bull.* 2011;97:105.

47. Saal JA. Natural history and nonoperative treatment of lumbar disc herniation. *Spine.* 1996;21:2S.

48. Patel A, Ogle AA. Diagnosis and management of acute low back pain. *Am Fam Physician.* 2000;61(6):1779-1786.

49. Nuhr M, Hoerauf K, Bertalanffy A, et al. Active warming during emergency transport relieves acute low back pain. *Spine.* 2004;29:1499.

50. Porter KM. Prehospital amputation. *Emerg Med J.* 2010;27: 940-942.

INTRODUCTION

This chapter will discuss the role of the EMS physician in the treatment of acute wounds and hemorrhage. As a first responder, a physician should be able to accurately characterize wounds, differentiate between stable and life-threatening hemorrhage, and effectively treat these wounds in a timely manner. We will start with a discussion of wound evaluation and treatment fundamentals. Then, we will cover the role of advanced hemorrhage control procedures, the use of hemostatic agents, and administration of blood products. An understanding of these fundamentals is essential to the EMS physician operating in the prehospital settings. These are especially important to providers operating in austere environments such as tactical medicine, urban search and rescue, and those tending to the entrapped victim.

OBJECTIVES

- Describe the initial prehospital evaluation and management of acute traumatic wounds.
- Describe the initial prehospital evaluation and management of open nonacute wounds.
- Describe the initial prehospital evaluation and management of active hemorrhage.
- Discuss prehospital use of tourniquets.
- Discuss prehospital use of hemostatic agents.
- Discuss prehospital use of blood, blood products, and factors for acute traumatic blood loss anemia.

ACUTE TRAUMATIC WOUNDS

Most wounds evaluated during EMS operations are acute traumatic wounds. These include a large spectrum of injuries ranging from abrasions to amputations. Evaluation of each of these wounds should include the same components. When first evaluating a wound, identify if there is a source of acute life-threatening hemorrhage. If present, address the source of hemorrhage first. The techniques for managing hemorrhage will be discussed later in this chapter. Wounds without life-threatening hemorrhage can be evaluated for the extent of tissue damage present and structures involved.

When evaluating extremity wounds, placing a temporary tourniquet similar to those used when placing a peripheral IV may be useful when evaluating a wound with non-life-threatening hemorrhage. Similarly, a blood pressure cuff may be used to temporarily control bleeding during wound evaluation. The temporary tourniquet is used only long enough to evaluate the extent of the wound and should not exceed a total of 15 to 20 minutes in duration.[1]

When evaluating the wound, note the depth, involved structures, and signs of contamination. If the wound involves major vascular structures, your priority should focus on hemorrhage control. If no major vascular structures are identified, continue to evaluate the wound for gross contamination.

The same components are required when evaluating wounds of the abdomen and thorax. Wounds involving the groin, axilla, and clavicles are at high risk for life-threatening hemorrhage. The close proximity of major vascular structures found within these areas make then more susceptible to injury. Wound packing and pressure dressings should be applied immediately to wounds with life-threatening hemorrhage in these locations. Additional techniques for hemorrhage control will be

discussed later in this chapter. If the wound involves deep structures of the abdomen or thorax, immediately treat the underlying injury (*pneumothorax, bowel evisceration, etc*) All other wounds should be evaluated for depth, involved structures, and contamination.

When operating in austere conditions, transportation to a definitive care facility may be delayed for several hours or days. Under these conditions, wounds may require closure in the field. If the patient is unable to be transported for an extended period of time, grossly decontaminate the wound by irrigating. This is accomplished by irrigating with tap water or normal saline.[2] Irrigation can effectively be completed using an 18- to 20-gauge angiocatheter, or blunt needle, and a 35- to 65-mL syringe. For larger wounds, various high-volume techniques can be employed to remove gross contamination. However, irrigation with a syringe and angiocatheter as described above is the most effective way to decontaminate a wound prior to closure.[3] If the patient will be quickly transported to definitive care, hemorrhage control alone is appropriate.

It is important to remember that the wound may not be completely decontaminated in the field. Closure of the wound should be consistent with techniques used for other contaminated wounds. Since suture is a foreign material, it can lead to an increased likelihood of infection. Sutures should be placed at further intervals, allowing for the least number of sutures possible, while allowing the approximation of the wound edges to control hemorrhage and promote healing. Both suture and staples placed in the prehospital environment are effective for wound closure.

OPEN NONACUTE WOUNDS

The evaluation of nonacute open wounds in the field requires further understanding of wound healing and signs of infection. Patients may present with postoperative wounds from recent surgery or subacute wounds from injuries incurred several days earlier. Subacute traumatic wounds will often be encountered during deployment to disaster areas or when working with rescue teams in austere conditions. Elderly patients and those with diabetes, venous stasis, lymphedema, previous radiation therapy, paraplegia, or other disability may also have chronic nonhealing wounds that may suffer infection or other complications.

It is appropriate to consider the individual phases of wound healing. Initially, involved tissues undergo vasoconstriction and localization of platelets. Both of these actions initiate the process of hemostasis. The wound will then express a variety of inflammatory changes. These will result in localized vasodilatation, and phagocytosis of retained bacteria and contaminants. Both hemostasis and the inflammatory phase occur within the first hour following injury. The proliferative phase results from the localized release of chemical markers, which stimulate cells to multiply and repair damaged tissue. Additionally, fibroblasts work to develop a collagen framework, forming a basis for the proliferative phase. Granulation tissue is the product of the collagen deposition, which begins approximately 12 hours after the injury. Eventually the wound margins will contract and remodeling will complete the healing process[4] (**Figure 57-1**). Wound can be closed at several points during the healing process. Primary closure describes wounds repaired within the first 6 hours. Closure by secondary intention describes wounds allowed to heal simply by following the natural phases of wound healing. These wounds will heal without sutures or staples. Closure by secondary intention is preferred for highly contaminated wounds. Delayed primary closure describes wounds closed with sutures or staples after an initial period of healing. These wound have been allowed to initiate the proliferative phase of healing prior to wound closure. These wounds are irrigated and left open for 2 to 4 days prior to closure with suture or staples.[1] Delayed primary closure is effective for treating contaminated wounds and allows for improved healing and aesthetic results.

Understanding the phases of wound healing and types of wound closure are essential to evaluating the open nonacute wound. Often, minor wounds evaluated after the first 6 hours of healing do not require further intervention. These wounds will require cleaning and decontamination, but have already established hemostasis. If these wounds do not involve deeper structures, further treatment is unnecessary.

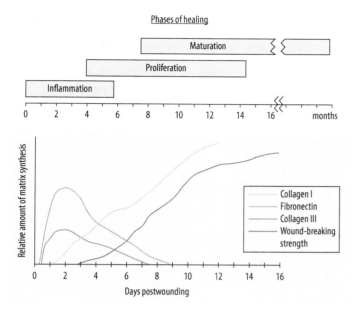

Phases of healing

FIGURE 57-1. Phases of wound healing. (Modified with permission from Brunicardi FC, Andersen DK, Billiar TR, et al. *Schwartz's Principles of Surgery*. 9th ed. McGraw-Hill; 2010.)

Nonacute wounds involving deeper structures require exploration prior to definitive treatment. If the wound complicates safe extraction or limits mobility, consider delayed primary closure for these patients. It is important to remember that contaminated wound should not be closed. If closure of a contaminated wound or one involving deep structures is necessary for safe extraction, the wound will need to be reopened and explored once definitive care can be established.

POSTOPERATIVE WOUND EVALUATION

When evaluating postoperative wound complications, focus on the anatomy of the structures involved. Some wounds are intentionally allowed to close by secondary intention due to extensive contamination or edema during a procedure. Wound dehiscences with bowel or omental evisceration are unique complications to abdominal incisions. These wounds should be evaluated for signs of infection and hemorrhage. Eviscerated organs should not be forced back into the abdominal cavity. This can lead to increased chance of infection or injury to the bowel. Dehiscence may result from excessive increase in intra-abdominal pressure. As a result, the viscera may have improved blood flow secondary to expansion allowed by the wound dehiscence. Eviscerated organs should be covered with saline soaked sterile gauze, and secured with a bulky dressing. These wounds will require emergency surgical intervention once definitive care is reached.

EVALUATION WOUND INFECTION

Infection is a frequent complication of subacute wounds. First, evaluate the wound for signs of erythema and warmth. If the area of erythema extends beyond the immediate margins of the wound, this should be noted and marked. Placing a marker line around the involved area will act as a baseline for the tracking a developing wound infection or cellulitis. Additionally, these wounds should be evaluated for the presence of purulent discharge. Fibrin and slough overlying healthy granulation tissue is often confused for purulent drainage and may appear as a white to yellow colored material located over the wound. However, fibrin and slough are typically adherent and will not express or wipe clear from the wound. Granulation tissue appears as a bumpy red soft tissue pattern in the wound base. When palpating the infected area, feel for areas of fluctance under and around the wound. Palpation over an abscess or fluid collection will often cause the expulsion of material from open

wounds. An abscess may still form within the subcutaneous tissue without direct extension to the open portion of the wound. Additional sutures may need to be removed when evaluating partially opened surgical wounds with possible abscess. It is prudent to never remove deep or subcutaneous sutures in the typical prehospital setting. This may lead to a variety of complications. However, superficial sutures may be removed to allow drainage of fluid collection when definitive treatment will be delayed for an extended period of time. Partially open wounds under strain from fluid collections, such as an abscess, hematoma, or seroma, may suffer catastrophic complications if not drained in a timely manner. Additionally, intentional drainage and irrigation of an abscess can definitively treat an early incisional wound infection.

ACTIVE HEMORRHAGE

The ability to control acute life-threatening hemorrhage is a cornerstone of prehospital trauma care. Patients presenting with acute life-threatening hemorrhage must be treated aggressively within the first few minutes of the injury. Extensive literature has been published using data collected from combat medical units. Uncontrolled hemorrhage accounts for a significant number of preventable deaths in the prehospital setting during military operations.[5] As a result, the military has placed great emphasis on treatment of acute life-threatening hemorrhage in the Tactical Combat Casualty Care Guidelines.[6]

EXTREMITY WOUNDS

A variety of treatment modalities are available to patients suffering acute extremity wounds. Abrasions and simple lacerations will be encountered frequently. These wounds may be irrigated with tap water or saline and dressed with simple bulky dressing. Wounds requiring closure should be evaluated using the criteria descried earlier in the chapter. Those patients suffering more extensive wound to extremities may require more aggressive intervention. Once the primary evaluation of the wound has been completed, the provider should have knowledge of the anatomical structures involved. Vascular injuries present the greatest threat to survivability. Both arterial and venous injuries pose a significant risk of blood loss. Additionally, those vascular injuries associated with unstable orthopedic injuries are at risk for deterioration during transportation. The initial treatment of acute life-threatening hemorrhage is the application of direct pressure. Wounds should be packed with gauze while maintaining sufficient direct pressure to control bleeding. Hemostatic agents or gauze impregnated with hemostatic agent can be applied directly to the open wound when direct pressure alone does not control the hemorrhage. Typically, blood soaked gauze should not be removed from the wound, since this may remove any formed clot from the wound. Additional gauze pads should be added over the initial gauze packing as necessary. When using gauze impregnated with hemostatic agent, it is necessary to completely remove the original gauze and replace with a new hemostatic dressing. This allows the hemostatic agent to have direct contact with the source of bleeding, increasing its efficacy. Once sufficient gauze has been employed to fill the wound, a pressure dressing should be applied. These can be constructed from elastic bandages or by using commercial products designed as pressure dressings. The elastic bandage should be applied with enough pressure to stop the active bleeding. As needed, additional pressure dressings can be placed over the wound to control hemorrhage. Orthopedic injuries should be stabilized to help with hemostatic control. When splinted, the EMS physician should still be able to evaluate and treat the source of hemorrhage.

In recent years, military experience and research have demonstrated the safety and effectiveness of tourniquets in the control of acute hemorrhage. Various designs are currently available to emergency medical providers (**Figure 57-2**). These range from simple constriction bands to pneumatic compression devices. They are applied proximal to the wound, with sufficient tension to stop pulsation to the distal extremity. Tourniquets should not be placed over joints, and are more effective

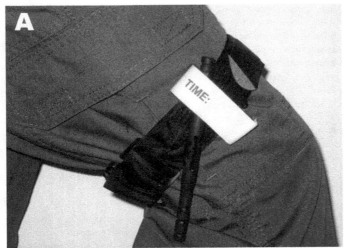

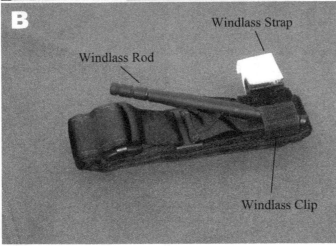

FIGURE 57-2. Combat application tourniquet (CAT), by Composite Resources. **A**: CAT deployed on the lower extremity. **B**: Parts of the CAT.

when placed over stable musculoskeletal structures. Marking the time of tourniquet application is mandatory.[7] Tourniquets can safely be removed from an extremity 2 hours after application with minimal occurrence of long-term injury.[8] Tourniquets should be used early in the treatment of life-threatening hemorrhage when clinically appropriate.

TRUNCAL WOUNDS

Wounds involving the torso provide a variety of complications specific to the location of the wound. The fundamentals of wound management are the same, but attention to anatomical structure involved is a key component. Wound to the thorax may involve cardiopulmonary structures as well as any of several major vascular structures. Open wounds involving the cardiopulmonary structures should be addressed immediately. Occlusive dressings are placed over all open chest wounds with suspected pulmonary involvement. The dressing is placed directly over the wound to provide complete closure of the chest wall defect. When needed, needle decompression or pericardiocentesis should be performed as described in Chapter 60.

Wounds involving the abdomen are often associated with significant intra-abdominal hemorrhage. Only a small amount of bleeding may be visible during the primary examination. Wounds over the flank may also be associated with significant retroperitoneal hemorrhage. These wounds should be packed with a bulky gauze dressing and secured with a pressure dressing when possible. Never remove blood soaked dressings as this

may remove any formed clot from the wound. Add additional gauze pads over the original dressing if continual bleeding is noted. Large wounds of the abdominal cavity may expose intra-abdominal structures. Do not replace eviscerated bowel into the abdominal cavity. Exposed abdominal viscera should be covered with saline soaked sterile dressings, then apply a dry gauze over the saline soaked gauze and secure the dressing.

Truncal wounds that involve vascular structures pose a significant risk of exsanguination. These wounds should be packed immediately with gauze. Additionally, Hemostatic agents or gauze impregnated with hemostatic agent can be applied when appropriate. Wound packing and continuous pressure are the key components of managing truncal vascular injuries. Wounds should be covered with pressure dressings whenever anatomical location of the wounds allow. Tourniquets have no defined role in the treatment of these wounds. There may be some effective use of tourniquet application for wound located proximal on the extremity near the groin or axilla, when no other treatment is effective.[7] Open wounds involving the subclavian and femoral vasculature require close monitoring. The application of a compressive dressing over the initial packing may be useful when treating abdominal wound near the pelvic girdle.

NECK WOUNDS

Wounds of the neck provide additional challenges because of the close proximity to vascular, airway, and neurological structures. These wounds can be immediately life threatening, and should be addressed immediately. Open wounds should be evaluated with close attention to regional anatomical structures. The location of the wound on the neck will indicate which deep structures may be involved. Large wounds involving the tracheal will require emergency airway procedures as described in the following chapter on airway emergencies. Vascular injuries will require similar treatment as those described above. Open wounds should be packed with gauze to fill the tissue defect. Hemostatic agents or gauze impregnated with hemostatic agent can also be used. A sufficient amount of pressure should be used to control bleeding, yet not compress airway structures. A pressure dressing should be applied when necessary to maintain hemostasis for compressible wounds. Routine cervical spine immobilization is not currently supported for penetrating wounds to the neck.[9] However, injuries caused by blunt force or penetration wounds with neurological deficit should be placed in precautionary cervical spine immobilization. Cervical collars should be utilized when indicated, if their application does not interfere with airway and hemorrhage control.

HEMOSTATIC AGENTS

DEVELOPMENT HISTORY

Hemostatic agents have been designed to provide temporary control of life-threatening hemorrhage due to penetrating trauma. The military saw a need for a more efficacious hemostatic dressing when injuries sustained from penetrating trauma were unable to be controlled with their standard Army Field Bandage. Hemostatic agents were initially designed for immediate "infield" control of severe hemorrhage. A limiting factor in their early use was the exothermic reaction of the first generation products. They are not a substitute for standard first-line hemorrhage control techniques. These agents are routinely used on patients not responding to initial management. As mortality from uncontrollable hemorrhage remains the number one cause of death in both civilian and military traumatic injuries, the role of these agents continues to grow.[10]

INDICATIONS/COMPLICATIONS

Hemostatic dressings are indicated for penetrating injury resulting in uncontrollable arterial or venous hemorrhage. They are not indicated in minor injuries or those responding to standard management. These agents have repeatedly demonstrated their ability to effectively control life-threatening hemorrhage and frequently prevent the need for tourniquet use or vessel ligation.[10,11] Early hemostatic agents produced a tissue damaging exothermic reaction. They have since been improved by limiting the temporary wound temperature to a maximum of 40°C.[12]

AGENT TYPES

The majority of commercially available hemostatic agents are produced in bandage form. However, there are several agents (Celox and TraumaDEX [Bleed-X], for example) that are available in a powder form. In this form, the agent is poured or applied with a commercial applicator directly into the wound. While showing favorable hemostatic outcomes, agents in powder form may require additional time to ensure complete removal from the wound,[13] therefore making these forms less desirable for some applications.

Advanced planning must take place when deciding on which hemostatic agent to select since it is likely to be cost prohibitive to carry multiple agents. We will explain the different mechanisms of action relied on by each agent to achieve hemorrhage control. The agents discussed in this section represent the most common of those currently being used in the prehospital environment. All of these agents have been tested and shown to achieve adequate hemorrhage control following the failure of traditional methods, or in cases of large bore arterial or venous injury (ie, liver lacerations, aortic injury, etc).[14-17]

Zeolite, a volcanic mineral, adsorbs water from the hemorrhage site in an exothermic reaction, allowing coagulation factors and platelets to collect and initiate clot formation.[11] QuikClot (Z-Medica, Wallingford, CT) uses zeolite technology and is FDA approved. It was originally developed in powder form, and is now available for civilian use in dressing form. QuikClot is the primary hemostatic agent used by the US Armed Forces.[15] In a recent study, swine sustaining lethal groin injuries, QuikClot achieved a 0% mortality rate.[10]

Chitosan, the active agent in several hemostatic agents, is derived from chitin, the structural component of the exoskeleton of crustaceans. Both HemCon (HemCon Medical Technologies, Inc, Portland, OR) and a new agent, Celox (MedTrade Products Ltd, Crewe, England) rely on chitosan as their active ingredient. Chitosan is effective by causing blood to gel when it comes in contact with it. The newly formed gel allows the dressing to adhere to the wound edges, forming a seal and stopping the hemorrhage.[18] Since no exothermic reaction is taking place when using chitosan products, heat injury is not a complication of these agents. Both HemCon and Celox are FDA approved and available for civilian use (**Figure 57-3**). A recent study proved the newer agent Celox to be as efficacious as the more established HemCon and QuikClot.[16]

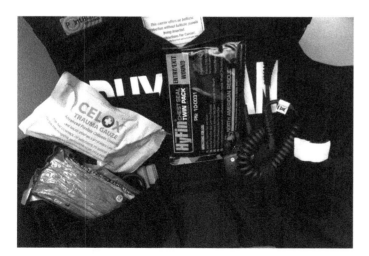

FIGURE 57-3. Conveniently carried items for addressing wounds and hemorrhage. Pictured here is an EMS physician's tactical vest with pockets containing items for immediate intervention of life-threatening wounds and hemorrhage: two Celox trauma gauze packets, 6-in hemorrhage control bandage, two chest seals, two tourniquets, two thoracostomy needles, #10-blade scalpel, trauma shears, and gloves.

TraumaDEX (Bleed-X) (Medafor Inc, Minneapolis, MN) is an example of a hemostatic agent containing the active ingredient, *poly-N-acetyl glucosamine*. This agent relies on a complex, biodegradable polysaccharide incorporated into microporous hemospheres to absorb water out of blood, leaving an increased concentration of coagulation factors and platelets to form a clot.[14] TraumaDEX (Bleed-X) is FDA approved and available in powder form by means of "injection" into a wound.

TRAUMATIC SHOCK IV THERAPY AND BLOOD TRANSFUSIONS

This section will be limited to identifying the need for blood transfusion following traumatic injury and determining the types of blood products available. A more complete discussion of shock may be found in Chapter 35. While initial trauma resuscitation is primarily directed toward maintaining the ABCs, the assessment and treatment of traumatic hypovolemic shock should be ongoing. Treatment of shock in this setting usually begins with crystalloid infusion to replace intravascular losses due to hemorrhage. Crystalloid resuscitation alone may be sufficient in the patient suffering from class I or II shock (mild to moderate shock). In patients suffering massive blood loss (~30%) in the cases of severe (stage III and IV) shock, attention must be paid to the fact that the oxygen-carrying capacity of the blood has likely diminished (**Table 57-1**). Development of traumatic blood loss anemia may occur and should influence the decision to begin an emergent blood transfusion. Identifying anemia in the field may be difficult due to environmental conditions, but one should pay close attention to vital signs, skin color/perfusion, and the patient's level of consciousness. One must remember that transfusions of packed red blood cells (PRBC) should not be used for volume replacement, but only for hemoglobin replacement with the goal of improving oxygen-carrying capacity. The decision for prehospital blood product administration must be made on a patient-by-patient basis but should be considered in all patients falling into the category of severe shock.[19]

A variety of blood products are available for emergent transfusion. PRBC are the first choice in severe shock as this blood product contains large amounts of hemoglobin to improve oxygen-carrying capacity. One must abide by state law and usually must coordinate with a local blood bank to obtain the ability to carry blood products in the prehospital setting. Blood must be stored in a refrigerated container with strict attention paid to temperature monitoring and recording. Once the physician has determined the need for an emergent blood transfusion, uncrossed O negative PRBC should be used. Since measuring of hemoglobin and hematocrit is not routinely performed in the prehospital setting, the end point of transfusion should be aimed at improving the clinical signs of traumatic blood loss anemia.

Although less important in the prehospital setting, platelet and clotting factor levels will diminish in the setting of massive blood loss and diluted with massive crystalloid infusions. Replacement of these blood products with platelet or fresh frozen plasma (FFP) should be considered. FFP is stored frozen and may take up to 90 minutes to thaw prior to use, which also limits its prehospital utility.

Activated recombinant factor VII has had favorable results when used in massive hemorrhage from traumatic injury.[20,21] Although not in mainstream prehospital use, synthetic alternatives to blood products do exist and research on them continues. Recombinant erythropoietin and hemoglobin-based red blood cell products are two examples of such substitutes.

Tranexamic acid (TXA) is another medical intervention under evaluation for the management of traumatic blood loss. Tranexamic acid is a synthetic derivative of lysine that binds sites on plasmin and plasminogen leading to inhibition of fibrinolysis. Some positive results with the use of TXA in trauma patients with significant hemorrhage have been reported.[22-24] The benefits of this therapy must be weighed against the potential complications. Additional studies and reports of use in the civilian prehospital setting are required to make more definitive determinations about its role in routine care of patients with hemorrhagic shock in the prehospital setting.

TABLE 57-1   Estimated Blood Loss Based on Patient's Initial Presentation

	Class I	Class II	Class III	Class IV
Blood loss (mL)	Up to 750	750-1500	1500-2000	>2000
Blood loss (% volume)	Up to 15%	15%-30%	30%-40%	>40%
Pulse rate	<100	100-120	120-140	>140
Blood pressure	Normal	Normal	Decreased	Decreased
Pulse pressure (mm Hg)	Normal/Increased	Decreased	Decreased	Decreased
Respiratory rate	14-20	20-30	30-40	>35
CNS/mental status	Slightly anxious	Mildly anxious	Anxious/confused	Confused/lethargic
Fluid replacement	Crystalloid	Crystalloid	Crystalloid and blood	Crystalloid and blood

Adapted with permission from ATLS: *Advanced Trauma Life Support for Doctors Student Manual*, 8th ed. Chicago: American College of Surgeons; 2008.

The EMS physician must also remember that blood transfusions do still carry with them a very small risk of infectious disease transmission. A detailed discussion of the risks of blood transfusion is beyond the scope of this chapter and should not prevent one from initiating an emergent transfusion in the acute blood loss setting.

KEY POINTS

- The EMS physician and provider should always address life-threatening hemorrhage before addressing other acute traumatic wounds.
- The EMS physician should evaluate acute open wounds for depth, involved structures, and presence of actual or potential contamination.
- The EMS physician should pay close attention to phases of healing, presence of possible infection, and postsurgical complications when evaluating nonacute open wounds.
- Tourniquets should be applied early and proximally when indicated for extremity wounds with acute life-threatening hemorrhage.
- Noncompressible wounds with hemorrhage should be managed with gauze packing and direct pressure.
- Hemostatic agents should be considered when traditional wound packing fails to control hemorrhage.
- Blood transfusions, utilization of synthetic blood products, and utilization of antifibrinolytic agents like tranexamic acid (TXA) should be considered as adjuncts to, or in some cases instead of, massive crystalloid fluid resuscitation.

REFERENCES

1. Jones TR, Wound Care in Stone CK, Humphries RL, et al. *Current Diagnosis and Treatment: Emergency Medicine.* 7th ed. Wound Care. McGraw-Hill; 2011.
2. Moscati RM, Mayrose J, Reardon RF, et al. A multicenter comparison of tap water versus sterile saline for wound irrigation. *Acad Emerg Med.* May 2007;14(5):404-409.
3. Singer AJ, Hollander JE, Subramanian MS, et al. Pressure dynamics of various irrigation techniques commonly used in the emergency department. *Ann Emerg Med.* 1994;24:36.
4. Barbul A, Efron DT, Kavalukas SL. *Wound healing in Brunicardi FC. Schwartz's Principles of Surgery.* 10th ed. Wound Healing. McGraw-Hill; 2015.
5. Martin M, Oh J, Currier H, et al. An analysis of in-hospital deaths at a modern combat support hospital. *J Trauma.* April 2009;66 (4 suppl):S51-S60; discussion S60-S61.
6. Military Health System. Tactical combat casualty care. Washington, DC. 2014. http://www.usaisr.amedd.army.mil/pdfs/TCCC_Guidelines_140602.pdf. Accessed May, 2015.
7. Kragh JF, Walters TJ, Baer DG, et al. Practical use of emergency tourniquets to stop bleeding in major limb trauma. *J Trauma.* February 2008;64(2 suppl):S38-S50.
8. Klenerman L. *The Tourniquet Manual: Principles and Practice.* London: Springer; 2003:20.
9. Brywczynski JJ, Barrett TW, Lyon JA, et al. Management of penetrating neck injury in the emergency department: a structured literature review. *Emerg Med J.* November 2008;25(11):711-715.
10. Pusateri AE, Holcomb JB, Kheirabadi BS, et al. Making sense of pre-clinical literature on advanced hemostatic products. *J Trauma.* 2006;60:674-682.
11. Alam HB, Burris D, DaCorta JA, Rhee P. Hemorrhage control in the battlefield: role of new hemostatic agents. *Mil Med.* 2005;170:63-69.
12. Alam HB, Uy GB, Miller D, et al. Comparative analysis of hemostatic agents in a swine model of lethal groin injury. *J Trauma.* 2003;54:1077-1082.
13. Kheirabadi BS, Scherer MR, Estep JS, et al. Determination of efficacy of new hemostatic dressings in a model of extremity arterial hemorrhage in swine. *J Trauma.* 2009;67(3):450-460.
14. Gegel BT, Burgert JM, Lockhart C, et al. Effects of Celox and TraumaDEX on hemorrhage control in a porcine model. *AANA J.* 2010;78(2):115-120.
15. Clay JG, Grayson K, Zierold D. Comparative testing of new hemostatic agents in a swine model of extremity arterial and venous hemorrhage. *Mil Med.* 2010;175:280-284.
16. Kozen BG, Kircher SJ, Henao J, et al. An alternative hemostatic dressing: comparison of CELOX, HemCon, and QuikClot. *Acad Emerg Med.* 2008;15(1):74-81.
17. Alam HB, Chen Z, Jaskille A, et al. Application of a zeolite hemostatic agent achieves 100% survival in a lethal model of complex groin injury in swine. *J Trauma.* 2004;56(5):974-983.
18. Dowling MB, Kumar R, Keliber MA, et al. A self-assembling hydrophobically modified chitosan capable of reversible hemostatic action. *Biomaterials.* 2011;32:3351-3357.
19. Feliciano DV, Mattox KL, Moore EE. *Trauma.* 6th ed. New York, McGraw-Hill; 2008.
20. Martinowitz U, Kenet G, Segal E. Recombinant activated factor VII for adjunctive hemorrhage control in trauma. *Transfus Altern Transfus Med.* 2001;3(5):30-36.
21. Geeraedts L, Kamphuisen PW, Kaasjager H, et al. The role of recombinant factor VIIa in the treatment of life-threatening haemorrhage in blunt trauma. *Injury.* 2005;36(4):495-500.
22. Shakur H, Roberts I, Bautista R, et al. Effects of tranexamic acid on death, vascular occlusive events, and blood transfusion in trauma patients with significant haemorrhage (CRASH-2): a randomised, placebo-controlled trial. *Lancet.* 2010;376(9734):23-32.
23. Morrison JJ, Dubose JJ, Rasmussen TE, et al. Military application of tranexamic acid in trauma emergency resuscitation (MATTERs) study. *Arch Surg.* 2012;147(2):113-119.
24. Roberts I, Perel P, Prieto-Merino D, et al. Effect of tranexamic acid on mortality in patients with traumatic bleeding: prespecified analysis of data from randomised controlled trial. *BMJ.* 2012;345:e5839.

CHAPTER 58

Burns

Alvin Wang
Ernest Yeh
William Hughes

INTRODUCTION

There are an estimated 1.2 million burn injuries per year in the United States. Of these, 50,000 patients are hospitalized and 4500 fire-related deaths occur. According to the 2012 Burn Repository Data, encompassing cases from 2002 to 2011, approximately 70% of patients who required admission were men with a mean age of 32 years. Children under 5 represented 19% of cases while patients older than 60 accounted for 12% of admissions. The overall mortality rate was 3.7%.[1]

Risk factors for mortality from burn include age greater than 60, burn greater than 40% BSA, and the presence of inhalation injury. Mortality was 0% with zero risk factors, 3% with one risk factor, 33% with two risk factors, and 90% with all three risk factors.[2] A variety of types of injury can result in a burn, requiring some variation in management strategies.

OBJECTIVES

- List types and causes of thermal, chemical, and electrical injuries.
- Describe the initial prehospital evaluation and management of thermal injuries.
- Describe the initial prehospital evaluation and management of exposure to acids and bases.
- Describe the initial prehospital evaluation and management of electrical injuries.
- Describe the initial prehospital evaluation and management of blast injuries.

THERMAL BURNS

DEPTH OF INJURY

The depth of injury is generally a function of pressure, temperature, and time of exposure. Contact burns can occur from contact with an extremely hot surface, usually for a brief period of time. These are most often occupational injuries. However, prolonged exposure to lower temperature objects can also cause deep tissue burns and generally occur in elderly patients or those with epilepsy.[3] First-degree burns are limited to the epidermis and cause erythema and pain similar to sunburn. Blisters do not form. Second-degree burns, also known as partial-thickness burns, involve epidermis and dermis. Blisters form early and if the area is denuded, the underlying dermis will be red and moist due to enhanced blood flow to this layer. The dermis will also retain its elasticity. Since nerve tissue remains viable, pain and proprioception remain intact. Third-degree burns, also known as full-thickness burns, involve all skin layers. The dermis will become charred and tough with the texture of leather. Sensation will be absent since the nerves are burned and the skin loses elasticity. Fourth-degree burns involve all skin layers and muscle or bone (**Figure 58-1**). These are usually seen in patients who were trapped or unconscious at the time of injury.

EVALUATION OF THE BURNED PATIENT

Of particular importance to EMS physicians who respond to the scene is scene safety. The responding physician must take care not to become a patient him or herself in the process of attempting to rescue the patient. Although the appearance and odor of the patient's wounds can easily become the focus of attention, the EMS physician must initially "ignore" the burn and treat any associated trauma in accordance with Advanced

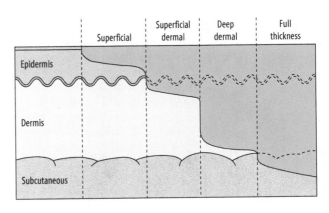

FIGURE 58-1. Depth of injury. (Reproduced from Hettiaratchy S, Papini R. Initial management of a major burn: II – assessment and resuscitation. *BMJ.* 2004;329(7457):101-103. With permission from BMJ Publishing Group, Ltd.)

Trauma and Life Support (ATLS) guidelines of the American Academy of Surgeons. Airway management, breathing, circulation, and environmental exposure must be initially addressed, followed by a complete history and physical examination. Estimation of burn surface area can be accomplished by using the "rule of 9s" (**Figure 58-2**) or the more accurate Lund and Browder chart [4] (**Figure 58-3**). An alternate method involves equating the patient's palmar surface area to 0.5% of the total BSA.

MANAGEMENT OF THE BURNED PATIENT

Once the initial primary and secondary surveys have been completed, attention should be turned toward stopping the burning process. In some cases, the patient's skin may still be smoldering and contaminated by products of combustion. Flooding quantities of water and a mild soap can be used. Appropriate analgesia must be provided during this process. Wounds should be covered with a clean dressing and, if available, a mild topical antibacterial agent. Silver sulfadiazine is a popular antibacterial agent, but bacitracin, polymyxin B, and neomycin may also be used. Broken bullae may be debrided or left intact. In cases where patients will be transported to a burn center, it may be more appropriate to avoid covering the burns in ointments that may need to be removed in order to allow for a burn surgeon to perform their evaluation.

Additionally, inhalation injury is present more frequently in patients with a serum carboxyhemoglobin greater than 10%, although a normal level does not exclude inhalation injury. Care must be taken to assess and reassess for signs and symptoms of inhalation injury.[5] Seventy percent of burn deaths are due to inhalation injuries.[6] (**Box 58-1**)

Inhalation burns can be characterized by their location above or below the glottis and by the presence of concomitant carbon monoxide (CO) poisoning and/or cyanide poisoning.[7-10] Injury above the glottis is associated with upper airway edema. Because the oropharynx is very efficient at removing heat from air, inhaled gases will be at almost normal temperature when entering the lungs. The oropharynx will be erythematous and soot may be present. Hoarseness should be taken as a sign of potential laryngeal edema and the larynx should be evaluated. Tissue edema frequently progresses during resuscitation and laryngeal obstruction can occur. Intubation for airway protection should occur early rather than later if laryngeal edema is suspected. Many patients will have normal respiratory parameters for the first 24 to 48 hours following their injury so decisions regarding airway protection should be made after a careful history and physical examination, combined with EMS physician's clinical suspicion.[11]

Subglottic inhalation injury occurs when noxious smoke particles are inhaled into the lungs. This results in mucosal edema, loss of ciliary function, bronchorrhea, vasoconstriction, and bronchospasm. Bronchial casts (analogous to skin eschar) may form, causing airway obstruction. Actual thermal damage can occur if hot liquid aspiration occurs or in cases of explosions where hot air is forced into the lungs. Steam

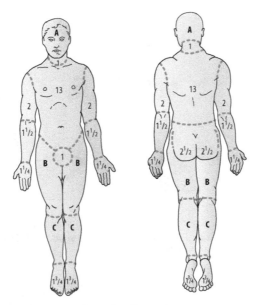
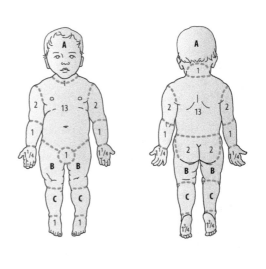

Relative percentages of areas affected by growth

	Age		
Area	**10**	**15**	**Adult**
A = half of head	5 $^1/_2$	4 $^1/_2$	3 $^1/_2$
B = half of one thigh	4 $^1/_4$	4 $^1/_2$	4 $^3/_4$
C = half of one leg	3	3 $^1/_4$	3 $^1/_2$

Relative percentages of areas affected by growth

	Age		
Area	**0**	**1**	**5**
A = half of head	9 $^1/_2$	8 $^1/_2$	6 $^1/_2$
B = half of one thigh	2 $^3/_4$	3 $^1/_4$	4
C = half of one leg	2 $^1/_2$	2 $^1/_2$	2 $^3/_4$

FIGURE 58-2. Rule of 9s. (Reprinted with permission from Demling RH. Burns & other thermal injuries. In: Doherty GM. eds. *Current Diagnosis & Treatment: Surgery.* 13 ed. New York, NY: McGraw-Hill; 2010:chap 14. Figure 14-2.

inhalation may be particularly damaging as the high moisture content of the air provides a much greater heat-carrying capacity. Although relatively rare, steam-related inhalational injury often progresses to respiratory failure within a few hours and is a poor prognostic factor.

Treatment of inhalation injury includes fluid resuscitation, airway protection, pulmonary toileting, bronchodilation, and mechanical ventilation if needed. Fluid requirements in patients with inhalation injury may be increased by 25% due to pulmonary edema. Routine intubation should be avoided, but progressive airway signs and symptoms should prompt consideration for early intubation. Mechanical ventilation parameters should be set in accordance with lung-protective ventilation strategies using a tidal volume of 6 mL/kg (ideal body weight), high PEEP, and permissive hypercapnea.[12] Bronchodilators can be used to treat airway hypersensitivity and may improve pulmonary edema. Many burn centers use nebulized heparin and mucolytics to prevent the formation of airway casts. Prophylactic steroids and antibiotics are not indicated.

Smoke generally contains 10% to 20% CO but because smoke exposure is relatively short, an individual's level may not be significant. Levels of 15% are often associated with neurologic impairment and levels higher than 60% may be fatal. The half-life of CO is 250 minutes at room air ($FiO_2 = 0.21$) but can be reduced to as low as 40 minutes with 100% oxygen. Individuals with smoke inhalation should be treated empirically with high flow oxygen prior to measurement of carboxyhemoglobin levels. Some EMS physicians may choose to use noninvasive carboxyhemoglobin monitors to guide therapy or transport destination, but at least one study has questioned the reliability of these devices.[13]

The presence of CO poisoning should lead the EMS physician to suspect associated cyanide toxicity. Cyanide is produced during the combustion of synthetic materials such as furniture foam and plastics. Because its half-life is short, treatment is rarely needed, but warranted if the patient remains persistently acidotic despite adequate resuscitation. Sodium thiosulfate and hydroxycobalamin are safe and effective treatments.

■ FLUID RESUSCITATION

Various resuscitation regimens have been devised and their use has dramatically reduced burn-related mortality.[3] Underresuscitation may result in the progression of partial-thickness burns to full-thickness burns and the development of multiorgan system failure. Conversely, overly aggressive fluid resuscitation may increase tissue and pulmonary edema, leading to respiratory compromise. The Parkland formula can be used to estimate the amount of crystalloid fluid required within the first 24 hours.[14,15]

$$\text{Fluid Required Over 24 h} = 4 \times \%\text{BSA} \times \text{Patient Weight (in kg)}$$

One-half of the calculated volume is given over the first 8 hours (from the time of injury, not from the time of resuscitation initiation) and the remaining half is given over the next 16 hours. % BSA includes only second-degree or higher burns. It is important to remember that this is only an estimate and fluid resuscitation should be individualized to maintain a urine output of 0.5 to 1 mL/kg/h. Fluid requirements may be increased if there is concomitant inhalation injury or electrical burn.[6] Ringer lactate is used most commonly, but 0.9% normal saline is equally acceptable, especially in the prehospital setting.

CHEMICAL BURNS

Chemical burns, although rare, may have devastating systemic effects and account for 30% of burn deaths.[3,16] Again, scene safety remains paramount and the responding EMS physician must ensure that he or she has donned the appropriate personal protective equipment. In addition, patients must be fully decontaminated before being brought into the emergency department to prevent contaminating other patients, staff members, and facilities. **Table 58-1** describes characteristics and treatment details for different types of acid.

% Total Body Surface Area Burn
Be clear and accurate, and do not include erythema
(Lund and Browder)

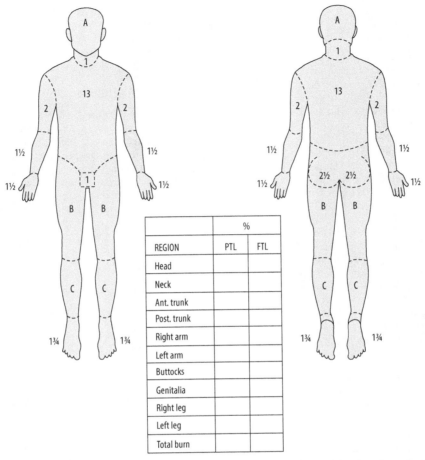

	%	
REGION	PTL	FTL
Head		
Neck		
Ant. trunk		
Post. trunk		
Right arm		
Left arm		
Buttocks		
Genitalia		
Right leg		
Left leg		
Total burn		

AREA	Age 0	1	5	10	15	Adult
A = ½ OF HEAD	9½	8½	6½	5½	4½	3½
B = ½ OF ONE THIGH	2¾	3¼	4	4½	4½	4¾
C = ½ OF ONE LOWER LEG	2½	2½	2¾	3	3¼	3½

FIGURE 58-3. Lund and Browder chart. (Reproduced from Hettiaratchy S, Papini R. Initial management of a major burn: II – assessment and resuscitation. *BMJ* 2004;329(7457):101-103. With permission from BMJ Publishing Group, Ltd.)

Box 58-1

Accessing for Inhalation Burns

Clues found on physical examination include:

- Singed nasal or facial hair
- Carbonaceous soot in the mouth or nose
- Facial burns
- Hoarseness when speaking

Historical clues for inhalation injury include burns occurring:

- While occupying an enclosed space
- Associated with an explosion
- Loss of consciousness

TABLE 58-1   Acid Burns

Substance	Characteristics	Treatment
Chromic acid[a]	Binds to hemoglobin resulting in decreased oxygen-carrying capacity	Surgical excision if >2% BSA May need exchange transfusion or dialysis
Formic acid[b]	Interferes with metabolic processes	Dialysis
Hydrofluoric acid[a]	Hypocalcemia, hypomagnesemia, hyponatremia resulting in seizures, hypotension, and ventricular fibrillation	Calcium gluconate gel (topical) Calcium gluconate injection (SQ) Electrolyte monitoring and repletion

[a]Herbert K, Lawrence JC. Chemical burns. *Burns*. December 1989;15(6):381-384.

[b]Matey P, Allison KP, Sheehan TM, Gowar JP. Chromic acid burns: early aggressive excision is the best method to prevent systemic toxicity. *J Burn Care Rehabil*. 2000;21(3):241-245.

Acid burns result in coagulative necrosis and can cause systemic absorption and toxicity even if only 1 to 2 %BSA is involved.[17] General principles involve decontamination by the removal of clothing and chemicals followed by copious irrigation with flooding quantities of cool water over 1 to 2 hours. Exceptions include exposure to elemental sodium, potassium, or lithium as these substances ignite when in contact with water. In addition, organic phenol is absorbed more rapidly when diluted.[16]

Alkali burns cause liquefaction necrosis and are generally more severe for a given amount of exposure. Prolonged irrigation (up to 8-24 hours) may be required and severe alkali burns are a poor prognostic factor.[18,19] Dilution is generally preferred to antidote administration because water is more readily available. Moreover, delay to irrigation is associated with extension in burn depth. Lastly, antidote administration may cause an exothermic reaction resulting in further injury.[17,20]

It would be impossible to list special considerations for every substance in this text, but various references exist to help guide medical treatment for various exposures. *Material data safety sheets* (MSDS) contain information on procedures for safe handling of that substance and includes physical data as well as information on toxicity, health effects, first aid, protective equipment requirements, and spill-handling procedures. In the United States, the Occupational Safety and Health Administration requirements dictate that MSDSs be available to employees in the vicinity of potentially harmful substances as well as to local fire departments and emergency planning officials. The savvy EMS physician should review the MSDS whenever possible in determining how best to care for their patient. In addition, CHEMTREC is a 24/7/365 call center resource which has a library of millions of MSDSs as well as rapid access to expert consultants including medical toxicologists. The phone number for CHEMTREC is +1 (800) 424-9300. Lastly, the American Association of Poison Control Centers sponsors 57 poison centers nationwide and is available 24/7/365. The phone number is (800) 222-1222.

ELECTRICAL INJURIES

Electrical burns (4% of burn admissions) are less common but have important acute management issues.[6] Electricity causes tissue damage by three mechanisms: direct cellular damage, thermal injury, and blunt trauma from associated falls.[21-24] Damage is proportional to the electrical current (amperes) of the source. The current that can be generated is proportional to the electrical potential of the electrical source (volts) and inversely proportional to the resistance (ohms) of the involved tissue. Skin resistance is reduced 40-fold by the presence of moisture and even further reduced by submersion in water.[25,26] Thermal energy (joules) is proportional to current, voltage, and time of contact.

▓ TYPE OF CURRENT

The type of current can also influence the amount of damage caused. Alternating current (AC), commonly found in high tension lines and home wiring, is three times more damaging than DC and accounts for the majority of injuries.[27] AC tends to cause repetitive muscular stimulation. Since the flexor muscles are stronger than the extensor muscles, AC electrocution tends to cause the hands to grip the electrical source, prolonging time of exposure. Conversely, direct current (DC), found in lightning, tends to cause a single muscular contraction and can often throw the victim clear of the electrical source.

▓ PATHWAY OF ELECTROCUTION

The pathway of entry and exit through the body can determine the amount of injury caused by electrocution. Vertical pathways are the most frequently lethal as it can involve the CNS as well as the heart and respiratory muscles. Horizontal pathways from one hand to the other can also involve the heart and spinal cord. Lower body injuries are generally less lethal but may cause extensive local injury.[27]

▓ LOW- VESRSUS HIGH-VOLTAGE INJURY

Domestic, low-voltage (less than 1000 V) electrocution typically causes small contact entry and exit wounds at the portal of entry and exit. Conversely, high-voltage injury (greater than 1000 V) is more likely to involve associated trauma from a fall, fracture from muscle contracture, rhabdomyolysis, cardiac rhythm disturbances, or compartment syndrome.[3] Moreover, arc injury can occur when electricity crosses a distance prior to contact. Temperatures in excess of 5000°F can be generated, resulting in severe thermal injuries.[28]

▓ LIGHTNING INJURY

Lightning generates more than 10 million V but the duration of exposure lasts only milliseconds, limiting damage. The pathognomic lightning injury is a necrotic, punctate full thickness burn with surrounding congestion and a feathering type of erythema known as Lichtenberg figures. The most common injury occurs in flashover phenomenon in which current travels over the entire surface of the body.[29] Fortunately, the only injury is superficial burns unless the clothing is ignited. Lightning can also cause blunt force trauma.[30] Expanding gas surrounding the advancing bolt of lightning can cause a shock wave with up to 20 atm of overpressure, resulting from high temperatures within the lightning bolt. Interestingly, the temperature can reach up to 30,000 K or up to five times the temperature of the Sun's surface. Many organ-specific injuries can occur as a result of lightning strike.[31] Asystole or ventricular fibrillation can occur.[28] Direct myocardial damage is less common; however, brain and spinal cord injuries can occur, leading to seizure, respiratory depression, coma, and paralysis.[31] Injury to the autonomic nervous system may produce fixed and dilated pupils, hypertension, and cool, pulseless extremities for the first few hours. Abdominal organ damage is rare, but can occur. More common is abdominal ileus and curling ulcers. Muscle and bone may undergo severe necrosis, leading to rhabdomyolysis and requiring surgical debridement. Tympanic membrane rupture is common as well as development of cataracts an early or late complication.

▓ MANAGEMENT OF ELECTRICAL INJURIES

The responding EMS physician should, as always, hold scene safety as a paramount concern. Care must be taken to avoid contact with live electrical sources and even seemingly de-energized electrical lines can become reenergized via back-feeding mechanisms as automatic circuit-breakers reset. Once scene safety is ensured, attention can be turned to traditional ATLS and burn resuscitation. An ECG should be obtained and dysrhythmias should be managed in accordance to ACLS guidelines. Spinal precautions should be taken in cases of neurologic deficit and/or history of a fall.[32] Moreover, severe muscular tetany may cause an occult fracture without external signs of trauma and these fractures should be splinted appropriately. Using surface burn area to estimate fluid resuscitation needs will generally result in underresuscitation. Fluid resuscitation calculations based on %BSA should be multiplied by a factor of 1.7 and the patient should be frequently reassessed for adequacy of urine output as well as development of rhabdomyolysis.[33] Liver, pancreatic, and renal function should be serially monitored.[34] A history of loss of consciousness or ECG abnormality generally warrants 24 hours telemetry monitoring.

BLAST INJURIES

EMS physicians and health care providers are increasingly faced with the possibility of needing to care for persons injured in explosions. Although many blast-related injuries can be managed in a manner similar to standard trauma and burn care, the blast pressure wave can cause unique injuries such as air emboli and blast lung. These injuries require meticulous initial assessment as early signs and symptoms may be subtle.

Again, scene safety is of paramount concern when responding to explosion. Whether the explosion was accidental or intentional, structural collapse and fire remain constant hazards at the scene of a blast. Moreover, in cases of terrorist blasts, the tactic of setting a second explosive device intended to target emergency responders is becoming quite common.[35]

Explosions result from the conversion of a solid or liquid into gas after detonation of an explosive material.[36] The expansion of gas causes a pressure wave and blast winds. Next, a period of low pressure develops before pressures finally normalize.[37] Blast injury occurs from the overpressure wave, projectiles thrown by the blast winds, and associated secondary mechanisms such as fire or structural collapse. Distance from the blast origin is a prime factor in determining the energy transmitted by the blast wave and is inversely and exponentially proportional to the cube power. That is to say that if the distance is doubled, the blast energy will actually be only one-eighth (2 to the third power).[38] The blast environment also has a significant impact on blast-related injury. Closed spaces result in higher blast wave overpressure and more serious injury compared to open spaces.[38]

Primary blast injuries occur via one of three mechanisms: spallation, implosion, and inertia. Spallation occurs when the pressure wave passes from a dense medium to a less dense medium.[39] Implosion occurs when gas, already contained within tissue, is compressed by the blast overpressure wave and subsequently expands as the overpressure wave passes.[40] Inertial forces are similar to the shearing forces experienced by the human body during blunt trauma such as motor vehicle collisions.[40]

Primary blast injury forces damage the human body at sites of air-tissue interface such as the pulmonary, gastrointestinal, and auditory systems.[40] The auditory system is the most frequently damaged because it is injured by the lowest amount of overpressure (35 kPA). Pulmonary and gastrointestinal tract injuries occur less frequently and require higher amounts of overpressure (75-100 kPA)[41] Tympanic membrane rupture occurs in up to 94% of patients with other primary blast injury.[42] Some experts advocate that patients without abdominal or pulmonary symptoms and intact tympanic membranes are at low risk to develop delayed complications.[41] However, a substantial portion of those with intact tympanic membranes do have evidence of blast lung injury as well.[43] Pulmonary edema and hemorrhage can result from direct alveolar trauma caused by blast overpressure. These inflammatory changes can develop over 12 to 24 hours, sometimes leading to delayed presentation. Spalling and implosive forces can lead to pulmonary contusion and alveolar tears.[43] These injuries can lead to hemothorax, pneumothorax, and pneumomediastinum.[44]

Blast lung syndrome is the combination of dyspnea, cough, and hypoxia that result from the impaired gas exchange and V/Q mismatch that occurs after blast injury to the lungs. The use of positive pressure ventilation (PPV) in patients with blast lung is associated with increased risk of air embolism due to alveolar tissue disruption and should only be used if other noninvasive strategies have been maximized and failed.[45] If PPV is required, lung-protective strategies should be utilized and PEEP should be avoided if possible.[46] The gastrointestinal system also has a substantial air-tissue interface and it is at substantial risk for bowel perforation caused by implosion forces. Spalling may also cause intramural intestinal edema and hemorrhage results in delayed perforation.[47] In severe cases, arterial disruption or air embolism may lead to intestinal ischemia.[48]

Secondary blast injury, caused by displacement of debris or shrapnel deliberately placed in terrorist devices, causes penetrating and blunt trauma seen commonly in civilian trauma.[49] Because the distance of fragment travel is much greater than the distance of harmful blast overpressure, secondary blast injuries are more common than primary blast injuries.[50] Secondary blast injury may result in abdominal solid organ injury.

Tertiary blast injuries occur when the patient is physically displaced by blast overpressure or blast winds and results in blunt trauma to the head, CNS, and musculoskeletal system as the victim impacts the ground or other object(s).

Quaternary blast injuries are all other associated injuries which could include flash blindness, burns, crush injury/compartment syndrome,

lung injuries from inhalation, exacerbation of a chronic medical illness (eg, angina, COPD), psychiatric illness (eg, PTSD), and others.

Musculoskeletal trauma from blast injuries is common and can result in traumatic amputation as well as immediate or delayed compartment syndrome.[51] In addition, secondary compartment syndrome can develop from fluid overresuscitation.[52,53] About 5% of patients injured in explosions will have a traumatic amputation.[54] This injury pattern occurs as blast overpressure causes bony fractures while blast winds disrupt soft tissues. These injuries can cause immediate mortality in 10% to 85% of patients.[55] The responding EMS physician should be prepared to manage these injuries with application of a tourniquet or performance of a fasciotomy if needed.

Management of blast injured patients can be exceptionally difficult as many treatment priorities can be in conflict.[56] Fluid resuscitation is often required due to acute hemorrhage, yet it can worsen pulmonary edema resulting from primary blast injury. Although intubation can be used as a treatment to improve ventilation, its use is associated with worsening of barotrauma and increased frequency of air embolism. Thus, overall immediate and delayed mortality for blast injured patients can be high depending on severity of initial injury.

KEY POINTS

- Estimation of burn surface area can be accomplished by using the "rule of 9s" (Figure 58-2) or the more accurate Lund and Browder chart (Figure 58-3). An alternate method involves equating the patient's palmar surface area to 0.5% of the total BSA.

- Acid burns result in coagulation necrosis and can cause systemic absorption and toxicity even if only 1% to 2 %BSA is involved.

- Alkali burns cause liquefaction necrosis and are generally more severe for a given amount of exposure.

- Electricity causes tissue damage by three mechanisms: direct cellular damage, thermal injury, and blunt trauma from associated falls.

- Inhalation injuries with thermal and blast injuries should be considered.

REFERENCES

1. American Burn Association. National Burn Repository®. Version 8.0. 2012. http://www.ameriburn.org/2012NBRAnnualReport.pdf.

2. Ryan CM, Schoenfeld DA, Thorpe WP, Sheridan RL, Cassem EH, Tompkins RG. Objective estimates of the probabilities of death from burn injuries. *N Eng J Med.* 1998;338:362-366.

3. Hettiaratchy S, Dziewulski P. Pathophysiology and type of burns. *Br Med J.* 2004;328:1427-1429.

4. Giretzlehner M, Dirnberger J, Owen R, Haller HL, Lumenta DB, Kamolz LP. The determination of total burn surface area: how much difference? *Burns.* September 2013;39(6):1107-1113.

5. Chen MC, Chen MH, Wen BS, Lee MH, Ma H. The impact of inhalation injury in patients with small and moderate burns. *Burns.* 2014 Dec;40(8):1481-1486.

6. Latenser BA, Miller SF, Palmer BQ, et al. National Burn Repository 2006: a ten-year review. *J Burn Care Res.* 2007;28(5):635-658.

7. MacLennan L, Moiemen N. Management of cyanide toxicity in patients with burns. *Burns.* 2015;41(1):18-24. pii: S0305-4179 (14)00210-1.

8. Antonio AC, Castro PS, Freire LO. Smoke inhalation injury during enclosed-space fires: an update. *J Bras Pneumol.* May-June 2013;39(3):373-381. doi:10.1590/S1806-37132013000300016.

9. Dries DJ, Endorf FW. Inhalation injury: epidemiology, pathology, treatment strategies. *Scand J Trauma Resusc Emerg Med.* April 19, 2013;21:31. doi:10.1186/1757-7241-21-31.

10. Huzar TF, George T, Cross JM. Carbon monoxide and cyanide toxicity: etiology, pathophysiology and treatment in inhalation injury. *Expert Rev Respir Med.* April 2013 ;7(2):159-170.

11. American Burn Association. Practice guidelines for burn care. *J Burn Care Rehab.* 2001;22:S1-S69.

12. Amato MBP, Barbas CSV, Medeiros DM, et al. Effective of a protective ventilation strategy on mortality in the acute respiratory distress syndrome. *N Eng J Med.* 1998;338:347-354.

13. Touger M, Birnbaum A, Wang J, et al. Performance of the RAD-57 pulse co-oximeter compared to standard laboratory carboxyhemoglobin measurement. *Ann Emerg Med.* 2010;56:382-388.

14. Theron A, Bodger O, Williams D. Comparison of three techniques using the Parkland Formula to aid fluid resuscitation in adult burns. *Emerg Med J.* September 2014;31(9):730-735.

15. Mitchell KB, Khalil E, Brennan A, et al. New management strategy for fluid resuscitation: quantifying volume in the first 48 hours after burn injury. *J Burn Care Res.* January-February 2013;34(1):196-202.

16. Vaglenova E. Chemical burns: epidemiology. *Ann Burns Fire Disasters.* 1997;10(1):16-19.

17. Seth R, Chester D, Moiemen N. A review of chemical burns. *Trauma.* 2007;9:81.

18. Gruber RP. The effects of hydrotherapy on the clinical course and pH of experimental cutaneous chemical burns. *Plast Reconstr Surg.* 1975;55:200.

19. Moran KD, O'Reilly T, Munster AM. Chemical burns: a ten-year experience. *Am Surg.* 1987;53(11):652-653.

20. Herbert K, Lawrence JC. Chemical burns. *Burns.* 1989;15(6):381-384.

21. Butler ED, Gant TD. Electrical injuries with special reference to the upper extremities: a review of 182 cases. *Am J Surg.* 1977;134:95-101.

22. DiVincenti FC, Moncrief JA, Pruitt BA. Electrical injuries: a review of 65 cases. *J Trauma.* 1969;9:497-507.

23. Hunt JL, Mason AD, Masterson TS, et al. The pathophysiology of acute electric injury. *J Trauma.* 1976;16:335-340.

24. Skoog T. Electrical injuries. *J Trauma.* 1970;10(10):816-830.

25. Fish R, Electric shock, Part I: physics and pathophysiology. *J Emerg Med.* 1993;11(3):309-312.

26. Jaffee RH. Electropathology: a review of the pathologic changes produced by electric currents. *Arch Pathol Lab Med.* 1928;5:835.

27. Jain S. Bandi V. Electrical and lightning injuries. *Crit Care Clin.* 1999;15:319.

28. Koumbourlis AC. Electrical injuries. *Crit Care Med.* 2002;30 (11 suppl):S424-S430.

29. Bernstein T. Electrical injury: electrical engineer's perspective and n historical review. *Ann NY Acad Sci.* 1994;720:1-10.

30. Lichtenberg R, Dries D, Ward K, et al. Cardiovascular effects of lightning strikes. *J Am Coll Cardiol.* 1993;21:531.

31. Pfortmueller CA, Yikun Y, Haberkern M, Wuest E, Zimmermann H, Exadaktylos AK. Injuries, Sequelae, and Treatment of Lightning-Induced Injuries: 10 Years of Experience at a Swiss Trauma Center. *Emergency Medicine International,* vol. 2012, Article ID 167698, 6 pages, 2012. http://www.hindawi.com/journals/emi/2012/167698/. Accessed May, 2015.

32. Baxter CR. Present concepts in the management of major electrical injury. *Surg Clin North Am.* 1970;50(6).

33. Luce EA, Gottlieb SE. "True" high-tension electrical injuries. *Ann Plast Surg.* 1984;12:321.

34. Kouwenhoven WB. Effects of electricity in the human body. *Electr Eng.* 1949;68(3);199-203.

35. Burke R. Explosive terrorism. In: Burke R, ed. *Counter-Terrorism for Emergency Responders.* 2nd ed. Boca Raton, FL: CRC Press; 2006.

36. Stuhmiller JH, Phillips YY III, Richmond DR. The physics and mechanisms of primary blast injury. In: Bellamy RF, Zjtchuk R, eds. *The Textbook of Military Medicine—Conventional Warfare: Ballistic, Blast, and Burn Injuries.* Washington, DC: Department of the Army, Office of the Surgeon General; 1991:241-70.

37. DePalma RG, Burris DG, Champion HR, Hodgson MJ. Blast injuries. *N Engl J Med.* 2005;352:1335-1342.

38. Nelson TJ, Wall DB, Stedje-Larsen ET, et al. Predictors of mortality in close proximity blast injuries during Operation Iraqi Freedom. *J Am Coll Surg.* 2006;202:418-422.

39. Schardin H. *The Physical Principles of the Effects of a Detonation. German Aviation Medicine, World War II.* Washington, DC: Department of the US Air Force, Office of the Surgeon General; 1950:1207-1224.

40. Phillips YY III, Zajtchuk R. The management of primary blast injury. In: Bellamy RF, Zajtchuk R, eds. *The Textbook of Military Medicine—Conventional Warfare: Ballistic, Blast, and Burn Injuries.* Washington, DC: Department of the Army, Office of the Surgeon General; 1991:295-335.

41. Yang Z, Wang Z, Tang C, Ying Y. Biological effects of weak blast waves and safety limits for internal organ injury in the human body. *J Trauma.* 1996;40(suppl):81-84.

42. Cohen JT, Ziv G, Bloom J, Zikk D, Rapoport Y, Himmelfarb MZ. Blast injury of the ear in a confined space explosion: auditory and vestibular evaluation. *Isr Med Assoc J.* 2002;4:559-562.

43. Crabtree J. Terrorist homicide bombings: a primer for preparation. *J Burn Care Res.* 2006;27:576-588.

44. Avidan V, Hersch M, Armon Y, et al. Blast lung injury: clinical manifestations, treatment, and outcome. *Am J Surg.* 2005;190:927-931.

45. Garner MJ, Brett SJ. Mechanisms of injury by explosive devices. *Anesthesiol Clin.* 2007;25:147-160.

46. Caseby NG, Porter MF. Blast injuries to the lungs: clinical presentation, management and course. *Injury.* 1976;8:1-12.

47. Mayorga MA. The pathology of primary blast overpressure injury. *Toxicology.* 1997;121:17-28.

48. Ho AM, Ling E. Systemic air embolism after lung trauma. *Anesthesiology.* 1999;90:564-575.

49. de Ceballos JP, Turegano-Fuentes F, Perez-Diaz D, Sanz-Sanchez M, Martin-Llorente C, Guerrero-Sanz JE. 11 March 2004: the terrorist bomb explosions in Madrid, Spain—an analysis of the logistics, injuries sustained and clinical management of casualties treated at the closest hospital *Crit Care.* 2005;9(suppl 1): 104-111.

50. Sebesta J. Special lessons learned from Iraq. *Surg Clin North Am.* 2006;86:711-726.

51. Born CT. Blast trauma: the fourth weapon of mass destruction. *Scand J Surg.* 2005;94:279-285.

52. Block EF, Dobo S, Kirton OC. Compartment syndrome in the critically injured following massive resuscitation: case reports. *J Trauma.* 1995;39:787-791.

53. Tremblay LN, Feliciano DV, Rozycki GS. Secondary extremity compartment syndrome. *J Trauma.* 2002;53:833-837.

54. Stansbury LG, Lalliss SJ, Branstetter JG, Bagg MR, Holcomb JB. Amputations in US military personnel in the current conflicts in Afghanistan and Iraq. *J Orthop Trauma.* 2008;22:43-46.

55. Frykberg ER, Tepas JJ III. Terrorist bombings. Lessons learned from Belfast to Beirut. *Ann Surg.* 1988;208:569-576.

56. Boston Trauma Center Chiefs' Collaborative. Boston marathon bombings: an after-action review. *J Trauma Acute Care Surg.* September 2014;77(3):501-503.

Resuscitation Procedures

Susan M. Schreffler
Deepali Sharma

INTRODUCTION

Emergency medical services primarily came into formal existence in the United States to serve one very important need: to provide field resuscitation to patients with severe cardiopulmonary conditions and major trauma. EMS physicians should be expert resuscitators evidenced by their mastery of all the techniques needed to provide the highest level of care. This is also the skill set needed to train and educate the EMS providers with which they work due to the obvious value of this basic prehospital intervention.[1,2]

PROCEDURES

- Cardiopulmonary resuscitation (CPR)
  - Standard CPR
  - Automated compression devices
  - External defibrillators
    - Automated external defibrillators
    - Multifunction monitor/defibrillators
- Airway and ventilatory management
  - Airway positioning
  - Airway adjuncts
    - Nasopharyngeal airways
    - Oropharyngeal airways
    - Bag-valve mask
  - NIPPV
    - Continuous positive airway pressure (CPAP)
    - Bilevel positive airway pressure (BiPAP)
  - Endotracheal Intubation
    - Direct laryngoscopy
    - Video-assisted laryngoscopy
    - Intubation adjuncts
      - Lighted stylets
      - Gum elastic bougie
  - Supraglottic airway devices
  - Rescue airway procedures
    - Percutaneous and surgical cricothyrotomy
    - Needle cricothyrotomy with transtracheal jet insufflation
    - Retrograde intubation

- Airway placement confirmatory devices
  - Colorimetric carbon dioxide detectors
  - Capnography
- Ventilators
- Vascular access
  - Peripheral venous access
  - Central venous access
  - Intraosseous access
    - Adult
    - Pediatric
  - Arterial lines
    - Radial
    - Femoral
  - Neonatal vascular access
    - Umbilical lines
    - Central lines
    - Peripheral access

CARDIOPULMONARY RESUSCITATION

Cardiopulmonary Resuscitation (CPR) is the manual or mechanical method of creating artificial circulation to temporarily provide vital organs, especially the brain and heart, with oxygenated blood until normal cardiopulmonary activity can be restored in a person in cardiac arrest.

▧ STANDARD CPR

Indications

Cardiopulmonary arrest

Essential Equipment

- Pocket mask or bag-valve mask
- Automatic external defibrillator or multifunction monitor/defibrillator

Technique

Step 1: Assess for responsiveness, absence of breathing, or presence of abnormal breathing/gasping.

Step 2: Apply automatic external defibrillator (AED) or multifunction monitor/defibrillator.
- If witnessed arrest or CPR initiated prior to arrival, use AED as indicated or multifunction monitor/defibrillator as indicated by rhythm interpretation.
- Ensure continued CPR during charging.[3]
- If unwitnessed arrest or defibrillation not indicated, go to Step 3.

Step 3: Assess circulation by checking for a pulse for 10 seconds.
- Adults and children: carotid/femoral
- Infants: brachial

Step 4: If no pulse, begin cycle of compressions to ventilations at a ratio of 30:2 (universally for all ages). In children, if two providers are available for resuscitation, a ratio of 15:2 should be used.

- Compressions:
  - *Adults and children*: Compress at least 5 cm (at least 2 in) at a rate no less than 100 **compressions/min.**
  - *Infants*: Compress 4 cm (1.5 in) at a rate no less than 100 compressions/min.
- *Rescue breathing*: Rescue breaths should be given once chest compressions have been initiated. Each breath should be delivered over 1 second with sufficient tidal volume to cause a visible chest rise.

Step 5: Continue compressions to ventilations at a ratio of 30:2 for 5 cycles. After 5 cycles: stop. Reassess pulse. Reanalyze rhythm. Use AED or multifunction monitor/defibrillator as indicated. If defibrillation is not indicated or the patient remains pulseless, return to Step 4.

Technique

- Failure to perform adequate compression depth and/or rate
- Inadequate chest recoil between compressions
- Failure to minimize frequency and duration of interruptions

AUTOMATED COMPRESSION DEVICES

Automated compression devices may be used to replace manual compression during CPR *in an adult patient*. Defibrillator pads must be applied to the patient before application of the automated compression devices. These devices may be programed to provide either 30:2 CPR or continuous chest compressions with interposed manual ventilations. There are two types of automated compression devices used in clinical practice: Physio Control LUCAS-2 and Zoll AutoPulse.

LUCAS Chest Compression System The LUCAS Chest Compression System is a piston-driven device that is designed to deliver consistent, uninterrupted, effective compressions at a consistent rate and depth (**Figure 59-1**).

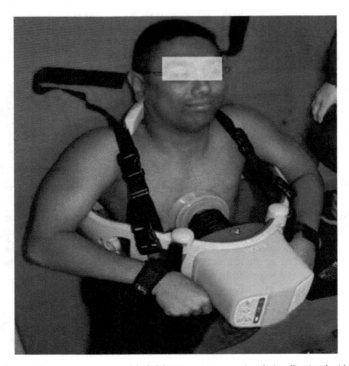

FIGURE 59-1. Physio control LUCAS-2 automatic compression device. (Reprinted with permission from Tintinalli JE, Stapczynski JS, Ma OJ, Cline DM, Cydulka RK, Meckler GD, eds. *Tintinalli's Emergency Medicine: A Comprehensive Study, 7th ed.* New York, NY: McGraw-Hill; 2011.)

Indications These devices may be considered when a nonpregnant *adult patient* with no traumatic injuries is found in cardiopulmonary arrest.[4,5]

Essential Equipment

- LUCAS-1 or LUCAS-2

Technique

Step 1: Unpack.

Step 2: Connect air (or battery).

- Confirm that the On/Off knob is in the *Adjust* position.
- If not already connect, attach the air hose to the connector.
- If using the air driven version—attach the connector to a portable air cylinder (or) a pressure regulator, open the air valve.

Step 3: Attach to the patient.

- Take the back plate out of the bag and approach the patient.
- Instruct those performing CPR to interrupt chest compressions.
- Work in a pair, one person on each side of the patient.
- Take a hold of the patient's arms. Take care to support the patient's head.
- Lift up the patient's upper body and lay the back plate below the armpits. Ensure that the patient's arms are outside of the back plate.
- Continue manual chest compressions.
- Take the upper part of the LUCAS out of the bag and pull up once on the release rings to check that the claw locks are open.
- Interrupt manual chest compressions.
- Place the upper part of the LUCAS over the patient's chest so that the claw locks of the support legs will engage with the back plate.
- Check by pulling upward that both support legs have locked against the back plate.

Step 4: Adjust device.

- To achieve effective compressions, ensure that the suction cup is centered over the sternum.
- Set the On/Off knob to *Adjust* position.
- Lower the suction cup with the height-adjustment handles until the pressure pad inside the suction cup touches the patient's chest without compressing the chest.
  - *If there is a distance between the pressure pad inside the suction cup and the sternum, LUCAS cannot be used.*

Step 5: Start mechanical chest compressions.

- Turn the On/Off knob to *Active* position. LUCAS device will initiate compressions.
- Check to ensure proper functioning.
- *When lifting the patient, stop compressions.* To stop compressions, turn the On/Off knob to the *Lock* position.

Step 6: Apply stabilization strap.

Step 7: Secure the patients arms to the straps on the support legs.

Technique

- Ineffective compressions if not positioned properly.
- If the patient is too large, the support legs cannot be locked to the back plate without compressing the patient.
- Only suitable for use in an adult patient.
- Contraindicated in patients with traumatic injury.
- Contraindicated in pregnant patients.
- Rib fractures, bruising, and soreness of the chest are not uncommon.[6]

AutoPulse Resuscitation System

The AutoPulse is a mechanical chest compression system with a load distributing band that provides improved circulation by squeezing the entire chest at a consistent, uninterrupted, effective rate and depth (**Figure 59-2**). The device uses a pressure sensor to calculate the amount of compression required for each specific patient.

Indications

The AutoPulse System is designed for adults with weight of no more than 136 kg with chest circumference of 76 to 130 cm and chest width of 25 to 38 cm. A patient weighing in excess of 136 kg may be suitable for the AutoPulse if they do not have a chest size of more than 130 cm.

Essential Equipment

- AutoPulse Resuscitation System
- AutoPulse batteries

Technique

There are two basic methods that can be applied:

1. *Log roll method*: at least three people required

   Step 1: Extend and then open the AutoPulse LifeBand and place the device next to the patient.

   Step 2: Log roll the patient away from the device.

   Step 3: Slide the AutoPulse device next to the patient and tuck the band on the patient side under the patient.

   Step 4: Log roll the patient back onto the device. Check alignment and adjust placement if necessary.

   Step 5: Close the LifeBand, fully extend, and then place on the patient's chest.

2. *Sit forward method*: at least three people required

   Step 1: Extend and then open the LifeBand and have the AutoPulse resting at the head of the patient.

   Step 2: Have two providers slip an arm under the patient's armpit and sit the patient forward.

   Step 3: Slide the AutoPulse down the bed, to the patient's buttocks.

   Step 4: Lay the patient back down on the board. Check alignment and adjust placement of necessary.

   Step 5: Close the LifeBand, fully extend, and then place on the patient's chest.

Technique

- Ineffective compressions if not positioned properly.
- Limited use based on weight and chest circumference.

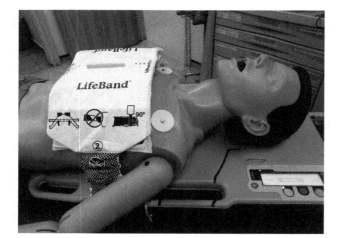

FIGURE 59-2. Zoll AutoPulse automatic compression device. (Reprinted with permission from Tintinalli JE, Stapczynski JS, Ma OJ, Cline DM, Cydulka RK, Meckler GD, eds. *Tintinalli's Emergency Medicine: A Comprehensive Study, 7th ed.* New York, NY: McGraw-Hill; 2011.)

- Only suitable for use in an adult patient.
- Contraindicated in patients with traumatic injury.
- Rib fractures and superficial skin injuries are not uncommon.

■ EXTERNAL DEFIBRILLATORS

Early defibrillation is the most important intervention in improving survivability in cardiac arrest; therefore, most EMS services carry external defibrillators. There are two types of external defibrillators: automated external defibrillator and multifunction monitor/defibrillator.

Indication

Defibrillation is performed when a patient in cardiac arrest is found to have the unsustainable rhythm of ventricular fibrillation or pulseless ventricular tachycardia.

Essential Equipment

- Automated external defibrillator or multifunction monitor/defibrillator
- Conductive pads

Automatic External Defibrillator

Automated external defibrillator (AED) is a simple computerized rhythm analyzing device that provides visual and audible instructions for the safe defibrillation of patients in cardiac arrest. It is used by many BLS agencies and first responder organizations.

Technique

Step 1: Power on device.

Step 2: Apply self-adhesive pads to the patient's chest.

Step 3: Press Analyze button.

Step 4: If indicated by AED, verify All Clear and press Shock button (may repeat up to three shocks).

Step 5: After three shocks or any "no shock indicated" signal, check for pulse. If no pulse, perform CPR.

Technique

- Ease of use and public availability may delay activation of 9-1-1 system.

Multifunction Monitor/Defibrillators

The multifunction monitor/defibrillator is a much more sophisticated device used by ALS agencies. Most of these devices have cardiac monitoring, pacing, cardioversion, and defibrillation capabilities. Defibrillation is facilitated using hands-off combination monitoring/defibrillation.

Technique

Step 1: Turn on the monitor/defibrillator.

Step 2: Apply ECG leads to the patient to analyze rhythm.

Step 3: Apply conductive pads to the patient's torso in the anterolateral position (**Figure 59-3**).

Step 4: If cardiac rhythm is conducive to defibrillation, prepare to deliver the electric charge to the patient.

Step 5: Select energy level and press Charge button.

Step 6: After ensuring All Clear, press the discharge/shock button to deliver the charge to the patient.

Step 7: Reevaluate the patient's cardiac rhythm. If still required, the unit can be recharged to deliver another electric charge to the patient if indicated.

Technique

- Failure to remove any fluid materials on the chest wall (conductive jelly, saline, sweat, urine, water) can result in arcing and thermal burns to the thorax.
- Repeated shocks may cause localized skin irritation/erythema.
- Failure to ensure an All Clear may lead to inadvertent electrical charge being delivered to rescue personnel.

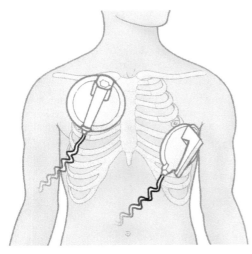

FIGURE 59-3. Anterolateral pad (paddle) position. (Reprinted with permission from Reichman EF. ed. *Emergency Medicine Procedures*. 2nd ed. New York, NY: McGraw-Hill; 2013.)

SYNCHRONIZED CARDIOVERSION

Synchronized cardioversion is performed at lower energies than defibrillation. In addition, it is important to set the monitor to a synchronization mode. This is important because inadvertent conversion of a perfusing rhythm to a nonperfusing rhythm is possible if the defibrillator is not set to the proper mode.

TRANSCUTANEOUS PACING

Transcutaneous pacing is a temporizing lifesaving procedure for symptomatic bradycardia.[7] It is important to note that this is used until a temporary transvenous or permanent pacemaker can be placed. Confirmation of capture can be difficult. If there is concern regarding the monitor confirmation, then the patients pulse can be assessed to confirm that the pulse corresponds to the pacer output. Furthermore, field ultrasound can be used for confirmation of ventricular capture.

AIRWAY AND VENTILATORY MANAGEMENT

Airway management is a fundamental lifesaving skill required of all prehospital providers. Basic airway management includes patient positioning and the use of airway adjuncts to establish or maintain a patent

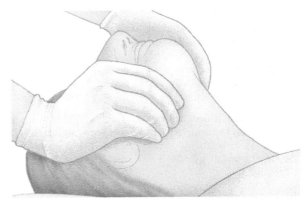

FIGURE 59-5. Jaw thrust. (Reprinted with permission from Reichman EF, ed. *Emergency Medicine Procedures*. 2nd ed. New York, NY: McGraw-Hill; 2013.)

airway. Basic airway management is the cornerstone skill from which advanced airway procedures progress.

AIRWAY POSITIONING

Indication

To establish and or maintain a patent airway by mechanically displacing the mandible and thereby lifting the tongue out of the oropharynx

Essential Equipment

- None

Technique

1) *Head-tilt chin lift*: in any patient without suspected cervical spine injury (**Figure 59-4**)

2) *Jaw thrust maneuver*: effective in patients with suspected cervical spinal injury (**Figure 59-5**)

   Step 1: Place the index and middle fingers of each hand posterior aspects of the mandible to push it upward.

   Step 2: Simultaneously, place the thumb of each hand on the chin and push downward to open the mouth.

NASOPHARYNGEAL AIRWAY

Indication

A nasopharyngeal airway (NPA) can be used to maintain a patent airway in patients with inadequate breathing who exhibit an intact gag reflex or clenched jaw (**Figure 59-6**).

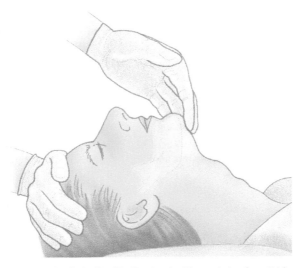

FIGURE 59-4. Head-tilt chin lift. (Reprinted with permission from Reichman EF, ed. *Emergency Medicine Procedures*. 2nd ed. New York, NY: McGraw-Hill; 2013.)

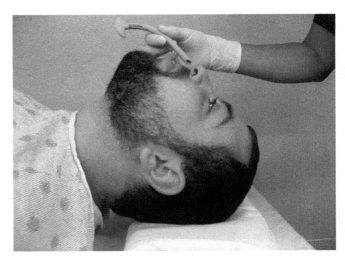

FIGURE 59-6. Nasopharyngeal airway. (Reprinted with permission from Reichman EF, ed. *Emergency Medicine Procedures*. 2nd ed. New York, NY: McGraw-Hill; 2013.)

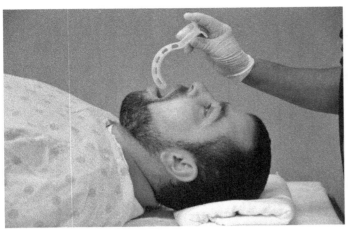 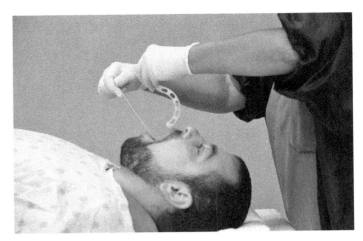

FIGURE 59-7. Oropharyngeal airway. (Reprinted with permission from Reichman EF, ed. *Emergency Medicine Procedures.* 2nd ed. New York, NY: McGraw-Hill; 2013.)

Essential Equipment

- Properly sized NPA
- Water-soluble lubricant or anesthetic jelly
- Suction system

Technique

Step 1: Open the airway with airway positioning technique.

Step 2: Choose the proper size NPA by measuring from nasal opening to ear lobe.

Step 3: Lubricate the NPA and insert into the nostril with the beveled side against the nasal septum.

Step 4: Gently advance and rotate 90° so the NPA is concave upward.

Step 5: Advance carefully along the floor of the nasopharynx until the flange rests against the nostril.

Technique

- Placement may lead to aspiration of gastric contents.
- Airway trauma may lead to epistaxis.
- Incorrect size or placement will compromise effectiveness.
- Insertion into a patient with a basilar skull fracture, may cause displacement of the device into the cranial vault.

OROPHARYNGEAL AIRWAY

Indication

An oropharyngeal airway (OPA) can be used to maintain a patent airway in patients with inadequate breathing who exhibit no gag reflex (**Figure 59**-7). Use of an OPA in a patient with an intact gag reflex may trigger vomiting and lead to aspiration of gastric contents. An OPA may also be used as a bite block to help prevent a patient from biting, occluding, and lacerating an endotracheal tube.

Essential Equipment

- Properly sized OPA
- Suction system

Technique

Step 1: Open the airway with airway positioning technique.

Step 2: Choose the proper size OPA by measuring from the corner of the mouth to the ear lobe.

Step 3: Adults—insert the OPA upside down until resistance is met, then rotate 180° and advance until flange is at the lips.

Pediatric patients—use a tongue depressor to hold the tongue down and guide the OPA into position right side up.

Technique

- Insertion of the OPA into a patient with an intact gag reflex can trigger vomiting and aspiration of gastric contents.
- Incorrect size or placement may exacerbate airway obstruction.
- Placement may cause oral trauma.

BAG-VALVE MASK (BVM)

Indications

Assisted ventilation for both adults and pediatric patients with the absence of spontaneous breathing or inadequate breathing

Essential Equipment

- Bag-valve mask with oxygen reservoir
- Oxygen supply and tubing

Technique

Step 1: Open the airway with airway positioning technique.

Step 2: Insert NPA or OPA to maintain patent airway.

Step 3: Ensure proper mask size—mask should completely cover the nose and mouth, but not leak.

Step 4: Create a good seal between the mask and the patient's face by using one or two person techniques and ventilate the patient (**Figure 59-8**).

NIPPV

Noninvasive positive pressure ventilation (NIPPV) is an effective noninvasive method of providing positive pressure ventilation for patients who need ventilator support but can still maintain their airway. NIPPV is commonly used in the prehospital setting for cases of acute pulmonary edema secondary to CHF, COPD, and asthma exacerbations.[8-10] NIPPV has been demonstrated to reduce the need for endotracheal intubations and relieve symptoms in these patient populations. The two methods of NIPPV used in the prehospital environment are continuous positive airway pressure and bilevel positive airway pressure (BiPAP). NPPV is contraindicated in the patient with apnea or agonal respirations, severe maxillofacial trauma, potential basilar skull fracture, severe epistaxis, or bullous disease.

Continuous positive airway pressure delivers continuous positive air pressure throughout the respiratory cycle. Bilevel positive airway pressure differs from CPAP in that it delivers two levels of positive pressure during the different phases of the respiratory cycle. BiPAP units can provide more relief, but are less practical for prehospital use because they are larger, more expensive and require more energy than CPAP.

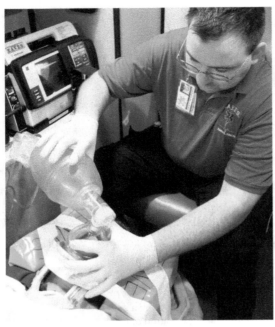 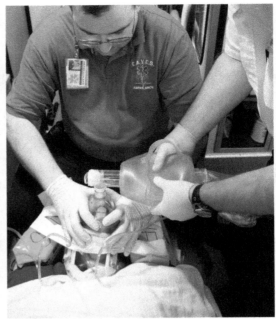

FIGURE 59-8. Bag-valve mask ventilation. (Left) EMS provider creates a seal with the one-handed c-hold. (Right) EMS provider creates the seal with the two-handed method while a second provider ventilates.

Continuous Positive Pressure Ventilation

Indication

Continuous positive pressure ventilation (CPAP) can be used in the prehospital setting for cases of acute cardiogenic pulmonary edema, COPD, asthma, traumatic respiratory distress, ARDS, and pneumonia in order to maintain a level of positive airway pressure. The patient must have spontaneous respirations and be able to maintain their own airway.

Essential Equipment

- CPAP unit—ideally it is small, relatively inexpensive, easily portable and tolerates leaks with independent setting for IPAP and EPAP.
- Oxygen supply.
- Power source.

Technique

Step 1: Ensure the patient has adequate respirations and is able to maintain their own airway.

Step 2: Select a proper size mask that is tight enough to allow a good, comfortable seal.

Step 3: Set IPAP at 8 to 10 and EPAP at 3 to 4 cm H_2O initially, using supplemental O_2 at 3 to 5 L/min.

Step 4: Monitor the patient's condition by assessing changes in vital signs (BP, pulse, heart rate), pulse oximetry, and patient comfort. Adjust setting with each IPAP/EPAP change, increasing EPAP at 1 to 2 cm incrementally with IPAP kept constant at a ratio (EPAP:IPAP) of 1:2.5.

Step 5: Continued hypercapnia is treated by increasing IPAP alone in 1- to 3-cm increments.

- Use caution when using NIPPV at pressures approaching 15 cm H_2O. High pressures (>15 cm H_2O) may cause excessive intrathoracic pressure reducing essential preload and afterload, resulting in hypotension.

Technique

- A good mask seal can prove challenging, requiring multiple adjustments.
- Gastric distension may lead to vomiting and aspiration.
- Increased intragastric pressure may lead to abdominal compartment syndrome.
- The patient may develop excessive secretions leading to airway compromise.

■ ENDOTRACHEAL INTUBATION

Endotracheal intubation is an advanced airway procedure during which an endotracheal tube is placed through the larynx into the trachea in patients who need definitive airway control. Endotracheal intubation is used to ensure airway patency, provide ventilations, and protect against aspiration. Prehospital endotracheal intubation is an area on which EMS physicians must focus.[11]

Direct Laryngoscopy (Figure 59-9)

Indications

Respiratory or other emergencies requiring definitive airway control

Essential Equipment

- PPE
- Suction catheter and source
- Bag-valve mask
- Oxygen
- Endotracheal tube and stylet
- 10 mL syringe
- Endotracheal tube holder or adhesive tape
- End-tidal CO_2 detector (capnography preferred)
- Stethoscope
- Laryngoscope with appropriate blades
- Alternative rescue devices (bougie, laryngeal mask airway, CombiTube, King)
- Surgical airway kit
- Medications for anesthesia, sedation, or rapid-sequence intubation

Technique

Step 1: Ensure all equipment is readily accessible and functioning.

- Inflate the cuff of the endotracheal tube to check for leaks.
- Insert the stylet into the endotracheal tube—ensure stylet does not extend beyond the end of the tube.

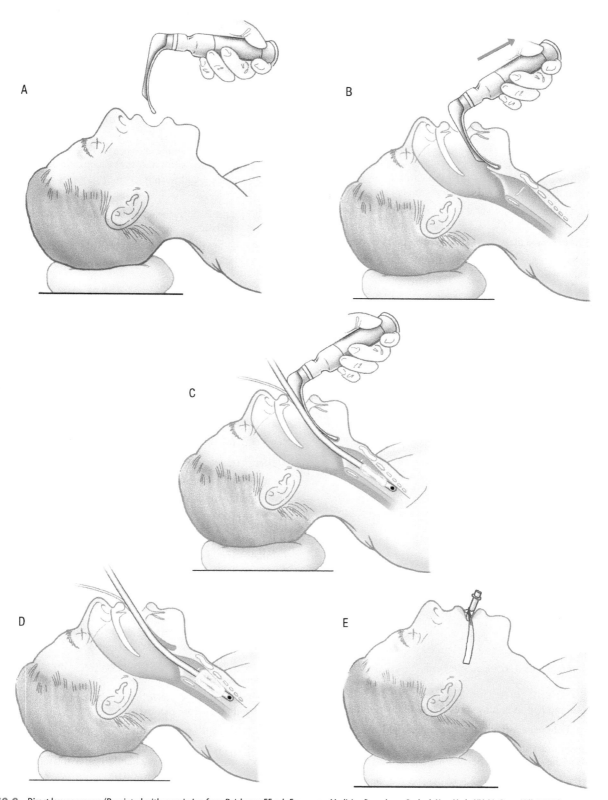

FIGURE 59-9. Direct laryngoscopy. (Reprinted with permission from Reichman EF, ed. *Emergency Medicine Procedures*. 2nd ed. New York, NY: McGraw-Hill; 2013.)

Step 2: Unless there are contraindications (suspected cervical spine injury), place the patient in "sniffing" position by placing a pillow or folded towel under the patient's occiput.

Step 3: Preoxygenate with 100% oxygen for 3 minutes using nonre-breather mask or bag-valve mask.

Step 4: While holding the laryngoscope in your left hand, open the patient's mouth with your right hand and inspect the oral cavity.

Step 5: Remove debris or dentures.

Step 6: Insert the laryngoscope blade with your left hand into the right of the patient's mouth, sweeping the tongue to the left.

Step 7: Advance the blade slowly and locate the epiglottis.

- If using a Macintosh blade, place the blade tip into the epiglottic vallecula.
- If using a Miller blade, place the blade tip posterior to the epiglottis.

Step 8: Elevate the laryngoscope upward and forward at a 45° angle to lift the mandible and expose the vocal cords.

- Pay special attention not to lever back against the patient's teeth; this can result in dental or and does not enhance the view of the cords

Step 9: Suction the airway as required.

Step 10: While maintaining your view of the vocal cords, insert the endotracheal tube into the right side of the patient's mouth.

Step 11: Pass the tube through the vocal cords until the balloon disappears into the trachea.

Step 12: Advance the tube until the balloon is 3 to 4 cm beyond the vocal cords.

Step 13: Inflate the endotracheal balloon with air, attach bag-valve mask, and start ventilations.

Step 14: Assess for proper tube placement using an end-tidal CO_2 detector (capnography or colorimetric), auscultation over the epigastrium, and auscultation of both lung fields for symmetry. Ultrasound (when available) may also be used, especially when auscultation is impractical (eg loud extrication scene, air medical transport).[12]

Step 15: Continue ventilations and secure the tube using a commercial tube holder or adhesive tape.

Technique

- Failure to recognize esophageal intubation.
- Failure to recognize mainstem bronchus intubation.
- Tube dislodgement can occur during patient movement.
- Oropharyngeal trauma from laryngoscopy or endotracheal tube placement.
- Vomiting and aspiration of gastric contents.
- Potential for laryngospasm and bronchospasm.

Video-Assisted Laryngoscopy (Figure 59-10)

The video laryngoscope is a high-resolution camera mounted to a laryngoscope blade that improves glottic visualization and is meant to increase the success rate of intubations.[13]

Indication Patients with the emergent need for definitive airway control

Essential Equipment

- Standard intubation equipment (see "Direct Laryngoscopy")
- Video-assisted monitor and laryngoscope blade

Technique

Step 1: Ensure all equipment is readily accessible and functioning.

- Inflate the cuff of the endotracheal tube to check for leaks.
- Insert the stylet into the endotracheal tube—ensure stylet does not extend beyond the end of the tube.

Step 2: Unless there are contraindications (suspected cervical spine injury), place the patient in "sniffing" position by placing a pillow or folded towel under the patient's occiput.

Step 3: Preoxygenate with 100% oxygen for 3 minutes using non-rebreather mask or bag-valve mask.

Step 4: While holding the laryngoscope in your left hand, open the patient's mouth with your right hand and inspect the oral cavity.

Step 5: Remove debris or dentures.

Step 6: Insert the laryngoscope blade with your left hand into the right of the patient's mouth, sweeping the tongue to the left.

Step 7: Watching the video monitor, advance the blade slowly, elevating the laryngoscope upward and forward lifting the mandible to expose the vocal cords.

- Pay special attention not to lever back against the patient's teeth; this can result in dental or and does not enhance the view of the cords.

Step 9: Suction the airway as required.

Step 10: While maintaining your view of the vocal cords on the video monitor, insert the endotracheal tube into the right side of the patient's mouth.

Step 11: Using the video monitor, advance the tube and watch as you pass the tube through the vocal cords until the balloon disappears into the trachea.

Step 12: Advance the tube until the balloon is 3 to 4 cm beyond the vocal cords.

Step 13: Inflate the endotracheal balloon with air, attach bag-valve mask, and start ventilations.

Step 14: Assess for proper tube placement by standard technique and secure in place.

Technique

See "Direct Laryngoscopy."

▌ SEMIRIGID FIBEROPTIC STYLET (FIGURE 59-11)

The semirigid fiberoptic stylets feature a metal stylet with a fiberoptic channel running through it that terminates in a lens, or in a video device improving glottic visualization and increases the success rate of intubations by placing the user's visual aspect at the terminal end of the endotracheal tube.[14]

Indication

Patients with the emergent need for definitive airway control

Essential Equipment

- Standard intubation equipment (see "Direct Laryngoscopy")
- Semirigid fiberoptic stylet device

Technique

Step 1: Ensure all equipment is readily accessible and functioning.

- Inflate the cuff of the endotracheal tube to check for leaks.
- Slide the endotracheal tube onto the semirigid fiberoptic intubation style and position the tube to ensure stylet does not extend beyond the end of the tube.

Step 2: Unless there are contraindications (suspected cervical spine injury), place the patient in "sniffing" position by placing a pillow or folded towel under the patient's occiput.

Step 3: Preoxygenate with 100% oxygen for 3 minutes using nonrebreather mask or bag-valve mask.

Step 4: While holding the device in the dominant hand, open the patient's mouth and inspect the oral cavity.

Step 5: Remove debris or dentures.

Step 6: Insert the device with the ETT loaded into the mouth in the midline and use your opposite hand to guide the tube at the mouth to keep it midline and moving smoothly.

Step 7: While looking through the eyepiece of on the video screen, following the airway in until the cords are in view.

- If the cords do not come immediately into view, the operator may have placed the device too deep into the oropharynx on the initial entry into the mouth. Simply back the device out until the cords are in view.

Step 9: Suction the airway as required.

Step 10: When the cords are in view, advance the device through the cords.

Step 11: When the view demonstrated the device is clearly through the cords, advance the endotracheal tube into the trachea.

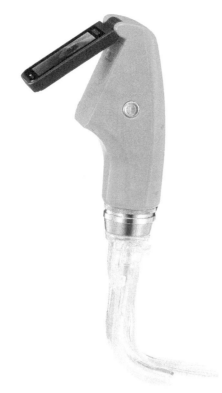

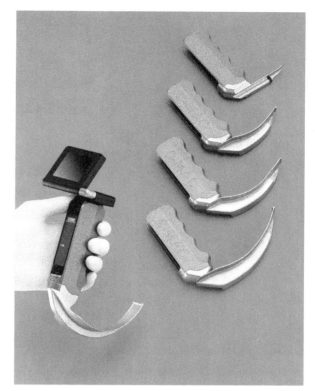

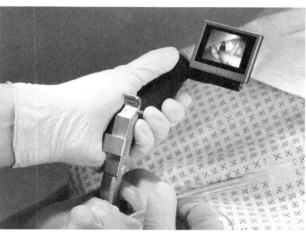

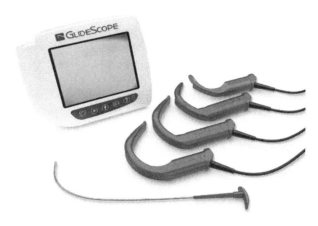

FIGURE 59-10. Video-assisted laryngoscopy. Many brands of video-assisted laryngoscopes of different design and cost are now available and in use in the field. (Reprinted with permission from Reichman EF, ed. *Emergency Medicine Procedures.* 2nd ed. New York, NY: McGraw-Hill; 2013.)

Step 12: The operator can actually watch for the balloon to pass into the trachea from the view from inside the ETT. Advance the tube until the balloon is 3 to 4 cm beyond the vocal cords.

Step 13: Inflate the endotracheal balloon with air, attach bag-valve mask, and start ventilations.

Step 14: Assess for proper tube placement by standard technique and secure in place.

Step 15: The device can then be quickly used to reenter the mouth and easily visualize the ETT in place.

Technique

If the device is placed too deep initially, the user may see only the esophagus. The user must take some care to follow the airway in from the mouth.

Lighted Stylet (Figure 59-12)

The lighted stylet is a semirigid stylet with a light on the end that can be used for the intubation of patients with a difficult airway when direct visualization is hindered.

Indication

Patients with the emergent need for definitive airway control and endotracheal intubation through direct visualization is obstructed

Essential Equipment

- Standard intubation equipment (see "Direct Laryngoscopy")
- Lighted stylet

Technique

Step 1: Position the patient for intubation.

Step 2: Preload an appropriately sized endotracheal tube onto the lighted stylet.

Step 3: Turn the stylet on and insert it into the patient's posterior pharynx while holding a "jaw thrust" position with the nondominant hand.

Step 4: Slowly advance the stylet and observe the patient's exterior, anterior neck. When the tip of the lighted stylet is within the trachea, a well-defined circle of light will be seen just below the hyoid bone, and above the thyroid cartilage. This is the ideal position for

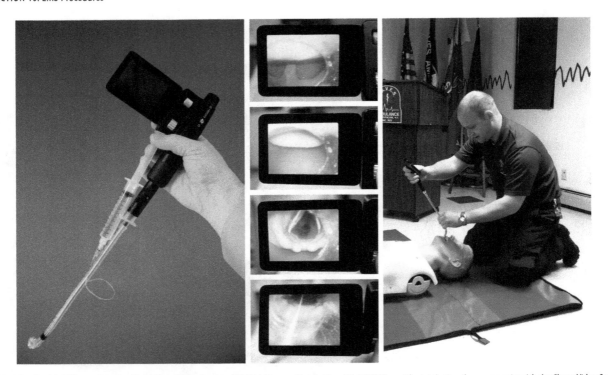

FIGURE 59-11. Semirigid fiberoptic stylet. (Left) Clarus Video System. (Middle) Stages of intubation. (Right) EMS provider intubating the mannequin with the Clarus Video System.

passing the tip of the endotracheal tube through the vocal cords (**Figure 59-13**).

Step 5: Advanced the endotracheal tube off the stylet.

Step 6: Inflate the endotracheal cuff, attach bag-valve mask, and initiate ventilations.

Step 7: Confirm tube placement by standard technique and secure in place.

Technique

- See "Direct Laryngoscopy."

Bougie (Endotracheal Tube Introducer) (Figure 59-14)

The bougie is a narrow diameter tracheal tube introducer that is used as an airway adjunct for difficult endotracheal intubations.

Indication

Patients with the emergent need for definitive airway control and endotracheal intubation through direct visualization is obstructed

Essential Equipment

- Standard intubation equipment (see "Direct Laryngoscopy")
- Bougie

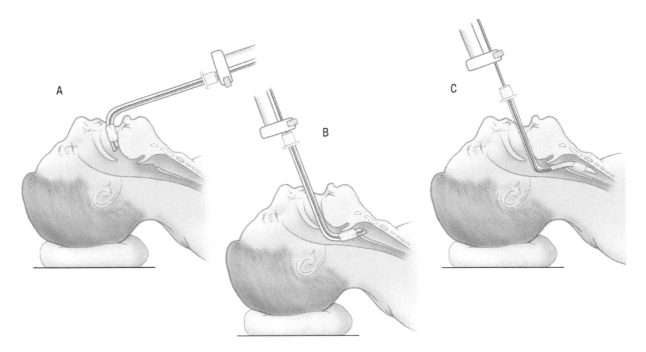

FIGURE 59-12. Lighted stylet intubation. (Reprinted with permission from Reichman EF, ed. *Emergency Medicine Procedures*. 2nd ed. New York, NY: McGraw-Hill; 2013.)

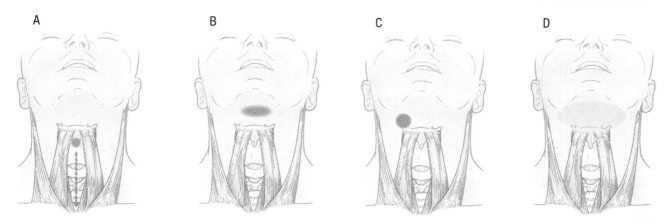

FIGURE 59-13. External view during lighted stylet intubation. (Reprinted with permission from Reichman EF, ed. *Emergency Medicine Procedures*. 2nd ed. New York, NY: McGraw-Hill; 2013.)

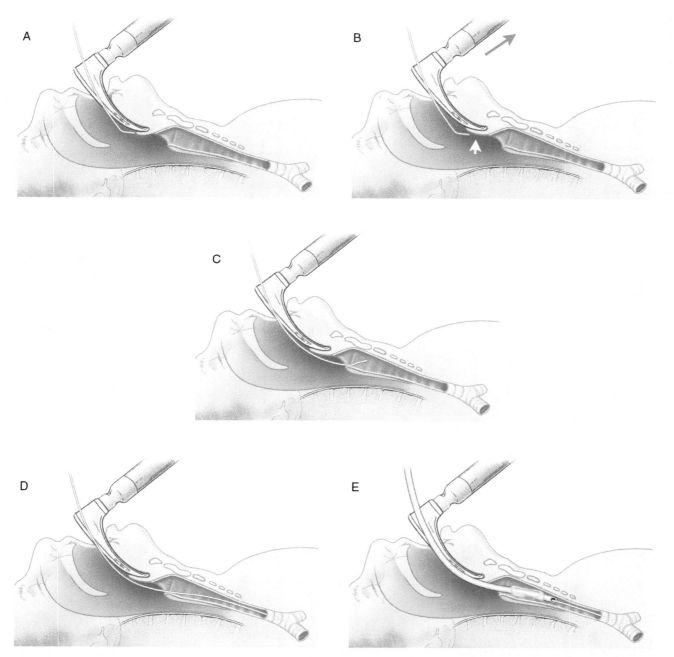

FIGURE 59-14. Bougie intubation. (Reprinted with permission from Reichman EF, ed. *Emergency Medicine Procedures*. 2nd ed. New York, NY: McGraw-Hill; 2013.)

Technique

Step 1: Once the best possible laryngeal view is obtained, pass the bougie into the patient's oropharynx and through the glottic opening. If unable to visualize the vocal cords, advance the bougie anteriorly under the epiglottis and feel for clicks as it slides along the tracheal rings.

Step 2: While maintaining the best laryngeal view, slide the endotracheal tube over the bougie, and advance it to the desired depth.

- If resistance is encountered while passing the tube, try rotating the bougie and tube 90°.

Step 3: Advanced the endotracheal tube off the stylet.

Step 4: Inflate the endotracheal cuff, attach bag-valve mask, and initiate ventilations.

Step 5: Confirm tube placement by standard technique and secure in place.

Technique

- Some operators will state that they do not feel the clicks of the endotracheal rings (this is variable) and may think they are not in place even if they are.

▨ SUPRAGLOTTIC AIRWAY DEVICES

Supraglottic devices are used in conjunction with a bag-valve mask for emergency airway maintenance when endotracheal intubation fails or no rapid sequence intubation (RSI) protocol exists.

Laryngeal Mask Airway (Figure 59-15)
Indications

Patients with an absent gag reflex who have impending or actual loss of airway patency or protection

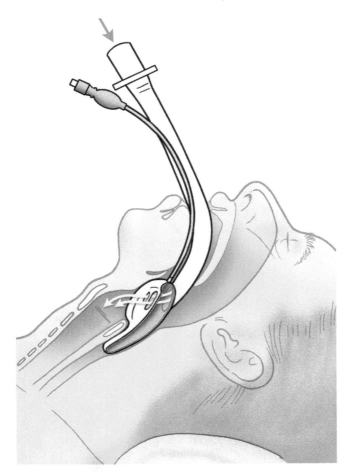

FIGURE 59-15. LMA placement. (Reprinted with permission from Reichman EF, ed. *Emergency Medicine Procedures.* 2nd ed. New York, NY: McGraw-Hill; 2013.)

Essential Equipment

- Properly sized laryngeal mask airway (LMA) for the patient
- Inflation syringe
- Suction system
- Endotracheal tube holder or tape
- Water-soluble lubricant

Technique

Step 1: Choose the correct size LMA based on manufacturer's recommendations.

Step 2: Visually inspect the device for damage.

Step 3: Inflate the cuff to verify patency.

Step 4: Deflate cuff completely so that the cuff walls are tightly flattened against each other, forming a spoon shape.

Step 5: Apply water-soluble lubricant to the posterior surface of the LMA.

Step 6: Inspect the patient's mouth and remove all debris or dentures before insertion.

Step 7: Preoxygenate and implement standard monitoring procedures.

Step 8: If not contraindicated (suspected C-spine injury), place the patient in the "sniffing position." If suspected C-spine injury, place the patient in neutral position.

Step 9: With the distal opening of the LMA facing anteriorly, insert the tip of the LMA into the patient's oropharynx.

Step 10: Under direct vision, press the tip of the cuff upward against the hard palate and flatten the cuff against it.

Step 11: Advance the LMA into the hypopharynx until resistance is met.

Step 12: Ensure the black line on the tubing is in line with the patient's upper lip.

Step 13: Inflate the cuff with the appropriate volume of air (refer to manufacturer's recommendations). A small outward movement of the tube is often noted as the device seats itself in the hypopharynx.

Step 14: Attach bag-valve mask and initiate ventilations.

Step 15: Confirm effective placement by $EtCO_2$ detection, auscultation of lung sounds, and misting in the tube.

Step 16: Secure tube using adhesive tape or a commercial tube holder device.

Technique

- Failure to provide adequate airway protection or ventilation
- Can induce vomiting and aspiration
- Oropharyngeal trauma from insertion

King Laryngeal Tube (King LT) (Figure 59-16)
Indications

Patients with an absent gag reflex who have impending or actual loss of airway patency or protection[15]

Essential Equipment

- Properly sized device (see manufacturer's recommendations)
- Inflation syringe
- Suction system
- Endotracheal tube holder or tape
- Water-soluble lubricant

Technique

Step 1: Choose the correct size device based on manufacturer's recommendations.

Step 2: Visually inspect the device for damage.

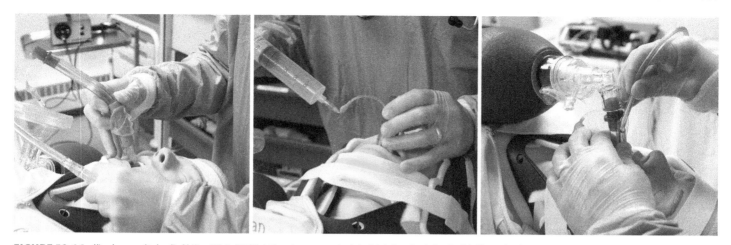

FIGURE 59-16. King laryngeal tube. (Left) King LTS-D. (Middle) After placement a single bulb is inflated to inflate both balloons. (Right) Some King laryngeal tubes have a channel to allow passage of orogastric tube and decompression of the stomach.

Step 3: Inflate the cuff with maximum amount of air to verify patency.

Step 4: Deflate cuff completely for insertion.

Step 5: Apply water-soluble lubricant to the beveled tip and posterior aspect of the tube. Do not introduce lubricant into the ventilation ports.

Step 6: Inspect the patient's mouth and remove all debris or dentures before insertion.

Step 7: Preoxygenate and implement standard monitoring procedures.

Step 8: If not contraindicated (suspected C-spine injury), place the patient in the "sniffing position." If suspected C-spine injury, place the patient in neutral position.

Step 9: While holding the King LT with the dominant hand, open the mouth with the nondominant hand, and apply a chin lift (if no cervical spinal injury suspected).

Step 10: Rotate the King LT laterally at 45° to 90° such that the blue orientation line is touching the corner of the mouth.

Step 11: Introduce the tip of the device into the oropharynx and advance behind the base of the tongue.

Step 12: As the tube tip passes under the tongue, rotate the tube back to midline (blue orientation line faces chin).

Step 13: Advance the King LT until the base of the connector aligns with the teeth or gums.

Step 14: Inflate the cuff with the appropriate volume of air (refer to manufacturer's recommendations). A small outward movement of the tube is often noted as the device seats itself in the hypopharynx.

Step 15: Attach bag-valve mask and initiate ventilations.

Step 16: Confirm effective placement by $EtCO_2$ detection, auscultation of lung sounds, and misting in the tube.

Step 17: Secure tube using adhesive tape or a commercial tube holder device.

Technique

- Failure to provide adequate airway protection or ventilation
- Can induce vomiting and aspiration
- Oropharyngeal trauma from insertion

COMBITUBE (FIGURE 59-17)

Indications

Patients >16 years old between 48 and 84 in in height with an absent gag reflex who have impending or actual loss of airway patency or protection[16]

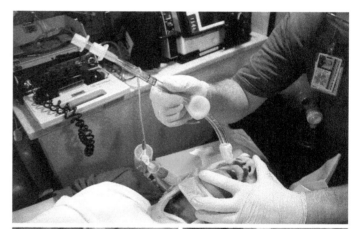
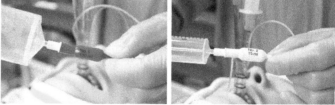
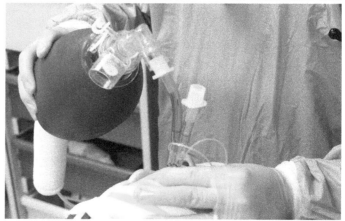

FIGURE 59-17. CombiTube placement. (Top) CombiTube. (Middle) After placement two separate balloons are inflated using two different sized syringes. (Bottom) Typically the longer blue tube will be ventilated and the shorter clear tube can be used to place an orogastric tube.

Essential Equipment

- CombiTube
- Two inflation syringes
- Suction system
- Endotracheal tube holder or tape
- Water-soluble lubricant

Technique

Step 1: Visually inspect the device for damage.

Step 2: Inflate both cuffs with maximum amount of air to verify patency.

Step 3: Deflate cuffs completely for insertion.

Step 4: Apply water-soluble lubricant to the beveled tip and posterior aspect of the tube. Do not introduce lubricant into the ventilation ports.

Step 6: Inspect the patient's mouth and remove all debris or dentures before insertion.

Step 7: Preoxygenate and implement standard monitoring procedures.

Step 8: If not contraindicated (suspected C-spine injury), place the patient in the "sniffing position." If suspected C-spine injury, place the patient in neutral position.

Step 9: Lift the mandible anteriorly, keeping the C-spine aligned as appropriate.

Step 10: Holding the CombiTube in the other hand, with its curve toward the hypopharynx, insert the tip into the oropharynx and advance it into the pharynx and esophagus.

Step 11: Advance gently until the black printed lines on the proximal end of the tubing straddles the teeth or gums.

Step 12: Inflate the proximal cuff with approximately 100 cc of air. The device will move slightly as it seats itself in the airway.

Step 13: Inflate the distal cuff with approximately 15 cc of air.

Step 14: Attach the bag-valve mask to the port labeled #1 (blue tube) and initiate ventilations.

Step 15: Auscultate lung sounds bilaterally.

- If lung sounds are present, epigastric sounds are absent and the chest rises, the device is positioned in the esophagus. Continue ventilations.
- If there is no chest rise and lung sounds are absent, or epigastric sounds are heard, attempt ventilation through the port labeled #2 (clear tube).
  - Auscultate breath sounds bilaterally again.
  - If breath sounds are present and the chest rises, the tube has been placed into the trachea. Continue ventilations.

Step 16: Ensure that the proximal and distal cuffs are inflated and continue ventilations.

Step 17: Secure tube using adhesive tape or a commercial tube holder device.

Technique

- Failure to provide adequate airway protection or ventilation
- Can induce vomiting and aspiration
- Oropharyngeal and esophageal trauma from insertion

SURGICAL AIRWAY PROCEDURES

When standard and rescue airway techniques fail, surgical airway techniques may be performed as a last resort. These are the "cannot intubate, cannot ventilate scenarios."[17] Surgical airway techniques may be the initial method of airway stabilization in patients with severe facial trauma or obvious obstructions to standard orotracheal intubations.

Indications

Patients requiring airway stabilization who have severe facial trauma, obvious obstructions to orotracheal intubation, or failed attempts at standard nonsurgical airway techniques

Essential Equipment

- Cricothyroidotomy
  - Cuffed endotracheal tube (size 5 or 6)
  - Scalpel (No. 11)
  - Hemostats
  - Tracheal hook
  - 4 ×4 gauze/sponges
  - Antiseptic swabs
- Percutaneous cricothyroidotomy using Seldinger technique
  - Commercial cricothyrotomy kit
  - Scalpel (No. 11)
  - 4 × 4 gauze/sponges
  - Antiseptic swabs
  - Syringe
  - Sterile water or saline
- Needle cricothyrotomy
  - Over-the-needle catheter, 16 or 18 ga, 8.5 cm (for pediatrics)
  - 10 mL Syringe
  - Scalpel (No. 11)
  - 4 × 4 gauze/sponges
  - Antiseptic swabs
  - Nasal cannula or oxygen tubing with Y-connector

Technique: Cricothyroidotomy (**Figure 59-18**)

Step 1: Position the patient supine, with the neck in a neutral position.

Step 2: Clean the patient's neck using antiseptic swabs.

Step 3: Identify the cricothyroid membrane, between the thyroid and cricoid cartilage.

Step 4: Using the nondominant hand, use the thumb and index or middle finger to stabilize the trachea.

Step 5: Make a stab incision through the skin between the two cartilages entering about 1 to 1.5 cm.

Step 6: Position the scalpel horizontally and make a 0.75-cm transverse incision through the cricothyroid membrane.

Step 7: Turn the scalpel 180° and extend the incision 0.75 cm off midline in the opposite direction and place the tracheal hook into the opening prior to removing the scalpel.*

Step 8: Remove the scalpel and using a tracheal hook, lift the caudal end of the opening to allow passage of a cuffed endotracheal tube directly into the trachea (No. 5 or No. 6).

Step 9: Inflate the cuff and attach the bag-valve mask and initiate ventilation.

Step 10: Confirm placement by assessing chest rise, presence of lung sounds, absence of epigastric sounds, and $ETCO_2$ detection (capnography preferred).

Step 11: Secure the tube in place with commercial device or adhesive tape.

Alternative Technique

Step 7(alt): Instead of placing the tracheal hook, place a bougie down into the airway heading caudally.

Step 8(alt): Now place a 6-0 cuffed endotracheal tube over the bougie and into the ostomy. Inflate the cuff and remove the bougie.

Step 9(alt): Attach the bag-valve mask and initiate ventilation.

Step 10(alt): Confirm placement by assessing chest rise, presence of lung sounds, absence of epigastric sounds, and $ETCO_2$ detection (capnography preferred).

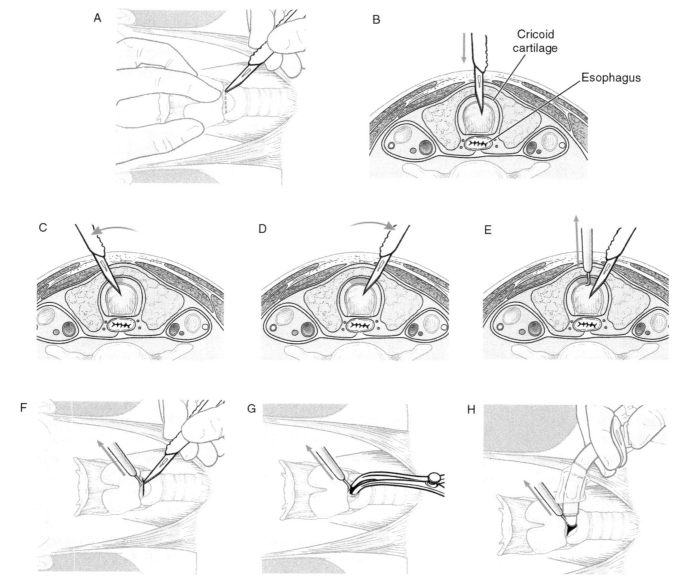

FIGURE 59-18. Surgical cricothyroidotomy. (Reprinted with permission from Reichman EF, ed. *Emergency Medicine Procedures*. 2nd ed. New York, NY: McGraw-Hill; 2013.)

Step 11(alt): Secure the tube in place with commercial device or adhesive tape.

Technique

- Entering with the scalpel too deep and injuring the esophagus
- Unrecognized misplacement of the endotracheal tube
- Aspiration of gastric contents
- Subglottic and laryngeal stenosis
- Placement can cause vocal cord injury, esophageal and tracheal lacerations
- Must monitor closely for mediastinal emphysema
- Performed in a very vascular region leading to the potential for hemorrhage

*Technique: Percutaneous Cricothyrotomy Using Seldinger Technique (*Figure 59-19*)*

Step 1: Position the patient supine, with the neck in a neutral position.

Step 2: Clean the patient's neck using antiseptic swabs.

Step 3: Identify the cricothyroid membrane, between the thyroid and cricoid cartilage.

Step 4: Using the nondominant hand, use the thumb and index or middle finger to stabilize the trachea.

Step 5: Attach the needle with the sheath in to the syringe and fill the syringe with a small amount of water or saline.

Step 6: Insert the needle into the cricothyroid membrane at a 45° angle caudally while applying negative pressure to the syringe. The presence of bubbles in the syringe will confirm that you are in the trachea.

Step 7: Once air is aspirated into the syringe, advance the catheter sheath over the needle into the trachea and remove the needle.

Step 8: Advance the guidewire through the sheath into the trachea and remove the sheath.

Step 9: Using a 15-blade scalpel, make a 0.5-cm vertical incision on both sides of the guidewire. *Do not cut wire.*

Step 10: Insert the dilator/airway tube combination over the guidewire and advance until it is flush against the skin.

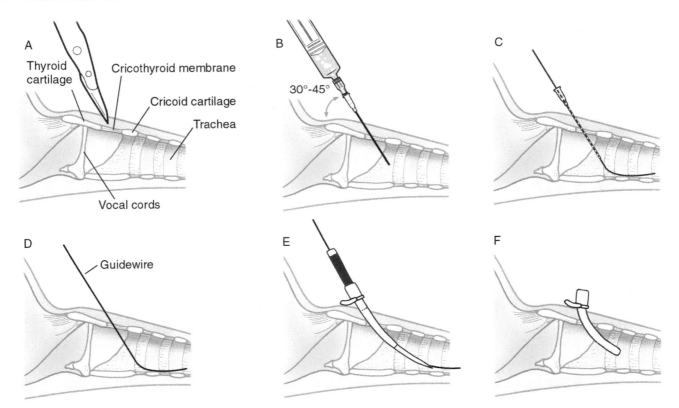

FIGURE 59-19. Percutaneous cricothyrotomy using Seldinger technique. (Reprinted with permission from Reichman EF, ed. *Emergency Medicine Procedures*. 2nd ed. New York, NY: McGraw-Hill; 2013.)

Step 11: Once the airway tube is in place, remove the dilator and guidewire.

Step 12: Inflate the cuff, attach bag-valve mask, and initiate ventilations.

Step 13: Confirm placement by assessing chest rise, presence of lung sounds, absence of epigastric sounds, and ETCO$_2$ detection (capnography preferred).

Step 14: Secure the tube in place with commercial device or adhesive tape.

Technique

- Unrecognized misplacement of the endotracheal tube
- Aspiration of gastric contents
- Subglottic and laryngeal stenosis
- Placement can cause vocal cord injury, esophageal and tracheal lacerations
- Must monitor closely for mediastinal emphysema
- Performed in a very vascular region leading to the potential for hemorrhage

Technique: Needle Cricothyrotomy With Transtracheal Jet Insufflation (**Figure 59-20**)

Step 1: Position the patient supine, with the neck in a neutral position.

Step 2: Clean the patient's neck using antiseptic swabs.

Step 3: Identify the cricothyroid membrane, between the thyroid and cricoid cartilage.

Step 4: Using the nondominant hand, use the thumb and index or middle finger to stabilize the trachea.

Step 5: Attach the needle with the sheath in to the syringe and fill the syringe with a small amount of water or saline.

Step 6: Insert the needle into the cricothyroid membrane at a 45° angle caudally while applying negative pressure to the syringe. The presence of bubbles in the syringe will confirm that you are in the trachea.

Step 7: Once air is aspirated into the syringe, advance the catheter sheath over the needle into the trachea and remove the needle.

Step 8: *Crucial step*: Reattach syringe and reconfirm tracheal position.

Step 9: Attach high-pressure manual jet ventilator to catheter (**Figure 59-21**).

Step 10: Begin ventilation at approximate ratio of 1 second insufflation to 5 seconds of exhalation; watch carefully that the chest falls after ventilation, signifying sufficient expiration.

Step 11: *Manually secure the catheter at all times* until more definitive airway control has been secured.

Technique

- Inadequate ventilation/hypoxia and hypercarbia
- Performed in a very vascular region leading to the potential for hemorrhage
- May lead to posterior tracheal wall/thyroid perforation or esophageal laceration.
- Placement can cause vocal cord injury, esophageal and tracheal lacerations
- Must monitor closely for mediastinal emphysema

▓ RETROGRADE INTUBATION

Equipment

- 68- to 80-cm spring guidewire with a J tip
- 16- to 18-gauge catheter over the needle (angiocatheter)
- Endotracheal tubes, various sizes
- Antiseptic swabs
- Sterile saline
- 10-mL syringes
- 18-gauge needles

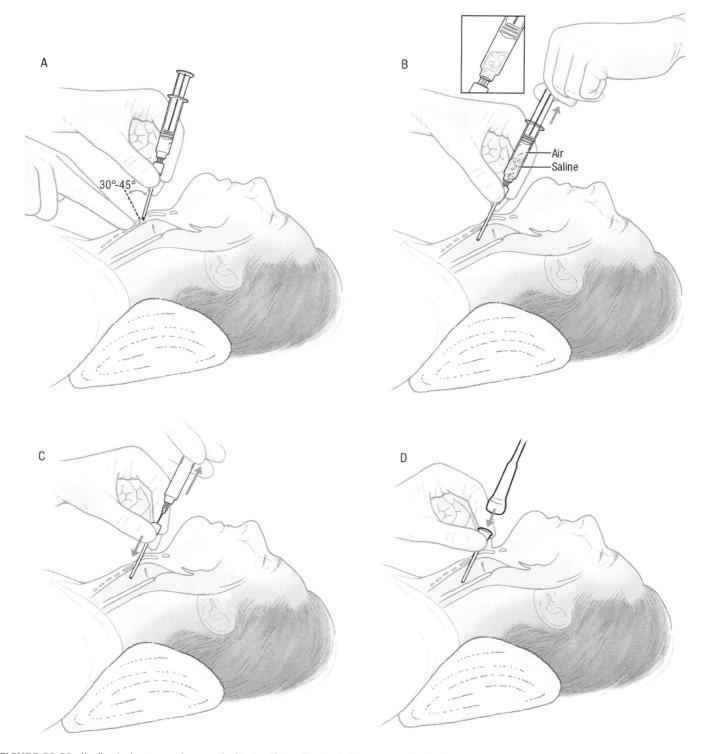

FIGURE 59-20. Needle cricothyrotomy with transtracheal jet insufflation. (Reprinted with permission from Reichman EF, ed. *Emergency Medicine Procedures*. 2nd ed. New York, NY: McGraw-Hill; 2013.)

- Hemostats, 2
- Magill forceps
- 20-mL syringe
- PPE
- Bag-valve device
- Oxygen source and tubing
- Suction source and tubing

- Yankauer suction catheter
- 1% lidocaine or spray anesthetic
- Adhesive tape or a commercial tube holder

Technique (**Figure 59-22**)

Step 1: Position the patient supine, with the neck in a neutral position.

Step 2: Clean the patient's neck using antiseptic swabs.

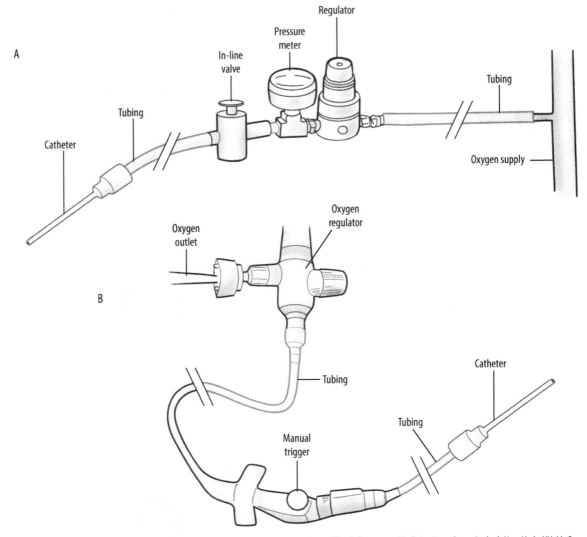

FIGURE 59-21. Transtracheal jet insufflation systems. (Reprinted with permission from Reichman EF, ed. *Emergency Medicine Procedures*. 2nd ed. New York, NY: McGraw-Hill; 2013.)

Step 3: Identify the cricothyroid membrane, between the thyroid and cricoid cartilage.

Step 4: Using the nondominant hand, use the thumb and index or middle finger to stabilize the trachea.

Step 5: Attach the needle with the sheath in to the syringe and fill the syringe with a small amount of water or saline.

Step 6: Insert the needle cephalad through the cricothyroid membrane at a 20° to 30° angle while applying negative pressure to the syringe. The loss of resistance signifies that the needle is in the larynx.

Step 7: Aspirated air into the syringe. The presence of bubbles in the syringe will confirm placement.

Step 8: Advance the catheter sheath over the needle into the trachea and remove the needle.

Step 9: Advance the guidewire through the sheath and into the oropharynx. The guidewire may exit the patient's mouth or nose. Retrieve the guidewire with the Magill forceps.

Step 10: Continue to advance the guidewire through the mouth (or nose) until 4 to 5 cm of wire remains protruding from the patient's neck.

Step 11: Carefully remove the catheter from the patient's neck while firmly holding the guidewire.

Step 12: Place a hemostat on the guidewire where it enters the patient's neck to ensure it does not get pulled into the trachea.

Step 13: Lubricate the endotracheal tube (ETT) liberally and insert the guidewire through the Murphy eye into the ETT.

Step 14: While holding the proximal end of the guidewire to maintain control, advance the ETT over the guidewire until resistance is met. The tip of the ETT should lie inside the cricothyroid membrane.

Step 15: Hold the proximal end of the guidewire firmly and release the hemostat.

Step 16: Pull the proximal end of the guidewire until it is seen disappear into the patient's neck and just into the trachea (5-6 cm).

Step 17: Advance the endotracheal tube until it is 20 to 21 cm (adult female) or 22 to 23 cm (adult male) at the teeth.

Step 18: Hold the endotracheal tube securely at the patient's lips and withdraw the guidewire through the patient's mouth.

Step 19: Inflate the endotracheal balloon with air, attach bag-valve mask, and initiate ventilations.

Step 20: Assess for proper tube placement using an end-tidal CO_2 detector (capnography or colorimetric), auscultation over the epigastrium, and auscultation of both lung fields for symmetry.

Step 21: Continue ventilations and secure the tube using a commercial tube holder or adhesive tape.

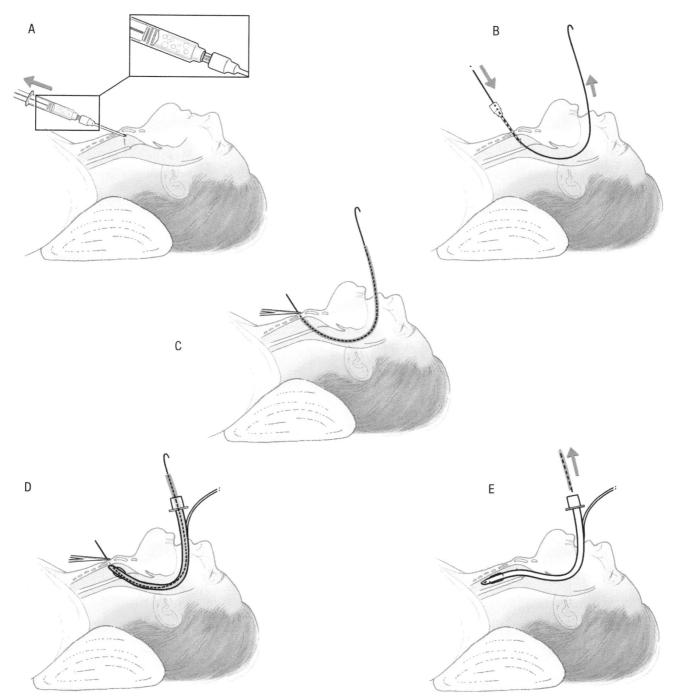

FIGURE 59-22. Retrograde intubation. (Reprinted with permission from Reichman EF, ed. *Emergency Medicine Procedures*. 2nd ed. New York, NY: McGraw-Hill; 2013.)

Technique

- Same as those associated with standard endotracheal intubation as well as needle cricothyrotomy (see those sections for further details).

▣ AIRWAY PLACEMENT CONFIRMATORY DEVICES

Once an advanced airway has been established by either nonsurgical or surgical methods, most commonly endotracheal intubation, supraglottic device placement, percutaneous or surgical cricothyrotomy, confirmation of placement can be augmented through end-tidal carbon dioxide (CO_2) detection. The devices available to determine end-tidal CO_2 range from continuous quantitative capnometers to a simple colorimetric device.

Colorimetric Carbon Dioxide Detector (EasyCap) The EasyCap is a commonly used single use device that changes color from purple to yellow in the presence of exhaled CO_2. It is placed directly in line on the end of the ETT. When adequate perfusion and unobstructed ventilation is present, colorimetric change from purple to yellow occurs. Colorimetric capnometers are 99% sensitive in ensuring ETT placement, but are not accurate enough for precise end-tidal CO_2 determinations.

Capnography Capnography displays real-time characteristic carbon dioxide waveforms. A persistent positive capnograph formation after clear and direct visualization of tube placement strongly supports proper tube placement.

Table 59-1 Conditions Associated With False Colorimetric or False Capnographic CO_2 Readings

False Negative Reading	Comments
Low pulmonary perfusion—cardiac arrest, inadequate chest compressions during CPR, massive pulmonary embolism	—
Massive obesity	—
Severe pulmonary edema	Secretions may obstruct the tube
False-positive reading	Comments
Recent ingestion of carbonated beverage	Will not persist beyond six breaths
Heated humidifier, nebulizer, or endotracheal epinephrine	Transient

Reprinted with permission from Tintinalli JE, Stapczynski JS, Ma OJ, Cline DM, Cydulka RK, Meckler GD, eds. *Tintinalli's Emergency Medicine: A Comprehensive Study, 7th ed*. New York, NY: McGraw-Hill; 2011.

Technique There are a few conditions associated with false colorimetric or capnographic CO_2 readings (**Table 59-1**).

VENTILATORS

Ventilators are pressure or volume cycled. Ventilators are routinely used in the emergency department setting, and less commonly used in the prehospital setting. Decisions with regard to mechanical ventilatory support include rate, mode, fraction of inspired oxygen minute ventilation, use of PEEP, continuous positive airway pressure, or bilevel pressure ventilation. Given the complexity of decisions required to properly use a ventilator, specialized training by prehospital providers is required. Ventilators are expensive. Coupled with specialized training needs, they are often cost prohibitive for many EMS agencies.

Ventilators are most commonly seen in aeromedical services. Aeromedical services are often involved in prolonged transport (transfers) and high acuity patient care. Aeromedical service personnel are usually highly trained critical specialists with training in ventilator use.

VASCULAR ACCESS

Vascular access provides the safe infusion of medications (short and long term), intravenous fluid hydration, blood products, and nutritional supplements.

PERIPHERAL VENOUS ACCESS

Peripheral venous access is intended for short duration use. Its ease of insertion, low cost, and low-complication risk make it the preferred method in the prehospital setting.[18]

Indication

Fluid resuscitation and medication administration

Essential Equipment

- PPE
- Angiocatheter—appropriate size 14 to 25 gauge
- Tourniquet
- Antiseptic solution/swabs—alcohol, chlorhexidine
- Gauze
- Tegaderm or transparent dressing
- Tape
- Blood collection tubes
- Saline lock set

Technique

Step 1: Select appropriate angiocatheter size based on intravenous (IV) site selection.

Step 2: Set up and "prime" saline lock.

Step 3: Apply tourniquet above IV site.

Step 4: Visualize and palpate vein.

Step 5: Cleanse IV site with antiseptic swab.

Step 6: Remove angiocatheter and inspect to verify there are no tears in the catheter sheath.

Step 7: Apply countertension at the IV site to stabilize the vein.

Step 8: Insert the angiocatheter through the skin at a 45° angle and then reduce the angle as you advance through the vein.

Step 9: Once the selected vein has been penetrated, "flash" will be observed as blood slowly fills the flash chamber.

Step 10: Once "flash" is observed, advance the needle slightly (0.5-1 cm) into the vein.

Step 11: Stabilize the catheter with your thumb and index finger and advance the catheter into the vein while simultaneously retracting the needle. Once the needle is fully retracted, it will lock in place.

Step 12: Remove tourniquet.

Step 12: Attach "primed" saline lock. Withdraw to verify blood return and flush with normal saline to ensure patency.

Step 13: Secure in place with Tegaderm, Venoguard, or adhesive tape.

Step 14: Place the needle into the sharps container.

Ultrasound-Guided IV Placement: Ultrasound-guided peripheral intravenous line placement is a useful and time-saving procedure. Indications for ultrasound-guided line placement include the following: failed traditional IV placement, the obese, edematous, or dehydrated patient where anatomy is difficult to visualize, significant burn injury, or sclerosed veins from repeat cannulizations or from intravenous drug use. In 2005, Costantino et al compared ultrasound-guided PIV access with the traditional blind technique and found that ultrasound-guided placement was more successful, required less time, reduced the number of needle punctures, and improved patient satisfaction.[19]

Success to ultrasound-guided peripheral line placement includes preparation, the appropriate equipment, the appropriate ultrasound probe, and cooperation of the patient. Angiocatheter needles of 1.88 to 2.5 in are recommended to avoid catheter dislodgment and infiltration. The high-frequency (7.5-10 MHz) linear probe is preferred over the curvilinear probe. The linear probe produced high resolution images of superficial structures. Appropriate vein choice is also critical to a successful cannulation. An article by Witting et al demonstrated higher success rates with picking a vein of a diameter of at least 0.4 cm and a depth no greater than 1.5 cm.[20]

Essential Equipment

- Angiocatheter needles (1.88-2.5 in).
- Ultrasound machine
- High-frequency linear probe
- Tegaderm
- Sterile gel
- Tourniquet
- Extension tubing
- Saline-filled syringes for flushes
- Skin preparatory materials (eg, Betadine, chlorhexidine, alcohol)
- Sterile gel

Technique

Step 1: Turn on the ultrasound machine.

Step 2: On a clean linear probe, place a Tegaderm to create a sterile field.

Step 3: Place a tourniquet in a high position of the arm.

Step 4: Using ChloraPrep create a large sterile field.

Step 5: Place sterile lubricant on the Tegaderm of the linear probe.

Step 6: Using the nondominant hand, locate the basilica vein on the medial aspect of the proximal arm.

Step 7: Center the vessel on the ultrasound monitor. One may utilize the horizontal or transverse approach for visualization and cannulization.

Step 8: Verification of the vein can be done with color Doppler. Further verification is done by determining the compressibility of the vessel. Veins collapse with compression and arteries maintain their contour.

Step 9: Using the dominant hand, insert the needle at a 45° angle to the skin. The insert point should be the same distance in front of the transducer as the depth of the vein.

Step 10: Upon insertion of the needle, visualization of the needle tip and following it through until a flashback of blood is noted in the angiocatheter is necessary. Look for the ring down artifact from the tip of the needle and the bull's eye sign on the ultrasound screen.

Step 11: US is two-dimensional; therefore, it may appear that one has cannulated the vessel when in reality, the needle is lateral to the vein.

Step 12: Upon entry into the vein, continue with usual and customary placement of a peripheral IV.

Technique

Cellulitis/infection at site—inoculating circulation with bacteria

Superficial thrombophlebitis, local tissue injury

Interstitial leakage

Limited access if massive edema, burn/injury site

Inadequate vascular flow if extremity with indwelling fistula or ipsilateral mastectomy

Easily occluded

Failure to check for flow into vein may lead to fluid extravasation.

Flow limited by small lumen of peripheral vein

CENTRAL VENOUS ACCESS

Central venous access is uncommon in the prehospital setting. If properly trained and the required equipment is available, a large bore intravenous central-line catheter may be placed into the internal jugular, subclavian, or femoral vein. Access of these large diameter veins allows for rapid fluid resuscitation, blood product and medication administration.

Indications

Patients who require rapid fluid resuscitation or blood products and peripheral venous access cannot be obtained

Essential Equipment
- PPE
- Site cleaning swabs (alcohol, chlorhexidine) and sterile sponges
- Anesthetic (lidocaine with epinephrine) and syringe with 22- to 24-gauge needle
- Steele introducer needle
- Guide wire
- Scalpel
- Dilator
- Triple lumen catheter
- IV caps and sterile saline flushes
- Sutures and scissors
- Sterile gauze
- Tegaderm dressing

- Ultrasound (if available)
- ECG monitoring

Technique (Seldinger Technique)

Step 1: Place the patient in the supine position and attach to ECG monitoring.

Step 2: Landmark the access site

- *Internal jugular (central approach)*: For a right-sided entry, turn the patient's head to the left. At the apex of the triangle formed by the two heads of the sternocleidomastoid muscle, locate the internal jugular vein lateral to the carotid artery. If no ultrasound guidance available, advance needle toward the ipsilateral nipple at a 30° to 45° angle to the skin, aspirating while advancing.
  - *Anterior approach*: Insert the needle at the anterior portion of the sternocleidomastoid at the level of the cricoid cartilage. The remainder of the approach and procedure is the same.
  - *Posterior approach*: Insert the needle at the posterior edge of the sternocleidomastoid at approximately 2 to 3 cm proximal from the clavicle.
- *Subclavian*: Turning the patient's head to the left, locate the midpoint of the clavicle; insert needle 1 cm lateral and inferior to the clavicle, at a 10° to 15° angle, diving under the clavicle and aiming for the suprasternal notch. Aspirating into the needle advance parallel to the skin 2 to 3 cm till venous return noted.
  - *Supraclavicular approach*: The supraclavicular approach is a second approach to the subclavian vein. Insert the needle 1 cm lateral to the lateral head of the sternocleidomastoid and 1 cm supraclavicular. Introduce the need and direct it toward the contralateral nipple. Aspirate as the needle is advanced and blood return should occur at approximately 2 to 3 cm upon entry into the skin. When placing the catheter, the length should be 2 to 4 cm less than compared to the infraclavicular approach.
- *Femoral*: Placing left hand such that thumb points toward pubic symphysis and index finger points to the iliac crest, locate the femoral artery at the corner formed by the thumb and finger. Insert needle at a 45° angle to the skin, 1 to 2 cm medial to the femoral artery pulse, aspirating while advancing.

Step 3: Don surgical cap, procedure mask, sterile gown. and sterile gloves.

Step 4: Set up equipment and prepare sterile field.

Step 5: Prepare skin by applying three rounds of sterilizing solution with three separate sponges. During each round, solution should be applied in an expanding circular motion.

Step 6: Isolate procedural field with sterile drapes.

Step 7: Locate vein with sterile ultrasound guidance.

Step 8: Anesthetize—using sterile fine gauge needle infiltrate the skin around the vascular access site, forming a skin wheal using local anesthetic. Consider sedation in the restless/combative patient.

Step 9: Place introducer needle—insert into the skin directed as per ultrasound guidance to the vein aspirating as you advance. Once venous blood flows into syringe, advance ½ cm into vein ensuring entire lumen of needle is in the vein.

Step 10: Assess for proper placement—aspirate again to ascertain low-pressure dark venous return, and/or confirm with ultrasound.

Step 11: Remove the syringe from the needle, leaving needle in vein.

Step 12: Insert guide wire into introducer needle—align guide wire and advance the wire 10 to 15 cm into the vein using a smooth steady motion. Watch ECG for PVCs or dysrhythmias while advancing the wire. If resistance is encountered, do not use force. Hold wire at all times once introduced into vein.

Step 13: Holding wire in place, remove introducer needle—control the wire above and below the needle as it is threaded out.

Step 14: Make skin incision to facilitate insertion of dilator and the catheter lumen, along the guide wire, through full thickness of dermis.

Step 15: Dilator insertion—holding onto the wire, thread dilator over the wire and insert into vein—the dilator enables passage of the catheter into the vein. Holding the wire steady, remove the dilator, leaving wire in place in the vein.

Step 16: Catheter placement—thread catheter over the wire and insert into vein, ensuring wire is held in place at all times.

Step 17: Remove the guide wire.

Step 18: Flush and cap the lumens.

Step 19: Secure catheter to skin using sutures and apply occlusive dressing.

Ultrasound-Guided Approach

- *Internal jugular with ultrasound:* Setup for the procedure should be done in the usual fashion. Once the operator is sterile and the area is prepped and draped in a sterile fashion, the ultrasound machine may be prepped for sterile use. Ultrasound gel is applied to the probe. A sterile sleeve is placed over the probe and extends several feet to cover the cord to allow for a sterile field. A sterile rubber band is applied to the base of the linear probe. Gel is then applied to the sterile probe and the anatomical landmarks are identified. The leg can be abducted and rotated to assist with displacement of the artery from the vein for better visualization. Place the linear probe inferior to the midinguinal ligament in the transverse position. The vessels should be clearly identified. The needle is then introduced while one continues to visualize the vessels under ultrasound guidance. Once the femoral vein is accessed, then ultrasound guidance stops momentarily. Maintaining the sterile field, postprocedure, the linear ultrasound probe is used for verification of placement of the ultrasound.

- *Subclavian with ultrasound:* Once the operator is sterile and the area is prepped and draped in a sterile fashion, the ultrasound machine may be prepped for sterile use. The linear probe is chosen and ultrasound gel is applied. A sterile sleeve is placed over the probe and extends several feet to cover the cord to allow for a sterile field. A sterile rubber band is applied to the base of the linear probe. Gel is then applied to the sterile probe and the anatomical landmarks are identified. The leg can be abducted and rotated to assist with displacement of the artery from the vein for better visualization. The needle is then introduced while one continues to visualize the vessels under ultrasound guidance. Once the femoral vein is accessed, ultrasound guidance stops momentarily. Maintaining the sterile field, postprocedure, the linear ultrasound probe is used for verification of placement of the ultrasound.

- *Femoral with ultrasound:* Setup for the procedure should be done in the usual fashion. Once the operator is sterile and the area is prepped and draped in a sterile fashion, the ultrasound machine may be prepped for sterile use. Ultrasound gel is applied to the probe. A sterile sleeve is placed over the probe and extends several feet to cover the cord to allow for a sterile field. A sterile rubber band is applied to the base of the linear probe. Gel is then applied to the sterile probe and the anatomical landmarks are identified. The leg can be abducted and rotated to assist with displacement of the artery from the vein for better visualization. Place the linear probe inferior to the midinguinal ligament in the transverse position. The vessels should be clearly identified. The needle is then introduced while one continues to visualize the vessels under ultrasound guidance. Once the femoral vein is accessed, then ultrasound guidance stops momentarily. Maintaining the sterile field, postprocedure, the linear ultrasound probe is used for verification of placement of the ultrasound.

Technique

- Failure to identify a pneumothorax (subclavian or internal jugular approaches).
- Contamination of the sterile field may lead to local infection inoculated into central circulation.
- Distorted local anatomy in trauma and radiation therapy patients decreases the success of placement.

- Increased risk of bleeding in a coagulopathic patient or an accidental arterial puncture.
- Cervical spine immobilization limits the use of jugular venous access.
- Femoral access has increased risk of infection and way limit patient's mobility.

INTRAOSSEOUS ACCESS

The long bones of the body are highly vascular. Intraosseous (IO) vascular access penetrates the bone marrow cavities of these long bones, providing access to the venous circulation. IOs can be used in all age groups.

Indications

Emergent need for vascular access in case of cardiac arrest, trauma, or shock when rapid peripheral access cannot be obtained

Equipment

- PPE
- Large-bore needle—size 13- to 18-gauge IO needle
- Skin sterilization solution/swabs—alcohol, chlorhexidine
- Lidocaine 1% local anesthetic
- IO drill and Syringe set
- IO infusion set
- Gauze
- Tape

Technique

Step 1: Select site intraosseous insertion site.

- *Adult:* site of placement include proximal humerus, distal tibia, distal femur, or sternum
- *Pediatric:* most commonly used site is the proximal tibia, just distal to the tibial tuberosity

Step 2: Cleanse and sterilize the site using an expanding circular motion.

Step 3: Landmark IO site and anesthetize the skin forming a wheal using 1% lidocaine, inserting Lidocaine into the needle path as well as the periosteum of the bone. Vapocoolant spray may also be used on the skin.

Step 4: Stabilizing the extremity, puncture the skin with IO needle till the bone, angling away from the growth plate. Applying steady pressure onto drill driver, penetrate the cortex, and access the marrow space. If using a manual IO drill, use rotating or twisting motion to penetrate the cortex.

Step 5: Disconnect drill driver from needle, holding needle steady, unscrew needle hub, and attach syringe to needle.

Step 6: Aspirate blood/marrow to confirm placement.

Step 7: Connect IV tubing to IO needle and infuse under pressure.

Step 8: Apply adequate gauze around IO site to stabilize needle, and tape firmly in place.

Pitfalls/Contraindications

- Potential for osteomyelitis.
- Intraosseous needles left in the marrow for longer than 72 hours are at a higher risk of local infection.
- Safe for short-term access only.
- Challenges to access if infection or burn injury at the insertion site.
- Presence of fracture or major injury to the extremity proximal to the insertion site is a contraindication to obtaining IO access at that extremity.
- Failure to stabilize extremity or use adequate pain control in the awake patient.
- Incorrect placement of the needle can cause injury to the growth plate with resultant growth deformity.
- Dislodging of needle from medullary space or "through and through" insertion and subsequent infusion can lead to large volume extravasation into surrounding tissue spaces.

ARTERIAL LINES

Arterial lines are used for continuous arterial blood pressure measurements and blood gas analysis.

Indication

When there is a need for continuous monitoring of blood pressure and frequent arterial blood sampling

Essential Equipment

- Personal protective equipment—gloves
- Antiseptic solutions and swabs
- Local anesthetic
- Arterial set, pressurized saline bag with heparin
- Transducer and recording equipment
- Sutures and scissors
- Gauze
- Tape and Tegaderm

Technique (Radial Artery)

- Ascertain site by palpating for arterial pulse and anesthetize the skin.
- Cleanse and sterilize the site using an expanding circular motion.
- Stabilize the limb and artery, stretching skin over pulse.
- Insert arterial needle.
  - Radial artery—45° to 60° angle
  - Femoral artery—90° angle
- Aspirate while advancing, on noting flash in hub, advance catheter.
- Connect to pressure tubing and assess for arterial waveform.

- Secure arterial line; if femoral with sutures; tape and secure with Tegaderm; secure IV tubing with tape.

Technique

- Failure to perform Allen test prior to cannulation, in event of poor ulnar perfusion, if radial artery gets occluded, arterial flow to the hand will be reduced
- Risk of hemorrhage, air emboli, or thromboemboli
- Accidental administration of medications into an arterial line may cause severe irreversible damage
- Risk of local infection
- Arterial vasospasm leading to partial or complete occlusion of artery

NEONATAL VASCULAR ACCESS

Central lines: for administration of hypertonic fluids, long-term IV medication, and parenteral nutrition. Procedure similar to adult central-line access, placement must be confirmed with radiograph.

Peripheral access: can be used for administration of isotonic fluids, medication, or blood products. Neonatal peripheral lines can be placed in the hand (dorsal arch or cephalic vein at wrist), elbow (cubital fossa), foot (dorsal arch, saphenous vein at ankle), leg (saphenous vein at knee), or scalp (superficial temporal).

- Use of EMLA cream 60 minutes prior to insertion is recommended.
- As compared to adult peripheral lines, neonatal peripheral lines are poorly supported by soft tissue, much more fragile and might often need recannulation. If placed in an extremity, splinting, immobilizing joint, and proper securing of the line to the extremity is a must. Most importantly, they should be replaced every 48 to 72 hours to avoid complications—sepsis, cellulitis, phlebitis.

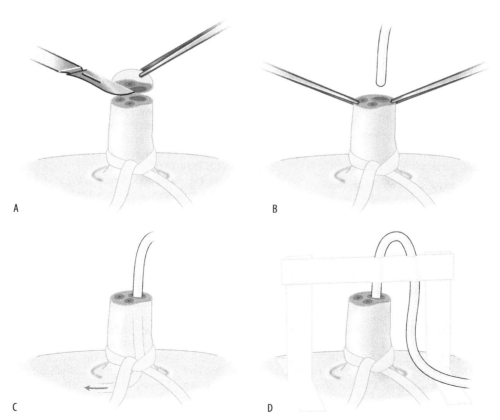

FIGURE 59-23. Umbilical vein cannulation. (Reprinted with permission from Tintinalli JE, Stapczynski JS, Ma OJ, Cline DM, Cydulka RK, Meckler GD, eds. *Tintinalli's Emergency Medicine: A Comprehensive Study*, 7th ed. New York, NY: McGraw-Hill; 2011.)

Umbilical lines: used in neonates for emergency resuscitation, medication infusions, exchange transfusions, and central venous access up to 1 week after birth providing CVP monitoring.

Umbilical Vein Catheterization (Figure 59-23)
Essential Equipment

- Personal protective equipment—sterile gloves, gown, and mask
- Sterile drapes and sheets
- Antiseptic solutions and swabs
- Umbilical catheter 3.5 to 5 F
- Clamps, forceps, and scalpel
- Suture (Silk 3.0), needle driver, scissors
- IV tubing and infusion solution
- Tape

Technique

Step 1: Cleanse and sterilize the site using an expanding circular motion.

Step 2: Drape the area and tape base of umbilical stump to stabilize.

Step 3: With scalpel cut the umbilical cord horizontally 1.5 to 2 cm from abdominal wall.

Step 4: Dilate the vein using forceps; remove any clots/thrombi; tighten umbilical tape to prevent bleeding from arteries.

Step 5: Prepare catheter by flushing with heparinized solution, and fill the lumen with infusion solution to avoid any air entry postinsertion into vein.

Step 6: Using the forceps to guide the catheter, insert catheter into umbilical vein aiming for the infant's right shoulder; once blood return is noted, advance an additional 1 to 2 cm, for a total of 4 to 5 cm in a full-term infant.

Step 7: To overcome resistance, the umbilical tape may be loosened or direction of insertion may be altered gradually. Do not force insertion if resistance does not decrease by previously noted maneuvers. Calculate insertion length by multiplying shoulder to umbilicus length by 0.6; this gives approximate position of the catheter past the ductus venosus to just below the right atrium.

Step 8: Secure catheter to umbilical cord with sutures and confirm placement of catheter with radiograph imaging.

Technique

- Identifying the incorrect vessel—vein versus artery
- Absolute contraindication in the presence of necrotizing enterocolitis, omphalitis, peritonitis
- Risk of hemorrhage, infection, perforation, air embolism
- Risk of portal vein thrombosis, hepatic abscess, or necrosis
- Dysrhythmias or pericardial perforation

REFERENCES

1. Strömsöe A, Svensson L, Axelsson ÅB, et al. Improved outcome in Sweden after out-of-hospital cardiac arrest and possible association with improvements in every link in the chain of survival. *Eur Heart J*. April 7, 2015;36(14):863-71.
2. Smith MW, Bentley MA, Fernandez AR, Gibson G, Schweikhart SB, Woods DD. Performance of experienced versus less experienced paramedics in managing challenging scenarios: a cognitive task analysis study. *Ann Emerg Med*. October 2013;62(4):367-379.
3. Cheskes S, Common MR, Byers PA, Zhan C, Morrison LJ. Compressions during defibrillator charging shortens shock pause duration and improves chest compression fraction during shockable out of hospital cardiac arrest. *Resuscitation*. August 2014;85(8):1007-1011.
4. Satterlee PA, Boland LL, Johnson PJ, Hagstrom SG, Page DI, Lick CJ. Implementation of a mechanical chest compression device as standard equipment in a large metropolitan ambulance service. *J Emerg Med*. October 2013;45(4):562-569.
5. Rubertsson S, Lindgren E, Smekal D, et al. Mechanical chest compressions and simultaneous defibrillation vs conventional cardiopulmonary resuscitation in out-of-hospital cardiac arrest: the LINC randomized trial. *JAMA*. January 1, 2014;311(1):53-61.
6. Smekal D, Lindgren E, Sandler H, Johansson J, Rubertsson S. CPR-related injuries after manual or mechanical chest compressions with the LUCAS™ device: A multicentre study of victims after unsuccessful resuscitation. *Resuscitation*. December 2014;85(12):1708-1712.
7. Sherbino J, Verbeek PR, MacDonald RD, Sawadsky BV, McDonald AC, Morrison LJ. Prehospital transcutaneous cardiac pacing for symptomatic bradycardia or bradyasystolic cardiac arrest: a systematic review. *Resuscitation*. August 2006;70(2):193-200.
8. Cheskes S, Turner L, Thomson S, Aljerian N. The impact of prehospital continuous positive airway pressure on the rate of intubation and mortality from acute out-of-hospital respiratory emergencies. *Prehosp Emerg Care*. October-December 2013;17(4):435-441.
9. Aguilar SA, Lee J, Dunford JV, et al. Assessment of the addition of prehospital continuous positive airway pressure (CPAP) to an urban emergency medical services (EMS) system in persons with severe respiratory distress. *J Emerg Med*. August 2013;45(2):210-219.
10. Williams TA, Finn J, Perkins GD, Jacobs IG. Prehospital continuous positive airway pressure for acute respiratory failure: a systematic review and meta-analysis. *Prehosp Emerg Care*. April-June 2013;17(2):261-273.
11. Diggs LA, Yusuf JE, De Leo G. An update on out-of-hospital airway management practices in the United States. *Resuscitation*. July 2014;85(7):885-892.
12. Hoffmann B, Gullett JP, Hill HF, et al. Bedside ultrasound of the neck confirms endotracheal tube position in emergency intubations. *Ultraschall Med*. October 2014;35(5):451-458.
13. Burnett AM, Frascone RJ, Wewerka SS, et al. Comparison of success rates between two video laryngoscope systems used in a prehospital clinical trial. *Prehosp Emerg Care*. April-June 2014;18(2):231-238.
14. Cooney DR, Cooney NL, Wallus H, Wojcik S. Performance of emergency physicians utilizing a video-assisted semi-rigid fiberoptic stylet for intubation of a difficult airway in a high-fidelity simulated patient: a pilot study. *Int J Emerg Med*. May 29, 2012;5(1):24.
15. Gahan K, Studnek JR, Vandeventer S. King LT-D use by urban basic life support first responders as the primary airway device for out-of-hospital cardiac arrest. *Resuscitation*. December 2011;82(12):1525-1528.
16. Wang HE, Szydlo D, Stouffer JA, et al. Endotracheal intubation versus supraglottic airway insertion in out-of-hospital cardiac arrest. *Resuscitation*. September 2012;83(9):1061-1066.
17. Wang HE, Mann NC, Mears G, Jacobson K, Yealy DM. Out-of-hospital airway management in the United States. *Resuscitation*. April 2011;82(4):378-385.
18. Engels PT, Passos E, Beckett AN, Doyle JD, Tien HC. IV access in bleeding trauma patients: a performance review. *Injury*. January 2014;45(1):77-82.
19. Costantino TG, Parikh AK, Satz WA, Fojtik JP. Ultrasonography-guided peripheral intravenous access versus traditional approaches in patients with difficult intravenous access. *Ann Emerg Med*. November 2005;46(5):456-461.
20. Witting MD, Schenkel SM, Lawner BJ, Euerle BD. Effects of vein width and depth on ultrasound-guided peripheral intravenous success rates. *J Emerg Med*. July 2010;39(1):70-75.

Acute Injury Management

CHAPTER 60

Danniel J. Stites
Andrew J. Harrell
Darren Braude

INTRODUCTION

Acute management of injuries in the field is one of the key components of routine emergency medical response. Although many controversies exist and will continue to arise concerning the indications for these interventions, when the decision is made to employ a procedure the technique should be performed properly. EMS physicians and medical directors must consider the impact of providers observing their technique and should always employ, and expect their providers to utilize, good technique. A step-by-step description of these interventions is included in this chapter.

PROCEDURES

- Spinal immobilization
  - From the ground
  - Standing takedown
  - Extrication device to long spine board
  - In-the-water immobilization
- Tourniquets
- Hemostatic bandages

GENERAL CONSIDERATIONS

The indications and need for spinal immobilization are highly controversial.[1] For instance, the NAEMSP/ACS-COT combined position paper questions the utility of long spine boards beyond initial extrication and some studies suggest that routine spinal immobilization of penetrating trauma patients who do not exhibit evidence of neurologic injury is unnecessary and potentially exposes the patient to unnecessary adverse effects.[2] Potential adverse effects include airway compromise, pain, pressure ulcers, and unnecessary radiographic imaging. This section will not address areas of controversy but will instead assume that spinal immobilization is necessary and indicated and that multiple techniques are potentially safe and acceptable when performing each skill and procedure (ie, log roll vs lift and slide). Of note, some EMS systems have replaced immobilization on a long spine board with spinal precautions on a firm mattress and utilize the long spine board primarily as a means of extrication. A recent study even showed better restriction in spinal movement when patients self-extricated wearing only a cervical collar.[3]

Indications Spinal immobilization may be performed in patients in whom there is significant concern for potential spinal cord injury. Concern for spinal cord injury may stem from mechanism, comorbid conditions, physical examination findings, or a combination of these factors. Some examples of patients who should be considered for spinal immobilization include patients with a high-energy mechanism of injury such as vehicle or motorcycle accidents, falls, and swimming/diving injuries in which prehospital clearance is impossible or impractical. Some examples of historical and physical examination findings that raise concern for spinal cord injury are complaints of neck pain, paresthesias, paralysis, and findings of midline tenderness or step-offs.

▩ FROM-THE-GROUND SPINAL IMMOBILIZATION TECHNIQUE

When victims are found down and/or are instructed to remain on the ground, spinal immobilization should take place from where they are found unless hazards prevent this approach.

Indication This technique may be considered when a patient requiring spinal immobilization is found lying supine or prone by EMS providers.

Essential Equipment

- Long spine board (LSB)
- Head immobilization device/tape/sandbags/towel rolls/ etc
- Semirigid cervical collar
- Straps/other devices to secure to LSB
- Sufficient manpower
- PPE

Technique

Step 1: First assume and maintain inline cervical spine alignment manually (**Figure 60-1**).

Step 2: Place semirigid cervical collar (**Figure 60-2**).

Step 3: The rescuer holding C-spine directs synchronous log roll of the patient w/ LSB placed (**Figure 60-3**).

Step 4: The patient and LSB rolled back as single unit (**Figure 60-4**).

Step 5: Patient's torso/pelvis/legs secured to LSB with straps first (**Figure 60-5**).

Step 6: Patient head immobilized w/ device to LSB last (**Figure 60-6**).

Pitfalls

- Failure to recognize spinal injury
- Failure to keep an awake patient informed of rescuer procedures and expectations
- Failure to maintain manual cervical spine control
- Failure to work as a team with all movements coordinated by the provider at the head of the patient
- Insufficient personnel to safely and effectively stabilize the patient
- Airway compromise

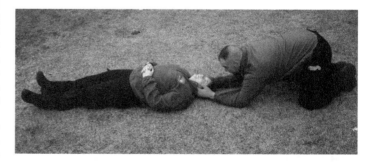

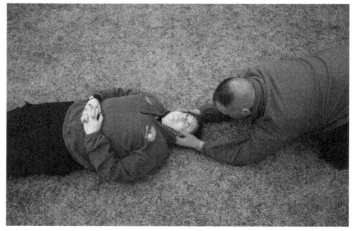

FIGURE 60-1. Manual immobilization of the C-spine.

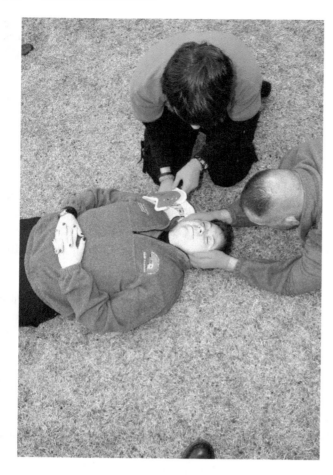

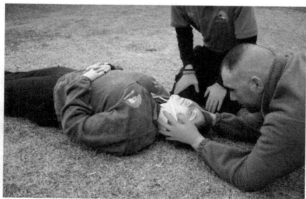

FIGURE 60-2. Placement of the C-collar.

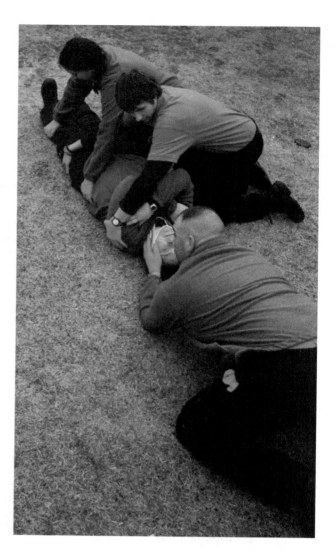

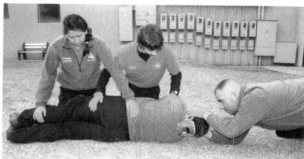

FIGURE 60-3. Log roll for inspection.

- Pain and discomfort
- Pressure ulcers from prolonged immobilization

■ STANDING TAKEDOWN SPINAL IMMOBILIZATION TECHNIQUE

While this remains a common technique in prehospital provider education, there is limited evidence beyond anecdotal accounts to support its use. In actual practice, ambulatory patients are often assisted to an LSB or mattress. Cervical spine immobilization can occur while the patient is standing, as illustrated below, prior to assisting the patient the a LSB or mattress.

Indication The standing takedown technique may be considered when a patient requiring spinal immobilization is found ambulatory or standing by EMS providers.

Essential Equipment

- Long spine board
- Head immobilization device/tape/sandbags/towel rolls/ etc
- Semirigid cervical collar
- Straps/other devices to secure to LSB
- Sufficient manpower
- PPE

Technique

Step 1: First assume and maintain inline cervical spine alignment manually from posterior approach to the standing patient (**Figure 60-7**).

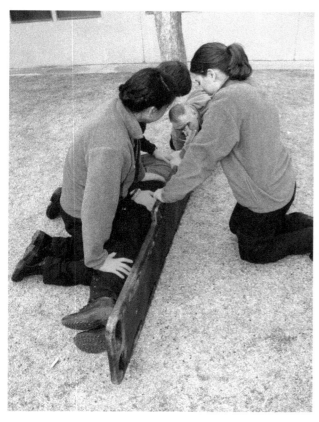
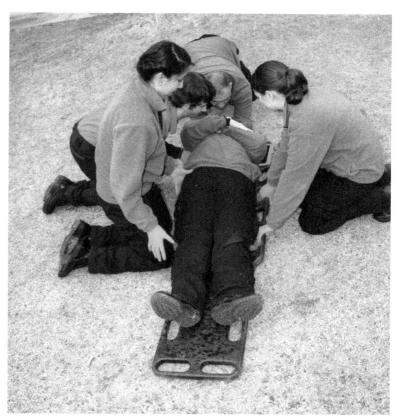

FIGURE 60-4. Log roll onto a long spine board.

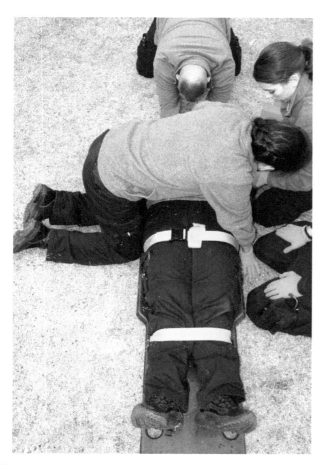
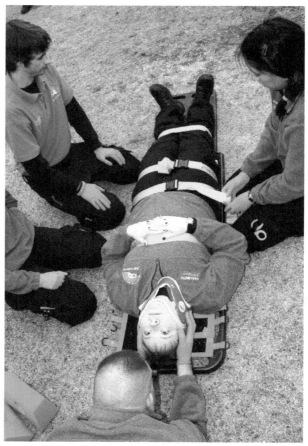

FIGURE 60-5. Strapping to the long spine board.

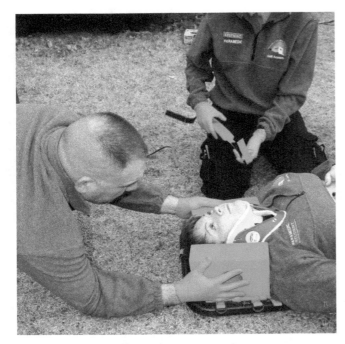

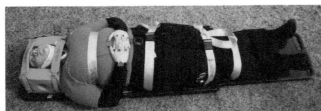

FIGURE 60-6. Head immobilized to the long spine board.

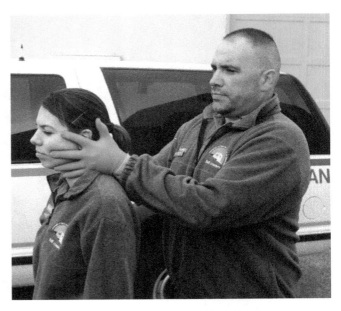

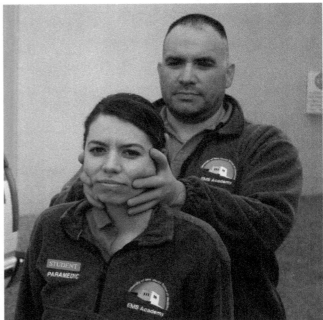

FIGURE 60-7. Standing takedown: inline cervical spine alignment.

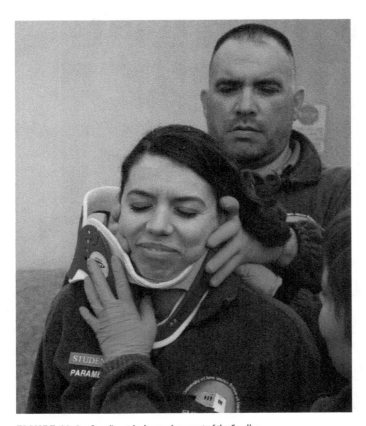

FIGURE 60-8. Standing takedown: placement of the C-collar.

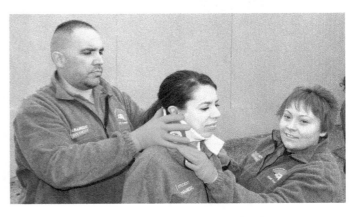

Step 5: C-spine rescuer directs backward lowering of the patient and LSB to ground surface (**Figure 60-11**).

Step 6: Patient torso/pelvis/legs secured to LSB w/ straps first (**Figure 60-12**).

Step 7: Patient head immobilized w/ device to LSB last (**Figure 60-13**).

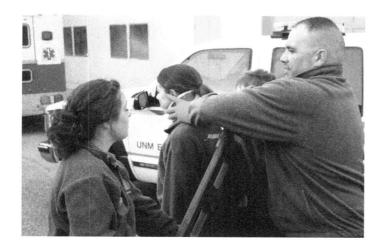

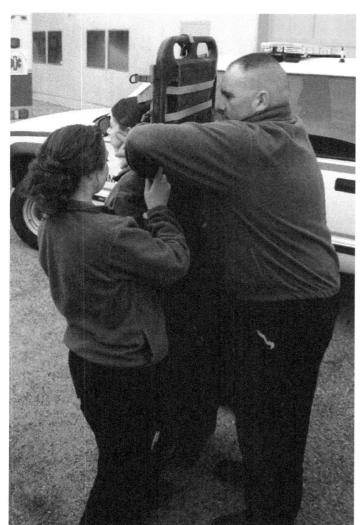

FIGURE 60-9. Standing takedown: placing the long spine board.

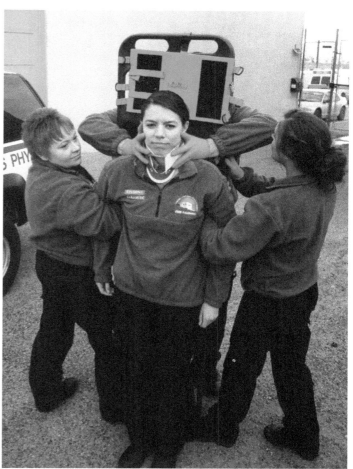

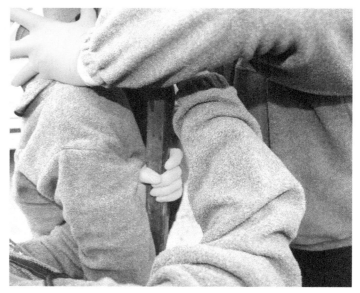

FIGURE 60-10. Standing takedown: support the patient.

Step 2: Place semirigid cervical collar (**Figure 60-8**).

Step 3: Place LSB upright between rescuer holding C-spine and patient's back (**Figure 60-9**).

Step 4: Additional rescuers grasp hand holds on LSB at level of patient's axilla to support the patient (**Figure 60-10**).

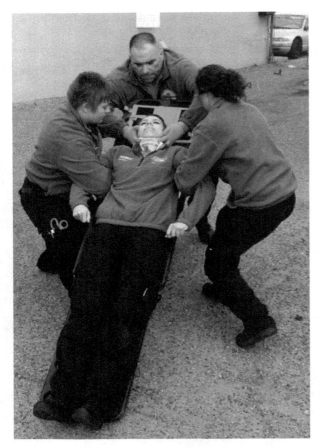

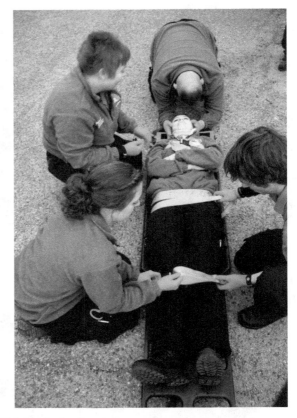

FIGURE 60-12. Standing takedown: securing to the long spine board.

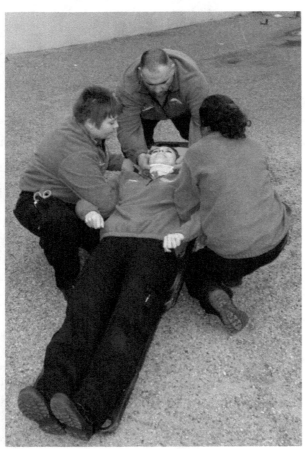

FIGURE 60-11. Standing takedown: backboard lowering.

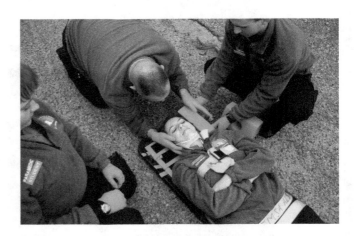

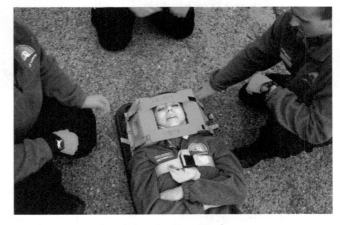

FIGURE 60-13. Standing takedown: head immobilization.

Pitfalls

- Failure to recognize potential spinal injury
- Failure to keep the patient informed of rescuer procedures and expectations
- Failure to maintain manual cervical spine control
- Failure to work as a team with all movements coordinated by the provider at the head of the patient
- Insufficient personnel to safely and effectively stabilize the patient

EXTRICATION DEVICE TO LONG SPINE BOARD SPINAL IMMOBILIZATION TECHNIQUE

A number of extrication devices designed to immobilize a patient from a closed space (usually seated in a motor vehicle) and aid in their extrication from that space and onto a long spine board. The most commonly references device is the Kendrick Extrication Device (K.E.D.).

Indication Used when a stable patient requiring spinal immobilization is found entrapped (ie, in a vehicle) with reduced access or within a confined space.

Essential Equipment

- Extrication device (K.E.D. is shown here) (**Figure 60-14**)
- Long spine board
- Head immobilization device/tape/sandbags/towel rolls/ etc
- Semirigid cervical collar
- Straps/other devices to secure to LSB
- Sufficient manpower
- PPE

Technique

Step 1: First assume and maintain inline cervical spine alignment manually from easiest approach to the injured patient (**Figure 60-15**).

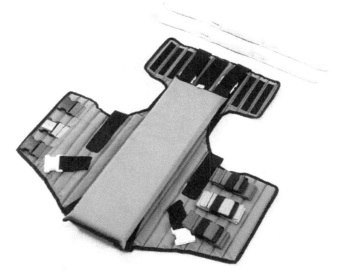

FIGURE 60-14. Kendrick Extrication Device (K.E.D.). (Reprinted with permission from Tintinalli JE, Stapczynski JS, Ma OJ, Cline DM, Cydulka RK, Meckler GD, eds. *Tintinalli's Emergency Medicine: A Comprehensive Study, 7th ed*. New York, NY: McGraw-Hill; 2011.)

Step 2: Place semirigid cervical collar (**Figure 60-16**).

Step 3: Additional rescuers place K.E.D upright behind the patient (**Figure 60-17**).

Step 4: Secure the patient firmly in K.E.D. utilizing color-coded strapping system (**Figure 60-18**).

Step 5: Secure head, chin, and leg straps (**Figure 60-19**).

Step 6: Extricate the patient utilizing K.E.D. haul straps and place on LSB (**Figure 60-20**).

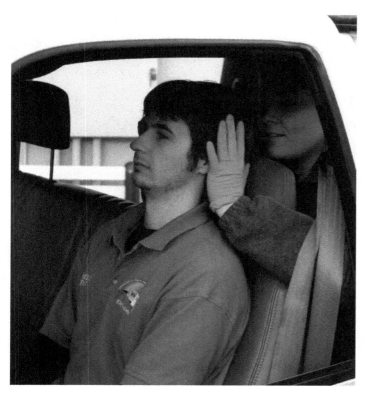

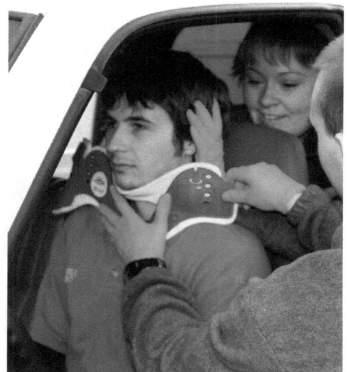

FIGURE 60-15. Extrication: inline C-spine immobilization.

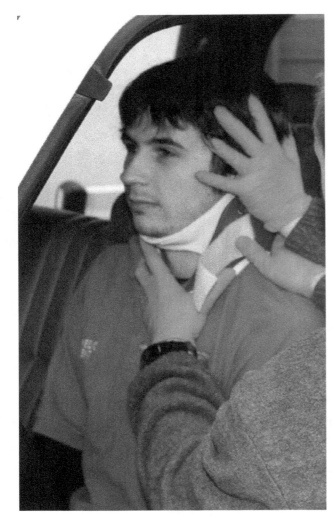

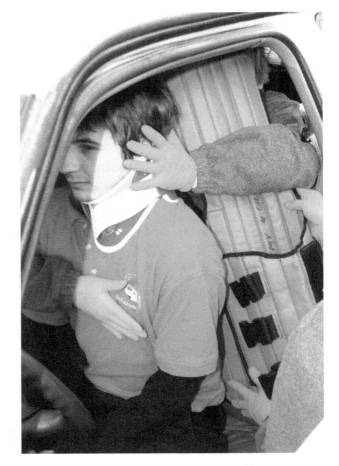

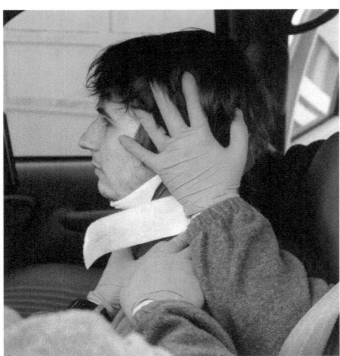

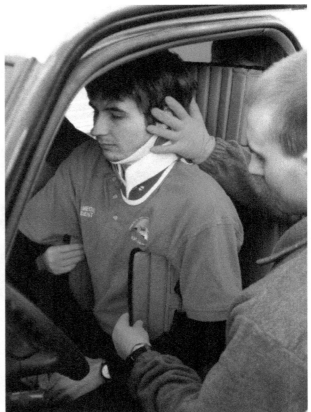

FIGURE 60-16. Extrication: placement of the C-collar.

FIGURE 60-17. Extrication: K.E.D. being placed.

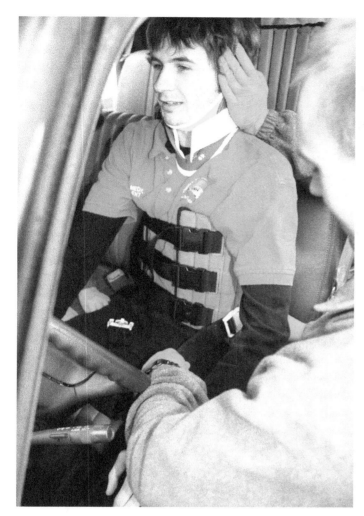

FIGURE 60-18. Extrication: securing torso.

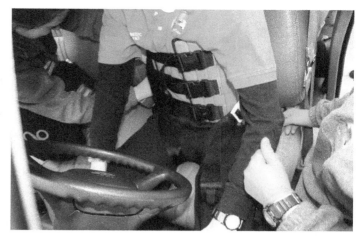

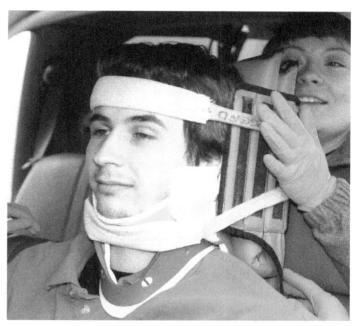

FIGURE 60-19. Extrication: securing the head, chin, and legs.

Step 7: Disconnect the leg straps, allowing the patient's legs to lay flat on the long spine board.

Step 8: Secure the patient in K.E.D. to LSB utilizing available patient restraint devices (**Figure 60-21**).

Pitfalls

- In unstable patients, in whom prolonged extrication time could be potentially fatal, the risks and benefits of expeditious extrication must be weighed. If expeditious extrication is performed, the cervical spine should not be ignored. Extrication even when performed quickly should still make every attempt to reduce spinal manipulation whenever possible.

- Forgetting to loosen or disconnect the leg straps when laying the patient on the LSB.

IN-THE-WATER SPINAL IMMOBILIZATION TECHNIQUE

Water rescue can take the form of different levels of technical rescue. The initial consideration of operational safety for rescuers should remain the primary concern in these situations. Presuming technical rescue is not required, or that the rescuers have the correct type and level of training, spinal immobilization may occur in otherwise safe conditions. Although deepwater backboard is possible, it may be impractical in most rescue operations and overall safety and maintaining the victim's airway above the water is the priority.

Indication For use when a patient requiring spinal immobilization is found in an aquatic environment.[4]

Essential Equipment

- Long spine board
- Head immobilization device/tape/sandbags/towel rolls/etc
- Semirigid cervical collar
- Straps/other devices to secure to LSB
- Sufficient manpower
- PPE

Technique

Step 1: Move the patient to a safe area to affect in-water immobilization—shallow, easiest to access—while maintaining cervical inline stabilization (**Figure 60-22**).

Step 2: Additional rescuers submerge LSB and move it under the patient, allowing it to rise up under the patient (**Figure 60-23**).

Step 3: The rescuer supporting the head holds the backboard and the patient while others secure the patient to LSB (**Figure 60-24**).

Step 4: Move head end of LSB toward egress point—shore, pool edge, boat transom (**Figure 60-25**).

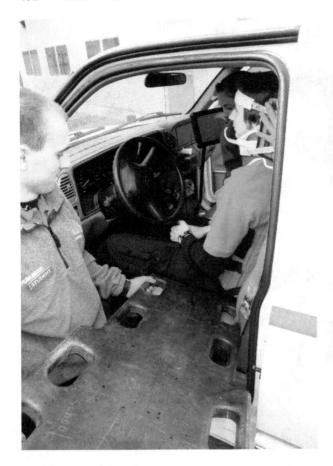

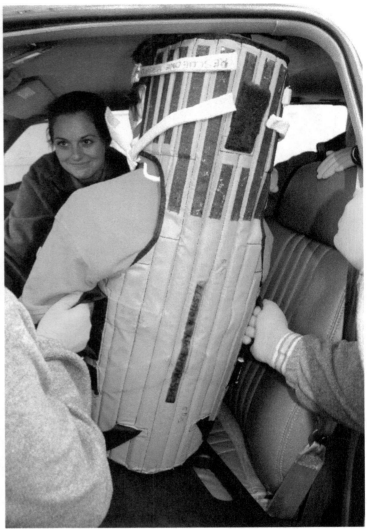

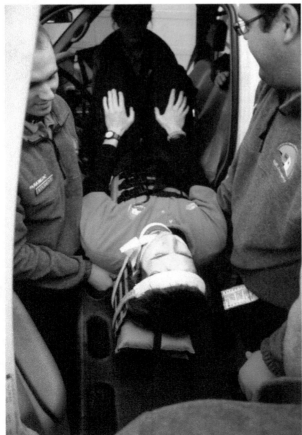

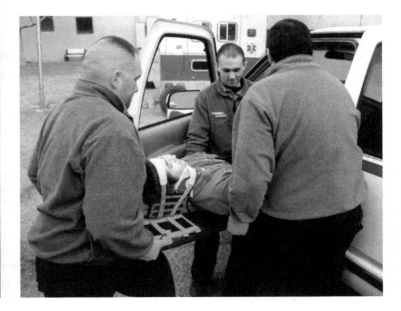

FIGURE 60-20. Extrication: extricating on the K.E.D.

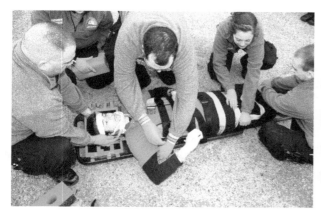

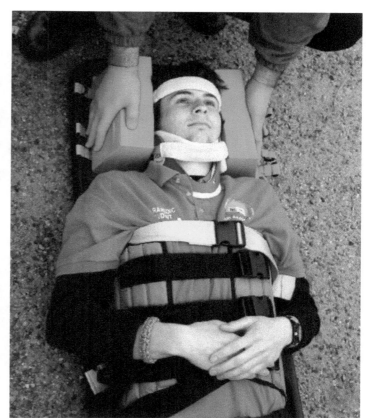

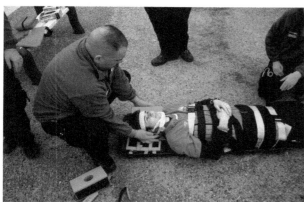

FIGURE 60-21. Extrication: securing to the long spine board.

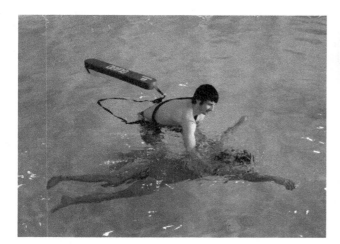

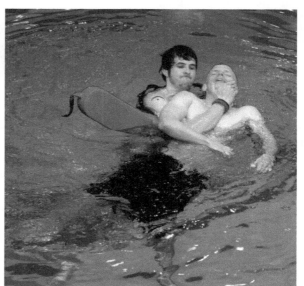

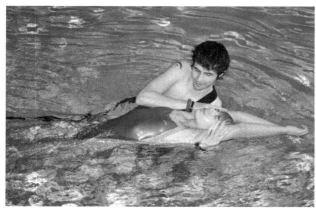

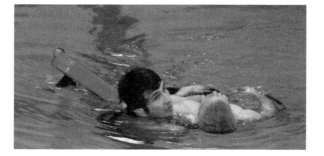

FIGURE 60-22. Water: move to a shallow, safe place.

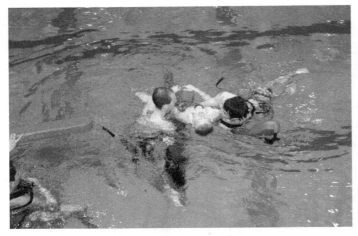

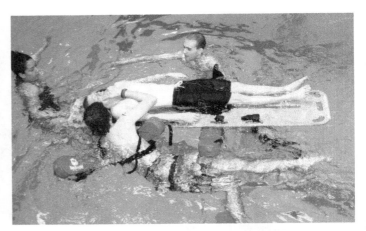

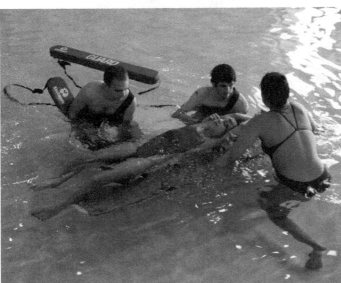

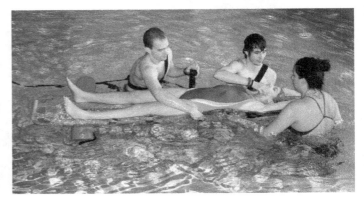

FIGURE 60-23. Water: submerging long spine board to move under the patient.

Step 5: Place head end of LSB on surface and slowly slide out of water (**Figure 60-26**).

Step 6: Ensure that the patient once removed from the water is moved an adequate distance from the water's edge to ensure the patient does not slide back into the water.

Pitfalls

- Failure to recognize potential spinal injury
- Failure to keep an awake patient informed of rescuer procedures and expectations
- Failure to maintain manual cervical spine control
- Failure to work as a team with all movements coordinated by the provider at the head of the patient
- Insufficient personnel to safely and effectively stabilize the patient
- Insufficient training in an aquatic environment
- Lack of proper gear or familiarity with that gear

LIFTING TECHNIQUES

Back injury is the most common occupational injury in EMS. Proper lifting technique and mechanics are essential to avoid injury.

EMS physicians and other providers should keep in mind: "If you are straining to lift an object or a person, get more help."

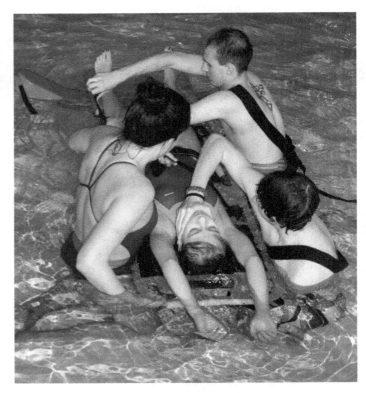

FIGURE 60-24. Water: securing to the long spine board.

Indication Patient movement requires planned team lifting.

Technique

Step 1: Plan a route and ensure the path is clear of potential obstacles/hazards.

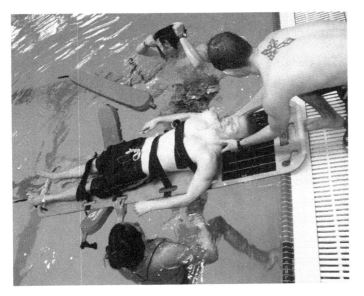
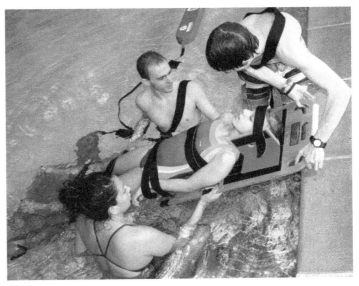

FIGURE 60-25. Water: move to egress point.

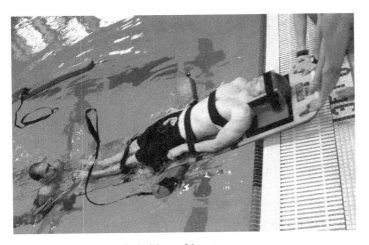
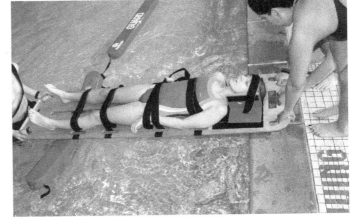

FIGURE 60-26. Water: slowly slide out of the water.

Step 2: Feet should be shoulder width apart.

Step 3: Bend at the knees.

Step 4: Keep your back straight and stomach muscles tightened.

Step 5: Keep the object close to your body.

Step 6: Lift with your legs.

Pitfalls

- Lifting a patient or object that is too heavy or cumbersome for the given number of rescuers
- Bending at the waist
- Twisting while lifting or carrying
- Failure to use specialized equipment when lifting or transporting bariatric patients
- Failure to plan ahead

TOURNIQUETS AND HEMOSTATIC AGENTS

Much has recently been published in medical literature about the resurgent use of field tourniquets and hemostatic agents from US military operations throughout the world with the US Army Institute of Surgical

Research at the forefront of this work. All providers should be familiar with the newest guidelines for information and changes consistent with the Tactical Combat Casualty Care (TCCC) Guidelines on tourniquet and hemostatic agent use. Much of the information gathered through military and tactical use regarding tourniquet and hemostatic gauze safety and complication rates can be extrapolated to the civilian EMS environment. The management steps here will focus on tourniquet use by civilian EMS.

TOURNIQUETS

Indication Tourniquets should be considered first-line intervention for life-threatening external hemorrhage amenable to tourniquet application or traumatic extremity amputation. In some circumstances of prolonged crush injury it may be appropriate to apply prior to extrication in order to avoid sudden systemic return of entrapped blood with low pH and high potassium. Tourniquet application is also required prior to intentional limb amputation for the rapid extrication of the moribund and otherwise hopelessly entrapped patient.

Essential Equipment

- TCCC-recommended tourniquet (**Figure 60-27**)
- PPE

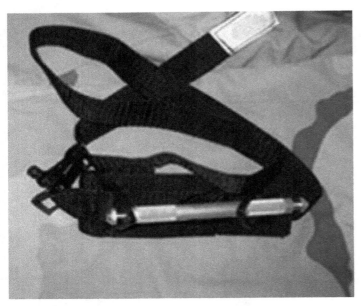

FIGURE 60-27. TCCC-recommended tourniquet. (Reprinted with permission from Tintinalli JE, Stapczynski JS, Ma OJ, Cline DM, Cydulka RK, Meckler GD, eds. *Tintinalli's Emergency Medicine: A Comprehensive Study, 7th ed.* New York, NY: McGraw-Hill; 2011.)

Technique

Step 1: Identify sources of bleeding anatomically amenable to tourniquet application.

Step 2: Apply tourniquet directly to exposed skin (preferable) 2 to 3 in above wound (**Figure 60-28**).

Step 3: Tighten tourniquet device to occlude blood flow checking for continued hemorrhage and/or distal pulse (Figure 60-28).

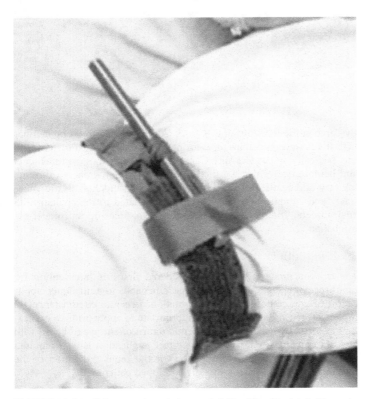

FIGURE 60-28. Tighten tourniquet device to occlude blood flow. (Reprinted with permission from Tintinalli JE, Stapczynski JS, Ma OJ, Cline DM, Cydulka RK, Meckler GD, eds. *Tintinalli's Emergency Medicine: A Comprehensive Study, 7th ed.* New York, NY: McGraw-Hill; 2011.)

Step 4: If bleeding continues after proper application and distal pulse *is still present*, apply a second tourniquet proximal to and beside the first device to eliminate pulse.

Step 5: Clearly expose tourniquet sites and mark time of application for receiving facility.

Pitfalls

- Lack of training and familiarity with device application and usage.

- Not fully tightening device—a properly applied tourniquet should *hurt*!

- Not securing locking mechanism to guard against tourniquet loosening unexpectedly.

- Failing to reevaluate device after application to inspect for complications or continued need.

■ HEMOSTATIC AGENTS

Indications Compressible bleeding site not amenable to tourniquet use or as adjunct to tourniquet removal/de-escalation

Essential Equipment

- TCCC-recommended hemostatic agent
- PPE

Technique Without Tourniquet Use

Step 1: Identify source of bleeding and recognize not compressible by tourniquet use.

Step 2: Perform blood sweep and attempt to directly visualize site of hemorrhage.

Step 3: Fully pack wound area with hemostatic dressing, maintaining direct pressure at site of hemorrhage during agent application.

Step 4: Maintain direct pressure for a minimum of *3 minutes* after application for full hemostatic effect to occur.

Step 5: Place pressure dressing—ace wrap, elastic bandage, etc—over hemostatic agent and wound to maintain firm pressure on injury site.

Step 6: Reevaluate to identify continued hemorrhage or recurrent blood loss.

Technique When De-Escalating Tourniquet

Step 1: Expose wound completely while proximal tourniquet in place.

Step 2: Perform blood sweep to remove any excess blood in wound while preserving any clot present in wound bed.

Step 3: Fully pack wound area with hemostatic dressing, maintaining direct pressure during agent application.

Step 4: Maintain direct pressure for a minimum of *3 minutes* after application for full hemostatic effect to occur.

Step 5: Place pressure dressing (ace wrap, elastic bandage, etc) over hemostatic agent and wound to maintain firm pressure on injury site.

Step 6: Release tourniquet slowly—but leave in place on injured extremity—and continually assess for rebleeding from the wound.

Pitfalls

- Lack of training and familiarity with hemostatic agent application and usage

- Failure to appropriately prepare wound area and apply/pack agent into wound

- Failure to maintain direct pressure for at least 3 minutes after agent application

- Failure to apply pressure dressing to agent and wound after packing and direct pressure

- Failure to utilize additional hemostatic agent if needed with rebleeding
- Failure to continually reevaluate wound for signs of recurrent hemorrhage
- Failure to reapply tourniquet if unable to maintain hemostasis after proper packing

CHEST DECOMPRESSION IN THE FIELD (CHAPTER 54)

Emergent field needle thoracostomy (NT) is currently used and indicated for cases of suspected tension pneumothorax (PTX) primarily in unstable blunt and penetrating trauma patients. Tube thoracostomy (TT) follows needle thoracostomy for definitive treatment and is performed prehospital in some systems by specially trained flight personnel or EMS field physicians in place of NT for PTX.[5]

NEEDLE THORACOSTOMY

Indications Suspected pneumothorax in the patient who acutely deteriorates or is found in extremis

Equipment

- IV catheter over needle, at least 3.25 in in length
- Antiseptic solution for site preparation
- One-way valve (aquarium air pump check valve, condom, glove tip, etc). Note: improvised one-way valves (aquarium air pump check valve, condom, glove tip, etc) have not been adequately studied; however, anecdotal experiences indicates that they may function as a barrier to air flow back into the chest cavity during inspiration.
- PPE

Technique

Step 1: Cover chest wound if present with three-sided or occlusive dressing (**Figure 60-29**).

Step 2: Identify the second intercostal space (ICS) at the midclavicular line on the affected side. The second rib is palpated just below the clavicle. The second ICS is just inferior to the second rib. Alternatively, it may be easier to identify the third rib, in which case the second ICS would lie just superior to the third rib. (**Figure 60-30**).

Step 3: Prepare the skin site with Betadine or alcohol swab if time permits (**Figure 60-31**).

Step 4: Advance the needle and catheter over the top of the third rib into the second ICS to avoid the neurovascular bundle lying under each rib and angling away from midline to avoid centrally located vascular structures (**Figure 60-32**).

Step 5: Slowly advance the needle until a gentle "give" is felt as the needle enters pleural cavity.

Step 6: Advance the needle until air is obtained in the syringe or alternatively advance the catheter while removing the needle listening for possible rush of air. Saline or water inside the syringe may make aid in the identification of air in the form of bubbles (**Figure 60-33**).

Step 7: Evaluate for signs of clinical improvement and continually reassess patient.

*Step 8: Apply a one-way (check) valve on the open proximal end of the catheter (**Figure 60-34**).*
Pitfalls

- Not utilizing a catheter long enough to gain entry into pleural space
- Not covering chest wall wounds with three-sided or occlusive dressings prior to NT
- Inappropriate NT in the patient not showing signs/symptoms of tension PTX

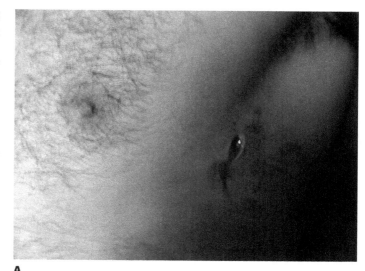

A

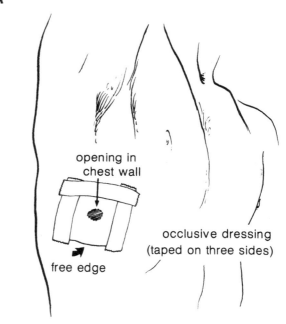

FIGURE 60-29. Application of the three-sided occlusive dressing. **A**: (Reprinted with permission from Tintinalli JE, Stapczynski JS, Ma OJ, Cline DM, Cydulka RK, Meckler GD, eds. *Tintinalli's Emergency Medicine: A Comprehensive Study, 7th ed*. New York, NY: McGraw-Hill; 2011.) **B**: (Reprinted with permission from Hall J, Schmidt G, Wood L. *Principles of Critical Care*. 2nd ed. McGraw-Hill; 1998.)

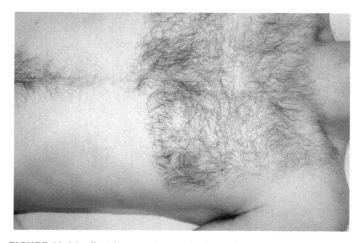

FIGURE 60-30. Chest decompression: anterior chest wall.

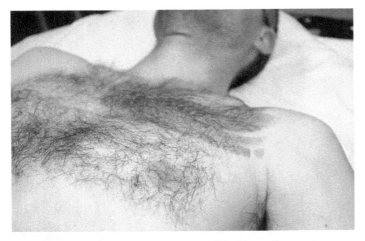

FIGURE 60-31. Chest decompression: prepare and identify second intercostal space.

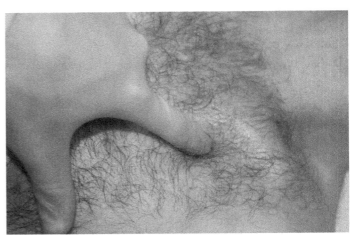

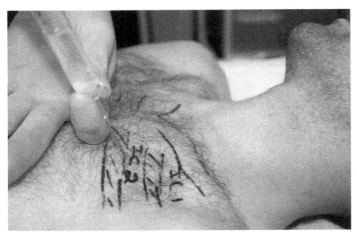

FIGURE 60-32. Chest decompression: placing needle into the second intercostal space.

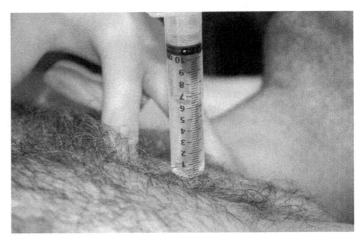

FIGURE 60-34. Chest decompression: improvised one-way valve.

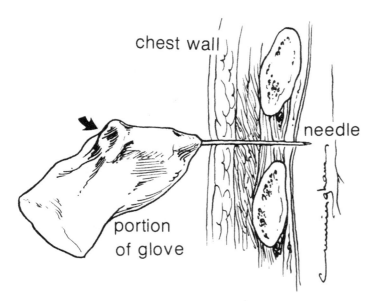

FIGURE 60-33. Chest decompression: Saline or water inside the syringe may make aid in the identification of air in the form of bubbles. (Reprinted with permission from Hall J, Schimdt G, Wood L. *Principles of Critical Care.* 2nd ed. McGraw-Hill; 2005.)

- Failure to identify recurrent tension PTX after initial decompression
- Damaging the neurovascular bundle that lies on the inferior border of each rib

■ TUBE THORACOSTOMY

Indications Suspected pneumothorax in the patient who acutely deteriorates or is found in extremis and the patient who has received NT by EMS for tension PTX

Equipment

- Chest tubes—adult 28-36F, child 16-24F
- Scalpel
- Tape
- Antiseptic solution
- Forceps
- Scissors
- Suture and needle driver
- Gauze pads
- Drainage apparatus w/ H_2O seal and suction
- PPE

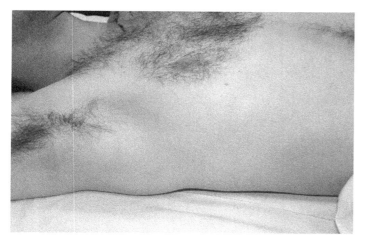

FIGURE 60-35. Thoracostomy: exposing the fifth ICS in the midaxillary line.

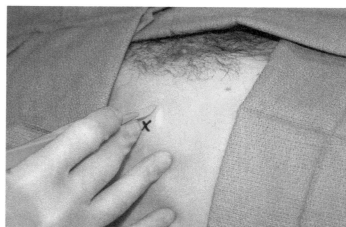

FIGURE 60-37. Thoracostomy: make 3- to 4-cm incision.

Technique

Step 1: Identify fourth or fifth intercostal space (fifth ICS is approximately at the level of the nipple in males), midaxillary line (MAL) on side of PTX (**Figure 60-35**).

Step 2: If time permits prepare the skin site with Betadine or alcohol and apply sterile towels to create a sterile field (**Figure 60-36**).

Step 3: Make a 3- to 4–cm-wide transverse incision onto fifth rib at the MAL (**Figure 60-37**).

Step 4: Bluntly dissect w/ gloved finger or forceps over top of fifth rib into fourth ICS (**Figure 60-38**).

Step 5: Considerable force may be required to enter pleural space and definitive pop likely upon entering pleural cavity. Spread tips of forceps in pleural cavity to widen access.

Step 5: Insert gloved finger into pleural space to verify proper position and to act as guide for the chest tube (**Figure 60-39**).

Step 6: With or without clamps on TT tip insert tube along tract and finger into pleural cavity, directing it posteriorly and superiorly (**Figure 60-40**).

Step 7: Secure the chest tube to the patient with suture, tape, and gauze dressing (**Figure 60-41**).

Step 8: Attach the chest tube to a suction/drainage device (**Figure 60-42**).

Pitfalls

- Time delay to transport and definitive care
- Poor sterile technique
- Not advancing chest tube far enough into chest cavity leaving drainage ports exposed outside of chest wall
- Damage to the neurovascular bundle that runs along the inferior portion of each rib
- Failure to position the chest tube inside the chest cavity
- Failure to appropriately secure the chest tube

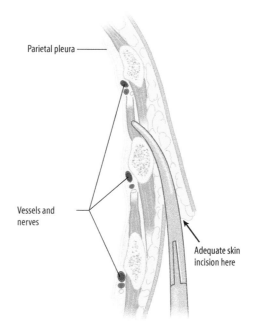

FIGURE 60-38. Thoracostomy: bluntly dissecting. (Reprinted with permission from Tintinalli JE, Stapczynski JS, Ma OJ, Cline DM, Cydulka RK, Meckler GD, eds. *Tintinalli's Emergency Medicine: A Comprehensive Study, 7th ed.* New York, NY: McGraw-Hill; 2011.)

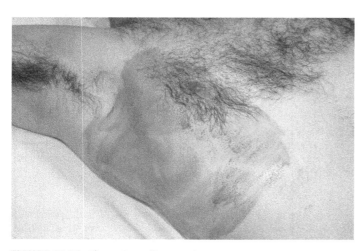

FIGURE 60-36. Thoracostomy: skin preparation.

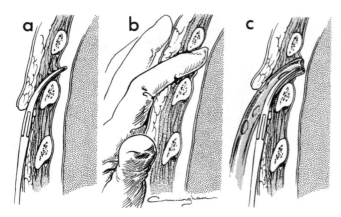

FIGURE 60-39. Thoracostomy: insert gloved finger into pleural space (Reprinted with permission from Hall J, Schimdt G, Wood L. *Principles of Critical Care.* 2nd ed. McGraw-Hill; 2005.)

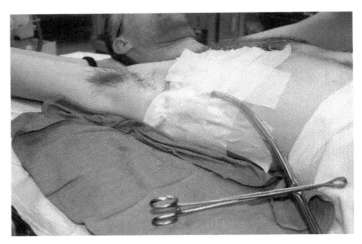

FIGURE 60-41. Thoracostomy: secure the chest tube.

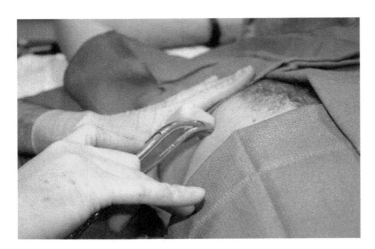

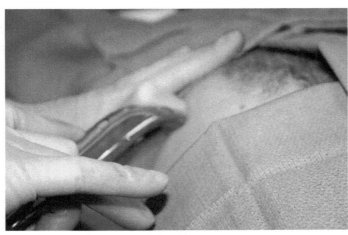

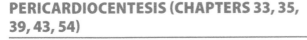

FIGURE 60-40. Thoracostomy: insert tube along tract.

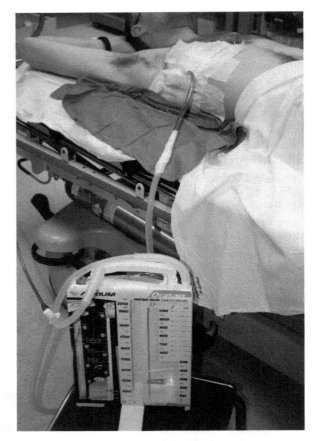

FIGURE 60-42. Thoracostomy: attach to drainage/suction.

PERICARDIOCENTESIS (CHAPTERS 33, 35, 39, 43, 54)

Pericardiocentesis is used primarily in acutely decompensated trauma patients who are in extremis and have signs and symptoms of tamponade physiology. Certain medical patients at risk for tamponade might also benefit from this procedure if other sources cannot be identified as causing their extremis. The steps below will start with the blind approach and then just add the steps needed for both ECG-assisted and US-guided pericardiocentesis. All types of pericardiocentesis carry some risk of adverse effects. The most common adverse effects are blood vessel injury, nerve injury, pneumothorax, hemothorax, ventricular or cardiac penetration, dysrhythmias, and liver injury.

◼ BLIND PERICARDIOCENTESIS

Indications Any acutely decompensated trauma or medical patient with a known or suspected cardiac tamponade. While there is no absolute contraindication in a hemodynamically unstable patient, care should be taken in patients with known history of a bleeding disorder.

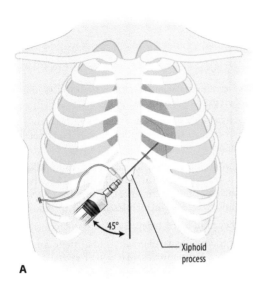

A

FIGURE 60-43. Needle angle for pericardiocentesis. (Reprinted with permission from Tintinalli JE, Stapczynski JS, Ma OJ, Cline DM, Cydulka RK, Meckler GD, eds. *Tintinalli's Emergency Medicine: A Comprehensive Study, 7th ed.* New York, NY: McGraw-Hill; 2011.)

Equipment

- 18- to 20-g Spinal needle or 3.25-in 14- to 16-g IV needle
- Large volume syringe (at least 20 cc or greater)
- Antiseptic solution
- PPE

Technique

Step 1: Prepare the subxiphoid area with antiseptic solution.

Step 2: The needle should enter the skin directly below or adjacent to the xiphoid process. The needle should be held at a 45° angle to the skin, aiming at the ipsilateral shoulder (**Figure 60-43**).

Step 3: The needle should be advanced, maintaining angle and direction, while pulling back on the syringe plunger.

Step 4: Stop advancing the needle when blood is obtained. Remove up to 50 cc of blood and reassess hemodynamic status. Removal of 25 cc or less in traumatic effusions often leads to improved hemodynamic status. If hemodynamic status does not improve, continue to remove blood in 25 cc increments until hemodynamic status improves. If hemodynamic status does not improve, after multiple attempts and blood return continues, it is possible that the needle has entered the ventricular space.

Step 5: Following hemodynamic improvement the needle may be removed and a sterile dressing placed over the needle insertion site.

Pitfalls

- Failure to recognize the signs and symptoms of pericardial tamponade in a timely fashion
- Inadequate needle length
- Improper approach, angle, or trajectory
- Ventricular rupture

ECG-ASSISTED PERICARDIOCENTESIS

Equipment

- Same as above plus single alligator clip electrode cable

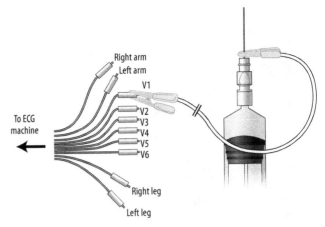

FIGURE 60-44. ECG lead on pericardiocentesis needle. (Reprinted with permission from Tintinalli JE, Stapczynski JS, Ma OJ, Cline DM, Cydulka RK, Meckler GD, eds. *Tintinalli's Emergency Medicine: A Comprehensive Study, 7th ed.* New York, NY: McGraw-Hill; 2011.)

Technique

Step 1: Attach the V_1 ECG monitor lead to the proximal portion of the needle (**Figure 60-44**).

Step 2: Utilize the same technique and approach as the blind technique (**Figure 60-45**).

Step 3: Proceed until blood is returned or ST elevation is noted on the monitor in lead V_1. ST elevation indicates that the needle has contacted the myocardium. Withdraw the needle and attempt to aspirate blood.

Step 4: Following hemodynamic improvement the needle may be removed and a sterile dressing placed over the needle insertion site.

Pitfalls

- Failure to recognize ST elevation on myocardial contact
- Poor electrical contact/conduction between the alligator clip and the needle or ECG lead
- Ventricular rupture

ULTRASOUND-GUIDED PERICARDIOCENTESIS[6]

Equipment

- Same as above plus US machine with appropriate probe

Technique

Step 1: Use the US to identify the point of maximal effusion (**Figure 60-46**).

Step 2: Prepare and sterilize the site of entry that will coincide with plane of the US. The projected path should attempt to minimize the number

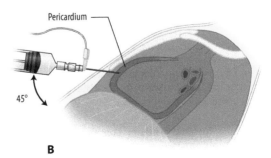

B

FIGURE 60-45. Advancing needle into pericardium.

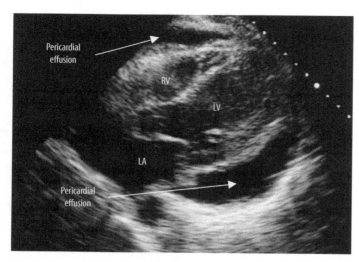

FIGURE 60-46. Ultrasound view of pericardial effusion. (Reprinted with permission from Palmeri ST, Cohen L, Shindler DM. Echocardiography. In: Pahlm O, Wagner GS, eds. *Multimodal Cardiovascular Imaging: Principles and Clinical Applications.* New York, NY: McGraw-Hill; 2011:chap 1.)

of structures encountered between the site of entry and the point of maximal effusion. If the projected path will transit a rib, it is important to remember to direct the needle over the superior margin of the rib to avoid damaging the neurovascular bundle that runs along the inferior margin of each rib.

Step 3: Advance the needle along the projected path, utilizing real-time US guidance until the tip of the needle enters the pericardium. After entering the pericardium the effusion may be drained as indicated in the blind technique until hemodynamic improvement occurs.

Step 4: Following hemodynamic improvement, the needle may be removed and a sterile dressing placed over the needle insertion site.

Pitfalls

- Misidentification of pericardial effusion or tamponade (commonly the anterior fat pad is inappropriately diagnosed as a pericardial effusion)
- Improper probe usage
- Inadequate depth of US image
- Ventricular puncture

FRACTURES AND JOINT INJURIES

The appropriate management of out-of-hospital extremity injuries including field reductions, splinting, and immobilization can significantly reduce the morbidity associated with these events. Specific steps to take when faced with fractures and dislocations of both upper and lower extremity injuries are covered in Section 10, while more detailed discussions of injury patterns are covered in the respective chapters listed in Section 9.

Indications for Splinting/Stabilization Without Reduction Splinting or stabilization of an extremity may be beneficial for any of the following conditions: obvious extremity or joint deformity/fracture/dislocation, point specific pain or crepitus, open injury, or partial amputation. Reduction in the field is not necessary if the patient has palpable distal pulses, good capillary refill, skin color, and is neurologically intact.

Equipment

Available splinting material whether commercial (plaster, fiberglass, malleable metal) or improvised

- Gauze or cotton padding
- Elastic bandage
- Tape
- Cravats
- PPE

Technique for Splinting/Stabilization

Step 1: Assess for neurovascular function distal to the injury (if neurovascular deficit exists go to the reduction section).

Step 2: Cover any visible wounds and pad the portion of the extremity that will be in contact with the splint. Ensure plenty of padding over bony prominences.

Step 3: Utilize the available splinting materials to immobilize the fracture or dislocation. Follow the manufacturer's directions when using commercially available splinting materials. Ensure the joints proximal and distal to the injury are also immobilized by the splint.

Step 4: Secure the splint using tape, an elastic bandage, or a cravat.

Step 5: Reassess the neurovascular function of the extremity following splint application. If a neurovascular deficit exists, remove the splint and begin at Step 1.

Pitfalls

- Failure to recognize neurovascular compromise
- Inadequate padding may lead to pressure sores
- Improper immobilization can lead to increased pain, neurovascular damage, or fracture displacement
- When using plaster or fiberglass, it is important to allow the splint to cure appropriately
- Failure to continually reassess the neurovascular function of the splinted extremity

Indications for Splinting/Stabilization After Reduction Reduction in the field is not necessary if the patient has palpable distal pulses, good capillary refill, skin color, and is neurologically intact.

Equipment

- Same as listed under "Indications for Splinting/Stabilization Without Reduction"

Technique

Step 1: Assess for neurovascular function distal to the injury (if no neurovascular deficit exists follow the steps to splinting listed under "Technique for Splinting/Stabilization").

Step 2: Determine the time interval until the patient will arrive at the hospital and whether field reduction is necessary (a transport time greater than 15 minutes is a general indication for field reduction).

Step 3: Determine the most likely location where the fracture or dislocation has occurred.

Step 4: Most fractures or dislocations can be reduced by slow steady traction along the long axis of the fractured bone (continuous traction may also be necessary). Joint dislocations may require longitudinal traction and a rotational force in the direction of normal alignment. If a fracture or dislocation is not easily reduced or requires more elaborate manipulation it is best to contact medical direction for further guidance.

Step 5: Following each reduction attempt the neurovascular status of the extremity should be reassessed.

Step 6: Once neurovascular function has been restored the extremity should be splinted. Follow the steps under "Technique for Splinting/Stabilization."

Pitfalls

- Failure to recognize neurovascular compromise
- Overly aggressive or jerky reduction attempts

- Unnecessarily delaying transport for repeated unsuccessful reduction attempts

- Failure to contact online medical direction in a timely fashion when faced with a complex or unfamiliar reduction

- Failure to continually reassess the neurovascular function of the splinted extremity

BURNS

Burns may result from many different causes and may vary from severe life-threatening injuries to very minor superficial injuries. EMS personnel should approach the scene of a burn cautiously and quickly remove the victim from the hazard only when it is safe to do so. Initial care of all burn victims should begin with careful attention to immediate causes of death. The approach to a burn victim should follow an approach as outlined in the "Approach to a Burn Victim."

TYPES OF BURNS

First degree

- Involves only the epidermis

- Painful

- Appear red

- Lacks blisters

Second degree

- Involves all of the epidermis and extends into the dermis

- Painful

- Appear moist, pink, white, or mottled

- Blisters may develop

- May be further subdivided into superficial and deep partial thickness

Third degree

- Involves all of the epidermis and dermis, may extend into the subcutaneous tissue

- Insensate

- Appear white or charred

- Also known as full thickness

Fourth degree

- Extends through the epidermis, dermis, and subcutaneous fat to involve underlying muscle and bone

Approach to a Burn Victim

Step 1: Safely and expeditiously remove the victim from the hazard area.

Step 2: Stabilize the cervical spine and immobilize the patient on a long spine board as clinically indicated.

Step 3: Assess the victim's airway. Consider intubation if there is any evidence of significant inhalational burns (airway edema, intraoral burns, soot in or around the mouth or nose) or other reason to believe there may be imminent airway compromise (coexisting neck or facial trauma).

Step 4: Assess the victim's ventilatory status and provide support as necessary.

Step 5: Quickly evaluate the patient for any other significant injuries, paying close attention to significant bleeding, and treat as clinically indicated with direct pressure, pressure dressing, or tourniquet.

Step 6: Remove any contaminated clothing and all clothing or jewelry that could potentially act as a tourniquet from resulting edema.

Step 7: Remove as much of the hazard as possible when clinically indicated. Using appropriate PPE and extreme caution brush off any dry chemicals that may potentiate the burn. If a chemical liquid is present, copiously irrigate the area to remove as much chemical as possible. Do not irrigate dry chemicals as this may potentiate the burn.

Step 8: Calculate the total body surface area (TBSA) burned. Many techniques, diagrams, and charts exist for the calculation of TBSA. The most commonly used are the Lund-Browder chart and the Rule of 9s. Another method is the palm method. This method supposes the size of the victim's palm is equal to 1% TBSA. Using this reference the TBSA of the burn can be extrapolated. When calculating TBSA, do not include areas of first-degree burns.

Step 9: Assess the hemodynamic status of the victim. Consider hypovolemic shock in patients with a large TBSA burn (>15%). If hemodynamically unstable patients, initiate fluid resuscitation immediately with normal saline or lactated Ringer solution. Intravenous access should be obtained if possible through intact skin but if necessary may be obtained through the burned area. If IV access is not possible, consider intraosseous access. A pressure bag applied to the fluid bag may be necessary to administer adequate, timely fluids through an IO.

Step 10: Cover the burned area with dry sterile dressings. Do not remove or deroof blisters or rub burn skin in an effort to either clean or warm the area. The use of antimicrobial ointments or creams and burn site cooling vary greatly and should be used in conjunction with the recommendations of the local burn center.

Step 11: In a hemodynamically stable patient with large TBSA burns and a transport time greater than 1 hour, consider initiating fluid resuscitation. The most commonly used method to guide fluid administration is the Parkland formula. It should be noted that controversy does exist with regard to virtually every fluid resuscitation formula.

Fluid Requirement for the first 24 hours = TBSA (%) × Weight (kg) × x 4 (mL)

Half of the fluid requirement as calculated by the Parkland formula should be given within 8 hours of the burn and the other half should be given over the next 16 hours. The patient should be monitored during fluid administration for signs of fluid overload.

Step 12: Continue to carefully monitor the patient for signs of airway or respiratory compromise, hypovolemia, and hypothermia, and consider transport to a designated burn center in the appropriate situation

Pitfalls

- Failure to continually reassess the neurovascular function of the splinted extremity

- Failure to remove clothing and jewelry

- Failure to recognize and treat coexisting injuries or conditions (trauma, carbon monoxide poisoning, or cyanide toxicity)

- Failure to maintain normothermia

- Prophylactic antibiotics are not indicated in the prehospital setting

- Delayed transport for IV access in patients with adequate blood pressure or short transport time

OPEN WOUNDS WITHOUT ACTIVE HEMORRHAGE (CHAPTER 57)

There are many considerations when determining the appropriate wound dressing. These considerations include the wound type, the underlying tissue, and the purpose of the dressing. Wound dressings are important for patient comfort, tissue preservation, limiting infections, and wound healing. The two major categories are occlusive and nonocclusive dressings.

Occlusive dressings seal the wound from exposure to the external environment. Occlusive dressings act as a barrier to prevent environmental pathogen infiltration. They also trap moisture in and around the wound, which allows the wound to heal and remain pliable. This pliability decreases reinjured that can be caused by movement if the wound were dry and cracked. Occlusive dressings generally have limited absorbent properties and are therefore of limited effectiveness on wounds with copious secretions, exudate or discharge. Occlusive dressings are commonly used for open chest wounds and can be combined with a moist sterile dressing for the management of intestinal evisceration.

Nonocclusive dressings allow air to reach the wound and are permeable to water and liquids in the environment. The most common nonocclusive dressings are gauze or cotton secured over the wound. Nonocclusive dressings are generally more absorbent than occlusive dressings and are therefore commonly used when the wound has copious secretions, exudate, or discharge. Nonocclusive dressings allow the wound to dry and may adhere to the wound. Wet to dry dressings utilize this adherence property to aid in wound debridement. In other circumstances, adherence may complicate healing by removing newly formed granulation tissue and causing painful dressing changes. Nonocclusive dressings are commonly used to cover IV sites, tracheostomy sites, drain sites, and partial- and full-thickness wounds. They may also be combined with other products (ABD, gauze, cotton, or foam pads) for added absorption.

Field decontamination before or during transport is appropriate if an open wound has visible gross contaminants (rocks, dirt, plants, other foreign material). Field decontamination can be accomplished with manual removal of any large particles followed by irrigation with copious amounts of water. Open chest and abdominal wounds should not be routinely irrigated.

REFERENCES

1. Bouland AJ, Jenkins JL, Levy MJ. Assessing attitudes toward spinal immobilization. *J Emerg Med*. October 2013;45(4):e117-e125.
2. White CC 4th, Domeier RM, Millin MG; Standards and Clinical Practice Committee, National Association of EMS Physicians. EMS spinal precautions and the use of the long backboard - resource document to the position statement of the National Association of EMS Physicians and the American College of Surgeons Committee on Trauma. *Prehosp Emerg Care*. 2014;18(2):306-314.
3. Engsberg JR, Standeven JW, Shurtleff TL, Eggars JL, Shafer JS, Naunheim RS. Cervical spine motion during extrication. *J Emerg Med*. January 2013;44(1):122-127.
4. Watson RS, Cummings P, Quan L, Bratton S, Weiss NS. Cervical spine injuries among submersion victims. *J Trauma*. October 2001;51(4):658-662.
5. Warner KJ, Copass MK, Bulger EM. Paramedic use of needle thoracostomy in the prehospital environment. *Prehosp Emerg Care*. April-June 2008;12(2):162-168.
6. Hatch N, Wu TS. Advanced ultrasound procedures. *Crit Care Clin*. April 2014;30(2):305-329.

CHAPTER 61

Obstetric Procedures

Edward A. Bartkus

INTRODUCTION

Babies have been born for millions of years without EMS intervention. This is one "emergency" that almost always turns out well. The CDC reported that, in 2009, there were 4,130,665 births in the United States (a birth rate of 13.5 per 1000 population), with 1.1% delivered out-of-hospital. The percent born preterm (<37 weeks' EGA) was 12.2%, and the percent born at a low birth weight (<2500 g) was 8.2%. In the United States, the overall infant mortality was 6.9 per 1000 live births, but 183.2 per 1000 babies born prior to 32 weeks' EGA.[1]

PROCEDURES

- Assessment of prehospital delivery likelihood
- Delivery (uncomplicated)
- Complicated delivery
  - Shoulder dystocia
  - Breech delivery
  - Umbilical cord prolapse
  - Uterine inversion
  - Postpartum hemorrhage (PPH)

ASSESSMENT OF PREHOSPITAL DELIVERY LIKELIHOOD

Ascertain the obstetric history (gravida and parity) using the $G_N P_{TPAL}$ numbering system. N is the total number of pregnancies; T is the number of term births (multiples, eg, twins only count as one birth); P is the number of preterm births (<37 weeks); A is the number of abortions (<20 weeks), and L is the total number of children who lived at least 28 days. Next, determine the estimated gestational age (EGA) of tis fetus in weeks—most accurately by a previous ultrasound, by dates from LMP, or distance from the symphysis to the fundus in centimeters (modestly accurate in the 20- to 36-week range; inaccurate in case of multiples, poly- or oligohydramnios).

Ascertain the presence of contractions (ctx), their time of onset, duration, and interval frequency. Stage 1 (from onset of labor to full cervical dilation) in a primiparous woman takes an average of 10 hours (95% complete by 25 hours); for a multiparous woman, the mean is 8 hours (95% by 19 hours). Stage 2 (full cervical dilation to delivery of the neonate) for a primiparous woman takes an average of 33 minutes (95% by 118 minutes); for a multiparous woman, a mean of 9 minutes, with 95% delivered by the end of 47 minutes. Primiparous women are likely to deliver when contractions are 3 to 5 minutes apart and last 40 to 90 seconds, increasing in strength and frequency for at least an hour. Delivery is imminent if contractions are 2 minutes or less apart, especially for a multiparous woman.[2]

Assess anticipated difficulties with prehospital delivery and/or need for neonatal resuscitation: preterm (<37 weeks' EGA; 12.18% in 2009), multiples (In 2009, twins occurred 33.2 times per 1000 births, triplet and higher order multiple birth rate was 1.53 per 1000 births), anticipated abnormal presentation/lie, lack of adequate prenatal care (none or first visit at >3 months' EGA; 6.6% of desired pregnancies, 14.5% of mistimed or unwanted pregnancies in 2002),[3] placenta previa (2.8 cases per 1000 singletons, 3.9 cases per 1000 twin pregnancies),[4] poly- or oligohydramnios, the presence of a cerclage, or the anticipated need for Cesarean section. A cerclage is a stitch that holds the cervix closed. It is commonly placed in a woman who has a weak (incompetent) cervix

that tends to dilate. The stitch works to hold the cervix closed, thus keeping dilation from occurring and preserving the pregnancy. Cervical cerclage is temporary and is removed before delivery of the infant. If labor progresses with it present, the stitch can cause cervical lacerations and hemorrhage. Rarely, a transabdominal cerclage is placed—this is permanent and all infants must be delivered via C-section. The cesarean delivery rate in 2009 was 32.3% of all births. Half of the women aged 40 and older (49.5%) delivered by cesarean compared with less than one in four women under age 20 (23.1%). This is also the case among women having singleton births (older women have higher rates of multiple births, which are more likely to be delivered by cesarean.

Perform a rapid, focused physical examination. Confirm the estimated gestational age by noting the symphysis to fundal height in centimeters. Remove all clothing from the lower half of the patient, and assess for dilation, effacement, and crowning.

DELIVERY (UNCOMPLICATED)

Obtain and prepare equipment for delivery (see **Table 61-1**). Calmness is first requirement of any delivery. Ninety-five to ninety-seven percent of all deliveries are vertex presentations—there is great probability the delivery will be uncomplicated. You will assist the mother—she will deliver the child. Cleanliness is second, and control is the third requirement. The cardinal movements are engagement, descent, flexion, internal rotation, extension, external rotation, and expulsion of the baby.

Essential Equipment

- PPE
- Plastic-lined under pad
- Drape sheet
- Towels
- Receiving blanket
- Two umbilical clamps or ties
- Scissors or scalpel
- Plastic bag for placenta with tie
- Cold pack

Technique

Step 1: Encourage the mother to take deep, slow breaths. Pain can be controlled to different extents through mental relaxation and by concentrating on deep breathing.

Step 2: Guide pushing, especially with crowning. Push between contractions (not at their peak) to attempt to slow down the birth. Have the mother blow out through her mouth at the peak of each contraction to help resist the urge to push. Stretching external vaginal opening with lubricated fingers may help decrease the likelihood of a tear.

Step 3: If the amniotic membrane is still intact and obstructing the delivery, pinch it to break a hole, and then tear it open.

TABLE 61-1 The APGAR Score

Sign	Score = 0	Score = 1	Score = 2
Skin color (**A**ppearance)	Blue or pale	Pink body and blue extremities	Completely pink
Heart rate (**P**ulse rate)	Absent	Slow (<100)	>100
Reflex irritability (**G**rimace)	No response	Grimace	Vigorous crying
Muscle tone (**A**ctivity)	Flaccid	Some extremity flexion	Active motion
Respiratory effort (**R**espiration)	Absent	Slow or irregular	Good and crying

Add the scores for each of the five signs to obtain the infant's APGAR score. The maximal possible score is 10. Scores less than 7 are considered low.

Reprinted with permission from Reichman EF. Emergency Medicine Procedures. 2nd ed. New York: McGraw-Hill, 2013.

Step 4: Place your hand on the advancing fetal head to control rate of expulsion, and support the baby's head as it emerges. Never pull or twist the head, as this can cause CNS injury.

Step 5: When the head has delivered, check for nuchal cord. If present, gently lift the cord over the baby's head or loosen it carefully so the baby can slip through the loop created by the cord (**Figure 61-1**).

Step 6: The baby's head will rotate to one side spontaneously. Gently guide the side of the baby's head downward so that anterior shoulder emerges with the next push (**Figure 61-2**).

Step 7: Lift the body upward gently to deliver the posterior shoulder, and the rest of the baby will follow very quickly—catch the feet between your fingers. (**Figure 61-3**) If the head comes out and the rest of the body does not after three pushes, have the mother pull her knees to her chest and push hard with each contraction. Consider an episiotomy as a last resort. (**Figure 61-4**)

Step 8: Hold delivered baby with both hands, slightly head down, at the level of the perineum. Dry and stimulate the child, noting the color, vigor of cry, and response to stimulation. Routine bulb suctioning of the oral and nasopharynx is no longer recommended unless airway obstruction is present. It is usually unnecessary and may result in vagal stimulation, causing apnea or bradycardia.

Step 9: Cord clamping should be delayed for at least 1 minute. Benefits of this additional blood flow include improved iron status, higher blood

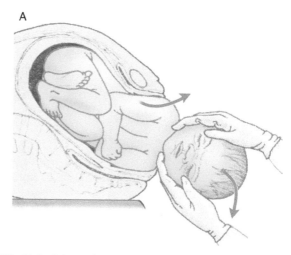

FIGURE 61-2. Delivery of the anterior shoulder. (Reprinted with permission from Reichman EF. *Emergency Medicine Procedures*. 2nd ed. New York: McGraw-Hill; 2013.)

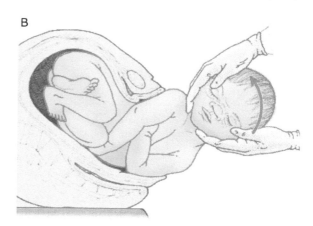

FIGURE 61-3. Delivery of the body. (Reprinted with permission from Reichman EF. *Emergency Medicine Procedures*. 2nd ed. New York: McGraw-Hill; 2013.)

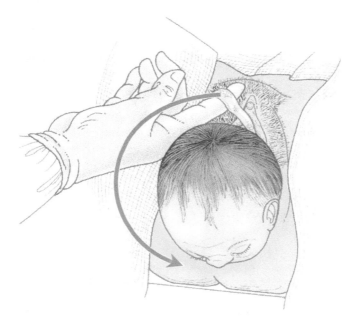

FIGURE 61-1. Reduction of a nuchal cord. (Reprinted with permission from Reichman EF. *Emergency Medicine Procedures*. 2nd ed. New York: McGraw-Hill; 2013.)

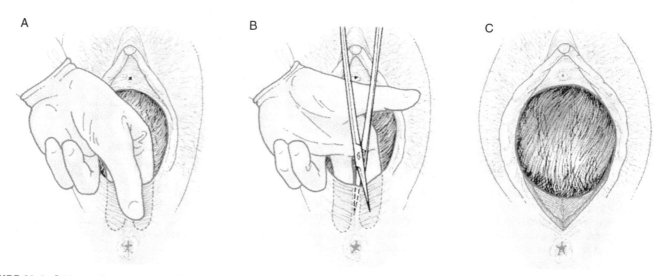

FIGURE 61-4. Episiotomy. (Reprinted with permission from Reichman EF. *Emergency Medicine Procedures*. 2nd ed. New York: McGraw-Hill; 2013.)

pressures after stabilization, and lower incidence of intraventricular bleeds.

Step 10: Ascertain the APGAR score (Table 61-1) at 1 and 5 minutes for the medical record, but resuscitation, if needed, should begin promptly and not awaiting the 1-minute score. Term babies should initially be resuscitated with room air and, when indicated, the administration of supplementary oxygen regulated by blending oxygen and air, if available. Chest compressions are started for a heart rate under 60. If the baby remains bradycardic after 90 seconds of resuscitation, increase the oxygen concentration to 100% until a normal heart rate is achieved.

Step 11: If oximetry is available, preductal measurements can be obtained from the right wrist or palm. At 1 minute, most babies will have an O_2 sat of 60% to 65%. It may take up to 10 minutes for a newborn to achieve normal preductal saturations of 85% to 95%.[5]

Step 12: When the child is stable, lay it on the mother's abdomen for warm skin-to-skin contact. There is no need to wait for the delivery of the placenta before beginning transport to the hospital. The placenta typically delivers about 15 minutes after the baby. Do not pull on the umbilical cord to hasten the expulsion.

Step 13: Uterine massage will help decrease postpartum hemorrhage, and an ice pack applied to the perineum will ease the pain and swelling.

COMPLICATED DELIVERY

Dystocia (difficult labor) is related to a problem of power, the passenger, or the passage.

▦ SHOULDER DYSTOCIA

Shoulder dystocia is caused by the impacted anterior shoulder of the fetus against the mother's symphysis pubis after the fetal head is delivered (**Figure 61-5**). The incidence correlates primarily to birth weight and maternal size. Maternal risk factors include a prepregnancy weight of greater than 180 lb (82 kg) or a weight gain of over 44 lb (20 kg). A history of diabetes mellitus (gestational or otherwise), advancing maternal

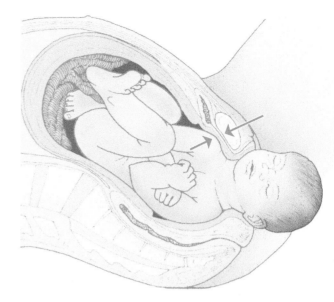

FIGURE 61-5. Shoulder dystocia. (Reprinted with permission from Reichman EF. *Emergency Medicine Procedures*. 2nd ed. New York: McGraw-Hill; 2013.)

age, short stature, abnormal pelvic size or shape, and previous pelvic trauma, all increase the risk from the maternal aspect. Other risk factors include a fetus that is postterm or has macrosomia and a prolonged first or second stage of labor, which results in significant molding.

McRoberts Maneuver Performing McRoberts maneuver can help dislodge the infant's shoulder: Pull the mother's legs back and out as far as possible to help enlarge pelvic outlet (**Figure 61-6**). Apply suprapubic pressure to help push down on and dislodge infant's shoulder (**Figure 61-7**).

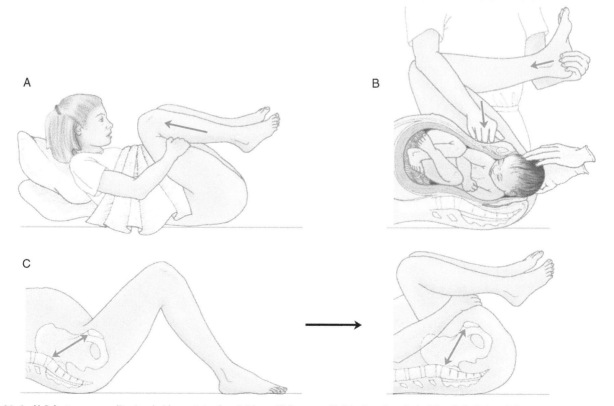

FIGURE 61-6. McRoberts maneuver. (Reprinted with permission from Reichman EF. *Emergency Medicine Procedures*. 2nd ed. New York: McGraw-Hill; 2013.)

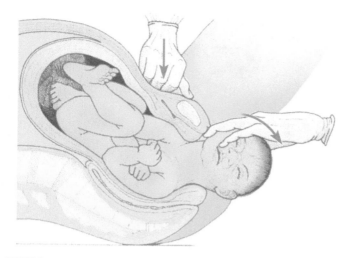

FIGURE 61-7. Application of moderate suprapubic pressure. (Reprinted with permission from Reichman EF. *Emergency Medicine Procedures.* 2nd ed. New York: McGraw-Hill; 2013.)

BREECH DELIVERY

Breech presentation is a term used to describe the situation in which the fetus's buttocks or legs present first (**Figure 61-8**). In a frank breech presentation, the most common type, both legs are extended upward, with both hips flexed and both knees extended. In a complete breech, the buttocks descend first, both hips are flexed, and one or both knees are flexed, resulting in one of both feet presenting with the buttocks. Breech presentations occur in 3% to 4% of all term pregnancies, with a higher incidence before 34 weeks' gestation. The morbidity rate is three to four times that of cephalad presentations. For the mother, perineal trauma is common. For the fetus, prolapsed cord, cord compression, and cord entanglement are common complications, and birth trauma is likely. A breech fetus is at higher risk of hypoxia, acidosis, and anoxia than an infant delivered in cephalad position.

Management Allow fetus to deliver on own, with no traction. Once the umbilical cord has delivered, help free the legs, if needed. Wrap the fetus in a towel and rotate so the shoulders are in an anterior-posterior position. As the shoulders become visible, either use a finger to hook each arm and apply gentle downward traction to remove each one or apply upward traction to facilitate the delivery of the poste-rior shoulder and then downward traction for the anterior shoulder

(**Figure 61-9**). After the shoulders have been delivered, rotate the body so the back is anterior. Next, use Mauriceau maneuver (**Figure 61-10**). Maintain flexion of the head by placing the index and middle fingers over the fetus's maxilla. With the body resting on the forearm of the same arm and the opposite hand supporting the head and shoulders, apply upward traction to the body while an assistant applies suprapu-bic pressure to encourage the delivery of the head with as little traction as possible.

UMBILICAL CORD PROLAPSE

There are two types of umbilical cord prolapse—overt and occult. An overt cord prolapse occurs when the cord enters the vaginal canal or presents externally before the fetus. An occult cord prolapse occurs when the cord slips into or near the pelvis and is occluded by a presenting part. The cord is not visible or palpable on examination. Cord prolapse occurs about once every 250 deliveries. Risk factors include premature rupture of membranes (PROM), transverse lie of the fetus in the uterus, breech presentation, a large fetus, multiparity, multiple gestations, preterm labor, and an unusually long umbilical cord. The major concern with prolapsed cord is cord compression and occlusion, resulting in fetal hypoxia, acidosis, anoxia, and/or death.

Assessment findings of an overt umbilical cord prolapse are straight-forward, but the occult prolapse can be much more insidious and requires a careful examination on the part of the EMS team. It is typi-cally characterized by fetal distress on monitoring equipment, including absence of short- and long-term variability, fetal bradycardia, or recur-rent variable decelerations that do not respond to maternal positioning, oxygen administration, or fluid administration.

If the umbilical cord presents externally or can be visualized in the vagina, use two fingers of a gloved hand to prevent any presenting part of a delivering fetus from occluding the cord. If the cord retracts spontaneously, let it do so, but never pull or replace a presenting cord in the uterus. Keep the cord free of pressure throughout transport—use Trendelenburg or knee-chest position to decrease pressure on the cord (recognizing that this is a very unstable position in a moving ambu-lance). Administer 100% oxygen via nonrebreather mask at 15 lpm, start an IV of normal saline, and administer a tocolytic agent, if available. Call ahead to the receiving facility to advise of the need for emergent obstet-rical assistance and possibly an immediate cesarean section.

UTERINE INVERSION

Uterine inversion is a rare complication of vaginal deliveries where the uterus partially or completely turns inside out. It is associated with signifi-cant blood loss and shock. Manual correction of this is required to save the

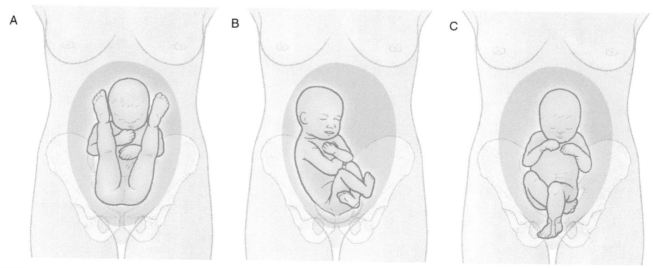

FIGURE 61-8. Breech presentation. (Reprinted with permission from Reichman EF. *Emergency Medicine Procedures.* 2nd ed. New York: McGraw-Hill; 2013.)

A

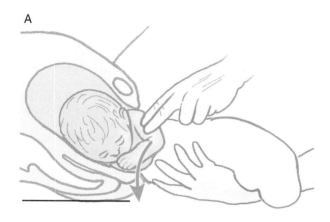

B

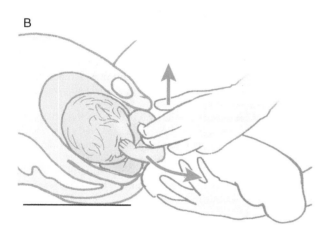

C

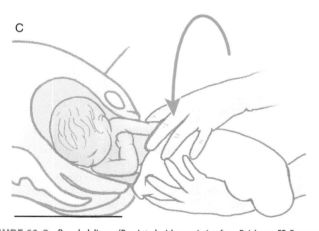

FIGURE 61-9. Breech delivery. (Reprinted with permission from Reichman EF. *Emergency Medicine Procedures*. 2nd ed. New York: McGraw-Hill; 2013.)

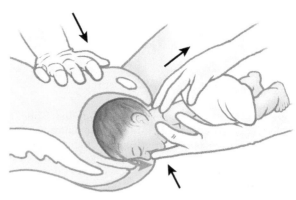

FIGURE 61-10. Breech presentation. (Reprinted with permission from Reichman EF. *Emergency Medicine Procedures*. 2nd ed. New York: McGraw-Hill; 2013.)

patient. Grasp the uterus and push it through the cervix toward the umbilicus then utilize your fist to place the uterus back in its normal position.

■ POSTPARTUM HEMORRHAGE

Postpartum hemorrhage (PPH) is defined as the loss of greater than 500 mL of blood after a vaginal delivery or more than 1000 mL of blood lost after a cesarean section. Normally, postlabor platelet aggregation and clot formation in the decidua is complemented by myometrial contraction that constricts and occludes blood vessels torn when the placenta disassociates from the uterine implantation site. Because blood flow to the uteroplacental boundary is about 600 mL/min, hemorrhage can be significant if uterine contraction does not occur. If uterine contraction is prevented, blood accumulates and clots in the uterus, further preventing uterine contraction and worsening the bleeding. PPH occurs in about 5% of all deliveries, and most hemorrhages occur within 24 hours of delivery. It is implicated in almost 30% of all pregnancy-related deaths.

Common causes of PPH are uterine atony, retained placental fragments (especially in cases of placenta accrete), and birth canal trauma. Risk factors for uterine atony include retention of placental fragments, overdistension of the uterus, multiparity, polyhydramnios, chorioamnionitis, prolonged or obstructed labor, use of general anesthesia, and magnesium tocolysis.

Uterine atony can be identified by a lack of uterine contractions and a flaccid uterus upon palpation. Vaginal bleeding should be apparent, but the external blood loss may not reflect the total blood loss, as much blood loss may be sequestered in the uterus (a typical term uterus holds 5 L). Evaluate the patient's hemodynamic status using signs and symptoms of shock, rather than estimates of total blood loss. Consider drawing blood samples for hemoglobin and hematocrit, type and crossmatch, and coagulation studies.

The primary goal of management is to preserve uteroplacental perfusion. Begin with vigorous uterine fundal massage. Administer high flow oxygen at 15 lpm via a nonrebreather mask and obtain large-bore peripheral IV access. If hypovolemic shock is present, initiate aggressive volume replacement with crystalloids and packed red blood cells. If available, add 10 to 20 USP units of oxytocin to 1000 mL of saline and run the solution at a rate to control uterine atony. Finally, consider packing the vagina to apply pressure internally.

REFERENCES

1. Centers for Disease Control and Prevention. National Center for Health Statistics. VitalStats. http://www.cdc.gov/nchs/vitalstats.htm. Accessed January 31, 2012.
2. Liao JB, Buhimschi CS, Norwitz ER. Normal labor: mechanism and duration. *Obstet Gynecol Clin N Am*. 2005:32(2):145-164.
3. Chandra A, Martinez GM, Mosher WD, Amba JC, Jones J. Fertility, family planning, and reproductive health of U.S. women: data from the 2002 National Survey of Family Growth. *Vital Health Stat 23*. 2005 Dec;(25):1-160.
4. Ananth CV, Demissie K, Smulian JC, Vintzileos AM. Placenta previa in singleton and twin births in the United States, 1989 through 1998: a comparison of risk factor profiles and associated conditions. *Am J Obstet Gynecol*. 2003;188:275-281.
5. Kamlin CO, O'Donnell CP, Davis PG, Morley CJ. Oxygen saturation in healthy infants immediately after birth. *J Pediatr*. May 2006;148(5):585-589.

CHAPTER 62

Pain Management, Sedation, and Anesthesia

Roy Ary

Tracy Leigh LeGros

Pain is the most common emergency complaint. The World Health Organization supports optimal pain treatment as a fundamental human right (http://who.int/mediacetre/news/notes/2007/np31/en/). Several prehospital studies have shown inadequate analgesia for these patients. Factors associated with failures in the management of prehospital pain include underestimation of pain, underdosing of analgesia medications, underfrequency of dosing, and inappropriate withholding of analgesia. The importance of prehospital analgesia has been outlined by the Emergency Medical Services Outcomes Project in the United States as follows: "the relief of discomfort might be the most important task EMS providers perform for the majority of their patients." This sentiment was also advocated by the National Association of EMS Physicians (NAEMSP), who issued a position paper stating that the relief of pain should be a priority for every EMS system. A more to the point assessment of prehospital undertreatment of pain was given in a Basket editorial: "The blame for 'oligoanalgesias' must be laid at the door of physicians in authority who have, through ignorance, underplayed the physiologic and psychological benefits of analgesia and overplayed the potential deleterious side effects of agents that are commonly available."

OBJECTIVES

- Describe the goals of prehospital analgesia and sedation.
- Discuss barriers to the administration of prehospital analgesia.
- Describe pain assessment and prehospital pain scales.
- Describe available pharmacological interventions.
- Describe available local and regional anesthesia.
- Discuss nonpharmacological interventions and therapies.
- Describe the development of analgesia and sedation protocols.

INTRODUCTION

Pain complaints present unique challenges to EMS providers. These patients may be difficult, distraught, evasive, and seemingly unreasonable. A full understanding of the differing types of pain, their presentations, and a concise, systematic approach to the treatment of these patients is paramount to optimizing their care. Furthermore, it is important to note that there are advanced life support agencies functioning without access to controlled substances for their patients. It is therefore important for EMS medical directors to understand the importance of these concepts. It is the responsibility of EMS physicians and medical directors to ensure that the problem of oligoanalgesia is addressed in CQI and education programs.

DEFINITION OF PAIN

Pain is the most common reason for patients to seek medical attention in the United States.[1] The International Association for the Study of Pain (IASP) defines pain as "an unpleasant sensory and/or emotional experience associated with actual or potential tissue damage. It usually motivates the patient to withdraw from the offending stimulus."[2] Pain is not only a sensory process, but also an affective, subjective phenomenon influenced by physiological processes and by diverse psychological and emotional processes. Most pain will resolve quickly once the stimulus is withdrawn. However, pain may at times persist despite stimulus removal

and apparent healing. At other times, pain may develop in the absence of any detectable stimulus or damage.

TYPES OF PAIN

There are two categories of pain: acute and chronic. Acute pain is associated with an injury or pathological illness that resolves with the resolution of the inciting cause. Acute pain is mediated through nerve fibers that fire in response to chemicals released with tissue damage. Chronic pain lasts longer than would be expected for a given injury or pathological condition. The main types of pain include nociceptive, neuropathic, phantom, and psychogenic pain.

▦ NOCICEPTIVE PAIN

Acute pain is mediated through nociceptors (pain receptors) that send impulses from the peripheral nerve fibers to the spinal cord and the cerebral cortex of the brain. These receptors respond to a broad range of noxious stimuli (thermal, mechanical, and chemical). Nociceptive pain may also be categorized into visceral, deep somatic, and superficial somatic pain.

Visceral pain: is usually caused by ischemia (low blood flow) and inflammation. Examples include appendicitis, ovarian torsion, and cardiac disease. It is diffuse and difficult to precisely locate and describe ("sick feeling," "deep," or "dull"). Visceral pain may actually present as referred pain to a more superficial location. Associated symptoms may include nausea and vomiting.

Deep somatic pain: occurs due to stimulation of the nociceptors in bones, tendons, ligaments, blood vessels, fasciae, and muscles (sprains and broken bones). It is also very difficult to localize and usually described as "dull" or "aching."

Superficial somatic pain: occurs due to stimulation of nociceptors in the skin and superficial tissue (cuts or bruises). It is a sharp pain that is easy to locate and describe.

▦ NEUROPATHIC PAIN

Neuropathic pain is usually caused by disorders of the peripheral or central nervous system. It may present with *dysesthesia* (unpleasant perception of sensory stimuli), or *allodynia* (pain due to stimuli not normally considered painful), *hyperalgesia* (intense response to a stimulus usually considered less painful), and paresthesias (pins and needle sensation). Neuropathic pain may be continuous or episodic in nature. It commonly presents as coldness, "pins and needles," numbing, or itching. Several common diseases may manifest neuropathic pain, including diabetes, multiple sclerosis, postsurgical patients, certain types of strokes, herpes zoster, HIV, nutritional deficiencies, malignancies, and fibromyalgia.

▦ PHANTOM PAIN

Phantom pain is a type of neuropathic pain caused by the loss of a part of the body that is no longer supplying sensory input to the brain. It is common in amputees (82% in upper limb; 54% in lower limb).[3] It is reported in 72% of patients within 1 week of amputation and in 65% of patients 6 months postamputation.[4,5] The pain may be such that even touching these patients with a blanket or strap evokes a pain response powerful enough to result in urination or defecation.

▦ PSYCHOGENIC PAIN

Psychogenic pain is caused by emotional, mental, or behavioral factors. It can be quite intense, and/or prolonged. It is also called psychalgia or somatoform pain. These patients are often "labeled" as hypochondriacs with fictitious pain. However, pain specialists consider this pain no less "real" or painful than other types of pain.

EPIDEMIOLOGY OF PAIN

Pain is the primary reason for emergency department visits (>50%) and becomes more common as a person ages.[6] However, there is no simple relationship between gender or age and pain.

PAIN IN CHILDREN

Pain in children was often ignored, with surgery and other procedures routinely performed on these patients because it was felt that pediatric patients had "immature" nervous systems that did not appreciate pain. Research on pain in children is still scarce. However, it is known that chronic pain syndromes in children are usually relapsing and remitting rather than the continuous pain often experienced by adults.[7]

PAIN IN WOMEN

Studies have shown that women are less likely than men to receive morphine analgesia for isolated extremity injuries. A similar study found that nurses are less likely to give analgesics to women than to men given identical clinical scenarios. A paramedic study showed no difference in the rate of paramedic-initiated analgesia, but there was a difference in the type of analgesia administered.

PAIN IN THOSE OF LOWER SOCIOECONOMIC STATUS

Multiples studies have shown that patients of lower socioeconomic status and minorities tend to receive less analgesia for their pain. A retrospective review of 953 patients receiving pain medication for lower extremity injuries found a clear trend in which each successively lower income group had a reduced likelihood of receiving analgesia. While this was not a statistically significant finding, the trend was pervasive and deserves further inquiry. Other studies have found that minorities also have their pain levels underestimated. A growing body of research reveals that there are extensive gaps in pain assessment and treatment among racial and ethnic populations, with minorities receiving less care for pain than non-Hispanic Caucasians

PAIN IN MIDDLE-AGED ADULTS

There are many types of pain associated with this group. The most common are headaches, chest pain, and back pain.

Headaches: This is the most common type of pain among all age groups. Tension headaches are by far the most common type (lifetime prevalence of 80%) and are more common in women and younger adults.[7]

Chest pain: Chest pain is the sine qua non of acute coronary syndrome (ACS). However, there is marked variability in pain intensity as well as other symptoms with ACS. Studies have shown that pain intensity peaks prior to hospital admission and many pain treatment strategies have been devised, including the use of nitrates, narcotics, β-blockers, and benzodiazepines. In the prehospital setting, there is currently *not* an optimal use, or combination of use, for these four most common therapies for ACS chest pain. There is also not much known about the impact that early and complete relief of chest pain has on the early phase of ACS, and few studies comparing pain-relieving strategies in the prehospital phase of ACS. However, Zedigh and colleagues found that prehospital interventions to decrease in chest pain within the first 30 minutes decreased heart rate and ST-segment elevations without decrements in systolic blood pressure or evidence of ST-segment depression.

Back pain: This is another common type of pain, one that is associated with many factors (physical, psychological, and social). It usually begins in the late teens to early forties, and plateaus in fifth decade of life, with an increased prevalence in those who smoke.[7]

Pain in geriatric patients: The most common pain in this group of patients is joint pain. The prevalence of hip and knee pain in those over 65 years of age is more than double that of younger adults.[7] The literature shows that both prehospital and emergency department staff *fail* to provide timely pain management for the elderly with femoral neck fractures. In these patients, communication issues and cognitive impairment comprise the majority of reported barriers to providing analgesia.

Pain in cancer patients: Cancer pain is caused by a variety of mechanisms and may involve the viscera, bone, or nerves. Patients with cancer experience greater pain in the later stages of their disease, and the treatment of their cancer may actually exacerbate their cancer pain.[7] There is significant evidence that the pain these patients experience is undertreated. The cancers cited most often as being associated with significant pain are bone, cervix, oral cavity, stomach, lung, genitourinary, pancreas, and breast.[7]

Pain in immunodeficient patients: Pain is a major problem for those with AIDs, especially in the later stages of the disease, and is comparable in intensity to that of cancer patients.[7] The incidence of pain in those with HIV is approximately 30%.[7] There is some gender and social bias in the treatment of these patients. In particular, women, less educated patients, and drug abusers are often undertreated.[7]

IMPORTANCE OF EARLY PAIN CONTROL

There are many reasons to treat pain adequately. Failure to do so may make it more difficult to treat future pain, increase the likelihood of developing chronic pain, and may lead to changes to a patient's behavior in response to future pain. Inadequate pain control may lead to an increased pain threshold, making it more difficult to treat subsequent episodes of pain.

THE "WIND-UP" PHENOMENON

There is a "wind-up phenomenon" that causes untreated pain to worsen. Nerve fibers become more adept at delivering pain signals to the brain. The intensity of the signals increases over and above what is needed to warrant attention. The brain becomes more sensitive to the pain. Thus, pain feels much intense even though the injury or illness is not worsening. Early analgesia minimizes this phenomenon.

PREEMPTIVE ANALGESIA

Preemptive analgesia or preventive analgesia is an evolving clinical concept. It involves the introduction of an analgesic regimen immediately upon recognition of pain or before the onset of noxious stimuli (ie, a planned procedure), with the goal of preventing sensitization of the nervous system to subsequent stimuli that could amplify pain. The importance of preemptive analgesia is that *untreated acute pain* has the potential to produce acute neurohumoral changes, neuronal remodeling, and long-lasting psychological and emotional distress, leading to a prolonged chronic pain states. Treatment should encompass the entire duration of the high-intensity noxious stimulation that can lead to establishment of central and peripheral sensitization caused by an injury.

PATIENT SATISFACTION

It is not surprising that patient satisfaction is higher when pain control is offered. Patients given analgesia are often "uptriaged" upon arrival to the emergency department, due to the perception that the patient's presentation is of a higher acuity. Conversely, patients not given analgesics in a prehospital setting are more likely to have a significant delay in receiving analgesics in the emergency department.

THE GOALS OF PREHOSPITAL PAIN MANAGEMENT, ANALGESIA, AND SEDATION

Success in patient treatment and therapies depends on the strength of the plan. All protocols should be developed, and reviewed with regularity, by a multidisciplinary team. This team should comprise paramedics, EMS supervisors, nurses, and physicians (medical control physicians, trauma surgeons, and emergency medicine specialists). The basic tenets of the plan should address these issues.

- Unanimous advocacy from leadership that patients should receive expeditious pain management
- Succinct, simple strategies and protocols that optimize pain assessment in all patients and require pain management intervention and recording of intervention following each assessment.
- EMS systems should develop policies and procedures for the safe utilization of pain medications

BARRIERS TO THE ADMINISTRATION OF PREHOSPITAL ANALGESIA

Paramount to the care of patients is to abide by the health care professional's responsibility to accept the patient's report of pain and to respond in a positive manner.[8] The development of any successful analgesia and sedation protocol must identify barriers to such care and develop protocols that mitigate these barriers.

▨ INABILITY TO ASSESS PAIN

The inability to assess pain is challenging. Hennes and colleagues found this to be the most common barrier, with paramedics listing it as their primary barrier in treating 87% of their pediatric patients and 90% of the adults. The use of pain assessments was dismally low for adolescents (5%) and children (2%) in the Hennes study. Several studies have confirmed the lack of pain assessment in pediatric patients. While 93% of prehospital providers had knowledge of adult analgesia indications for extremity fractures, only 50% thought that analgesia was needed for children with these injuries. These statistics were similar for adults and children with burns. Moreover, medical control leadership in the mandatory use of pain assessments for all patients has been clearly shown to improve compliance with the administration of analgesia and has been advocated in the NAEMSP position paper.

▨ CALCULATION OF LOW PAIN SCORES

All pain concerns should be addressed. Some providers equate low pain scores as an indication not to medicate. Situational or experiential factors also come into play. Some providers believe they can ferret out true pain from "false" pain based on patient behavior, communication, and the interpretation of physical and hemodynamic parameters. Below are factors providers may use to gauge the need for analgesia.

Patient behavior and cooperation: Observation of the patient's behavior and level of cooperation is used as an indicator for pain.

Nonverbal communication: Signs such as facial expressions, guarding, and withdrawing from examination were also seen as important.

Physical signs: Signs such as diaphoresis, swelling, deformity, or abnormalities in vital signs are also seen as important. Some paramedics question the patient's pain claim if their physical examination and vital signs do not correspond.

▨ DIFFICULT VASCULAR ACCESS OR VASCULAR ACCESS NOT REQUIRED

Difficult vascular access is a known barrier to analgesic administration. One study found this reason cited as a barrier to the administration of morphine analgesia in 80% of both their adult and pediatric patients. These same providers cited "vascular access not required" as a barrier in 67% of both their adult and pediatric patients. Often providers find it easier to simply transport these patients and allow the emergency staff to obtain access and address painful conditions. However, delaying analgesia or sedation to a patient until arrival to the hospital only delays care. Other routes of analgesics administration should be considered such as oral, intranasal, intramuscular, or interosseus routes. A retrospective review of the time to analgesia for patients with painful extremity injuries found that only 12% received prehospital analgesia (average time 23 minutes). The other 88% received their first parenteral analgesia in the emergency department (113 minutes later). These results mirror a similar study of lower extremity fractures in which the mean time for the EMS treated group was 28 minutes versus 146 minutes for the ED treated group. Clearly, delaying pain management until arrival to the ED is not an optimum strategy.

▨ RECORD KEEPING OR OTHER CARE ADEQUATE

Prehospital providers undertake an inordinate amount of tasks, even during routine transports. Record keeping, application of monitors, the obtaining of intravenous access, continual patient assessments, and reports to medical control/hospital of destination are just some of these. Paramedics also have to explain treatments and treatment options, obtain

histories, allergies, medications, and engage in specific care such as splinting, hemorrhage control, elevation, and wound care. It is not surprising that the barrier of "other care adequate" and "record keeping" receive mention as significant barriers to analgesia and sedation. However, as previously stated, pain is the most common reason for patients to seek emergency care. Mandatory pain assessments with expected provider actions should be part of the quality assurance studies of EMS organizations.

▨ POSSIBLE DRUG SEEKING

The perception of drug seeking behavior may significantly reduce administration of analgesic medications. In the Hennes study, 81% of paramedics listed drug seeking as their reasoning for withholding analgesia. More impressively, these same paramedics (65%) also voiced drug seeking as a reason to withhold pain medications in children.

▨ PROVIDER BELIEF THAT PATIENTS OFTEN EXAGGERATE OR OVERREPORT PAIN

Providers' personal bias may play a role in their perception of a patient's pain and subsequently affect the overall administration of an analgesic. One study queried paramedics as to how they recognize pain. The overall response was that there is no classic sign and that experience was their guide.[9] Overall, the majority of the paramedics in this study do not perceive all patients to be honest and feel that some exaggerate their pain.[9] Some paramedics consider the "on a Scale of 1 to 10" to be too subjective to utilize as an indicator for analgesic medications. Others felt this overexaggerated behavior was a justification for calling an ambulance or to be seen quicker.[9] Additionally, 83% of providers considered the cultural background of the patient to have a major impact on the patient's pain experience. Some cultures are thought to be more vocal and emotional in expressing their pain.

▨ PROVIDER INADEQUACY IN ADEQUATELY ASSESSING AND TREATING PAIN

A paramedic's perception of the patient's pain determines the treatment that is rendered. A provider's belief that they can objectively determine a patient's pain level and treat accordingly (withhold or provide analgesia or sedation) is *false*.[10] Medical care providers, prehospital or otherwise, cannot see, feel, or define the pain that is experienced by a patient. Caregivers, prehospital providers, and others have been shown to underestimate patient pain levels. In the Hennes study, 37% of paramedics thought they administered morphine to adults with chest pain (actual number 4%); 24% reported giving morphine for extremity fractures (actual 12%); and 89% thought they gave morphine for burns (actual 14%). Now this may be related to the provider's desire to meet establish goals on self-surveys. However, disparities such as these are concerning, and require further investigation.

▨ FEAR OF OBSCURING THE DIAGNOSIS OR OF COMPLICATIONS

This is a concern for many paramedics, and some would rather not treat a patient's pain if they consider the pain to be a crucial element in diagnosis.[9] Pain and its resultant anxiety are counterproductive to diagnostic and therapeutic interventions. Uninterrupted pain also adversely affects immune function, wound healing, and is associated with diagnosis-specific adverse events, such as blood pressure elevations in head-injured patients. Early studies and texts created a concern that analgesic administration blunts accurate examinations and delays or obscures diagnosis (eg, acute abdominal conditions). This is incorrect. Severe pain precludes proper examination. Diagnostic tenderness is usually not affected by analgesia. Early pain management allows better cooperation and facilitates examination, and several studies have demonstrated that it is a safe practice to administer opioids in patients suspected to harbor critical illness.

▨ PATIENT RELUCTANCE TO REQUEST PAIN MEDICATION

There is a certain degree of reluctance on the part of patients to complain of pain or to ask for pain medication. McEachin found that two-thirds of patients were not aware that EMS providers could give analgesics. The remaining third did not ask for analgesia despite knowledge of the availability of these medications. The same study found that 93% felt that their pain was poorly assessed and 66% felt their pain was not well managed. EMS providers should take the lead in advocating for early pain management for their patients. Pain assessment scales could guide the EMS provider in the appropriateness of analgesia.

FACTORS INVOLVED IN THE DECISION TO ADMINISTER PREHOSPITAL ANALGESIA

Paramedics consider the types of illnesses (limb trauma, cardiac pain, back pain, labor, abdominal pain, sickle cell crises, and fractures), travelling time, nature of the roads, and hospital delays in their decision-making process.[9]

FACTORS INVOLVED IN THE DECISION TO WITHHOLD PREHOSPITAL ANALGESIA

The type of injury or illness also influences a paramedic's decision to withhold pain treatment. The paramedic's perception of patient honesty is a key factor. Additionally, some paramedics feel that they can psychologically help patients control pain. They feel it is essential to take control of the situation, relieve anxiety, and gain the patient's trust. For these providers, it is considered possible to "talk the patient down through their pain and reduce their pain *without the need for drugs.*"[9]

PAIN ASSESSMENT

Pain is a complex, multidimensional experience determined not only by the injury severity, but also by previous pain experience, personal beliefs, motivations, and environmental factors. There is no objective measurement of pain. Self-reporting is the most valid. Caregivers cannot perceive the pain experienced by their patients, therefore, they must rely on self-reports, pain assessment scales, verbal and nonverbal communication, injury mechanisms, previous experiences, and empathy. Reports of pain may not correlate with the observed disability or physical examination findings. Pain assessment scales are important in providing a quantitative assessment of the pain as well as response to interventions. In spite of their repeated validation as an important tool that improves patient care, pain scales continue to be underutilized. Pain scales aid in

real-time assessment and the care of patients and are vital for quality improvement that allows real time analyses of efficacy of interventions or changes in practice patterns.

THE VISUAL ANALOG PAIN SCALE (VAS)

The VAS is one of the most commonly used pain measurement tools. It consists of a 10-cm slide ruler device that is bounded on each end by perpendicular marks and descriptors. Patients are asked to move the slide rule along the scale to indicate the severity of their pain. The VAS has been shown valid for research purposes as well as a reliable measure of pain severity (**Figure 62-1**).

THE NUMERICAL RATING SCALE (NRS)

The NRS is a rapid and simple pain severity tool, in which patients are asked to rate their pain on a scale of 0 to 10. The advantages of this scale lies in its simplicity, reproducibility, easy comprehensibility, and sensitivity to small changes in pain. Patients prefer the NRS to the VAS. The NRS can be administered verbally without requiring cognitive translation into a mark on a 10-cm scale (**Figure 62-2**).

WONG-BAKER FACES

Wong-Baker FACES can measure pain in infants and young children using self-report scales or scales using physiological and behavioral measurement. Caregivers and parents tend to underestimate the severity of pain in pediatric patients. Pain scales for pediatric patients need to be tailored to the patient's stage of development. In infants, pain assessment is inferred by behavioral responses (crying and facial grimacing) and physiological parameters (vital signs). In toddlers and young children, pictorial pain scales such as Wong-Baker FACES are useful. Older children can use NRS, VDS, or perhaps even VAS to assess their pain (**Figure 62-3**).

Verbal Descriptor Scales (VDS) The VDS is the simplest for the patient to use. Patients are asked to choose a word that describes their

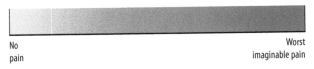

FIGURE 62-1. Visual analog scale. (Reprinted with permission from Tintinalli JE, Stapczynski JS, Ma OJ, Cline DM, Cydulka RK, Meckler GD, eds. *Tintinalli's Emergency Medicine: A Comprehensive Study, 7th ed.* New York, NY: McGraw-Hill; 2011.)

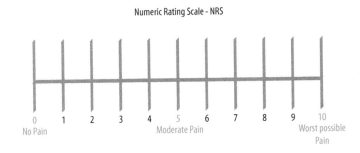

FIGURE 62-2. Numeric rating scale.

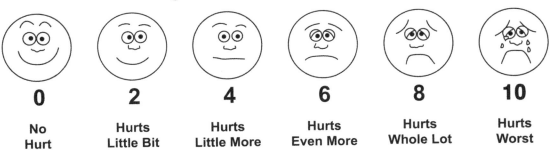

FIGURE 62-3. Wong-Baker FACES pain scale (Wong-Baker FACES Foundation (2015). Wong-Baker FACES® Pain Rating Scale. Retrieved [Date] with permission from http://www.WongBakerFACES.org.)

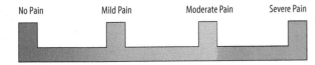

FIGURE 62-4. Verbal descriptor scale.

pain. It ranges from "None…Mild…Moderate…Severe" although other descriptors can be used. The VDS appear to be favored by older patients. There seems to be more interindividual variability with the VDS. The verbal descriptor scale is useful in patients who are unable to rate their pain on the NRS. Tanabe validated the VDS in a study of ED patients (**Figure 62-4**).

PHARMACOLOGICAL INTERVENTIONS

The prehospital provider has a wide variety of pharmacological and non-pharmacological interventions to employ in the pain management and sedation of their patients. This section deals with the medications and techniques that can be used for these purposes. The medical control director, field supervisors, and providers must all be intimately aware of the actions, indications, and contraindications of these drugs and techniques.

NONOPIATE ANALGESICS

These are a group of drugs that primarily inhibit prostaglandin synthesis. They are usually the first-line drugs in the management of mild to moderate pain. The analgesic effects have a therapeutic ceiling, meaning escalating doses do not enhance pain relief. Specific advantages of these drugs are a lack of tolerance, lack of dependence, low abuse potential, and a lack of respiratory depression and sedation. They do have some problematic side effects, including gastrointestinal bleeding, and acute renal failure. This group includes acetaminophen (APAP), salicylates (ASA), cyclooxygenase (COX)-specific inhibitors, and the nonsteroidal anti-inflammatory agents (NSAIDs).

Acetaminophen: Acetaminophen is a well-known antipyretic and analgesic agent. It has a low side-effect profile and can be used safely at appropriate dosages. It can be a first-line therapy in the management of mild to moderate pain. The recommended dose in adults is 325 to 1000 mg by mouth (PO) or rectum (PR). In July 2011, the FDA decreased the recommended dose from 4000 mg to 3000 mg daily secondary to the potential for hepatic damage with chronic use. In infants and children, the dose is 10 to 15 mg/kg PO/PR. The toxic effect of APAP is hepatotoxicity. Chronic APAP use by those with liver disease (cirrhosis, hepatitis, and alcoholism) can result in hepatotoxicity even at recommended dosages.

Salicylates: These drugs are nonsteroidal anti-inflammatory agents that are derivatives of salicylic acid. Aspirin, also known as acetylsalicylic acid (ASA), is the best-known agent in this group. Several salicylates are used therapeutically, including aspirin, methyl salicylate (oil of Wintergreen), salsalate, diflunisal, and others. None are more effective than another. All have similar antipyretic and analgesic effects. They are COX inhibitors that inhibit platelet aggregation and gastric prostaglandin synthesis. Because of these properties, they are useful in the prevention of heart attacks, strokes, and blood clot formation. These drugs are also classified as NSAIDs because they inhibit the cyclooxygenase enzyme. However, ASA's effect on this COX enzyme is irreversible, and the anti-platelet effects will last until platelets are regenerated (days). Therefore, when patients are advised against the use of NSAIDs due to bleeding, they should also be advised to discontinue ASA. These drugs carry the risk of gastrointestinal bleeding, tinnitus, renal failure, and anaphylactic reactions.

NSAIDs: Nonsteroidal, anti-inflammatory agents (NSAIDs) are non-selective COX inhibitors. All have a similar mechanism of action and a therapeutic ceiling of analgesia. None have more superior analgesia than

another for pain relief. It is noted that some patients, however, do respond more favorably to one class more than another. The dose required to treat an inflammatory condition is typically higher than the analgesic doses. NSAIDs have no respiratory depression, sedation, dependence, or tolerance associated with their use. Side effects are frequent and can be severe. Dyspepsia will develop in 10% to 20% of patients. Gastrointestinal bleeding is common, with the lowest risk with ibuprofen and the highest risk with ketorolac. Most are administered orally, with the exception of indomethacin (also given PR), and ketorolac (also given IV). There is no evidence of improved analgesic efficacy with IV use over PO use. The parenteral route should only be used if the patient is unable to tolerate oral therapy.

Nitrous Oxide: Nitrous oxide (N_2O) is a colorless, odorless, and rapidly absorbed, inhalable gas that produces central analgesia and sedation. It has been used in clinical practice as a moderate analgesic and mild sedative in the hospital and prehospital setting, primarily for procedural sedation. It can be used alone or with other agents. It is typically self-administered to prevent hypoventilation and loss of airway protective reflexes. Usually the agent is given as a 50/50 O_2-N_2O mixture. It can be used safely in prehospital pain management and for painful procedures such as fracture and dislocation reductions. A 16-year study of over 2700 patients found that significant pain relief occurred in 80% of patients treated with N_2O. Nitrous oxide has side effects, most of which are mild, but include dizziness, nausea, and drowsiness (most common). It is also a mild cardiac depressant and causes mild elevation in the venous resistance. However, there is little effect on ventilatory drive.

Tramadol: Tramadol is a central acting phenanthrene alkaloid codeine, an opioid prodrug with a weak affinity for the *mu* opioid receptor. It is used to treat moderate to moderately severe pain. It also has an effect on the reuptake of serotonin and norepinephrine in the CNS, which makes it practical in the management of chronic pain. The dosage is 50 to 100 mg PO. It is often used by providers as an alternative to opioid analgesics because of suspected drug-seeking or maladaptive patient behavior. Side effects are frequent, and include dizziness, nausea, headache, and somnolence. Seizures can occur, especially in those patients taking antidepressants (SSRIs, TCAs, MAO inhibitors) and in those with a previous history of seizures. Because of the lack of superior efficacy in the treatment of moderate to severe pain and the side-effect profile of the drug, the use of tramadol in the prehospital setting should be limited.

OPIATES

Opioid analgesics are sometimes referred to as the opiates or narcotic analgesics. They have a long history of use in the treatment of pain, dating back to 4000 BC. Throughout their history, their sedative and abuse potential has been well evidenced. Despite these drawbacks, no other class of drugs in history has been so long utilized. Opioids act by binding to the opiate receptors within the central and peripheral nervous systems. The pain alleviating effects occur on the CNS *mu* receptor sites. They are appropriate drugs for moderate to severe pain. Perhaps because of their abuse potential, these drugs are often underdosed and underutilized in the treatment of acute, painful injuries. Other factors related to the lack of use appropriate use of opioids include poor understanding of the their pharmacological properties, fear of obscuring diagnoses, fear of potential side effects, fear of disciplinary action for their use (even for legitimate medical purposes), and a fearing of causing addiction or acquiescing to a drug-seeking patient. However, these drugs have many advantages. They are inexpensive, minimally sedating, readily available, with short half-lives, a rapid onset of action, limited cardiovascular side effects, easy control of administration, and reversibility. The disadvantages of opioids include respiratory and CNS depression. In the event of these adverse effects, opioids may be reversed with naloxone or nalmefene. Intranasal opioids are commonly used in the prehospital and emergency department settings, in both children and adults. Opioids should be titrated in short fixed intervals, with additional doses given as needed, and the monitoring for adverse effects.

Morphine (Roxanol): Morphine is the naturally occurring active ingredient in opium, obtained from the poppy plant. It is the gold standard analgesic to which all others are compared. Morphine has been extensively studied in the prehospital setting and has a good safety profile, rapid onset of action, and a duration of action of 3 to 5 hours. Morphine acts on the CNS *mu* receptors, resulting in analgesia, euphoria, miosis, decreased gastrointestinal motility, and respiratory depression (hypoxia and hypercapnia). The large disadvantage of this drug is that it increases histamine release, resulting in pruritus, but more importantly, loss of vascular tone, bronchospasm, nausea, and vomiting. Additionally, injectable morphine contains sodium bisulfite, which may also cause bronchospasm in patients with asthma and those with allergic reactions. The effective dosing of morphine is 0.1 mg/kg every 3 to 5 minutes. Adults tolerate 10 mg dosing well. The maximum single dose is 10 mg. Morphine may be given IV, IM, or SQ with equal efficacy. In the absence of an IV, the SQ route is less painful. Regimented dosing (every 5 minutes until pain symptoms resolve) is safe and effective in the prehospital setting. Morphine has lost status to newer, designer opioids with better CV stability and no histamine release.

Hydromorphone (Dilaudid): Hydromorphone is a semisynthetic mu receptor agonist that is 5 to 10 times as potent as morphine. As with morphine, it is a very good analgesic for moderate to severe pain, with similar adverse effects, onset of effect, and duration of action. Following IV dosing, drug levels rise rapidly; however, there is a delay in the CNS effects. In the opioid naive patient, a reasonable starting dose is 0.03 mg/kg (2 mg IV). The duration of action is 3 to 4 hours. Hydromorphone may be given IV, IM, or SQ.

Meperidine (Demerol): Meperidine is a synthetic opioid that is still used despite its multiple disadvantages. As with other mu receptor agonists, it has dose-dependent analgesia, and was commonly used by physicians due to their familiarity with the drug. The recommended dose of meperidine is 0.5 to 1.0 mg/kg. It is 8 to 10 times *less powerful* than morphine. Analgesia begins within 15 minutes of either PO or IV administration, with a peak effect in 1 to 2 hours. It can produce tachycardia due to vagolytic activity. It has been the opioid of choice for the treatment of severe abdominal pain because it was believed to cause less spasm at the sphincter of Oddi in those patients with suspected cholecystitis. However, this advantage has been disputed, as there have been no human studies validating this effect. Meperidine is also contraindicated in those patients taking MAO inhibitors, as it can cause severe respiratory depression, excitation, seizures, and hyperthermia. Because of its atropine-like structure, it may cause tachycardia and xerostomia. Importantly, meperidine accumulates in renal disease, and induces histamine release. As there are better opioid alternatives, the use of meperidine in the hospital and prehospital setting is discouraged.

Fentanyl (Sublimaze): Fentanyl is the most popular opioid in the world. It is attractive for prehospital use because of its short duration of action. Fentanyl is a synthetic opioid analgesic that is 50 to 80 times more potent than morphine. The analgesic dosing for fentanyl is 1.0 to 1.5 µg/kg, titrated to affect every 3 to 5 minutes. Fentanyl has an onset of action of 1 to 2 minutes, with maximum effects within several minutes. It is almost a pure analgesic, with very little sedation. One study enrolling 2000 patients found that only one required naloxone for respiratory depression. Importantly, it does not release histamine. Fentanyl does not induce vasodilation or myocardial depression. It is also the agent of choice for those with reactive airways disease. The disadvantages of fentanyl include bradycardia, hypotension, increased intracranial pressure, antidiuretic hormone release, nausea, vomiting, pruritus, and chest wall rigidity. Chest wall rigidity occurs with larger doses, rapid administration, and is well documented to occur in neonates and children. The etiology of chest wall rigidity is unknown. If this occurs, the provider should first administer naloxone. If symptoms persist, rapid sequence intubation should be performed. Fentanyl should not be administered to children <6 months of age, as it stimulated the central vagus nucleus in the brainstem, resulting in prolongation of the refractory period of the AV node and significant bradycardia. Fentanyl, despite these side effects, is an excellent analgesic for hospital and prehospital use.

Nalbuphine (Nubain): Nalbuphine is a semisynthetic narcotic agonist-antagonist analgesic (kappa receptor agonist and *mu* receptor antagonist). Nalbuphine has a class B pregnancy classification; however, caution is advised because of its antagonistic properties. It can precipitate withdrawal symptoms in opioid-dependent patients. Nalbuphine has minimal hemodynamic effects and does not release histamine. Sedation is the most common side effect. Dosing is 10 mg for adults (SQ, IM, or IV), with an onset of effect of 5 to 10 minutes and a duration of action of 3 to 6 hours. It has a ceiling effect on analgesia and respiratory depression at approximately 30 mg.

Butorphanol (Stadol): Butorphanol is available in parenteral form and as a nasal spray. The transnasal form has been used to treat migraine headaches. It has similar effects as nalbuphine, but should be avoided in patients with heart failure or advanced coronary disease, as it may decrease myocardial contractility and cause increases in pulmonary wedge pressure, heart rate, and systemic vascular resistance. The dosing is 1 to 2 mg IV/IM/SQ. The elderly clear the drug more slowly, so half dosing is recommended.

Buprenorphine (Buprenex): Buprenorphine is a semisynthetic opioid with partial activity (but high affinity) for the *mu* receptor from which it slowly dissociates. It has similar effects to morphine in terms of analgesia. There is a ceiling effect on respiratory depression with escalating doses. Buprenorphine at a dose of 0.4 mg is the equivalent of 10 mg of morphine IM, but has a longer duration of action. The dose for analgesia is 0.3 mg IM or IV. With IM administration, the initial effects are seen within 15 minutes with a peak at 1 hour. With IV administration, the onset of effects and the peak is shorter. The medication does have a sublingual form that produces effective pain relief. Opiate addiction is often treated with a sublingual formulation with naloxone added to prevent diversion and surreptitious use.

SEDATIVE-HYPNOTICS

These drugs include ketamine, benzodiazepines, propofol, and etomidate. The key thing to remember is that when treating acute pain, the isolated use of sedatives without analgesia is to be discouraged.

Ketamine (Ketalar): Ketamine is a phencyclidine derivative (NMDA blocker and glutamate inhibitor) anesthetic agent that dissociates cortical activity from the brainstem rather than depressing CNS function. It is an intense coanalgesic, sedative, and amnestic, and has been termed "the safest anesthetic agent in the world." It has been used in pediatric procedural sedation for decades. Moreover, because it maintains all vital signs and protective airway reflexes, it is used in the most rural clinics of the third world and in disaster medicine without cardiac or pulse oximetry monitoring, IV access, or supplemental oxygenation. In disaster and combat, ketamine is used in surgery with minimal personnel and without monitoring equipment. A recent review of prehospital ketamine use found it to be an ideal drug that is safe, effective, and more appropriate than other drugs currently in use. The advantages of this drug are that it has a low cost and a large therapeutic window. Ketamine also *has no histamine release*, and outstanding cardiovascular stability. Ketamine may raise BP and pulse minimally, weakly releases norepinephrine, and is a potent bronchodilator. One of the biggest advantages of ketamine is that dissociation is not dose related. This makes adequate sedation reliably and safely achieved with a single dose and without the requirement of IV access. To date, there has never been reported case where IV access averted or would have averted an adverse outcome. There has always been concern related to the use of ketamine in trauma patients with head injuries due to concerns about raising intracranial pressure. However, more recent studies have shown that ketamine may have a neuroprotective role, and its use in ventilated patients may provide superior cerebral circulation. A ketamine review of over 70,000 patients found one significant cardiovascular complication—"Hypoxic Cardiac Arrest Secondary to Respiratory Depression… In a Debilitated Adult (1971)." Ketamine also has psychotropic effects and must be avoided in those with psychiatric disease. Ketamine is also contraindicated in those <3 months of age. It will increase oral and/or bronchial secretions, usually in those <5 years old which is blunted with atropine or glycopyrrolate. Ketamine also causes laryngospasm in the very young and usually resolves within minutes. Additional side effects include hypertonus (purposeless movements that are benign but impressive), and a patchy erythematous torso rash in 5% to 20 % of patients. This rash is not an allergic reaction. It disappears within 20 minutes requires no treatment and does not recur. However, the most discussed side effect of ketamine use is the emergence reaction" that occurs in 10% of children and up to 50% of adults. It is one of the most feared complications, but is relatively benign. Administering ketamine very slowly and recovering in a dark room with minimal stimulation helps prevent this emergence reaction. Benzodiazepines should be administered if symptoms develop.

Despite the long list of contraindications, ketamine has been found to be safe and effective in the prehospital setting, with little significant complications reported. Ketamine can be administered SQ, PO, PR, IV, IM, transdermally, nasally, intrathecally, and via epidural injection. Ketamine also has many favorable characteristic for the treatment of burn patients. The dosing for ketamine is 1 mg/kg IV and 4 to 5 mg/kg IM. Its onset of action is 30 to 60 seconds (IV) and 3 to 5 minutes (IM). Ketamine's duration of effect is 10 to 15 minutes (IV) and 20 to 30 minutes (IM).

Benzodiazepines: Benzodiazepines are useful in the prehospital setting for procedural sedation or with another agent for analgesia. They are anxiolytics, amnestic, sedative agents *without analgesic properties.* These agents are commonly used for RSI, treatment of seizures, behavioral emergencies, and as an induction agent for anesthesia. Benzodiazepines are classified by their duration of action. The three most common agents are midazolam, lorazepam, and diazepam. They have minimal cardiac effects, and they decrease cerebral blood flow and cerebral metabolic rate. They raise seizure threshold and are often used as anticonvulsants. When used in combination with opioids, benzodiazepines have a synergistic effect in lowering blood pressure and producing respiratory depression. Benzodiazepines should be used sparingly patients on barbiturates or with COPD. Benzodiazepine-associated hypotension is dose related, more likely to occur in the elderly, and may be mitigated by ensuring patient euvolemia. These drugs are to be avoided in those with head injury, shock, or drug/alcohol use. Because these drugs are hepatically metabolized, caution is advised for use in patients with liver disease. The rescue agent for benzodiazepines is flumazenil. Flumazenil use must be avoided in those with benzodiazepine dependence, however, as it may precipitate life-threatening withdrawal symptoms. Midazolam, lorazepam, and diazepam are discussed in detail below. Although all of these drugs are effective sedatives, *diazepam and lorazepam have no advantage over midazolam if the goal is to produce a short, titratable state of anxiolysis and sedation.* Both have longer half-lives than midazolam; both are more difficult to titrate than midazolam and less well suited for procedural sedation. Moreover, diazepam has more respiratory depression, phlebitis, hypotension and longer sedation than midazolam.

Midazolam (Versed): Midazolam is an ultrashort acting benzodiazepine that produces anxiolysis, sedation, anterograde and retrograde amnesia, and is an anticonvulsant. It is three to four times more potent than diazepam and has better IM absorption. Midazolam is water soluble (no vascular irritation), but may cause apnea when used with fentanyl (usually requires minimal interventions such as airway readjustment or bagging). Midazolam may be given IV, IM, and intranasally. Intranasal midazolam has been shown to be highly effective for pediatric sedation in the hospital setting. Dosing for midazolam is 0.05 to 0.1 mg/kg IV or IM. When used in combination with opioids, the dosing is 0.02 mg/kg IV or IM.

Lorazepam (Ativan): Lorazepam has a longer onset and duration of action than midazolam. It is often used as the first-line agent in the treatment of seizures. It is also commonly used to calm agitated patients. Lorazepam has been shown to work very well in combination with haloperidol to control acute psychosis or combative behavior. For sedation, lorazepam dosing is 0.05 mg/kg IV or IM (maximum dose 4 mg). For

the acutely agitated or combative patient, dosing of 2 mg PO/IV/IM is sufficient to produce tranquilization.

Diazepam (Valium): Diazepam has an intermediate onset of action and a fairly prolonged duration of effect. It is frequently used in the prehospital setting because it can be given PO, IM, PR, and IV. Compared to midazolam, it has a slower onset of action, more side effects, lesser amnestic effects, and less potency. As with other benzodiazepines, respiratory depression and sedation is a concern. Adult dosing for diazepam is 2 to 4 mg IV/IM (maximum dose is 5-10 mg). The onset of action is 3 to 5 minutes (IV) with effects lasting 90 minutes. Pediatric dosing is 0.04 to 0.2 mg/kg IV/IM (maximum dosing is 0.6 mg/kg every 8 hours).

Propofol (Diprivan): Propofol is a unique alkylphenol agent that is highly lipid soluble, profoundly sedating, and very short acting. It is a sedative, amnesic, anxiolytic, antiemetic, anticonvulsant, euphoric, and hypnotic drug without analgesia effects. It is also a potent vasodilator without any histamine release. It is rapidly metabolized by the liver and has a rapid onset and offset of action. Sedation occurs within1 minute of administration and recovery occurs within 5 to 15 minutes. The disadvantages of propofol include no analgesia, significant injection pain, myoclonus, respiratory depression and apnea that is related to dose and the speed of administration. Avoid propofol in those with increased intracranial pressure, COPD, and pulmonary hypertension. Propofol blocks sympathetic tone and allows parasympathetic vagal responses to predominate (blunting reflexive tachycardia). Propofol may also produce neurological events, such as posturing, myoclonus, and seizure-like activity. Importantly, propofol contains egg, soy, and EDTA. However, the egg component is lecithin (most egg allergies are to the egg albumin). Additionally, there is a difference between generic and trade name formulation. Diprivan uses ethylenediaminetetraacetic acid as an antibacterial agent. *The generic form uses a sulfite* (avoid with sulfite allergies). Dosing is 0.5 to 1.5 mg/kg IV given as an initial bolus, followed by 0.5 mg/kg IV (or a continuous infusion of 50-200 μg/kg/min titrated to effect). The effective dose varies (no apparent weight relationship) but use dose reduction in the elderly. Propofol can be safely combined with opioids and is effective but has significant side effects requiring vigilant reassessments. Recent studies have combined the use of propofol and ketamine. The addition of ketamine (intense coanalgesic, dissociative sedative with amnestic properties) counteracts the adverse hemodynamic and respiratory effects of propofol. The dosing for "ketofol" is 1:1 (10 mg/mL ketamine + 10 mg/mL propofol in the same syringe) given in 1 to -3 mL aliquots.

Etomidate (Amidate): Hypnotic, carboxylated imidazole derivative with anesthetic properties. It produces anxiolysis, sedation, and amnesia that is equal to barbiturates with fewer cardiovascular side effects. The advantages of etomidate include high dosing predictability (more predictable than benzodiazepines); fast onset (1 minute) and fast offset (5-15 minutes), and no histamine release (offers high hemodynamic stability). Etomidate also lowers intracranial and intraocular pressures, and is often used for the RSI of head injured patients. The disadvantages to etomidate include myoclonus, hypoxia, injection pain, nausea, vomiting, and decreased seizure thresholds. Etomidate is contraindicated in those patients at risk for seizures, or with adrenal insufficiency, as its use has been shown to negatively affect the adrenocortical stress response. This drug should also be avoided in children <10 years old. Etomidate dosing for RSI is 0.2 to 0.6 mg/kg IV over 30 to 60 seconds. The dosing for procedural sedation is 0.2 mg/kg titrated to a moderate sedation endpoint (maximum dosing is 0.6 mg/kg).

Haloperidol (Haldol): Haloperidol is a high potency antipsychotic drug with low anticholinergic side effects, but high frequency of extrapyramidal side effects. It has been used to chemically restrain acutely psychotic and agitated patients. It provides excellent sedation when combined with a benzodiazepine. It can be given IM or IV, has a rapid onset of action, and minimal respiratory depressive effects. The disadvantages are the extrapyramidal side effects: inability to initiate movement, inability to remain motionless, motor spasms of the neck, jaw or eyes, motor restlessness, muscle rigidity, and tremors. Haloperidol dosing is 5 mg IM, titrated to effect.

Barbiturates: Barbiturates are one of the oldest classes of sedatives/hypnotic drugs. They provide sedation, hypnosis, and amnesia with good titratability, an onset of action of <1 minute, and rapid recovery. Barbiturates are highly lipophilic and cross the blood-brain barrier readily. These agents do, however, have significant disadvantages. Barbiturates cause respiratory depression in a dose-dependent fashion (avoid in those with COPD or asthma). Centrally mediated peripheral vasodilation, combined with *histamine release,* leads to transient drops in systolic BP of 10% to 30% (partially attenuated by a rise in heart rate). Barbiturates may cause profound cardiovascular depression secondary to negative inotropic effects as well. These drugs also lack a reversal agent. They have been replaced by newer agents. They are also effective anticonvulsants. Patients with porphyria should not be given barbiturates because they stimulate porphyrin synthesis. The two most common used barbiturates for sedation are the ultrashort acting agents: thiopental and methohexital.

Thiopental (Pentothal): Thiopental has an action onset of <1 minute, and a duration of action of 5 to 20 minutes. Dosing is 1 to 3 mg/kg slow IVP (decrease in the elderly and those with renal insufficiency). Importantly, rectal dosing for children is well tolerated (20-25 mg/kg PR) and does not result in apnea or respiratory depression (ideal for laceration repair).

Methohexital (Brevital): Methohexital is the shortest acting of the barbiturates and is twice as potent as thiopental. Dosing is 0.75 to 1.0 mg/kg. The onset of action is within 1 minute and the duration of action is <10 minutes.

Chloral hydrate (Somnote): The American Academy of Pediatrics recommends oral chloral hydrate for children undergoing diagnostic imaging. It is safe, with little respiratory depression, and may be given PO or PR. Chloral hydrate does not lower the blood pressure or heart rate, but may decrease cardiac contractility and the threshold for dysrhythmias. It may also produce a paradoxical agitation or prolonged sedation in special needs children. For this reason, it is recommended for use in those pediatric patients undergoing imaging *but not procedures.* The disadvantages of chloral hydrate are aspirations and deaths have been reported, the onset of action may be up to 1 hour, there are no analgesic properties, and children on tranquilizers or other sedatives may respond poorly. The dose is 25 to 100 mg/kg PO/PR with redosing every 30 minutes as needed (maximum dose is 100 mg/kg).

LOCAL AND REGIONAL ANESTHESIA

▇ TOPICAL APPLICATIONS

Topical applications are a safe and effective method of pain control. The advantages are the painless route of administration and application on almost any body surface area. The primary disadvantage is a slow onset of action.

TAC: TAC is a mixture of tetracaine, adrenaline (epinephrine), and cocaine. This topical application has been replaced by other mixtures.

LET: This topical application contains 4% lidocaine 0.1% epinephrine, and 0.5% tetracaine. LET is an excellent and safe topical anesthetic agent. It can be premixed and stored in a refrigerated unit. It is applied to wounds by soaking a cotton ball in LET and securing the cotton ball to the wound. Blanching of the skin around the wound indicates adequate anesthesia.

EMLA: EMLA is a Eutectic Mixture of Local Anesthetics (2.5% lidocaine and 2.5% prilocaine). It is approved by the FDA only for use on intact skin, although its successful use in open wounds has been reported in the medical literature. Approximately 1 hour of topical application of EMLA is required to achieve local anesthesia, a characteristic that limits its usefulness in emergency cases. Infants younger than 3 months are at a theoretically higher risk for development of methemoglobinemia from EMLA owing to inadequate levels of methemoglobin reductase.

Liposomal lidocaine: ELA-Max is a relatively new proprietary mixture of 4% liposomal lidocaine approved by the FDA for the temporary relief of pain from minor cuts and abrasions. Its onset of action is much shorter than that of EMLA (only 30 minutes) and it carries a much lower risk of methemoglobinemia because it does not contain prilocaine. This formulation may replace EMLA for most topical indications.

▇ LOCAL ANESTHETIC AGENTS

Tetracaine: Tetracaine is an ester agent. It is most commonly used in the ED for corneal anesthesia and as a component of LET.

Lidocaine: Lidocaine is the most commonly used local anesthetic agent. Its low cost, rapid onset, duration, and toxicity profile make it ideal for most routine applications. The maximum dose of lidocaine is 4 to 4.5 mg/kg. Therefore, a 70-kg patient should receive no more than 300 mg, or 30 mL of a 1% solution. The maximum dose may be increased to 7 mg/kg when lidocaine is given with epinephrine, but the increase will also cause an increase in the sympathomimetic side effects (tachycardia and hypertension) and a theoretically higher risk of infection due to diminished blood supply to the affected area. The pain of injection can be reduced by either warming lidocaine to body temperature prior to administration[4] or buffering it with sodium bicarbonate (1 mL sodium bicarbonate to 9 mL of 1% lidocaine).

Bupivacaine: Bupivacaine is slightly more potent than lidocaine and lasts longer. However, its onset of action is later. The maximum dose of bupivacaine is 2.5 mg/kg. A 70-kg patient should receive no more than 175 mg, or 35 mL of a 0.5% solution. This amount can be increased to 3 mg/kg if this agent is given with epinephrine. Owing to bupivacaine's high potency and protein binding, the risk of systemic toxicity with its use is much greater than with use of lidocaine.

Mepivacaine: Mepivacaine is structurally similar to lidocaine, with a similar onset of action and a slightly longer duration. As with bupivacaine, this longer duration of action is associated with a slightly higher risk of toxicity. The toxicity of mepivacaine is between that of lidocaine and bupivacaine, corresponding to its intermediate duration of action.

Ropivacaine: Ropivacaine is a relatively new amide local anesthetic approved by the US Food and Drug Administration (FDA) in 1996. Being the s-isomer of bupivacaine, ropivacaine is very similar in terms of onset of action, slightly less potent, and slightly shorter duration of action; however, it is associated with a 70% lower likelihood of cardiac toxicity. It also costs almost twice as much as bupivacaine.

▇ REGIONAL NERVE BLOCKS

Regional nerve blocks are used for areas that are not amenable to local infiltration, such as the palms, the soles, and the fat pads of fingers and toes. Other advantages include avoidance of local tissue distortion, and the ability to anesthetize large areas with fewer injections and less anesthetic agent (reducing the likelihood of toxicity and overall patient discomfort).

General technique: The provider should first explain the procedure and the benefits and risks to the patient, obtain verbal consent, and assess for any allergies. The general procedure is simple: (a) prepare the skin with povidone-iodine or other antiseptic skin solution; (b) identify the area's landmarks; (c) induce a superficial skin wheal at the injection site to reduce the discomfort of further manipulation; (d) advance the needle to the target area while asking the patient to report any paresthesias; (e) if the patient does report paresthesias, the needle is within the nerve sheath (withdraw the needle 1-2 mm); (f) draw back on the syringe; (g) aspirate to ensure that the needle is not in a vessel; and (h) inject the agent slowly. The agent of choice is usually lidocaine. Bupivacaine may be preferable when longer duration of action is desired.

Types of regional nerve blocks: The emergency medicine literature expounds upon many types of regional nerve blocks. The emerging use of ultrasound has made many of these blocks easy to perform. The value of regional nerve blocks is substantial. They provide safe and rapid analgesia for patients that may have contraindications to other forms of analgesia. Military corpsmen have been using these techniques with great success in the field. A selected few regional nerve blocks are described below.

Hematoma block: The hematoma of a fracture can be locally anesthetized to relieve the pain associated with relocation of a displaced fracture. This block is most commonly used for metacarpal fractures. In most cases 2 mL of agent is usually sufficient. In this case, if aspiration of blood confirms placement of the needle within the hematoma, care should be taken to avoid anatomic locations of known vessels.

Digital nerves: Each finger has two sets of nerves, called the dorsal and palmar digital nerves which travel in the 2, 4, 8, and 10 o'clock positions around the digit. These four branch from two root nerves at the metacarpal-metatarsal heads. The most common approach for the digital nerve block is the proximal-most aspect of the finger or toe, where the nerves travel in the most consistent path. A skin wheal is formed on the dorsal surface of the finger or toe. The needle is then directed to the 2, 4, 8, and 10 o'clock positions, respectively. After aspiration is performed, 0.5 to 1 mL of agent is injected at each site. Epinephrine and other vasoconstricting agents should not be used in this location because of the risk of critical ischemia associated with their use.

Bier block: A Bier block involves the IV injection of regional anesthesia in a tourniqueted extremity. Its use is relatively uncommon in the controlled setting of the emergency department, but has the advantage of the creation of a bloodless field. Peripheral IV access should be established in the target extremity at least 10 cm distal to the tourniquet. Additionally, access should be established in a backup extremity in case resuscitation access is needed.

NONPHARMACOLOGICAL INTERVENTIONS

Pain is not only a sensory process, but also an affective and subjective phenomenon influenced not only by physiological processes, but by diverse psychological and emotional processes as well. Nonpharmacological techniques can be used as an adjunct to other pain relieving modalities in controlling pain. These nonpharmacological interventions include psychological, verbal, and physical interventions. There is a growing body of literature showing that psychological techniques ameliorate pain. There has been reluctance on caregivers to apply these techniques for several reasons. The first is that many believe that psychological techniques are ineffective. The second is that few providers receive any training their application. Health care providers are much more comfortable providing a medication for pain control. It is also important to remember that the use of these techniques requires the cooperation of the patient. If the patient is resistant or unaccepting, the success of the technique dramatically drops. Verbal interventions can be employed by health care providers in the form of explanation of what is occurring to the patient, what will be done, and also by offering words of comfort and support. Family members may also provide this intervention to the patient. Physical interventions are much more commonly used by prehospital personnel and are important in the relief of pain.

■ COGNITIVE THERAPIES

Emotional support and information speaking: These techniques have positive therapeutic effect, and can be taught to even basic paramedic personnel. Patients can find comfort in the words from another individual. Careful use of appropriate wording is important. Good communication skills can ease the uncertainty of injury. For children, having the child's primary caregiver present reduces the stress and anxiety of both the parents and the patient. Verbally providing information about the patient's condition may be comforting to both.

Music: Music holds promise as an adjuvant pain management tool, and in mild cases may supplement or even replace pharmacological interventions before, during, and after painful procedures. However, music therapy for pain should not be considered a first-line treatment. A Cochrane review found that listening to music reduces pain intensity levels and opioid requirements.

Distraction: Distraction is the best studied and most effective of the psychological techniques. Engaging in thoughts or activities that distract attention from pain is one of the most commonly used and highly endorsed strategies for controlling pain. The process of distraction appears to involve competition for attention between a highly salient sensation (pain) and consciously directed focus on some other information processing activity. Distraction is a highly effective technique in the pediatric population in conjunction. Virtual reality (VR) is a relatively new technology that enables individuals to immerse themselves in a virtual world. This multisensory technology has been used in a variety of fields, and most recently has been applied clinically as a method of distraction for pain management during medical procedures.

Guided imagery: Guided imagery is a technique that uses the imagination of the patient to control pain. It can use a voice to guide the patient to an individual imaginary place away from the pain. This is accomplished using a pleasant imaginary scenario involving places, sounds, smells, tastes, and feelings. Sensory focusing is a process, where instead of avoiding thinking about pain, the patient is asked to think of the pain as a physical object in which they can manipulate. The patient is asked to imagine the pain getting smaller and more manageable. As in guided imagery, the patient must participate in the process for the technique to be effective.

Humor: Humor in medicine is not a new concept. One area of great promise is the use of humor to moderate a patient's response to pain. In recent years, there also have been claims that humor and laughter possess unique characteristics for coping with pain and stress. Theoretically, explanations include the release of endorphins, the lowering of tension, as well as the distraction that results from humor. Laughter is less important, it is believed, than the emotional involvement in the humor. Studies have found that emotionally engaging in video segments were equally effective in increasing pain tolerance, whether the videos were funny, sad, or frightening. The primary mechanism, therefore, has been the interpretation of the video as being a compelling and emotional distraction from the pain.

■ BEHAVIORAL TECHNIQUES

Psychological strategies for coping with pain have not been as utilized as pharmacological methods. Fear, anxiety, and depression account for substantial psychological stressors in patients experiencing pain. Relaxation and biofeedback work by helping control physiological responses that contribute to pain production.

Relaxation techniques: These are simple techniques that can be easily taught and used in the prehospital setting for pain control or for a painful procedure. Relaxation may enhance the sense of efficacy with other modalities in the treatment of pain. Relaxation techniques are used to lower arousal, including the unnecessary muscle tension that can increase pain via the sympathetic nervous system. Relaxation techniques are an integral part of the psychological therapy of chronic pain. One method employed is *diaphragmatic breathing* and relaxing the upper chest. For children this technique can be employed by asking them to blow away the pain which can be facilitated by bubble wands, pinwheels, or imaginary candles.

Coping techniques: The patient's ability to control their pain depends on their specific ways of dealing with pain, adjusting to a painful condition, and reducing the distress caused by the pain. Coping actions are employed purposefully and intentionally, and can be assessed in terms of overt and covert behavior. Overt coping strategies include rest, medication, and use of relaxation. Covert coping strategies include various means of self-distraction, self-reassurance that the pain will diminish, information seeking, and problem solving. Coping strategies are thought to alter both the perceived pain intensity and one's ability to manage and tolerate pain.

■ PHYSICAL THERAPIES

Thermal applications: Cold application is a simple and inexpensive therapy which has been accepted for decades as an effective nonpharmacologic intervention for pain management. It increases the pain threshold, as well as decreases the inflammatory reaction and spasm. Cold is commonly used in the treatment of acute soft tissue injuries, and has been shown to reduce pain effectively in the postoperative period. The use of cryotherapy, that is, the application of cold for the treatment of injury or disease, is widespread in sports medicine today. It is an established method when treating acute soft tissue injuries, but there is a discrepancy between the scientific basis for cryotherapy and clinical studies. Prolonged application at very low temperatures should be avoided, as serious side effects, such as frostbite and nerve injuries, may occur. Local warming is an effective treatment for nausea, vomiting, and pain during ambulance transport.

Positioning/repositioning/elevation: Immobilization of fractures provides comfort. Elevation of an injured body part may alleviate some of the intensity of pain. Backboards used for spinal immobilization should be padded, as unpadded backboards are, themselves, a source of significant discomfort.

Immobilization/splinting/traction: Immobilization has been used for thousands of years to treat painful injuries. Care must be taken, however, as immobilization can lead to decreased sensation to involved areas. There is no advantage to immobilization of the cervical spine in soft tissue injury compared to control subjects without immobilization. If there is a radicular pain associated with the injury, there is no evidence supporting cervical immobilization beyond 48 to 72 hours. Lumbar supports have a role in preventing reinjury of the back , but provide little preventive benefit.

DEVELOPMENT OF ANALGESIA AND SEDATION PROTOCOLS

Specific protocols differ in every region of the country. Any attempt to elevate one protocol over others would be moot. Most EMS services have standard protocols that are complaint based, and most have instructions to contact medical control for further pain orders as needed. However, it is interesting to note that many of these complaint categories may not contain, within their algorithms, the administration of analgesia or sedation. Categories such as wound care, extremity fractures, and chest pain contain analgesia within their protocols. However, some protocols, even those for abdominal pain may specifically say, "Pain medications should NOT be administered to anyone complaining of abdominal pain unless ordered by medical control." The term "unless ordered" may leave significant leeway to not address pain complaints. Moreover, *routine trauma care protocols* provide succinct algorithms on when to go to the trauma center, how often to take the vitals, the need for two intravenous access, but have *no mention* of any pain control for patients meeting trauma center criteria. The same is true for the *crush injury* and *hemorrhage* protocols these authors have reviewed. All protocols should be reviewed, by a multidisciplinary team, to ensure that all painful conditions are treated expeditiously and appropriately. The treatment of pain *will not* alter examination findings or obscure diagnoses.

IDENTIFICATION OF BARRIERS

The most important initial step in the development of sedation and analgesia protocols is the identification of barriers to treatment. Many studies over the last decade have addressed the identification of barriers, and many have been reviewed here.

PROVIDER EDUCATION

In order to overcome these barriers, a multidisciplinary education plan is required. The plan should incorporate the following: (a) knowledge of the differing types of pain; (b) instruction on how pain affects patients of all ages; (c) a comprehensive pharmacological education regarding available medication, their dosages, indications, and contraindications; (d) education regarding nonpharmacological adjunctive treatments; (e) mandatory pain assessments for all patients; and (f) training in

providers perceptions regarding cultural, gender, age-related factors in the patients under their care.

QUALITY IMPROVEMENT AND ASSESSMENTS

These are not only required for all EMS services, but their use in quantitatively and qualitatively assessing proper analgesia and sedation is essential. As previously mentioned, providers self-assessment of the care they render may be far different from what is actually provided. Patient surveys, emergency department patient follow-up reports, and comparison of perceived versus actual pain management administered may be utilized. All information gathered needs to be fed back to the provider in a nonjudgmental and instructive manner, with the focus on optimizing patient outcomes and relieving pain symptoms.

REFERENCES

1. Turk DC, Dworkin RH. What should be the core outcomes in chronic pain clinical trials? *Arthritis Res Ther.* 2004;6(4):151-154.
2. Bonica JJ. The need of a taxonomy. *Pain.* 1979;6(3):247-248.
3. Kooijman CM, Dijkstra PU, Geertzen JH, Elzinga A, Van der Schans CP. Phantom pain and phantom sensations in upper limb amputees: an epidemiological study. *Pain.* 2000;87(1):33-41.
4. Jensen TS, Krebs B, Nielson J, Rasmussen P. Phantom limb, phantom pain and stump pain in amputees during the first 6 months following limb amputation. *Pain.* 1983;17(3):243-256.
5. Jensen TS, Krebs B, Neilsen J, Rasmussen P. Immediate and long-term phantom limb pain in amputees: incidence, clinical characteristics and relationship to pre-amputation limb pain. *Pain.* 1985;21(3):25-278.
6. Cordell WH, Keen KK, Giles BK, Jones JB, Jones JH, Brizendine EJ. The high prevalence of pain in emergency medical care. *Am J Emerg Med.* 2002;20(3):165-159.
7. *Macrae WA. Epidemiology of pain. In:* Jaggar S, Holdcroft A, eds. *Core Topics in Pain.* Cambridge University Press; 2005:99-103, chap 14.
8. McCaffrey M, Beebe M. *Pain: Clinical Manual for Nursing Practice.* London: Mosby; 1994.
9. Jones G, Machen I. Prehospital pain management: the paramedic's perspective. *Accid Emerg Nurs.* 2003;11(3):166-172.
10. Leduc T, Paris P. Relieving the pain. *J EMS.* December 1996:74-82.

BIBLIOGRAPHY

Abuhl FB, Reed DB. Time to analgesia for patients with painful extremity injuries transported to the emergency department by ambulance. *Prehosp Emerg Care.* October-December 2003.; 7(4):445-447.

Adams R, White B, Beckett C. The effects of massage therapy on pain management in the acute care setting. *Int J Ther Massage Bodywork.* 2010;3(1):4-11.

Albanese J, Amaud S, Rey M, Thomachot L, Alliez B. Martin C. Ketamine decreases intracranial pressure and electroencephalographic activity in traumatic brain injury patients during propofol sedation. *Anesthesiology.* 1997;87:1328-1334.

Alonso-Serra H, Wesley K. Prehospital pain management [position paper]. *Prehosp Emerg Care.* 2003;7:482-488.

Am J Emerg Med. 2003;10:190-195.

Am J Emerg Med. 2008;26: 985-1028.

Aourell M, Skoog M, Carleson J. Effects of Swedish massage on blood pressure. *Complement Ther Clin Pract.* 2005;11(4):242-246.

Barker R, Kober A, Hoerauf K, Latzke D, Adel S, Kain ZN, Wang SM. Out-of-hospital auricular acupressure in elder patients with hip fracture: a randomized double-blinded trial. *Acad Emerg Med.* 2006;13(1):19-23.

Baskett PJ. Acute pain management in the field. *Ann Emerg Med.* 1999;34:784-785.

Battaglia J, Moss S, Rush J, et al. Haloperidol, lorazepam, or both for psychotic agitation? A multicenter, prospective, double-blind, emergency department study. *Am J Emerg Med.* 1997;15(4):335-340.

Bennett HJ. Humor in medicine. *South Med J.* 2003;96(12):1257-1261.

Bijur PE, Silver W, Gallagher EJ. Reliability of the visual analog scale for measurement of acute pain. *Acad Emerg Med.* 2001;8:1153-1157.

Bonanno FG. Ketamine in war/tropical surgery (a final tribute to the racemic mixture). *Injury.* 2002;33:323-327.

Borland M, Jacobs I, King B, et al. A randomized controlled trial comparing intranasal fentanyl to intravenous morphine for managing acute pain in children in the emergency department. *Ann Emerg Med.* 2007;49:335-340.

Bounes V, Charpentier S, Houze-Cerfon CH, Bellard D, Ducasse JL. Is there an ideal morphine dose for prehospital treatment of severe acute pain? A randomized, double-blind comparison of 2 doses. *Am J Emerg Med.* 2008;26, 148-154.

Bredmose PP, Lockey DJ, Grier G, et al. Prehospital use of ketamine for analgesia and procedural sedation. *Emerg Med J.* 2009;26: 62-64.

Brogan G, Giarrusso E, Hollander J, et al. Comparison of plain, warmed and buffered lidocaine for anesthesia of traumatic wounds. *Ann Emerg Med.* 1995;26:121-125.

Brooks PM. *N Engl J Med.* 1991;324:1716-1725.

Bursch B, Zelter LK. *Nelson Textbook of Pediatrics.* 2004:358-366.

Ceber M, Sailhoglu T. Ketamine may be the first choice for anesthesia in burn patients. *J Burn Care Res.* 2006;27:760-762.

Cepeda MS, Carr DB, Lau J, Alvarez H. Music for pain relief. *Cochrane Database Syst Rev.* 2006 Apr 19;(2):CD004843.

Chang A, Bijur P, Meyer R, Kenny M, Solorzano C, Gallagher J. Safety and efficacy of hydromorphone as an analgesic alternative to morphine in acute pain: a randomized clinical trial. *Ann Emerg Med.* 2006;48:164-172.

Chestnut RM, Marshall LF, Klauder MR, et al. The role of secondary brain injury in determining outcome from severe head injury. *J Trauma.* 1993;34:216-222.

Chia Y-Y, Chow L-H, Hung C-C, et al. Gender and pain upon movement are associated with the requirements for postoperative patient-controlled IV analgesia: a prospective survey of 2,298 Chinese patients. *Can J Anesth.* 2002 49:249-255.

Cohen FL. Postoperative pain relief: patients' status and nurses' medication choices. *Pain.* 1980;9:265-274.

Cohen SP, Christo PJ, Moroz L. Pain management in trauma patients. *Am J Phys Med Rehabil.* 2004;83(2):142-161.

Considine J, Hood K. Emergency department management of hip fractures: development of an evidence-based clinical guidelines by literature review and consensus. *Emerg Med.* 2000;4:329-6.

Crystal C, Blankenship R. Local anesthetics and peripheral nerve blocks in the emergency department. *Emerg Med Clin North Am.* 2005;23:477-502.

Dillard JN, Knapp S. Complementary and alternative pain therapy in the emergency department. *Emerg Med Clin North Am.* 2005;23(2):529-549.

Drayer RA, Henderson J, Reidenberg M. Barriers to better pain control in hospitalized patients. *J Pain Symptom Manage.* 1999;17(6): 434-440.

Ducharme J. Acute pain and pain control: state of the art. Ann Emerg Med. 2000 Jun;35(6):592-603. Review. Erratum in: *Ann Emerg Med.* 2000;36(2):171.

Dunwoody CJ, Krenzischek DA, Pasero C, Rathmell JP, Polomano RC. Assessment, physiological monitoring, and consequences of inadequately treated acute pain. *J Perianesth Nurs.* February 2008;23 (1 suppl):S15-S27.

Eidelman A, Weiss J, Lau J, et al. Topical anesthetics for dermal instrumentation: a systematic review of randomized, controlled trials. *Ann Emerg Med.* 2005;46:343-351.

Evers AS, Crowder CM. General anesthetics. In: Hardman JG, Limbird LE, Gilman AG, eds. *Goodman & Gilman's The pharmacological Basis of Therapeutics.* New York: McGraw-Hill; 2001: 337-365.

Fitzgerald M, Millar C, MacIntoch N, et al. Hyperalgesia i preterm infants. *Lancet.* 1988;1(8530):292.

Fuchs-Lacelle S, Hadjistavropoulos T, Lix L. Pain assessment as intervention: a study of older adults with severe dementia. *Clin J Pain.* 2008.

Gallagher J, Esses D, Lee C, Lahn M, Bijur P. Randomized clinical trial of morphine in acute abdominal pain. *Ann Emerg Med.* 2006;48:150-160.

Gennis P, Miller L, Gallagher EJ, Giglio J, Carter W, Nathanson N. The effect of soft cervical collars on persistent neck pain in patients with whiplash injury. *Acad Emerg Med.* 1996;3(6):568-73.

Gerson LW, Emond, JA, Camargo CA. US emergency department visits for hip fracture, 1992-2000. *Eur J Emerg Med.* 2004;11: 323-328.

Green SM, Krauss B. Clinical practice guidelines for emergency department ketamine dissociative sedation in children. *Ann Emerg Med.* 2004;44(5):460-471.

Green SM, Li J. Ketamine in adults: what emergency physicians need to know about patient selection and emergence reactions. *Acad Emerg Med.* 2000;7:278-281.

Hartstein BH, Barry JD. Mitigation of pain during intravenous catheter placement using a topical skin coolant in the emergency department. *Emerg Med J.* 2008;25(5):257-261.

Havel CJ, et al. *Acad Emerg Med.* 1999;6:989-997.

Hennes H, Kim MK, Pirrallo RG. Prehospital pain management: a comparison of providers' perceptions and practices. *Prehosp Emerg Care.* 2005;9(1):32-39.

Herlitz J, Richter A, Hjalmarson A, Holmberg S. Variability of chest pain in suspected acute myocardial infarction according to subjective assessment and requirement of narcotic analgesics. *Int J Cardiol.* 1986;13:9-22.

Herlitz J, Richter A, Hjalmarson A, Howgren C, Holmberg S, Bondestam E. Chest pain in acute myocardial infarction. A descriptive study according to subjective assessment and morphine requirement. *Clin Cardiol.* 1986;9:423-428.

Hijazi Y, Bodonian C, Bolon M, Salord F, Boulieu R. Pharmacokinetics and haemodynamics of ketamine in intensive care patients with brain or spinal cord injury. *Br J Anaesth.* 2003;90:155-160.

Holdgate A, Shepherd SA, Huckson S. Patterns of analgesia for fractured neck of femur in Australian emergency departments. *Emerg Med Australasia.* 2010;22, 3-8.

Hudak DA, Dale JA, Hudak MA, DeGood DE. Effects of humorous stimuli and sense of humor on discomfort. *Psychol Rep.* 1991:69(3 pt 1):779-786.

Humphries Y, Melson M, Gore D. Superiority of oral ketamine as an analgesic and sedative for wound care procedures in the pediatric patient with burns. *J Burn Care Rehabil.* 1997;18:34-36.

Jensen MP, Turner JA, Romano JM, Karoly P. Coping with chronic pain: a critical review of the literature. *Pain.* 1991;47(3):249-283.

Johansson P, Kongstad P, Johansson A. The effect of combined treatment with morphine sulphate and low dose ketamine in a prehospital setting. *Scand J Trauma Resusc Emerg Med.* 2009, 17:61-66.

Johnson JC, Atherton GL. Effectiveness of nitrous oxide in a rural EMS system. *J Emerg Med.* 1991;9(1-2):45-53.

Kanowitz A, Dunn TM, Kanowitz EM, Dunn WW, Vanbuskirk K. Safety and effectiveness of fentanyl administration for prehospital pain management. *Prehosp Emerg Care.* 2006;10(1):1-7.

Kaptchuk TJ. Acupuncture: theory, efficacy, and practice. *Ann Intern Med.* 2002;136(5):374-383.

Keck JF, Gerkensmeyer JE, Joyce BA, Schade JG. Reliability and validity of the Faces and Word Descriptor Scales to measure procedural pain. *J Pediatr Nurs.* 1996;11(6):368-374.

Ketcham DW. Where there is no anaesthesiologist: the many uses of ketamine. *Trop Doctor.* 1990;20:163-166.

Kober A, et al. *Anesth Analg.* 2002;95:723-727.

Kober A, et al. *Anesthesiology.* 2003;98:1328-1332.

Kober A, et al. *J Urol.* 2003;170:741-744.

Kober A. *Anesth Analg.* 2003;96:1447-1452.

Kremer E, Atkinson JH, Ingelzi RJ. Measurement of pain: patient preference does not confound pain measurement. *Pain.* April 1981;10(2):241-248.

Leporte JR. *Drug Saf.* 2004;27:411-420.

Lewis, et al. *Br J Clin Pharmacol.* 2002;54:320-326.

Lord B, Cui J, Kelly AM. The impact of patient sex on paramedic pain management in the prehospital setting. *Am J Emerg Med.* 2009;27, 525-529.

Luger TJ, Lederer W, Gassner M, et al. Acute pain is under assessed in out-of-hospital emergencies. *Acad Emerg Med.* 2003;10:627-632.

Mace SE, et al. *Pain Management and Sedation.* New York: McGraw-Hill; 2006:400.

Macoux FX, Goddrich JE, Dominick MA. Ketamine prevents ischaemic neuronal injury. *Brain Res.* 1988;452:329-355.

Manegazzi. *Ann Emerg Med.* 1991;20:348-350.

March LM, Chamberlain AC, Cameron ID, et al. How best to fix a broken hip. Fractured Neck Femur Outcomes Project Team. *Med J Aust.* 1999;170:489-494.

Maunuksela EL, Olkkola KT, Korpela R. Measurement of pain in children with self-reporting and behavioral assessment. *Clin Pharmacol Ther.* 1987;42(2):137-141.

McClean SA, Maio RF, Domeier RM. The epidemiology of pain in the prehospital setting. *Prehosp Emerg Care.* 2002;6(4):402-405.

McCormack HM, Horne DJ, Sheather S. Clinical applications of visual analogue scales: a critical review. *Psychol Med.* November 1988;18(4):1007-1019.

McEachin CC, McDermott JT, Swor R. Few emergency medical services patients with lower-extremity fractures receive prehospital analgesia. *Prehosp Emerg Care.* 2002;6(4):406-410.

McGrath PA, Brigham MC. The assessment of pain in children and adolescents. In: Turk DC, Melzack R, eds. *Handbook of Pain Assessment.* New York: Guildford Press; 1992:295-314.

McLean SA, Maio RF, Domeier RM. The epidemiology of pain in the prehospital setting. *Prehosp Emerg Care.* 2002;6:402-405.

Michael GE, Sporer KA, Youngblood GM. Women are less likely than men to receive prehospital analgesia for isolated extremity injuries. *Am J Emerg Med.* 2007;25, 901-906.

Nadler SF. *J Am Osteopath Assoc.* 2004;104:6-12.

Nelson BP, Cohen D, Lander O, et al. Mandated pain scales improve frequency of ED analgesic administration. *Am J Emerg Med.* 2004;22:582-585.

Nicolaou DD, et al. *Emergency Medicine. A Comprehensive Study Guide.* New York: McGraw-Hill; 2004:275-280.

Ong CKS, Lirk P, Seymor RA, Jenkins B. The efficacy of preemptive analgesia for acute postoperative pain management: a meta-analysis. *Anesth Analg.* 2005;100:757-773.

Owens VF, Palmieri TL, Comroe CM, et al. Ketamine: a safe and effective agent for painful procedures in the pediatric burn patient. *J Burn Care Res.* 2006;27:211-216.

Paris P, Yealy D. Pain management. In: Marx JA, ed. *Rosen's Emergency Medicine: Concepts and Clinical Practice.* St Louis, MO: Mosby; 2002:2555-2577.

Paris PM. Analgesia. In: Keuhl AE, ed. *Prehospital Systems and Medical Oversight.* 3rd ed. 659-664.

Ped Em Care. May 2008;24(5):300-303.

Persson LC, et al. *Spine.* 1997;22:751-758.

Pfenninger E, Grunert A, Bowdler I, Kilian J. The effects of ketamine on ICP during haemorrhage shock under conditions of both spontaneous breathing and controlled ventilation. *Acta Neurochir.* 1985;78:113-118.

Porter K. Ketamine in prehospital care. *Emerg Med J.* 2004;21(3):351-354.

Read D, Ashford B. Surgical aspects of operation Bali Assist: initial wound surgery on the tarmac and in flight. *ANZ J Surg.* 2004;74:986-991.

Reid C, Hatton R, Middleton P. Case report: prehospital use of intranasal ketamine for paediatric burn injury. *Emerg Med J.* 2011;28:328-329.

Renn CL, Dorsey SG. *AACN Clin Issues.* 2005;16:277-290.

Ricard-Hibon A, Chollet C, Belpomme V, Duchateau FX, Marty J. Epidemiology of adverse effects of prehospital sedation analgesia. *Am J Emerg Med.* 2003;21(6):461-466.

Rickard C, O'Meara P, McGrail M, et al. A randomized controlled trial of intranasal fentanyl vs intravenous morphine for analgesia in the prehospital setting. *Am J Emerg Med.* 2007;25:911-917.

Roy M, Peretz I, Rainville P. Emotional valence contributes to music-induced analgesia. *Pain.* 2008;134(1-2):140-147.

Rudman N, Mcllmail D. Emergency department evaluation and treatment of hip and thigh injuries. *Emerg Med Clin North Am.* 2000;18:29-66.

Rupp T, Delaney KA. Inadequate analgesia in emergency medicine. *Ann Emerg Med.* 2004;43(4):494-503.

Salam G. Regional anesthesia for office procedures. Part 1: head and neck surgeries. *Am Fam Physician.* 2004;69:585-590.

Scheiber S, Galai-Gat T. Uncontrolled pain following physical injury as the core-trauma in post-traumatic stress disorder. *Pain.* 1993;54(1):107-110.

Schofield P. Assessment and management of pain in older adults with dementia: a review of current practice and future directions. *Curr Opin Support Palliat Care.* 2008;2:128-132.

Schwedler M, Miletich DJ, Albrecht RF. Cerebral blood flow and metabolism following ketamine administration. *Can Anaesth Soc J.* 1982;29:222-226.

Shaprio HM, Wyte SR, Harris AB. Ketamine anaesthesia in patients with intracranial pathology. *Br J Anaesth.* 1972;44:1200-1204.

Silka PA, Roth MM, Moreno G, et al. Pain scores improve analgesia administration patterns for trauma patients in the emergency department. *Acad Emerg Med.* 2004;11:264-270.

Stewart RD. Nitrous oxide sedation/analgesia in emergency medicine. *Ann Emerg Med.* 1985;14(2):139-148.

Stuber M, Hilber SD, Mintzer LL, Castaneda M, Glover D, Zeltzer L. Laughter, humor and pain perception in children: a pilot study. *Evid Based Complement Alternat Med.* 2009;6(2):271-276.

Svenson J, Abernathy M. Ketamine for prehospital use: new look at an old drug. *Am J Emerg Med.* 2007;25:977-980.

Tentillier E, Ammirati C. Prehospital management of patients with severe head injuries. *Ann Fr Anesth Reanim.* 2000;19:275-281.

Thomas SH, Silen W, Cheema F, et al. Effects of morphine analgesia on diagnostic accuracy in emergency department patients with abdominal pain: a prospective randomized trial. *J Am Col Surg.* 2003;196(1):18-31.

Thomas SH. Prehospital trauma analgesia. *J Emerg Med.* 35(1):47-57.

Thompson DR. Narcotic analgesic effects on the sphincter of Oddi: a review of the data and therapeutic implications in treating pancreatitis. *Am J Gastroenterol.* 2001;96(4):1266-1272.

Turturro M. Pain, priorities, and prehospital care. *Prehosp Emerg Care.* 2002;6:486-488.

Vassiliadis J, Hitos K, Hill CT. Factors influencing prehospital and emergency department analgesia administration to patients with femoral neck fractures. *Emerg Med.* 2002;14:261-266.

Vermeulen B, Morabia A, Unger P-F, et al. Acute appendicitis influence of early pain relief on the accuracy of clinical and US findings in the decision to operate—a randomized trial. *Radiology Mar.* 1999;210(3):639.

Wedmore I, Johnson T, Czarnik J, et al. Pain management in the wilderness and operational setting. *Emerg Med Clin North Am*. 2005;23:585-601.

Weksler N, Ovadia L, Muati G, et al. Nasal ketamine for paediatric pre-medication. *Can J Anaesth*. 1993;40:119-121.

Wiechman Askay S, Patterson DR, Sharar SR, Mason S, Faber B. Pain management in patients with burn injuries. *Int Rev Psychiatry*. 2009:21(6):522-530.

Woody GE, Senay EC, Gellar A, et al. *Drug Alcohol Depend*. 2003;72:163-168.

Zedigh C, Alho A, Hammar E, et al. Aspects on the intensity and the relief of pain in the prehospital phase of acute coronary syndrome: experiences from a randomized clinical trial. *Coron Artery Dis*. 2010;21:113-120.

Zempsky W, Cravero JP. American Academy of Pediatrics Committee on Pediatric Emergency Medicine and Section on Anesthesiology and Pain Medicine: relief of pain and anxiety in pediatric patients in emergency medical systems. *Pediatrics*. 2004;114:1348-1356.

Zimmer G. Acute pain management. In: Tintinalli J, Kelen G, Stapczynski J, eds. *Emergency Medicine: A Comprehensive Study Guide*. New York, NY: McGraw-Hill; 2004:257-264.

CHAPTER 63 Field Diagnostics

Norma L. Cooney
Derek R. Cooney

INTRODUCTION

Diagnostic evaluation of patients in the field continues to see new advancements. In addition to performance of a high-quality history and examination, EMS physicians should be able to perform a number of diagnostic procedures in the field. The procedures detailed below are core EMS physician skills; however, there are a number of equipment specific diagnostic maneuvers that are beyond the scope of this chapter due to variability in equipment manufactures. In addition to the diagnostics covered in this text EMS physicians should be familiar with use of the monitor functions of their agencies' monitor/defibrillators, thermometers, and any point-of-care testing devices the agency cares: blood glucometers, lactate meters, and minianalyzers.

FIELD DIAGNOSTIC PROCEDURES

Below is a list of field diagnostic techniques covered in this chapter.

- Performing a prehospital 12-lead ECG
- Waveform capnography
- Prehospital ultrasound
- Compartment pressure monitoring

12-LEAD ELECTROCARDIOGRAM

Indications

- Chest pain
- Back, neck, jaw, or arm pain without chest pain
- Upper abdominal pain or reflux symptoms
- Syncope (or near syncope)
- Palpitations or unexplained tachycardia
- Dyspnea of uncertain origin
- Diaphoresis of uncertain origin
- Anxiety (+/− sense of impending doom)
- Suspected electrolyte abnormalities (DKA, CRF, adrenal insufficiency)
- Found down for unknown period
- Crush injuries and compartment syndrome
- Environmental injury (hypothermia, hyperthermia, electrical injury, dysbarism, submersion/postdrowning)
- Generalized weakness

Essential Equipment

- Monitor/defibrillator with 12-lead capability

Technique

- Proper placement of the leads is important to avoid incorrect diagnosis and negative changes on the ECG (**Figure 63-1**).
- Place V1 electrode at the fourth intercostal space to the right of the sternum.
- Place V2 electrode at the fourth intercostal space to the left of the sternum.
- Place V3 electrode in the middle of V2 and V4.
- Place V4 electrode at the fifth intercostal space at the midclavicular line.

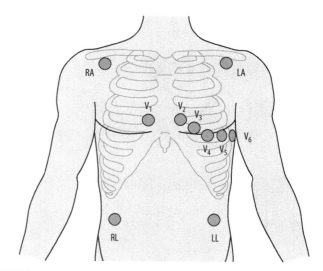

FIGURE 63-1. 12-Lead ECG lead placement.

- Place V5 electrode at the anterior axillary line at the same level of V4.
- Place V6 electrode at the midaxillary line at the same level as V4 and V5.
- Place RL electrode below the torso but above the ankle.
- Place LL electrode below the torso but above the ankle.
- Place the RA electrode below the right shoulder and above the right elbow.
- Place the LA electrode below the left shoulder and above the left elbow.

Interpretation

A thorough understanding of the electrophysiology of the heart is important for interpretation of the ECG. Recognition of basic and lethal rhythms is essential. Diagnosis directs therapy which in certain cases is lifesaving. The scope of this book does not lend itself to teach ECG readings and interpretation. EMS physicians must have a mastery of basic 12-lead interpretation inclusive of rhythms identification and evaluation of ischemia, MI, conduction delays, and signs of toxicological findings.

WAVEFORM CAPNOGRAPHY

Indications

- Capnography is a measure of the partial pressure of carbon dioxide (CO_2) in the respiratory gases. The role of waveform capnography in the prehospital medicine setting is to assist with diagnosis, provide guide to respiratory status of the patient, and to trouble shoot ventilator issues. Indications are as follows: Evaluation of proper endotracheal tube placement
- Evaluation of patient's breath-by-breath ventilation respiratory status
- Ability to determine deterioration or maintenance of airway either pre- or postintubation

Essential Equipment

Waveform capnograph or capable monitored defibrillator with module (**Figure 63-2**)

Technique

- Connect patient end of the tubing to endotracheal tube or nasal canula device.

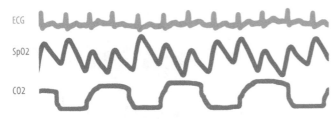

FIGURE 63-2. Waveform capnography on the monitor with ECG and SpO_2.

TABLE 63-1 Conditions That Affect End-Tidal CO_2 ($ETCO_2$)	
Increase in $ETCO_2$	Decrease in $ETCO_2$
Increased cardiac output	Decreased cardiac output
Hypoventilation	Hyperventilation
Hyperthermia	Hypothermia
Bicarbonate administration	Cardiac arrest
Insufflation of CO_2 for laparoscopic surgery	Pulmonary embolism
	Fat or air embolism
	Disruption of ventilation system (eg, disconnect, circuit leak)
	Accidental extubation
	Endotracheal tube obstruction

Reprinted with permission from: Tintinalli JE, Stapczynski JS, Ma OJ, Cline DM, Cydulka RK, Meckler GD, eds. *Tintinalli's Emergency Medicine: A Comprehensive Study Guide.* 7th ed. New York: McGraw-Hill; 2011.

- Connect monitoring end of the cannula to the waveform capnographer or capnography module for the monitor defibrillator.

Interpretation

- Confirmation of placement of ETT and continued ventilator monitoring of an intubated patient.

  - A standard respiratory waveform should be noted. Continuous monitoring is indicated. Loss of waveform indicates loss of endotracheal tube placement of cardiac decompensation in most cases. The airway and cardiovascular status should be immediately evaluated (**Table 63-1**).

- Evaluation of cardiopulmonary resuscitation.

  - If no waveform during CPR, rule out esophageal intubation.
  - Optimize chest compression for effective CPR so that $ETCO_2$ values are between 10 and 20 mm Hg. If it is 10 mm Hg or less after initiation of ACLS, poor outcomes are expected.

- After intubation, look for CO_2 waveforms during chest compressions. A flat tracing should alert for a misplaced ET tube.

PREHOSPITAL ULTRASOUND

Newer, more portable, ultrasound devices can be carried in helicopters and ambulances and may provide another noninvasive evaluation tool to providers and physicians in the field.

■ EFAST—EXTENDED FOCUSED ASSESSMENT WITH SONOGRAPHY FOR TRAUMA

Indications

Ultrasound has become a standard of care in the diagnostic evaluation of the trauma patient. The eFAST examination is the point-of-care (POC) test used to evaluate seriously injured trauma patients. The most common indication is for thoracoabdominal trauma.

- Identify free fluid in the abdominal cavity.
- Identify a pneumothorax.
- Identify a pericardial fluid/tamponade.

Essential Equipment

- Ultrasound machine
- Low-frequency curvilinear probe for better penetration of tissues in the abdomen
- High-frequency linear probe for better resolution in the thoracic cavity
- Ultrasound gel

Technique

Step 1: Lay the patient in the supine position.

Step 2: Use the low-frequency probe (exchange of probes delays obtaining diagnostic information).

Step 3: Perform the examination in a stepwise fashion, going in a clockwise or counterclockwise fashion is recommended.

Step 4: *Scan the lung.* Place the probe in the second or third intercostal space in the midclavicular line in the sagittal position. Gently slide the probe superiorly and inferiorly to look for lung sliding and comet tails (vertical artifacts from the pleural line). Then place the probe laterally at the sixth intercostal space. In M-mode, the lung sliding pattern is referred to as the seashore sign. On M-mode, the lung pulse (heartbeats pulsations of the expanded lung present when no lung sliding evident) is equivocal to lung sliding. Perform this on both sides of the lungs (**Figure 63-3**).

Step 5: *Scan the hepatorenal space.* Place the probe at the right lateral midaxillary line at the inferior portion of the ribs (**Figure 63-4**). Keep the probe pointed cephalad. Scan superiorly and inferiorly. In order for the most optimal visualization, direct the probe in an oblique direction. This visualizes the kidney in a normal anatomic position. First, look for free fluid between the kidney and the liver in the potential space known as Morrison pouch (**Figure 63-5**). Then, attempt to appreciate the integrity of the solid organ for possible solid organ laceration.

Step 6: *Scan the bladder.* Place the probe over the bladder in the longitudinal and transverse planes (**Figure 63-6**). Scan the bladder in all directions to evaluate for an intact bladder and evaluate for free fluid in the pelvis, seen posterior to the bladder in the rectovesicular space (**Figure 63-7**).

Step 7: *Scan the splenorenal space.* Place the probe in the left midaxillary line just beneath the thoracic ribs and slightly posterior (**Figure 63-8**). Direct the probe marker cephalad. Scan superiorly and inferiorly. The left kidney is slightly higher than the right kidney in comparison. In order for the most optimal visualization, direct the probe in an oblique direction. This visualizes the kidney in a normal anatomic position. First, look for free fluid between the kidney and the spleen (**Figure 63-9**). Then, attempt to appreciate the integrity of the solid organ for possible solid organ laceration.

Step 8: *Scan the pericardial space.* Place the probe in the subxiphoid space and rotate the probe approximately 30° to the right (**Figure 63-10**). Direct the probe slightly posteriorly. Look for a hypoechoic region (black stripe) between the pericardial sac and the myocardium (**Figure 63-11**).

Interpretation

- Free fluid noted in the peritoneal cavity mandates an immediate surgical consult on arrival to the trauma center. In the context of trauma and unstable vital signs, trauma patients would potentially be taken

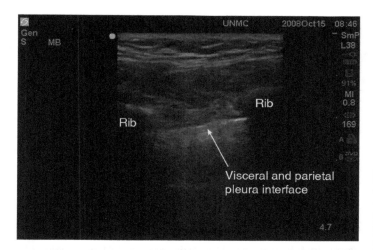

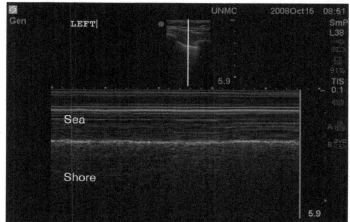

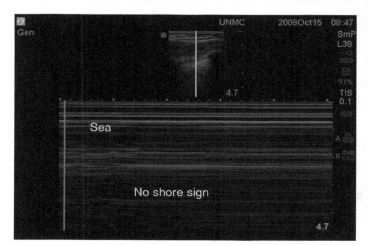

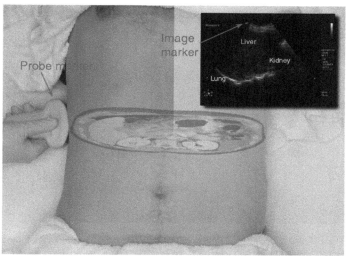

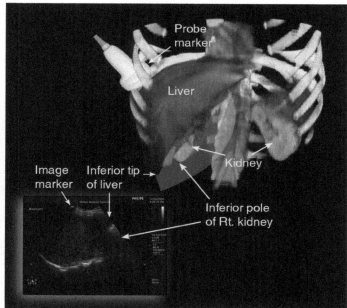

FIGURE 63-4. Probe positioning for evaluating the hepatorenal space. Imaging of the hepatorenal recess. **A**: US probe placement with the corresponding US screen image. **B**: A view of the US beam (green) as it passes through the liver and kidney with the corresponding US image. (Reproduced with permission from Reichman EF, ed. *Emergency Medicine Procedures*. 2nd ed. New York, NY: McGraw-Hill; 2013.)

FIGURE 63-3. Lung slide. Imaging a pneumothorax. **A**: Rib shadowing is seen on both sides of the intercostal space. The echoic interface of the parietal and visceral pleura demonstrates the "sliding-lung" sign. **B**: The "sea-shore" sign. It is visible when the lung and chest wall are in contact with each other. Note the bright echogenic stripe of the pleural interface between the chest wall ("sea") and the lung ("shore"). **C**: The "sea-shore" sign and the pleural interface are absent when a pneumothorax is present. (Reproduced with permission from Reichman EF, ed. *Emergency Medicine Procedures*. 2nd ed. New York, NY: McGraw-Hill; 2013.)

immediately for exploratory surgery and so a trauma notification should be called to the receiving facility.

- Pericardial effusion/tamponade. If the patient has tamponade, immediate pericardiocentesis should be performed; otherwise careful monitoring and notification should be made to the receiving facility.

■ CONFIRMATION OF ENDOTRACHEAL INTUBATION

Indications

Ultrasound can be used to confirm and/or guide endotracheal intubation in patients when visualization is difficult and/or capnography is not available. This can be done real time or as a secondary confirmatory technique after intubation is complete.

Essential Equipment

- Ultrasound machine
- High-frequency linear probe
- Ultrasound gel

Technique

Ultrasound findings of the intubated patient will show the tracheal wall with two parallel echogenic lines that are representative of the

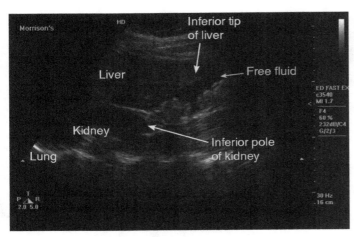
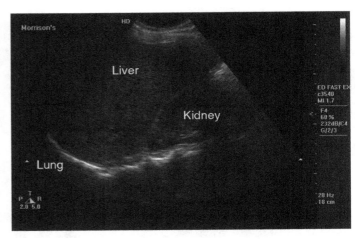

FIGURE 63-5. Hepatorenal view: Morrison pouch. A positive FAST examination of the hepatorenal recess. **A**: An echolucent fluid stripe in Morrison pouch. **B**: A normal examination for comparison. (Reproduced with permission from Reichman EF, ed. *Emergency Medicine Procedures*. 2nd ed. New York, NY: McGraw-Hill; 2013.)

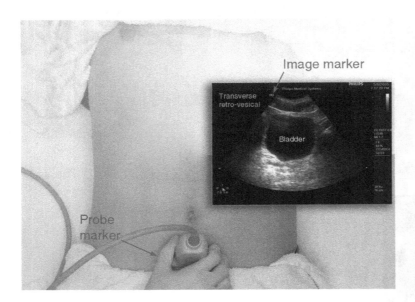
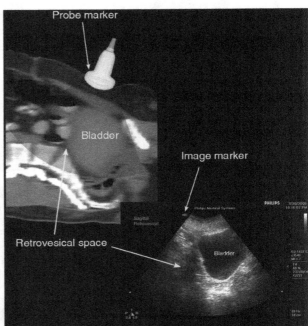
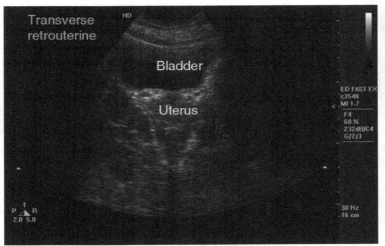
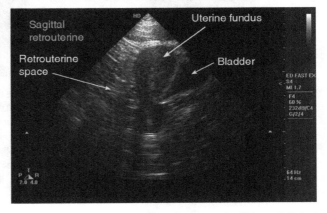

FIGURE 63-6. Bladder view. Imaging of the rectovesical and the rectouterine spaces. **A**: Transverse US probe placement for the rectovesical view with the corresponding US image. **B**: Sagittal view, and probe orientation, of the rectovesical space displaying the US beam path (pink) and the corresponding US image. **C**: Transverse view of the rectouterine space. **D**: Sagittal view of the rectouterine space. (Reproduced with permission from Reichman EF, ed. *Emergency Medicine Procedures*. 2nd ed. New York, NY: McGraw-Hill; 2013.)

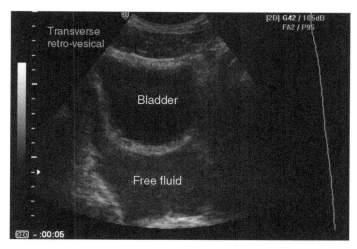
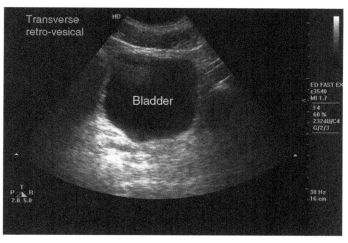

FIGURE 63-7. Fluid in the pelvis. A positive FAST examination of the rectovesical space. **A**: Transverse view of an echolucent fluid area. **B**: A normal examination for comparison. (Reproduced with permission from Reichman EF, ed. *Emergency Medicine Procedures*. 2nd ed. New York, NY: McGraw-Hill; 2013.)

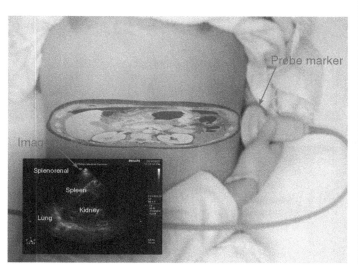
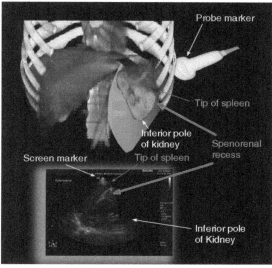

FIGURE 63-8. Splenorenal view. Imaging of the splenorenal space. **A**: US probe placement with the corresponding US screen image. **B**: View of the US beam (green) as it passes through the spleen and kidney. (Reproduced with permission from Reichman EF, ed. *Emergency Medicine Procedures*. 2nd ed. New York, NY: McGraw-Hill; 2013.)

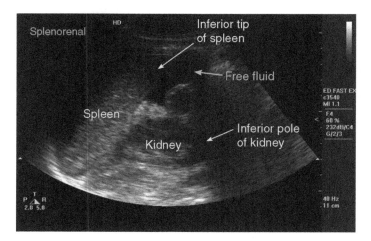
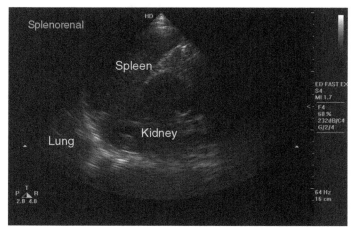

FIGURE 63-9. Fluid in the splenorenal space. A positive FAST examination of the splenorenal space. **A**: An echolucent fluid stripe. **B**: A normal examination for comparison. (Reproduced with permission from Reichman EF, ed. *Emergency Medicine Procedures*. 2nd ed. New York, NY: McGraw-Hill; 2013.)

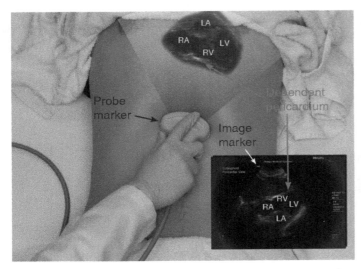

FIGURE 63-10. Pericardial view. Imaging of the pericardial space. US probe placement for the subxiphoid view with the corresponding US image. (RV, right ventricle; RA, right atrium; LV, left ventricle; LA, left atrium). (Reproduced with permission from Reichman EF, ed. *Emergency Medicine Procedures*. 2nd ed. New York, NY: McGraw-Hill; 2013.)

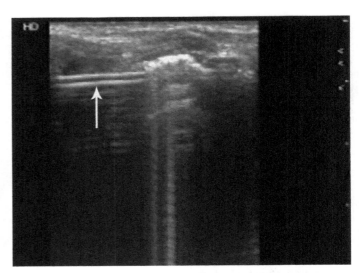

FIGURE 63-12. Longitudinal (long axis) view of an endotracheal tube within the trachea. The endotracheal tube appears as two closely spaced echogenic parallel lines. (Reproduced with permission from Ma OJ, Mateer J, Blaivas M. *Emergency Ultrasound*. 2nd ed. New York: McGraw-Hill; 2007.)

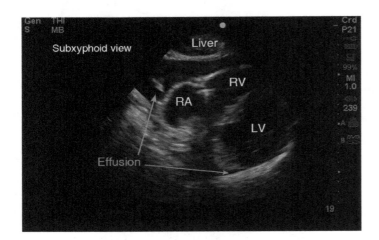

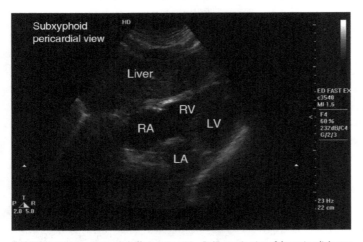

FIGURE 63-11. Pericardial effusion. A positive FAST examination of the pericardial space. **A**: A large echolucent area of fluid in the inferior-posterior aspect of the pericardial space and a small amount of fluid in the more superior area of the pericardial space. **B**: A normal examination for comparison. (Reproduced with permission from Reichman EF, ed. *Emergency Medicine Procedures*. 2nd ed. New York, NY: McGraw-Hill; 2013.)

inner and outer structures of the endotracheal tube. Visualization of the tube can be done in two planes. Along the short axis, the ETT will appear curved (**Figure 63-12**). Along the longitudinal axis, the ETT will appear to be linear (**Figure 63-13**). The long axis technique was described by Raphael and Conard using a foam or saline filled balloon.[1] Under visualization the tube will be seen moving into position. This does not replace the standard evaluation and evaluation of intubation via visualization through the cords, fogging of the ETT, capnography, or waveform capnography, however, should be considered an adjunctive tool to assist during difficult intubations. To ensure that there is not an esophageal intubation, the probe moved to left of the midline to examine the esophagus. If an esophageal intubation occurs, ultrasound will show a stented open esophagus. In the transverse view the tube will be located lateral and posterior to the glottis (**Figure 63-14**). When used during intubation with the transducer transversely placed over the suprasternal notch (known as the

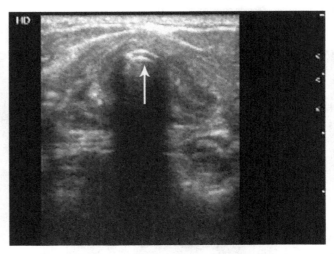

FIGURE 63-13. Transverse (short axis) view of an endotracheal tube within the trachea. The endotracheal tube appears as two closely spaced curved echogenic parallel lines. (Reproduced with permission from Ma OJ, Mateer J, Blaivas M. *Emergency Ultrasound*. 2nd ed. New York: McGraw-Hill; 2007.)

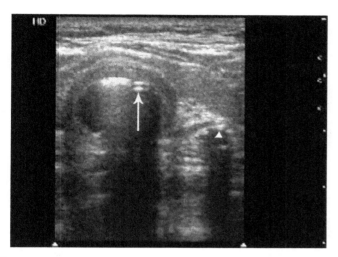

FIGURE 63-14. Transverse (short axis) view of an endotracheal tube within the esophagus. The endotracheal tube appears as two closely spaced curved echogenic parallel lines. The tube is notably lateral and posterior to the glottis. (Reproduced with permission from Ma OJ, Mateer J, Blaivas M. *Emergency Ultrasound*. 2nd ed. New York: McGraw-Hill; 2007.)

T.R.U.E. method) it was found to be 98.2% accurate at identifying the placement of the tube.[2] T.R.U.E. stands for tracheal rapid ultrasound examination. A similar study by Adi et al showed a similar result with an accuracy of 98.1%.[3]

INFERIOR VENA CAVA ULTRASOUND

Ultrasound can be used to evaluate volume status in patients who may be suffering from shock. The size and collapsibility of the inferior vena cava provides insight into the volume status of the patient.

Indications

Patients showing signs of shock or in whom volume status is questioned

Essential Equipment

- Ultrasound machine
- Low-frequency curvilinear probe
- Ultrasound gel

Technique

The low-frequency curvilinear probe is placed in the transverse position in the midline in the subxiphoid position to locate the IVC. The probe is then rotated to show the IVC in the longitudinal plane. The heart and the hepatic vein will be visible. The diameter of IVC should be measured 1 cm from the junction of the IVC and the hepatic vein. In a healthy normovolemic individual the IVC will collapse by 50% during inspiration. The diameter of the IVC of an adult typically measures between 15 to 20 mm during exhalation and 0 to 14 mm during inhalation.[4]

Interpretation

The IVC collapsibility index is defined as the IVC diameter during expiration—the IVC diameter during inspiration divided by the IVC diameter during expiration: (IVCd EXP—IVCs INSP)/ IVCd EXP. When the index is close to 0, then the central venous pressure is high and the patient is likely to fluid overloaded, and when the index is near 100, then the CVP is low and the patient is volume depleted.[4] Atkinson et al combined this approach with evaluation of the cardiac evaluation with ultrasound and have devised a methodology for attempting to better differentiate causes of shock utilizing ultrasound (**Table 63-2**).[5]

OBSTETRICAL EVALUATION (LIMITED)

Obstetrical POC ultrasound in the prehospital medicine setting can be utilized to appreciate the current state of the fetus. In the first trimester, visualization of the intrauterine pregnancy is limited from the transabdominal approach. As the pregnancy progresses, the intrauterine pregnancy can be better visualized transabdominally. In the prehospital setting, transabdominal ultrasound is the most feasible approach to ultrasound as this is noninvasive. Therefore, visualization of the very early pregnancy can be difficult if not impossible to detect without the use of a transvaginal probe.

Indications

- First trimester transabdominal ultrasound is used for confirmation of intrauterine pregnancy and is usually of benefit after approximately 8 weeks. As the first trimester pregnancy evolves, an intrauterine pregnancy can be appreciated and cardiac motion can typically be detected.
- Second trimester ultrasound is used for confirmation of pregnancy and detection of cardiac activity and rate.
- Third Trimester is used to confirm a live intrauterine pregnancy with cardiac activity with rate and to determine the position of the head.

Essential Equipment

- Ultrasound machine
- Low-frequency curvilinear probe
- Ultrasound gel

Technique

A transabdominal curvilinear lower frequency 3.5- to 5-MHz ultrasound probe is used. This allows for a broader visual field and a better appreciation of the pelvic structures. In the transabdominal approach, the resolution is low, and as such the small pelvic structures are difficult to appreciate. The midline sagittal view is best for evaluating the uterus

TABLE 63-2	Abdominal and Cardiac Evaluation With Sonography in the Hypotensive Patient		
Category of Shock	Cardiac Function	IVC	Treatment
Septic	Hyperdynamic left ventricle / Hypodynamic in late sepsis	Narrow IVC, collapses with inspiration	IV fluid, pressors
Cardiogenic	Hypodynamic left ventricle	Dilated IVC, little or no collapse with inspiration	Ionotropic medications
Hypovolemic	Hyperdynamic left ventricle	Narrow IVC collapses	Evaluation of cause, IV fluids, and blood replacement
Obstructive (cardiac tamponade)	Pericardial effusion / Diastolic collapse right ventricle	Dilated IVC, no collapse with inspiration	Pericardiocentesis
Obstructive (pulmonary embolus)	Dilated right ventricle / Dilated right atrium	Dilated IVC minimal collapse	Thrombolytics

Reprinted with permission from: Atkinson PR, McAuley DJ, Kendall RJ, et al. Abdominal and cardiac evaluation with sonography in shock (ACES): an approach by emergency physicians for the use of ultrasound in patients with undifferentiated hypotension. *Emerg Med J*. February 2009;26(2):87-91. With permission from BMJ Publishing Group, Ltd.

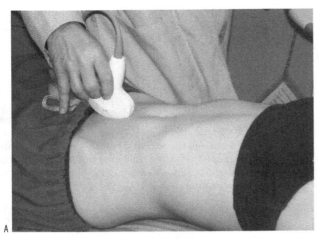
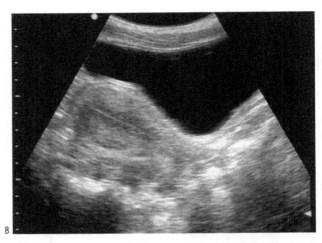

FIGURE 63-15.   Midline longitudinal (sagittal) view of the pelvis. **A:** The probe is placed superior to the pubic bone with the probe indicator pointing cephalad. **B**: Corresponding ultrasound image. (Reproduced with permission from Ma OJ, Mateer J, Blaivas M. *Emergency Ultrasound*. 2nd ed. New York: McGraw-Hill; 2007.)

(**Figure 63-15**). The probe is placed superior to the pubic bone with the probe indicator pointing cephalad. For best orientation purposes, the indicator should be on the left side of the monitor. Hence, the left side of the monitor correlates with the body's cephalad orientation. The point of reference should be the bladder which is located anterior to the uterus. The uterus should then be able to be visualized as well as the endometrial stripe. The ovaries can then be appreciated with slight deviation of the probe laterally to each respective side. The transverse view is obtained by laying the probe in the transverse plane angled caudad and with the probe indicator to the patient's left. (**Figure 63-16A**) Sweeping the pelvis by angling the probe from caudad to cephalad and back provides views of the bladder, uterus, ovaries, and cervix. (**Figure 63-16B-D**)

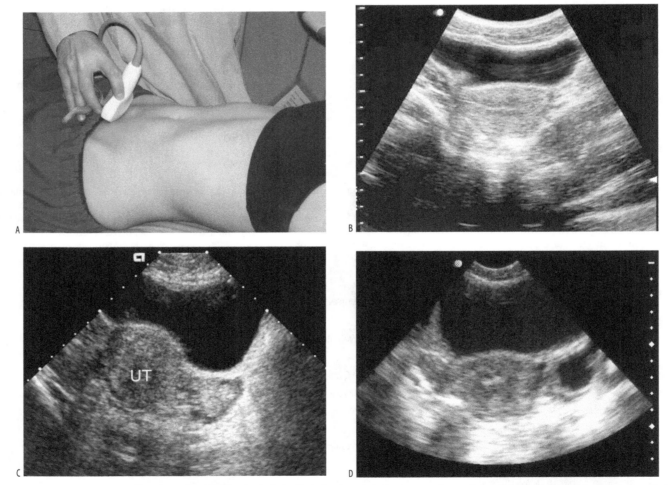

FIGURE 63-16.   Transverse views of the pelvis. **A**: The transverse view is obtained by laying the probe in the transverse plane angled caudad and with the probe indicator to the patient's left. **B-D**: Sweeping the pelvis by angling the probe from caudad to cephalad and back provides views of the bladder, uterus, ovaries, and cervix. (Reproduced with permission from Ma OJ, Mateer J, Blaivas M. *Emergency Ultrasound*. 2nd ed. New York: McGraw-Hill; 2007.)

In the second and third trimesters, ultrasound should be focused and goal directed. Indications in these two trimesters include trauma, vaginal bleeding, premature labor, and abdominal pain. Detection of fetal cardiac activity is crucial. Evaluation for abruption and previa in the prehospital setting is advanced. However, fetal position is crucial. Malposition of the fetus would direct the prehospital provider to discourage pushing with contractions. Prehospital notification regarding the critical status of the fetus and mother could then be conveyed to the receiving hospital.

The leading cause of nonobstetrical mortality is trauma,[6] and it occurs in 6% of pregnant patients.[7]

Interpretation

First trimester: An ectopic pregnancy is an obstetrical emergency. Visualization of an ectopic pregnancy is difficult from the transabdominal approach; therefore, exclusion of an ectopic cannot reliably be made in pregnancies less than 6 weeks' gestation. Confirmation of an intrauterine pregnancy typically rules out an ectopic pregnancy. However, although rare, it is important to note that spontaneous heterotopic pregnancies (EPs) occur. A heterotopic pregnancy is defined as an intrauterine and extrauterine pregnancy occurring simultaneously. The incidence of this in a healthy female with no history of pelvic inflammatory disease (PID) or the use of assisted reproductive technologies is between 1/8000 and 1/30,000.[8] The occurrence of an ovarian HP is a singular event as it comprises only 2.3% of all HPs.[9] It is important to note that if an ectopic pregnancy is suspected, the ultrasound operator should look for free fluid in the hepatorenal space, free fluid surrounding an empty uterus, and free fluid in Morrison pouch (hepatorenal view).

At 6 weeks of gestational age, a double decidual sac sign may be seen transabdominally. The inner line represents the decidua capsularis and the outer line represents the decidua parietalis. The potential space that exists between the two layers contains a small amount of endometrial fluid. This can be seen prior to the identification of a yolk sac from the transabdominal views.[10] The double decidual sign is only present in about half of intrauterine pregnancies and is not 100% accurate and is typically noted on transvaginal views. The yolk sac which is a ring-like structure within the gestational sac is considered to be the first definitive sign of an intrauterine pregnancy (**Figure 63-17**). From 6 ½ to 7 weeks, a heartbeat can be detected and viability can be assessed.

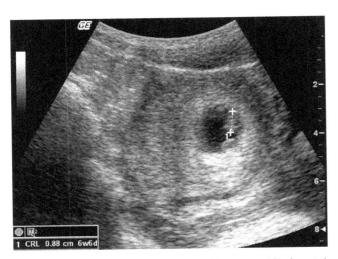

FIGURE 63-17. Yolk sac. The yolk sac which is a ring-like structure within the gestational sac is considered to be the first definitive sign of an intrauterine pregnancy. (Reproduced with permission from Ma OJ, Mateer J, Blaivas M. *Emergency Ultrasound*. 2nd ed. New York: McGraw-Hill; 2007.)

Second trimester: In the second trimester, abortions (miscarriages) are less common. If a spontaneous abortion occurs, bleeding is the most common presentation. Etiologies for second trimester abortions include chromosomal abnormalities, malformations of the uterus such as uterine septum, problems with an incompetent cervix, and autoimmune diseases such as lupus or antiphospholipid syndrome. From the prehospital medicine ultrasound standpoint, a transabdominal ultrasound confirms cardiac activity and fetal movement. These are the two areas of ultrasound focus.

Third trimester: The third trimester complications include placenta previa, placental abruption, and malpresentation (breech or transverse Lie). The common symptom of placenta previa is bright red, sudden, profuse, and painless vaginal bleeding, which usually occurs after the 28th week of pregnancy. An ultrasound is about 95% accurate in determining whether placenta previa is present.

Placental abruption is another condition that can result in fetal death. In this condition, the placenta separates from the uterus prior to labor. This can result in serious bleeding and cardiovascular shock to the mother. Occurrence is in less than 1% of births.

Malpresentation of the fetus in the breech or transverse lie position is also a known complication of third trimester pregnancy. In the ninth month of pregnancy, the fetus typically situations him or herself in the head down position. This is known as vertex or cephalic presentation. In approximately 3% of pregnancies, the fetus has a breech presentation. On rare occasion, the fetus will have a transverse presentation.

FRACTURE IDENTIFICATION

Indications

Early identification of long bone fractures is important for treatment, management, and optimal care of the patient. The benefits to POC US are many including the portability, compactness of equipment, and cost-effectiveness in the diagnosis. Diagnosis of a fracture can be done at bedside with confidence in the diagnosis. Study done by Grechenig et al showed the ability to diagnose a fracture as small as 1 mm.[11] Bellevue Hospital conducted a study showing the accuracy and ability to diagnose long bone fractures with significant reliability.[12]

Technique

- The US probe should be placed at the area of the maximal point of tenderness.

- The ultrasound may detect foreign bodies or subperiosteal hematomas.

The linear high-frequency (5.0-10 MHz) transducer is recommended for the utilization and diagnosis of most fractures in the prehospital medicine setting. Identification of long bone and sternal fractures are the most applicable and pertinent to this practice of medicine. Disruptions of the cortical surface of the bone are best appreciated on the long axis. A sternal fracture will be visualized as a discrete cortical discontinuity of the anterior sternum (**Figure 63-18**). In addition, movement of the sternal fracture fragments with respiration may be visualized during respiration. One of the pitfalls of a sternal fracture is the visualization of the sternomanubrial junction. This sternomanubrial junction appears smooth and with a hypoechoic joint space in contrast to the cortical irregularity noted on the sternal fracture.

Identification and diagnosis of fractures in the prehospital medicine setting have been shown to assist with earlier pain medication administration and notification to the receiving hospitals.

Interpretation

The large variation in acoustic impedance between soft tissue and bone allows for ultrasound diagnosis of fractures. The linear high-frequency transducer is placed in the transverse orientation. The location and depth of the bone of concern is assessed. Once the bone has been identified, the transducer is oriented in the long axis of the bone. The transducer is moved along in the superior and inferior directions of the extremity to evaluate for any irregularities within the cortex.

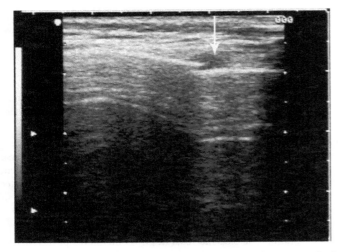

FIGURE 63-18. Ultrasound of the sternum (long axis). A sternal fracture is visualized as a discrete cortical discontinuity of the anterior sternum. (Reproduced with permission from Ma OJ, Mateer J, Blaivas M. *Emergency Ultrasound.* 2nd ed. New York: McGraw-Hill; 2007.)

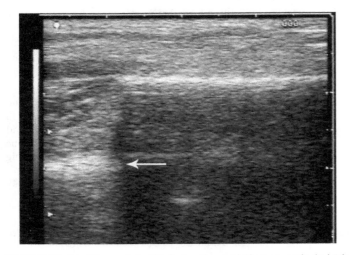

FIGURE 63-19. Ultrasound of a tibia fracture (long axis). The arrow marks the bright edge of the cortex of the proximal tibia. The distal fragment is displaced and the bright line of the cortex can be seen approximately 1 cm above the arrow. (Reproduced with permission from Ma OJ, Mateer J, Blaivas M. *Emergency Ultrasound.* 2nd ed. New York: McGraw-Hill; 2007.)

The cortical bone will be visualized as a very bright white density (**Figure 63-19**). Effusions or hematomas are seen as a hypoechoic area.

COMPARTMENT PRESSURE MONITORING

Measurement of compartment pressures may be necessary in patients with prolonged entrapment of a limb by machinery, farm accident, building collapse, blast, or other compression or crush injury.

Indications

- Evaluation for compartment syndrome

Essential Equipment

- Povidone iodine or chlorhexidine solution
- Sterile drapes or towels
- 4 × 4 gauze
- 18-gauge needle, 1½ in long
- Manometer

- 20-mL syringe
- Sterile saline
- Three-way stopcock
- Intravenous extension tubing

Technique

A simple manometer can be used to check compartment pressures using readily available medical supplies (**Figure 63-20**).

Step 1: Attach an 18-gauge needle to one end of intravenous tubing.

Step 2: Attach the other end of the IV extension tubing to a three-way stopcock.

Step 3: Prep the site(s) using sterile technique.

Step 4: Insert the needle into a sterile bottle of normal saline.

Step 5: Insert a second 18-gauge needle into the sterile saline bottle.

Step 6: Connect a 20-mL syringe to the stopcock.

Step 7: With the stopcock turned open to the syringe and IV tubing, aspirate normal saline to one-half of the length of the tubing.

Step 8: Keep the system closed to the third port of the stopcock.

Step 9: Attach intravenous tubing from the third port of the stopcock to a blood pressure cuff.

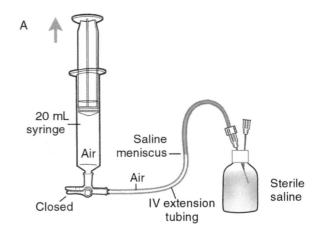

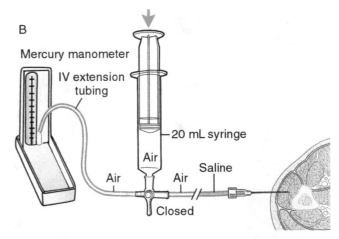

FIGURE 63-20. Needle manometer technique for compartment pressure. **A**: The air-saline meniscus will be convex shaped away from the patient when the pressure in the compartment is greater than the system. **B**: The air-saline meniscus will disappear as the compartment pressure equalizes with the pressure within the system. (Reproduced with permission from Reichman EF. ed. *Emergency Medicine Procedures, 2e.* New York, NY: McGraw-Hill; 2013.

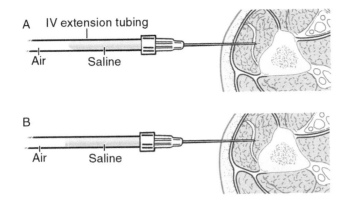

FIGURE 63-21. Air-saline interface. **A**: The air-saline meniscus will be convex shaped away from the patient when the pressure in the compartment is greater than the system. **B**: The air-saline meniscus will disappear as the compartment pressure equalizes with the pressure within the system. (Reproduced with permission from Reichman EF, ed. *Emergency Medicine Procedures.* 2nd ed. New York, NY: McGraw-Hill; 2013.)

Step 10: Remove the syringe from the stopcock while it is closed and aspirate 15 mL of air. Reconnect the syringe to the system.

Step 11: In the prepped and sterile field, place the 18-gauge needle into the desired compartment. Open the system so all three ports are open. Keep the needle in line with the air-saline meniscus to obtain an accurate reading.

Step 12: Inject sterile saline slowly using the 20-mL syringe until the air-saline meniscus is flat.

Step 13: Read the manometer for compartment pressure.

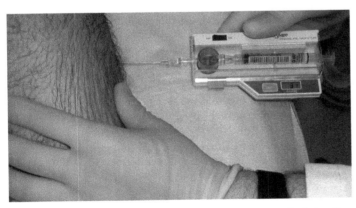

FIGURE 63-22. Stryker intracompartmental pressure monitor system. The device utilizes an 18-gauge 2.5-in side-ported needle, a purpose-specific diaphragm chamber, and a 3-mL syringe (filled with saline) to direct compartment pressures into the digital handheld monometer. (Reproduced with permission from Reichman EF, ed. *Emergency Medicine Procedures.* 2nd ed. New York, NY: McGraw-Hill; 2013.)

Interpretation

The air-saline meniscus will be convex shaped away from the patient when the pressure in the compartment is greater than the system. (**Figure 63-21A**) The air-saline meniscus will disappear as the compartment pressure equalizes with the manometer system. (**Figure 63-21B**) Normal pressures run from 0 to 8 mm Hg. Pressures over 30 mm Hg should prompt evaluation for compartment syndrome and possible fasciotomy.

Commercially Available Device

The Stryker intracompartmental pressure monitoring system simplifies this technique with an all-in-one design. The device utilizes an 18-gauge 2.5-in side-ported needle, a purpose-specific diaphragm chamber, and a 3-mL syringe (filled with saline) to direct compartment pressures into the digital handheld monometer (**Figure 63-22**).

REFERENCES

1. Raphael DT, Conard FU 3rd. Ultrasound confirmation of endotracheal tube placement. *J Clin Ultrasound.* September 1987;15(7): 459-462.
2. Chou HC, Tseng WP, Wang CH, et al. Tracheal rapid ultrasound exam (T.R.U.E.) for confirming endotracheal tube placement during emergency intubation. *Resuscitation.* October 2011;82(10):1279-1284.
3. Adi O, Chuan TW, Rishya M. A feasibility study on bedside upper airway ultrasonography compared to waveform capnography for verifying endotracheal tube location after intubation. *Crit Ultrasound J.* July 4, 2013;5(1):7.
4. Lyon ML, Verma N. Ultrasound guided volume assessment using inferior vena cava diameter. *Open Emerg Med J.* 2010;3:22-24.
5. Atkinson PR, McAuley DJ, Kendall RJ, et al. Abdominal and Cardiac Evaluation With Sonography in Shock (ACES): an approach by emergency physicians for the use of ultrasound in patients with undifferentiated hypotension. *Emerg Med J.* February 2009;26(2):87-91.
6. Varner MS. Maternal mortality in Iowa from 1952-1986. *Surg Gynecol Obst.* 1989;168:555-562.
7. Pearlman MD, Tintinalli JE, Lorenz RP. Blunt trauma in pregnancy. *N Eng J Med.* 1990;323:1609-1613.
8. Kamath MS, Aleyamma TK, Muthukumar K, Kumar RM, George K. A rare case report: ovarian heterotopic pregnancy after in vitro fertilization. *Fertil Steril.* 2010;94(5):1910.e9–1910.e11.
9. Tal J, Haddad S, Nina G, Timor-Tritsch I. Heterotopic pregnancy after ovulation induction and assisted reproductive technologies: a literature review from 1971 to 1993. *Fertil Steril.* 1996;66(1):1-12.
10. Lazarus E. What's new in first trimester ultrasound. *Radiol Clin N Am.* 2003;41:663-679.
11. Grechenig W, Clement HG, Fellinger M, Seggl W. Scope and limitations of ultrasonography in the documentation of fractures—an experimental study. *Arch Orthop Trauma Surg.* 1998;117:368-371.
12. Waterbrook AL, Adhikari S, Stolz U, Adrion C. The accuracy of point-of-care ultrasound to diagnose long bone fractures in the ED. *Am J Emerg Med.* September 2013;31(9):1352-1356. doi:10.1016/j.ajem.2013.06.006. Epub 2013 Jul 26.

INTRODUCTION

Field surgical procedures are for the most part relatively uncommon with few cases reported and published. Barriers to reporting likely include a preponderance of poor or unfavorable outcomes and the perceived risk of litigation in these high acuity scenarios. Although some hospital-based surgical "go teams" exist,[1,2] it is more likely that an EMS physician will be responding to these incidents in most communities. Rather than task a system to make available an additional trauma surgeon it is seemingly more appropriate for EMS physicians (of all primary training backgrounds) to maintain their education and training in these potentially lifesaving procedures. The following text is meant as an introduction to these procedures as they are likely to be performed in the austere and limited environment of the prehospital setting and in no way meant to substitute for, or replace the need for, EMS physicians to study and train on these techniques in the controlled environment of the anatomy lab or operating theater.

FIELD SURGICAL PROCEDURES

- Extremity amputation
- Thoracotomy
- Escharotomy
- Fasciotomy
- Perimortem cesarean section

FIELD SURGERY KIT

EMS Physician Basic Instrument Kit (Centurion SUT17530)

1 Fenestrated drape

4 Cloth towels

1 Spinal needle, 20 gauge × 3 ½ in

1 Needle, 18 gauge ×1 ½ in

1 Needle, 27 gauge × 1 ¼ in

2 Syringes, 10 mL

20 Gauze sponges

1 Safety scalpel with #11 blade

1 Safety scalpel with #15 blade

1 Safety scalpel with #21 blade

1 Tracheal hook

1 Tracheal dilator

1 Forcep, 1:2 teeth

1 Curved scissors

1 Needle holder, 6 in

1 Needle holder, 8 in

3 Curved hemostats

3 Straight hemostats

Additional Instruments

2 Gigli saw handles

4 Gigli saw blades

1 Safety scalpel with #10 blade

1 Rib spreader

4 Tourniquets (CAT or SOFT-T style)

1 Disposable OB kit

2 W35 skin staplers

2 Syringes, 20 mL

Optional Instruments

2 Army navy retractors

1 Curved (Metzenbaum) scissors

2 Russian forceps, 5½ in and 8 in

1 Bladder retractor

Other instruments as preferred by EMS physician/team

FIELD AMPUTATION

Field extremity amputation is a relatively uncommon procedure for any EMS physician to have to consider; however, there is a documented need for this capability in the prehospital setting.[3-10] Because of the potential for an awake patient to possibly require such a drastic and potentially painful intervention, it is appropriate for the EMS physician to ensure the availability of sedatives (eg, ketamine, midazolam, etomidate) and analgesics (eg, fentanyl, morphine) on the scene, by either carrying them with them or having them available by other means within the system.

Indication

When the entanglement of an extremity (or extremities) precludes timely rescue and patient care that is deemed necessary to sustain life, and it is believed that survival of the patient without the amputation of the extremity is doubtful, the choice must be made between life and limb. In cases where immediate rescue from the entanglement is not necessary for life preservation, care and time should be taken to exhaust all options for disentanglement before field amputation is considered. In some cases, where traumatic amputation is nearly complete and the patient has signs of potential life-threatening injuries it may be appropriate to consider field amputation if the partially amputated limb is unlikely to be salvaged. In this case the procedure is to complete, rather than perform, the amputation.

In cases where a living victim is entrapped by a deceased victims remains, it may be necessary to perform a dismemberment (by the same technique) in order to rescue the living victim.

Equipment

- Face mask with an eye shield or goggles
- Povidone iodine or chlorhexidine solution
- 2 Straight hemostats
- Gauze pads
- 2 Gigli saw handles
- 1 Gigli saw blade
- 1 Safety scalpel with #10 blade
- 1 Curved scissors
- 1 Tourniquet (CAT or SOFT-T style)

Technique

After establishing intravenous access and addressing issues of sedation and analgesia, attempt one more disentanglement procedure by rescue personnel. If this fails or patient condition precludes it, optimize airway and ventilator management and proceed with the amputation.

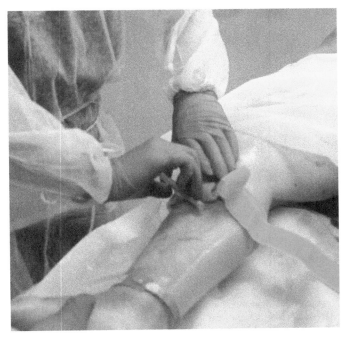

FIGURE 64-1. Tourniquet placement. Place a tourniquet to the proximal limb. Here a combat application tourniquet (CAT) is used.

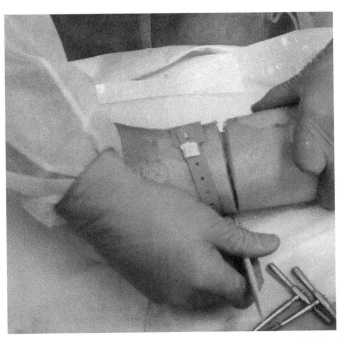

FIGURE 64-3. Sharp division of tissues. The circumferential wound is extended through the deep tissues and down to the bones.

Step 1: Place a tourniquet to the proximal limb and mark the time (**Figure 64-1**).

Step 2: Choose a location as distal as possible and perform a prep with antiseptic solution if time and environment allow.

Step 3: Incise the skin circumferentially with the #10 Scalpel blade, cut through the subcutaneous tissue, and open the fascia (**Figure 64-2**).

Step 4: At this point some EMS physicians might proceed by identifying muscle groups and attempting to divide with scissors, identify likely blood vessels, and apply clamps.[11] Alternatively, the muscle groups and vessels can be divided sharply with the #10 Scalpel

blade if the tourniquet is properly in place (**Figure 64-3**). If there is any question of hemostasis, then clamping major arteries may be appropriate.

Step 5: (Optional) Wrap two gauze pads or sterile towels around the extremity at the incision site and apply a clamp to hold the ends of each together and use to gain purchase of the bone and retract the surrounding soft tissues.

Step 6: Place the Gigli saw wire around the bone(s) (**Figure 64-4**), connect the saw handles, and with smooth long strokes divide the bone(s) (**Figure 64-5**).

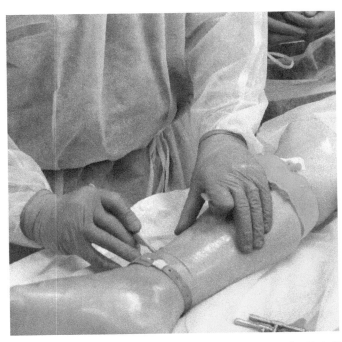

FIGURE 64-2. Circumferential skin incision. Incise the skin circumferentially with the #10 Scalpel blade, cut through the subcutaneous tissue.

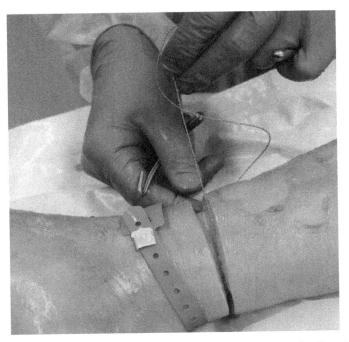

FIGURE 64-4. Placing the Gigli saw wire. The Gigli saw wire is slid underneath and looped back and then hooked onto the handles

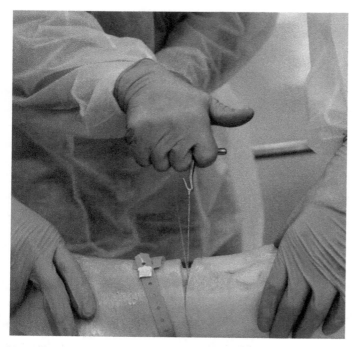

FIGURE 64-5. Dividing the bones.

Step 7: Evaluate the stump and address bleeding if present (**Figure 64-6**).

Step 8: Apply a padded dressing the wound and allow rescue of the patient to be completed and the patient transported to the trauma center.

Step 9: If it can be recovered, transport the amputated limb to the hospital.

Patients undergoing field amputation should receive tetanus prophylaxis and broad spectrum antibiotics to reduce risks of infection.

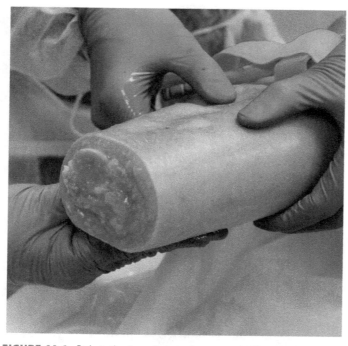

FIGURE 64-6. Evaluate the stump. Evaluate the stump and address bleeding if present address by tightening the tourniquet, then apply clamps only if necessary. The patient is now able to be rescued and transported. Apply a dressing and transport.

Complications

- Intentional loss of offending limb
- Loss of life/death
- Hemorrhage
- Nerve damage
- Operator/assistant injury

PREHOSPITAL THORACOTOMY

Although emergency resuscitative thoracotomy is traditionally considered a somewhat heroic measure with relatively poor outcomes the practice of prehospital thoracotomy continues.[12,13] A number of successful cases have been reported individually and in series and the practice is considered routine in some services when criteria are met.[14-17] These authors advocate for the continued practice and review of outcomes associated with this presumably earliest possible intervention scenario. However, some consideration should be given to the risk to providers and the potential for a delayed transport to the hospital.

In a paper by Seamon et al a statistical comparison was made between penetrating trauma victims transported by private care or the police and those transported by EMS and survival rates were worse in the EMS group (4 patients [5.1%] vs 19 patients [18.6%] patients).[18] Despite the expected difference in response time and over time from injury to arrival to the hospital that should be expected when not awaiting EMS arrival, the authors ascribe this mortality benefit to the lack of prehospital procedures and advocate for a "scoop and run" approach. The so-called Philadelphia model cannot be supported based on this limited data; however, common sense would dictate that procedures, when done in this population of patients, should probably occur en route to the hospital. Therefore, if the same can be asserted for prehospital thoracotomy, the potential for injury to the operator and assistants during an attempt to perform this procedure in a moving vehicle should be considered prior to initiating the procedure. It is impossible to speculate on whether the same result would be found if thoracotomy was one of the potential procedures provided to the study population.

Indication

- For thoracic exploration in patients with penetrating chest trauma who have lost vital signs acutely
- Control hemorrhage within the chest
- Relieve a pericardial tamponade surgically or one that cannot be decompressed by needle thoracotomy
- To cross-clamp the aorta and redistribute the cardiac output to the brain and heart
- To perform open cardiac massage

Equipment

- Face mask with an eye shield or goggles
- Povidone iodine or chlorhexidine solution
- Sterile towels
- Sterile gloves and gown
- #10 Scalpel blade
- Curved (Mayo) scissors, 8¾ and 6¾ in
- Curved (Metzenbaum) scissors, 5½ in
- Toothed forceps
- Satinsky vascular clamp
- Rib retractor, 12 in spread
- Suction source
- Suction tubing

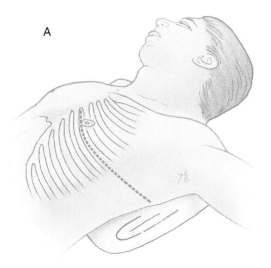

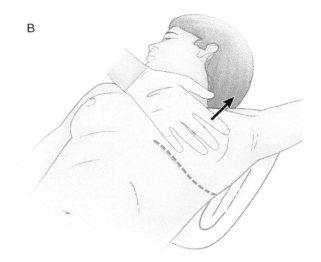

FIGURE 64-7. Landmarks for initial thoracotomy incision. (Reprinted with permission from Reichman EF, eds. *Emergency Medicine Procedures.* 2nd ed. New York, NY: McGraw-Hill; 2013.)

- Yankauer suction catheter
- 2-0 silk suture on a large curved needle
- Hemostats, needle driver, 10 in
- Gauze 4 × 4 squares
- Gigli saw

Technique

The patient should be first intubated and oxygenation and ventilation should be maximized.

Step 1: Identify landmarks of the fourth and fifth intercostal space below the nipple in males and below the inframammary fold in the female (**Figure 64-7**).

Step 2: Make an incision from the sternum to the left posterior axillary line (**Figure 64-8A**).

Step 3: Bag-valve-mask ventilation is temporarily stopped to allow for entrance to the thoracic cavity. If intubated, consider advancement of the ETT into the right mainstem bronchus to avoid lung injury during the left-sided thoracotomy.

Step 4: Extend the incision through the subcutaneous tissues down to the intercostal muscles. Mayo scissors may need to be used to incise the intercostal muscles.

Step 5: Insert middle finger through the incision and separate the lung from the chest wall. Move the fingers in the cephalad and caudad position while simultaneously cutting the remainder of the intercostal muscles (**Figure 64-8B**).

Step 6: Resume ventilation.

Step 5: Insert the rib spreader and open (**Figure 64-8C**).

Step 6: Exploration of the left side of thoracotomy procedure. If myocardial puncture wound located, carefully open the pericardial sac while avoiding the phrenic nerve and apply a temporizing measure (0 silk suture, or stable, or Foley with balloon—inflate balloon and clamp external end of Foley) (**Figure 64-8D**). If no evidence of origin of patient arrest, proceed to right side thoracotomy.*

Step 7: Extend the incision onto the right chest wall with the #10 Scalpel blade and then extend the incision using a curved Mayo scissor and continue to the right posterior axillary line.

Step 8: Use a Gigli saw to cut sternum (pass a clamp under the sternum and grasp one end of the Gigli saw blade and pull back under sternum, then connect the saw handles and with smooth long strokes to divide the sternum. Alternatively, a trauma sheer may be used. The internal mammary arteries will be severed and bleed. Apply hemostats for hemostasis. They can be tied off later with suture.

Step 9: Place the rib spreaders in the middle to open the chest wall (Figure 64-9f) or the anterior chest wall may be held open by assistants with appropriate PPE.

Step 10: Lift the anterior chest wall with care to adherent structures and bleeding.

Step 11: Explore the thoracic cavity for source of injury and apply temporary repair with 0 silk suture, stapler, or vascular clamp.

Step 12: Perform open cardiac message as appropriate.

*Alternatively a "clam shell" thoracotomy may be initiated from the beginning if there is a need for immediate full view, or if the penetrating trauma is to the right chest, it may be appropriate to complete the left and right side thoracotomies, cut the sternum, and free the anterior chest wall without first exploring the left chest (**Figure 64-9**).

Patients undergoing field thoracotomy should receive tetanus prophylaxis and broad-spectrum antibiotics to reduce risks of infection if they experience ROSC.

Complications

- Death
- Hemorrhage
- Vascular injury
- Organ injury
- Phrenic nerve injury
- Operator injury

ESCHEROTOMY

The relative simplicity of this procedure lends itself to potential successful performance in almost any clinical environment, including the back of a moving ambulance in a patient with an inability to ventilate.

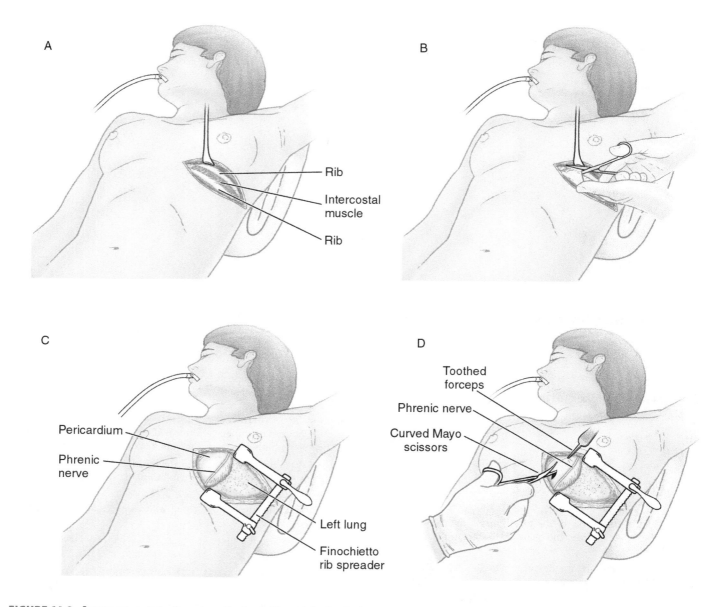

A

Rib

Intercostal muscle

Rib

B

C

Pericardium

Phrenic nerve

Left lung

Finochietto rib spreader

D

Toothed forceps

Phrenic nerve

Curved Mayo scissors

FIGURE 64-8. Emergency resuscitative thoracotomy. (Reprinted with permission from Reichman EF, eds. *Emergency Medicine Procedures.* 2nd ed. New York, NY: McGraw-Hill; 2013.)

However, the potential pain and discomfort to the patient, and risk to providers, should not be underestimated and care should be taken in performing the procedure when indicated.

Indication

- Cardiopulmonary compromise secondary to restrictive effects primarily from full-thickness burns. The burns do not need to be circumferential to cause this complication and escharotomy should be performed to alleviate this impending life threat. Analgesia and sedation should be considered and provided when appropriate.

Equipment

- Glove, gown, and face mask
- Povidone iodine or chlorhexidine solution
- #10 Scalpel blade on a handle
- Gauze 4 × 4 squares
- Local anesthetic solution if available
- Needles and syringes

Technique

Step 1: Make a skin incision along the appropriate plane with a #10 scalpel blade extending approximately 2 cm beyond the eschar tissue to allow for tissue expansion (**Figure 64-10**).

Step 2: Do not make incision depth greater than the depth of the dermis.

Step 3: Run your gloved finger along the incision line to ensure adequate separation of tissues.

Complications

Bleeding

Injury to deep structures including blood vessels, nerves, muscle, and connective tissues

Subsequent compromise of tissue leading to infection

Tissue ischemic secondary to inadequate release of tissues

Operator injury

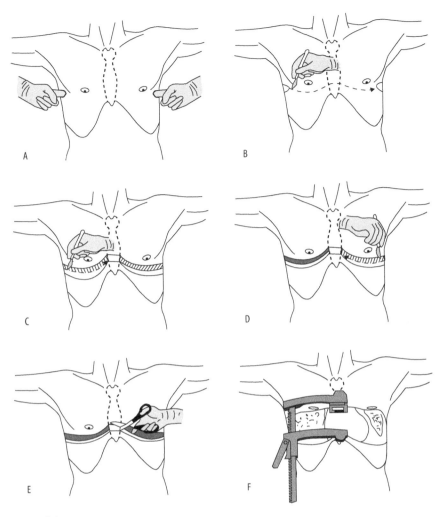

FIGURE 64-9. Clam shell thoracotomy technique.

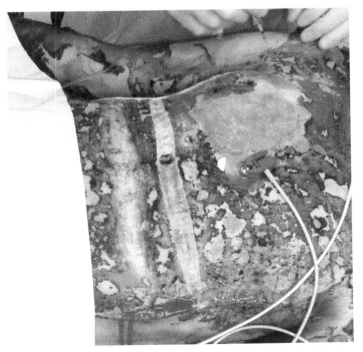

FIGURE 64-10. Escharotomy. The H-pattern of the escharotomy is meant to allow chest wall expansion.

FASCIOTOMY

When neurovascular compromise is suspected due to compartment syndrome, fasciotomy should be performed after identifying the correct compartment.

Indication

- Compromise of blood flow to the distal tissues to the extent of ischemia
- When compartment pressure measuring device is available the following criteria should be considered:
  - Absolute compartment pressures >30 mm Hg.
  - Absolute compartment pressure >20 mm Hg if the patient is hypotensive combined with any clinical signs of compartment syndrome.
  - ΔP or "delta P" of less than 30; delta P is defined as the difference between the diastolic blood pressure and the absolute or measured compartment pressure.

Equipment

- Povidone iodine or chlorhexidine solution
- Face mask and cap
- Sterile gloves and gown
- Sterile drapes or towels
- Equipment for compartment pressure measurement
  - Needle (Whitesides) manometer technique
  - Stryker monitor system

- 4 × 4 Gauze squares
- #10 Scalpel blade on a handle
- Tissue forceps
- Metzenbaum scissors
- Curved forceps
- Surgical retractors (if available)
- Dressings
- Splint material

Technique

There are numerous compartments within the body that may require fasciotomy. A full and complete understanding of the anatomy of the anatomic structures is imperative in order to perform a fasciotomy without compromising the musculature, and neurovascular structures. The most common location for requiring fasciotomy is the leg which has four compartments (anterior, lateral, deep posterior, and superficial posterior). A tibial fracture is the most common mechanism of injury that precludes compartment syndrome. The other compartments of the body that may necessitate fasciotomy include the thigh (**Figure 64-11**), which contains three compartments (anterior, medial, and posterior), arm, forearm, digits, hand, and foot.

Complications

- Bleeding
- Muscle laceration and/or injury
- Tendon laceration and/or injury

A

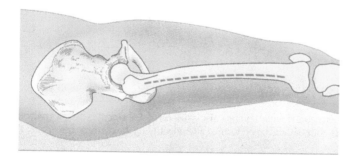

B

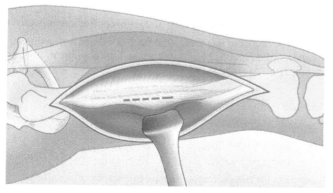

FIGURE 64-11. Fasciotomy of the thigh. (Reprinted with permission from Reichman EF, eds. *Emergency Medicine Procedures.* 2nd ed. New York, NY: McGraw-Hill; 2013.)

- Vascular lacerations and/or injury
- Increased compartment pressures in adjacent compartments
- Infection

PERIMORTEM CESAREAN SECTION

Since 1986 perimortem cesarean section has been recommended and the mark for the goal of delivery has been 4 minutes. Although the literature does not reflect that this goal is often reached reviews seem to show that the earlier the procedure is performed, the better for the child and the mother.[19,20] Additionally, it has been shown that in a simulated model of a pregnant mother in cardiac arrest, even moving the patient from the room decreased effectiveness of CPR and the authors recommended that perimortem cesarean section be performed in the location where the mother arrested.[21] Despite these findings it is uncommon to find reports of prehospital perimortem cesarean section.[22-24] Based on the current available literature it is reasonable to consider performing a prehospital perimortem C-section if the procedure can be performed within less than 10 minutes of arrest. No data exist to reasonably predict outcomes and therefor EMS physicians must judge each situation based on the circumstances.

Indication

- Maternal arrest with the possibility of maternal salvage
- Maternal arrest with the possibility of fetal salvage

Equipment

- #10 Surgical scalpel blade
- #15 Surgical scalpel blade and handle
- 1 Curved (Mayo) scissors
- 1 Curved (Metzenbaum) scissors
- 1 Forcep, 1:2 teeth
- 1 Curved scissors
- 1 Needle holder, 6 in
- 1 Needle holder, 8 in
- 3 Curved hemostats
- 3 Straight hemostats
- Two army-navy retractors
- Needle drivers, 8 and 6 in long
- Povidone iodine or chlorhexidine solution
- Sterile drapes
- Sterile gloves
- Two skin staplers
- Bulb syringe
- Clean towels or blanket for baby
- Two sterile umbilical cord clamps
- Neonatal resuscitation equipment

Technique

- Step 1: With a #10 Scalpel blade make a midline vertical incision that extends approximately 1 cm below the umbilicus to approximately 2 to 3 cm above the pubic symphysis (**Figure 64-12A**).
- Step 2: Cut down through the recuts abdominal muscle down to the sheath.
- Step 3: Use retractors (if available) for better visualization of the rectus sheath.
- Step 4: Using forceps, pick up the rectus sheath and use the Mayo scissors to create a midline hold. Extend the hole caudad and cephalad with the scissors (Figure 64-12).

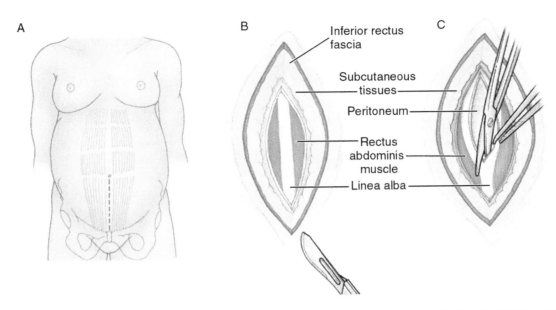

FIGURE 64-12. Perimortem C-section incision. (Reprinted with permission from Reichman EF, eds. *Emergency Medicine Procedures*. 2nd ed. New York, NY: McGraw-Hill; 2013.)

- Step 5: Lift up on the peritoneum and incise with the curved scissors (**Figure 64-13A**). Expose the uterus (**Figure 64-13B**). Use a retractor (if available) for better visualization.

- Step 6: Palpate uterus to determine positioning of the head.

- Step 7: Make approximately a 3-cm midline vertical incision in the uterus. Visualization of the amniotic sac should occur (**Figure 64-14A**).

- Step 8: Insert one finger into the uterus and extend the incision with the scissors to the fundus while letting the finger guide and protect the fetus (**Figure 64-14B**).

- Step 9: In the same manner, extend the incision inferiorly (**Figure 64-14C**).

- Step 10: Rupture the amniotic sac with a blunt instrument.

- Step 11: Insert your hand between the fetal head and the pubic symphysis (**Figure 64-15A**).

- Step 12: Gently flex the head while applying anterior and superior traction (**Figure 64-15B**).

- Step 13: Deliver the head of the fetus (**Figure 64-15C**).

- Step 14: Suction the mouth and nose (**Figure 64-15D**).

- Step 15: While a second provider should be applying pressure to the fundus of the uterus, apply gentle upward traction of the head. Once the shoulders are delivered, the remainder of the fetus will follow (**Figure 64-15E**).

- Step 16: For fetal positioning in the breech position or transverse lie, deliver the feet first. It is important to grasp the fetus by the pelvic bones to assist with deliver and not the abdomen.

- Step 17: Clamp the umbilical cord at the proximal and distal ends. Clamp approximately 10 to 15 cm away from the fetus and the second clamp 2 to 3 cm distally from the first clamp.

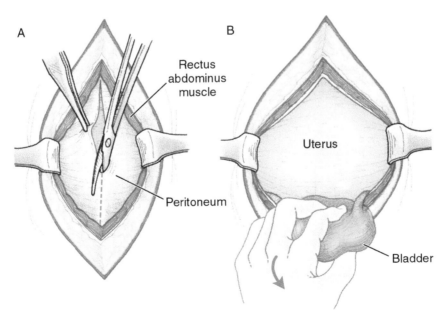

FIGURE 64-13. Exposure of the uterus. (Reprinted with permission from Reichman EF, eds. *Emergency Medicine Procedures*. 2nd ed. New York, NY: McGraw-Hill; 2013.)

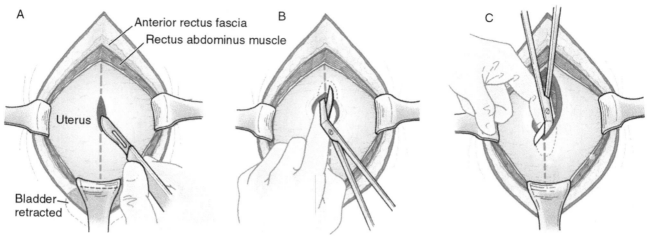

FIGURE 64-14. Uterine incision. (Reprinted with permission from Reichman EF, eds. *Emergency Medicine Procedures*. 2nd ed. New York, NY: McGraw-Hill; 2013.)

- Step 18: Cut the umbilical cord.
- Step 19: Begin resuscitative measures for the newborn.
- Step 20: Explore the inside of the uterus for a second fetus and to rule out any signs of hemorrhagic source.

- Step 21: If the mother is still alive, deliver the placenta.
- Step 22: If the mother is alive, clamp any obvious bleeders, pack the abdomen with wet gauze and continue resuscitative efforts for mother and newborn.

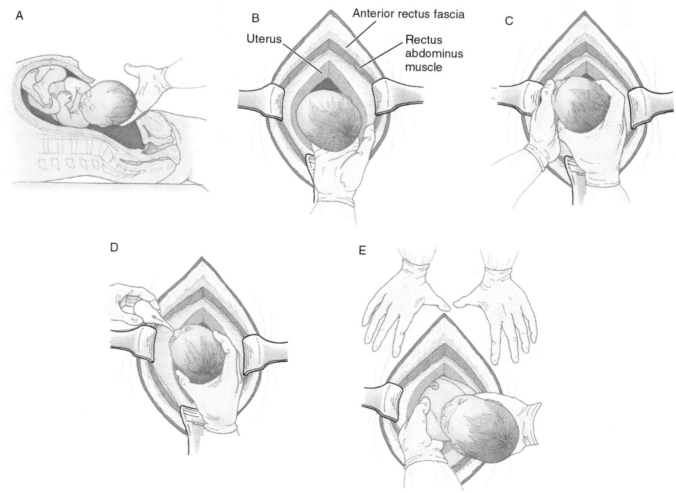

FIGURE 64-15. Delivering the infant. (Reprinted with permission from Reichman EF, eds. *Emergency Medicine Procedures*. 2nd ed. New York, NY: McGraw-Hill; 2013.)

Complications

- Maternal hemorrhage
- Maternal organ injury
- Fetal injury
- Sepsis

OTHER SURGICAL PROCEDURES

Surgical airway management (Chapter 59)
Thoracostomy (Chapter 59)

REFERENCES

1. Raines A, Lees J, Fry W, Parks A, Tuggle D. Field amputation: response planning and legal considerations inspired by three separate amputations. *Am J Disaster Med.* Winter 2014;9(1):53-58.

2. Scott C, Putnam B, Bricker S, et al. The development and implementation of a Hospital Emergency Response Team (HERT) for out-of-hospital surgical care. *Prehosp Disaster Med.* June 2012;27(3):267-271.

3. Foil MB, Cunningham PR, Hale JC, Benson NH, Treurniet S. Civilian field surgery in the rural trauma setting: a proposal for providing optimal care. *J Natl Med Assoc.* 1992;84:787-789.

4. Ebraheim NA, Elgafy H. Bilateral below-knee amputation surgery at the scene: case report. *J Trauma.* 2000;49:758-759.

5. Sharp CF, Mangram AJ, Lorenzo M, Dunn EL. A major metropolitan "field amputation" team: a call to arms... and legs. *J Trauma.* 2009;67:1158-1161.

6. Ho JD, Conterato M, Mahoney BD, Miner JR, Benson JL. Successful patient outcome after field extremity amputation and cardiac arrest. *Prehosp Emerg Care.* 2003;7:149-153.

7. Stewart RD, Young JC, Kenney DA, Hirschberg JM. Field surgical intervention: an unusual case. *J Trauma.* 1979;19:780-783.

8. Jaslow D, Barbera JA, Desai S, Jolly BT. An emergency department-based field response team: case report and recommendations for a "go team". *Prehosp Emerg Care.* 1998;2(1):81-85.

9. Kampen KE, Krohmer JR, Jones JS, Dougherty JM, Bonness RK. In-field extremity amputation: prevalence and protocols in emergency medical services. *Prehosp Disaster Med.* January-March 1996;11(1):63-66.

10. Macintyre A, Kramer EB, Petinaux B, Glass T, Tate CM. Extreme measures: field amputation on the living and dismemberment of the deceased to extricate individuals entrapped in collapsed structures. *Disaster Med Public Health Prep.* December 2012;6(4):428-435. doi:10.1001/dmp.2012.70. Review. PubMed PMID: 23241475.

11. Porter KM. Prehospital amputation. *Emerg Med J.* December 2010;27(12):940-942.

12. Athanasiou T, Krasopoulos G, Nambiar P, et al. Emergency thoracotomy in the pre-hospital setting: a procedure requiring clarification. *Eur J Cardiothorac Surg.* August 2004;26(2):377-386.

13. Wright KD, Murphy K. Cardiac tamponade: a case of kitchen floor thoracotomy. *Emerg Med J.* November 2002;19(6):587-588.

14. Lockey DJ, Davies G. Pre-hospital thoracotomy: a radical resuscitation intervention come of age? *Resuscitation.* December 2007;75(3): 394-395.

15. Coats TJ, Keogh S, Clark H, Neal M. Prehospital resuscitative thoracotomy for cardiac arrest after penetrating trauma: rationale and case series. *J Trauma.* April 2001;50(4):670-673.

16. Craig R, Clarke K, Coats TJ. On scene thoracotomy: a case report. *Resuscitation.* January 1999;40(1):45-47.

17. Keogh SP, Wilson AW. Survival following pre-hospital arrest with on-scene thoracotomy for a stabbed heart. *Injury.* September 1996;27(7):525-527.

18. Seamon MJ, Fisher CA, Gaughan J, et al. Prehospital procedures before emergency department thoracotomy: "scoop and run" saves lives. *J Trauma.* July 2007;63(1):113-120.

19. Benson MD, Padovano A, Bourjeily G, Zhou Y. Perimortem cesarean delivery: injury-free survival as a function of arrest-to-delivery interval time. *Obstet Gynecol.* May 2014;123(suppl 1):137S.

20. Einav S, Kaufman N, Sela HY. Maternal cardiac arrest and perimortem caesarean delivery: evidence or expert-based? *Resuscitation.* October 2012;83(10):1191-200.

21. Lipman SS, Wong JY, Arafeh J, Cohen SE, Carvalho B. Transport decreases the quality of cardiopulmonary resuscitation during simulated maternal cardiac arrest. *Anesth Analg.* January 2013; 116(1):162-167.

22. Bloomer R, Reid C, Wheatley R. Prehospital resuscitative hysterotomy. *Eur J Emerg Med.* August 2011;18(4):241-242.

23. Brun PM, Chenaitia H, Dejesus I, Bessereau J, Bonello L, Pierre B. Ultrasound to perimortem caesarean delivery in prehospital settings. *Injury.* January 2013;44(1):151-152.

24. Kaye R, Shewry E, Reid C, Burns B. The obstetric caseload of a physician-based helicopter emergency medical service: case review and recommendations for retrieval physician training. *Emerg Med J.* 2014;31(8):665-668.

PART III

Special Operations and Disaster Medicine

CHAPTER 65

Fire Ground Operations and Rehab

Andrew R. Poreda

Derek R. Cooney

INTRODUCTION

Firefighters tackle a wide variety of challenging operational scenarios and suffer significant stress and physiological demands during the discharge of their duties.[1] Because the majority of modern fire department emergency calls are for EMS, it is possible for physicians to be less familiar with the fire and rescue operations of the department they work with. EMS physicians must be aware of the unique operational challenges of firefighting and the potential role that the physician plays on the fire ground and their duties as the fire department physician.

OBJECTIVES

- Understand basic fire ground operations, including training requirements, fitness requirements, firefighter protective gear, and various tasks performed on the fire ground.
- Understand basic fire ground rehabilitation, including the need for rehab, firefighter physical fitness, the rehab station itself, and common medical/traumatic injuries.

FIRE AND RESCUE OPERATIONS

While on the fire ground the firefighter may be asked to perform a multitude of tasks, including fire suppression, search and rescue, ventilation, and salvage and overhaul (**Box 65-1**).[2] Fire suppression is the actual spraying of water and/or chemicals onto and around the fire, extinguishing it. Search and rescue is a systematic search of the entire building for victims. It consists of a primary search, which is rapid but thorough, and a secondary search, which is a more thorough search performed only after the fire is under control. Ventilation is the removal of heated air, smoke, and gases from the structure that is then replaced with cooler air. Ventilation increases firefighter visibility and decreases hot, toxic gases created by the fire. Finally, salvage and overhaul is an attempt to minimize property damage from the fire and the associated suppression activities, while also trying to detect hidden fires and determine the point and cause of origin.

FIREFIGHTER TRAINING REQUIREMENTS

Becoming a firefighter is arduous journey that begins at the state and local levels. Training requirements are on a state-to-state basis, with additional training provided by the local jurisdiction. There is, however, the National Fire Protection Association (NFPA), which is a national organization created to "reduce the world wide burden of fire and other hazards on the quality of life by providing and advocating consensus codes and standards, research, training, and education."[3] NFPA 1001 is the standard for firefighter training which describes the various tasks and knowledge that each firefighter should have.[4] The ProBoard Fire Service Professional Qualifications System is a national organization that certifies firefighters

---

Box 65-1

Fire and Rescue Operations

Engine company operations

- Rescue operations
- Establishing a water supply
- Lead initial fire attack with hose lines
- Manning of backup fire hose lines
- Ensuring exposure protection (spraying adjacent structures to keep them cool)
- Use of heavy duty water streams for attack and containment (master stream)
- Tactical use of building fire protective systems
- Overhaul (searching for hidden areas of heat or fire after fire attack is over)

Truck/ladder company operations

- Rescue operations
- Ventilation (tactical opening of roof, windows, doors, walls to allow heat out)
- Laddering (placing ladders for rescue and egress)
- Forcible entry (making entry into the building or opening for engine company)
- Ladder-pipe operation (for ladder truck)
- Utility control (managing electric and gas supplies)
- Salvage of property
- Checking fire extension and overhaul

Rapid intervention team (RIT)

- Search and rescue for firefighters
- Aid in escape/evacuation of firefighters
- Provide rescue air supply
- Aid in continuous scene safety assessment

Other department services

- Advanced rescue operations (vehicle, high angle, swift water, open water, confined space, dive team, etc)
- Hazardous materials
- Fire and injury prevention
- Fire investigation
- Codes enforcement

---

according to NFPA standards and has been adopted by 30 states, thus allowing firefighters to transfer their credentials across state lines.

Firefighting is a physically demanding job,[5] with an average heart rate of 179 during the most demanding tasks.[6] As such, the International Association of Fire Fighters (IAFF) and the International Association of Fire Chiefs (IAFC) have created the Candidate Physical Ability Test (CPAT), a screening test which is designed to "ensure that all fire fighter candidates possess the physical ability to complete critical tasks effectively and safely."[7] The CPAT recreates a similar VO_2 Max (a measure of their maximum oxygen consumption, and thus overall physical fitness) to that seen in firefighter simulations.[8] Also, the higher a candidate's VO_2 Max, the more likely they are to pass the

CPAT[9]; thus the CPAT appears to be an effective screening tool for firefighter physical fitness.

FIREFIGHTER PROTECTIVE EQUIPMENT

Firefighters are required to wear personal protective equipment (PPE) while performing their duties. NFPA 1971, NFPA 1981, NFPA 1851, and NFPA 1852 describe firefighter PPE and their maintenance. A complete description of PPE is outside the scope of this chapter; however, **Box 65-2** lists the basic components.[10]

While protecting the firefighter from extreme conditions, PPE does present some limitations to the user. The SCBA itself limits peripheral vision by as much as 28%[11]; limits communication, mobility,[12] and increases weight. The SCBA also has a limited air supply, with time frames depending on the type of cylinder and manufacturer. As a result of the thermal and moisture barriers of the coat and trousers, firefighter PPE also creates "microclimates" that are warmer and wetter, with temperatures of 48°C (118°F) and 100% relative humidity surrounding the firefighter.[13] PPE increases energy consumption and decreases VO_2 Max, mostly as a result of the extra weight the firefighter is now carrying plus the gears' inability to dissipate heat.[14-16] All of this extra heat, humidity, restrictions in vision and mobility, and weight puts an additional mental, cardiovascular, and thermoregulatory strain on the firefighter.[17,18]

Box 65-2

Basic Firefighter Personal Protective Equipment

- Helmet—provides impact protection

- Hood—protects the ears, neck, and face from heat, not otherwise protected by the coat and SCBA

- Coat and trousers—a three-layer garment made of an outer shell, a moisture barrier, and a thermal barrier

- Gloves—protects from heat and cold; resistant to punctures, cuts, and liquid absorption

- Boots—puncture resistant

- Eye protection—protects from flying particles and splash; 80% of eye injuries to firefighters is the result of not wearing eye protection.

- Hearing protection—protects from high levels of noise created by sirens, alarms, and the various tools used on scene, which has been recorded as high as 120 db.

- Self-contained breathing apparatus (SCBA)—protects from oxygen deficiency and hot, toxic gases; consists of a harness, air cylinder, regulator, and face piece

- Personal alert safety system (PASS) alarm—a notification system for a downed or disorientated firefighter.

REHAB[19] AND INJURY PREVENTION

THE NEED FOR REHAB

The need for firefighter rehab at the scene is easily explained when you consider the morbidity and mortality of firefighting. Each year, tens of thousands of firefighters are injured during the course of their duties; this includes training, responding to or returning from an emergency, or at the fire ground. In 2002 alone, there were an estimated 80,800 injuries to firefighters.[20] The most common injuries include sprains, strains, and open wounds, with the most common causative factor being overexertion.[21] As expected, larger incidents lead to more injuries.[22]

Unfortunately, many firefighters also lose their lives as a result of their job. The most recent data from 2009 showed that 90 firefighters died as a result of firefighting duties, including those that suffered a heart attack or stroke within 24 hours of an emergency response or training activity.[23] The most common cause of death includes cardiac arrest, trauma, asphyxiation, and motor vehicle accidents (see **Figure 65-1**), with most deaths caused by overexertion.[24,25] The typical line-of-duty death is a low-ranking male volunteer firefighter, at a structure fire, and is caused by overexertion.[25,26] Interestingly, the most common cause of death changes based on age; younger firefighters are more likely to die from trauma, while older firefighters are more likely to die from cardiac arrest.[25,26] Additionally, firefighters are more likely to die from cardiac arrest responding to the alarm and during fire suppression than during other nonemergent duties,[26] probably a result of the increased cardiovascular demand of fire suppression activities.[27] Firefighters are also more likely to die from cardiac arrest if they smoke, have hypertension, have coronary artery disease (CAD), or are over 45 years old.[28] Some of these same risk factors actually predict death from cardiac arrest as well, including smoking, CAD, and hypertension.[29] Lastly, firefighting as an occupation does not appear to have higher rates of CAD, but seems to be the result of conventional and usually modifiable CAD risk factors, including age, smoking, diastolic blood pressure, and family history.[30]

FIREFIGHTER FITNESS FOR DUTY AND PHYSICAL FITNESS

The way to prevent morbidity and mortality is to adequately screen firefighters during the initial medical clearance, and to encourage physical fitness and overall well-being.[31] NFPA 1582 was created for the purpose of firefighter medical screening. It includes a comprehensive list of medical disorders that pose a "significant risk to safety and health of the person or others."[32] These include medical disorders like craniofacial abnormalities, low visual acuity, recurrent syncope, uncontrolled seizures, etc. The initial and annual medical workup recommended by the NFPA includes a CBC, BMP, LFTs, lipid panel, urine analysis, audiology screening, pulmonary function testing, ECG, mammography or PSA testing, routine immunizations, HIV testing, colon cancer screening, a chest x-ray every 5 years, and heavy metal screening if needed.[33]

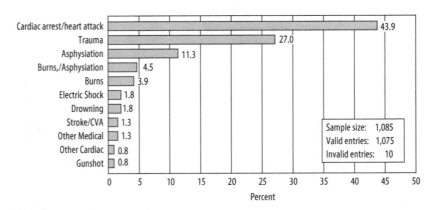

Cause	Percent
Cardiac arrest/heart attack	43.9
Trauma	27.0
Asphysiation	11.3
Burns,/Asphysiation	4.5
Burns	3.9
Electric Shock	1.8
Drowning	1.8
Stroke/CVA	1.3
Other Medical	1.3
Other Cardiac	0.8
Gunshot	0.8

Sample size: 1,085
Valid entries: 1,075
Invalid entries: 10

FIGURE 65-1. Cause of fatal firefighter injuries from 1990-2000 (From US Fire Administration. Firefighter fatality: retrospective study. http://www.usfa.dhs.gov/downloads/pdf/publications/fa-220.pdf. Accessed August 12, 2011)

Given the extreme cardiovascular workload experienced by firefighters, a minimum VO_2 Max has been recommended by the NFPA, along with multiple other sources.[3,33,34] In addition, routine cardiac stress tests have been advocated for firefighters with two or more risk factors for CAD (ie, smoking, diabetes, hypertension, hyperlipidemia, physical inactivity, obesity, or strong family history).[32,33] Screening for CAD in firefighters has been shown to reduce overall medical costs.[31] A recent study recommends that these cardiac stress tests be limited by exhaustion or age-predicted maximum heart rate, as opposed to the 85% submaximal tests that are commonly used for screening purposes.[35]

By virtue of the screening process, firefighters generally have a higher level of physical fitness than the general population[36] and firefighter physical fitness is associated with an improved metabolic profile.[37] Firefighting taxes all aspects of physical fitness[38]; and physical fitness influences performance of firefighter tasks,[39] as firefighters with higher physical fitness completed tasks quicker.[40] Unfortunately, a firefighter's self-perception of their own physical fitness is not associated with their actual physical fitness.[41] Therefore, the NFPA created standard 1583 to help define physical fitness programs for fire department members[42-44] (**Box 65-3**). One study showed that the physical fitness of firefighters could be substantially improved in as little as 16 weeks.[45]

Maintaining medical well-being is also discussed in NFPA 1582. Unfortunately as firefighters age, they have a similar rate of decline in cholesterol, hypertension, and body composition as compared to the general public.[37] But they also have a higher prevalence of obesity, high LDL, and low HDL cholesterol as they age.[46] This higher rate of obesity has been linked to higher rates of CAD risk factors in firefighters as well.[47] Furthermore, obesity was even more prevalent when assessed by percentage body fat, debunking the myth that firefighters were misclassified as obese simply because they were muscular.[48] As such, some authors

---

Box 65-3

NFPA 1583 Fitness Program Components

- Aerobic capacity
- Body composition
- Muscular strength
- Muscular endurance
- Flexibility

Box 65-4

Nine Components of Rehab

1. Relief from climactic conditions
2. Rest and recovery
3. Active and/or passive cooling or warming
4. Rehydration
5. Calorie and electrolyte replacement
6. Medical monitoring
7. Medical treatment by EMS
8. Accountability
9. Release to work

---

have recommended that annual medical screening should "proactively target cardiovascular risk factors."[47]

■ THE REHAB STATION

The fire ground rehab station is specifically set up to provide rest for firefighters who have been working for extended periods of time. NFPA 1584 was created to describe the rehabilitation process, which focuses on nine key areas[49] (**Box 65-4**):

Relief from Climactic Conditions The site must be distant from the operation, must allow a place to remove PPE prior to entering, it must be protected from the prevailing environment, and with no exhaust fumes nearby. It must be large enough for the incident, and provide areas for medical monitoring and transport. **Figure 65-2** shows the layout of a suggested rehab station.[50]

Rest and Recovery The NFPA recommends that firefighters rest for at least 20 minutes after using two 30-minute SCBA bottles, one 45-minute or one 60-minute SCBA bottle, or after 40 minutes of intense workout without an SCBA.[50] This time frame is just a recommendation and can be adjusted as needed. Interestingly a few articles have come out recently showing that 30 minutes may be insufficient time for recovery,[44] and that actual recovery time may be as much as 120 minutes![50]

Active and/or passive Cooling or Warming Firefighters with cold-related stress are encouraged to add clothing or blankets, while firefighters with heat-related stress should remove PPE, drink fluids, and apply

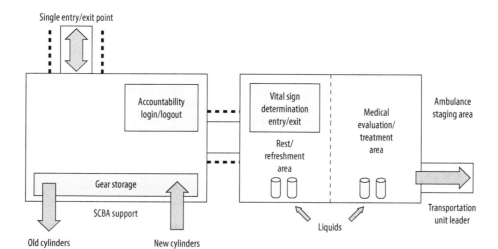

FIGURE 65-2. Suggested layout of the rehabilitation station. (Reproduced with permission from Dickinson ET, Wieder MA, eds. Emergency Incident Rehabilitation, 2nd ed. Upper Saddle River, NJ: Pearson Education; 2004.)

active and/or passive cooling techniques. One study has recently shown that forearm water immersion is superior to a fan with a mister, which is superior to removing PPE.[51] Recent advances in firefighter cooling techniques include an ice-vest; however, one study suggests it is not beneficial when combined with forearm immersion.[52] Despite work to develop cooling garments and study of cooling techniques, more research in this area is necessary.[53]

Rehydration Firefighters that were dehydrated prior to working had higher cardiovascular strain than those adequately hydrated.[54] Fluid replacement combined with forearm immersion increased working time by 100%, when compared to passive cooling and no hydration.[55] Another study showed that working time was increased, while heart rate and core temperature were decreased with fluids.[56] Thus, the NFPA recommends that firefighters should consume fluids to satisfy thirst and to continue hydrating after the incident.[50]

Calorie and Electrolyte Replacement The NFPA recommends that there be an area for firefighters to wash their hands and face, and that food be available, especially during incidents of more than 3 hours.[50]

Medical Monitoring NFPA recommends that there be at minimum a BLS crew available medical care. Additionally, the crew should be alert for signs of heat/cold stress, including chest pain, shortness of breath, weakness, dizziness, nausea, and headache. They also recommend that any members who are treated for heat-related injuries be removed from active duties.[50] Medical treatment of firefighters should be in accordance with local protocols.

Medical Treatment by EMS When a firefighter becomes a patient, it is necessary that EMS assets are available to initiate treatment and transport if necessary. Ideally, local protocols should address firefighter treatment after failure of rehab, or when immediate medical interventions are needed.

Accountability All members entering/leaving the rehab area should be tracked according to local accountability standards.[50]

Release to Work EMS personnel should evaluate firefighters prior to their release from the rehab area. Furthermore, if one crew member is seriously injured or killed, all crew members should be removed from duty for medical and mental health evaluation.[50] The psychological aspects of firefighting will be covered later in this chapter.

Finally, an article by Barr, et al gives an excellent review of the extreme physiologic stressors of firefighting, and I refer you to that for a more thorough review of the topics covered thus far.[57]

▓ COMMON MEDICAL AND TRAUMATIC EMERGENCIES

Common medical emergencies at the scene of a fire include sudden cardiac arrest, heat stress, and cold stress. Please refer to Chapters 29 and 33 for specific treatment of these common problems.

Common traumatic emergencies at the scene of a fire include musculoskeletal injuries, burns, and inhalation injuries. Please refer to Chapters 51 to 53, and 56 for treatment of musculoskeletal injuries. Please refer to Chapters 54 and 56 for treatment of burn-related injuries. Interestingly, a certain pattern of burn injuries has been described in firefighters; known as "nozzleman" burns (**Figure 65-3**), these are burns of the bilateral lower extremities as a result of prolonged contact with hot surfaces and heated water.[58]

The products of combustion and thus inhalation injuries include myriad of chemicals that depend greatly on the materials present and the conditions under which they are combusted. Common products of combustion include particulate matter, carbon dioxide, carbon monoxide (CO), nitrogen dioxide, hydrogen chloride, hydrogen cyanide (HCN), sulfur dioxide/sulfuric acid, acrolein, formaldehyde and acetaldehyde, and benzene.[59] A review of all of these chemicals is beyond the scope of this chapter; however, we will focus on two: CO and CN. CO is present in virtually all fire environments and is a product of incomplete

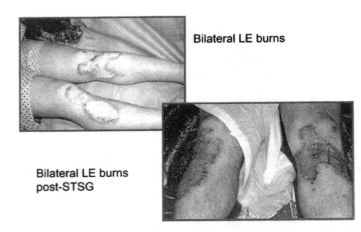

FIGURE 65-3. An example of "nozzleman burns" (From Rabbitts A, Alden NE, O'Sullivan G, et al. Firefighter burn injuries: a 10-year longitudinal study. *J Burn Care Rehabil.* 2004;25:430-434. Reproduced with permission.)

combustion.[60] The National Institute for Occupational Safety and Health (NIOSH) has listed the "immediately dangerous to life or health" (IDLH) concentration of CO at 1200 parts per million (ppm).[60] One recent study found that CO poses a greater threat to victims than does oxygen deprivation or heat, and that all CO levels recorded at the ceiling of live-fire simulations exceeded the IDLH level.[61] Treatment of CO poisoning includes removing the victim from the source, applying supplemental oxygen via a nonrebreather, and considering transporting to a facility with hyperbaric oxygen capabilities.[62] CN is derived primarily from the combustion of nitrogen-containing polymers such as nitriles, polyamides, nylons, and polyurethane.[60] NIOSH has listed the IDLH as 50 ppm,[63] and treatment of CN poisoning focuses on the administration of antidotes such as hydroxycobalamin, or a cyanide antidote kit (a combination of amyl nitrate, sodium nitrite, and sodium thiosulfate).[64] Unfortunately, the products of combustion are also present during the overhaul stage of firefighting.[65] One study showed significant changes in spirometric lung function in firefighters who did not wear SCBA during overhaul.[66] Given these findings and the multitude of toxic chemicals still present after the fire is out, firefighters should continue to wear SCBA during overhaul.

POSTINCIDENT CARE OF FIREFIGHTERS

▓ PSYCHOLOGICAL CARE

Posttraumatic stress disorder (PTSD) is listed in the DSM-IV as a member of the anxiety disorders. PTSD is characterized by the reexperiencing of an extremely traumatic event accompanied by symptoms of increased arousal and by avoidance of stimuli associated with the trauma for at least 1 month.[67] The prevalence of PTSD is estimated to be 22.2% in American firefighters, while the general population has a lifetime prevalence of 6.8%.[68,69] Firefighters routinely witness extremely traumatic events on a regular basis as part of their duties. In fact, firefighters report that the highest areas of stress include a catastrophic injury to self or coworker, gruesome victim incidents, rendering aid to seriously injured vulnerable victims, minor injury to self, and exposure to death and dying.[70] Risk factors for developing PTSD in firefighters include preexisting negative appraisals (ie, those who exaggerate negative thoughts),[71] those who have high hostility, those with low self-efficacy, and those who catastrophize about negative events.[72,73] The treatment of PTSD focuses on either pharmacotherapy, psychotherapy, or a combination of the two.[74]

Critical incident stress management (CISM) is a "comprehensive, integrative, multicomponent crisis intervention system" that was initially developed by Mitchell in the early 1980's.[75,76] It focuses on seven components, one of which includes critical incident stress debriefing (CISD), which is a structured group discussion designed to mitigate acute symptoms, assess the need for follow-up, and provide a sense of closure.[76] There is an ongoing debate as to the effectiveness of CISM/CISD in treating acute stress.[77-80] Opponents of CISM/CISD argue that the initial studies are weak and have serious methodological flaws, it does little to prevent PTSD, and may in fact cause harm by worsening the symptoms[79,80] Proponents of CISM/CISD state that studies that showed harm did not test CISM/CISD, but rather tested single-session debriefing which is not in the context of the full, seven- component CISM model.[78,80] Two Cochrane reviews show that there is no evidence that single-session individual psychological debriefing prevents PTSD, and that multiple session interventions aimed at all individuals should not be used.[81,82] The American Psychiatric Association states that psychological debriefings or single-session techniques are not recommended, as does the United Kingdom's National Institute for Clinical Excellence.[75,83] The NFPA also has guidelines for the psychological well-being of firefighters. NFPA 1500 is the minimum standard for occupational health and safety and includes a section regarding member assistance and wellness programs. The NFPA recommends that the member assistance program assist members with substance abuse, stress, and personal problems, while the wellness program should be focused on preventing health problems and enhancing overall well-being.[84] The NFPA also includes a section on critical incident stress programs, and states that a program should be designed to relieve stress created by the incidents.[85] Unfortunately it gives little advice to the physician on how to implement any of these above-mentioned programs, and what makes an effective program.

Fortunately, it appears the physician may be able to count on firefighters to report their own diagnosis of PTSD. One recent study used the PTSD Checklist to screen firefighters for PTSD after the 9/11 attacks, and found a sensitivity of 85%.[85] The PTSD Checklist was initially designed to screen Vietnam War veterans for PTSD, and it must be followed by a formal psychological interview to confirm the diagnosis[86]; however, it does appear to be an appropriate screening tool for firefighters. Given all of this information, it is this author's opinion that single-session debriefing be abandoned and instead be replaced with appropriate psychological screening for PTSD, and combined with long-term psychological care.

LONG-TERM AFFECTS OF FIREFIGHTING

A few studies have looked at the long-term consequences of firefighting, which have mostly circled around the respiratory effects, and the risks of developing cancer. Firefighting has been associated with acute decrements in lung function, as measured by spirometry within 2 hours of a fire.[87] This study also suggested that the change in lung function is not merely due to airway hyperresponsiveness from preexisting conditions.[88] These acute changes in lung function also seem to correlate with the severity of smoke exposure.[88] Another recent study has shown that the incidence and point prevalence of sarcoidosis is increased in firefighters; however, it created only minimal impairment.[89]

Multiple studies have also attempted to show the link between cancer and firefighting. Early studies were limited due to the size of the studies and the rates of specific cancers. One recent study combined these smaller cohort studies, which showed no significant risks of developing cancer.[90] However, subcohort analysis did show significant rates of colon, kidney, brain, and leukemia based on duration of employment.[91] Two large case-control studies from Massachusetts and California showed higher rates of colon and brain, and testicular, melanoma, brain, esophageal, and prostate cancer, respectively.[91,92] However, another study has shown that there is no convincing evidence that employment as a firefighter is associated with increased all-cause, CAD, cancer, or respiratory disease mortality.[93] This study does mention that brain cancer mortality was consistently high, yet not statistically significant. More studies are needed to better define which cancers firefighters may be at risk for developing.

- Firefighting is a physically and psychologically demanding job.
- The most common cause of firefighter death during an incident is from heart attack, and areas of prevention should focus on overall firefighter physical fitness and the reduction of cardiac risk factors.
- NFPA 1582 is the standard for assessing personnel for fitness for duty.
- NFPA 1583 outlines the recommended components of a fitness program.
- NFPA 1584 details the nine components of a rehab program.
- Critical incident stress management (CISM) is a "comprehensive, integrative, multicomponent crisis intervention system" which includes seven components, one of which includes Critical incident stress debriefing (CISD), which is a structured group discussion designed to mitigate acute symptoms, assess the need for follow-up, and provide a sense of closure.
- There may be some increased risk of pulmonary disease and cancer in firefighters; however, further study is needed.

REFERENCES

1. Young PM, Partington S, Wetherell MA, St Clair Gibson A, Partington E. Stressors and coping strategies of UK firefighters during on-duty incidents. *Stress Health*. 2014;30(5):366-376.
2. Hall R, Adams B. eds. *Essentials of Fire Fighting*. 4th ed. Stillwater, OK: Oklahoma State University; 1998.
3. NFPA. About NFPA. http://www.nfpa.org/categoryList.asp?categoryID=143&URL=About%20NFPA. Accessed August 2, 2011.
4. NFPA 1001: Standard for Fire Fighter Professional Qualifications. 2008 Edition.
5. Gledhill N, Jamnik VK. Characterization of the physical demands of firefighting. *Can J Sport Sci*. 1992;17(3):207-213.
6. Holmer I, Gavhed D. Classification of metabolic and respiratory demands in fire fighting activity with extreme workloads. *App Ergonomics*. 2007;38:45-52.
7. IAFF. Wellness-fitness initiative. http://www.iaff.org/hs/CPAT/cpat_index.html. Accessed August 2, 2011.
8. Williams-Bell FM, Villar R, Sharratt MT, et al. Physiological demands of the Firefighter Candidate Physical Ability Test. *Med Sci Sports Exer*. 2009;41(3):653-662.
9. Sheaff AK, Bennett A, Hanson ED, et al. Physiological determinants of the candidate physical ability test in firefighters. *J Strength Cond Res*. 2010;24(11):3112-3122.
10. Owen CG, Margrain TH, Woodward EG. Etiology and prevalence of eye injuries within the United Kingdom fire service. *Eye*. 1995;9(suppl):54-58.
11. Samo DG, Bahk JK, Gerkin RD. Effect of firefighter masks on monocular and binocular peripheral vision. *J Occup Enivron Med*. 2003;45:428-432.
12. Park K, Hur P, Rosengren KS, et al. Effect of load carriage on gait due to firefighting air bottle configuration. *Ergonomics*. 2010;53(7):882-891.
13. Rossi R. Fire fighting and its influence on the body. *Ergonomics*. 2003;46(10):1017-1033.
14. Baker SJ, Grice J, Roby L, et al. Cardiorespiratory and thermoregulatory response of working in fire-fighter protective clothing in a temperate environment. *Ergonomics*. 2000;43(9):1350-1358.
15. Dreger RW, Jones RL, Petersen SR. Effects of the self-contained breathing apparatus and fire protective clothing on maximal oxygen uptake. *Ergonomics*. 2006;49(10):911-920.

16. Bruce-Low SS, Cotterrell D, Jones GE. Effect of wearing personal protective clothing and self-contained breathing apparatus on heart rate, temperature and oxygen consumption during stepping exercise and live fire training exercises. *Ergonomics*. 2007;50(1):80-98.

17. Young PM, Gibson AS, Partington E, Partington S, Wetherell MA. Psychophysiological responses in experienced firefighters undertaking repeated self-contained breathing apparatus tasks. *Ergonomics*. December 2014;57(12):1898-1906.

18. Greenlee TA, Horn G, Smith DL, Fahey G, Goldstein E, Petruzzello SJ. The influence of short-term firefighting activity on information processing performance. *Ergonomics*. 2014;57(5):764-773.

19. US Fire Administration. Emergency incident rehabilitation. http://www.usfa.dhs.gov/downloads/pdf/publications/fa_314.pdf. Accessed August 31, 2011.

20. US Dept of Commerce, National Institute of Standards and Technology. The economic consequences of firefighter injuries and their prevention. Final report. http://fire.nist.gov/bfrlpubs/NIST_GCR_05_874.pdf. Accessed August 12, 2011.

21. Walton SM, Conrad KM, Furner SE, et al. Cause, type, and workers' compensation costs of injuries to fire fighters. *Amer J Industrial Med*. 2003;43:454-458.

22. Fabio A, Ta M, Strotmeyer S, et al. Incident-level risk factors for firefighter injuries at structural fires. *J Occup Environ Med*. 2002;44(11):1059-1063.

23. US Fire Administration. Firefighter fatalities in the United States in 2009. http://www.usfa.dhs.gov/downloads/pdf/publications/ff_fat09.pdf. Accessed August 12, 2011.

24. US Fire Administration. Firefighter fatality: retrospective study. http://www.usfa.dhs.gov/downloads/pdf/publications/fa-220.pdf. Accessed August 12, 2011.

25. CDC. Fatalities among volunteer and career firefighters—United States, 1994-2004. *MMWR Morb Mortal Wkly Rep*. 2006;55(16):453-455.

26. Kales SN, Soteriades ES, Christophi CA, et al. Emergency duties and deaths from heart disease among firefighters in the United States. *N Engl J Med*. 2007;356(12):1207-1215.

27. Smith DL, Manning TS, Petruzzello SJ. Effect of strenuous live-fire drills on cardiovascular and psychological responses of recruit firefighters. *Ergonomics*. 2001;44(3):244-254.

28. Kales SN, Soteriades ES, Christoudias SG, et al. Firefighters and on-duty deaths from coronary heart disease: a case control study. *Env Health*. 2003;2:14.

29. Geibe JR, Holder J, Peeples L, et al. Predictors of on-duty coronary events in male firefighters in the United States. *Amer J Cardio*. 2008;101:585-589.

30. Glueck CJ, Kelley W, Wang P, et al. Risk factors for coronary heart disease among firefighters in Cincinnati. *Amer J Indus Med*. 1996;30:331-340.

31. National Institute for Occupational Safety and Health. NIOSH fire fighter fatality investigation and prevention program: leading recommendations for preventing fire fighter fatalities, 1998-2005. http://www.cdc.gov/niosh/docs/2009-100/pdfs/2009-100.pdf. Accessed August 13, 2011.

32. NFPA 1582: Standard on Comprehensive Occupational Medical Program for Fire Departments. 2007 Edition.

33. Swank AM, Adams KJ, Barnard KL, et al. Age-related aerobic power in volunteer firefighters, a comparative analysis. *J Strength Cond Res*. 2000;14(2):170-174.

34. Sothmann MS, Saupe K, Jasenof D, et al. Heart rate response of firefighters to actual emergencies. Implications for cardiorespiratory fitness. *J Occup Med*. 1992;34(8):797-800.

35. Angerer P, Kadlez-Gebhardt S, Delius M, et al. Comparison of cardiocirculatory and thermal strain of male firefighters during fire suppression to exercise stress test and aerobic exercise testing. *Amer J Cardiol*. 2008;102:1551-1556.

36. Davis SC, Jankovitz KZ, Rein S. Physical fitness and cardiac risk factors of professional firefighters across the career span. *Res Quarterly Exer Sport*. 2002;73(3):363-370.

37. Donovan R, Nelson T, Peel J, et al. Cardiorespiratory fitness and the metabolic syndrome in firefighters. *Occup Med*. 2009;59:487-492.

38. Rhea MR, Alvar BA, Gray R. Physical fitness and job performance of firefighters. *J Strength Cond Res*. 2004;18(2):348-352.

39. Del Sal M, Barbieri E, Garbati P, et al. Physiologic responses of firefighter recruits during a supervised live-fire work performance test. *J Strength Cond Res*. 2009;23(8):2396-2404.

40. Elsner KL, Kolkhorst FW. Metabolic demands of simulated firefighting tasks. *Ergonomics*. 2008;51(9)1418-1425.

41. Peate WF, Lundergan L, Johnson JJ. Fitness self-perception and VO2 max in firefighters. *J Occup Environ Med*. 2002;44:546-550.

42. NFPA 1583: Standard on Health-Related Fitness Programs for Fire Department Members. 2008 Edition.

43. Perroni F, Tessitore A, Cortis C, et al. Energy cost and energy sources during a simulated firefighting activity. *J Strength Cond Res*. 2010;24(12):3457-3463.

44. Hilyer JC, Brown KC, Sirles AT, et al. A flexibility intervention to reduce the incidence and severity of joint injuries among municipal firefighters. *J Occup Med*. 1990;32(7):631-637.

45. Roberts MA, O'Dea J, Boyce A, et al. Fitness levels of firefighter recruits before and after a supervised exercise training program. *J Strength Cond Res*. 2002;16(2):271-277.

46. Byczek L, Walton SM, Conrad KM, et al. Cardiovascular risks for firefighters: implications for occupational health nurse practice. *AAOHN J*. 2004;52(2):66-76.

47. Soteriades ES, Hauser R, Kawachi I, et al. Obesity and cardiovascular disease risk factors in firefighters: a prospective cohort study. *Obes Res*. 2005;13:1756-1763.

48. Poston WSC, Haddock K, Jahnke SA, et al. The prevalence of overweight, obesity, and substandard fitness in a population-based firefighter cohort. *J Occup Environ Med*. 2011;53(3):266-273.

49. NFPA 1584: Standard on the Rehabilitation Process for Members During Emergency Operations and Training Exercises. 2008 Edition. http://www.nfpa.org/codes-and-standards/document-information-pages?mode=code&code=1584.

50. Horn GP, Gutzmer S, Fahs CA, et al. Focus on firefighter physiology: physiological recovery from firefighting activities in rehabilitation and beyond. *Prehosp Emerg Care*. 2011;15:214-225.

51. Selkirk GA, McLellan TM, Wong, J. Active versus passive cooling during work in warm environments while wearing firefighting protective clothing. *J Occup Environ Hygiene*. 2004;1:521-531.

52. Barr D, Reilly T, Gregson W. The impact of different cooling modalities on the physiological responses in firefighters during strenuous work performed in high environmental temperatures. *Eur J Appl Physiol*. 2011;111:959-967.

53. McEntire SJ, Suyama J, Hostler D. Mitigation and prevention of exertional heat stress in firefighters: a review of cooling strategies for structural firefighting and hazardous materials responders. *Prehosp Emerg Care*. April-June 2013;17(2):241-60.

54. Brown J, Derchak A, Bennett A, et al. Impact of pre-participation hydration status on structural firefighter cardio-respiratory response to standard training activities. *Med Sci Sports Exer*. 2007;39(5): Supp 153.

55. McLellan TM, Selkirk GA. The management of heat stress for the firefighter: a review of work conducted on behalf of the Toronto fire service. *Indus Health*. 2006;44:414-426.

56. Selkirk GA, McLellan TM, Wong J. The impact of various rehydration volumes for firefighters wearing protective clothing in warm environments. *Ergonomics*. 2006;49(4):418-433.

57. Barr D, Gregson W, Reilly T. The thermal ergonomics of firefighting reviewed. *Applied Ergonomics*. 2010;41:161-172.

58. Rabbitts A, Alden NE, O'Sullivan G, et al. Firefighter burn injuries: a 10-year longitudinal study. *J Burn Care Rehabil*. 2004;25:430-434.

59. Lees, P. Combustion products and other firefighter exposures. *Occup Med*. 1995;10(4):691-706.

60. CDC. IDLH : carbon monoxide. http://www.cdc.gov/niosh/idlh/630080.html. Accessed August 27, 2011.

61. Cone DC, MacMillan D, Parwani V, et al. Threats to life in residential structure fires. *Prehosp Emerg Care.* 2008;12:297-301.
62. Tomaszewski C. Carbon monoxide. In: Nelson LS, Hoffman RS, Lewin NA, et al, eds. *Goldfrank's Toxicologic Emergencies.* 9th ed. New York, NY: McGraw-Hill; 2011.
63. CDC. IDLH : Hydrogen cyanide. http://www.cdc.gov/niosh/idlh/74908.HTML. Accessed August 27, 2011.
64. Kirk MA, Holstege CP, Isom GE. Cyanide and hydrogen sulfide. In: Nelson LS, Hoffman RS, Lewin NA, et al, eds. *Goldfrank's Toxicologic Emergencies.* 9th ed. New York, NY: McGraw-Hill; 2011.
65. Bolstad-Johnson DM, Burgess JL, Crutchfield CD, et al. Characterization of firefighter exposures during fire overhaul. *AIHAJ.* 2000;61:636-641.
66. Burgess JL, Nanson CJ, Bolstad-Johnson DM, et al. Adverse respiratory effects following overhaul in firefighters. *J Occup Environ Med.* 2001;43:467-473.
67. American Psychiatric Association. *Diagnostic and Statistical Manual of Mental Disorders.* 4th ed, text rev. Washington, DC: American Psychiatric Association, 2000.
68. Corneil W, Beaton R, Murphy S, et al. Exposure to traumatic incidents and prevalence of posttraumatic stress symptomatology in urban firefighters in two countries. *J Occup Health Psych.* 1999;4(2):131-141.
69. Kessler RC, Berglund P, Delmer O, et al. Lifetime prevalence and age-of-onset distributions of DSM-IV disorders in the National Comorbidity Survey Replication. *Arch Gen Psych.* 2005;62(6):593-602.
70. Beaton R, Murphy S, Johnson C, et al. Exposure to duty-related incident stressors in urban firefighters and paramedics. *J Traumatic Stress.* 1998;11(4):821-828.
71. Bryant RA, Guthrie RM. Maladaptive self-appraisals before trauma exposure predict posttraumatic stress disorder. *J Consulting Clin Psych.* 2007;75(5):812-815.
72. Heinrichs M, Wagner D, Schoch W, et al. Predicting posttraumatic stress symptoms from pretraumatic risk factors: a 2-year prospective follow-up study in firefighters. *Amer J Psych.* 2005;162:2276-2286.
73. Bryant RA, Guthrie RM. Maladaptive appraisals as a risk factor for posttraumatic stress: a study of trainee firefighters. *Psych Sci.* 2005;16(10):749-752.
74. American Psychiatric Association Practice Guidelines: treatment of patients with acute stress disorder and posttraumatic stress disorder. http://www.psychiatryonline.com/pracGuide/PracticePDFs/ASD_PTSD_Inactivated_04-16-09.pdf. Accessed August 31, 2011.
75. A primer on critical incident stress management (CISM). http://www.icisf.org/who-we-are/what-is-cism. Accessed August 31, 2011. http://www.icisf.org/a-primer-on-critical-incident-stress-management-cism/.
76. Robinson R. Reflections on the debriefing debate. *Inter J Emerg Ment Health.* 2008;10(4):253-260.
77. Tuckey MR, Scott JE. Group critical incident stress debriefing with emergency services personnel: a randomized controlled trial. *Anxiety Stress Coping.* January 2014;27(1):38-54.
78. Bledsoe BE. Critical incident stress management (CISM): benefit or risk for emergency services. *Prehosp Emerg Care.* 2003;7:272-279.
79. Wessely S, Deahl M. Psychological debriefing is a waste of time. *Brit J Psych.* 2003;183:12-14.
80. Raphael B, Wooding S. Debriefing: its evolution and current status. *Psych Clin N Amer.* 2004;27:407-423.
81. Rose SC, Bisson J, Churchill R, et al. Psychological debriefing for preventing post traumatic stress disorder (PTSD). *Cochrane Data Sys Reviews.* 2002;(2):CD000560.
82. Roberts NP, Kitchiner NJ, Kenardy J, et al. Multiple session early psychological interventions for the prevention of post-traumatic stress disorder. *Cochrane Data Sys Reviews.* 2009;(3):CD006869.
83. Mayor S. Psychological therapy is better than debriefing for PTSD. *Brit Med J.* 2005;330:689.
84. NFPA 1500: Standard on Fire Department Occupational Safety and Health Program. 2007 Edition. http://www.nfpa.org/codes-and-standards/document-information-pages?mode=code&code=1500.
85. Chiu S, Webber MP, Zeig-Owens R, et al. Performance characteristics of the PTSD checklist in retired firefighters exposed to the World Trade Center disaster. *Ann Clin Psych.* 2001;23(2):95-104.
86. McDonald SD, Calhoun PS. The diagnostic accuracy of the PTSD checklist: a critical review. *Clin Psychol Rev.* 2010;30(8):976-987.
87. Sheppard D, Distefano S, Morse L, et al. Acute effects of routine firefighting on lung function. *Amer J Indus Med.* 1986;9:333-340.
88. Musk AW, Smith TJ, Peters JM, et al. Pulmonary function in firefighters: acute changes in ventilatory capacity and their correlates. *Brit J Indus Med.* 1979;36:29-34.
89. Prezant DJ, Dhala A, Goldstein A, et al. The incidence, prevalence, and severity of sarcoidosis in New York City firefighters. *Chest.* 1999;116:1183-1193.
90. Youakim S. Risk of cancer among firefighters: a quantitative review of selected malignancies. *Arch Environ Occup Health.* 2006;61(5):223-231.
91. Kang D, Davis LK, Hunt P, et al. Cancer incidence among male Massachusetts firefighters, 1987-2003. *Amer J Indus Med.* 2008;51:329-335.
92. Bates MN. Registry-based case-control study of cancer in California firefighters. *Amer J Indus Med.* 2007;50:339-344.
93. Haas NS, Gochfeld M, Robson MG, et al. Latent health effects in firefighters. *Int J Occup Environ Health.* 2003;9:95-103.

CHAPTER 66

Tactical Medical Support

INTRODUCTION

Tactical emergency medical support, or TEMS, was patterned after the successful military model of specially trained medics embedded within remotely deployed fighting units. While the military took full advantage of specialized medical support years ago, it was not until the late 1980s that civilian law enforcement began to embrace the concept of integrated medical care.[1]

OBJECTIVES

1. Briefly describe the origins of tactical emergency medical support (TEMS).

2. Describe various models of the provision of TEMS along with advantages and disadvantages of each.

3. Explain basic concepts of tactical operations.

4. List ways in which the medical element in tactical operations enhances mission success.

5. List specific medical threats that must be managed during tactical operations.

6. List unique considerations specific to a TEMS program.

TACTICAL EMERGENCY MEDICAL SUPPORT

Most EMS providers are taught to stage away from a scene where their personal safety may be in jeopardy. Police action, by definition, is inherently unsafe, making civilian EMS providers unable to deliver expeditious care in areas of high threat. Several high-profile incidents, however, have reinforced the need for EMS providers trained to function "inside the perimeter" where a scene may not be totally secure. In February 1997, two heavily armed robbers entered the Bank of America in North Hollywood and engaged law enforcement officers in a long and bloody firefight. Ultimately, one of the robbers committed suicide while the other was shot by police as he tried to flee and later died at the scene. Surviving family members soon afterward brought suit against the Los Angeles Police Department alleging that his death was due, in part, to lack of timely medical care.[2] One of the more vivid illustrations of the value of embedded tactical medical support came in October 2007 when a SWAT officer was shot in the neck during a high-risk warrant service. Two physicians with the Dallas Police Department were immediately at the injured officer's side where it was determined he was without a patent airway. The tactical physicians achieved hemostasis and performed a surgical airway saving his life.[3]

Being a tactical medical provider, however, is more than simply taking an on-duty medical crew and donning them with ballistic helmets and vest. Highly specialized medical training should precede any provider's deployment for real-world missions with a law enforcement team.[4] Dozens of civilian and government-sponsored training programs in tactical medicine exist, but students seeking such training should carefully examine the curriculum choosing schools that focus on medicine in the tactical environment as opposed to schools that seem to center on weapon manipulation and tactical techniques. While important, these fundamentals of tactical movement should be learned and practiced with the student's own team.

The configuration of tactical medical support varies greatly across the country. Some agencies still depend on EMS standby far away from the incident scene in the cold zone. While this model certainly reduces the burden of training needs on the part of the medical provider, it defeats the advantage of utilizing proximate and immediately available medical expertise in times of critical injury. In 1994, the National Tactical Officers Association released its official position statement on the provision of TEMS stating: "…the ultimate goal should be that TEMS providers are deployed within the operational perimeter in proximity to tactical operations. Doing so permits rapid access to casualties, the opportunity to provide medical countermeasures, and enables TEMS providers to make recommendations to team leaders."[5] Integrated TEMS providers should complete a recognized tactical medical course along with an agency-specific basic SWAT school. This will allow the medical staff to seamlessly fit into the tactical movement of the team, become familiar with a team's capabilities and region-specific tactics, and cultivate the necessary trust among officers so that they may feel comfortable seeking medical advice or care from TEMS providers and so providers can recognize subtle changes in an officer's behavior or mannerism that might be recognized as an early indicator of illness or injury.

Yet another variation on medical support exists in the form of cross-trained commissioned officers who are sent to EMT or paramedic training. This model provides for a fully functional SWAT officer with the added capability of medical training. While this model may seem attractive at first, one must consider that maintaining a dual skill set can be time consuming and cost prohibitive. Not only must the officer maintain law enforcement certifications and training, he must also attain regular civilian medical employment to retain assessment skills and technical acumen. The EMS physician must consider all options in consultation with the SWAT commander when designing a new tactical medical support program.

BASIC CONCEPTS OF TACTICAL OPERATIONS

Tactical law enforcement operations typically involve assignments that are beyond the scope of enforcement of standard patrol officers. Types of police actions that necessitate tactical operations include high-risk warrant service, barricaded subjects, hostage situations, and even executive/dignitary protection details.

SWAT response to any given assignment or threat involves a multi-layer response utilizing surveillance techniques, patrol officers, detectives, tactical long riflemen, and a medical support element. Operations may be planned weeks in advance or be escalated into direct action quickly depending on the dynamics of the given circumstance. Such situations have a unique set of challenges making the operation even more demanding. For example, the protective equipment itself is necessary but can be cumbersome. Ballistic helmet, vest, gloves, and gas masks add to the weight the officer must bear while still trying to maintain maximum flexibility and efficiency of movement (**Figure 66-1**). These

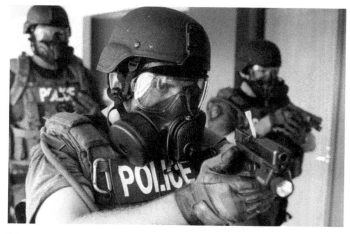

FIGURE 66-1. Gas masks and other protective gear add to the physiologic stress of maintaining mobility in a high-threat environment. (Photo by Patrick Lanham * Lanham Photography)

stressors contribute to emotional stressors already in place in a high-threat environment. It also taxes the physical stress which may be exacerbated when tactical operations must be conducted in extremes of heat or cold. Tactical medical staff must take these unique considerations in mind when anticipating medical threats and when preparing for a given response to a tactical incident.

The medic is not without his own stressors, however. When providing medical care in a high-threat environment, significant operational limitations exist that are not typical of the classical health care environment. For example, a patient assessment may need to be performed with limited lighting if not total darkness at times as a light signature could betray a team's location or diminish night vision adaptation. The tactical medic must also function while maintaining noise discipline and in environments where auscultation may be impossible due to the need for hearing protection or due to background noise. Medical care must also be provided using principles of cover and concealment, which may necessitate care being delivered in alternate positions that are less than ideal. In fact, medical care may even need to be performed remote from the actual victim in the form of instructions over a phone or across any type of barricade.[6]

INTEGRATING THE MEDICAL ELEMENT IN TACTICAL OPERATIONS

Tactical teams spend a great deal of time training. As such, much like the military experience, a great source of morbidity for specialty teams is during training exercises, making it important for a tactical medical presence to be in attendance for all training sessions in addition to actual operations.[7] Medical staff should be comfortable evaluating and managing common musculoskeletal complaints and should also have baseline medical records of the team members paying particular attention to status of immunizations, overall health, and level of fitness. Not only does this enhance the value of an integrated medical element, it also facilitates the development of trust between medical providers and law enforcement personnel.[8]

Upon obtaining this information, the tactical medic should also take advantage of the opportunity to educate the officers in basic buddy aid and self-aid. By serving as a single point of contact for the medical needs of the team, the medic may serve as the medical conscience for the commander.[9] It is in this role that the medical element should be present for the planning stage of an operation. Issues for consideration are numerous (see **Box 66-1**).

MEDICAL OPERATIONS IN A TACTICAL INCIDENT

In a departure from routine civilian medical care, medical care in the tactical environment has unique constraints and requirements which may alter the manner and location of provided treatments. Initial treatment of a casualty may be minimal at the site of injury and while under effective fire. During this "Care Under Fire" stage, removing the casualty from harm and ending the threat is of primary importance. Expanded care is performed after the provider and casualty are no longer under direct threat but only with equipment which can be carried by the medic. Care begins to resemble routine civilian medicine once evacuation has begun, and definitive care is undertaken well removed from the threat environment. Full description of the tactical role of the medical element is a large topic, and readers should seek instruction from a number of dedicated texts and courses on the subject for full operational methods.

Tactical operations can expose the medical provider to a wide range of possible illness and injury patterns. Criminal activity is not limited to a particular time, location, or environment, and, therefore, SWAT operations must be carried out across any possible spectrum of circumstances. This requires the medical support element to be prepared and experienced in the treatment of a very broad set of possible maladies in both officers and civilians. In addition to the expected traumatic injuries possible during any violent physical encounter, persons in a tactical

Box 66-1
Threats to the Team

Environmental

CBRNE

Psychological

Blunt/ballistic trauma

Resources required to mitigate threats

Adequate number of tactical medical staff
- Size of area of operations
- Complexity and dynamics of mission
- Potential for multiple casualties
- Anticipated duration of operation
- Possible need for HAZMAT resources

Patient care areas
- Operational safe area/zones of operation
- Casualty collection points

Special needs of hostages or suspects
- Underlying medical conditions
- Implanted medical devices or hardware

Transportation routes
- Best ingress and egress plans
- Traffic concerns

Destination choices
- Availability of trauma centers
- Specialty resources anticipated
- Knowledge of hospital diversion plans

environment are prone to heat and cold stress, a host of medical illnesses, chemical and biologic agents, as well as some unique injury patterns from specialized tools used by SWAT teams.

Regardless of the possible suspect danger encountered by the tactical team, the environment in which they operate is a significant and constant threat to both their operational readiness and health. While the key maneuvers in ending a potentially violent situation may last only several seconds, the overall time of deployment is hours to even days. During this time, officers will be exposed to the elements in full tactical equipment likely consisting of a Nomex or similar suit, heavy body armor, helmet, APR mask or respirator, ammunition loadout, and specialized breaching tools. This equipment can weigh in excess of 40 lb and does not allow effective evaporative cooling. In some situations, officers may be wearing occlusive chemical suits, which severely limit their homeothermic mechanisms. These factors make heat illness a very real threat to the team members. Dehydration, heat cramps, heat exhaustion, and even heat stroke can affect team members even in seemingly inactive duties. Medical staff should reinforce oral hydration guidelines and be vigilant for any suggestion of early heat illness. Oral hydration requirements can reach 0.5 to 1 L/h with moderate activity in hot and humid environments.[10] Adequate rest-work cycles should also be ensured during prolonged deployments to help avoid both environmental and mental stresses. CBRNE environments mandate rotation of personnel to ensure a minimum amount of time is spent in chemical/biologic occlusive suits and respirators, and medics should provide pre and postentry medical exams to ensure operators are fit to return to duty. Full protocols are beyond the scope of this text; however, suggested standards can be found in OSHA hazardous material operations and NFPA regulations.[11] While heat illness is often the more common malady faced by team members, cold injury is also a significant threat. Much of a deployment may be spent outside in a concealed position awaiting a moment of entry. Wet conditions greatly accelerate heat loss due to water's significantly greater heat capacity and conductance compared to air. In addition, adaptive responses are less effective and hypothermia becomes more profound if the rate of cooling is slow. This is especially critical with marksmen/observers who may be in a fixed position for prolonged periods of time and must maintain a high degree of mental activity. Uniform selection must take into account these factors and hypothermia must be avoided. Decreased body temperature has significant detrimental effects on critical thinking, reaction time, muscle power, coordination, and morale.[12-15] All these effects can seriously decrease the capability of the tactical element. Lastly, dehydration is still a threat in cold environments due to a combination of decreased perceived need for fluids as well as increased renal filtration from peripheral vasoconstriction.

The tactical environment poses a number of traumatic threats to police, suspects, and civilians. Lacerations and puncture wounds are common and come from a number of possible sources. Broken glass, metal, and debris created during the breaching and entry to the area pose a threat. Additionally, animal bites both from civilian animals and police working dogs can occur. In addition to the visible lacerations and punctures caused, bites also raise the possibility of infectious complications such as cellulitis, myositis, abscess formation, and tetanus, as well as localized rhabdomyolysis and compartment syndrome caused by the prolonged powerful bite of a police dog which is subduing a suspect. Falls with associated blunt trauma are likewise a threat in this environment. Rappelling and helicopter operations may be a part of agency tactics and can increase the risk of closed head injury and significant deceleration injury.

The act of engaging with potentially violent suspects presents an obvious threat to officers and civilians. Criminals and terrorists can use a variety of possible weapons against police and civilians. Edged weapons such as ice picks and knives can inflict serious wounds, even though soft ballistic armor. The medical element must be skilled in treating ballistic injuries, and these may range from low-velocity small-caliber handgun munitions to high-velocity large-caliber rifle and shotgun projectiles. Despite the formidable protection offered by modern body armor, vulnerable areas do exist and officers are not immune to ballistic injury. Significant injuries can be sustained to the face, neck, and proximal extremities. Additionally, there is substantial energy transferred to the wearer of soft body armor during a gunshot. This is known as "behind armor blunt trauma" and can cause serious injury. A .357 magnum handgun round defeated by soft ballistic armor delivers five times the energy of a major league fastball to the wearer, and the vest can deform up to 4.4 cm against the wearer by NIJ standards. This can break ribs, lacerate solid organs, and cause *commotio cordis* and resulting in ventricular arrhythmia. Tactical medical providers should have the capacity for defibrillation to treat this eventuality.

Military data have shown that the largest proportion of potentially salvageable injuries involves airway loss, extremity hemorrhage, and tension pneumothorax,[16] and modern tactical casualty care has involved ways of rapidly and effectively dealing with these injuries while under austere conditions. Airway loss secondary to trauma is a significant threat in this environment and one of the prime responsibilities of the medical element (**Figure 66-2**). While EMT-paramedic and physician level providers are adept at endotracheal intubation for airway control, the time and setup needed is sometimes not practical in a high threat environment. In addition to intubation, providers should become proficient with blind airway devices and techniques for cricothyroidotomy to rapidly secure an airway. Effective techniques have been developed by military and other groups to allow rapid field cricothyroidotomy even using night vision goggles under little to no light.[17] Needle decompression for treatment of tension pneumothorax is well within the scope of practice of readers of this text and should be available and practiced.

Hemorrhage control is another pillar of tactical medical care. Many of the hemorrhage control techniques used in an emergency room setting are not applicable in the tactical environment, where equipment at the

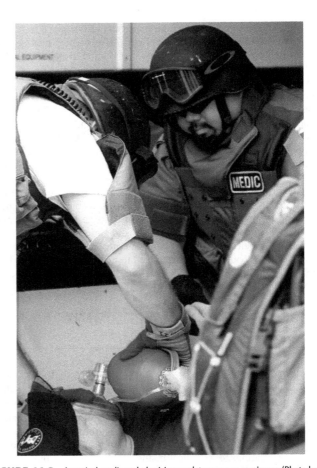

FIGURE 66-2. A tactical medic and physician work to manage an airway. (Photo by Ray Kemp * 9-1-1 Imaging.)

site of injury will be minimal, access to the casualty will be limited due to hostile individuals, and mission goals must be met to prevent further loss of life. In this environment, the tourniquet has reemerged as a simple, potentially lifesaving piece of equipment. Military experience and research has shown that correct application of a proper modern tourniquet provides rapid control of extremity hemorrhage while still under direct threat and may even allow operators to remain mission capable. There are several modern tourniquets available, and reviews of their ease of application, weight, occlusion effectiveness, and subjective use can be found in a number of military and civilian sources for those looking to choose a product for field use.[18,19] Regardless of the model chosen, they should be carried by each officer, be readily available for self-application, and be trained with regularly to ensure proper use. Another evolving technology for use in rapid hemorrhage control under austere conditions is the hemostatic dressing. These have undergone significant civilian and military testing to stop arterial and venous bleeding which is not amenable to tourniquet placement. The literature on individual dressings is widespread, and while several have proven effective on stopping significant animal models of proximal extremity hemorrhage, there have been a number of problems including excess heat production, burns, significant embolism/thrombosis, and local tissue damage which have caused some dressings to fall from favor.[20] Medical directors should be familiar with this volume of literature prior to choosing a dressing for use in the field.

Further trauma can be a result of burn and blast injury both from deliberate incendiary devices as well as accidental ignition of environmental hazards. Improvised explosives and deliberate fires are common tools of terrorist and criminal suspects. In addition, the manufacture of many drugs of abuse and chemical weapons produce flammable and potentially explosive environments which may be entered by tactical teams while executing warrants or other high-risk entry work. These vapors can be ignited from routine sparks caused during forced entry or by the muzzle flash of a weapon, resulting in fire or explosion.

Aside from traumatic injury, there are a number of other hazards facing those in tactical operations. The constellation of chemical, biological, radiologic, and nuclear (CBRN) threats are all part of the tactical arena. Chemical agents ranging from simple irritants to sophisticated nerve agents must be planned for by the medical element. Treatment of these agents is covered elsewhere in this text; however, the tactical medical element should be familiar with the available treatments and antidotes to chemical weapons. Biologic agents and low-grade nuclear dispersal devices ("dirty bombs") may also be encountered.

Police and tactical teams work on a force continuum to control suspects, which ranges from verbal commands to lethal force. Between these two extremes, several tools have emerged which allow control of potentially dangerous suspects without resorting to deadly force. These are known as less lethal technologies, and they present specialized injury patterns which must be handled by the tactical medical team. Of those agents commonly encountered and used by law enforcement, oleoresin capsicum (OC) and CS/CN gases will be some of the most frequently utilized. Oleoresin capsicum, or "pepper spray," is an extract of the common pepper species. It causes Substance P–mediated pain, erythema, and edema to skin, as well as lacrimation, injection, and blepharospasm of the eyes. Corneal abrasions can occur in a significant minority of those exposed, 7% in one study,[21] but this appears to be due to rubbing of the eyes rather than direct chemical erosion.[22] Respiratory irritation and bronchospasm in those with reactive airway disease may occur. Pain relief is primarily time dependent, and other agents such as milk, Maalox, topical lidocaine, and baby shampoo were not found superior to water irrigation for pain relief.[23] CS and CN gases produce similar skin burning and mucosal irritation with shorter length of effect. Treatment is generally supportive and decontamination is carried out with water primarily.

Conducted electrical devices (CEDs) are another less lethal option for law enforcement officers. Most widespread in use is the TASER, which uses a charge of 50,000 V at 20 cycles/s, causing tetany of major muscle groups. While its primary control is through this resultant incapacitation, it can also be quite painful. This is delivered in repeatable 5-second durations through a pair of barbs attached to 35 foot wires. It is in use with over 17,800 law enforcement agencies with an estimated 2,370,000 human deployments in the field.[24] TASER use avoids other pain compliance measures and can spare the use of lethal force. It has been shown to significantly reduce the odds of both officer and suspect injuries in retrospective studies of 24,000 use-of-force incidents in 12 departments.[25] It has also shown to reduce the incidence of injury compared to physical control measures by over sixfold.[26] CEDs have been associated with less than 1% of in-custody deaths.[27] However, concern has been raised for their safety, particularly their potential ability to cause cardiac injury. This has led to a volume of available literature on safety, including over 20 published studies and an AAEM position paper.[28] Bozeman et al found no evidence of arrhythmia during ECG monitoring of 84 subjects during TASER deployment.[29] Ho and colleagues have studied a number of deployment scenarios designed to mimic real world use and have found no evidence of EKG, electrolyte, or cardiac biomarker abnormalities in a series of studies.[30,31] In a prospective trial of 426 consecutive TASER deployments by a major metropolitan SWAT team, Eastman showed that use spared lethal force in 5.4% of situations. There was only one serious injury, which was a delayed death 12 hours after deployment. The suspect's condition was consistent with excited delirium with altered mental status, hyperthermia, and bizarre behavior.[32] A prospective multicenter observational trial by Bozeman et al[33] characterized the injury patterns seen in over 1200 uses. Most suspects had no injury (78.1%), though mild injuries such as contusions, painful puncture wounds and chipped teeth were seen in 21.6%. There were two closed head injuries from falls, and two delayed deaths consistent with excited delirium.

Treatment of CED injuries should focus on the specifics surrounding the deployment and monitoring for significant symptoms. Excited delirium and toxicologic illness are common causes for CED use, and

they should be monitored and treated. Special attention should be given to the fall caused by the momentary incapacitation and the mental status of the patient following. Barb extraction techniques mirror methods used for fish hook removal, and can usually be accomplished in the field, though barbs to the face, neck, and genitalia should be treated as impaled objects. Most CED deployments do not result in significant injury, with most requiring no specialized medical care. Serious injury or admission is rare.[26] Existing evidence does not support routine screening tests or admission for observation in asymptomatic persons.[28] However, symptoms such as chest pain should be investigated considering the patient's underlying risk factors and history. Medical review after CED deployment can help refine departmental usage policy.

Impact weapons are another law enforcement tool for controlling violent suspects. These can range from simple batons to rubber and bean bag munitions fired from shotguns or 37-mm launchers. These are generally a last resort prior to lethal force, and while considered less lethal, they can cause significant injury. Bean bag munitions are generally fired at the legs and abdomen and deliver energy equivalent to a major league fastball. Pain and bruising are the common result, but serious injuries such as hemo/pneumothorax, splenic rupture, cardiac contusion, solid organ contusion, and penetrating fatal chest injury have been reported in the literature.[34]

Noise flash diversionary devices, commonly termed *flash bangs*, are a common tool of the tactical team to distract and disorient potentially violent suspects. These devices burn rapidly to emit a loud noise and bright flash, which allows a tactical team a precious few seconds' advantage when confronting suspects. Their roughly 2 million candle power flash is enough to temporarily blind those in close proximity without causing permanent damage. The device produces a 200-dB concussion and 15 psi overpressure at the site of ignition. This is louder than a jet engine and equivalent to an extra atmosphere of pressure. This is enough to cause TM rupture and pulmonary overpressure injury. However, the pressure wave decays exponentially and is below the threshold for injury at a distance of 5 ft which is their minimum deployment distance. Injuries are rare, but officers or suspects exposed at close proximity can experience significant blast injury similar to any other overpressure device.

UNIQUE CONSIDERATIONS IN A TEMS PROGRAM

There are many models for providing medical support of special operations law enforcement teams. Tactical medical staff may be drawn from surrounding ambulance services, fire departments, or from within the law enforcement agency itself.[35] Regardless, potential candidates must be screened for several reasons. First, what is their motivation for joining the team? Nothing will kill a new tactical medical program faster than a health provider saying "Hi, I'm your new medic. Where's my gun?" Make sure medical providers who wish to practice TEMS are doing so for the right reasons. Additionally, TEMS providers, particularly physicians, must understand that the primary task of any special operations team is successful completion of the law enforcement mission. Medical considerations often must run secondary to tactical priorities. This can be difficult for new tactical personnel to understand, but it *must* be understood.[36,37]

IMPLEMENTING A TEMS PROGRAM

Although many nationally recognized organizations endorse the provision of TEMS, some police agencies remain fearful of "liability." It has been suggested that the absence of medical support within a law enforcement agency, specifically a special operations unit, carries more risk than the delivery of such medical support. Thus, TEMS remains a growing subspecialty of emergency medical services.[37]

Many common questions arise during the developmental stage of a TEMS unit not the least of which is: "What is the best model for a tactical medical program?" (See **Box 66-2**). Because of the wide diversity of local and regional law enforcement practices, the assortment of EMS systems within a given locale, and the broad variety of statutory and regulatory

Box 66-2

Issues in Developing a TEMS Program

Insurance coverage

- Malpractice—who provides and who funds it
- Liability—different from malpractice coverage
- and often overlooked
- Workman's comp—coverage of illness or death
- During training or actual operations
- Exclusions of coverage—will tactical duties
- Reduce or negate current insurance coverage

Employment status

- Law enforcement employee?
- Commissioned
- Civilian/noncommissioned

Paid vs volunteer status

Composition of TEMS unit

- BLS, ALS, or mixed capability
- Selection criteria/standards
- Training standards

Funding agreements

- Equipment needs
- Uniform allowance
- Training needs

To arm or not to arm the medics

- Local laws
- Needs of the team
- Collaborative discussion and decision
- Possibility of role confusion if armed
- Clear safety protocols if not armed

Medical control agreements

- Hospital negotiations
- Physician involvement
- Local governing bodies

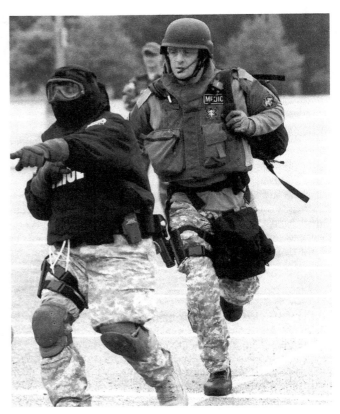

FIGURE 66-3. A tactical physician is being directed to the scene of a downed officer. (Photo by Patrick Lanham * Lanham Photography.)

value to the medical program and also allows the physician to practice without the need for obtaining medical control authorization. The administrative experience possessed by many physicians also augments the development of the program's structure and gives credibility to the head of the law enforcement agency when acting as a liaison to police or government administration.

The physician may be an active tactical medical provider or assume a more traditional medical director role to tactical EMT or paramedic staff on the team (Figure 66-3). In this way, proximate and thorough medical oversight of tactical medical care is accomplished. As the value of this oversight is realized, it is not uncommon for the physician's role to become expanded within the police agency to include AED programs, first-aid classes, and as an expert consultant for in-custody injuries/deaths or any medical matter that may relate to the duties of the agency.[39]

boundaries in each state, there is no single model that will fit every agency's needs. The medical provider and tactical commander must work together at addressing the optimum configuration of medical support in ensuring mission success.

Whether or not the tactical medical staff is armed, firearms training should be a regular and mandatory part of instruction. This includes training on all armaments to include less-lethal weapons. While it is important that the medic must be able to use any weapon in the course of tactical operations if necessary or if commanded, the weaponry knowledge is most commonly used to render any tool in the arsenal safe should an officer be injured especially if accompanied by altered mental status.[38]

ROLE OF THE PHYSICIAN IN A TEMS PROGRAM

While the term *medic* has been used throughout this chapter, the word *physician* may be substituted in any context as some teams utilize physicians as the primary tactical medical provider (**Figure 66-3**). However, there are certain considerations that are unique to the tactical physician. The level of training and education of a physician immediately lends

KEY POINTS

- TEMS is widely accepted as a standard element in modern tactical teams.
- Specialized training is required prior to a TEMS provider deploying with a team.
- Function and role of TEMS within a tactical team is a law enforcement decision, not medical.
- TEMS should be integrated into routine training as well as operational planning in order to maximize the benefit of the tactical medical element.
- Operational effectiveness of a TEMS program depends on the provider's intimate knowledge of tactics, weapons utilized, anticipated medical threats, a baseline medical knowledge of each team member, and a close working relationship with command staff and local governing officials.

REFERENCES

1. Heck, JJ, Isakov, AP, Bozeman, WP. Tactical emergency medical support. In: Hauda WE, DeAtley C, Bogucki S, eds. *Emergency Medical Services: Clinical Practice and Medical Oversight.* Vol 4. Dubuque, IA: Kendall-Hunt Publishing; 2009:203.
2. CNN Transcripts. Federal Lawsuit Examines if LAPD Could Have Done More to Save Bank Robber After Deadly Shootout. Atlanta, GA. 2000. http://transcripts.cnn.com/TRANSCRIPTS/0002/27/sun.03.html.
3. PoliceOne.com. Dallas SWAT doctors credited with saving officer's life during raid. San Francisco, CA. 2007. http://www.policeone.com/SWAT/articles/1365650-Dallas-SWAT-doctors-credited-with-saving-officers-life-during-raid.
4. Heiskell LE, Carmona RH. Tactical emergency medical services: an emerging subspecialty of emergency medicine. *Ann Emerg Med.* 1994;23:778.
5. National Tactical Officers Association. Inclusion of tactical emergency medical support (TEMS) in tactical law enforcement operations. *Tactical Edge.* 1994;12:86.
6. Vayer JS, Hagmann JH, Llewellyn CH. Refining Prehospital Physical Assessment Skills: A New Teaching Technique. *Ann Emerg Med.* 1994;23:786.
7. Jones BH, Perrotta DM, Chervak ML, et al. Injuries in the military: a review and commentary focused on prevention. *Am J Prev Med.* 2000;18:71.
8. Young, SE, Pierluisi GJ. Operational performance and preventive medicine. In: Schwartz RB, McManus, JG, Swienton, RE. eds. *Tactical Emergency Medicine.* Philadelphia, PA: Lippincott Williams & Wilkins; 2008:131.
9. Sztajnkrycer M, Báez A, Eberlein C. Resident And Faculty Involvement In Tactical Emergency Medical Support: A Survey Of U.S. Emergency Medicine Residency Programs. *The Internet Journal of Rescue and Disaster Medicine.* 2004 Volume 5 Number 1. https://ispub.com/IJRDM/5/1/13623. Accessed May, 2015
10. Sawka MN, Wenger CB, Montain SJ, et al. Heat stress control and heat casualty management. Washington, DC: Headquarters, US Department of the Army and Air Force; 2003:13. TB MED 507/AFPAM 48-152.
11. EMS Sector Standard Operating Procedures Supplement 13. *NFPA Hazardous Materials Response Guidebook.* 3rd ed. Quincy, MA: NFPA; 1997.
12. Pendergast DR. The effect of body cooling on oxygen transport during exercise. *Med Sci Sports Exer.* 1988;20(suppl):S171-S176.
13. Reeves, DL, Winsborough, MM, Bachrach, AJ. Neurophysiological and behavioral correlates of cold water immersion. In: Bove AA, Bachrach AJ, eds. *Underwater and Hyperbaric Physiology IX: Proceedings of the Ninth International Symposium on Underwater and Hyperbaric Physiology.* Bethesda, MD: Undersea and Hyperbaric Medical Society; 1987:589-598.
14. Coleshaw SRK, van Someren RNM, Wolff AH, et al. Impairment of memory registration and speed of reasoning caused by mild depression of body core temperature. *J Appl Physiol.* 1983;55:27-31.
15. Davis FM, Baddeley AD, Hancock TR. Diver performance: the effects of cold. *Undersea Biomed Res.* 1975;2:195-213.
16. Holcomb JB, Stansbury LG, Champion HR, wade C, Bellamy RF. Understanding combat casualty care statistics. *J Trauma.* 2006;60:397-401.
17. MacIntyre A, Markarian MK, Carrison D, Coates J, Kuhls D, Fildes JJ. Three step cricothyoidotomy. *Military Medicine.* 2007;172(12):1228-1230.
18. Walters T, US Army Institute of Surgical Research. Testing of battlefield tourniquets. Presented at: Advanced Technology Applications for Combat Casualty Care 2004 (ATACCC) Conference, published in the Conference Proceedings; August 16-18, 2004; St Petersburg, FL.
19. Hill J, Montgomery L, Hopper K, Roy LA: Evaluation of Self-Applied Tourniquets for Combat Applications, Second Phase. Washington, DC, Naval Sea Systems Command, Public Release, 2007. http://archive.rubicon-foundation.org/xmlui/bitstream/handle/123456789/6870/ADA480501.pdf?sequence=1. Accessed May, 2015.
20. Lawton G, Granville-Chapman J, Parker PJ. Novel hemostatic dressings. *JR Army Med Corps.* 155(4):309-314.
21. Brown L, Takeuchi D, Challoner K. Corneal abrasions associated with pepper spray exposure. *Am J Emerg Med.* 2000;18:271.
22. Zollman TM, Bragg RM, Harrison DA. Clinical effects of oleoresin capsicum (pepper spray) on the human cornea and conjunctiva. *Ophthalmology.* 2000;107:2186.
23. Barry JD, Hennessy R, McManus JG. A randomized controlled trial comparing treatment regimens for acute pain for topical oleoresin capsaicin (pepper spray) exposure in adult volunteers. *Prehosp Emerg Care.* 2008;12:432-437.
24. TASER. Statistics and Facts. TASER Website. https://www.taser.com/press/stats. Accessed May, 2015.
25. McDonald JM, Kaminski RJ, Smith MR. The effect of less-lethal weapons on injuries in police use-of-force events. *Am J Pub Health.* 2009;99:2268-2274.
26. Haileyesus T, Annest JL, Mercy JA. Non-fatal conductive energy device-related injuries treated in US emergency departments, 2005-2008. *Inj Prev.* 2010;17(2):127-130. doi:10.1136/ip.2010.028704.
27. US Bureau of Justice statistics 2002.
28. Vilke GM, Bozeman WP, Chan TC. Emergency department evaluation after conducted energy weapon use: review of the literature for the clinician. *J Emerg Med.* 2011;40:598-604.
29. Bozeman WP, Barnes DG, Winslow JE III, Johnson JC, Phillips CH, Alson R. Immediate cardiovascular effects of the Taser X26 conducted electrical weapon. *Emerg Med J.* 2009;26:567-570.
30. Ho JD, Dawes DM, Heegaard WG, Calkins HG, Moscati RM, Miner JR. Absence of electrocardiographic change after prolonged application of a conducted electrical weapon in physically exhausted adults. *J Emerg Med.* 2011;41(5):466-472.
31. Ho JD, Dawes DM, Bultman LL, Moscati RM, Janchar TA, Miner JR. Prolonged TASER use on exhausted humans does not worsen markers of acidosis. *Am J Emerg Med.* 2009;27:413-418.
32. Eastman AL, Metzger JC, Pepe PE, et al. Conducted electrical devices: a prospective, population based study of medical safety of law enforcement use. *J Trauma.* 2008;64:1567-1572.
33. Bozeman WP, Hauda WE 2nd, Heck JJ, Graham DD Jr, Martin BP, Winslow JE. Safety and injury profile of conducted electrical weapons used by law enforcement officers against criminal suspects. *Ann Emerg Med.* 2009 Apr;53:(4)480-489.
34. de Brito D, Challoner KR, Sehgal A, et al. The injury pattern of a new law enforcement weapon: the police bean bag. *Ann Emerg Med.* 2001;38:383-390.
35. Wipfler III EJ, Campbell JE, Heiskell LE. History and role of the tactical medical provider. In: Wipfler III EJ, Campbell JE, Heiskell LE, eds. *Tactical Medicine Essentials.* Sudbury, MA: Jones and Bartlett; 2012:13.
36. DeLorenzo RA, Porter RS. Care of ballistic and missile casualties. In: DeLorenzo RA, Porter RS, eds. *Tactical Emergency Medicine.* Upper Saddle River, NJ: Prentice Hall; 1999:49.
37. Vayer JS, Schwartz RB. Developing a tactical emergency medical support program. *Top Emerg Med.* 2003;25:285.
38. Rinnert KJ, Hall WL. Tactical emergency medical support. *Emerg Med Clin N Am.* 2002;20:934.
39. Gildea JR, Janssen AR. TEMS physician involvement and injury patterns in tactical teams. *J Emerg Med.* 2008;35:413.

CHAPTER 67

Wilderness Medicine

Jeremy Joslin
J. Matthew Sholl
Garreth C. Debiegun

INTRODUCTION

Although many definitions of wilderness medicine have been suggested, one of the most used definitions derives from transport time, and is usually described as longer than one or two hours away from definitive care. This definition suggests an inclusive nature of wilderness medicine which can be superimposed upon other subsets of prehospital care such as austere, expedition, rural EMS, and disaster medicine. In defining it as such, wilderness medicine encompasses quite an area of significance that extends into the very core of emergency medical services.

Much like tactical EMS, wilderness medicine has seen a surge in academic progress recently, and shares the same sense of pride and accomplishment that comes from practicing in a rich, maturing subspecialty. Indeed, advances in the science of wilderness medicine can be applicable to everyday EMS care—from a remote rescue dispatch to an urban medical call.

OBJECTIVES

- Define wilderness medicine and describe various types and facets.
- Discuss wilderness search and rescue and discuss essential personnel, specialized techniques/equipment, and proper interface with IC and EMS.
- Discuss basic principles of operational EMS in austere environments.
- Contrast philosophies concerning readiness versus improvisation with equipment and supplies examples.
- Describe types of wilderness medicine practitioners.
- Discuss wilderness medicine training, certifications, societies, and fellowship status.
- Define expedition medicine and describe applications of this type of operational medicine.
- Discuss planning process for medical support of expeditions.
- Discuss operational concerns that may arise during the expedition and how to respond to these challenges.
- Briefly discuss contractual arrangements and terms that are important to successful medical support of expeditions.

DEFINITION OF AND FACETS UNIQUE TO WILDERNESS MEDICINE

Although a commonly used definition of wilderness medicine is described above, in practice, the subspecialty tends to be defined using an additional, circumstantial descriptor which helps exclude some of the overlapping scope of other EMS subsets. These descriptors can be based on a type of location such as "in the woods" or "on a mountain," a type of activity such as hiking or skiing, or a specifically prolonged transport time usually defined as one to two hours.

Further characterization can be made based on the interaction of several of these factors. Commonly, patients are recreating in the wilderness at the time of the illness or injury. For example, snow blindness (UV keratitis) might occur in a mountaineer who has spent significant time on a glacier without eye protection. Although it would be rare, UV Keratitis could conceivably occur in a nonwilderness setting and may not be considered wilderness medicine. Thus this situation is defined as

wilderness medicine by the type of injury, the location, and the activity during which it occurred. Many other "typical" wilderness medicine problems can be considered where the illness or injury most commonly occurs in a nonurban area.

Wilderness medicine may also be defined by the need to improvise or use a specialized body of knowledge. For example, the makeshift connection of a Foley catheter to a latex glove creating a hydration reservoir and proctoclysis system which was used to save the life of a critical patient trekking in the Himalayas describes the quintessential anecdote of wilderness medicine practice with improvisation.[1]

In summary, there are many factors to consider when defining wilderness medicine, but the most commonly considered ones are location, activity, time to care, and type of injury. Thus a more robust definition has been put forth that wilderness medicine involves "injuries and illnesses caused by the interaction between humans and their natural environment occurring in potentially austere and threatening environments."[2] Despite these definitions describing wilderness medicine as being borne from the wilderness, there also do exist several common sets of illness and injury germane to wilderness medicine even though they are frequently encountered in the urban setting. The common theme among these involves the direct interaction of humans with their environment. Typical examples are hypothermia, hyperthermia, lightning, and drowning. Toxic exposures to plants and animal-related injuries may also occur in a nonwilderness environment. Animal bites and stings fall under the rubric of wilderness medicine, and are commonly felt to be under the purview of the wilderness medical practitioner.

■ WILDERNESS MEDICINE AS A UNIQUE TYPE OF PREHOSPITAL CARE

Given these varying definitions of wilderness medicine as well as the clear overlap with other areas of prehospital care, what makes wilderness medicine unique? There are situations that may be encountered in typical prehospital care, but are more common in the wilderness setting (lightning strike, hypothermia, etc). There are also situations that will never be encountered in urban EMS whereas they are common in wilderness medicine (snow blindness, HAPE). The elements that comprise this austere medical practice environment are some of the key aspects that make wilderness care unique (**Box 67-1**).

EQUIPMENT

While national and state guidelines list specific equipment that should be stocked on any registered ambulance there is no definitive list for the wilderness rescuer. Furthermore much of the equipment that is considered commonplace or even essential to typical prehospital care may be difficult or impossible to utilize in the wilderness setting. A typical example of this is tanked oxygen which is administered to a majority of EMS transported patients; however, bringing oxygen to a patient in the wilderness is rarely possible. Only small tanks are light enough to be transported and these would be empty so quickly as to be nearly useless in most scenarios. Another classic example is electronics. While GPS and computer documentation is commonplace in the urban or suburban prehospital setting, in the wilderness such limitations as waterproofing and the need for extra batteries often prove prohibitive. The importance of documentation in the backcountry should not be underestimated simply because of the low-tech manner in which it need be performed.

Box 67-1

Unique Factors That Define Wilderness Medicine

- Lack of resources
- Effect of environment on the patient
- Effect of environment on the rescuers
- Transport logistics

ENVIRONMENT EFFECTS

The austere environment may naturally wreak havoc on supplies and equipment, rescuers responding to a patient, and the physiology of the patient as well. In fact, the environment may be an even more important factor on medical supplies, many of which are not designed to withstand extremes of environment. For example, intravenous fluids are of limited benefit in a cold winter type environment due to freezing or their effects on patient core temperature. Conversely many medications degrade with heat and may not function in a hot desert type environment.

Consider the effects of environment on a patient. A middle-aged male who sustains a femur fracture from a fall in an urban setting is rapidly covered with blankets and then moved to a heated ambulance. Wet clothes are removed and warm blankets are added at the hospital. In the wilderness the same patient is forced to lie in the snow for many minutes or even hours awaiting the assistance of his climbing partners. He is then placed on an insulating pad and covered with down, but may spend hours generating his own heat before he is evacuated and offered external warming. Meanwhile blood loss and impending shock are complicated by early hypothermia which provides further physiologic insult to his initial injury.

Environmental factors affect rescue personnel as well. Cold hands lack dexterity, making technical skills such as IV starts or laceration repairs very difficult. Extremes of temperature limit work performance of rescue personnel who must spend time and energy caring for themselves to prevent hyper- or hypothermia in the rescuers. This need to consider the health and safety of the rescuers often takes significant time during a rescue and requires considerable pre-rescue preparation.

EVACUATION AND TRANSPORT

As can be expected, transport times are significantly protracted and can be divided into two portions: evacuation and transport. The primary portion, evacuation, is the wilderness-specific portion and is laid out in **Figure 67-1**; this is followed by a more traditional ground or air-based transport to the hospital. Oftentimes the difficulty of moving the patient imparts extra risk to the providers, such as a patient injured on a mountain that requires rappelling to descend. Because of the added complexity, more resources and certainly more time are required for evacuation than urban- or suburban-based transport.[3] This added time has given birth to the concept of the "Golden Day," which replaces the traditional "Golden Hour" that is so central to front-country EMS (Figure 67-1).

Similar to EMS transport priorities, evacuations can be described by their priority and acceptable risk to effect that evacuation. Emergent evacuation is the type most familiar to the EMS or prehospital provider as it references the situation when a patient must be brought from the backcountry to definitive care as soon as possible and even a relatively high risk rescue may be acceptable. This may range from patients with environmental injuries (HACE) to toxin exposures (snake bites) to medical problems (ACS/MI). A convenient evacuation is undertaken when a patient has a condition that warrants termination of their involvement in the trip and further care in the urban setting but may occur in a more time convenient manner such as after a storm or in the comfort of daylight. Typical examples of these situations are nonimproving gastroenteritis or an expanding cellulitis.

The number of rescuers is often fewer than one would desire, and the need for rescuers is typically much higher. It is estimated that it will take 6 to 12 rescuers per mile to transport a patient who requires carrying. Thus a 2-mile transport would require at a minimum 12 rescuers, and 4 miles would require 24 to 48 rescuers. Such rescuers may be search and rescue (SAR) team members who are typically volunteers and will be driving in from various locations. Alternatively, the number of rescuers may be limited to the trip or event with which the victim was traveling. In either case, obtaining more rescuers may not be feasible.

Regardless of the number of personnel available the amount of prior preparation required is often much higher than that for street-based prehospital providers. While the medical knowledge may be similar, other skill sets are required to keep the providers functional. These may include rope handling skills, ski skills, avalanche knowledge, desert survival, river travel experience, or boat handling skills on the ocean. The intricate interplay between rescue skills, medical capabilities, as well as operational and survival abilities is also a defining element of wilderness medicine. Training in these specialized rescue skills must be maintained in addition to medical training.[4]

IMPROVISATION VERSUS READINESS

With limitations in both personnel and equipment, rescuers need to consider contrasting values of being fully prepared for every possible scenario versus being able to improvise new uses for other equipment that is otherwise being carried. One prehospital care example of this balance is emergency management of the airway. Should a rescue team carry a full endotracheal intubation kit complete with laryngoscopes of various sizes and several endotracheal tubes? Or should they only carry a Combitube, King LT, LMA, or other supraglottic device? An expedition leader with very limited ability to carry equipment may ultimately choose a single ETT and a scalpel. An extreme example would be the physician who packs a safety pin which could be used to anchor the tongue to the lower lip, thus theoretically preventing airway occlusion by the posterior tongue.[5] Similar questions arise with cervical spine immobilization. A SAR team may choose to carry a single adjustable-size cervical collar rather than a range of sizes, whereas an expedition leader may choose to carry a single SAM-splint and use this to improvise a cervical collar.[6]

Consider a patient who sustains traumatic injuries in an avalanche while backcountry skiing. The patient is a 5- to 6-hour transport from the trailhead and the injury occurs late in the day at 3:15 PM with sundown only 1:15 away. The patient's travel group must affect the rescue unaided and decides to dig a snow cave and spend the night in the mountains rather than attempt a transport in the middle of the night while battling cold temperatures and limited visibility. This is clearly the best tactical decision but a pure medical decision would advocate following ATLS guidelines and extricating the patient as soon as possible. The operational goals of providing care in the wilderness can sometimes seem opposed to the medical goals leading to an oft-cited edict: Good medicine can sometimes be bad tactics.[7]

Why is wilderness medicine valuable to the physician with no interest in the wilderness and what can be learned from this for application to front-country-based prehospital care? It is a central tenet of wilderness medicine to practice with limited access to resources in austere settings. These two difficulties mean that wilderness physicians must be experts at operational skills and creative problem-solving skills, which are two qualities that may be particularly useful in other EMS settings (such as tactical support, disaster response, etc).Further, many nonwilderness prehospital providers such as EMS dispatchers may interact with patients in austere or isolated settings, such as the patient who uses a cell phone to dial 9-1-1 from the mountains or the EMT responding to a patient in a remote location.[8]

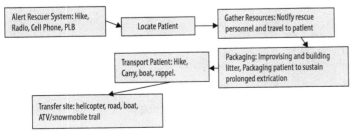

FIGURE 67-1. Rescue and evacuation.

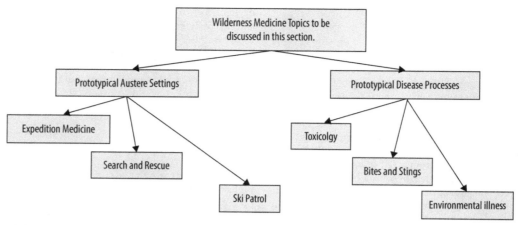

FIGURE 67-2. Prototypical austere settings and prototypical disease processes.

WILDERNESS MEDICINE SYSTEMS AND PRACTICE VENUES

Wilderness medicine may be categorized by both austere settings and specific diseases in nonaustere settings. Within austere environments, we will consider the three most commonly encountered venues: expedition medicine, search and rescue, and ski patrol. Within nonaustere settings we will briefly touch on a few key wilderness medicine topics: toxicology, bites and stings, and environmental injuries (**Figure 67-2**).

EXPEDITION MEDICINE

Expedition medicine is probably the prototypical clinical application of wilderness medicine and is often practiced by physicians of varying specialties depending on whom the expedition may be able to hire for medical care. Providing care in an expedition setting necessitates use of elements from multiple other medical specialties including austere or disaster medicine, international and travel medicine, prehospital and transport medicine, sports medicine, emergency medicine, EMS medicine, primary care, and, of course, wilderness medicine topics.[9] Incorporating this wide knowledge base and putting it to practice, expedition medicine relies heavily on both appropriate medical knowledge as well as good operational skills with tactical decision making.[10] In fact, a thorough understanding of the prehospital care system in the location of the expedition is critical to plan for any potential rescues or evacuations and plan contingencies. Given the heavy reliance on operational and tactical skills necessary for expedition medicine it should be clear that the EMS-trained physician is naturally well suited to this role.

Being contracted to provide expedition medical care may entail acceptance of varying expectations of your practice. You may be an expedition team member who partakes in the adventure as a regular group member but with the added expectation of taking responsibility for medical problems as they arise (**Figure 67-3**).

This is frequently what people envision when they think of expedition medicine. More congruent with the practice of the EMS physician is to offer a priori guidance to a team that is planning their expedition, in much the same way an EMS service medical director would. Some expeditions may request online medical control only, allowing EMTs, paramedics, or midlevels to provide the hands-on care with only remote guidance by the physician using satellite phone or radio to communicate between the expedition and the on-call physician. Lastly, practicing expedition medicine may entail stationing at a single remote, but highly trafficked location and administering care as patients travel by; this is the model employed at Mount Everest base camp and in much of the Himalayas.

PLANNING AND CONTRACTS

Describing how to completely plan an expedition is beyond the scope of this book, but some specific steps and processes will be explored. Contracts are of a critical importance in expedition medicine as they are in event medicine because they help all parties (physician, expedition planners, and participants) know what to expect and define what level of service the physician will provide (**Box 67-2**).

Specific planning begins as the location and expedition members are identified. Demographics and basic medical information of expedition members should be obtained. This allows for the prediction and planning of medical contingencies. A group that involves only teenagers is unlikely to experience a cardiac event and aspirin or cardiac medications may not be packed, but allergy and extra trauma supplies may be packed instead. Furthermore, if a particular group member has a history of seizures the physician may choose to travel with alternative formulations of benzodiazepines such as rectal diazepam or intranasal midazolam. In addition, equipment particular to the needs of the environment can be packed such as dexamethasone and acetazolamide in the mountains or acetic acid in a marine environment.

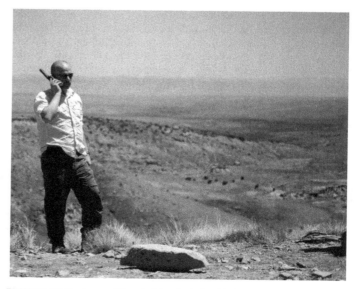

FIGURE 67-3. An expedition physician checks in with event management by satellite phone.

Key Considerations of a Contract

- Ensure that both organizers and participants realize the limited scope of medical care that can be provided due to environment, geography, terrain, as well as bulk and weight of supplies and equipment.

- Agree upon plans for the purchase, packaging, and transport of supplies and equipment

- Address compensation to the physician as well any costs incurred by personal transportation to and from the expedition. These arrangements typically follow the model put forth by cruise medicine physicians which either employs a physician full time for finite period of time (1 to 6 months) or offers the physician free participation in the expedition in exchange for medical coverage. It is uncommon for a physician to receive specific compensation as is common in the American fee-for-service model.

- Describe evacuation contingencies. Are all participants required to carry evacuation insurance? Where does the responsibility of the physician end after the evacuation handoff? Several national and international organizations offer evacuation insurance. Ones to consider are Divers Alert Network (DAN), which will also cover cost of hyperbaric chambers, Wilderness Medicine Society (underwritten by Global Rescue), and the American Alpine Club.

- Articulate malpractice insurance policies and payments which can be complex when dealing with international travelers and foreign medical providers. If traveling out of state, but within the United States, medical licensure laws should be reviewed and considered. Although many countries do not regulate the practice of medicine, be cognizant of the many that do as penalties may be severe. Improper licensure may directly affect liability policy coverage

- Strongly consider an indemnification clause that limits your liability for actions by the expedition organizer or other operational decisions beyond your control.

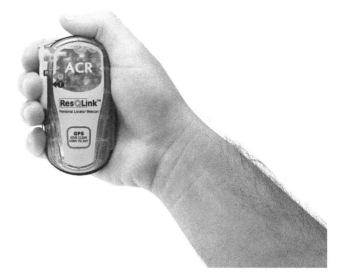

FIGURE 67-4. The ResQLink personal locator beacon. The ResQLink personal locator beacon (or PLB) is a full-powered, GPS-enabled rescue beacon designed for anglers, pilots, and backcountry sportsmen.

Medical contingencies should be mitigated by specific planning. A specific evacuation plan should be drafted for any injured participants. This will be specific to the environment and activities. For example, on a prolonged river trip a patient may be affixed to a boat and floated out of the environment whereas in a mountain environment a carry out, ski out, or helicopter trip may be required. As previously stated, this requires knowledge of the prehospital system in the location of the expedition and how the expedition will interface with this. Evacuation plans and protocols should include a list of what roles will be filled by whom (incident commander [IC], safety officer, logistics section, etc) as well as who will make decisions about the need to evacuate. This is important because often the incident commander may be the trip leader who has the most knowledge of the operational factors in an evacuation but may have limited medical knowledge, for example may not understand the need to evacuate a woman of childbearing age with abdominal pain and a missed menses. In addition, it may be important to plan for times when the trip physician is not available such as during summit attempts, dives, or satellite phone malfunction, this is akin to off-line medical control.

▓ COMMUNICATIONS

There are generally three modalities of communication that are utilized: radio frequency based, cell phone based, and satellite based. Radio frequency–based communication is the oldest and has the benefit of being the most time proven method as well as often being most energy efficient. However, it is limited by "line of site" range and may require government permits or license to operate on certain bandwidths or with enough power to cover reasonable distances (eg, HAM radio). Satellite communication includes sat phones but also messaging systems such as SpotDeLorme in Reach that pair with smart phones. Satellite-based communication has the benefit of working on most of the planet (though there are a few known dead spots) but are heavy users of power, require a clear view of the sky, and can be expensive. Finally cell phones are well known to most people and have an increasingly impressive range of coverage including rural areas on all continents but especially in the developing world and can even be used from areas near to Mount

Everest base camp. Personal locator beacons are small devices which can be activated to send out a radio signal to a satellite when the owner requires assistance (**Figure 67-4**). These originated as EPIRBs (emergency position indicating radio beacon) in marine settings and have expanded to land-based versions that operate on radio frequency, satellite, or a combination of the two.

SEARCH AND RESCUE

Some search and rescue (SAR) teams are essentially EMS agencies which have been extended even further from the hospital, and can incorporate nearly the same operations as a street-based EMS agency while performing in a more austere setting.[11] Other SAR agencies contribute significant search skills and assets to a region, but provide first-aid level medical care only.[12] A physician's role may vary from that of medical director, medical control, or rescuer. Physicians can function as regular members of a search team, hiking the ground in search of lost patients, or may be brought to the patient for pure medical care while other rescuers handle technical matters. Discussion of operation as a member of a SAR team is beyond the scope of this chapter and involves myriad skills such as search techniques, lost person profiling, and technical rescue skills such as rope handling.

As a medical director or medical control, the SAR physician must interface with EMS and possibly the incident commander and so should be fluent in their language and needs. The role of the medical director should be discussed in advance to include what exact role the director will fill, who is authorized to act under that director, and how the scope of practice for the wilderness providers will vary from that of other prehospital providers. It is common for wilderness providers to have an expanded scope of practice above that of other prehospital providers; the medical director must specifically state what this is and how it relates to the local EMS system.

Insurance is an important consideration for the SAR medical director and mostly focuses on malpractice both of a medical but also of a technical rescue nature. As with EMS medical direction, the SAR medical director must be closely involved in discussions about what medical equipment the team carries, and also should be aware of what nonmedical equipment the team carries that may be improvised to serve medical purposes. Decisions of equipment to carry will later dictate what practice protocols are followed.

SKI PATROL

The role of wilderness medicine as it relates to ski patrol is similar to that of SAR. It may range from that of a more SAR-based patrol, for example, Tuckerman's Ravine Ski Patrol in New Hampshire that occasionally may have to carry or fly a patient out, to a more EMS-based type patrol that staffs only EMTs with no special training and can drive a patient on a snowmobile in much the same way ambulance personnel would.[13,14] Again issues of contract, insurance, equipment, protocols, and EMS interfacing all must be considered and make ski patrol medical direction a merging of wilderness and typical EMS medicine.

TOXINOLOGY

Toxinology is a specific subset of toxicology that handles only toxins naturally produced by plants or animals. Furthermore, it considers not just the nature of the chemical, but also the plant or animal that produces this and the venom apparatus that delivers toxin. Plant-based toxinology may be relevant to the wilderness physician who cares for campers who enjoy foraging for food, or lost persons who forage out of desperation to survive. More commonly toxinology is relevant to the wilderness provider as patients become exposed via bites or stings. This area is ripe for further research and has a large knowledge base to be learned by the wilderness or toxicology physician. This includes identification of specific animals (eg, coral snake vs other similar appearing snakes), as well as identification of toxinologic syndromes (dry snake bite vs symptomatic ones), and knowledge of appropriate treatments. All of these require general knowledge and experience as well as some specific local wisdom. A classic example of local knowledge includes the old adage "red on yellow kill a fellow, red on black venom lack" which helps differentiate poisonous coral snakes from nonpoisonous look-a-likes but holds true only in North America. Identification of toxinologic syndromes and knowledge of treatment is critical making decisions such as who should be evacuated and what prehospital treatment should be applied where antivenom is not available.

EDUCATION

Courses directed specifically toward EMS providers include the Wilderness First Aid, Wilderness First Responder (WFR), or Wilderness EMT (WEMT) courses. Each may be taught within a standard First Responder or EMT curriculum or may be taught after the student completes a stand-alone FR or EMT class. Both courses generally add knowledge specific to wilderness illnesses and injuries, expand on the EMT or FR's physical examination and patient monitoring skills, as well as cover general EMS skills tailored to the wilderness environment. While there are some commonalities, each agency teaching these topics offer variability in the subject matter and content[15] and few, if any, combine these topics with comprehensive wilderness operational, survival, and wilderness skills. These courses, especially the Wilderness EMT course, may act as an introduction to wilderness medicine and could offer the EMS physician insight into the nuances of wilderness care.

A physician interested in practicing wilderness medicine would need to augment these courses with additional education.[16]

Many educational organizations have developed "advanced" courses, aimed at the medical practitioner with a higher skill set (ie, paramedics, nurses, and physicians) (**Table 67-1**). These courses are variable in duration and content but attempt to address the needs of a medical provider with advanced scope of practice. Again, there exists no minimum industry standard for these curricula and none of the courses embed significant amount of the additional skills necessary to truly practice in a wilderness environment.[15]

The *Wilderness Medical Society*, along with subsections of other national societies such as the National Association of EMS Physicians (NAEMSP), the American College of Emergency Physicians (ACEP), and others have generated significant interest and energy in wilderness medicine.[17] The Wilderness Medical Society in particular has generated numerous educational resources for the interested physician that includes the following:

- An annual conference with several topic-specific courses and lectures.
- The Fellow of the Academy of Wilderness Medicine (FAWM) program which requires 100+ hours of didactics mixed with experiential accomplishments. This is separate from institutional-based fellowship training programs.
- A quarterly published newsletter.
- The *Wilderness & Environmental Medicine* journal.
- The Diploma in Mountain Medicine (DiMM) which is based largely on the European model of mountain medicine and is intended to better integrate operations, survival, and rescue skills for the advanced level provider.[18]

The Wilderness Medical Society also advertises multiple wilderness medicine electives for medical students. Many of these experiences involve wilderness educators as well as resident and attending level physicians. The electives are highly variable in their duration, location (classroom vs experiential), and curricula. Presently, activities are ongoing to catalog the content of these curricula and to suggest minimum content for all wilderness medicine electives in an effort to standardize the content and learning. These courses may be open to interested EMS medicine fellows. A list of wilderness medicine electives may be found on the Wilderness Medical Societies Web site[16]

The additional skills necessary for the wilderness physician to safely and effectively practice in an austere wilderness environment may otherwise be difficult to learn in traditional medical education. The interested EMS physician or wilderness physician may be more successful in learning these skills from agencies that teach courses pertinent to the targeted environment (ie, mountaineering courses, dive courses, etc), or specific rescue courses (such as avalanche or swift water rescue). Another laudable means to learn these additional skills is through direct relationships with existing search and rescue teams or other agencies that practice wilderness skills. Finally, some physicians enter into wilderness medicine with significant personal experience in the wilderness setting.

TABLE 67-1	Some Wilderness Medicine Courses		
Course	Urban Equivalent	Typical Duration	Typical Participants
WFA	American Red Cross first aid	16 hours	Lay persons for personal care
WFR	First responder	75 hours	Professional guides
WEMT	EMT—intermediate	Full EMT course + 40-hour module	EMTs and professional rescue personnel
AWLS	ACLS	22 hours	RNs, paramedics, NPs, Pas, MDs, DOs looking for wilderness training

8. Hallagan LF, Reid T, DeLappe R. EMS in rural settings: a program to advance EMS in Yellowstone National Park. *Wilderness Environ Med.* 1997;8:253-254.
9. Adema G, Davis D, Stinson M. A seven-year experience in expedition medicine: the Juneau Icefield Research Program. *J Emerg Med.* 2003;24(3):257-264.
10. Iserson KV. Medical planning for extended remote expeditions. *Wilderness Environ Med.* December 2013;24(4):366-377.
11. Russell. Wilderness emergency medical services. *Emerg Med Clin N Am.* 2004;22:561-573.
12. Declerck MP, Atterton LM, Seibert T, Cushing TA. A review of emergency medical services events in US national parks from 2007 to 2011. *Wilderness Environ Med.* 2013 Sep;24(3):195-202.
13. Sagalyn EB, McDevitt MC, Ernst R. Utah ski patrol: assessing training types and resources. *Wilderness Environ Med.* 2014;25(4):450-456.
14. Constance BB, Auerbach PS, Johe DH. Prehospital medical care and the National Ski Patrol: how does outdoor emergency care compare to traditional EMS training? *Wilderness Environ Med.* June 2012;23(2):177-189.
15. Welch T, Clement K, Berman D. Wilderness first aid: is there an "industry standard?" *Wilderness Environ Med.* 2009;20:113-117.
16. Morton PM, Marshall JP. Wilderness medicine education for the physician. *Emerg Med Clin N Am.* 2004;22:539-559.
17. Warden CR, Millin MG, Hawkins SC, Bradley RN. Medical direction of wilderness and other operational emergency medical services programs. *Wilderness Environ Med.* March 2012;23(1):37-43.
18. Wilderness Medical Society website. http://www.wms.org. Accessed August 28, 2012.

KEY POINTS

- The EMS physician should be knowledgeable about wilderness medicine, defined as "injuries and illnesses caused by the interaction between humans and their natural environments occurring in potentially austere and threatening environments."
- EMS care in the wilderness setting often involves search, rescue, on-scene treatment or stabilization, care during extrication, and evacuation to definitive care.
- Wilderness medicine may encompass scheduled, planned events such as expedition medicine, or may involve unscheduled emergency rescue situations such as search and rescue or avalanche response.
- The EMS physician must balance between states of complete readiness and the ability to improvise care based on the availability of limited resources in the wilderness environment.
- The EMS physician who practices wilderness medicine should have a strong ability to "improvise, adapt, and overcome" in order to meet the many challenges that are faced in the myriad of wilderness medicine care environments.
- The EMS physician may need to be personally familiar with and capable of performing skills such as rope handling, skiing, desert survival, and other skills unique to the wilderness environment.
- The Wilderness Medicine Society serves as an excellent clearinghouse of wilderness medicine training opportunities.

REFERENCES

1. Grocott MP, McCorkell S, Cox ML. Resuscitation from hemorrhagic shock using rectally administered fluids in a wilderness environment. *Wilderness Environ Med.* 2005;16:209-211.
2. Sholl JM, Curcio EC. An introduction to wilderness medicine. *Emerg Med Clin N Am.* 2004;22: 265-279.
3. Johnson L. An introduction to mountain search and rescue. *Emerg Med Clin N Am.* 2004;22:511-524.
4. Schmidt TA, Federiuk CS, Zechnich A, Forsythe M, Christie M, Andrews C. Advanced life support in the wilderness: 5-year experience of the Reach and Treat team. *Wilderness Environ Med.* 1996;3:208-215.
5. London S. Using pins and pens for wilderness care. *ACEP News,* December 2010.
6. McGrath T, Murphy C. Comparison of a SAM splint-molded cervical collar with a Philadelphia cervical collar. *Wilderness Environ Med.* 2009;20:166-168.
7. Frank Butler Jr MD, CAPT US Navy, SEAL.

Mass Gatherings

Joshua M. Mularella
Oliver M. Berrett
Jeremy Joslin
Melissa Kohn

INTRODUCTION

Mass gathering medical care generally refers to the organized care provided for groups of at least 1000 people, including both spectators and participants, although some authors put this number as high as 25,000.[1-3] The event types range considerably from large community events such as parades, fundraisers, festivals, and fairs to political rallies, religious events, sporting competitions, and outdoor and indoor performances such as music concerts. However, to define a mass gathering simply by the number of participants is inadequate.[1] A more conceptual definition has been suggested by Arbon, which endorses the idea that a mass gathering is a collection of people that because of its inherent features including density of people, location, or environment may limit medical access.[1] Mass gatherings occur in nearly every conceivable location and condition and hence pose unique challenges to the medical provider for planning purposes and provision of medical care.

HISTORY

Despite a long social history of mass gatherings in the United States, the first medical literature reviewing health care in mass gatherings surfaces in the 1960s when volunteer health care providers supported antiwar demonstrators.[4] During the ensuing decades, a reservoir of case reports provided information for medical planning and provision at specific mass events such as stadiums, concerts, and the Olympics. In 1990, ACEP released a guide for medical care for crowds,[5] and in 2000, NAEMSP released a National Position Paper titled "Mass Gathering Medical Care," which called for a rigorous scientific evaluation of medical care delivery in place and the adequacy of care, an assessment of injury patterns, and minimum standards for preparation and delivery of medical care.[6] The statement also introduced the concept of the medical action plan and the medical director's checklist.[7]

CURRENT NEED

Hundreds of millions of people attend mass gathering events every year in the United States alone.[8]

Consistent in the literature is the fact that even though large-scale mass gatherings are composed of relatively "well" proportion of the population, injuries are generated more frequently at mass gathering events than in the general population.

OBJECTIVES

- Describe types of mass gatherings and discuss varying needs based on type.
- Describe common medical conditions and complaints at mass gathering events.
- Discuss factors that can lead to widespread illness and development of an MCI.
- Describe the role of the event medical director.
- Describe types of personnel utilized in event medical support.
- Describe event medical support planning and essential factors of consideration (eg, number of participants, access, communication, supplies, local medical resources, etc).

- Describe environmental factors that play a role in event planning and operational adjustments.
- Discuss contractual arrangements and terms that are important to successful medical support of mass gathering events.
- Discuss CQI and research initiatives specific to mass gathering events.
- Provide a basic event medical planning checklist/medical needs assessment form.
- Provide lists of common equipment for large-scale events.

BACKGROUND

MASS GATHERINGS

Medical incidents at mass gatherings and events can be separated into primary care, emergency care, and major incident.[9] The medical components should include accessible primary care stations inside the event, response elements embedded within, and transportation staged in a well thought-out location nearby. Gatherings also provide vulnerability to participants by the simple nature of a crowd effect, density, relative anonymity of would-be criminals and have recently served as targets for terrorists[10] (Atlanta Olympics, Boston Marathon). This increasing threat of targeted, large-scale violence at mass gatherings requires even more preventative foresight and catastrophe preparation.

Provision of medical care at a mass gathering event can be complex as it integrates multiple aspects of medicine including public health, primary care, and emergency medical services. Management of any medical incident at an event requires coordination with the other logistical elements intrinsic to the event itself including security, event coordinators and staff, and the participants or public.[11] In addition, Arbon describes three elements that affect the health of participants including environmental factors, the psychosocial component of the crowd, and the biomedical aspect which includes the overall baseline health of participants and may include widespread involvement of drugs or alcohol.[12]

TYPES OF GATHERINGS

The most common types of mass gatherings are sporting events, concerts, and various festivals, fairs, and religious gatherings. Sporting events most often cited in the literature include the Olympic Games and those played at the collegiate or professional level.[13-21] Many of these are held in fixed stadiums with nonmoving crowds and difficult access to care. Other athletic events such as triathlons, endurance races, and other long distance events are more spread out, requiring medical assets to be staged throughout the course.[22]

Similar to stadium-based sports, concerts generally have fixed and nonmobile crowds unless multiple stages exist. Rock concerts in particular have been associated with higher patient presentation rates due to drugs, alcohol, and mosh pits.[23-26] Fairs and festivals, on the other hand, are generally spread out with a large number of participants over multiple days and therefore pose their own unique problems in regard to planning and staffing.[27-32]

INJURIES AND COMPLAINTS

Most patient complaints can be categorized as either traumatic, medical, or support. As mentioned previously, certain events (ie, rock concerts) are more likely to produce specific types of patient complaints (ie, orthopedic injuries). Several mass gatherings have been described in the literature, documenting specifically the rates of patient presentations and chief complaints. A retrospective review of the New York State fair over a 5-year period showed an average patient presentation rate (PPR) of 4.8/10,000. The three most common complaints were dehydration (11.4%), abrasions/lacerations (10.6%), and falls (10.2%) (**Table 68-1**).[30]

Other events, such as concerts, would be expected to have more traumatic injuries. A review of 405 major concerts in the 1990s showed that rock concerts had approximately 2.5 times more patients than nonrock

TABLE 68-1	Top 3 Complaints at the New York State Fair (2004-2008)
Dehydration	11.4%
Abrasions/lacerations	10.6%
Falls	10.2%

concerts.[24] However, the distribution between traumatic injuries and medical complaints were the same. Other events that produce traumatic injuries include outdoor races, demonstrations, and rallies, events that include active participation such as climbing or fighting, and events that utilize dangerous elements such as pyrotechnics.[8,27]

There are many characteristics that can be used to predict the types of injuries to expect. In a 2002 review of the literature, Milsten et al identified the most common variables affecting injury rates and injury types which included venue size and participant numbers, among others (**Box 68-1**).[8] Duration of the event, venue type, and location are also major variables in predicting patient load. Events held indoors vary based on spectator mobility.

A study reviewing injuries at an Olympic venue showed higher rates for *mobile crowds vs seated crowds*.[8,13] Indoor events should be evaluated for points of egress and other barriers. Venues held outside have many contributing factors. Environmental exposure to excesses of heat and cold are major contributors to health problems at mass events.[7,8,12] Preparations for exposure should be taken seriously. Leonard points out the following common-sense fact: whatever is in or around the venue that can produce injury should be expected to produce injury (ie, if there is water, anticipate drownings; if there is elevation, consider falls; if proximity to insects or animals, expect bites, etc).[5,8]

Certain crowd demographics can also predict injury patterns and rates and should be considered when planning. The age of the population—older crowds are generally more frail and have preexisting health problems. The mood of the crowd- the density of the participants, and the consumption of drugs and/or alcohol have been shown to affect injury patterns and rates, as mentioned previously.[5,8,12]

Two additional vulnerabilities of mass gatherings merit special preparation. Congregations of people are vulnerable to public health risks including exposure to contagious pathogens via respiratory transmission, food preparation and distribution, contaminated water sources, and inadequate sewage management.[14] Khan describes the preparations made to treat a feared influenza epidemic during the Hajj pilgrimage and represents an example of promoting public health stewardship during a temporary mass event.[31] Terrorist plots frequently target groups of people to maximize injury. Recent domestic examples include the Atlanta Olympic bombing and the Boston Marathon bombing. Coordination among event planners and responders should take these risks into consideration and allocate appropriate contingencies for mass casualties.[10,33]

MEDICAL ACTION PLAN

In 1990, the American College of Emergency Physicians (ACEP) developed a step-by-step guide for providers to aid in the preparation of the

Box 68-1
Most Common Variables Affecting Injury Rate/Type
Weather
Event type
Event duration
Age
Crowd mood and density
Attendance

Box 68-2
Components of a Medical Action Plan
1. Physician medical oversight
2. Medical reconnaissance
3. Negotiations for event medical services
4. Level of care
5. Human resources
6. Medical equipment
7. Treatment facilities
8. Transportation resources
9. Public health elements
10. Access to care
11. Emergency medical operations
12. Communications
13. Command and control
14. Documentation
15. Continuous quality improvement

medical component of mass gatherings.[5] A decade later the National Association of Emergency Medical Services Physicians (NAEMSP) published *Mass Gathering Medical Care: The Medical Director's Checklist.*[7] Foresight and preparation are paramount to providing safe and an effective medical delivery and developing a medical action plan will streamline the process.

The medical action plan is an essential organizational tool for the preparation of medical delivery at mass gathering events. The plan should be used in all stages of organization and in the execution of medical care. It will require the approval of the medical director and must strictly follow all applicable laws and protocols. Fifteen components comprise the medical action plan (**Box 68-2**).

Medical Oversight Medical oversight should be provided by a physician capable of caring for the acutely ill patient, preferably have EMS training or experience. The medical director assumes the mantle of responsibility for all medical operations during the event and thus must understand the applicable laws pertaining to medical administration, interpret the medicolegal implications, and participate in the assessment of risk. An agreement in the form of a contract should be drafted for the medical component and the event leadership that contains such details clearly spelled out. The medical director should determine the appropriate level of care, and be available for consultation to assess staffing needs, estimate medical supply volumes, and develop the formulary. The contract should contain other important details including deadlines and negotiated terms such as payment and liability agreements.[6,34]

Reconnaissance The planning stages for the event should commence months or weeks prior to an event depending on the size, scale, and complexity of the event. Events that are complicated by large-scale, heightened security concerns, and complex venues or event design may require a year or more to plan. In the early stages, reconnaissance of the venue site and medical resources should be conducted. The venue should be inspected to identify potential risks and sources of injury. The information gathered from the site will guide planning strategies regarding intraevent transport and communications, to determine location options for command structure, treatment, and mobile staging sites, as well as to plan emergency egress, mass casualty related points and establish landing zones or other transport hubs. Medical reconnaissance should help identify medical resources and staff onsite or that is otherwise provided, estimate needed medical supplies and volumes, serve to introduce leadership of participating parties if applicable, and establish an interface with local EMS systems.[8]

Negotiations The medical director should meet with event organizers prior to the event to discuss the medical plan and ensure buy-in by those involved. Topics of discussion include equipment/supplies, staffing, communication equipment, potential compensation, and medicolegal issues such as liability coverage.

Level of Care As indicated earlier, a fundamental part the medical action plan is determining the level care appropriate for the event. Several studies show that events tend to consist primarily of "well" people and that the majority of injuries are low acuity.[1,8,15,27] However, acute emergencies may arise anytime which makes it essential for the responders to assess, stabilize, and treat or transfer. A venue's interface with existing EMS systems may dictate how autonomous the medical operation should plan to be. An early paper describing medical provisions at the Winter Games in Calgary showed that ALS level providers were not needed in the urban areas because of the proximity and accessibility of the city EMS system; however, ALS level providers were essential in the rural areas.[15] ALS and physician level care may be required in austere locations where transport time is unreasonably long.[27] The medical director should exercise discretion in selecting the level of care based on resource availability and other contributing factors and should match the standard of EMS care available in the surrounding area.

Medical Equipment Medical equipment, supplies, and formularies should be thoughtfully planned in advance. Although some literature describes the need of specific items such as cardiac defibrillators,[35,36] resources are generally scarce overall. There are numerous generic event medical supply lists in textbooks and in other medical literature which may help. These lists can serve as a starting point and be tailored to a specific event. Preparatory steps start with reviewing the treatment level, protocols, and expense allowance. Anticipating the expected needs and volumes of the event is a notoriously difficult aspect of planning. Practical supplies such as paper, pens, and folders should be considered in the inventory as well as personal comfort items such as sunscreen and insect repellant.[34]

Treatment Facilities Some events will require modest medical facilities consisting of mobile providers working out of a medical bag or an ambulance. Large venues and prolonged events will likely require a specified, onsite treatment location such as a tent or room that can serve as the triage and treatment site. An onsite treatment facility must be clearly marked, and its location widely known to the providers, event staff, and participants. The on-site location should maximize accessibility for providers and patients, and provide maximal proximity to off-site transport.

Communications Communications is the most vulnerable part of the medical action plan and therefore proper planning is important. EMS personnel at mass gathering events typically rely on the radio capabilities of local EMS agencies (eg, UHF vs digital) and therefore extra radios and batteries should be available. Staff should be trained on radio operations and the use of clear speech. Phone service (land line, cell, satellite) can serve as a backup to radio transmission or serve as the primary means of communication . Text messaging in particular can be useful when high ambient noise renders audio transmission unreliable.[37]

Medical Command and Control The organizational structure of medical provision should integrate with the larger administrative command system and clearly outline authority and responsibility. Some authors encourage using the unified command model, particularly if multiple EMS and/or law enforcement agencies are involved.[34] The medical command center should be accessible and clearly marked. The location could be either on- or off-site depending on the layout of the event site, but for reasons of convenience, it is ideal to be adjacent to other organization centers (security). The center should have at least one person present at all times.

The advantages for onsite medical control are well described. Having a physician onsite is beneficial for the safe release of patients back into the crowd.[38] Onsite physicians also reduce the number of off-site transports and decrease the patient burden on the local EMS systems.[29,38] Physicians are usually responsible for developing protocols at events and if on-site are able to reexamine or modify treatments as needed.[39] Finally, physicians have the expertise and the authority to render definitive medical decisions and appropriate refusals of care.[34,39]

Documentation Prior to an event the medical director should establish the method for documenting patient interactions. Often the local EMS patient care report (PCR) is used but, if an event is large enough, a customized form may be more desirable. At a minimum the PCR should include the following: patient's name, contact information, chief complaint, impression, treatment, and disposition.

All records should be kept on file for at least as long as mandated by state law. For minors of some states, this may mean the clock does not start until the age of maturity. Immediately after an event, the medical director or their designee should conduct an organized audit of patient care. In the case of emergencies or mass casualty incidents where a PCR may not be available, whatever information is at hand (triage tags) should be used. Review of these records allows for changes and recommendations for future events.

EVENTS

PERSONNEL

Care provided at mass gatherings varies widely in both preparation and staffing depending on the size and nature of the event. The medical director's checklist provides the most guidance to date on this topic.[7] Also, several states have passed legislation mandating minimum levels of staffing. For example, New York State Sanitary Code Part 18 requires specific thresholds for staffing based on expected numbers of participants (**Table 68-2**).

The first step in planning for any event is the appointment of the medical director. There are few prerequisites to be an EMS medical director but at the very least they should hold a valid state medical license and be familiar with local EMS protocols. A familiarity with emergency medicine and ACLS is preferred. This individual should draft the event medical action plan.

TABLE 68-2	New York State Sanitary Code Part 18.4 Emergency Health Care Requirements for Mass Gatherings		
Attendees	On-Site Facility	On-Site Ambulance	Physician
5-15K	1: 2 EMTs	1: 1 EMT	Available in 15 min
15K-30K	2: 2 EMTs each	1: 1 EMT	Available in 15 min
30K-50K	2: 2 EMTs each	2: 1 EMT each	1 on-site
>50K	2: 2 EMTs each	3: 1 EMT each	1 on-site

This represents the legal minimum by the State. Many events exceed this minimum as deemed necessary by the event medical coordinator.

One of the necessary sections of this plan is whether the medical director will provide direct or indirect oversight at the event. Direct medical oversight is preferred for several reasons. It is clear that a physician on-site can reduce hospital transports and advocate for EMS with the event organizers.[6,29,38-40]

The medical action plan should identify an appropriate number of staff on hand at an event including physicians, physician extenders, paramedics, EMTs, nurses, and support personnel. The exact number and distribution of staff will vary depending on the event. The medical plan should also include descriptions of patient transportation not only within the event itself but to area hospitals if necessary. Mutual aid agreements should be established to provide more staff and supplies should conditions warrant.

An outbreak of medical illness at mass gathering events is not common but should be considered and plans prepared. Respiratory and GI-related illnesses spread quickly at mass gatherings due to the close proximity of participants.[31,41] The decision to stockpile medications depends on medical reconnaissance.

◼ PREPLANNING CONSIDERATIONS

The two primary factors to consider when developing the medical action plan are the attendees themselves and external influences (ie, weather, food, shelter, etc). The estimated size of the crowd itself is proportional to patient volume and can therefore be used to plan for medical staffing and supplies.[42] Not all events are created equal, however. Sporting events and rock concerts have a higher propensity for alcohol/drug use and violence and therefore tend to have higher patient presentation rates.[20,21,23,43]

Several authors have attempted to forecast patient presentation rates using more external variables in addition to crowd size and mobility such as temperature, humidity, and day of the week with variable results.[9,33,43-45]

KEY POINTS

- Common variables affecting injury rate and type are weather, event type, event duration, age, crowd mood and density, attendance.
- There are 15 key components to a medical action plan.
- An on-site treatment location should maximize accessibility for providers and patients, and provide maximal proximity to off-site transport.
- Communications is the most vulnerable part of the medical action plan and therefore proper planning is important.
- The medical plan should also include descriptions of patient transportation not only within the event itself but to area hospitals if necessary.
- Mutual aid agreements should be established to provide more staff and supplies should conditions warrant.

REFERENCES

1. Arbon P. Mass-gathering medicine: a review of the evidence and future directions for research. *Prehosp Disaster Med.* 2007;22(2):131.
2. De Lorenzo RA. Mass gathering medicine: a review. *Prehosp Disaster Med.* 1997;12(01):68-72.
3. Michael JA, Barbera JA. Mass gathering medical care: a twenty-five year review. *Prehosp Disaster Med.* December 1997;12(4):305-312.
4. Chused TM. Medical care during the November 1969 antiwar demonstrations in Washington, DC. An experience in crowd medicine. *Arch Intern Med.* January 1, 1971;127(1):67.
5. Leonard R, Petrilli R, Calabro J, Noji E. *Provision of Emergency Medical Care for Crowds [Monograph].* Dallas, TX: American College of Emergency Physicians; 1990.
6. Jaslow D, Yancy A II, Milsten A. Mass gathering medical care. *Prehosp Emerg Care.* January 2000;4(4):359-360.
7. Jaslow D, Yancy A, Milstein A. *Mass Gathering Medical Care: The Medical Director's Checklist for the NAEMSP Standards and Clinical Practice Committee.* Lenexa, KS: National Association of Emergency Medical Services Physicians; 2000.
8. Milsten AM, Maguire BJ, Bissell RA, Seaman KG. Mass-gathering medical care: a review of the literature. *Prehosp Disaster Med.* 2002;17(3):151-162.
9. Zeitz KM, Schneider DPA, Jarrett D, Zeitz CJ. Mass gathering events: retrospective analysis of patient presentations over seven years. *Prehosp Disaster Med.* 2002;17(3):147-150.
10. Stratton SJ. Violent sabotage of mass-gathering events. *Prehosp Disaster Med.* 2013 Aug;28(4):313.
11. Ranse J, Hutton A. Minimum data set for mass-gathering health research and evaluation: a discussion paper. *Prehosp Disaster Med.* 2012;27(6):543-550.
12. Arbon P. The development of conceptual models for mass-gathering health. *Prehosp Disaster Med.* 2004;19:208-212.
13. Baker WM, Simone BM, Niemann JT, Daly A. Special event medical care: the 1984 Los Angeles Summer Olympics experience. *Ann Emerg Med.* 1986 Feb;15(2):185-190.
14. Meehan P. Public health response for the 1996 Olympic Games. *JAMA.* May 13, 1998;279(18):1469-1473.
15. Thompson JM, Savoia G, Powell G, Challis EB, Law P. Level of medical care required for mass gatherings: the XV Winter Olympic Games in Calgary, Canada. *Ann Emerg Med.* April 1991;20(4):385-390.
16. Bock HC, Cordell WH, Hawk AC, Bowdish GE. Demographics of emergency medical care at the Indianapolis 500 mile race (1983-1990). *Ann Emerg Med.* October 1992;21(10):1204-1207.
17. Carveth SW. Eight-year experience with a stadium-based mobile coronary-care unit. *Heart Lung.* October 1974;3(5):770-774.
18. Pons PT, Holland B, Alfrey E, Markovchick V, Rosen P, Dinerman N. An advanced emergency medical care system at National Football League games. *Ann Emerg Med.* April 1980;9(4):203-206.
19. Shelton S, Haire S, Gerard B. Medical care for mass gatherings at collegiate football games. *South Med J.* November 1997;90(11):1081-1083.
20. Spaite DW, Meislin HW, Valenzuela TD, Criss EA, Smith R, Nelson A. Banning alcohol in a major college stadium: impact on the incidence and patterns of injury and illness. *J Am Coll Health.* November 1990;39(3):125-128.
21. Wolfe J, Martinez R, Scott WA. Baseball and beer: an analysis of alcohol consumption patterns among male spectators at major-league sporting events. *Ann Emerg Med.* 1998;31(5):629-632.
22. Friedman LJ, Rodi SW, Krueger MA, Votey SR. Medical care at the California AIDS Ride 3: experiences in event medicine. *Ann Emerg Med.* 1998;31(2):219-223.
23. Erickson TB, Aks SE, Koenigsberg M, Bunney EB, Schurgin B, Levy P. Drug use patterns at major rock concert events. *Ann Emerg Med.* 1996;28(1):22-26.
24. Grange JT, Green SM, Downs W. Concert medicine: spectrum of medical problems encountered at 405 major concerts. *Acad Emerg Med.* 1999;6(3):202-207.
25. James SH, Calendrillo B, Schnoll SH. Medical and toxicological aspects of the Watkins Glen rock concert. *J Forensic Sci.* January 1975;20(1):71-82.
26. Janchar T, Samaddar C, Milzman D. The mosh pit experience: emergency medical care for concert injuries. *Am J Emerg Med.* 2000;18(1):62-63.
27. Bledsoe B, Songer P, Buchanan K, Westin J, Hodnick R, Gorosh L. Burning Man 2011: mass gathering medical care in an austere environment. *Prehosp Emerg Care.* 2012;16(4):469-476.
28. Bortolin M, Ulla M, Bono A, Ferreri E, Tomatis M, Sgambetterra S. Holy Shroud Exhibition 2010: health services during a 40-day mass-gathering event. *Prehosp Disaster Med.* 2013;1-6.

29. Boyle MF, De Lorenzo RA, Garrison R. Physician integration into mass gathering medical care: the United States Air Show. *Prehosp Disaster Med.* 1993;8(02):165-168.

30. Grant WD, Nacca NE, Prince LA, Scott JM. Mass-gathering medical care: retrospective analysis of patient presentations over five years at a multi-day mass gathering. *Prehosp Disaster Med.* 2010;25(2):183-187.

31. Khan K, Memish ZA, Chabbra A, et al. Global public health implications of a mass gathering in Mecca, Saudi Arabia during the midst of an influenza pandemic. *J Travel Med.* 2010;17(2):75-81.

32. Ounanian LL, Salinas C, Shear CL, Rodney WM. Medical care at the 1982 US Festival. *Ann Emerg Med.* May 1986;15(5):520-527.

33. Arbon P, Bridgewater FHG, Smith C. Mass gathering medicine: a predictive model for patient presentation and transport rates. *Prehosp Disaster Med.* 2001;16(03):150-158.

34. Grange JT. Planning for large events. *Curr Sports Med Rep.* 2002; 1(3):156-161.

35. Crocco TJ, Sayre MR, Liu T, Davis SM, Cannon C, Potluri J. Mathematical determination of external defibrillators needed at mass gatherings. *Prehosp Emerg Care.* 2004;8(3):292-297.

36. Motyka TM, Winslow JE, Newton K, Brice JH. Method for determining automatic external defibrillator need at mass gatherings. *Resuscitation.* June 2005;65(3):309-314.

37. Lund A, Wong D, Lewis K, Turris SA, Vaisler S, Gutman S. Text messaging as a strategy to address the limits of audio-based communication during mass-gathering events with high ambient noise. *Prehosp Disaster Med.* 2013;28(1):2-7.

38. Brunko M. Emergency physicians and special events. *J Emerg Med.* August 1989;7(4):405-406.

39. Parrillo SJ. Medical care at mass gatherings: considerations for physician involvement. *Prehosp Disaster Med.* 1995;10(04):273-275.

40. Grange JT, Baumann GW, Vaezazizi R. On-site physicians reduce ambulance transports at mass gatherings. *Prehosp Emerg Care.* 2003;7(3):322-326.

41. Wharton M, Spiegel RA, Horan JM, et al. A large outbreak of antibiotic-resistant shigellosis at a mass gathering. *J Infect Dis.* December 1990;162(6):1324-1328.

42. De Lorenzo RA, Gray BC, Bennett PC, Lamparella VJ. Effect of crowd size on patient volume at a large, multipurpose, indoor stadium. *J Emerg Med.* 1989;7(4):379-384.

43. Milsten AM, Seaman KG, Liu P, Bissell RA, Maguire BJ. Variables influencing medical usage rates, injury patterns, and levels of care for mass gatherings. *Prehosp Disaster Med.* 2003;18(4):334-346.

44. Zeitz KM, Zeitz CJ, Arbon P. Forecasting medical work at mass-gathering events: predictive model versus retrospective review. *Prehosp Disaster Med.* 2005;20(3):164-168.

45. Perron AD, Brady WJ, Custalow CB, Johnson DM. Association of heat index and patient volume at a mass gathering event. *Prehosp Emerg Care.* 2005;9(1):49-52.

International Deployment

Gerard DeMers
Gary M. Vilke

- Discuss cultural, legal, and other nonmedical operational concerns that must be addressed in the predeployment planning and during deployment operations.
- Describe unique medical conditions related to disasters in international venues.

INTRODUCTION

Emergency medicine service (EMS) personnel have opportunities to deploy in a variety of settings from urban international disaster response to sustained humanitarian missions for developing areas of the world. Types of deployments are listed in **Table 69-1**. Terms to describe these missions vary but generally offer some combination of direct clinical care to refugees, displaced persons or host country citizens, medical education information exchange, including consulting and training, establishing public health programs, health care team development, building or rebuilding health care infrastructure, and medical support to other deploying professionals. Missions may be short in duration, require multiple rotations over time, or require months to years of direct sustained medical support. Medical operations are usually conducted as a component of multidisciplinary teams or organizations, and other services offered may include food and water distribution or civil engineering programs. Each stage of response may need medical support, and personnel responsibilities may be well defined or fluid depending on needs. Clinical or administrative medical roles may be necessary depending on the circumstances. There are multiple ways for EMS personnel to participate in international deployments.

OBJECTIVES

- Describe types of need prompting international deployment.
- Describe different ways to participate in international deployments.
- Describe planning for readiness to deploy to international venues.
- Discuss how to determine what supplies may be available locally, when planning insertion into locations that are difficult to access.
- Describe health risks and other potential hazards inherent to international deployment to a disaster area.

INTERNATIONAL DEPLOYMENT OPPORTUNITIES

Involvement in international missions may be on an individual basis. Alternatively, personnel may participate through private/not-for-profit groups, EMS agency team, hospital team, government or nongovernment organizations (NGOs), or through interagency operations. Becoming involved in these missions is a matter of personal and professional preference. Some issues to consider when joining a medical mission: Are the sponsoring organization's views and beliefs supportable? Are capabilities and resources provided to meet mission goals? Is the safety profile for the mission acceptable? Protecting personnel against violence and dangerous conditions is a key consideration.

Ground operations for humanitarian missions may be complex and involve multiple agencies. Key operational players in regions vary and may include international governmental agencies, both military and civilian, international organizations (IOs), NGOs, and host nation (HN) agencies. See **Table 69-2** for examples. Each of these operational agencies may have a niche area of focus or response and are funded by a range of sources ranging from private donation to competitive governmental grants. An example of an NGO that fills a specific niche is Operation Smile that provides surgical correction and educational services for children and adults with congenital facial abnormalities such as cleft palates. Coordination of these agencies is sometimes problematic and may lead to overlap in services, diversion of care from other needed areas, or conflict between agencies. These operational players may have political views or agendas that may be congruent or in conflict with other organizations on the ground.

The Office for the Coordination of Humanitarian Affairs (OCHA), an office that operates under the United Nations (UN), facilitates humanitarian agency response when multiple agencies are working in the same area. OCHA serves to provide a cross-organizational coordination of humanitarian activities in partnership with national and international actors. It utilizes "cluster" meetings, which are organizations with similar

TABLE 69-1	Medical Mission Types				
Mission Types	Etiologies	Rotation Duration	Security Concerns	Associated Factors	
Environmental disasters	Earthquakes, hurricanes, floods, drought, etc	Short to long	Potential risk	• Disrupted infrastructure • Local health capabilities may be compromised	
Man-made disasters	Terrorism, industrial accidents, aircraft crash, etc	Short	High security risk	• May be prone to secondary attacks or incidents	
Complex humanitarian disasters response	Conflicts (political, religious, land, and/or ethnic disputes) often associated with environmental disasters	Short to long	High security risk	• Political vacuum • Displaced population • High morbidity and mortality • 50% of the affected population are children • Disrupted infrastructure	
Medical information exchange/education/mentoring	Educator shortage	Short	Lower risk	• Cultural or language barriers impact delivery	
Clinical care delivery (direct patient care)	Provider shortage	Short to long	Lower risk	• Sustainability • Standard versus sufficiency of care	
Public health programs	No organized public health infrastructure	Short to long	Lower risk	• Immunization programs • Water and sanitation • Vector control • Disease surveillance and outbreak control	

TABLE 69-2 Key Player Examples in Humanitarian Missions

Organization	Affiliation/Type	Services Provided
Peace Corps	NGO	Education; health, business, agriculture, environment, and communications development
Amnesty International	NGO	Humanitarian rights advocacy
Médecins Sans Frontières (MSF)*	NGO	Medical care delivery, advocacy
International Rescue Committee (IRC)	NGO	Medical care delivery, resettlement of refugees, advocacy
Operation Smile	NGO	Medical/surgical care delivery, education
International Red Cross/Crescent	IO	Medical care delivery, policy, advocacy
United Nations Office for the Coordination of Humanitarian Affairs (OHCA)	IO	Agency response coordination, advocacy, financing, policy development
World Health Organization (WHO)	IO	Health surveillance, policy and procedure development, coordination
US Military	Governmental	Medical, engineering, education, security
US AID	Governmental	Financing, coordinating aid efforts
Office of Foreign Disaster Assistance (OFDA)	Governmental	Disaster assessment and response
Urban Search and Rescue (USAR)	Government/Private	Search and rescue
Disaster Medical Assistance Teams (DMAT)	Governmental	Disaster medical response
Center for Disease Control (CDC)	Governmental	Disease surveillance, treatment recommendations

*MSF = Doctors Without Borders

NGO = non-governmental organization, IO = international organization

focus, logistics support, and financing management to maximize effective utilization of resources in regions where the OCHA is involved in operations. Some agencies may choose not to cooperate with other agencies, such as the military, in order to preserve a perception of neutrality. An example of this would be Médecins Sans Frontières (MSF or "Doctors Without Borders"). Military and civilian agencies have different doctrines guiding their missions, organization structures, and strengths and weaknesses, which can lead to challenges with interagency missions. Each agency has different organizational structures, chain of commands, and financial sources. Some may only participate in long-term missions and others focus on short-term interventions in disaster settings.

A disaster is any event that results in a precipitous or gradual decline in the overall health status of a community with which it is unable to cope adequately.[1] Often disasters are described as an event that adversely affects a region where the needs exceed available resources. Disasters often overwhelm local health care capabilities and illustrate need for acute global health response. As demonstrated by numerous catastrophes over the last decade (ex: 2015 earthquake in Napal, 2014 mudslide in Afghanistan, 2011 tsunami in Japan, 2010 mudslides in the Philippines, 2010 earthquake in Haiti, 2004 tsunami affecting Thailand) natural disasters are occurring with alarming frequency worldwide. Twenty-four-hour news cycles and social media may sway public opinion to affect missions. Long-term "disasters," like famine, lasting years or decades receive less media coverage and may arise from man-made or natural events such as wars, political instability, drought, or persecution. These conditions may lead to population displacement within the host country or to surrounding countries where communities often are not receptive to the presence of immigrants.

Outcomes from short- or long-term disasters depend on the magnitude of the event and the susceptibility of the affected population. There are a number of host country aspects impacting humanitarian medical operations including extent of poverty, limited resources, including personnel and equipment, differential access by the population to health care when these services are available, urbanization and overcrowding, malnutrition, limited access to potable water, and disease outbreaks.[1] Disasters may be a short distinct event with fairly quick recovery, recurrent or periodic, or can be long term in nature without a defined recovery period. Duration of recovery from disasters depends on a number of factors including predisaster civil infrastructure and state of host country's health system, amount and duration of damage sustained to region, and number of mass casualty incidents (MCI).

This chapter will outline concerns in predeployment, deployment, and postdeployment phases of international operations. Planning in each phase is critical to minimize challenges and frustrations that can occur during these operations. Flexibility is certainly needed in potential settings of limited resources, variable training of international coworkers, encountering diverse cultural habits, respecting foreign laws and rules, language barriers, and differences in standards of care.

PREDEPLOYMENT PREPARATION

MEDICAL READINESS AND TRAVEL HEALTH

Medical personnel who travel as part of humanitarian missions to provide medical aid may be tasked to leave suddenly without much preparation, with limited information and few medical supplies. This is typically the case for medical support of acute disasters and less commonly an issue for long-standing humanitarian operations. The major focus for these missions is often on helping others and less on personal health and safety. However, becoming a casualty during the mission makes the unprepared person a liability rather than an asset. There may be an austere environment with little infrastructure support available during your mission. Even if basic needs are covered by a sponsoring organization, one needs to be ready to be self-sufficient, often for a number of days.

Health screening, dental, and medical clearance ought to be completed for all deploying health care personnel. Preexisting medical conditions and pregnancy may preclude deployment to high-risk areas with limited medical capability to treat complications. Being prepared for international deployment is very important and often requires significant lead time for scheduling travel clinic appointments along with acquiring prophylactic medications and equipment. Vaccinations also need some lead time for building an immunity response. Most travel medicine sources recommend preparing a minimum of 4 to 8 weeks prior to the trip.[2] Having up to date vaccinations in advance can simplify the process. See **Table 69-3** for suggested vaccinations and travel medications. Dates and duration of trip, location, expected activities, and accommodations during the mission will be necessary to plan accordingly. Bringing a medical records summary and medical condition bracelet with known allergies is suggested.

Utilizing medical intelligence, information that defines known health risks for destination countries or regions, personnel can mitigate endemic disease risks.[3] This information is used to provide risk assessments to educate and to guide prophylaxis against vector-borne disease, diarrheal illnesses, and other regional conditions. Working abroad in austere and endemic disease environments requires behavior modification for many daily activities such as eating, drinking, and exposure to the environment as each may involve health risks that need to be avoided to prevent disease. Health concerns are of much greater importance when

TABLE 69-3	Predeployment Immunizations and Travel Medications	
Immunizations		**Travel Medications**
Routine	Travel related[a] Hepatitis A	Malaria[b]
Diphtheria[c]	Hepatitis B	Chloroquine, atovaquone/proguanil, doxycycline, mefloquine, primaquine
Tetanus[c]	Typhoid	
Pertussis[c]	Rabies	Antiretroviral
Measles[d]	Meningococcal disease	(In case of needle stick injuries)
Mumps[d]	Polio	Antidiarrheal
Rubella[d]	Japanese encephalitis	Quinolone, azithromycin
Varicella	Yellow fever	Altitude
Pneumococcus		Acetazolamide
Influenza		Motion sickness
		Scopolamine, dimenhydrinate
		Prophylaxis and self-treatment

[a]Dependent on mission location and exposure risk
[b]Malarial prophylaxis depends on regional resistance patterns
[c]Td or Tdap
[d]MMR

traveling to these areas. Behavior modification can serve to limit exposures to mosquitos and from potentially contaminated water or high-risk foods. "Boil it, peel it, or forget it" is recommended to reduce the chances for getting diarrheal illness. Do not eat raw foods, things that are not cooked, or that cannot be peeled. High-risk food sources include buffets, salads or other undercooked foods, street vendors, unpasteurized dairy products, and nonbottled, unfiltered, or carbonated water. When local dining options are unavailable, eating food that is cooked and served hot is safest. Bottled water may not be available so a water filter and chemical water purification method or boiled water should be utilized. Treated water should be used to wash dishes, brush teeth, and prepare food. Even with food and water precautions, you should still bring an antidiarrheal medication and antibiotic for treatment if symptoms occur. There are a variety of resources that provide regional information about known diseases and health concerns posing risk to deployed personnel. Please see **Table 69-4** for a list of some available resources.

Some deploying areas may have significant tuberculosis (TB) and HIV/AIDS infection rates among populations. Respiratory and body fluid precautions with personal protective equipment (PPE) should be utilized as indicated during procedures and in clinical care. In high-risk areas, fit-tested masks or N-95 respirators should be used when potential exposures may occur.[4] Tuberculin skin testing (TST) should be completed before deployment and 8 to 10 weeks after return.[5] Risk assessments are also important to evaluate posttravel illness, which are discussed in the Postdeployment section.

Packing essential items for work and leisure in austere environments are critical for the individual success in the deployment. Equipment such as a complete supply of daily and "as needed" medications and personal hygiene materials should be brought, with a small backup supply in case of prolonged deployment without replenishment. Personnel should not deploy to endemic malarial areas without malaria chemoprophylaxis, permethrin-impregnated bed netting, and DEET mosquito

TABLE 69-4	Travel Resources
1.	Centers for Disease Control (CDC) (www.cdc.gov/travel)
2.	Health information for international travel—CDC Yellow Book
3.	World Health Organization (WHO) (www.who.int/int)
4.	International travel and health—WHO Green Book
5.	International Society for Travel Medicine (www.istm.org)
6.	State Department (www.travel.state.gov)
7.	CIA World Factbook (www.cia.gov/library/publications/the-world-factbook/)
8.	SPHERE Guidelines (www.sphereproject.org/)

repellent. Several sets of comfortable and sturdy work clothing should be brought along with work supplies such as personal protective equipment including nitrile gloves, masks, and procedural protection goggles. Often these items are not available from the hosting agency or are often in short supply. Recommended personal items are listed in **Table 69-5**. There are often items that cannot be brought on a deployment depending on the host agency and this should be confirmed with the agency prior to departure. Some of these frequently discouraged or contraindicated items are listed in Table 69-5.

TABLE 69-5	Recommended Deployment Items

Personal Gear List

- Recommendations only
  - *Clothing:*
    - Underwear and socks
    - Rugged travel clothing
    - Shower clothes and sandals
    - Bandana*
    - Rain gear*
    - Team uniforms (×3-4 sets)
    - Boots
    - Off-duty shoes
    - Light jacket/windbreaker or team sweatshirt(s)
    - Head gear (ie, team cap)
  - *Personal items:*
    - Baby wipes (travel size)*
    - Personal medications (bring extra supply)
    - Toothbrush and paste
    - Bathroom tissue
    - First-aid kit with moleskin*
    - Hand sanitizer (travel size)*
    - Sunscreen and lip balm*
    - Insect repellant (DEET 25%-50%/permethrin for clothing)
    - International cell phone and charger*
    - International electrical converters
    - Lock and cable set*
    - Foot powder*
    - Watch*
    - Ear Plugs*
    - Camelback, water bottle*
    - Daypack or small bag/ fanny pack
    - Sleeping bag/sack, sleeping pad, travel pillow, and ground cloth
    - Bed netting (pretreated with permethrin)
    - Snacks*
    - Towel/hand towel
    - Comb/brush*
    - Deodorant/antiperspirant*
    - Shaving gear
    - Eye glasses (include spare pair), contacts, sunglasses
    - Shampoo/conditioner/soap/lotion
    - Sewing kit*
  - *Personal entertainment:* *
    - Reading material
    - MP3 player with headset
    - Extra phone/device batteries
    - Small camera

(continued)

TABLE 69-5 Recommended Deployment Items *(Continued)*

- *Tools/equipment:*
  - Work gloves/latex free gloves
  - Masks (N95 or equivalent)
  - Stethoscope
  - Otoscope/ophthalmoscope*
  - Eye shields
  - Light source (headlamp, angle head light, flashlight, etc)
  - Utility knife/utility tool
  - Water filter and purification kit
- *Items to be carried on person*
  - Medical licenses and certifications
  - Small notebook and pen
  - Driver's license and "official" ID
  - Extra local currency (small bills for tipping)

Prohibited items:
- Alcoholic beverages
- Firearms, ammunition
- Mace or pepper spray

Not recommended:
- Personal computers
- Expensive photo equipment
- Any expensive electronic equipment
- Excessive personal gear
- Personal electric devices requiring electricity

BACKGROUND RESEARCH FOR THE MISSION

Readiness to deploy to international venues involves planning for the individual as well as the team. Personnel should have appropriate and up-to-date licensure and credentialing for the role(s) that they will be filling prior to deployment. Copies of these documents should be kept on person during the mission. Individuals deploying with a new organization should learn about its philosophy, including mission and vision, policies, capabilities, required credentials, services provided, funding sources, prior mission reports, and relationship with other organizations. Becoming familiar with the current mission goals, destination, population that will receive care, travel arrangements, and team composition is important. Other considerations are contract agreements, liability coverage, scope of practice limitations, and if personal insurance is provided. The mission will dictate what supplies and equipment is brought. Once that is determined, personnel should get acquainted with the inventory to know its capabilities and limitations.

An orientation to the country and situation where the team will deploy is important. This orientation should include background information on local conditions, laws, government, customs, currency, and security issues. Personnel must abide by local laws or be subject to the host country's legal system. Knowing local customs and beliefs is important in order to effectively deliver culturally appropriate services and care. Accepted practices in your country may not be appropriate in mission settings. It is optimal to have prior experience working with other team members prior to the mission, but this is not always possible. An experienced team is also preferable to orient new members with little international experience. Recording your experience with a journal and photos is strongly recommended, though you should always ask permission to photograph patients.

There are many distinctions when practicing medicine in everyday settings in industrial countries contrasted to disaster situations or in humanitarian missions. Personnel should be specifically trained in the practice of medicine and unique medical issues that are unique to

disasters and humanitarian missions. On-the-job training in austere field conditions is not optimal. An example of potential scenario would be dealing with mass casualty triage and stabilization in a non-English speaking country with different accepted customs and norms. Care provided by personnel may be refused if not delivered in a culturally appropriate manner. Medical intelligence can be used as a guide to prepare personnel for appropriate treatment of endemic diseases. Many global health diseases are not encountered routinely and recognition of disease patterns will improve patient care. In clinical missions in tropical settings, a handbook of tropical medicine for reference is an invaluable reference. Other clinical subject areas that are particular to global medicine include disaster medicine, refugee medicine, and tropical medicine, which will be discussed in the following section.

OPERATIONAL PLANNING

Prior to departure either the individual or the sponsoring organization should do a needs assessment for the mission. This assessment outlines the what, who, where, how, why, and when the mission will be conducted to maximize effective delivery of services for the host country. Steps include determining the magnitude of the disaster/humanitarian mission and defining the specific health and nutritional needs of an affected population (especially in context of host country language and cultural norms).[6] This allows the team to prioritize issues and to understand if scope of care provided will be congruent with local needs. Identifying existing and potential public health problems that may be addressed by the mission or that may pose a threat to the deploying team will maximize impact and safety.

Evaluating the capacity of the local response (including assets and logistics) is useful to prevent diversion of care away from these resources and integrating wherever possible to efforts and to maximize training of host nationals. Establishing priorities and objectives for action by the deploying team with aim of working through the local health care channels will serve to avoid duplication of efforts. Determining external resource needs and prioritizing actions will mitigate unrealistic expectations. Often everything that gets planned may not be feasible with time, personnel, or resource constraints. Determine how execution of mission objectives will be conducted for each step through duration, scope, and exit strategy.[6] Knowing your role and that of your sponsoring agency will avoid overstepping responsibilities during the mission.

Security during the mission should be planned early and involves knowing what potential and actual threats are present in the mission location. A threat assessment evaluates threats to the team in a potential host country from environmental, political, civil, military, or economic instability concerns (eg, crime). Relief workers have also been threatened and targeted for kidnappings, hostages, or killed regardless of affiliation.[7-9] It may be necessary to have hired or host country security forces protecting personnel during the mission. While all unexpected threats to relief teams cannot be planned for, it is important to maximize safety even in higher risk locations. Collaborations or integration with host country and/or other organizations often occurs during missions and knowing the backgrounds of these agencies is also important to ensure safe interactions.

LOGISTICS PLANNING

Funding expenses for missions encompasses supply, transportation, communication, shelter/hotels, and a variety of other items or services. Funding may be provided by sponsor agency, contract, direct and indirect donations, grants, or may be the responsibility of individuals. Methods of payment for expenses and items should be determined prior to departure to plan accordingly. Contact other team members and coordinate logistics for appropriate supplies and to get tips on preparation. Self-sufficiency for individuals and teams cannot be emphasized enough as reliable supplies in destination countries often are not ensured. Personal diagnostic equipment such as a stethoscope, ophthalmoscope, otoscope, and flashlight are invaluable in the austere work environment. Adhering to work and personal hygiene may be difficult in some environments so bringing personal hand sanitizer and soap is strongly recommended. Medical equipment and supplies may include pharmaceuticals, extra medical disposables (gloves, masks [N-95], procedural supplies), and nonmedical equipment as determined by mission parameters. Supplies may be purchased or they may be donated. Do not bring expired medications or other expired perishable items. Also do not rely on local sources for pharmaceuticals due to high prevalence of counterfeit medications in local pharmacies.[10] The safest solution to ensure reliability of medications is to bring along adequate supplies for the mission or have a secure method for delivery from verified medical supply companies. Special items, such as decontamination supplies, may be requested as needed dependent on the mission. Advanced planning or requests may be needed to coordinate acquisition and delivery of these items to the target location. Whenever possible it is helpful to determine what supplies are available locally to avoid duplication and to augment necessary materials where needed, though this information is often not available prior to arrival.

Transportation to the host country and to destination site should be coordinated among team members, especially when planning insertion into locations that are difficult to access. Special arrangements may be needed such as chartering a small aircraft, boat, or vehicle that may only be available at limited times for remote area access. Having local language proficiency will go a long way to smooth transit by facilitating negotiations for in country transportation and to simply get accurate directions. If team members do not speak indigenous dialects or if English is not used, local English-speaking guides may be hired and may act as day-to-day routine interpreters during travel.

Having an evacuation plan through commercial air or air ambulance should be prearranged for unexpected contingencies. Setting up travel and evacuation insurance should be completed prior to departure in case of injury or illness that requires emergent return to medical facilities outside of the region. Most conventional insurance policies do not cover travel or evacuation insurance.

Communication and translation services should be set up prior to arrival at the mission site though often is coordinated after arrival. International cellular or satellite phones may be needed for communication between multiple sites, with other agencies, or stateside. Translation services will likely have to be arranged through volunteer, contract, or via host community liaisons. Attempts should be made to hire individuals proficient in medical translation and with knowledge of any local dialects that may be encountered.

Organizing local human resources (medical and nonmedical) can improve work efficiency, increase staffing, and may serve a dual purpose for education of locals during clinical events. Local volunteers may only need the means and direction to support relief operations. Potential roles may be to identify leaders to organize food and water distribution and assist with sanitation program enforcement. Identifying and incorporating community health workers (individuals with rudimentary health care experience) can increase local interest in the mission as these individuals are often highly regarded in their communities.

DEPLOYMENT

The first priority of deployment is personal health protection. Personnel often place more focus on treating numbers or working without breaks, which can lead to undue stressors during the mission. There are unique medical and nonmedical issues facing participants in a foreign aid missions. Circadian rhythm dysfunction, better known as jet lag, is likely to occur if multiple time zones (more than 5) are crossed to reach the work site.[2] Jet lag is worse when traveling west to east. Adapting to the new time zone requires behavioral modification by forcing yourself to adapt to new eating and sleeping hours. A few suggestions to facilitate the transition are not napping during the day, limiting alcohol and caffeine consumption, and using sleeping pills as needed only for 2 days.

Work stress and shift length are also details to keep in mind to avoid burnout and frustration during the mission.[11] Personal and team health is important for disease prevention during medical missions. Monitor yourself and your colleagues along with ensuring an equitable distribution of workload will aid in meeting mission goals and avoiding burnout. Keeping a watchful eye for vector-borne diseases and reminding colleagues to use prophylaxis like malaria treatment, mosquito netting, TB masks, and PPE are also important.

Medical conditions encountered are typically dependent on whether the mission is disaster versus humanitarian, patient access to medical services, and actual setting. At-risk populations in disaster and humanitarian settings are children less than 5 years, pregnant women, and the elderly.[1] Services provided also depend on the scope of care for the medical providers to treat deployed team members, host nations, other organizations, or some combination offered. The medical aspects of international relief missions are only one component of potential interventions. Larger missions include aspects beyond medical delivery of care. Standards and recommendations were updated in 2011 with the Sphere Project revision, which outlines minimum recommended requirements for care of affected populations in disasters or humanitarian settings.[12]

Measures of mission success are sometimes difficult to quantify though it is crucial to assess effectiveness and provide meaningful measures of progress. The purpose of these measures is to observe trends to show progress or no progress with interventions. Measures should be timely so that changes or problem areas may be acted upon promptly in real time. They may include effectiveness of tasks, disease and injury rates, transition of care to other organizations or to nationals through education, or overall mission accomplishments (not just number of patients seen). Data should be measured consistently to see trends and compare different areas. Measures should provide enough detail to enable observers to establish whether the situation is changing and to determine a cost-benefit analysis of interventions. Analyzing trends may highlight specific areas that require additional resources or that may not need further intervention. Resources provided for these missions should be cost-effective and sufficient to meet the goals of the mission. The only way to determine effective utilization of these resources is by measuring their impact.[13]

Elements common to disaster and humanitarian settings include the following issues and considerations. Exposure to elements can lead directly to death and increase caloric requirements so adequate temporary shelters may be needed for displaced populations. When resources are available, relief workers must consider mechanisms for equitable distribution of food. Nutrition requirements for malnourished host nationals may be addressed with a minimum of 2000 kcal/person/day. Targeted supplemental and therapeutic feeding programs should be made available for vulnerable and the severely malnourished. Minimum requirement of potable water is 3 to 5 L/person/day and 15 L/person/day for routine needs. A high priority in any displaced population living in crowded conditions is to improve sanitation and access to noncontaminated water sources. Appropriate and early management of severe diarrhea and dehydration should be addressed with goal of preventing outbreaks. Vitamin A deficiency is common in the malnourished and contributes significantly to measles case fatality in unvaccinated populations. Vitamin A supplementation and measles, mumps, and rubella (MMR) vaccination are simple lifesaving interventions. Establish disease surveillance and a health information system necessary to monitor effectiveness of health interventions and realign priorities.[12,14] Develop appropriate treatment algorithms for prevalent diseases based on treatment standards among the local population.

■ DISASTERS

Health risks to team members in disasters depend on the nature of the incident. Examples of physical hazards may be illustrated by the aftermath of an earthquake and include aftershocks, debris, unstable buildings at risk of collapse, fires, and disrupted gas or electrical lines. Other hazards include loss of sanitation systems and poor hygiene from loss of water supply, leading to diarrheal outbreaks. Close quarters of displaced populations also predisposes to respiratory illness outbreaks.

An "all hazards approach" that addresses common planning issues and precautions should be used to mitigate risks to personnel and in treating host nationals; while this chapter cannot describe all of the possible conditions that may be encountered in disasters, an "all-hazards" approach will help address the widest range of potential concerns.[15] Disaster medicine encompasses niche areas and heavily relies on triage to best utilize available resources. The type and phase of disaster, which are described below, will provide the mechanism for the majority of injuries or illnesses encountered (eg, earthquakes may lead to acute mechanical injuries such as fractures and dislocations, lacerations, or crush injuries and may require specialty care of rhabdomyolysis including emergent dialysis for acute renal failure).[16] Delayed presentation of casualties complicates routine management of soft tissue injures or fractures. Victims suffering open wounds in unsanitary environments are predisposed to extensive tissue infections and tetanus. Wound management for these cases potentially includes surgical debridement, antibiotics, and tetanus immune globulin/vaccination.

Stages of acute disasters may be broken down into phases: acute emergency phase (0-1 month), late or recovery phase (1-6 months), and rehabilitation and development phase (6+ months).[6] The acute emergency phase is characterized by an initial chaotic environment, limited available information, disruption of infrastructure, and potentially high morbidity and mortality rates. Host nation resources may be destroyed or become rapidly overwhelmed, leading to requests for outside assistance. This phase is where rapid assessments are conducted to determine needs and scope of support required. Political and logistical requests rerouted through governmental and private channels. Nearby states within the affected country or neighboring countries may provide medical teams that assist quickly due to proximity. Lead time for traveling from countries further away and potential disruption of local airports may delay distant teams by days or weeks. Determining where to position relief teams is also crucial for optimal operations rather than haphazard deployments without planning or coordination. This phase is characterized by rapidly trying to assess source and extent of damage, number of casualties, and optimal locations for staging response.[14]

Deployments in this phase may involve several areas that prehospital providers are uniquely qualified including triage and management of mass casualties that overwhelm local resources. Care may be directed at stabilization and transfer to higher level of care or be limited to what can be provided in the staged treatment area. Medical or surgical team capabilities are usually determined prior to deployment to the disaster area and they may be employed to augment local hospitals or set up at portable hospitals if local infrastructure is destroyed. Deployed teams may also be part of urban search and rescue (USAR) or aeromedical evacuation units that transport casualties to unaffected surrounding facilities or distant medical sites.

The recovery phase targets interim care during improvement and expansion of relief interventions usually guided by available surveillance data. Transition to established communication and supply lines for medical services occurs in this phase. Building local medical capacity and capability are goals for eventual host nation assumption of medical care for nationals. By this time there is expected to be a gradual decline in affected population mortality rate. Redeployment or departure of relief teams generally occurs during this phase. The rehabilitation phase is where the health profile of affected region approaches predisaster baseline for the indigenous population. The emphasis shifts from relief operations to self-sufficiency.

■ HUMANITARIAN OPERATIONS

Humanitarian operations may be conducted in any climate though many long-term operations are conducted in the tropics where tropical diseases are routinely encountered. Delivery of care for humanitarian operations can vary dependent on the setting such as village clinics, urban or regional hospitals (either government or private), or refugee encampments. There are unique medical and nonmedical issues facing participants in a humanitarian mission. Categories of tropical illnesses include direct infectious, vector-borne, animal-associated, and environmental diseases. Representative samples of tropical conditions that may be encountered are listed in **Table 69-6**. Untreated chronic illnesses along with their complications, diseases related to lack of childhood immunizations, nutritional deficiencies, and problems of untreated acute or chronic injuries are likely to be encountered. Simple interventions such as encouraging breast-feeding, vaccination programs, and providing health education can address some of these issues.

Refugee medicine has many unique aspects including overcrowding, disease outbreak control, and lack of timely access to health care. Displaced persons and refugees may be encountered in large numbers with little or no prior contact with medical services. A sudden influx of refugees or displaced persons into camps can easily overwhelm capabilities to provide adequate living area, potable water, sewage disposal, and medical care. Communicable diseases from the new immigrants can serve as nidus for disease outbreaks. Medical personnel can evaluate the potential risk of disease transmission and provide information to identify practical control measures. Prior planning for such contingencies is crucial since displaced populations may be encountered without advance notice. The medical component of relief teams plays a key role in the management of refugees.

After the basics of care for refugee medicine are addressed by providing security, food, water, sanitation, and shelter longer term medical services can be initiated. Medical services for refugee camps include pediatrics, infectious disease, OB/GYN, preventive medicine, geriatrics, and psychiatry.[12] Common diseases presenting in refugee camps are associated with crowding and hygiene. Examples disease outbreaks, such as diarrheal illnesses, tuberculosis, meningococcal meningitis, and measles are significant causes of morbidity and mortality. Endemic vector-borne disease, such as malaria, can be mitigated through distribution of bed netting to residents and vector control. Additional concerns that may be encountered are assaults, rapes, sexually transmitted diseases, burns, growth and developmental delays due to chronic illness and malnutrition, among others.[12]

In addition to routine medical care, preparing and reducing risk for outbreaks of disease is paramount among camp residents. Surveillance and rapid response to outbreaks can prevent medical resources from being overwhelmed. Develop clinical case definitions of potential diseases encountered for an active surveillance program. Case finding of early disease presentations in the camp through "house visits" should be preemptively treated before illness spreads to other residents. Develop emergency outreach procedures and teach treatment protocols among physician extenders, such as community health workers. Mass immunization campaigns should be initiated early in unvaccinated initial populations in setting up refugee camps and in new arrivals.[12]

POSTDEPLOYMENT

Self-health for personnel is equally important in the postdeployment period. Continuing malaria prophylaxis as directed minimizes chances of acquiring malaria, although it does not eliminate the risk. Other travel-related diseases might manifest up to several months after return so it is recommended to monitor for concerning signs and symptoms. Persistent or recurrent fever without likely source such as an upper respiratory infection, persistent diarrhea, rash, unexplained weight loss, abdominal pain, persistent cough are some examples that warrant a medical evaluation. Be sure to relay the travel, work, and potential exposure history to the health provider so that they may consider tropical diseases in the differential diagnosis. As mentioned a TST should be completed 8 to 10 weeks on return from a high-risk area.[2]

Presenting experiences about deployments serves several functions. Educating colleagues about the mission and cases seen are opportunities to provide learning about rarely encountered conditions and situations. This presentation could spark interest in your colleagues to join similar missions in the future. Providing lessons learned to the sponsoring organization with debriefs can improve future missions.

TABLE 69-6   Conditions Encountered in Tropical Settings

Condition	Clinical Features	Vector/Transmission	Treatment
Diarrheal diseases (variety of viral/bacterial pathogens)	• Dehydration, electrolyte abnormalities • Growth retardation	• Fecal-oral	Oral rehydration solution, IVF if available
HIV/AIDS	• Flu-like symptoms with acute seroconversion • Later opportunistic infections depending on viral load and immunity	• Blood, body fluid exposure, vertical transmission	Highly active antiretroviral therapy (HAART)
Tuberculosis (*M tuberculosis*)	• Fever, cough, hemoptysis, chest pain, weight loss	• Aerosol or respiratory droplets	Four-drug anti-TB Rx
Malaria (*P falciparum* (most life-threatening form of malaria), *P vivax*, *P ovale*, and *P malariae*)	• Nonspecific and varied presentation • Cyclic fever, malaise, anemia, cough.	• *Anopheles* mosquito	Antimalarial Rx depending on species and resistance patterns
Viral hemorrhagic fever (VHF) (multiple species—eg, dengue, Marburg, Lassa, etc)	• Fever, joint pain, malaise • More severe infection including hemorrhagic fever	• Various routes of transmission (mosquito, body fluid)	Supportive Isolation precautions
Meningococcal Meningitis (*N meningitides*)	• Fever, nuchal rigidity, altered mental status, petechial rash, • Rapidly progressive fatal disease	• Aerosol or respiratory droplets	β-Lactam or third generation cephalosporin or chloramphenicol Vaccinate at-risk population and antibiotic prophylaxis for contacts
Leishmaniasis (cutaneous, mucosal, and visceral)	• Nonhealing sores that lasts weeks to months • Kala azar: sometimes fever, weight loss, weakness, anemia, hepatosplenomegaly • Symptoms may not appear for weeks to months after getting bitten	• Sand fly	Antimonial Rx for cutaneous and amphotericin B for visceral/mucosal
Filariasis (*W bancrofti*)	• Dependent on worm burden: may be asymptomatic • Acute manifestations: • Adenolymphangitis filarial fever, tropical pulmonary eosinophilia • Chronic disease: lymphedema (limb or genitalia)	• Mosquito-borne	Diethylcarbamazine (DEC), ivermectin (good for treating microfilariae but no effect on adult worm), albendazole Supportive for chronic disease
Rabies	• Rapidly fatal ascending encephalopathy • Hydrophobia, hypersalivation, altered mental status	• Small mammals—dogs, bats, etc • Aerosol, bite	*Immediate* and *thorough* washing of all bite wounds and scratches with *soap* and *water*. Postexposure prophylaxis (both HRIG *and* HDCV)
Schistosomiasis (*S haemotobium*, *S mansoni*, *S japonicum*)	• Swimmer's itch: cutaneous self-limited infection with pruritic papular rash lasting 12 hours to 1 week. • Katayama fever: fever, chills, myalgias, arthralgias, dry cough, diarrhea, headache, LAD, and hepatosplenomegaly • Chronic infection depends on species and worm burden-intestinal, hepatic and urinary	• Snail. • Contact with contaminated fresh water	Supportive for swimmer's itch, praziquantel for systemic infection.
Tetanus (*C tetani*)	• Spastic paralysis • Respiratory failure	• Spores enter "wound"; germinate to release tetanospasmin	Irrigate wound Tetanus toxoid Tetanus immune globulin for high-risk wounds or unimmunized
Typhoid/paratyphoid (*S typhi*)	• Fevers, headache abdominal pain, constipation, diarrhea, altered mental status	Fecal-oral	Chloramphenicol, β-lactams, or trimethoprim-sulfamethoxazole, and fluoroquinolones
Typhus (*R prowazeki*)	• Fever, chills, headache, rash and generalized pain • Complications such as vascular collapse, gangrene, acute respiratory distress syndrome, and coma can occur.	Body louse	Tetracycline, chloramphenicol
Measles	• Exanthem, high fever, runny nose, coryza, cough, red eyes, and Koplik spots	Aerosol droplet exposure	Supportive care Complications and susceptible to secondary infections in malnourished populations
Relapsing fever (*B recurrentis*)	• Fever usually last 4–6 days and alternate with afebrile periods • Severe joint pain, chills, jaundice, nose or other bleeding	Body louse	Tetracycline, doxycycline, or erythromycin
Leptospirosis	• Fever, malaise, headache, cough, jaundice, renal failure	Exposure to contaminated fresh water from urine of small infected mammals	Doxycycline

CONCLUSION

International deployment for disaster response and humanitarian missions can be an immensely rewarding experience. Prior planning and training for these missions will improve the experience for health care personnel and for host nationals. Operational and logistics groundwork can also facilitate mission success. Medical intelligence can guide training, predeployment vaccinations, and preparation for medical missions. Promoting self-health to mitigate disease risk and stress is key in the deployment and postdeployment phases. Medical conditions experienced in disaster and humanitarian settings are very different than those experienced in industrialized settings. Many governmental and nongovernmental agencies provide a variety of services in international settings. Medical personnel have many opportunities to join these global health missions and should maximize their impact by being well prepared.

KEY POINTS

- Preplanning for international deployment includes many variables and is crucial to success.
- Personal health safety must be considered at every stage: planning, deployment, and postdeployment.
- Acute disasters may be broken down into phases: acute emergency phase (0-1 month), late or recovery phase (1-6 months), and rehabilitation and development phase.

REFERENCES

1. Wisner B, Blaikie P, Cannon T, Davis I. *At Risk: Natural Hazards, People's Vulnerability, and Disasters.* 2nd ed. London: Routledge; 2004.
2. Hill DR, Ericsson CD, Pearson RD, et al. The practice of travel medicine: guidelines by the Infectious Diseases Society of America. *Clin Infect Dis.* December 15, 2006;43(12):1499-1539.
3. Leder K, Steffen R, Cramer JP, Greenaway C. Risk assessment in travel medicine: how to obtain, interpret, and use risk data for informing pre-travel advice. *J Travel Med.* 2015;22(1):13-20.
4. Harrop T, Aird J, Thwaites G. How to minimise risk of acquiring tuberculosis when working in a high prevalence setting: a guide for healthcare workers. *BMJ.* March 16, 2011;342:d1544.
5. Szep Z, Kim R, Ratcliffe SJ, Gluckman S. Tuberculin skin test conversion rate among short-term health care workers returning from Gaborone, Botswana. *Travel Med Infect Dis.* July-August 2014;12(4):396-400.
6. Auf der Heide E. *Disaster Response: Principles of Preparation and Coordination.* St Louis, MO: Mosby; 1989.
7. Sheik M, Gutierrez MI, Bolton P, Spiegel P, Thieren M, Burnham G. Deaths among humanitarian workers. *BMJ.* 2000;321:166-168.
8. Rowley EA, Crape BL, Burnham GM. Violence-related mortality and morbidity of humanitarian workers. *Am J Disaster Med.* 2008;3(1):39-45.
9. Fast L. Mind the gap: documenting and explaining violence against aid workers. *Eur J Int Rel.* 2010;16(3):365-389.
10. Newton PN, Green MD, Fernández FN, Day NP, White NJ. Counterfeit anti-infective drugs. *Lan Inf Dis.* 2006;6(9):602-613.
11. Aitken P, Leggat P, Harley H, Speare R, Leclercq M. Human resources issues and Australian Disaster Medical Assistance Teams: results of a national survey of team members. *Emerg Health Threats J.* 2012;5.
12. Steering Committee for Humanitarian Response. *The Sphere Project: Humanitarian Charter and Minimum Standards in Disaster Response.* Geneva, Switzerland: Sphere Project; 2011.
13. Health disaster management: guidelines for evaluation and research in the Utstein Style. Volume I. Conceptual framework of disasters. *Prehosp Dis Med.* 2003;17(suppl 3):1-177.
14. Auf der Heide E. The importance of evidence-based disaster planning. *Ann Emerg Med.* January 2006;47(1):34-49.
15. Paton D, Johnston D. Disasters and communities: vulnerability, resilience and preparedness. *Dis Prev Man.* 2001;10(4):270-277.
16. Sever MS, Vanholder R, Lameire N. Management of crush-related injuries after disasters. *N Engl J Med.* 2006; 354:1052-1063.

CHAPTER 70

Army Emergency Medical Response

Jimmy L. Cooper

Peter J. Cuenca

INTRODUCTION

The first formally trained ambulance service owes its existence to military operations. The first formal emergency medical service is traced back to the middle ages during the crusades of the 11th century. The Knights of Saint John received instruction in first-aid treatment from both Arab and Greek doctors. These Knights of Saint John then acted as the first formally trained prehospital medical personnel, treating soldiers on both sides of the war on the battlefield and bringing in the wounded to nearby tents for further medical treatment.[1] The military again played a significant role in the development of prehospital care in 1487 during the Siege of Malaga, in Spain. This was the first recorded use of an ambulance—a horse drawn cart with a trained attendant.[2] In the 1700s, Napoleon Bonaparte appointed Baron Dominique-Jean Larrey to develop the first systematic collection of wounded on the battlefield. In 1797, Larrey created "ambulance volantes" or light with carriages with trained personnel to collect, transport, and treat injured.[3] Larrey developed all of the precepts of emergency medical care that are used today by all modern EMS systems: rapid access to the patient by trained personnel, field treatment and stabilization, and rapid transportation back to the medical facility while providing medical care en route.[4]

OBJECTIVES

- Describe the factors that make military EMS unique.
- Describe provider types and skill sets.
- Describe basic principles of care under fire.
- Describe essential equipment for care under fire.
- Describe basic principles of patient extraction, forward treatment, and treatment destinations.
- Describe the roles of EMS physicians in military EMS.
- Discuss the approach to care of noncombatants and enemy combatants.
- Describe the interoperability issues in military-civilian EMS deployment for domestic disasters.

MILITARY AND THE HISTORY OF EMS

At the beginning of the 1860s, the United States created the first field ambulance and attendant. The first recorded use of a field ambulance and attendant was during the Civil War. During the US Civil War, both sides attempted to emulate the medical practices of the Napoleonic wars. During the Battle of Bull Run, the ambulance service was being coordinated by the Quartermaster Corps. It was then transferred to Surgeon General Jonathan Letterman, MD, to organize, and he reinstated all of Larrey's concepts greatly increasing the survival rate of the wounded. In 1862, due to the unexpected size of casualty lists during the battle of Manassas where it took 1 week to remove the wounded from the battlefield, Dr Jonathan Letterman, Head of Medical Services of the Army of the Potomac, revamped the Army Medical Corps. His contribution included staffing and training men to operate horse teams and wagons to pick up wounded soldiers from the field and to bring them back to field dressing stations for initial treatment. This was our Nation's first Ambulance Corps. Dr Letterman also developed the three-tiered evacuation system.[5-7] Dr Jonathan Letterman is known today as the Father of Modern Battlefield Medicine.

ROLES OF CARE

The fundamental characteristic of the modern *army health services* (AHS) is the distribution of medical resources and capabilities to facilities at various echelons of command, diverse locations, and progressive capabilities, which are referred to as roles of care. As a general rule, no role is bypassed except for medical urgency, efficiency, or expediency. The rationale for this organization principle is to ensure the stabilization/survivability of the casualty through advanced trauma management and far forward resuscitative surgery prior to movement between military treatment facilities (MTFs). This strategy is tactical in nature and only addresses Roles of Care I and II.[8,9]

■ ROLE I

Role I is the first level of medical care a soldier receives and is also referred to as unit-level medical care. This role of care includes immediate lifesaving measures, disease and nonbattle injury (DNBI) prevention, combat and operational stress control preventive measures, patient location and acquisition, medical evacuation (MEDEVAC) from supported units (point of injury or wounding), company aid posts, or casualty collection points to supporting MTFs; treatment is provided by designated combat medics' treatment squads/teams. The major emphasis at this level of care is for the patient to return to duty or to stabilize him/her and allow for his/her evacuation to the next role of care. The measures at Role I include maintaining the airway, stopping bleeding, preventing shock, protecting wounds, immobilizing fractures, and other emergency measures as indicated.[8,9]

Nonmedical personnel performing first-aid procedures assist the combat medic in his/her duties. Each individual soldier is trained to be proficient in a variety of specific first-aid procedures including aid for chemical casualties with particular emphasis on lifesaving tasks. This training enables the common soldier to apply immediate first aid to alleviate potential life-threatening situations. Self and buddy aid is repeatedly identified as absolutely essential for ensuring casualty survival. If the casualty is to survive, lifesaving actions such as the application of a tourniquet often cannot be delayed until the arrival of a medic. The person most likely to provide immediate aid is not the medic but another soldier. Combat leaders understand modern battlefield trauma care concepts and realize that tactical treatment strategies may vary somewhat from trauma care in the civilian sector. All army combatants on the battlefield are trained, equipped, and completely ready to save lives by performing such basic measures such as stopping the bleeding and opening the airway. Greater awareness of the importance of *tactical combat casualty care* (TCCC) on the part of unit commanders is now being reported as a major factor in avoiding these preventable deaths.[8-11]

The combat lifesaver (CLS) is a nonmedical soldier selected by the unit commander for additional training beyond basic first-aid procedures. In accordance with (IAW) AR 350-1, each squad, crew, or equivalent-sized deployable unit has at least one member trained and certified as a combat lifesaver. Combat lifesavers must be recertified every 12 months at unit level. The primary duty of this individual does not change. Functioning as a combat lifesaver is a secondary mission undertaken when the tactical situation permits. CLS training is provided by medical personnel assigned, attached, or in a medical platoon of a maneuver unit. The senior 68W combat medic designated by the commander manages the training program. The Army Medical Department Center and School (AMEDDC&S) proponent for CLS utilized TCCC principles as the foundation of for the CLS course. The CLS course is focused on training soldiers in those skills that save lives in combat: bleeding control, treatment of chest injuries, airway management and the tactical context of care, safe patient extraction, and movement techniques that avoid additional injuries.[10]

The 68W combat medic is the first individual in the medical chain that makes medically substantiated decisions based on military occupational specialty (MOS)–specific training. Combat casualty care is the primary mission of the 68W. The enhanced technical proficiency and medical competency of the 68W combat medic save lives on the battlefield. The current combat medic training program incorporates TCCC principles. TCCC principles have continued to be the primary focus of the combat medic training program. More than 60% of the curriculum is dedicated toward battlefield medicine. The combat medic is uniquely skilled and capable of providing advanced combat casualty care. The 68W MOS critical tasks consist of the treatment skills required to address the three leading causes of battlefield death. These casualty care skills are related to combat trauma assessment, bleeding control, advanced airway management, and needle decompression.[10,12]

68W Advanced Initial Training (AIT) is located at the AMEDDC&S, Fort Sam Houston, Texas. This course is the basic course to teach 68W combat medics critical medical treatment skills and tasks. It is a 16-week course with 17 iterations annually, consisting of 450 students per class for a total of 7600 students each year. The course consists of 7 weeks of Emergency Medical Technician-Basic course, 1 week of limited primary care, 5 weeks of Tactical Medicine, and 3 weeks of Combined Situational and Field Training Exercises. The primary changes to the 68W Program of Instruction from 2001 to 2009 were the incorporation of National Registry Emergency Medical Technician-Basic (NREMT-B) and TCCC. Significant focus has been on Tactical Medicine and battlefield lifesaving care.[13]

Role I begins from point of wounding/injury and ends at the level of the Battalion Aid Station (BAS). At the BAS, a physician, physician assistant, and nurse practitioner are trained and equipped to provide advanced trauma management to the combat casualty. Combat medics support these health care providers. The BAS also conducts routine sick call when the tactical situation permits. Based on input from recent operational experience with 68W combat medics function at the BAS, the army identified the need and resulted in focused additional training of 68Ws on basic principles and techniques of sick call, medication administration, and wound care. 68W combat medics also gained additional training on orthopedics, respiratory illnesses, ear-nose-throat (ENT) disease, and abdominal illness and injuries.[10]

ROLE II

Role II medical treatment is provided by the combat medic, physician or physicians' assistant at the level of the brigade support medical company, the area support medical company, or the forward surgical team (FST) associated with one of the medical companies. At this role, care is rendered and evaluation is made to determine evacuation priority. The Role II MTF has the capability to provide packed red blood cells, limited x-ray, laboratory, dental support, combat and operational stress control, and preventive medicine. The Role II MTF provides a greater capability to resuscitate trauma patients than is available at Role I. Role II assets are located in the following locations:

- Medical company (brigade support battalion), assigned to modular brigades which include the heavy brigade combat team (BCT), infantry BCT, the Stryker BCT, and the medical troop in the armored cavalry regiment.

- Medical company (area support) which is an echelons above brigade asset and provides direct support to the modular division and supports echelons above brigade units.

- Preventive medicine and combat and operational stress control assets are also located in the brigade support medical support company and area support medical company.

Patients who can return to duty (RTD) within 72 hours (1-3 days) or within theater evacuation guidelines are held for treatment. Patients, who are nontransportable due to their medical condition, may require resuscitative surgical care from a forward surgical team collocated with a medical company/troop. A detailed discussion of the FST composition and capabilities is contained in Army Field Manual 4-02.25, employment of forward surgical teams, tactics, techniques, and procedures. The goal is to reach surgical care within 1 hour of injury. FSTs provide immediate, life-sustaining resuscitation and surgery until the patient can reach a higher-level facility for definitive treatment and longer-term care.

Doctrinally, FSTs consist of 20 personnel, including at least three general surgeons, an orthopedic surgeon with supporting nursing personnel consisting of nurse anesthetists, critical care, operative, and emergency nurses, and their health care support personnel. FST personnel are capable of rapid assembly and takedown of the operation. The unit comprises two operating tables and a blood supply. The FST logistically supports up to 30 operations over 72 hours before needing resupply. Forward surgical teams offer a highly effective combination of proximity and capability for patients who cannot be evacuated rapidly to a combat support hospital. Role II provides MEDEVAC from Role I MTFs and also provides Role I medical treatment on an area support basis for units without organic Role I resources.

ROLE III

At Role III, the patient is treated in a medical treatment facility staffed and equipped to provide care to all categories of patients, to include resuscitation, initial wound surgery, and postoperative treatment. This role of care expands the support provided at Role II. Patients who are unable to tolerate and survive movement over long distances receive surgical care in a hospital as close to the supported unit as the tactical situation permits. This role includes provisions for the following:

- Evacuating patients from supported units

- Providing care for all categories of patients in an MTF with the proper staff and equipment

- Providing support on an area basis to units without organic medical assets

ROLE IV

Role IV medical care is found in continental US (CONUS)–based hospitals and other safe havens. Mobilization requires expansion of military hospital capacities and the inclusion of Department of Veterans Affairs (VA) and civilian hospital beds in the National Disaster Medical System (NDMS) to meet the increased demands created by the evacuation of patients from the area of operations. The support-base hospitals represent the most definitive medical care available within the AHS.

In addition, it discusses the difference between MEDEVAC and casualty evacuation (CASEVAC), as well as coordination requirements for and the use of nonmedical transportation assets to accomplish the CASEVAC mission.[13]

TACTICAL COMBAT CASUALTY CARE

War has historically provided an opportunity for medical advancement and innovation. Military medical personnel face the challenge of managing a high volume of severe multisystem injuries, relative to what is encountered in civilian practice. Combat casualty care providers face injury and illness in an austere, wartime environment with unpredictable evacuation times and limited supplies and staff. The frequency of multiple or mass casualties may overwhelm available resources. In addition, medical providers not only care for injured members of the military, but for injuries and illnesses suffered by the local population and enemy combatants. Such challenges have fostered innovation in all aspects of tactical medical training. Since 2001, significant changes in medical training have been implemented for soldiers (warrior tasks and battle drills [WTBD] perform immediate lifesaving measures), combat lifesavers, and 68W combat medics.

An effective combat trauma management strategy depends on an understanding of the epidemiology of death on the battlefield. This is the cornerstone of developing the tactical medical strategy and is essential to ongoing evaluation. This type of analysis defines the direction of future training and research and identifies areas in need of improvement. Modern combat casualty care evolved from investigation of casualty data from Vietnam. Analysis of the Wound Data and Munitions Effectiveness Team (WDMET) database of Vietnam casualties reveal that the majority (85%) of deaths on the battlefield are nonsurvivable (**Figure 70-1**). These

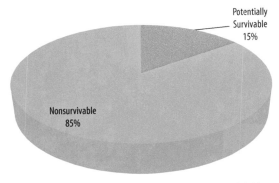

FIGURE 70-1. Percentage of survivable versus nonsurvivable battlefield injuries. (Data from Wound Data and Munitions Effectiveness Team. The WDMET Study. Bethesda, MD: University of the Health Sciences; 1970.)

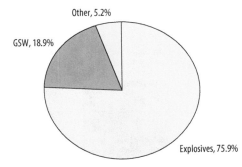

FIGURE 70-2. Percentage of US Military battle injuries in OEF/OIF by mechanism of injury. OEF, Operation Enduring Freedom; OIF, Operation Iraqi Freedom. (Courtesy Joint Theater Trauma Registry.)

casualties have fatal injuries, irretrievable even with the best current tactical medical training, equipment, and treatment. There exists a subset of combat deaths (15%) that are preventable and potentially survivable. The tactical medical training strategy is designed to provide deploying soldiers and health care providers with sufficient medical skills and equipment to treat these potentially survivable life-threatening injuries in all phases of combat.[14,15]

BATTLEFIELD INJURIES AND CAUSES OF DEATH

To improve treatment and develop training for military medical personnel in the combat theater, mechanisms of injury and patterns of combat deaths and treatment provided in the prehospital arena need to be analyzed to direct health care interventions. Critical review of deaths due to trauma is essential for the evolution of the tactical medical training strategy. This is not meant to detract from the accomplishments of combat medics. In some instances, a medic may not have been present when the injuries occurred. The delivery of care on the battlefield is dictated as much by the tactical situation as by the traditional medical necessity. While a casualty may sustain an injury that is considered treatable and from which the soldier should not have died, if this same injury occurs during a fire fight that prohibits a medic or soldier from reaching the casualty, then the injury is potentially survivable but not necessarily "preventable."

The Wound Data and Munitions Effectiveness Team study of Vietnam casualties provided one of the first objective databases to study combat casualties and preventable causes of death. Building on the WDMET concept, the Joint Theater Trauma Registry (JTTR) was developed by the US Army Institute of Surgical Research in partnership with the US Air Force and US Navy, in response to a Department of Defense directive to capture and report battlefield injury.[16] The JTTR is designed to facilitate the collection, analysis, and report of combat casualty care data along the continuum of care, and to make this data accessible to health care providers engaged in the care of individual patients. In addition the JTTR serves as a system analysis and quality improvement tool. Data from medical charts, hospital records, and transport records is gathered, reviewed, and coded. This comprehensive clinical database contains over 40,000 entries to include more than 10,000 battle injuries.[17] With this information, important combat epidemiological questions can now be answered.

Injury patterns and deaths from current theaters indicate that most combat-related injuries occur as a result of penetrating trauma caused by explosions, followed by gunshot wounds. Only a small percentage of battle injuries are related to motor vehicle accidents and other causes (**Figure 70-2**).

Explosions combine primary blast, blunt, and penetrating mechanisms to create multisystem, high-energy injuries with extensive soft-tissue damage, wound contamination, and bleeding from multiple sites. Battle injury patterns demonstrate that the highest rate of injury is to the extremities, followed by the head/neck, torso, and spine/back.

The WDMET has directed military medical research and tactical trauma training in the development of modern combat casualty care. This database identified the primary causes of preventable death on the battlefield: extremity bleeding (9%), chest injuries (5%), and airway obstruction (1%)[14,15] (**Figure 70-3**).

Recent studies confirm many of the WDMET findings, with evidence that compressible bleeding, chest injuries, and airway compromise remain the leading causes of preventable battlefield death in OIF and OEF.[18,19] TCCC is designed to provide both medical and nonmedical soldiers with medical skills to treat these preventable causes of battlefield death.

Combat presents a unique environment and a unique set of constraints on prehospital medicine. Military providers must recognize this unique environment and adjust accordingly to provide care in combat. The inadequacy of applying a civilian prehospital trauma model to tactical situations has long been recognized.[20,21] The TCCC program was initiated by the Naval Special Warfare Command, and later continued by the US Special Operations Command (USSOCOM). This effort developed a set of tactically appropriate battlefield trauma care guidelines that provide combat casualty providers with trauma management strategies that combine good medicine with good tactics.[22] Since then, it has been implemented across all services. Tactical Combat Casualty Care guidelines recognize that trauma care in the tactical environment has three goals:

(1) Treat the casualty.

(2) Prevent additional casualties.

(3) Complete the mission.

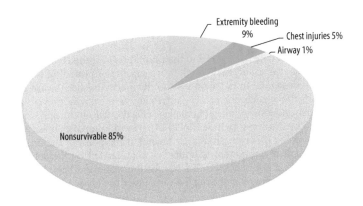

FIGURE 70-3. Primary causes of preventable battlefield death. (Data from Wound Data and Munitions Effectiveness Team (WDMET) database of Vietnam casualties.)

Tactical Combat Casualty Care: Principles

- Phased care in combat based on tactical situation

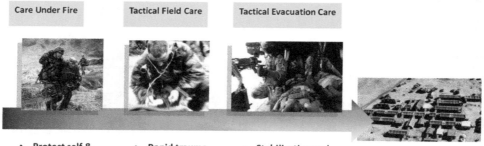

FIGURE 70-4. Principles of tactical combat casualty care.

Using an evidenced-based methodologies approach, TCCC was developed to deal with the unique challenges of battlefield medicine (**Figure 70-4**). The Committee on TCCC is a multiservice and civilian group of trauma specialists, operational medical officers, and combat medical personnel. Its chartered purpose is to monitor updates in the field of operational medicine and update guidelines accordingly.[23]

TCCC is the standard of care for battlefield treatment. Care in combat is focused not just on injuries suffered by the soldier but on the tactical situation surrounding the event. Phased care in combat is a new way to approach care for battlefield casualties. Applying civilian trauma principles in a tactical environment is not only frequently ineffective but may lead to more casualties. Following the principles of Care Under Fire, Tactical Field Care, and Tactical Evacuation Care has saved the lives of soldiers and care providers. The AMEDD has adopted the TCCC principles into all facets of military medical training. These principles are not just for medical providers. These lifesaving principles are incorporated into every soldier's training with warrior tasks and battle drills. In addition, every combat lifesaver is taught TCCC care principles. It was incorporated into the 68W Health Care Specialist Program of Instruction (POI) and has continued to be the primary focus of combat medic initial and sustainment training programs. The guidelines divide casualty care during combat into three distinct phases as follows: Care Under Fire, Tactical Field Care, and Tactical Evacuation Care. The correct intervention must be performed at the correct time in the continuum of operational medicine.

CARE UNDER FIRE

Combat casualty care providers and their units are presumed to be under effective hostile fire, and the care they are capable of providing is very limited. The essential initial action is to return effective fire toward the threat with the specific intent of neutralizing or otherwise preventing hostile personnel from continuing to place effective fire on the unit. Care is rendered by the first responder (WTBD perform immediate lifesaving measure, combat lifesaver, or combat medic) at the point of the injury. Available medical equipment is limited to that carried by the soldier: improved first- aid kit (IFAK), CLS bag, or the medic aid bag. A summary of actions conducted during the care under fire phase includes:

1. Return fire and take cover.

2. Direct or expect casualty to remain engaged as a combatant if appropriate.

3. Direct casualty to move to cover and apply self-aid if able.

4. Try to keep the casualty from sustaining additional wounds.

5. Casualties should be extricated from burning vehicles or buildings and moved to places of relative safety. Do what is necessary to stop the burning process.

6. Airway management is generally best deferred until the Tactical Field Care phase.

7. Stop life-threatening external bleeding if tactically feasible:

   - Direct casualty to control bleeding by self-aid if able.

   - Use a CoTCCC-recommended tourniquet for bleeding that is anatomically amenable to tourniquet application.

   - Apply the tourniquet proximal to the bleeding site, over the uniform, tighten, and move the casualty to cover.

Once these tasks have been accomplished and the unit is no longer under effective hostile fire, this phase of TCCC is complete.

TACTICAL FIELD CARE

Care rendered by the medic once the medic and the casualty is no longer under effective hostile fire. It also applies to situations in which an injury has occurred, but there has been no hostile fire. Available medical equipment is still limited to that carried into the field by medical personnel. Critical to this phase is to treat the three preventable causes of battlefield death: bleeding control, chest injuries, and airway obstruction.

Uncontrolled bleeding remains the largest single cause of combat deaths and accounts for 60% of the preventable causes of battlefield death.[21] Review of Vietnam data attributes over 2500 deaths to preventable extremity bleeding.[14,15] Bleeding must be immediately and aggressively addressed with tourniquets, blood clotting agents, and rapid evacuation. As such, the control of bleeding remains a priority in all phases of TCCC and includes employment of hasty (rapidly applied over clothing) tourniquets as the primary means of controlling significant extremity bleeding.[24,25] After extraction from hostile fire, dressings with blood clotting properties and direct pressure are applied to bleeding sites on the torso that are not amenable to tourniquet application.[26] The recognition of bleeding as the major cause of preventable death has led to a paradigm shift in the approach to the bleeding patient.

Chest injuries causing lung collapse is a potentially life-threatening condition and may rapidly progress to tension, an immediate life threat. The WDMET database showed this injury caused 3% to 4% of all combat deaths and 33% of the preventable causes of death.[27] Recent OIF/OEF studies confirm this injury to be the second most common cause of preventable battlefield death. Temporary treatment consists of needle thoracentesis using a 3.25-in 14-gauge intravenous catheter into the chest. Tube thoracostomy should follow at the earliest possible juncture.[28,29]

Analysis of combat deaths in OIF/OEF revealed airway obstruction to be the third leading cause of preventable battlefield deaths. Approximately 1% to 2% of combat deaths are caused by airway obstruction which is preventable with advanced airway techniques.[30] The combat casualty provider must be able to provide basic and advanced airway support and control. This includes use of basic airway, bag-valve-mask ventilator support, definitive airways, and using a portable mechanical ventilator. The TCCC guidelines recommend surgical cricothyroidotomy as the preferred method to establish a definitive airway during tactical field care for airway obstruction. Time to evacuate to a medical treatment facility may vary considerably.

TACTICAL EVACUATION CARE

Care rendered once the casualty has been picked up by an aircraft, vehicle, or boat. Additional medical personnel and equipment may have been prestaged and available at this stage.

US Army flight medic training and capabilities are significantly lagging behind the accepted civilian standard. In-flight medical care during rotary wing medical evacuation has remained relatively unchanged since the Vietnam War. The US Army flight medic, as a currently trained Emergency Medicine Technician-Basic, has completed the 68W Combat Medic Course and the Flight Medic Course which is a total of 58 classroom hours and an additional 106 hands-on hours of instruction. The current US civilian standard for a paramedic has Emergency Medical Technician-Basic as a prerequisite, and includes 1000 to 1200 hours of instruction, broken down to 500 to 600 hours of classroom/practical laboratory, 250 to 300 hours of clinical, and 250 to 300 hours of field internship. Equipment and training for US Army flight medics are rudimentary compared to civilian standards. No current doctrinal capability exists for intratheater critical care transport of patients following emergency surgery at the forward surgical team . This capability is at present filled by taking nurses from the combat support hospital (CSH) or FST to transport critically ill patients from facility to facility. No standardized quality assurance, patient documentation, or

medical oversight systems exist. Civilian helicopter transport systems have intense oversight from physicians with specific training in prehospital and en route critical care. Army MEDEVAC oversight is from the local flight surgeon who may have minimal experience in prehospital or in-flight critical care.

The US Army Medical Department Center and School (AMEDDC&S) established a medical evacuation integrated capability development team (ICDT) in March 2010 as a result of over 40 after action report comments concerning the medical skill level of flight medics, and a mortality study being conducted by the US Army Institute of Surgical Research. The ICDT discussed and analyzed all capability gaps associated with the flight medic and the lack of a dedicated critical care transport team/skill set for postsurgical patients who require critical care–trained health care professionals. This resulted in a decision brief to the CG, AMEDDC&S, who approved an expanded flight medic training program to close the identified skill gaps with implementation of an EMT-paramedic and required flight critical care skills.

BATTLEFIELD EXPERIENCE

Comparing OEF/OIF to Vietnam, the mortality rate of combat-sustained injury has decreased by 40%.[31] The survival rate in OIF/OEF exceeds 90%.[32] Data are mounting to support the widespread availability of TCCC as a dominant factor in reducing preventable deaths, in addition to rapid evacuation and improved body armor. This has resulted in an estimated 1000 battle-injured lives saved in the current conflict[33] (**Figure 70-5**).

Over the past century, the killed in action (KIA) rate has not changed significantly remaining between 20% and 25%.[31] The KIA rate refers to the percentage of casualties who die *before* reaching a medical facility out of all seriously injured casualties (**Figure 70-6**).

In OIF/OEF, the KIA rate has decreased to 13.8%.[14] Of those KIA, most are nonsurvivable (85%) and irretrievable with the current tactical trauma management. Approximately 15% of combat deaths are preventable. Recent studies report that compressible bleeding (8%), chest injuries (3%-4%), and airway obstructions (2%-3%) remain the leading causes of preventable battlefield death in OIF and OEF. Tourniquet usage has increased and exsanguinations from isolated extremity wounds are no longer the problem that they presented in Vietnam and at the outset of the current conflict. Less than 2% to 3% of combat deaths were due to isolated hemorrhaging extremity wounds amenable to tourniquet, compared to 9% combat deaths in Vietnam.[15] Continued training utilizing TCCC principles is warranted.[34]

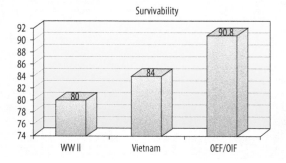

	World War II	Vietnam War	OIF/OEF
% Case Fatality Rate	19.1%	15.8%	9.4%

Survivability

FIGURE 70-5. The mortality rate of combat-sustained injury has decreased since World War II. Survivability is over 90%. (Data from Holcomb JB. Understanding combat casualty care statistics. *J Trauma.* 2006;60(2):397-401.)

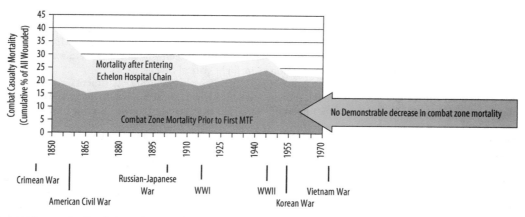

FIGURE 70-6. Combat casualty mortality. Blue shading indicates the part of total casualties that became mortalities before entering the echelon chain (that has been differentiated by the black shading). (Courtesy Defence Advanced Research Projects Agency [DARPA].)

KEY POINTS

- Much of civilian trauma care has evolved out of military medical practices

- The Army Health Service defines Roles of Care to describe the distribution of medical resources and capabilities provided at different locations and environments.

- Role I is unit level medical care that includes maintaining airway, stopping bleeding, preventing shock, protecting wounds, immobilizing fractures, and other emergency measures as indicated.

- Role II is provided by a combat medic, physician, or physicians' assistant at a medical treatment facility capable of initial stabilization and evacuation.

- Role III is provided in a medical treatment facility staffed and equipped to provide care to all categories of patients, to include resuscitation, initial wound surgery, and postoperative treatment.

- Role IV is provided in a hospital in the continental United States and other safe havens.

- The Vietnam casualty data from WDMET revealed that 15% of battlefield deaths were preventable.

- Tactical Combat Casualty Care (TCCC) is designed to target causes preventable death in the field. The phases include Care Under Fire, Tactical Field Care, and Tactical Evacuation Care.

- Mortality has significantly reduced over time for those who make it to the echelon hospital chain.

- Overall mortality rate of combat-sustained injury has dropped significantly since the Vietnam data.

REFERENCES

1. Hecht BK, Lee D. First aid: from witchdoctors & religious knights to modern doctors. Medicine.net.com. http://www.medicinenet.com/script/main/art.asp?articlekey=52749.

2. Boyd D, Edlich R, Micik S. *Systems Approach to Emergency Medical Care.* Norwold, CT: Appleton-Century-Crofts; 1983.

3. Richardson RG. *Larrey: Surgeon to Napoleon's Imperial Guard.* London, England: John Murray; 1974.

4. Welling DR, Rich NM, Hutton JE, Burris DG. Applying the principles of Larrey's flying ambulance: an international military medevac mission. HCP Live. May 25, 2007. http://www.hcplive.com/publications/surgical-rounds/2006/2006-12/2006-12_07.

5. General Orders No. 147, August 2, 1862. In: United States War Department, ed. *War of the Rebellion: A Compilation of the Official Records of the Union and Confederate Armies.* Washington, DC: Government Printing Office; 1880.

6. Munson E. Transportation of federal sick and wounded. In: Miller FT, ed. *Photographic History of the Civil War.* New York: Review of Reviews Co; 1911.

7. Faust, PL. Ambulance corps. In: Faust PL, ed. *Historical Times: Illustrated Encyclopedia of the Civil War.* New York: Harper & Row Publishers; 1986:9-10.

8. 2010 Army Posture Statement, Addendum F, Army Force Generation (ARFORGEN). The Army's core process. https://secureweb2.hqda.pentagon.mil/vdas_armyposturestatement/2010/addenda/Addendum_F-Army%20Force%20Generation%20(ARFORGEN).asp.

9. FORSCOM, US Army. Contingency Expeditionary Force (CEF) Strategy White Paper. AR 525-29. Army Force Generation. March 14, 2011.

10. US Army. Medical Education and Demonstration of Individual Competence. TC 8-800. September 15, 2014.

11. Hooper TJ, Nadler R, Badloe J, Butler FK, Glassberg E. Implementation and execution of military forward resuscitation programs. *Shock.* May 2014;41(suppl 1):90-97.

12. US Army. Army Geospatial Enterprise Concept of Operations for Battle Command-Generating Force Enterprise Activities, Draft v. 1.0. September 23, 2010.

13. US Army. The Army Training Strategy: training in a time of transition, uncertainty, complexity and austerity. October 3, 2012.

14. Bellamy RF. The causes of death in conventional land warfare: implications for combat casualty care research. *Mil Med.* 1984;149(2):55-62.

15. Bellamy RF. Combat trauma overview. *Textbook of Military Medicine;* Office of The Surgeon General at TMM Publications Borden Institute Walter Reed Army Medical Center Washington, DC. 1995:1-42.

16. Eastridge BJ. Trauma system development in a theater of war: experiences from Operation Iraqi Freedom and Operation Enduring Freedom. *J Trauma.* 2006;61(6):1366-1373.

17. Beekley AC, Bohman H, Schindler D. *Combat Casualty Care: Lessons Learned from OEF and OIF.* Eric Savitsky, Brian Eastridge, Borden Institute (U.S.) Office of the Surgeon General, eds. Borden Institute. Fort Detrick, MD.

18. Holcomb JB. Causes of death in US Special Operations Forces in the global war on terrorism 2001-2004. *Ann Surg.* 2007;245(6):986-991.

19. Kelly JF. Injury severity and causes of death from Operation Iraqi Freedom and Operation Enduring Freedom: 2003-2004 vs 2006. *J Trauma.* 2008;64(2):S21-S27.

20. Butler F. Tactical combat casualty care in special operations. *Mil Med*. 1996;161(suppl):3-16.

21. Butler F. Tactical combat casualty care 2007: evolving concepts and battlefield experience. *Mil Med*. 2007;172(11):S1-S19.

22. Butler F. Tactical combat casualty care: combing good medicine with good tactics. *J Trauma*. 2003;54(5):S2-S3.

23. Tactical combat casualty care guidelines. http://www.usaisr.amedd. army.mil/pdfs/TCCC_Guidelines_140602.pdf.

24. Kotwal RS, Butler FK, Gross KR, et al. Management of junctional hemorrhage in tactical combat casualty care: TCCC guidelines? proposed change 13-03. *J Spec Oper Med*. Winter 2013;13(4):85-93.

25. Kragh JF Jr, Burrows S, Wasner C, et al. Analysis of recovered tourniquets from casualties of Operation Enduring Freedom and Operation New Dawn. *Mil Med*. July 2013;178(7):806-810.

26. Achneck HE. A comprehensive review of topical hemostatic agents: efficacy and recommendations for use. *Ann Surg*. 2010;251(2):217-228.

27. McPherson J. Prevalence of tension pneumothorax in fatally wounded combat casualties. *J Trauma*. 2006;60(3):573-578.

28. Givens ML. Needle thoracostomy: implications of computed tomography chest wall thickness. *Acad Emerg Med*. 2004;11(2):211-213.

29. Harcke HT. Chest wall thickness in military personnel: implications for needle thoracentesis in tension pneumothorax. *Mil Med*. 2007;172(12):1260-1263.

30. Mabry RL. Fatal airway injuries during Operation Enduring Freedom and Operation Iraqi Freedom. *Prehosp Emerg Care*. 2010;14:272-277.

31. Holcomb JB. Understanding combat casualty care statistics. *J Trauma*. 2006;60(2):397-401.

32. Gawande A. Casualties of war: military care for the wounded from Iraq and Afghanistan. *N Engl J Med*. 2004;351(24):2471-2475.

33. Defense Health Board memorandum for: Ellen P. Embrey, Deputy Assistant Secretary of Defense, Performing the Duties of the Assistant Secretary of Defense for Health Affairs. Tactical Combat Casualty care and Minimizing Preventable Fatalities in Combat. August 2009.

34. TRADOC, US Army. The U.S. Army Learning Concept for 2015. PAM 525-8-2. January 20, 2011.

Technical Rescue Operations

Derek R. Cooney

INTRODUCTION

Rescue of patients from environments and circumstances that pose uniquely high levels of risk or that require the use of specialized techniques and equipment fall into a special category of medical operations. Although the average EMS physician, or prehospital provider, will not routinely encounter these circumstances, operational medical effectiveness requires some basic knowledge of these rescue types, their hazards, and specific medical challenges.

OBJECTIVES

- Define technical rescue and the major types of technical rescue.
- Describe principles of medical support of general and specific types of technical rescue.
- Describe a practical approach to medical support of general and specific types of technical rescue.
- Discuss EMS physician–specific responsibilities.

TECHNICAL RESCUE

The NFPA standard 1670 defines *rescue* as "those activities directed at locating endangered persons at an emergency incident, removing those persons from danger, treating the injured, and providing for transport to an appropriate health care facility" and *technical rescue* as "the application of special knowledge, skills, and equipment to safely resolve unique and/or complex rescue situations."[1] Although the technical aspects of the rescue described here may be beyond the ability and training of most EMS physicians, the medical aspects of the rescue, and the safety concerns for the rescuers, make this an essential area of awareness for EMS physicians and medical directors. In contrast to rescue, *recovery* operations (retrieval of property or victims' remains) are nonemergency operations and should only be carried out in situations where risk assessment is favorable and operational planning has been completed in a thorough and deliberate manner with all alternatives considered.

In addition to being aware of the capabilities of the agencies operating in the EMS system, EMS physicians should also consider their community and the special features that may call for technical rescue operations. The existence of a mine or caves, open water or rivers, mountainous features, open wells, tall buildings, or other potentially challenging features should be considered. Partnering with municipal agencies, such as the department of public works, department of water, waste management, city planning, and emergency management can aid the medical director and other EMS system leaders engage in the necessary needs assessment.

NEEDS ASSESSMENT

A needs assessment is used to identify the level of response that should be expected of the system and at an agency level (**Box 71-1**). The first step is to perform a *hazard analysis and risk assessment* in order to determine the potential needs of the community. The next step is to consider the *resources and capabilities* of each agency and of the system as a whole. It is possible that a community or system may have identifiable hazards that require technical rescue capability that the system cannot support because of a lack of resources. This should lead to active pursuit of grants, training, or mutual aid agreements with agencies/systems that have the resources available. When considering the development of capabilities to provide a particular technical rescue operation, it is also important to consider the hazard that it is meant to mitigate. In some cases, the

---

Box 71-1

Needs Assessment

- Hazard analysis/risk assessment
- System/agency resources and capabilities analysis
- Hazard-based risk/benefit analysis
- Operational level analysis

risk of rescue attempts may outweigh the potential for rescue. Confined space rescue in some environments may not be worth the risk when the likelihood of survival of the victim is low and the risks to rescuers are high, thus presenting an unfavorable *risk/benefit analysis*. The final consideration, after accounting for the other three, is to determine the *operational level* that is most appropriate. Not every agency should be expected to provide the maximum level of response to every hazard they may encounter; however, it may be appropriate to provide one of the three operational levels for every potential rescue operation that the agency may face during their duties.

OPERATIONAL LEVELS

There are three levels of operationally definable levels provider in the technical rescue environment: *awareness, operations, technician* (**Box 71-2**). Agencies providing rescue services should have written standard operating procedures (SOPs) to address any and all rescue operations to be performed by members of the agency. In addition, these SOPs should address the scope of the agency and the providers at the various levels. *Awareness* level providers are providers who have been deemed to have the minimum level of skill and capacity to respond to a technical rescue. *Operations* level providers are trained to the level required to identify hazards and intervene through the use of equipment and limited techniques. *Technician* level providers are capable of providing advanced techniques and are expected to also be able to coordinate and supervise a technical rescue operations.

FIRST RESPONDERS

Many times, the first on-scene provider(s) may be trained and equipped to the awareness level and should not attempt to initiate technical rescue. EMS physicians who arrive in this capacity should first perform a scene size-up, establish or communicate with command, and then assist in denying entry of less than operations and technician level providers. During this period there should be some attempt to contact victims and perform nonentry rescue procedures. Setting up safety zones should be initiated in order to limit hazards and everyone on-scene should be made aware of *lockout* (method for keeping equipment from being set in motion and endangering workers)[1] and *tagout* (method of tagging, labeling, or otherwise marking an isolation device during hazard abatement operations to prevent accidental removal of the device)[1] procedures. The incident commander should be made aware of the potential resource and rescue needs so that these resources and personnel can be requested. EMS physicians on rescue scenes should work with command and the safety officer to ensure highest level of possible provider and victim safety, including proper PPE for rescuers and victims, air supply/ventilation, and proper medical monitoring/rehab. Knowledge of the

---

Box 71-2

Operational Levels

- Awareness
- Operations
- Technician

technical rescue teams and special operations assets in the community/system is essential.

TRAINING

Personnel require specialized training, equipment, and knowledge to be considered proficient in the various types of technical rescue. Training levels correspond with the operational levels: awareness, operations, technician. It is important to note that in many cases, at the technician level a provider is considered technically proficient in skills but still requiring direction. On the other hand, a provider considered to be a *technical specialist* is technically proficient in skills and also does not require direction and is able to practice independently because they have obtained a level of special expertise in a particular area and are effectively a subject matter expert. As with all other complex skill sets, technician training and status does not necessarily confer proficiency in technical rescue. This requires practice/frequency of operation and continued study and application (NFPA 1670 4.1.5).[1]

OPERATIONAL MEDICINE IN TECHNICAL RESCUE

Medical personnel, including EMS physicians, need to be trained to the operations level or higher if they are to be expected to enter the "hot zone" to perform patient assessment, initiate advanced medical care, and assist with planning of patient extrication. In order for an EMS physician to become a medical expert within a technical rescue operation, they will have to receive the same training as other providers and must spend time training with the full team. In order for the physician to be of the most benefit to the team, they must also be accessible (occupational health, trust issues on scenes), personally train and train with the medical component of the team (to ensure proficiency and trust), and prepare to provide continuous medical surveillance of team members.

PREPLANNING

Size-up and incident management planning occur on the scene of the incident, take into account the specifics of the incident, result in an incident action plan, and are ultimately a function of the command structure. Preplanning is a multifaceted, multidisciplinary function of leadership within agencies and the system as a whole. The preplan for the system should include training events, development of a medical cache, acquisition and maintenance of special operations and safety equipment, and any and all PPE needed for potential operations. The level of preplanning should include medical oversight and involvement of the EMS physician for the development and delivery of medical education/training for medical and nonmedical team members, recognition of the need for medical care by all team members (eg, CPR and first aid), and occupational health for team members (acute and long term). Each known hazard/site within the community should also have a site-specific preplan that includes all operations components (including medical).

IMPLEMENTATION

The planning and implementation phase of the incident begins at the time of the first call and continues through size-up and all the way through until rehab and after action. Initial components of the action plan include gathering important intelligence about the situation (ie, hazards, potential/known victims, potential for rescue/survival, immediately available resources, delay for specialized technical rescue resources if needed). The EMS physician's roles include participation in planning medical and safety aspects of incident response, advising command regarding medical aspects that will have a bearing on rescue/extrication efforts, and coordinating/facilitating patient care and comfort during the rescue. Some direct responsibilities of the physician may include acute care of victims, clinical medical record-keeping, acute care for team members (human and canine), coordination with area EMS/transport agencies (ground and air) and definitive medical care entities (hospitals), and emergency management agencies as necessary. The EMS physician

should be appropriately prepared to coordinate and/or participate in the transfer of care of patients (victims and/or team members as applicable) to definitive care entities and ensure/provide rehab[2,3] for team members during and after the operations are complete.

REHAB AND AFTER ACTION

The same nine components of rehab detailed in Chapter 65 apply for rehab in technical rescue operations.[4] In addition to compiling and reviewing medical records and rehab charts, the EMS physician should follow up on any occupational injuries/illness of team members and prepare a summary for the hot-wash and/or after action report. A detailed review of the medical aspects of the operation should be conducted and adjustments should be made to medical caches, protocols, and policies based on the outcomes. Medical supplies should be restocked and equipment restored and maintained to ensure readiness for the next event.

TYPES OF TECHNICAL RESCUE

NFPA 1670 lists 12 types of technical rescue (**Box 71-3**).[1] In all cases of involvement with technical rescue the proper operation-specific PPE and safety equipment should be used and personnel engaging in the operation should be well trained and qualified and be in appropriate physical and mental health prior to participation.

ROPE RESCUE

Rope rescue scenes are typically those in which the patient is located in an inaccessible location, such as down a steep embankment or on the outside of a structure. *High-angle* rescue refers to rescue operations in which the rope supporting the weight of the rescuer is being used over a surface that is at greater than a 45° pitch/slope (**Figure 71-1**). *Low-angle* rescue is when the rope is still required and holds the weight of the rescuer, but the slope of the ground or working surface is less than 45°. Both high and low angle rope rescue operations are potentially dangerous. Medical personnel participating in a rope rescue need to be trained to the operations level or higher and be prepared to be lowered or transported/supported by ropes to perform patient assessment, initiate advanced medical care, and assist with planning of patient extrication. Safety concerns include issues related to high-angle dangers (falls, edge safety, risk of head injury) and any other hazard that makes a rope operation appropriate. Annual training and verification of proficiency is important in all tasks and skills defined by the NFPA under Chapter 5 of the NFPA 1670 standard.[1] **Box 71-4** lists some of the unique requirements called for by the standard. Due to the demands of the work, rescuers require significant personal

---

Box 71-3

Technical Rescue

- Rope rescue
- Structural collapse search and rescue
- Confined space search and rescue
- Vehicle search and rescue
- Water search and rescue
- Wilderness search and rescue
- Trench and excavation search and rescue
- Machinery search and rescue
- Cave search and rescue
- Mine and tunnel search and rescue
- Helicopter search and rescue
- Tower rescue
- Animal technical rescue

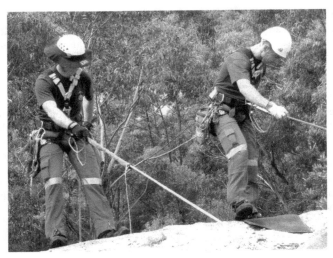

FIGURE 71-1. Rescuers training on rope rescue techniques. (Reproduced with permission from Dr. John Lyng.)

Box 71-4

Rope Rescue: Some Organizational Requirements

Operations Level

1. Establishing the need for, selecting, and placing edge protection

2. Selecting, using, and maintaining rope rescue equipment and rope rescue systems

3. Configuring all knots, bends, and hitches used by the organization

4. Selecting anchor points and equipment to construct anchor systems

5. Constructing and using single-point anchor systems

6. Constructing and using multiple-point anchor systems with regard to the potential increase in force that can be associated with their use

7. Selecting, constructing, and using a belay system

8. Selecting and using methods necessary to negotiate an edge or other obstacle that includes protecting all personnel working nearby from accidental fall

9. Ascending and descending a fixed line

10. Self-rescue

11. Selecting, constructing, and using a lowering system in both the low- and high-angle environments

12. Securing a patient in a litter

13. Attaching a litter to a rope rescue system and managing its movement

14. Selecting, constructing, and using rope-based mechanical advantage haul systems in both the low- and high-angle environments

15. Negotiating a loaded litter over an edge during a raising and lowering operation

Technician Level

1. Accessing a patient using techniques that require rescuers to climb up or down natural or man-made structures, which can expose the climber to a significant fall hazard

2. Using rope rescue systems to move a rescuer and a patient along a horizontal path above an obstacle or projection

3. Performing a high-angle rope rescue of a person suspended from, or stranded on, a structure or landscape feature

4. Understanding and applying the principles of the physics involved in constructing rope rescue systems, including system safety factors, critical angles, and the causes and effects of force multipliers

5. Performing a high-angle rope rescue with a litter using tender(s) to negotiate obstacles, manipulate or position the patient, or provide medical care while being raised and lowered

Reproduced with permission from NFPA 1670-2014, Standard on Operations and Training for Technical Search and Rescue Incidents, Copyright © 2013, National Fire Protection Association. This reprinted material is not the complete and official position of the NFPA on the referenced subject, which is represented only by the standard in its entirety.

---

fitness and technical proficiency. This type of rescue is very technical and requires study and practice with rope work, knot tying, and complete mastery of the mechanical advantage systems, rope rescue systems, fall protection system, edge protection, harnesses, and all other rope hardware and software. In order to ensure patient care needs can be met, it may be necessary to plan on a modular equipment/supply load out so that the rescuer(s) can deliver care without the burden of having to take significant amounts of unnecessary equipment to the patient.

■ STRUCTURAL COLLAPSE SEARCH AND RESCUE

Structural collapse presents many complexities for rescuers (**Figure 71-2**). A number of important size-up features need to be considered: type of structure (light, wood frame vs. steel, and concrete) and cause of collapse (natural disaster, fire, explosion, impact of a vehicle, engineering failure). Control of at-risk utilities and shoring and stabilization of the structure in order to prevent secondary collapse are important components of this type of operation. Medical providers training to be part of an urban search and rescue (USAR) team or to provide other structural collapse search and rescue should be well trained and in good physical condition.[5] Candidates should be screened for claustrophobia, as this may be a disqualifying condition in some cases. Rescuers may need to perform a significant number of tasks and interventions in a confined space with a number of potential hazards. Advanced search, stabilization, patient packaging, and extrication techniques are necessary. Search patterns may be strategically designed based on collapse patterns with anticipated void types where victims might be found alive. Acoustic search devices, thermal imaging cameras, and highly trained canine teams are sometimes needed to located victims. Concerns over fire protection and hazardous materials are real. Special patient concerns include crush injuries/syndrome,[6] compartment syndrome, rhabdomyolysis,[7] hypo- and hyperthermia, dehydration, traumatic amputation, and severe hemorrhage. In some cases the EMS physician may need to consider emergency field amputation or dismemberment of the body of a deceased victim in order to save the patient.[8] USAR teams organized at the state and national level follow a standard model of organization and are expected to provide 24-hour capability and be self-sufficient for 72 hours (**Figure 71-3**).[9] Due to the complexity and risks of structural collapse search and rescue, the organizational requirements and level of rescuer/provider training and preparedness are significant (**Box 71-5**).

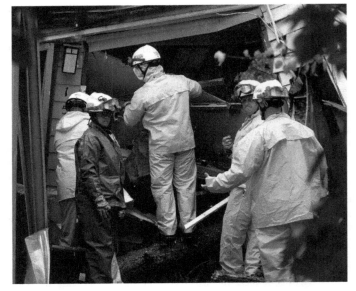

FIGURE 71-2. USAR team investigates a structural collapse. USAR team members investigate a light wood-framed residential structure after collapse caused by a natural disaster. (FEMA News Photo.)

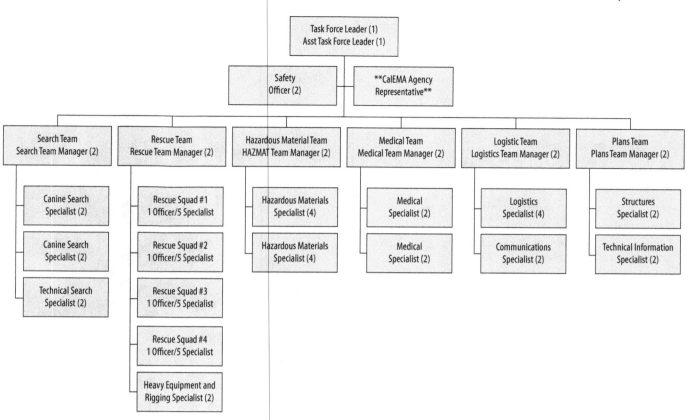

FIGURE 71-3. California USAR Task Force organizational chart.

CONFINED SPACE SEARCH AND RESCUE

Confined spaces are any environment that has limited entry and egress, is not designed for continuous human occupancy, and may be oxygen deficient or contain an asphyxiant or dangerous airborne contaminant. Additional hazards in this environment may be the risk of entrapment (eg, tunnel collapse) or engulfment (eg, grain in a grain silo). One of the primary considerations for the EMS physician is ensuring nonentry by any personnel that is not properly trained and equipped with SCBA or surface-side air. Prevention of the rescuer injury and death is a key concern for response to a confined space incident. Rescuer death and injury from confined space rescue attempts is a well-known threat and yet in 2010 New York suffered the loss of another firefighter during a rescue attempt in a confined space when he was asphyxiated trying to rescue a public works worker who was down a sewer manhole[10] (**Figure 71-4**). The lack of SCBA during these rescue attempts is likely due to the apparent urgency of the rescue and the lack of suitable access while wearing a standard air bottle in the usual fashion. During the initial size-up the location, type of space, and use of the space should be considered and any on-scene workers or employees with knowledge of the operations of the space should be questioned. All attempts should be made to stop asphyxiants and flammable or otherwise harmful substances from entering the area and ventilation efforts should be made if possible.[11] Air metering should be performed and hazardous materials response requested when appropriate. If there is any question of air quality, SCBA or surface-side air should be worn and should be donned prior to approaching the entrance to the space. Medical personnel must have been trained to operations level or higher and be properly equipped and dressed out for entry into the confined space to perform patient assessment, initiate advanced medical care and, assist with planning of patient extrication. Situation-appropriate packaging and transport equipment (eg, SKED, webbing, harness, etc) should be taken into the space if known to be necessary and if operationally appropriate. Additional risks include bite and stings from snakes and stinging insects, heat, loud noise, visibility, water,

hazardous materials, psychological stresses, and physiological stresses of the operation. Continuous medical surveillance of team members is particularly important during confined space rescue operations and a rehab operation should also be set up.

VEHICLE SEARCH AND RESCUE

Significant rescue effort may be needed to free a patient from a motor vehicle collision. Because the patient may need immediate medical intervention, and/or because disentanglement and extrication may represent a prolonged effort, it is important that EMS providers and physicians are well versed with vehicle search and rescue operations and are able to provide medical interventions in a safe and effective manner. Scene safety includes a number of variables to consider: vehicle stability, potential for fire/explosion, electrical shock (especially in hybrid and electric cars), inadvertent airbag deployment, hazardous materials, traffic and roadway hazards, crowd control, and injury from damaged vehicles and debris. Additional hazards may be related to the accident scene (eg, downed electrical lines, collapse risk if vehicle hit a structure, high-angle risks if the vehicle is down a steep embankment) (**Figure 71-5**). Prior to attempting care of the patient, medical providers should confirm that the vehicle is adequately stabilized, they have clearance from fire/rescue personnel to enter the work area, and are wearing appropriate vehicle rescue PPE. Eye and hearing protection should not be omitted and should be considered for the patient as well. Helmet should also be worn. Having some awareness of the types of tools and techniques used by the fire/rescue agency is a crucial component of preplanning for medical response to these scenes. EMS physicians on the scene should ideally wear clearly marked specialized PPE (helmet, protective tech rescue pants/jacket/coveralls) that provides protection and identification. The EMS physician should maintain a global perspective on patient care and protection as well as rescue. Instituting medical interventions to allow safe extrication of the patient may mean providing sedation and/or pain management above and beyond routine protocol doses and in some cases may even require

---

Box 71-5

Structural Collapse and Rescue: Some Organizational Requirements

Awareness Level

1. Recognizing the need for structural collapse search and rescue

2. Identifying the resources necessary to conduct structural collapse search and rescue operations

3. Initiating the emergency response system for structural collapse incidents

4. Initiating site control and scene management

5. Recognizing the general hazards associated with structural collapse incidents, including the recognition of applicable construction types and categories and the expected behaviors of components and materials in a structural collapse

6. Identifying the 13 types of collapse patterns and potential victim locations

7. Recognizing the potential for secondary collapse

8. Conducting visual and verbal searches at structural collapse incidents, while using approved methods for the specific type of collapse

9. Recognizing and implementing a search and rescue/search assessment marking system, building marking system (structure/hazard evaluation), victim location marking system, and structure marking system (structure identification within a geographic area), such as the ones used by the FEMA Urban Search and Rescue System

10. Removing readily accessible victims from structural collapse incidents

11. Identifying and establishing a collapse safety zone

12. Conducting reconnaissance (recon) of the structure(s) and surrounding area

Operations Level

1. Sizing up existing and potential conditions at structural collapse incidents

2. Recognizing unique collapse or failure hazards

3. Conducting hasty primary and secondary search operations (low and high coverage) intended to locate victims trapped on, inside, and beneath collapse debris

4. Accessing victims trapped inside and beneath collapse debris

5. Performing extrication operations involving packaging, treating, and removing victims trapped within and beneath collapse debris

6. Stabilizing the structure and performing rescue shoring operations in order to stabilize the structure, if necessary.

Technician Level

1. Evaluating existing and potential conditions at structural collapse incidents

2. Recognizing unique collapse or failure hazards

3. Conducting search operations intended to locate victims trapped inside and beneath collapse debris

4. Accessing victims trapped inside and beneath collapse debris

5. Performing extrication operations involving packaging, treating, and removing victims trapped within and beneath collapse debris

6. Stabilizing the structure and performing rescue shoring operations in order to stabilize the structure

Reproduced with permission from NFPA 1670-2014, Standard on Operations and Training for Technical Search and Rescue Incidents, Copyright © 2013, National Fire Protection Association. This reprinted material is not the complete and official position of the NFPA on the referenced subject, which is represented only by the standard in its entirety.

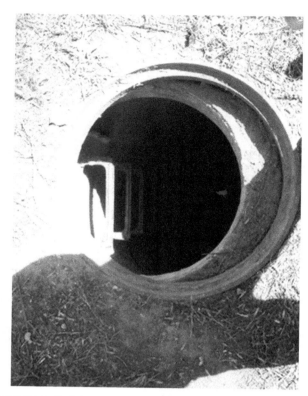

FIGURE 71-4. Manhole where two men died from asphyxiation. From a case report by the state of New York. A firefighter attempted to save a village public works worker without using SCBA and both men died of asphyxiation before they could be rescued. (Reprinted with permission from Douglas Dubner. From the New York State Department of Public Health, Case Report 10NY060. Available at: https://www.health.ny.gov/environmental/investigations/face/10ny060.htm.)

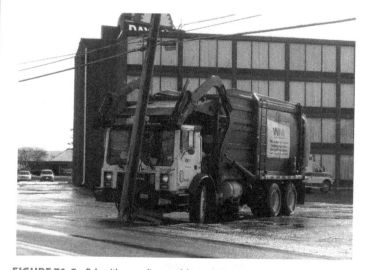

FIGURE 71-5. Pole with power line struck by truck. The driver of the vehicle suffered only minor injuries, but his care was delayed due to concerns around the instability of the high voltage electrical pole that had been driven through. (Reproduced with permission from Dr. Derek Cooney.)

intubation. Having a procedure for carrying and safely storing controlled substances and paralytics, as well as field surgery instruments and other advanced medical equipment, is a key component to responding as an EMS physician to vehicle rescue operations.

WATER SEARCH AND RESCUE

Water search and rescue operations are known to be particularly hazardous and at time deadly to rescuers.[12-14]

A water *rescue* operation is one where a living victim is known (or suspected) to require assistance getting safely free of an environment where the water is deep enough to cause drowning and any of the following exist:

risk for hypothermia, dangerous current, waterborne hazardous materials, obstacles that could cause injury or entrapment, widespread flooding. A water *recovery* operation is one in which the victim is known or presumed to be dead (eg, has not been witnessed to surface >90 minutes) or hopelessly beyond rescue. In addition to open-water rescue, there are four other types that require specialized skill: *swift water rescue, ice rescue, surf rescue, and dive rescue.* First response actions to an immediate open water emergency have been "Reach, Throw, Row, Go" for a significant time and this mnemonic is based on sound common sense. In cases where a rescuer is present and the body of water is still and controlled (like a swimming pool) this strategy may still be sound. Ideally the rescuer would be wearing a personal floatation device even in uncomplicated circumstances. However, for formal operations appropriate PPE is required including an appropriately rated and well-fitted PFD and rescue helmet (especially when there is any risk of swift water or current).

The simplest rescue mantra of "Reach, Throw, Row, Go" is good common sense for untrained providers because it instills some level or awareness. *Reach*—the first step is to attempt a rescue while still firmly on solid ground. If the victim is within reach of a pole, then this should be used to reach to them. *Throw*—the next step would be to throw a floatation device to the victim. Typically this would be a ring or other easily deployed floatation device of the designed and rated for rescue, and that has a water rescue (floating) rope attached so that the victim can be pulled into shore, side of the pool, dock, etc. *Row*—once solid ground options have been exhausted (or do not apply), then utilization of a watercraft is the next step. This mode of rescue requires a greater level of skill and the ability to safely operate a watercraft. In small boats (as is implied by "row") there is the risk of capsizing and the potential for both the victim and rescuer to drown. Bringing about a victim is difficult work and requires some skill and coordination with the victim unless using a watercraft and equipment designed for the task. Another option is to combine *row* with *throw* by throwing the victim a rescue device and bring them to the edge of the boat without bringing them aboard. *Go*—is the last and riskiest component to this method and should only be performed by highly accomplished swimmers with formal lifeguard training. Entering the water in many ways may result in creating a second victim. Victims themselves may drown their rescuer by accident due to panic. This four-part method is primarily for lifeguarding at pools and smaller still water lakes and ponds and is not appropriate for an organized water search and rescue operation. However, the common sense approach of limiting risk to the rescuer is sound.

EMS physicians should be aware that water rescue requires highly technical maneuvers with purpose build equipment (even the boats) and that other types of rescue teams should not be allowed to attempt a water rescue. Even if some of the rope rescue hardware and software seem familiar, the conditions of swift water (**Figure 71-6**), ice, and surf rescue require different training and techniques. When considering dive rescue operations it should be made very clear that this type of rescue is not appropriate for swift water. In addition, only trained and certified public

safety/rescue divers with proper maintenance of their skills, equipment, and dive medical clearance should be involved in dive rescue operations. Divers with recreational diver certification should not be allowed to engage in dive rescue operations. Although most rescue divers are not working at great depth, there is still a risk of dive accidents, which could lead to decompression illness and arterial gas embolism, both requiring immediate treatment in a hyperbaric oxygen chamber. EMS physicians should be aware of the closest available hyperbaric center that provides emergency treatment services. Divers Alert Network (DAN) provides a 24-hour emergency resource for health care professionals and divers: +1 (919) 684-9111/DiversAlertNetwork.org.

Inflatable rescue boats can aid in rescue on open water, rivers, swift water, and even in some cold-water/ice rescue operations. They are relatively lightweight and portable and can achieve operations in shallow waters. The lower sides allow for boat-side rescue and the inflatable nature of the boat allows it to withstand swamping to a greater degree because of the inherent buoyancy of the design. Some rigid-hulled rescue boats also take advantage of this feature with an added "air tube" around the hull. These are referred to as "semirigid" or "rigid inflatable." Rigid inflatables are extremely stable in the water and do not typically capsize like a standard hull row boat might. Recreational boats with standard hulls designed for cruising, fishing, and skiing are not appropriate for this type of operation and commandeering a boat is typically unwise.

Some online introductory courses exist that can aid EMS physicians in gaining initial awareness of the hazards of water search and rescue operations and should be shared with the first responders they work with unless they are otherwise trained (eg, http://www.boat-ed.com/waterrescue/).

WILDERNESS SEARCH AND RESCUE

Wilderness search and rescue operations are multidisciplinary operations that require significant expertise from the medical component. EMS physicians functioning as a component of these operations should have specialized training and experience in order to provide the best possible physician support. Wilderness search and rescue teams should be supported by an appropriately qualified EMS physician.[15] Other aspects of the specific medical concerns in this environment are detailed in Chapter 67.

TRENCH AND EXCAVATION SEARCH AND RESCUE

Any time a trench or excavation is being used, there is the risk of a trench emergency. Soil-pile slides, shoring collapse, cave-ins, and falling rock can all lead to life-threatening emergencies. This unique type of confined space emergency offers many challenges to rescuers. After performing a size-up and setting up a safety perimeter to avoid worsening the collapse, the scene should be assessed for any potential living victims. If any are located, it may be possible to lower breathing air or oxygen, protective equipment, and water. Heavy equipment, shoring, cribbing, air bags, and rope rescue techniques may all be required to affect a rescue. As with confined space rescues care should be taken to divert all water and hazardous materials away from the area. Some other clinical concerns include the potential for hypothermia, traumatic asphyxia, multisystem trauma, airway compromise, crush syndrome, and head injury.

MACHINERY SEARCH AND RESCUE

Sedation and analgesia for victim to facilitate extrication is an important role for EMS physicians to consider, in addition to bleeding control, and potential treatments for the prevention of crush syndrome.[16-18] While many industrial entrapment patients can be extricated by disassembly of the machinery by responders from industry, the medical sector must plan for the contingency that this is not possible or not possible without critical harm to the victim. The extreme alternative is field amputation and EMS physicians must plan and prepare for this contingency in advance. Farm-related injuries can have many of the same clinical features and concerns.[19]

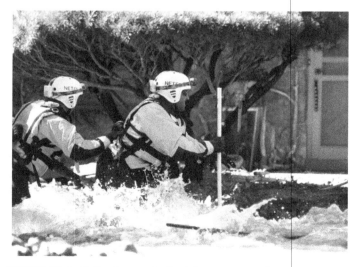

FIGURE 71-6. Swift water poses significant danger to rescuers. Rescuers move across a swift water hazard. (FEMA News Photo.)

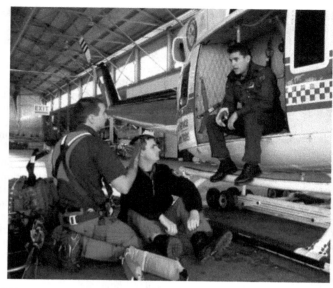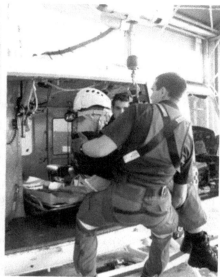

FIGURE 71-7. EMS physician training on air medical rescue techniques. Here an EMS physician (fellow) is being provided hands-on awareness training in preparation for an operational tour with the helicopter retrieval service provided by the Ambulance Service of New South Wales. (Reproduced with permission from Dr. John Lyng.)

CAVE SEARCH AND RESCUE

Caving or spelunking can result in significant injury and at times death. The majority of injuries noted in a recent study by Stella-Watts et al; 1356 victims were identified with 74% of injuries being the result of a fall.[20] The majority were extremity injures with 41% of the injuries being fractures; however, head injuries accounted for 15%. The rescue challenges are significant and include skills and awareness involved in rope rescue, confined space rescue, wilderness rescue, and in some cases water rescue.

MINE AND TUNNEL SEARCH AND RESCUE

Mine and tunnel emergencies include all the elements of confined spaces, structural collapse, and trench collapse. There is a significant risk of hazardous materials in these types of operations and there may even be the need for rescue from machinery. The enhanced concern during caisson operations and pressurized drilling is the risk of decompression illness for workers in these environments and hyperbaric oxygen therapy may be needed to prevent significant neurological injury, further complicating the rescue. In addition to the usual confined space consideration for asphyxiation, significant attention should be played to air quality and safety for rescuers in this environment. Specialized mine rescue training courses are available.[21]

HELICOPTER SEARCH AND RESCUE

The use of rotor-wing aircraft for search and rescue has applications in wilderness and water rescue environments most commonly. Air medical operations are detailed in Chapter 18. Water and wilderness rescue using specialized aircraft with rescue winch capability requires significant training for all members of the team (**Figure 71-7**).

TOWER RESCUE

Rescue from towers (radio towers, cellular towers, etc) is highly technical work. Failure of technique, procedures, or equipment can lead to extreme falls. It is recommended that all operational member of the team be trained and able to show competency in all of the areas listed in **Box 71-6**.[1] This type of rescue involves all of the same high-angle rescue hazards in addition to concerns specific to high voltage and extreme height.

ANIMAL TECHNICAL RESCUE

Although EMS physicians are not expected to serve in the place of veterinarians during rescue operations, it is important that they be aware of

---

Box 71-6

Tower Rescue Operations Level Skill Set

1. Job hazard analysis used on tower sites
2. 100% fall protection
3. Tower anchorages
4. Use of energy-absorbing lanyards
5. Use of work-positioning lanyards
6. Self-retracting lifelines
7. Vertical lifelines for fall arrest
8. Ladder climbing safety systems (cable and rail)
9. Horizontal lifelines
10. Use of a preclimb checklist
11. Tower ladder/peg climbing techniques
12. Transferring between the ladder and the tower structure
13. Selection and use of appropriate rescue equipment and techniques for a given tower rescue situation

Reproduced with permission from NFPA 1670-2014, Standard on Operations and Training for Technical Search and Rescue Incidents, Copyright © 2013, National Fire Protection Association. This reprinted material is not the complete and official position of the NFPA on the referenced subject, which is represented only by the standard in its entirety.

---

some of the technical concerns that affect the animal victims and their human rescuers. Animals in strange and unfamiliar environments, especially when injured and deprived of their usual access to food and water, may find rescuers and equipment threatening and it is important to be aware of potential behavior and posture clues specific to the animal type being rescued. Animal rescue training is required to ensure proper positioning, rigging of harnesses and lines, use of packaging equipment, and recognition of behavioral ques. Training also includes tactics concerning injury avoidance and when and how to attempt containment. Chemical restraint is indicated in some circumstances, however, if the EMS physician should be working and/or communicating closely with a veterinarian or the animal control team if they intend to assist with this aspect of rescue. Basic resuscitation of animals is also an appropriate skill for the EMS physician and other team members to acquire.

- A technical rescue *needs assessment* for each agency and the system should be performed and serve as guidance in development of response plans and resource development.

- The four components to performance of a needs assessment: *hazard analysis/risk assessment, resources and capabilities analysis, risk/benefit analysis, operational level analysis.*

- The NFPA defines standards for operational levels (*awareness, operations, technician*) for the different types of technical rescue.

- EMS physicians working with technical rescue teams should be aware of the level of response being provided and have, themselves, an awareness level training and competency in that area of technical rescue.

- Lockout, tagout, and other scene safety principles should be practiced by all responders and team members. A safety officer should be assigned and should ensure adherence to all safety and operational standards.

REFERENCES

1. NFPA 1670. *Standard on Operations and Training for Technical Search and Rescue Incidents.* 2014 ed. Quincy, MA: National Fire Protection Association; 2014.

2. McEntire SJ, Suyama J, Hostler D. Mitigation and prevention of exertional heat stress in firefighters: a review of cooling strategies for structural firefighting and hazardous materials responders. *Prehosp Emerg Care.* April-June 2013;17(2):241-260.

3. Horn GP, DeBlois J, Shalmyeva I, Smith DL. Quantifying dehydration in the fire service using field methods and novel devices. *Prehosp Emerg Care.* July-September 2012;16(3):347-355.

4. NFPA 1584. *Standard on the Rehabilitation Process for Members During Emergency Operations and Training Exercises.* 2008 ed. Quincy, MA: National Fire Protection Association; 2008.

5. Roth PB, Gaffney JK. The federal response plan and disaster medical assistance teams in domestic disasters. *Emerg Med Clin North Am.* May 1996;14(2):371-382.

6. Hu Z, Zeng X, Fu P, et al. Predictive factors for acute renal failure in crush injuries in the Sichuan earthquake. *Injury.* May 2012;43(5):613-618.

7. Malinoski DJ, Slater MS, Mullins RJ. Crush injury and rhabdomyolysis. *Crit Care Clin.* January 2004;20(1):171-192.

8. MacIntyre A, Kramer EB, Petinaux B, Glass T, Tate CM. Extreme measures: field amputation on the living and dismemberment of the deceased to extricate individuals entrapped in collapsed structures. *Disaster Med Public Health Prep.* 6(4):428-435.

9. Urban Search and Rescue Program. California Fire Service and Rescue Emergency Mutual Aid System. California Emergency Management Agency. http://www.caloes.ca.gov/FireRescueSite/Documents/CalOES%20-%20Fire%20and%20Rescue%20-%20Urban%20Search%20and%20Rescue%20-%2020141201.pdf. Accessed May, 2015.

10. A department of public works worker and a volunteer firefighter died in a sewer manhole (Case Report 10NY060) https://www.health.ny.gov/environmental/investigations/face/10ny060.htm.

11. Dorevitch S, Forst L, Conroy L, Levy P. Toxic inhalation fatalities of US construction workers, 1990 to 1999. *J Occup Environ Med.* July 2002;44(7):657-662.

12. Volunteer fire fighter drowns after being thrown from his swiftwater rescue boat – West Virginia. Death in the line of duty. NIOSH Firefighter Fatality Investigation Program. January 25, 2011. http://www.cdc.gov/niosh/fire/pdfs/face201009.pdf.

13. A fire fighter drowns after attempting to rescue a civilian stranded in flood water – Colorado. Death in the line of duty. NIOSH Firefighter Fatality Investigation Program. April 30, 2002. http://www.cdc.gov/niosh/fire/pdfs/face200102.pdf.

14. Career fire fighter dies while diving for a civilian drowning victim - Rhode Island. Death in the line of duty. NIOSH Firefighter Fatality Investigation Program. October 8, 2009. http://www.cdc.gov/niosh/fire/pdfs/face200832.pdf.

15. Warden CR, Millin MG, Hawkins SC, Bradley RN. Medical direction of wilderness and other operational emergency medical services programs. *Wilderness Environ Med.* March 2012;23(1):37-43.

16. Cohen B, Laish I, Brosh-Nissimov T, et al. Efficacy of urine alkalinization by oral administration of sodium bicarbonate: a prospective open-label trial. *Am J Emerg Med.* December 2013;31(12):1703-1706.

17. Scharman EJ, Troutman WG. Prevention of kidney injury following rhabdomyolysis: a systematic review. *Ann Pharmacother.* January 2013;47(1):90-105.

18. Sanadgol H, Najafi I, Rajabi Vahid M, Hosseini M, Ghafari A. Fluid therapy in pediatric victims of the 2003 bam, Iran earthquake. *Prehosp Disaster Med.* September-October 2009;24(5):448-452.

19. Simpson SG. Farm machinery injuries. *J Trauma.* February 1984;24(2):150-152.

20. Stella-Watts AC, Holstege CP, Lee JK, Charlton NP. The epidemiology of caving injuries in the United States. *Wilderness Environ Med.* September 2012;23(3):215-222.

21. Mine rescue training. Mine Safety & Health Program. Colorado School of Mines. http://inside.mines.edu/MSH-underground-SaR.

CHAPTER 72

Hazardous Materials Response

Derek R. Cooney

- Describe PPE types and appropriate use of each.
- Describe decontamination operations.
- Describe the resources, equipment, and methods available for product/hazard identification.
- Describe factors impeding medical operations in a hazardous materials environment.

INTRODUCTION

A hazardous material is defined as "a substance (either matter - solid, liquid, gas - or energy) that when released is capable of creating harm to people, the environment, and property..." and may mean little to most EMS providers and medical directors in their daily practice, despite that they are all around us.[1] In addition to the recognition that hazardous materials are common components of our personal and occupational lives, it is important to consider the potential of a large-scale hazardous materials (HAZMAT) incident in any EMS system. Most EMS physicians are well versed in the occupational component of hazardous materials as it pertains to the Occupational Safety and Health Administration (OSHA) regulations that apply to the work environment but may not be fully prepared to respond in support of a hazardous materials incident operation and may not even be familiar with the principles laid out in 29 CFR 1910.120 (Hazardous Waste Operations and Emergency Response: HAZWOPER) or the availability of various publications on the topic provided by OSHA, NIOSH, FEMA, and the EPA. HAZMAT incidents occur in all areas affecting every community (**Figure 72-1**). This chapter will serve as a primer aimed at the EMS physician as a component of the response to a HAZMAT incident.

OBJECTIVES

- Discuss basic principles to the approach to a hazardous materials incident.
- Discuss some specific concerns based on different types of hazards.

ROLES OF THE EMS PHYSICIAN

Response to serious, large-scale, hazardous materials incidents is not a common operational event for the average EMS physician. Special training and experience are key components to a successful hazardous materials operation. Although most EMS physicians are not HAZMAT technicians there are still roles for a physician responding to these events (**Box 72-1**). Because of the importance of these physician-specific roles, those EMS physicians that are HAZMAT technicians should not become involved in the operation inside the hot or warm zones unless there is a specific and unusual medical intervention that can only be provided by the physician. The EMS physician is expected to serve as a medical content expert in all areas of prehospital care and toxicology is no exception. Serving as on-scene medical control for the sick and injured victims of a serious HAZMAT-associated incident allows providers to provide toxin-specific care without complicated radio communication and it also allows for rapid communication of special needs (eg, antidotes and secondary decontamination preparation) to the receiving hospital(s) and emergency management officials who can locate and potentially mobilize certain stockpiles. When medical and traumatic conditions coexist with a serious HAZMAT exposure, the EMS physician may also aid providers in prioritizing care goals (ie, rapid treatment and transport verses standard decontamination). In cases of mass casualty HAZMAT exposures, the physician may also aid in adjusting the triage values of patients who may normally be deemed immediate (red tag) in the standard triage

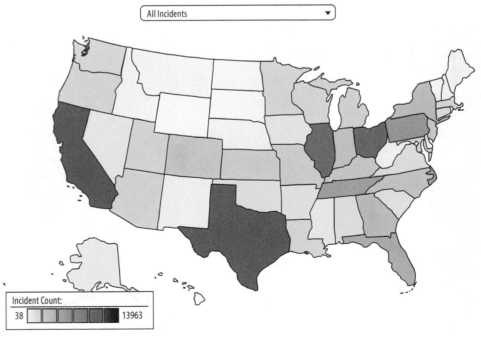

U.S. Department of Transportation
Pipeline and Hazardous Materials Safety Administration
Office of Hazardous Material Safety
2005–2014 Incident Map

All Incidents ▼

Incident Count:
38 ▭▭▭▭▭▭ 13963

Source: HAZMAT Intelligence Portal, U.S. Department of Transportation. Data as of 9/1/2014.

FIGURE 72-1. US Department of Transportation Pipeline and Hazardous Materials Safety Administration Office of Hazardous Material Safety 2005–2014. (Reprinted from http://phmsa.dot.gov/HAZMAT/library/data-stats/incidents. Accessed September 1, 2014.)

Box 72-1

Roles of the EMS Physician at a Serious HAZMAT Incident

1. Serve as on-scene medical control
2. Provide expertise in toxicology and treatment priorities
3. Assist in triage and treatment in mass casualty incidents
4. Provide additional support of health and safety of providers through rehab operations

Box 72-2

Potential Types of HAZMAT Exposure

1. Agriculture/farm accidents
2. Industrial accidents
3. Transportation accidents/spills
4. Fires (residential and commercial)
5. Criminal activity (drug labs, arsonist supplies, and bomb making)
6. Terrorism
7. Chemical suicide

(START and JumpSTART), but due to their exposure are unlikely to survive regardless of intervention. In some cases a nonbreathing expectant (black tag) individual may be deemed immediate (red tag) if the toxic exposure is known to be a that is easily reversed (eg, aerosolized fentanyl) (SALT triage). In addition to this role as a content expert, every operational activity that places a heavy physiological demand on the rescuers (like fire ground, tactical, and HAZMAT operations) should have some attention paid to provider rehabilitation (rehab). The EMS physician may need to serve as an advocate for, and play some part in, establishing a rehab station/revolution during the operation. In order to allow for success in these roles, the EMS physician must be involved in the preplanning for these types of events and have a working familiarity with key operational stakeholders. The EMS physician and/or medical director should be involved in disaster and operational response planning and actively seek out training and drill opportunities.

SERIOUS HAZARDOUS MATERIALS INCIDENTS

Serious exposures and/or large-scale incidences can occur in a number of circumstances and locations in a community (**Box 72-2**). Such exposures are significant as they may represent the ongoing presence of an environment that poses and immediate danger to life and health (IDLH). Agricultural and industrial environments are common places to encounter large amounts of hazardous materials in use and in storage. Farm and factory accidents can lead to large-scale exposure and the potential for numerous and/or very serious human exposures. Transportation of hazardous materials occurs through every community with roads, railroad tracks, pipelines, or waterways (**Table 72-1**, **Figure 72-2**). Large capacity containers are common in all forms of local, interstate, and international transportation of these substances. Other important exposures to consider are those encountered during fires (residential and commercial)

TABLE 72-1 Hazardous Materials Incidents by Mode of Transportation in 2012

Mode of Transportation	Incidents
Waterway	70
Railway	662
Highway	13,242
Air	1,460
Total	15,434

Data from HAZMAT Intelligence Portal, U.S. Department of Transportation Pipeline and Hazardous Materials Safety Administration.

and during EMS calls, especially where clandestine drug labs operate or bomb-making activity has been planned or performed. Acts of terrorism, both foreign and domestic, represent significant HAZMAT threats, especially when rescue and medical treatment goals may cause tunnel vision among emergency personnel. Another HAZMAT treat to the public and responders is the intentional creation of toxic gas or other dangerous materials for the purpose of suicide and EMS physicians should be well versed in these trends.

HAZARDOUS MATERIALS

The Department of Transportation (DOT) has defined classes of hazardous materials in an effort to categorize like materials and establish general patterns of handling and hazard mitigation. The DOT defined nine

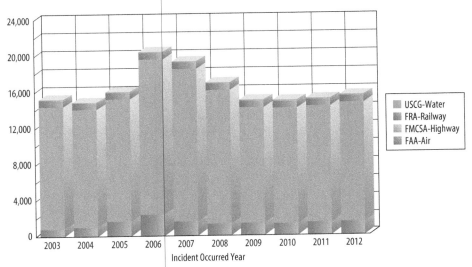

FIGURE 72-2. Hazardous materials incidents by mode of transport 2003–2012. (Data from the HAZMAT Intelligence Portal, U.S. Department of Transportation Pipeline and Hazardous Materials Safety Administration.)

categories depicted in **Table 72-2**. Another way to consider hazardous materials is by their general category describing the key type of hazard when exposed to humans: chemical, biological, radiological/nuclear, and explosive (CBRNE). Hazard risks from different classes or types of materials are also described under the DOT class as having one of more of five hazard risks. These are thermal, radioactive, asphyxiation, chemical, etiological, and mechanical (TRACEM).[2] Thermal refers to heat damage (eg, burns). Radioactive refers to all radiological injuries (acute and chronic). Asphyxiation risk is due to a materials ability to cause displacement of oxygen, or the rendering of the lungs incapable of exchanging gases. Chemical risk refers to a materials activity when interacting with substances that make it react in a hazardous way, or to the reaction it has when in contact with humans (eg, creation of toxic fumes during a reaction, chemical burns). Etiological risk refers a substances potential to cause disease (eg, cancer). Mechanical risk is any associated mechanical force or injury applied to humans relative to the other properties of the substance (eg, shrapnel from the explosion of the container, blast wave from an explosion).

■ CHEMICAL

Gases (DOT Class 2) pose at times extreme danger due to their ability to rapidly expand if heated or otherwise improperly released. Flammable and combustible liquids (DOT Class 3) may cause significant heat release, or result in a boiling liquid expanding vapor explosion (BLEVE).

Flammable and combustible solids (DOT Class 4) may pose significant risk due to their ability to burn in the correct conditions, and many of them are unstable in wet environments, like when sprayed with a hose or washed from a patient with wet decontamination techniques. Oxidizers (DOT Class 5) are also potentially exothermic in that they can cause rapid reactions in the presence of oxygen, or by removing it from the air. Toxins (DOT Class 6) can take many forms and can be very potent in concentrations found in industrial usage. Strict decontamination practices are required to avoid secondary contamination. Corrosives (DOT Class 8) are acids and bases and are very dangerous to skin, eyes, lungs, and may react violently when exposed to certain substances. Miscellaneous (DOT Class 9) can be any hazardous substance not meeting the other definitions. In many cases the substance is hazardous in certain situations during transport, due to temperature or its potential effects on drivers or pilots if they were exposed during operation of the vehicle.

Clandestine drug labs pose a unique, potentially occult, threat to rescuers and prehospital providers. The chemicals used in the "cooking" of methamphetamine, for example, present significant hazards, as do the by-products of the "cook" (**Box 72-3**).[3] Typically responders should be on the alert when a collection of chemicals, cleaners, or other industrial use materials are found in the kitchen or living spaces, especially when cooking equipment, scales, and industrial/chemistry glass implements are also noted. Low technology setups are also common and may be in the bathroom, closet, or even in a bag or the trunk of a car.

TABLE 72-2	**DOT Hazardous Materials Classification**	
Class	Characteristics	TRACEM Risk(s)
1—Explosives *Examples: dynamite, fireworks*	• Detonates of deflagrates by contact with spark, flame, or friction • Usually contains nitrogen	T—heat energy due to detonation A—fire may deplete available oxygen E—blood and body part exposure M—shock wave, shrapnel, falls, crush
2—Gases *Examples: propane, anhydrous ammonia,*	• Significant expansion and contraction depending on pressure and temperature	T—cryogenic gases, and gases rapidly expanding, can cause severe cold injury A—may displace oxygen
3—Flammable/combustible liquids *Examples: gasoline, kerosene*	• Flammable = flashpoint <100°F (37.7°C) • Combustible = flashpoint 100–200°F (37.7-93.3°C)	T—large amount of heat energy released C—hydrocarbons and carcinogens M—shrapnel from containers
4—Flammable/combustible solids *Examples: white phosphorus, grain silo dust, combustible metals*	• Fine particulate matter with low ignition temperatures • Substances that undergo spontaneous combustion • Organic material undergoing decay	T—fire and exothermic reactions C—produce caustic vapors M—shrapnel from containers
5—Oxidizers *Examples: ammonium nitrate, hydrogen peroxide*	• Chemicals that can release oxygen or use oxygen in the air • React easily with other chemicals • May react at or just above room temperature	T—exothermic reactions C—toxic by-products during reactions M—shrapnel from containers from explosive failure
6—Toxic and infectious substances *Examples: pesticides, cyanide, ricin, HIV*	• Poisons, biotoxins, infectious agents, medical waste • Toxic effects are based on concentration, length of exposure, and individual sensitivity • Published LD50 and LC50 values	C—toxic by inhalation, absorption, ingestion, injection E—may be utilized in terrorism
7—Radioactive *Examples: Cesium-137, Cobalt-60, Plutonium-239, Technetium-99m*	• Specific activity greater than 0.002 microcuries per gram (μCi/g) • Nuclear materials, industrial sources, nuclear medicine materials	T—thermal burns R—biological effects are related to type and dose of exposure
8—Corrosive *Examples: sulfuric acid, hydrofluoric acid, lye*	• Corrodes steel or aluminum faster than 0.246 in (6.25 mm) a year at a temperature of 131°F (55°C) • Burns and irritation • Lungs very susceptible	T—exothermic reaction C—injures by reacting with the tissues
9—Miscellaneous *Examples: dry ice, PCBs, molten sulfur*	Potentially hazardous depending on the situation	TRACEM—dependent on specific materials

A, asphyxiation; C, chemical; E, etiological; M, mechanical; R, radioactive; T, thermal.

Hazardous Materials of Clandestine Drug Lab Precursors

Acetic anhydride (*irritant, corrosive*)

Anhydrous ammonia (*rapid asphyxia*)

Benzene (*blood disorders; carcinogen*)

Chloroform (*altered mental status [AMS]*)

Cyclohexane (*irritant*)

Ethyl ether (*irritant, AMS*)

Ethanol (*flammable*)

Hydrogen cyanide (*rapid asphyxia*)

Hydrochloric (*irritant; corrosive*)

Hydriodic acid (*irritant; corrosive*)

Hypophosphorous acid (*corrosive*)

Iodine (*oxidizer; corrosive*)

Lead acetate (*blood disorders*)

Lithium aluminum hydride (*water reactive, explosive*)

Mercury chloride (*irritant; corrosive*)

Methylamine (*corrosive*)

Petroleum ether (*AMS*)

Phenylacetic acid (*irritant*)

Piperdine (*corrosive*)

Red phosphorus (*reactive; explosive*)

Safrole (*carcinogenic*)

Sodium metal (*water reactive; corrosive*)

Sodium hydroxide (*corrosive*)

Thionyl chloride (*water reactive; corrosive*)

By-products

Phosphine gas (*poison gas; flammable gas*)

Hydriodic acid (*corrosive*)

Hydrogen chloride gas (*poison gas; corrosive*)

Phosphoric acid (*corrosive*)

Yellow or white phosphorus (*reactive; explosive; poison*)

Cryogenic liquids (*frost bite*)

Water reactive metals (*reactive; explosive*)

Flammable solvents (*flammable*)

Some Infectious Agents Bacterial

Anthrax (*Bacillus anthracis*)

Plague (*Yersinia pestis*)

Tularemia (*Francisella tularensis*)

Brucellosis (*Brucella melitensis, Brucella suis, Brucella abortus, Brucella canis*)

Q Fever (*Coxiella burnetii*)

Viral

Smallpox (*Variola virus*)

Eastern equine encephalitis (*EEE virus*)

Hemorrhagic fever (*Ebola virus*)

Acquired immune deficiency syndrome (*human immune virus*)

Chronic viral hepatitis (*hepatitis C virus*)

Toxins

Staphylococcal enterotoxin B (some *Staphylococcus*)

Ricin (castor beans)

Botulinum (*Clostridium botulinum*)

Mycotoxins (*Fusarium, Myrotecium, Cephalosporium, Trichoderma, Verticimonosporium, Stachybotrys*)

■ BIOLOGICAL

Biological hazardous material can include medical waste (DOT Class 6), laboratory waste (DOT Class 6), or even infectious agents (DOT Class 6). In the case of a planned act of violence these may be attached to a bomb or otherwise may have been weaponized for use in bioterrorism (**Box 72-4**). Infectious agents and bioterrorism are covered in Chapter 48.

■ RADIOLOGICAL/NUCLEAR (DOT CLASS 7)

Radiological and nuclear hazards are of constant concern for law enforcement, national security agencies, and emergency management organizations. EMS physicians must know the basics of response to radiological emergencies.

Radiation Types The broad classification of radiation that affects our view of medical threat is that of nonionizing and ionizing. Ionizing radiation is biologically significant due to the fact that it has a high frequency and short wave length, and carries enough kinetic energy to liberate an electron and ionize the affected atom or molecule. Direct damage or indirect damage through the formation of free radicals leads to dysfunction in DNA and molecular machinery. Acute and long-term effects are related to the dysfunction that follows the exposure including cell killing, mutations, chromosomal aberrations, oncogenic transformation, and alteration of gene expression. Stochastic effects are accumulative and include risk of cancer, decline in microvasculature leading to radiation-induced soft tissue wound healing issues, and teratogenesis. Nonstochastic effects include burns, hair loss, cataract, hemopoietic syndrome, gastrointestinal syndrome, and central nervous system dysfunction.

Ionizing Radiation There are different types of ionizing radiation to consider: α, β, γ, x-ray, and neutrons. α Particles are positively charged particles with a high linear energy transfer and a very short penetrance and are very dangerous if ingested. β Particles are high energy electrons emitted from a nucleus and vary in energy. β Particles are not as efficient as α particles at ionizing, but penetrate up to 2 to 3 m in air, but cannot penetrate deeper than the skin. γ Radiation is emitted from the nucleus and penetrates many meters through air and may require lead or concrete shielding. X-rays are emitted from outside the nucleus and are usually created by bombarding a target with electrons until target electrons change energy shells. They can also be emitted from a radioactive material and have similar penetrating effectiveness to that of γ radiation. Neutrons are uncharged particles that have deep penetration and are present inside nuclear reactors (**Figure 72-3**).

Units of Measure The most basic way to measure radiation would be to consider exposure, which tells us only the ionization component and is typically relayed in roentgen or coulomb. Radiation risk to humans is usually discussed in terms of absorbed dose and equivalent dose. Absorbed dose is the absorption of radiation energy per unit mass of the absorber of ionizing radiation and the equivalent dose represents the biologic risk of damage from that dose. The units associated with absorbed dose are the Gray (Gy = 1 J/kg) and the rad (rad = 100 erg/g) and the units for equivalent dose (absorbed dose X radiation weighting factor) are rem and sievert (Sv = 100 rem). The rad (radiation absorbed

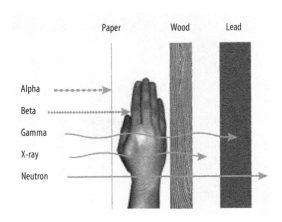

Paper   Wood   Lead

Alpha

Beta

Gamma

X-ray

Neutron

FIGURE 72-3. Ionizing radiation. (Reproduced with permission from Canadian Nuclear Safety Commission. Working Safely with Nuclear Gauges. Ottawa, Canada: Canadian Nuclear Safety Commission; 2007: Figure 2.)

dose) is equal to 0.01 J/kg. The rem (radiation equivalent in man) is equal to the biological damage expected from absorption of 0.01 J/kg.

$$1\,Gy = 100\,rad$$
$$1\,mGy = 100\,mrad$$
$$1\,Sv = 100\,rem$$
$$1\,mSv = 100\,mrem$$

These units are extremely helpful and easily equate to controlled exposures in the medical setting (such as radiology or nuclear medicine) and in nuclear power facilities where excessive monitoring and safety programs have led to detailed understanding of the risks to humans. Unfortunately, in the HAZMAT response scenario, this is no likely to be the case and the EMS physician is more likely to be given information in the form of counts per minute (CPM) from radiological survey meters. This is the time for consultation of a health physics expert because there is not really a direct conversion to dose rate. Typically, the radiological survey meter (Geiger counter) displaying CPM is relaying the number of atoms in the radioactive material that are detected to have decayed in 1 minute based on a calibration to Cesium-137 (Cs-137) and therefore 120 CPM on the meter (for Cs-137) is about 1 μSv/h (microsievert per hour) or 0.001 mSv (0.1 mrem). The usual cutoff for detection of the presence of radiological contamination is >100 CPM. This means there is likely more than background radiation present. In order to estimate, the dose rate (dose per minute) is essential to consult with a health physics expert. If a health physics technologist is present and can estimate dose/minute, then this may be used to calculate estimated dose and in ALARA calculations for rescuers (http://www.radprocalculator.com/ALARA.aspx). It is important to note that rescuers with an estimated potential risk of receiving over 25,000 mrem should be involved in life-saving activities and be made aware of the risks. They must be volunteers at this level of exposure. In addition, it is important to consider that the risk of ingested radioisotopes represents a much higher risk from internal exposure when compared to external exposure to radiation. This risk should be relayed to all rescuers and, as with all HAZMAT operations, no eating, drinking, or touching of the face or mucous membranes should occur in areas where primary or secondary contamination may be present.

Exposure and Contamination It is important to recognize that exposure and contamination mean very different things. *Exposure* refers to the radiation absorption of a person who has been in the presence of a radioactive source or material. *Contamination* refers to a situation in which the person has the radioactive material on their person or inside of them. Internal contamination (from ingestion, inhalation, absorption, or injection/impalement/shrapnel) is more dangerous than external contamination due to incorporation of substances into organs and bone and

due to prolonged exposure from the contamination that cannot be easily removed. External decontamination takes time to be done carefully and techniques to limit the spread of contamination take precedence (after medical treatment concerns). A primary decontamination should occur in the field; however, patients requiring transport and treatment should be decontaminated at the hospital during or after treatment. Exposure to a radiological material does not result in the patient becoming radioactive and uncontaminated patients can be cared for without threat to the health and safety of rescuers and providers.[4]

ALARA ALARA stands for *as low and reasonably achievable*, and refers to the strategy of utilizing three factors to limit exposure to the lowest possible amount during the operation. With the aid of a health physicist, the time, distance, and shielding for operational tasks may be determined. Because dose is determined by the total absorption as a factor of *time*, limiting the time has a major impact on reducing risk. Due to the drop of in dose with *distance* based on different materials type of radiation and energy this is also a major component of limiting risk. *Shielding*, although seemingly important to most rescuers, is not a practical component of PPE in most scenarios. The donning of lead aprons would have a significant negative impact on rescue operations without significant reduction in overall health risk. Examples of shielding that make more sense include placing shielding over the source when possible and taking cover behind objects that may block some of the harmful radiation (walls, buildings, vehicles). ALARA calculations should be a component of all radiological emergency rescue operations and safe limits only exceeded when there is obvious risk to life that can be remedied by rescue, and when rescuers are aware and consent to the risk.

Sources of Radiological Material Although there is significant concern among members of the public over radiological material used and stored at nuclear energy facilities and those moved over the roads and railways, these materials are closely tracked and regulated by governmental agencies: The US Nuclear Regulatory Commission (NRC), the US Environmental Protection Agency (EPA), the Food and Drug Administration (FDA), the US DOT and state governments. During emergencies involving this industry immediate emergency response and mobilization of assets (both governmental and industry related) will likely occur. However, there are other sources of radiological material in the community that are less well controlled despite regulatory guidance. Food irradiators (Cesium-137), welding/industrial radiography equipment (Iridium-192), oncology services (Cobalt-60, Iodine-131, Technetium-99m), nuclear medicine services (Iodine-131), and medical imaging (Technetium-99m) are all potential sources if radiological materials. Industrial sources can be extremely dangerous and may not be particularly well maintained or secured in some cases. This leads to concerns over the theft and use of these sources in criminal activity (assassination, murder, assault) and terrorism with high- or low-level explosives as a contamination delivery method (dirty bomb). Nuclear detonation is unlikely, however, there are small thermonuclear devices still unaccounted for.

PPE Providers, rescuers, and EMS physicians should obtain appropriate levels of radiological emergency training in the proper equipment, and protective clothing procedures. Dosimeters are very helpful tools during this type of operation and are crucial to personal safety and in assisting medical command personnel in making important operational decisions. The Oak Ridge Institute for Science and Education (ORISE) Radiation Emergency Assistance Center/Training Site (REAC/TS) maintains educational materials and training courses for emergency responders, physicians, and other health care providers and key personnel (https://orise.orau.gov/reacts).

Antidotes *Uptake prevention*—Washing mucous membranes and increasing bowel motility can reduce uptake of certain radioisotopes. Some agents will bind radioisotopes in the gut and hasten fecal elimination, thus avoiding uptake and the need for urinary elimination. *Dilution and blocking*—overwhelming receptors and diluting out the radionucleotides results in washout and delay/prevention of end-organ uptake and increased elimination by the body's normal physiological mechanisms (eg, administering potassium iodine to dilute and compete against radioactive iodine for binding sites on the thyroid). *Mobilization*—enhancing elimination through altering physiological parameters is sometimes employed for specific contaminations (eg, urine – alkalization increases elimination of uranium and acidification increases elimination of radiostrontium). *Chelation*—in specific radionucleotide ingestions, in specific circumstances it may be beneficial to use chelation therapy. However, chelators may have a number of undesirable effects and should only be given on recommendation of a qualified expert. Selection and delivery of antidotes require expertise and consultation with health physics experts. Sustained events may offer time for this type of consultation. The EMS physician should then relay this information to receiving hospitals and emergency management and health department officials in cases of widespread contamination.[5]

Key Resources in a Radiological Emergency

- Radiation Emergency Assistance Center/Training Site (REAC/TS) 1-865-576-1005
- US Department of Energy Radiological Assistance Program Regional Coordinating Offices (**Figure 72-4**)
- Local hospital radiation safety office that is usually on-call for emergencies and is a member of the Nuclear Medicine Department
- Local nuclear energy facility that may send their survey and response team if available

■ EXPLOSIVES (DOT CLASS 1)

The effects of explosives and the approach to the scene of a known detonation are discussed in Chapter 77 in greater detail. It is important to note that in addition to the effects of the blast, there are also the concerns related to the unspent explosives, by-products, or combustion, and the potential for intentional dispersal of a hazardous material by way of explosives. When evaluating a scene of a detonation, and patients exposed to that scene, it is important to consider the possibility of the presence of chemical, biological, and radioactive materials. Recognition of explosive materials and their packaging can also aid in improving the safety of any emergency response operation. It is possible that explosives may be present on the scene of a fire or medical emergency and basic knowledge of their appearance may serve to save the lives of the physician and fellow responders. Immediate notification of the bomb squad

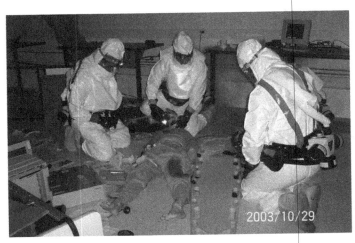

FIGURE 72-4. U. S. Department of Energy Radiological Assistance Program Regional Coordinating Offices. (Reprinted with permission from Blumen IJ, Rhee JW. Radiation emergencies. In: Strange GR, Ahrens WR, Schafermeyer RW, Wiebe RA, eds. *Pediatric Emergency Medicine.* 3rd ed. New York, NY: McGraw-Hill; 2009:chap 143.)

and tactical withdrawal from the scene is necessary in order to mitigate risk to responders. Some providers may choose to take a calculated risk if rapid rescue is necessary for immediate care of life-threating conditions in already identified patients who can be rapidly extracted from the area. There is always the possibility of the existence of a "secondary device" and/or booby traps planted at the scene when terrorism or other criminal activity is at the root of an incident.

COMPONENTS OF A HAZARDOUS MATERIAL RESPONSE OPERATION

Every organization and every member of a response system must be familiar with their system/agency operational parameters, usually referred to as standard operating procedures (SOGs). Although SOGs will vary between systems and agencies, response to a HAZMAT incident should include the same basic components. The orchestration of personnel from fire, EMS, law enforcement, HAZMAT, and emergency management, and other governmental and commercial entities requires a specific locally designed plan in order to reach the level of detail required for interoperability and safe practices. These plans should include components relating to the following key operational components: isolation and protection, identification, decontamination, rescue and medical care, containment, and investigation (**Box 72-5**).

ISOLATION AND PROTECTION

The first concern is isolation of the incident and protection of life, property, and the environment. David Lesak developed a system known by its pneumonic, GEDAPER.[6] Incident commanders for HAZMAT operations are expected to follow these steps when attempting to gain initial control and operational effectiveness at the scene: gathering information, estimating course and harm, determining strategic goals, assessing tactical options and resources, planning and implementing actions, evaluating, reviewing. Although the physician is not likely to be the incident commander, they should understand the process that is occurring and know that they may be asked to participate. The first component of isolation and protection is to manage the scene from a safety perspective.

■ SCENE MANAGEMENT

Upon arrival all personnel should exercise caution and avoid taking unnecessary risks. In general, providers should approach the scene uphill and upwind and take care to note environmental clues: wind direction, unusual odors, leakage, vapor clouds, fire and other hazards. Before making an approach, use binoculars to observe the scene from safe distance. When approaching, avoid driving through leakage or vapor clouds and do not enter incident area until it has been determined that it is safe. If trained and equipped, providers may attempt to detect and identify materials involved (technician level and above only). Based on indicators and available detection data, the next step is to assess risk to self and other rescuers including the potential for fire or explosion. Safe distances and zones (hot, warm, cold) should be established, along

---

Box 72-5

Components of a HAZMAT Response

1. Isolation and protection
2. Identification
3. Decontamination
4. Rescue and medical care
5. Containment
6. Investigation

with a command post, decontamination corridor(s), and triage areas. Law enforcement should assist in control of the area and establish clear routes for ambulances and additional rescue and operations vehicles.

COMMAND

In all cases, the responsibility for safety of all potentially endangered persons is considered a command responsibility. Prior to the establishment of zones, areas for protected operation are defined, followed shortly by establishment of hot, warm, and cold zones by HAZMAT technicians and personnel (**Figure 72-5**). These zones will remain in effect for the remainder of the incident.

Hot zone: directly contaminated area and any surrounding area exposed to gases, vapors, mist, dust, or runoff. Responders and vehicles outside this zone except for trained personnel wearing the proper protective clothing.

Warm zone: the larger area that surrounds hot zone represents a safer working environment that still requires protective clothing. Initial triage, decontamination, and most other EMS activities performed in this zone for higher acuity patients.

Cold zone: surrounds the warm zone and is restricted to emergency personnel, but by definition requires a much lower level of personal protective equipment (PPE). This is the location of the command post, staging, rehabilitation area, and other support personnel.

The decontamination area should be set up as a corridor from the perimeter of the hot zone and extending through the warm zone from the edge of the hot zone and up to the edge of the cold zone. Ideally the decontamination corridor should be close to a water source, downwind from the command post and upwind from the Hot Zone, located away from environmentally sensitive areas, and the medical monitoring/rehabilitation area should be located near the terminal end.

PROTECTION OF RESCUERS

Avoidance of life-threatening exposures to rescuers is a key component of any hazardous materials response operation. Some operational considerations are proper identification, knowing permissible exposure limits, monitoring weather and other environmental conditions, utilizing appropriate personal protective equipment , instituting effective decontamination practices, and ensuring control of the scene. Positioning of vehicles, command posts, decontamination corridor and staging of ambulances and other rescuers are also important considerations. Training for responders as defined by NFPA 472 outlines the different levels of training needed for different levels of providers, as well as outlines the following tactical objectives: incident response planning, communication procedures, response levels, site safety, control zones, PPE, incident mitigation, decontamination, and medical monitoring.[7] The four levels or training include first-responder awareness, first-responder operations, hazardous material technicians, hazardous materials specialists, and on-scene incident commander. NFPA 472 helps define the minimum skills, knowledge, and standards for training outlined in HAZWOPER and discusses EMS provider training and response preparation.[8] Provider rehabilitation should also be a medical consideration. Chapter 65 contains a section of firefighter rehabilitation that applies to HAZMAT operation rescuers as well.

PERSONAL PROTECTIVE EQUIPMENT

Standard precautions should be considered in any patient care situation. If there is a risk of splash, then mask, gloves, and gown (if available) should be worn. In cases where contact with known, unknown, or penitentially present hazardous materials is possible, the appropriate level of HAZMAT suit should be donned. There are generally four levels of protection. Levels A, B, and C are chemical/HAZMAT suits and the fourth level (D) is standard operations attire (with standard precautions) or any other appropriate and available protection. Level D is usually what first

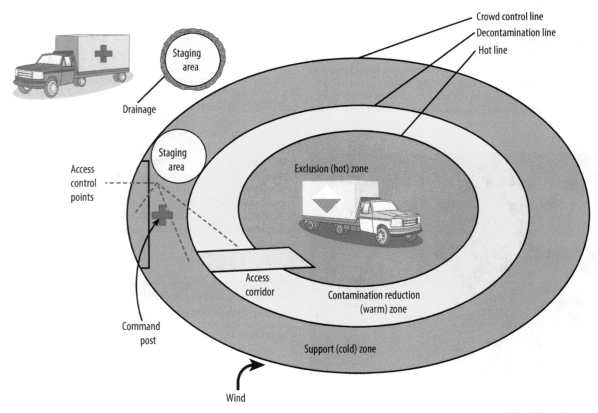

FIGURE 72-5. HAZMAT scene management. (Reprinted with permission from Kaufman BJ. HAZMAT incident response. In: Nelson LS, Lewin NA, Howland M, Hoffman RS, Goldfrank LR, Flomenbaum NE, eds. *Goldfrank's Toxicologic Emergencies.* 9th ed. New York, NY: McGraw-Hill; 2011:chap 130.)

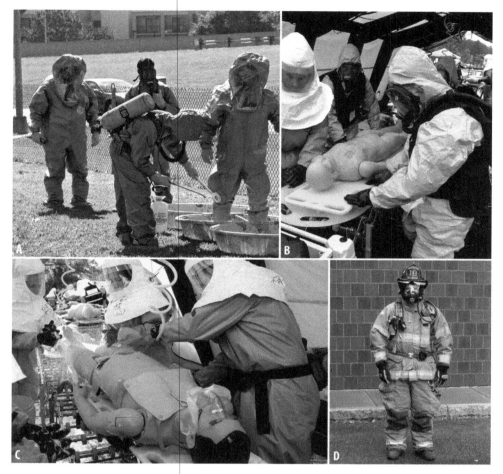

FIGURE 72-6. Personal protective equipment: Levels A, B, C, and D. **A**: Providers in gray suits are in Level A protection while those in green are in Level B. **B**: Providers in silver are in Level B and provider in tan is in Level C. **C**: Providers in tan are in Level C. **D**: Provider in D is in Level D—turnout gear does not provide significant protection from hazardous chemicals.

responders will have available on their initial arrival at the scene. Levels A to C will arrive with HAZMAT team members (**Figure 72-6**).

Level A: Indicated when the greatest level of protection is required due to the danger of exposure to unknown chemical hazards or levels above the IDLH or greater than the AEGL-2. Protects against respiratory and skin risk. Self-contained breathing apparatus (SCBA) or special supply line with escape bottle is required for use of Level A suits. The suit is a totally encapsulating chemical protective suit that provides protection against chemical agents in the air and from direct contact. Wearing the suit without SCBA or supplied air can cause suffocation. This level is reserved for trained HAZMAT technicians.

Level B: Indicated when the greatest level of protection is required due to the danger of exposure to unknown chemical hazards or levels above the IDLH or greater than the AEGL-2. Protects against respiratory risk, but has a lesser protection for the skin. Self-contained breathing apparatus or special supply line with an escape bottle is required to reach the level of protection of a Level B suit.

Level C: Indicated when there is an identified substance with known concentrations that allow for the use of powered air purifying respirator (PAPR) or an air purifying respirator (APR). Level C suits are usually used for decontaminating at the scene or for secondary decontamination. The suit and hood are chemical resistant.

Level D: This level of protection really includes EMS uniforms, flight suits, turnout gear, and standard precautions. Standard gloves, eye shields, masks, and protective clothing (even firefighting gear) are not considered chemical resistant and offer little to no hazardous material protection. This level is only appropriate for cold zone work.

HAZARDOUS MATERIAL IDENTIFICATION

Hazardous materials identification is a key step in response to an incident and if done correctly, can provide significant operational guidance to rescue, HAZMAT, and medical components of the response. A number of resources have been developed by governmental, regulatory, and professional organizations. The existence of multiple identification and labeling systems can complicate the identification for those not possessing proper training, knowledge, and access to reference materials. The EMS physician must have some operational understanding of these systems, but more importantly, must know how to access and utilize references during an event. The physician's role as medical content expert may be underserved without this basic knowledge.

▓ LABELING

Significant resources and development have resulted in labeling and identification methods that are now also a regulatory requirement, not just in the United States, but in many developed countries. EMS physicians must understand the basic configurations of these labeling systems in order to utilize the many available resources described later in this chapter.

DOT Hazard Label The US Department of Transportation hazard warning label for the identification of hazardous materials is represented by classes (**Figure 72-7**). Each substance is assigned a class and many times further categorized into a subclass. These allow identification of hazards to responders and the public during accidents. These can be used to derive operational guidance when used in conjunction with guidebooks and databases described later in the chapter. Specifications

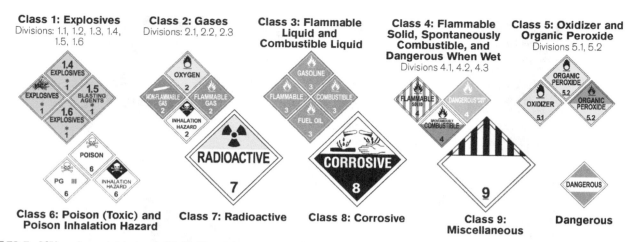

FIGURE 72-7. DOT hazardous materials placards. (Modified from Federal Motor Carrier Safety Administration. http://www.fmcsa.dot.gov/sites/fmcsa.dot.gov/files/docs/Nine_Classes_of_Hazardous_Materials-4-2013.pdf.)

described in 49 CFR 172 require labeling of shipping packages, tank trucks, tractor trailers, and railroad cars.

CHRIS Code The US Coast Guard utilizes a three-letter code system to identify individual chemicals. These can be used in conjunction with the Chemical Hazards Response Information System (CHRIS) manual, or the online Hazard Assessment Computer System (HACS), or by telephone to technical support personnel located at Coast Guard headquarters.

NFPA 704 The National Fire Protection Agency (NFPA) has developed a graphical and text designation that appears as a diamond-shaped placard that is usually found on, or inside, buildings. The placard is coded with colors and numbers that indicate the level of the chemical's health, flammability, and instability hazards, along with special hazards such as water and air reactivity (**Figure 72-8**).

United Nations Numbers The United Nations (UN) Committee of Experts on the Transport of Dangerous Goods has adopted a four-digit number that identifies chemicals with similar characteristics. These can be found on shipping papers and sometimes on placards or labels. The system was adopted from a US DOT system and the numbers are known as UN numbers or North American (NA) numbers or DOT numbers.

Safety Data Sheet The Occupational Safety and Health Administration requires that safety data sheet (SDS), formally the materials safety data sheets (MSDS), be available to employees for potentially harmful substances handled in a workplace. This document is typically supplied by the manufacturer. It contains information pertaining to the handling, storage, and emergency response to exposure. The SDS is also required to be made available to local fire departments, emergency responders, and local and state emergency planning officials.

■ HAZARDOUS MATERIALS REFERENCES
Guidebooks

Emergency Response Guidebook (Department of Transportation): This guidebook, also known as "the orange book" was developed for first responders to use during the initial phase of a dangerous goods/hazardous materials transportation incident. It is intended for firefighters, police, and other emergency services personnel who may be the first to arrive at the scene of a transportation incident involving a hazardous material. The guidebook is conveniently sized and is also available as a PDF or as an application for smart phones and mobile devices.

NIOSH Pocket Guide to Chemical Hazards: The pocket guide is a source of general industrial hygiene information on several hundred chemicals/

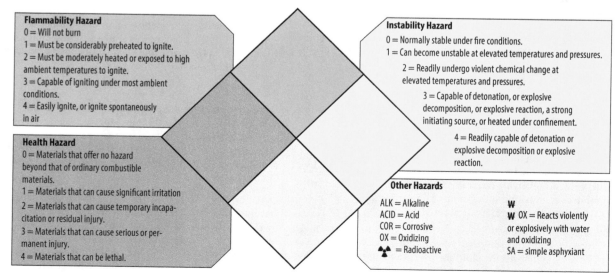

FIGURE 72-8. NFPA 704.

classes found in the work environment. Key data provided for each chemical/substance include name (including synonyms/trade names), structure/formula, CAS/RTECS Numbers, DOT ID, conversion factors, exposure limits, IDLH, chemical and physical properties, measurement methods, personal protection, respirator recommendations, symptoms, and first aid. Free copies and a downloadable version can be obtained from the CDC Web site.

Call Centers

CHEMTREC: 24-hour emergency assistance center that provides critical information for identification and operational response to hazardous materials events. (800) 424-9300

American Association of Poison Control Centers: Poison centers provide medical management advice and have toxicologists on-call for consultation. Poison centers may be able to connect the EMS physician with important stakeholders with access to antidote stockpiles. In some situations, a medical toxicologist may be available to aid medical care at receiving facilities. (800) 222-1222

National Response Center: Provides information and federal response to large-scale spills. Contacting the hotline can potentially lead to mobilization of significant assets: Federal On-Scene Coordinators (FOSC), Regional Response Team (RRT), Coast Guard National Strike Force (NSF), Coast Guard Public Information Assist Team (PIAT), EPA Environmental Response Team (ERT). (800) 424-8802.

Databases and Other Information

Wireless Information System for Emergency Responders (WISER): An on-line database that provides information on the identification, chemical properties, health risks, and operational response to hazardous materials. A desktop version as well as smart phone and mobile applications versions are also available (http://wiser.nlm.nih.gov/).

Computer-Aided Management of Emergency Operations (CAMEO): An on-line database from the EPA that provides information on the identification, chemical properties, health risks, and operational response to hazardous materials. There is also an interface that allows mapping with air dispersion modeling. A desktop version as well as smart phone and mobile applications versions are also available (http://www.epa.gov/oem/content/cameo/).

Public Health Emergency Preparedness and Response: Information site that provides facts, description, and emergency response information from CDC related to the bioterrorism, chemical emergencies, radiological emergencies, mass casualties, natural disasters and severe weather, and outbreaks and epidemics (http://emergency.cdc.gov/hazards-specific.asp).

The Emergency Response Safety and Health Database (ERSH-DB): Developed by NIOSH and provides information on high-priority chemical, biological, and radiological agents that could be encountered by personnel responding to a terrorist event (http://www.cdc.gov/niosh/ershdb/).

Toxicology Data Network (TOXNET): A search engine designed by the National Library of Medicine that allows access to several databases on toxicology, hazardous chemicals, environmental health, and hazardous materials releases (http://toxnet.nlm.nih.gov/).

DETECTION

▓ HAZARD LEVELS

EMS physicians may be informed of certain values during detection work. These should be interpreted by qualified HAZMAT personnel and the meanings/risks relayed to the physician and other providers to allow proper medical operational planning to occur.

IDLH—immediately danger to life and health

LD-50—lethal dose, 50% of individual will die at this exposure dose

ppm/ppb—parts per million/parts per billion of air concentration

PEL—permissible exposure limit below which operations may proceed

TLV-C—threshold limit value-ceiling level

TLV-STEL—threshold limit value-short-term exposure limit

LEL—lower explosive limit

LFL—lower flammable limit

▓ DETECTION EQUIPMENT

A number of specialized pieces of detection equipment may be employed at the scene. These should be operated by qualified personnel and the results require interpretation in consultation with HAZMAT technicians and the correct databases or medical experts (ie, toxicologist or health physicist).

Combustible gas indicators (CGI): measure concentrations of gas in the area and can be used to establish the presence of a concentration. Using known values for the lower explosive limit (LEL) or lower flammable limit (LFL) of certain substances, HAZMAT technicians determine the level of risk.

Gas meters: oxygen meters may be used to check for asphyxiant gases or oxygen-poor environments. Carbon monoxide and hydrogen sulfide meters are also available.

Photoionization detectors: detect the presence and concentration of volatile organic vapors. Although they detect the presence of a volatile substance, they do not provide identification.

Ion mobility spectroscopy (IMS) meters: used to detect explosives, drugs, chemical agents, nerve agents, and mustard agents: Improved chemical agent monitor (ICAM), Advanced Portable Detector (APD) 2000,

Radiological survey meters: radiation survey meters, namely the Geiger-Müller counter (Geiger counter) measures α, β, and γ radiation.

Laser spectroscopy detection equipment: recent advance in technology has led to specialized equipment with various processing and filtering methods that utilize algorithms and include databases of known chemical and explosive compounds, allowing identification without taking samples. This advanced equipment is not typically available and would likely only be available with response from specialized teams.

DECONTAMINATION

Decontamination takes place at the scene and likely prior to entry into a health care facility in many cases. Dry and wet decontamination may be required. Prioritizing medical care over decontamination will occur and may limit the type level of decontamination. At the scene, a decontamination corridor is set up moving from the hot zone to the cold zone. Only simple lifesaving interventions should occur prior to decontamination (airway management, control of major hemorrhage, certain antidotes). Providers in proper protective suits provide dry and wet decontamination of victims and rescuers in an assembly line fashion. After removal of clothes (at least down to undergarments) and all dry contamination are removed (to best level), a detergent and water solution with a pH of 8 to 10 is used to clear the individual from head to toe (when standing). Removal of clothing may remove 80% to 90% of contamination. Copious rinsing follows. Nonambulatory patients should be decontaminated front and back, head to toe. For victims, care is needed to ensure not to injure skin and wounds and they must be protected from cold at the end. Every reasonable effort to protect privacy should occur. Rescuers in suits should undergo a nine-step technical decontamination (**Figure 72-9**). In some cases, it may be operationally necessary to do a mass decontamination with spray from a fire engine or ladder truck. This technique can provide a *gross decontamination* of a large group of ambulatory victims in cases of nonwater reactive substances that do not pose a significant threat to the environment. Secondary decontamination may be required at the hospital and EMS providers may need to assist in the decontamination upon arrival.

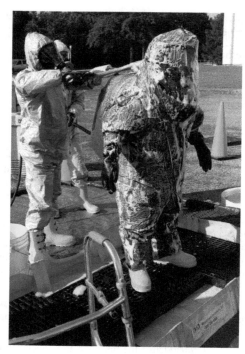

FIGURE 72-9. Decontamination.

RESCUE AND MEDICAL CARE

Rescuers must maintain order and persist with a well laid out plan in order to achieve operational success and avoid rescuer injury and/or death. When triaging mass casualties it is important to consider moving green tag patients to a safe area within the hot zone if the potential continued exposure does not pose a significant risk. Ideally, decontamination should occur as soon as possible, in order of those most severely in need. Moving a large group through the decontamination corridor can be difficult, even when they are ambulatory. Providers must determine whether a cursory decontamination and movement of triage activities to the warm zone is beneficial. After this step, those who are most severely injured (immediate) can be have treatment initiated and transport if decontamination has reduced the risk enough for providers to do so in Level D protection in an enclosed space (no dangerous off-gassing). Those who are not injured, or who have only minor injuries, can undo further decontamination and progress down the corridor to the cold zone. Patients who are expectant, and the deceased (gray, black, navy), should likely stay in the zone they are found until viable patients have been initially decontaminated and treated. If comfort care is available, it should be done in the hot or warm zone prior to decontamination until there is space in the decontamination corridor, warm zone, and eventually the cold zone. In the case of such a large number of victims, it may be appropriate to request and attempt deployment of additional decontamination assets.

Medical care of these patients should first focus on life threats, and traumatic and medical conditions may take precedent. Hazardous materials–related illness should be treated based on the best available information (identification data and physical symptoms) and be focused on acquiring and administering an antidote if one exists and is clinically relevant.

BIOLOGICAL EFFECTS

All organ systems may be affected by hazardous materials, in a number of different ways, based on the properties of the substance (**Box 72-6**).[9]

ACUTE EXPOSURE

Acute and chronic exposures to hazardous materials cause health effects and may present in different ways. Due to the nature of a HAZMAT response operation, the overwhelming majority of medical effects considered by the responding EMS physician will be due to acute exposures. Although acute exposure includes those lasting up to 14 days, most are much more brief and concentrations may vary from small to extremely high. Clinical symptoms from exposures can be immediate, or may also present much later.[10]

◼ CARDIOVASCULAR

Cardiovascular collapse can occur in severe exposures to some chemicals. Both excitatory and depressant effects may occur depending on the substance(s) involved. Hydrocarbons can cause sensitivity of the myocardium to catecholamines (β-agonists, pressors), leading to ventricular ectopy and dysrhythmias (ventricular tachycardia, ventricular fibrillation). Hypoxia from direct effects of the solvents on the lung, or from aspiration, may lead to worsening of the effects. Supportive care with oxygen, airway management, fluid resuscitation and keeping the patient as calm and comfortable as possible are the key elements of care.[11]

◼ RESPIRATORY

Irritant gases may lead to rapid induction of inflammation of the linings of the respiratory tract. Pulmonary edema and asphyxia can also occur. With significant exposures, upper airway obstruction may occur. Depending on the particular properties of the substance, it may result in different symptoms and time of onset. Chlorine and ammonia are water soluble and will typically affect the upper airways. Substances that are not as soluble (or insoluble) in water typically affect the lower airway. Phosgene gas has mild effects acutely and victims can develop noncardiac pulmonary edema at 12 to 36 hours after exposure. Indirect effects to the respiratory system include the risk of aspiration from central nervous system depressants and substances that induce seizures or vomiting. Supportive care should include oxygen, airway management, and consideration for transfer to a center with advanced critical care, pulmonary services, and extracorporeal membrane oxygenation (ECMO) capability.[12]

◼ GASTROINTESTINAL

Direct gastrointestinal irritation may lead to vomiting and diarrhea, leading to dehydration. If ingested, caustics can cause bleeding and potential perforation of the alimentary tract. In most cases, ingestion of unknown or specific chemicals does not warrant use of charcoal, gastric lavage, or whole bowel irrigation, and in some cases these interventions are strictly contraindicated. Supportive care with fluid hydration,

---

Box 72-6

Examples of Substances With Different Biological Effects[9]

Irritants (eyes, lungs, skin)	Chlorine and ammonia gas
Respiratory agents (lungs)	Hydrogen sulfide (H_2S)—paralyzes the breathing
Sensitizers (lungs, skin)	Chromates in printing ink pigments
Hematopoietic agents (blood)	Benzene and aniline damage the blood cells
Anesthetics (CNS)	Methanol, isopropyl alcohol (IPA), toluene
Hepatotoxic agents (liver)	Chlorinated hydrocarbons
Nephrotoxic agents (kidneys)	Cadmium
Simple asphyxiants (blood)	Methane, ethane, propane, butane, pentane, nitrogen, carbon dioxide
Chemical asphyxiants (blood)	Carbon monoxide, cyanides
Corrosives	Acids and bases
Carcinogen	Benzene and asbestos

oxygen and airway management are the most appropriate prehospital interventions.

NERVOUS SYSTEM

Central Some chemical exposures cause direct suppression of the central nervous system (CNS). Anesthetic gases, alcohols, opioids, and organic solvents can all act on the CNS. Altered mental status, headache, weakness, dizziness, stupor, and coma, as well as respiratory depression are all concerns with CNS depressants. Some chemicals cause CNS excitation leading to agitation, delirium, seizures, and hyperthermia. Supportive care, airway management, inhibition of seizures, and use of antidotes when appropriate are the main prehospital care considerations.

Peripheral Peripheral nervous system (PNS) effects from exposure to certain chemicals can lead to alteration of sensation (paresthesia), loss of distal tone and findings of weakness in major muscle groups (can be ascending), decrease or loss of reflexes may all occur acutely or progressively over the next several days. Supportive care and airway management if respiratory muscle fatigue is noted are the main prehospital care considerations.

RENAL

A number of hazardous chemicals can cause nephrotoxicity leading to direct effects on the kidneys. Others may lead to rhabdomyolysis, also potentially leading to kidney failure. In some cases, aggressive fluid resuscitation may be adequate therapy; however, alkalization or acidification of the urine may be indicated in specific exposures.

HEPATIC

Hepatotoxicity does not typically become clinically apparent for several days. Some chemical exposures have direct toxic effects on the liver that can lead to liver failure, delirium, clotting defects, and death. Supportive care at the scene may not have any effect on the outcome of some exposures of this type.

HEMATOLOGICAL

Some exposures directly affect hemoglobin, binding oxygen sites and changing the properties of the hemoglobin leading to ineffective oxygen delivery to end organs. Some lead to hemolysis or even bone marrow suppression. In cases of carbon monoxide exposure or induction of methemoglobinemia, oxygen therapy and transport to the hospital for aggressive therapy is key. Mixed poisonings may occur with carbon monoxide exposure, such as cyanide in the case of structure fires. In this case both exposures should be treated. Some organic solvents, in addition to their other toxic properties, release CO during metabolism (eg, methylene chloride).

METABOLIC

Acidosis and electrolyte abnormalities secondary to chemical exposures can be severe and lead to myocardial dysfunction and dysrhythmias. Supportive care with oxygen and fluids is the first-line care for these patients. In cases where ECG changes are noted and hyperkalemia is strongly suspected, glucose, insulin, albuterol, calcium, and bicarbonate may be initiated. This should be based on ECG findings and the proper exposure history. In some uncommon circumstances, point-of-care testing may be available to evaluate electrolytes, lactate levels, blood gases, and pH.

DERMAL

Irritants and corrosives can cause immediate burns. Acids typically cause more superficial burns in comparison to strong bases that are known for penetrating deeply into tissues that may last for hours. Other chemicals may readily penetrate skin and become systemically absorbed (like organophosphates) and result in illness without obvious direct effect on the skin itself. Decontamination of the skin with water and mild detergents is usually the first step in prehospital care of dermal exposures.

OCULAR

Irritants and caustics are particularly problematic for the eyes of exposed individuals. Direct injury from the chemicals may cause severe, deep burns (eg, strong bases) and in some cases blindness may be caused by chemical exposure. Washing the eyes with copious amounts of saline and transport to a facility with ophthalmology services is likely the most important prehospital care.

CHALLENGES TO CARE

Movement in chemical protective suite and the utilization of respiratory protection may limit providers' and EMS physicians' ability to provide care to victims. Typically only simple immediate lifesaving maneuvers are attempted by rescuers in Class A and even Class B suits. Rapid primary decontamination of seriously ill victims is usually recommended in order to deliver these patients to the warm or cold zone to allow medical care to be provided without need of these higher level suits, thus improving the capabilities of care providers.

TREATMENT WITH ANTIDOTES

Choosing to treat hazardous materials victims with an antidote depends on proper identification of the substance causing the condition. In cases where a particular substance is suspected, the toxidrome should match the exposure. When this is not the case, EMS physicians should consider the coexistence of other medical conditions and the possibility of trauma. Toxidromes are described in more detail in Chapter 46. Common antidotes are listed in **Table 72-3**. It is important to note that most antidotes will not be available in the prehospital setting without activation of HAZMAT teams, emergency management, or the utilization of disaster response plans for the mobilization of a stockpile or cache. In addition to local or regional caches developed as the result of disaster planning, the DHHS has a program known as CHEMPACK. The CHEMPACK program is a function of the CDC's Division of Strategic National Stockpile (SNS) which can provide antidotes to nerve agents and was envisioned as a medical countermeasure in the event of an attack on civilians with nerve agents.

CONTAINMENT

The scene must be contained and bystanders and other nonresponders must be kept clear of the area and the scene. Law enforcement will usually be best suited for securing the scene in this fashion. Defining the zones and enforcing them is an important component. Unfortunately, if planning and execution of the scene security are not done properly, this may hinder the movement of ambulances and patients. Containment for ecological and waste management purposes is important; however, it is possible for injuries and exposures to occur during these components as well.

INCIDENT INVESTIGATION

Evidence collection and sampling is out of the realm of the EMS physician and only qualified HAZMAT technicians are to perform these tasks. However, it is important to consider that clothing and other contaminated items being discarded at during decontamination or treatment may be considered evidence and when possible should be arranged by victim and law enforcement to take custody of these items. This is especially true when terrorism is suspected. Radiologic contamination should be collected by the proper authorities as well and may lead to additional patient care information. EMS physicians and providers may be asked to make statements after completion of patient care activities.

TABLE 72-3	Some Hazardous Materials Antidotes		
Hazardous Material	Antidote	Adult Dose	Pediatric Dose
Organophosphates	Atropine	1-2 mg IV bolus	0.02-0.04 mg/kg IV bolus; minimum dose
Nerve Agents		Titrate to effect (TTE)	of .1 mg; TTE
Carbamates	Pralidoxime (2-PAM)	1-2 g slow IV infusion over 10 minutes, then 500 mg/h IV infusion	20-40 mg/kg IV infusion over 10 minutes, then 5-10 mg/kg/h IV infusion
Hydrofluoric acid (HFA) skin burns	Calcium gluconate 2.5%-10% topical gel or solution	Topical application	Topical application
Systemic HFA	Calcium gluconate 10%	10-20 mL (1-2 amps) slow IV bolus	0.2-0.3 mL/kg slow IV bolus
Fluoride poisoning		Repeat dosing may be required	Repeat dosing may be required
	Calcium chloride 10%	5-10 mL (0.5-1 amps) slow IV bolus	0.1-0.2 mL/kg slow IV bolus
		Repeat dosing may be required	Repeat dosing may be required
Cyanides	USA cyanide antidote kit Amyl nitrite	By inhalation	By inhalation
	USA cyanide antidote kit Sodium nitrite	10 mL (1 amp) IV over 5 minutes	0.12-0.33 mL/kg IV over 5 minutes, up to a maximum of 10 mL (1 amp)
	USA cyanide antidote kit Sodium thiosulfate	50 mL (1 amp) IV bolus over 10 to 20 minutes	1.6 mL/kg IV over 10 to 20 minutes, up to a maximum of 50 mL (1 amp)
	Hydroxo-cobalamin	5 g IV	70 mg/kg over 15 minutes not to exceed a single dose of 5 g
Aromatic amines	Methylene blue	1-2 mg/kg IV over 5 minutes	1-2 mg/kg IV over 5 minutes
Arsine		Repeat dosing may be required	Repeat dosing may be required
Chlorobenzene			
Chromates			
Nitrates/nitrites			
Simple asphyxiants	Oxygen	100% by inhalation	100% by inhalation
Systemic asphyxiants		Hyperbaric O_2 therapy at 2.5-3.0 ATA	Hyperbaric O_2 therapy at 2.5-3.0 ATA
Carbon monoxide			
Hydrazines	Pyridoxine	25 mg/kg IV	25 mg/kg IV

KEY POINTS

- NFPA 472 and 473 detail important operational guidelines concerning personnel protective equipment and training for a hazardous materials operation.

- The *Emergency Response Guidebook* is an important tool for the EMS physician when responding to, or given medical control for, a HAZMAT operation.

- CHEMTREC, poison control center, and the National Response Center are important call centers that may be used by EMS physicians when engaged in a serious hazardous materials operation.

- WISER and CAMEO are highly useful tools that can offer operational and medical guidance and come in online and mobile applications, making them potentially available during an event.

- Some antidotes exist for specific exposures, but may not be available in the prehospital environment.

- Utilization of local stockpiles and CHEMPACK may need to be activated in some exposures, or when large numbers of patients require antidotes or other exposure-specific drug therapy.

- Decontamination, supportive care, and transport to a hospital with the appropriate capabilities are key interventions.

REFERENCES

1. Cengage Learning, Delmar. *Firefighter's Handbook: Firefighting and Emergency Response*. 3rd ed. Cengage Learning; Clifton Park, NY. March 24, 2008:847.
2. Office of Fire Prevention and Control, State of New York Department of State. *HAZMAT Technician-Basic Student Manual*. New York State Division of Homeland Security and Emergency Services. Washington DC. September 2005.
3. Drug Enforcement Administration. Guidelines for law enforcement for the cleanup of clandestine drug laboratories. 2005 Edition. http://www.justice.gov/dea/resources/img/redbook.pdf. Accessed October 1, 2013.
4. REAC/TS. The medical aspects of radiation incidents. The Radiation Emergency Assistance Center/ Training Site. https://orise.orau.gov/files/reacts/medical-aspects-of-radiation-incidents.pdf. Accessed October 1, 2013.
5. Man-li TSE. Antidotal treatment for radioactive materials. *Federation of Medical Societies of Hong Kong. The Hong Kong Medical Diary*. April 2011;16(4).
6. Lesak DM. *Hazardous Materials: Strategies and Tactics*. Prentice Hall; San Francisco, CA. June 2, 1998.
7. Noll G. NFPA 472: Using NFPA 472 to develop a competency-based HAZMAT/WMD emergency responder training program. *NFPA J.* 102(2):54-59.
8. NFPA 473: Standard for Competencies for EMS Personnel Responding to Hazardous Materials Incidents. National Fire Protection Association, 2008.
9. Online HAZMAT School. Hazardous material toxicology. Hazwoper Refresher #936. https://classes.HAZMATschool.com/course_content/936/dynframeset.html?3-8hr-refresh-toxicology.html. Accessed October 1, 2013.
10. Borak J, Olson KR. *Managing Hazardous Materials Incidents: Medical Management Guidelines for Acute Chemical Exposures*. U.S. Department of Health and Human Services. Washington DC. July 1996.
11. Levine MD, Gresham C. Hydrocarbon toxicity treatment & management. eMedicine, Medscape. March 2013. http://emedicine.medscape.com/article/821143-overview. Accessed October 1, 2013.
12. de Lange DW, Sikma MA, Meulenbelt J. Extracorporeal membrane oxygenation in the treatment of poisoned patients. *Clin Toxicol (Phila)*. June 2013;51(5):385-393.

CHAPTER 73

Cruise Ship, Airline, and Resort Medicine

Ricky C. Kue

INTRODUCTION

The operational environment of commercial travel can be as challenging as any other for the EMS physician to provide quality emergency medical care. As an aging population remains mobile and continues to travel, the importance of planning and preparation for emergency medical care has become more important than ever. Planning for and providing emergency medical care in commercial travel environments such as a cruise ship or passenger airline require a thorough understanding of the limitations those environments produce.

OBJECTIVES

- Describe the cruise ship medical operations and the EMS physician role onboard.
- Discuss unique challenges in patient management at sea.
- Describe airline medical operations and the EMS physician role as medical director for airline operations.
- Discuss unique challenges in patient management in the air.
- Discuss basic jurisdictional and FAA regulations pertaining to in-flight medical emergencies.
- Describe the process of flight diversion for a medical emergency.
- Describe typical resort medical operations and the concept of "concierge medicine" for resort guests.
- Discuss licensure and liability issues for EMS physicians practicing travel medicine.

Consider the example of delivering clinical care during an in-flight medical emergency requires the EMS physician to not only understand the pathophysiology of a given medical condition, but also appreciate operational considerations such as altitude and flight physiology, providing medical care within the equipment and resource-limited environment, and consider the overall impact of deciding whether or not to divert a flight.

Provision of medical care onboard a cruise ship is no less challenging. It is typically the medical officer's responsibility to plan for medical care and potential onboard disasters, respond to emergencies, monitor and respond to potential epidemiologic events, oversee ancillary medical staff, and be the overall "medical conscience" for the command staff of a vessel. The challenge in making the decision to divert to a nearby port or have a patient medically evacuated from sea requires proper forethought and planning on the part of the medical officer. Resort medicine can be challenging since many of the typical services provided may not be emergent in nature depending on the type of resort; however, at any moment a medical emergency can be encountered and the EMS physician must be ready to respond especially since many resorts may be located somewhere advanced medical care is not available.

Consider other aspects of EMS medicine which have similar planning and operational considerations to airline cruise ship and resort medicine. Operational preplanning for anticipated illnesses and preventive health services in the urban search and rescue, fireground support, or tactical medical environment is performed to minimize injury or illness to team members as well as maximize the overall success of the mission. This approach has great relevance to medical care planning for cruise ship or airline medicine. Delivering medical care in the unique physical environment such as a passenger airline draws on practices and principles of helicopter and air medical transport which may be all too familiar to the EMS physician. Regardless of the operational environment, the EMS physician must appreciate the balance he or she must maintain between providing state-of-the-art emergency medical care and seeing that the nonmedical objectives are successfully met. The objectives of this chapter are to provide the EMS physician a basic understanding of the cruise ship, airline, and resort medicine as it pertains to his or her role as a provider or medical director.

CRUISE SHIP MEDICINE

Passenger travel onboard luxury cruise lines continue to be a popular vacation choice. The US Department of Transportation (DOT) Maritime Administration estimates that approximately 10.6 million passengers were carried on North American–based cruise ships during 2010. This number is up from 9.9 million passengers who traveled in 2009.[1] These numbers were over the estimated capacity for both 2009 and 2010, representing over 100% occupancy rates and a considerable degree of cruise ship travel by the general public. Cruise ships have grown in size with current luxury vessels capable of carrying up to 5400 passengers. Over the past 5 years, the average size of ships has increased by approximately 14.2% to 2272 passengers. Some of the largest passenger capacity vessels can carry up to 5400 passengers.[1] Providing health care at sea can be considered part wilderness medicine, travel medicine, and preventive health medicine. The EMS physician must consider the limitations in medical resources, diagnostic equipment, and available consultation when evaluating patients as well as the operational challenges that occur when a medical evacuation is needed. Preventive health becomes extremely important in the closed population of a cruise ship and the risk of rapidly spreading infectious diseases. In this manner, the best medical care is sometimes preventative.[2] Considering the diverse passenger population and worldwide locations most cruise ships travel, cruise line medical operations have had to adapt and meet the challenge of providing medical while being miles out to sea. There is no particular personal demographic to describe patients encountered at sea. Cruise ship passengers can be viewed as a cohort of the general population at large with similar chronic illnesses and comorbidities. Travel for days at a time at sea can pose a challenge for passengers with complex medical conditions. Although most cruise line passengers are advised to medically prepare for a trip by securing adequate personal medications, medical clearance by a personal physician when necessary, updating specific immunizations, etc, it is still up to the medical department onboard to prepare to encounter any type of medical or surgical emergency.

Studies have been published in the literature attempting to describe the epidemiology of illness and injury encountered while at sea. A quick review of the available literature demonstrates that medical complaints remain the most common types of reason for accessing medical services on a cruise ship over traumatic injuries.[3-6] In two studies specifically looking at cruise ship infirmary visits, respiratory diseases were the most common reason for visit. Other common visit diagnoses included nervous system/sensory organ systems including motion sickness, gastrointestinal, dermatologic, and cardiovascular diseases.[3,4] Traumatic injuries remained less common than medical illnesses and in both of the aforementioned studies represented less than 20% of all ship infirmary visits. Of the traumatic injuries, the most common include sprains, soft tissue contusions, and wounds and fractures.[3,4] One study examining the frequency of accidents and injuries occurring at sea found similar results over 3 years with wounds, contusions, joint sprains, and bony fractures as the most common types of injuries. The most common mechanism was due to a slip or fall typically within a passenger cabin compartment or bathroom.[5] Considering maritime health care for nonpassenger cruise ships, similar injury patterns are reported in the literature among sea goers such as merchant mariners and typically encompass more medical and urgent care complaints than serious traumatic or work-related injuries.[7]

Preventive health considerations and rapidly spreading infectious diseases deserve special mention when considering the overall delivery of health care onboard a cruise ship.[8-11] Numerous case reports and media attention on diseases such as viral gastroenteritis spreading through ships and ruining vacationers have made preventive health an important aspect of the ship medical officer's duties. Common sources of viral infectious outbreaks include food handling and water sources onboard the ship. A review of recent foodborne and waterborne outbreaks reveal commonly encountered bacterial pathogens such as *E Coli*, *Salmonella*, and *Shigella*, whereas common viral pathogens are mainly attributed to noroviruses.[12,13] Most, if not all of these, outbreaks can be traced back to some type of storage or mishandling issue which results in inappropriate pathogen growth. The cruise ship environment is especially susceptible to these outbreaks due to the relative proximity passengers and crewmembers have to each other onboard the closed physical space of a ship. This makes hand-washing and other sanitary strategies important. Limited space at sea also means limited supplies of noncontaminated food or water to sustain passengers and crewmembers until a ship can return to shore. Finally, treatment for large victim numbers becomes challenging given the limited resources of most ship infirmaries. As one could imagine, a significant epidemiological event could easily overwhelm the staff and resources of a ship's medical department.

In efforts to better plan and prepare for epidemiological catastrophes onboard a cruise ship, the CDC has available resources to help ship clinicians with preventing and managing these incidents. In 1975, the CDC developed the Vessel Sanitation Program (VSP) to help the cruise line industry minimize the risk of acute diarrheal diseases among passenger and crewmembers sailing into the United States. Overall, the incidence of acute diarrheal diseases onboard cruise ships has declined from 1999 to 2000 as part of these efforts.[14] The CDC also publishes the *Vessel Sanitation Program Operations Manual* which is regularly updated and acts as a general resource for ship medical officers in preventing such outbreaks.[15] The CDC also provides informational bulletins for clinicians on specific pathogens that ship medical officers may encounter such as Noroviruses.[16] It is important that the EMS physician understand his or her role not only as a clinician but also as a preventive health officer whose duties may also include supervising food and water handling and storage, monitoring of sanitary conditions in other ship areas such as food storage and preparation areas or bathrooms.

Maritime health care pose some unique challenges and operational considerations for the EMS physician to manage. Operationally, almost all ships follow a similar chain of command. The EMS physician would likely see themselves serving the role as a medical officer within the medical department of a ship. The medical officer typically oversees the medical department unless there is a chief medical officer. A cruise ship is typically divided into its different functional departments. Two common departments are the deck department and the engineering department. The deck department typically commands and navigates the ship. The *captain* of the ship is considered the overall commander of the vessel with subordinate officers such as the *first officer, second officer, third officer*, etc, as the next chain of command. The *medical officer* typically functions as a special staff member to the captain providing guidance and insight with respect to medical and health issues. At sea, one of the most challenging decisions to make for the medical officer is whether or not a ship must initiate a medical evacuation at sea or divert the ship to a nearby port due to passenger or crewmember illness or injury. Such decisions are not taken lightly and must be weighed against the overall well-being of this ship if a diversion is to be made. Although this decision can be costly, it should always be a consideration if risk to life is significant. The EMS physician should also consider the fact that aeromedical evacuation from sea is not usually his or her final decision; rather it is left to the flight surgeon or medical officer and pilot of the responding agency such as the US Coast Guard.[17] Effective transfer to definitive care may not always involve emergent evacuation at sea by helicopter. In fact, sometimes, knowing what available resources at particular ports of call is essential in planning medical care during a given voyage. Communications capability while at sea is another crucial aspect of medical care the EMS physician should be familiar with. This may include satellite or radio communications. Ultimately, any of the above decisions is made in conjunction

with the captain of the ship as he or she has ultimate operational control of the vessel.

The role of the EMS physician as ship medical officer will often include multiple job roles from preventive health officer and sanitation officer to both primary care and acute care clinician as mentioned previously. Provision of good medical care onboard begins with proper medical preplanning by the medical department. Medical preplanning for a cruise includes taking into consideration travel location and ports of call, knowing the endemic diseases and illnesses, planning for appropriate vaccinations and adequate treatment supplies for endemic diseases, and gathering as much medical information about passengers and crewmembers as possible. Major cruise lines maintain medical departments that include ground or shore operations to perform these preplanning activities as well as monitoring and quality improvement functions. The EMS physician may find themselves functioning as the medical director for a cruise line and function in this administrative capacity. This may include oversight of training and clinical care by physician extenders, nurses, paramedics, and EMTs. It is also important that training for medical scenarios onboard the ship while at port and at sea occurs regularly to maintain the response readiness of the medical department. Along with knowing endemic diseases, it is also important to research regional weather patterns and its impact on ship operations. High winds and rough seas will greatly affect passenger comfort as well as increase the likelihood of fall injuries on deck. Weather can also affect food storage considerations and vector-borne illnesses as well. Knowing local medical facilities and capabilities will also help guide the medical officer in making the most informed decision on diversion and medical referral/evaluation at port.

Preventive health services such as food handling and storage inspections, water treatment and wastewater management, and other sanitary functions are just as valuable as clinical duties. These supervisory activities begin at port prior to departure and throughout the cruise to minimize the chance of any epidemiological outbreaks. As mentioned previously, the uncontrolled outbreak of a highly contagious disease such as Norovirus gastroenteritis can significantly affect cruise operations. Preventive health includes routine surveillance for such diseases while at sea so appropriate measures can be taken before a critical mass of individuals are affected. Responding to emergent medical and surgical conditions is also an important aspect of cruise medicine. As with any planning for emergency medical care, the EMS physician should consider the most common illnesses and injuries as well as the most severe ones to prepare for. According to previously published studies, common life-threatening conditions mirror those seen in most emergency departments and include asthma exacerbation, angina, myocardial infarction, syncope, congestive heart failure, and stroke.[4] Data suggest that the overwhelming majority of patients remain onboard the ship and can be managed accordingly. It is relatively rare that a diversion must be made for medical disembarkation or an immediate aeromedical evacuation be initiated. Most complex complaints can be managed with follow-up arranged at a port-of-call with subsequent evacuation.[3,5]

When considering care of particular diseases and injuries, the EMS physician should consider research and technology used in other aspects of prehospital care pertinent to the cruise ship environment. The EMS physician may wish to consider having available fibrinolytic therapy for time-sensitive conditions such as ST-segment elevation MI or acute ischemic stroke. Specific transport equipment and monitoring systems used in EMS may be better suited for the cruise ship environment for patient movement from tight quarters or operational areas of the ship such as an engine room multiple levels below deck to safely move patients to the infirmary. Application of diagnostic modalities such as bedside emergency ultrasonography can be extremely useful on a ship. Most modern ship infirmaries are capable of providing limited radiographic capabilities as well. The ability to utilize telemedicine with shore-based consultants can also be beneficial.

Relatively little formal guidance is available for EMS physicians in planning and providing for cruise ship medical care. Although there are currently no authoritative or regulatory organizations that oversee the provision of medical care at sea, attempts by some are being made to standardize the care being delivered. The cruise line industries have worked on self-regulating their medical activities at sea.[17] The American College of Emergency Physicians has also published health care guidelines for cruise ship medical facilities to help define what standards of care should be.[18] This document provides some basic standards in which cruise ship medical facilities should maintain to provide optimal medical care.

COMMERCIAL AIRLINE MEDICINE

Provision of medical care at an altitude of 30,000 ft in a passenger airline can truly test the capabilities of an EMS physician. Commercial air travel is a common travel modality with roughly 600 million passengers serviced domestically every year.[19] It is inevitable that medical emergencies will occur in-flight given the diverse population that currently uses commercial air travel. Medical advances have allowed individuals to live longer with complex medical conditions, some of which may be greatly affected by the physiology of flight. The occurrence of in-flight medical emergencies has been studied previously. In 2000, a Federal Aviation Administration (FAA) study of 1132 in-flight medical events occurring on domestic flights during 1996 and 1997 found a rate of 13 events per day.[20] A 2013 study showed a 1/604 rate of medical emergency/flight.[21] This estimate is considered by most to be an underestimate of the true number of medical events since this study only looked at those which involved ground-based medical support. Interestingly, this study also found that 69% of all in-flight medical emergencies were attended by a health care professional: physicians volunteered in about 40% of cases, nurses in 25% and paramedics in 4%. The overall agreement between the in-flight provider diagnosis and hospital diagnosis was about 79% and the passenger's condition improved in 60% of cases.[22] Officials from British Airways reported on their experience with in-flight medical emergencies during 1999 and reported 3386 medical incidents averaging about one per 11,000 passengers. Approximately, 70% of these were attended to by cabin crew only, about 1000 required the assistance of a health care professional onboard[23] and in the study by Peterson et al, a physician passengers aided in care in about 48% of cases. The 10 most common complaints seen from the 2000 FAA report included chest pain, syncope, asthma exacerbation, head injury from overhead compartment contents, abdominal complaints, diabetic-related complaints, allergic reactions, psychiatric problems, obstetrical and gynecological complaints. One study of European in-flight emergencies found syncope to be the most commonly encountered in-flight medical emergency.[24] This is similar to findings from another FAA study in 2009 which looked at the frequency of specific in-flight medical emergencies.[25]

The cabin environment of a commercial airliner in itself is a physiologic stressor to the human body. Unlike the cabin environment of a typical rotor-wing aircraft during air medical transport, the cabin of most fixed-wing aircrafts is pressurized for passenger comfort since the typical flight altitudes of an airline well exceed that of a rotor-wing aircraft. Typical flying altitudes of a commercial airliner are approximately 25,000 to 35,000 ft above ground level (AGL). At these altitudes, the barometric pressures of gas can be as little as one-fourth of that at sea level. This is referred to as the "physiologic deficient zone" which is considered by most aviation medicine specialists to be between 10,000 and 50,000 ft. In this zone, hypoxia can develop due to a lower partial pressure of available oxygen, expansion of trapped gas and air according to Boyle law, which leads to dysbarism and noticeable physiologic changes that occur in the body due to the reduced pressures at this altitude. Trapped gas expansion can lead to conditions such as ear block, sinus block, barodontalgia, and decompression sickness. To avoid these situations, most commercial airliners pressurize their cabin to a more comfortable "altitude." Although the FAA requires commercial airlines to pressurize cabins to 10,000 ft, most cabins are typically pressurized to an altitude of approximately 5000 to 8000 ft. For most healthy adults, physiological changes to this altitude produce minor if not negligible symptoms. At these pressures, the partial pressure of oxygen is reduced from 95 to approximately

56 mm Hg in healthy passengers, which corresponds to about a 4% reduction in the oxygen saturation.[22,26] However, for passengers with significant chronic diseases such as respiratory or cardiovascular disease, a cabin pressure of 8000 ft may still be significant enough to produce acute symptoms or disease. The cabin environment can be dryer than ambient air and can trigger exacerbation of asthma and reactive airway diseases in susceptible individuals.

Providing medical care during a commercial flight raises certain legal and regulatory issues such as duty to act, malpractice liability, and airline obligation to provide medical care. To address these issues, the US Congress passed legislation known as the *Aviation Medical Assistance Act* in 1998, which directs the FAA to assess regulations related to onboard aircraft medical equipment including the availability of automated external defibrillators (**Table 73-1**), mandate appropriate flight attendant medical training, and have air carriers in good faith report monthly to the FAA in-flight medical incidents especially any in-flight deaths.[22,26] In addition to setting mandates and reporting mechanisms, the Aviation Medical Assistance Act also addresses liability concerns for air carriers and health care providers when delivering medical care akin to most "Good Samaritan" laws. Essentially, the act states that an air carrier is not considered liable for damages in any action brought in a federal or state court arising out of the carrier's actions in soliciting medical assistance from a passenger or out of any acts of omission by the assisting passenger so long as the passenger is not an employee or agent of the carrier and as long as the carrier believes the assisting passenger is medically qualified. It also declares that the assisting passenger is not liable for damages during the provision of medical care except for gross negligence or willful conduct. A key point to consider for intervening health care providers is that he or she must be a volunteer, rendering care in good faith in accordance with his or her scope of practice and receive no monetary compensation.

With regard to cabin crew, most flight attendants have some level of medical training to respond to medical emergencies including basic first aid, CPR, and the use of an automated external defibrillator. As a general rule, when an in-flight emergency occurs, the cabin crew have a duty to

TABLE 73-1 Typical On-Board Emergency Medical Kits Mandated by the FAA

Type of Equipment	Items	Quantity
Diagnostic	Stethoscope	1
	Sphygmomanometer	1
Airway	Oropharyngeal airway	Various sizes
	Mask for CPR	Various sizes
	Bag-valve mask	1 Device
IV Infusion	Syringes and needles	1 × 5 mL
		2 × 10 mL
	Infusion kit	1 Set
	Norma saline (0.9%)	1 × 500-mL bag
Resuscitation (as of 2004)	FDA-approved AED	1
Medications	Nitroglycerin (0.4-mg tab)	10
	Diphenhydramine (50-mg INJ)	2 ampules
	Diphenhydramine (25-mg tab)	4
	Dextrose (50% INJ)	1 ampule
	Epinephrine (1:1000 INJ)	2 ampules
	Epinephrine (1:10000 INJ)	2 ampules
	Aspirin (325-mg tab)	4
	Lidocaine (20-mg INJ)	2 ampules
	Bronchodilator inhaler	1 MDI

act and will solicit assistance from medically qualified passengers with more complex cases. Similar to the chain of command which exists on cruise ships, there is a chain of command onboard a commercial airline. The overall command of an aircraft is performed by the *pilot-in-charge* (PIC) who is typically assisted by a first officer. If any incidents (whether or not it is medical in nature) occur in-flight, the PIC is appropriately updated so that he or she can determine the best course of action understanding that the PIC must also consider the safety of the remaining passengers, crew, and aircraft. Most airline carriers have a ground-based medical consultation service which provides the flight crew with medical direction. These ground-based services are usually in communication via radio and available 24/7 to air carriers. These consultants take into consideration aircraft location, altitude, and heading, patient assessment and condition, and will provide the PIC a medical assessment of the situation so that he or she can determine the best course of action. These services will also use the resources of onboard medical assistance to best determine the severity of situation as well. Ultimately, it is important for any onboard health care provider who is assisting the flight crew with a medical emergency to understand these operational considerations in the decision-making process. It is far more common for the flight crew and PIC to act on the clinician's advice rather than to dispute it.

The EMS physician may find themselves functioning as a medical director or consulting physician at a ground-based medical support service. Air carriers do employ physicians as part of their aviation medical departments to seek guidance on training, equipment, and response planning for in-flight medical emergencies. As with most other types of operational and wilderness medicine preplanning, it is important to appreciate the environment in which a medical emergency may arise as well as the available resources at hand. Ground-based services will need to consider the operational aspects of the air carriers they service including the general aircrafts within the fleet, flying patterns, locations of major hubs, and in-flight resources such as staff and equipment. Whether the EMS physician is ground based or happens to be the passenger of a flight during a medical emergency, some considerations in medical care should be taken. Complaints related to hypoxia can be addressed with supplemental oxygen or a change in altitude/cabin pressure. The latter is typically done in conjunction with the PIC. Most other specific complaints such as allergic reaction or asthma exacerbation can be addressed expectantly with the available onboard medical resources. If there is any threat to life or clinical deterioration, then a discussion with the ground consultation and PIC should occur on the possibility of diverting to the nearest airport for further medical care. This is also true for time-sensitive conditions such as ST-segment elevation MI or stroke. Although most air carriers are not required to have advanced electro-cardiograph capabilities, some carriers do have telemedicine capabilities which should be identified early on during the incident. Considering that some AEDs have monitoring capabilities, it is imperative that the responding provider be familiar with the onboard AED capabilities. The occurrence of in-flight cardiac arrest has been described in the literature in which asystole and PEA were the most common rhythms identified from AED data. Ventricular fibrillation or tachycardia was identified in about 25% of cases reviewed.[27] Termination of resuscitation (TOR) is a challenging decision to make given the public nature of a cardiac arrest in-flight. TOR guidelines have been published and support the idea of terminating efforts based on certain criteria.[28] When examining the circumstances of an in-flight cardiac arrest and whether or not to terminate efforts, consider that a resuscitation of prolonged duration will likely have poor outcomes regardless of continued efforts, place passengers and crew at risk for personal injury, and prolong the view of an active arrest to other passengers. Physical limitations of cabin space in aisle ways and common areas may be all that is available to flight crew and assisting passengers. Performance of CPR may be challenging given the limited space and patient movement may present as a challenge given the tight quarters of typical coach class cabins.

Flight diversion for an in-flight medical emergency can have operation and financial cost consequences. Although most medical providers would argue that there should not be any cost associated with patient lives, operational considerations in performing a flight diversion are not small. Factors such as emergent/unscheduled landings, potential need to dump fuel, landing with an overweight aircraft, altered flight patterns, landing in poor weather or unfamiliar conditions add risk to the overall safety and well-being of the remaining passengers onboard.[27] Typically, the decision to perform diversion is not solely left to the onboard medical provider. Not all providers onboard have the specialty training to appreciate the operational significance of medical decision making or have enough clinical practice to be comfortable in managing all cases with the available resources onboard. The PIC will usually make contact with ground-based consultation services for their recommendations in addition to the recommendations from onboard providers to decide the safest course of action. Understanding that there are more things at stake than just the well-being of a single individual, the PIC is the individual who has final authority on flight diversion. One airline company that studied its rate of airline diversion for medical emergencies found based on a 1-year study period that they had an equivalent of 210 diversions for every one million flights with one diversion occurring for every 12.6 medical incidents.[29] To better assist clinicians for in-flight medical emergencies, the Aerospace Medical Association publishes medical guidelines for airline travel and outlines the prescreening process for passengers who may not be considered "airworthy" as well as some of the common in-flight emergencies encountered.[30] For EMS physicians who choose to provide medical direction and/or advisement on Airline Medicine programs, some attention should also be paid to recent increasing interest in prevention of current and emerging infectious diseases.[31-34]

RESORT AND CONCIERGE MEDICINE

Access to immediate medical care is not always the first thing travelers consider when selecting their destination of travel. However, more and more individuals are now considering the availability of medical services at their location and have even considered locations that offer particular health services at the destination. In an attempt to define "resort medicine," the major challenge comes when considering what type of care is being delivered. Traditionally, most resort medicine services include immediate availability to medical care in the event of minor illness or injury. This can be viewed as another type of urgent care medicine which happens to provide preferred access to a particular resort or hotel. Some resorts have now begun to offer more comprehensive, nonurgent medical services as part of the resort experience. This type of medical care is more akin to the current "concierge" or retainer medicine model of care. In this case, the primary medical care delivered is not emergency medicine or urgent care medicine. Rather, it is the provision of comprehensive medical diagnostics and preventive medical services for a fee. It is important for the EMS physician involved with either types of resort medicine to understand the type of care he or she is providing. While emergency medicine and urgent care medicine is a more familiar practice to the EMS physician, the delivery of comprehensive primary care at such health spas or resort may be more complex and have different implications.

Concierge or retainer medicine has become increasingly popular with the public due to its "on-demand" style of access to medical care. It has often been described as consumer-focused care where a patient can access medical care with providers who limit their overall patient load and provide more access for these patients as well as more focused care with longer visits based on a collected fee. Benefits of such practices include same-day or next-day visits, 24-hour phone call access to providers, detailed annual wellness and physical exams, and access to immediate specialty consultation.[35] Resorts that provide comprehensive health care as part of their experience can be considered a form of concierge medicine. It is important to recognize the EMS physician's role in such a setup. Is he or she there to coordinate or provide emergency or urgent medical care needs or are they a part of the comprehensive medical evaluation team? If it is the latter, then he or she should be comfortable with primary health care management. If the medical care is for urgent or emergency complaints that arise during the course of a visitor stay, then the EMS physician should be aware of his or her capabilities while providing medical care and subsequent follow-up, as well as the local prehospital and medical resources in the event a guest needs referral and evaluation at a higher level of care. An important aspect of concierge medical care is also to determine with the resort or facility that will provide for medical liability coverage. That is to say, does the resort provide some type of comprehensive liability coverage or does the clinician provide for his or her own malpractice? Similarly, it is important for the provider to determine at what scope of practice he or she will function in. The provider should consider the equipment as well as facility space he or she needs when providing concierge medical care. Additional questions should be considered when participating in resort medical care and are noted in **Box 73-1**.

There are currently no guidelines or regulatory oversight over providers that deliver concierge medicine. These issues are typically determined by the individual provider with their malpractice policy carrier to determine the degree of coverage based on what the provider requests to perform. This factor is important since one would not want to deliver care he or she is not trained to provide. Ethical issues exist with provision of concierge medicine since this type of care is inherently designed to provide preferential access and care to member patients and raise questions on whether particular screening exams are actually performed based on published preventive health guidelines.[36] Whether the EMS physician is providing emergency medical care or primary care at a resort, it is still important to consider factors such as geographic location, weather patterns, endemic diseases, and local medical resources as part of the medical planning.

KEY POINTS

- Medical care begins with good planning—understand the geography, location, endemic diseases, local medical resources, and operational aspects and resource limitations of cruise ship or airline environment.
- Infectious disease outbreaks onboard a ship can be significant; proper preventive health and sanitary monitoring functions are just as important for the EMS physician as are clinical duties.
- Medical evacuation while at sea may not always be the best option for a patient; consider onboard resources for care, medical resources at nearby ports, and the possibility of diversion to the closest port or return to home port.
- Most in-flight medical emergencies are handled onboard and do not require diversion.
- Air carriers have medical ground-based consultation services as part of their response to in-flight medical emergencies.
- Be familiar with the available equipment and medications available in an airline onboard emergency medical kit.
- The Airline Medical Assistance Act of 1998 provides for "good Samaritan" liability protection for qualified health care providers assisting with in-flight medical emergencies.

- Any decision to divert an airline flight or cruise ship off course for a medical emergency is ultimately the decision of the captain (pilot-in-charge).
- When providing resort medical care, be sure to know if you are providing urgent medical care for emergencies or providing comprehensive primary medical care as part of guest experience.
- Confirm that there is adequate medical malpractice coverage for specifically the scope of practice being provided as part of a resort medicine practice. It is important to stay within this scope of practice and to properly refer to higher level of care when indicated.

REFERENCES

1. United States Department of Transportation Maritime Administration. North American cruise statistical snapshot 2010. Washington, DC. 2011. http://www.marad.dot.gov/documents/North_American_Cruise_Statistics_Quarterly_Snapshot.pdf.
2. Putnam J. Maritime health care. *Br J Sports Med.* 2005;39:693-694.
3. DiGiovanna T, Rosen T, Forsett R, et al. Shipboard medicine: a new niche for emergency medicine. *Ann Emerg Med.* 1992;21:1476-1479.
4. Peake DE, Gray CL, Ludwig MR, et al. Descriptive epidemiology of injury and illness among cruise ship passengers. *Ann Emerg Med.* 1999;33:67-72.
5. Dahl E. Passenger accidents and injuries reported during 3 years on a cruise ship. *Int Marit Health.* 2010;61:1-8.
6. Schutz L, Zak D, Holmes JF. Pattern of passenger injury and illness on expedition cruise ships to Antarctica. *J Travel Med.* July-August 2014;21(4):228-234.
7. Kue R, Cukor J, Fredrickson A. Providing student health services at sea: a survey of chief complaints onboard a maritime academy training ship. *J Amer Coll Health.* 2009;57:457-463.
8. Schlaich C, Gau B, Cohen NJ, Kojima K, Marano N, Menucci D. Infection control measures on ships and in ports during the early stage of pandemic influenza A (H1N1) 2009. *Int Marit Health.* 2012;63(1):17-23.
9. Mouchtouri VA, Bartlett CL, Diskin A, Hadjichristodoulou C. Water safety plan on cruise ships: a promising tool to prevent waterborne diseases. *Sci Total Environ.* July 1, 2012;429:199-205.
10. Mitruka K, Felsen CB, Tomianovic D, et al. Measles, rubella, and varicella among the crew of a cruise ship sailing from Florida, United States, 2006. *J Travel Med.* July 2012;19(4):233-237.
11. Lim PL. Influenza and SARS: the impact of viral pandemics on maritime health. *Int Marit Health.* 2011;62(3):170-175.
12. Rooney RM, Cramer EH, Mantha S, et al. A review of outbreaks of foodborne disease associated with passenger ships: evidence for risk management. *Public Health Rep.* 2004;119:427-434.
13. Rooney RM, Bartram JK, Cramer EH, et al. A review of outbreaks of waterborne disease associated with passenger ships: evidence for risk management. *Public Health Rep.* 2004;119:435-442.
14. Cramer EH, Blanton CJ, Blanton LH, et al. Epidemiology of gastroenteritis on cruise ships, 2001-2004. *Am J Prev Med.* 2006;30:252-257.
15. Centers for Disease Control and Prevention. Vessel sanitation program operations manual. Atlanta, GA. 2005. http://www.cdc.gov/nceh/vsp.
16. Centers for Disease Control and Prevention. CDC factsheet noroviruses. Atlanta, GA 2004. http://www.cdc.gov/nceh/vsp/default.htm.
17. Clutter P, van Boheemen S. Cruise ship nursing: an international experience. *J Emerg Nurs.* 2007;33(1):65-68.
18. American College of Emergency Physicians. Healthcare guidelines for cruise ship medical facilities. Irving, TX. 2011. http://www.acep.org/Content.aspx?id=29980.
19. Bureau of Transportation Statistics: TranStats. Washington, DC. 2011. http://www.transtats.bts.gov/.

20. DeJohn CA, Veronneau SJ, Wolbrink AM, et al. The evaluation of in-flight medical care aboard selected U.S. air carriers: 1996 to 1997. Federal Aviation Administration, Office of Aviation Medicine Technical Report no. DOT/FAA/AM-0013; 2000; Washington, DC.

21. Peterson DC, Martin-Gill C, Guyette FX, et al. Outcomes of medical emergencies on commercial airline flights. *N Engl J Med*. May 30, 2013;368(22):2075-2083.

22. Gendreau MA, DeJohn CA. Responding to medical events during commercial airline flights. *N Engl J Med*. 2002;346:1067-1073.

23. Dowdall N. "Is there a doctor on the aircraft?" Top 10 in-flight medical emergencies. *BMJ*. 2000;321:1336-1337.

24. Sand M, Bechera FG, Sand D, et al. Surgical and medical emergencies on board European aircraft: a retrospective study of 10189 cases. *Critical Care*. 2009;13:R3.

25. DeJohn CA, Veronneau SJ, Hordinsky JR. The status of inflight medical care aboard selected US air carriers. Federal Aviation Administration, Office of Aviation Medicine. Phoenix, AZ. 2009. http://www.faa.gov/data_research/research/med_humanfacs/aeromedical/aircraftaccident/medicalemergency/.

26. Goodwin T. In-flight medical emergencies: an overview. *BMJ*. 2000;321:1338-1341.

27. Brown AM, Rittenberger JC, Ammon CM, et al. In-flight automated external defibrillator use and consultation. *Prehosp Emerg Care*. 2010;14:235-239.

28. Millin MG, Khandker SK, Malki A. Termination of resuscitation of nontraumatic cardiopulmonary arrest: resource document for the national association of EMS physicians position statement. *Prehosp Emerg Care*. 2011;15:547-554.

29. Delaune EF, Lucas RH, Illig P. In-flight medical events and aircraft diversions: one airline's experience. *Aviat Space Environ Med*. 2003;74:62-68.

30. Aerospace Medical Association Medical Guidelines Taskforce. Medical guidelines for airline travel, 2nd edition. *Aviat Space Environ Med*. 2003;74:A1-A19.

31. Khan K, Eckhardt R, Brownstein JS, et al. Entry and exit screening of airline travellers during the A(H1N1) 2009 pandemic: a retrospective evaluation. *Bull World Health Organ*. May 1, 2013;91(5):368-376.

32. Selent M, de Rochars VM, Stanek D, et al. Malaria prevention knowledge, attitudes, and practices (KAP) among international flying pilots and flight attendants of a US commercial airline. *J Travel Med*. December 2012;19(6):366-372.

33. Priest PC, Jennings LC, Duncan AR, Brunton CR, Baker MG. Effectiveness of border screening for detecting influenza in arriving airline travelers. *Am J Public Health*. August 2013;103(8):1412-1418.

34. Centers for Disease Control and Prevention (CDC). Public health interventions involving travelers with tuberculosis—U.S. ports of entry, 2007-2012. *MMWR Morb Mortal Wkly Rep*. August 3, 2012;61(30):570-573.

35. DeMaria AN. Concierge medicine: for better or for worse? *J Amer Coll Cardiol*. 2005;46:377-378.

36. Portman RM, Romanow K. Concierge medicine: legal issues, ethical dilemmas, and policy challenges. *J Health Life Sci Law*. 2008;1:3-38.

Disaster Preparation and Response

ICS and NIMS

Molly A. Furin

INTRODUCTION

The current Incident Command System developed out of difficulties faced by firefighters four decades ago. During the 1970s, a series of forest fires ravaged southern California threatening populated areas. Despite adequate resources and personnel, many people were injured or killed and significant property damage was sustained.[1,2] Out of tragedy came the defined need for a better, more systematic approach.

OBJECTIVES

- Review the history of the creation of ICS.
- Describe NIMS and its relation to ICS and disaster response.
- Discuss the attributes and benefits of ICS.
- Outline the structure of ICS and positions within ICS with a special focus on roles pertinent to a physician.

BACKGROUND

Reviews of the events and management of the tragic California fires of the 1970s revealed several significant problems. Multiple organizations were forced to work together during the incidents. They typically had disparate organizational structures which made establishing and maintaining leadership problematic. Too many workers were reporting to one supervisor, leading to an unwieldy span of control. Planning and resource allocation were poorly coordinated within and between organizations. Intra-agency communication was not well established, and differences in terminology used by various agencies led to misunderstandings and vague reporting.[3] Incident information was unreliable and incident objectives were nonspecific.[4] Overall, it was resource and personnel management and organization which contributed to failures during the incidents, and firefighter leadership worked to change these problems.

FIRESCOPE

Fire Fighting Resources of Southern California Organized for Potential Emergencies (FIRESCOPE), a cooperative task force between local, state, and federal agencies, developed the seeds of the current Incident Command System.

INCIDENT COMMAND SYSTEM

The Incident Command System (ICS) is an organizational and management tool utilized during disaster situations and emergency response operations. FIRESCOPE recognized the need for a system to coordinate the multiple organizations responding to an incident. The system would need to be capable of incorporating agencies from diverse geographical locations with varying skills and leadership structures. It would need to use language and positions which could be universally recognized by the

group. A management structure based on the division of labor emerged, and while there have been several versions of ICS, the basic principles and attributes remain essentially unchanged. As it became recognized that the characteristics of wildfire fighting paralleled many of the characteristics of other disasters, ICS began to be applied more widely. It is now considered the standard among emergency management and its utilization is strongly encouraged by the federal government. The Hospital Incident Command System has developed from the core of the original ICS retaining many of its attributes. EMS physicians may encounter ICS while responding to a major disaster or while working in their own emergency departments. EMS physicians must be aware of the properties and structure of ICS and which positions they may be called upon to fill. They must also be advocates for the utilization of ICS as the national standard in emergency services delivery.

NATIONAL INCIDENT MANAGEMENT SYSTEM

In addition, ICS is a critical component of the National Incident Management System (NIMS). NIMS was designed in order to enable multiple agencies from different jurisdictions to work together during emergencies or disasters. NIMS is both flexible, as it is adaptable to incidents of all type and scale, and extremely structured in order to coordinate the incident management.[5] In the wake of the terrorist attacks of 2001 and the hurricane seasons of 2004 and 2005, the federal government recognized the importance of intra-agency coordination and made this a priority in homeland security. NIMS is a national guideline for managing emergency incidents based on five components: preparedness, communication and information management, resource management, command and management, and ongoing management and maintenance.[6] ICS, multiagency coordination systems, and public information are the elements which form the command and management component.

HOMELAND SECURITY PRESIDENTIAL DIRECTIVE 5

Homeland Security Presidential Directive 5, issued in March 2004, requires all federal departments and agencies to utilize NIMS. Compliance with NIMS became a condition for federal preparedness assistance.

THE NATIONAL RESPONSE FRAMEWORK

The National Response Framework (NRF) is an additional component of national disaster response planning. The NRF replaced the former National Response Plan. NRF is not an operational plan, but as its name suggests, a framework to guide responses to disasters and incidents of national significance. It is a blueprint which delineates the nation's response efforts. The principles of the NRF enable the country to respond to an emergency in a coordinated fashion. While NIMS outlines the approach to managing an incident, NRF describes the principles which enable a unified national approach to a disaster. NRF is intended to be an "all-hazards" model, so that it may be utilized in responding to any type and size incident from small scale to large. The five fundamental principles of NRF are engaged partnerships, tiered response, scalable, flexible, and adaptable operational capabilities, unity of effort through unified command, and readiness to act (NRF Web site). NRF also provides Emergency Support Function Annexes, which provide operational and procedural guidance based on the type of resource. ESF #8, Public Health and Medical Services, incorporates medical and mental health.

ATTRIBUTES OF ICS

With the development of ICS, 14 beneficial characteristics emerged. These factors often improved upon flaws in prior incident management (**Box 74-1**).

COMMON TERMINOLOGY

Establishing common terminology enables diverse entities from different specialties and jurisdictions to communicate effectively. It eliminates problems of group-specific lingo or terms and regional slang. Organizational positions and functions as well as resource descriptions are referred to by universal terms.

MODULAR ORGANIZATION

The organizational structure of the ICS develops based on the size, type, and complexity of the incident. It develops from the top down and can adapt to meet the needs of all types of hazards. Since it is expandable, it is able to change or grow depending on the nature of the incident. ICS should be employed even at smaller incidents. One issue with implementing ICS is that many providers feel uncomfortable with the principles and have little experience within the system. Frequently using and training with ICS facilitates its use in a larger or more complex emergency.[7]

MANAGEMENT BY OBJECTIVES

ICS requires that overall incident objectives and specific assignments and plans be developed. Objectives should be measurable and strategies to achieve those objectives must be created. Results must be documented to monitor progress.

INCIDENT ACTION PLANNING

Incident action planning refers to the process of communicating the overarching objectives for the incident. The incident action plan (IAP) refers to the formal documentation of the incident objectives. Priorities, tactics, and strategies will be included.[8]

MANAGEABLE SPAN OF CONTROL

Span of control emerged as a significant issue during the wildfires in southern California in the 1970s. The current ICS model limits the span of control for each individual position. The ideal span of control is three to seven subordinates. A larger span of control becomes unmanageable, contributing to poor leadership and supervision.

Box 74-1

Attributes of ICS

1. Common terminology
2. Modular organization
3. Management by objectives
4. Incident action planning
5. Manageable span of control
6. Incident facilities and locations
7. Comprehensive resource management
8. Integrated communications
9. Establishment and transfer of command
10. Chain of command and unity of command
11. Unified command
12. Dispatch/deployment
13. Accountability
14. Information and intelligence management

INCIDENT FACILITIES AND LOCATIONS

Specific types of facilities are designated by the ICS as well as suggested locations. Common facilities include the Incident Command Post, where the command staff centralize, and bases and camps for resources and personnel. Other facilities such as staging areas and triage areas may be established as the incident demands.

COMPREHENSIVE RESOURCE MANAGEMENT

Resource management is a critical element of incident management. Every resource, including personnel, and its utilization must be documented and its status kept current. Comprehensive resource management enables effective functioning at the incident and aids leadership in deciding the best manner in which to use resources. It assists in planning strategies for long-term events and cuts wastefulness.

INTEGRATED COMMUNICATIONS

Communications are designed to be interoperable and a plan to coordinate communications is created. Errors based on lack of information or miscommunications are decreased, and the response team functions more smoothly when all sectors remain well informed.

ESTABLISHMENT AND TRANSFER OF COMMAND

The initial establishment of command is paramount to the entire response effort. The primary response team is usually the first to take command. Systems for establishing command and how and when to transfer that command are necessary. Command may be transferred when more qualified individuals or services arrive or when the nature of the incident changes. A briefing process is standard when command needs to be transferred. ICS very clearly prescribes the process of formally transferring command.

CHAIN OF COMMAND AND UNITY OF COMMAND

Relationships are clearly delineated in the ICS which is a hierarchical system.[9] Chain of command refers to the ranking of personnel within the system. Each individual has a specific position within the organization with an orderly line of authority. Unity of command means that each individual has one and only one supervisor. Therefore, each person knows from whom he or she should be receiving orders and to whom he or she should report. These specific lines of authority reduce confusion among personnel and ensure that all orders are generated from the top of the chain and work their way down. Within ICS all decision making and commands are from the top down. Information tends to be collected by those on the ground and works its way from the bottom up.

UNIFIED COMMAND

Unified command occurs when multiple different agencies work together as the incident command. Decisions are made jointly between the various organizations, maintaining a unified leadership for the entire incident response. All partners in the unified command structure share decision making and power equally.[4] Unified command can be useful when several jurisdictions are involved in an incident, when multiple different types of agencies need to respond to an incident, or both. Unified command is typically preferable if the incident is complex and is not clearly the domain of one particular type of response agency. It enables different groups from different jurisdictions to function seamlessly on the response team. Both planning and resource management decisions are shared by the members of the unified command team.

DISPATCH/DEPLOYMENT

History has shown that many difficulties arise with convergent volunteerism, when resources volunteer themselves or dispatch without orders to do so. ICS controls which resources are deployed and the timing of deployment. The control of resources and personnel aids in accountability and overall safety of the incident response.

ACCOUNTABILITY

ICS strives to maintain full accountability for every resource responding to an incident. Five principles form the basis of accountability: check-in/check-out procedures, the incident action plan, unity of command, span of control, and resource tracking. Check-in/check-out enables command staff to know exactly what resources are at the scene. The incident action plan outlines all response operations and requires an accurate status of all resources. Unity of command aids in accountability by having each individual assigned to a supervisor. Span of control enables leaders to appropriately communicate with and direct their personnel. Resource tracking requires that all supervisors account for all resources, formally documenting their status. Together, these five processes enable an accurate picture of personnel and materials available at an incident.

INFORMATION AND INTELLIGENCE MANAGEMENT

ICS requires and facilitates the gathering, communication, and utilization of all information and intelligence related to the incident. The flow of information is frequently from individual responders or emergency personnel up to the command staff. An appropriate flow of communication and management of information ensures coordination of effort during the response. It also assists command staff in obtaining an accurate picture of the entire response effort, enabling effective incident management.

The current ICS addresses many of the weaknesses encountered by FIRESCOPE. In addition, it is designed to be universally applicable. The system works to coordinate vertically across disciplines and horizontally between all levels of government. It is an all-hazards approach to incident management, and should be employed at incidents and preplanned events of all nature and size.

STRUCTURE OF ICS

The ICS is a hierarchical, modular structure (**Figure 74-1**).[10] At the top of the structure is the incident commander, followed by the command staff: public information officer, safety officer, and liaison officer. The command staff supports the incident commander and carries out necessary functions to assist the incident commander. Below the command staff are the general staff, which may consist of up to four or five sections. The general staff are the functional areas of the incident management team. These sections are operations, logistics, planning, financial/administration, and intelligence/investigations. During the early stages of an incident, ICS may consist of the incident commander alone. The system expands as the incident grows and personnel become available, adapting to the needs of the particular emergency.

COMMAND STAFF

The incident commander is the person who is responsible for the overall incident management. The incident commander has authority at the scene and is responsible for delegating tasks. The Incident Command Post is established by the incident commander. Additional responsibilities include ensuring incident safety, determining objectives and goals for the incident, approving the *incident action plan*, and coordinating all command and general staff activities.[2] It is important to note that while command must develop the incident goals, they should not be directly involved in strategies or tactics unless there are insufficient personnel to establish the operations and planning sections. Strategic development is usually the domain of the planning section, and tactical decisions are made by the operations section. Incident commanders offer direction and guidance based on their authority and knowledge.

PUBLIC INFORMATION OFFICER

The public information officer maintains the flow of information at an incident. He or she must review the incident and develop appropriate information for media release, and must schedule media briefings over the course of the incident. The public information officer also makes information available to incident personnel. All information to be released to the public must be approved by the incident commander. In incidents that involve multiple command posts, the public information officer will lead or participate in the Joint Information Center, the purpose of which is to coordinate the dissemination of information so that a consistent message is delivered to the public.

SAFETY OFFICER

The safety officer strives to keep all incident personnel safe and free from injury. Safety officers review the incident action plan to check

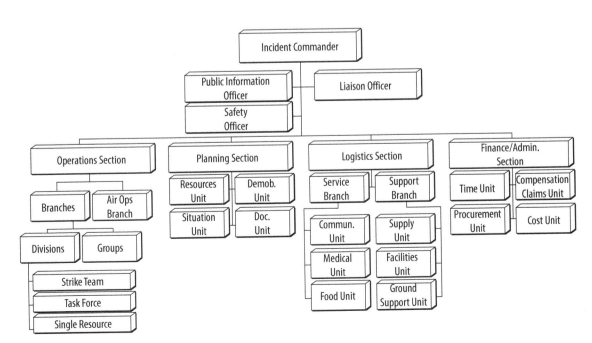

FIGURE 74-1. Incident Command System structure.

for unsafe practices, and they have the authority to stop any hazardous activities which they find. It is the job of the safety officer to approve the medical plan for the incident. This is one role which may be filled by an emergency physician who possesses the appropriate training, or the emergency physician will consult and assist the safety officer with any occupational health and safety issues.

LIAISON OFFICER

Another role which may accommodate an emergency physician is the liaison officer. The liaison officer is the point of contact for all agency representatives and coordinates all activities between agencies. The liaison officer must be aware of all available resources, capabilities, and limitations. Medical personnel may fit into this role well in certain types of incidents. A physician may be the person who is most knowledgeable about local hospitals, emergency medical services, and public health. As a liaison officer, he or she may be best suited to contact and work with these different agencies.

At times it may be appropriate for additional command staff positions to be formulated. These positions may be legal counsel or a medical advisor. A medical advisor may be utilized in order to keep the incident commander fully informed during specific types of incidents. Situations where a medical advisor may be useful include acts of bioterrorism, incidents requiring medical or mental health services, or mass prophylaxis.[2] In these situations the knowledge set of a physician may facilitate the goals of the incident commander.

GENERAL STAFF

The general staff form the functional units of the ICS. Each section is headed by a chief. Branches are the next organizational level and branch directors are their leaders. Divisions or groups follow, both lead by supervisors. Divisions are defined by geographical area, whereas groups are defined by functional areas.

OPERATIONS SECTION

The operations section is a fundamental module in the ICS since it undertakes all tactical activities. The operations section's functions are to reduce immediate hazards, save lives, and preserve property. Operations may be divided based on either a functional or geographical approach. When divided by function, groups are formed, and when divided by geography, divisions form. Task forces may operate which consist of a group of various types of resources working together with one leader and common communications. Strike teams are formed of combinations of the same type of resources, also with a single leader. Single resources are an individual piece of equipment, personnel, or a unified group which work under one supervisor.[2] Together these resources will carry out the operations necessary based on the type of emergency. The operations section chief manages all tactical operations and develops the tactical portions of the incident action plan. He or she also controls the utilization of resources for active operational activities.

PLANNING SECTION

All data relevant to the incident is compiled and evaluated by the planning section. The planning section is responsible for disseminating all information to the appropriate persons. Specialized data collection systems may be established as needed. The planning section incorporates relevant material from the various plans into the incident action plan. It also maintains the status of all resources and writes a demobilization plan. Often the planning section divides into four units. The resources unit records the status of all resources at the incident. It works to anticipate the needs for additional resources as well. Resource status, frequently shortened to "res-stat," is a summary of this information. The situation unit collects and analyzes any information on the incident status. A summary of this information is referred to as "sit-stat" or situation status. Demobilization planning begins as early as possible in an incident, and the demobilization unit ensures an organized plan for demobilization. The documentation unit records all documents relevant to the incident. It is crucial to document all events as they occur. At the completion of an incident, the only information which will be recalled is that which is documented. Scribing, carrying a notebook at all times, and photography all aid in accurately recounting the events of an emergency. For the medical professional, the 214 form should be completed daily in order to record it as accurately as possible.

LOGISTICS SECTION

Logistics fulfills all service support requirements. The logistics section provides facilities, housing, food, supplies, communication, security, and transportation needed by personnel. The section is divided into units in order to fulfill these needs. The supply unit orders and stores necessary resources and supplies. The ground support unit provides transportation and writes a traffic plan. Facilities are established and maintained by the facilities unit. Food and water are provided by the food unit. The communications unit obtains and organizes communication systems needed at the scene. The medical unit is responsible for the health and medical needs of all personnel at the scene. This is distinct from EMS or the medical aspect of the operations section, which is treating victims. The medical unit may be led by an emergency physician, or a physician may participate in its functioning. Specific medical needs and disaster-specific hazards should be anticipated by the medical unit. Personnel may be at risk for different injuries or medical problems based on the type of incident and the work that needs to be done.

The financial aspects of incident management can be overwhelming.

FINANCE/ADMINISTRATION SECTION

Finance and administration forms another section of the general staff. This section is responsible for finances related to the incident, as well as recording personnel time, addressing compensations and claims, establishing vendor contracts, and informing incident leaders regarding financial issues. Especially during large or long-term incidents, where funding is being received from myriad sources and payment must be made to many agencies and vendors, a finance and administration section is crucial. This section helps the incident commander to anticipate further monetary needs and aids in budgeting resources. It is often broken down into four units. The compensation/claims unit concerns itself with injuries and property damage related to the incident. Costs are tracked and analyzed by the cost unit. The procurement unit arranges and maintains vendor contracts. Recording time for the incident is the responsibility of the time unit.

While operations, planning, logistics, and finance/administration are the four major sections which are typically formed in ICS, a fifth section, intelligence/investigations, may be necessary. At times these functions may be added to the planning or operations sections or may be the responsibility of command staff. When this section is established, its duties are to gather and share incident-related intelligence.[6] Intelligence may include collecting information in a criminal investigation or may involve disseminating information and countermeasures in incidents such as public health events.

As the ICS system expands, multiple facilities must be established in order to house staff and resources. The types and numbers of facilities will depend on the nature of the incident. The incident command post should be present at every event. It houses the incident commander, command staff, and general section chiefs. The incident command post should be housed near the actual scene, as it is responsible for directing tactical operations. Central communications should also be part of the incident command center. An incident base is a location for support activities.[6] It may store equipment or personnel. Satellites to the incident base, which are needed to service more distant sites, are called camps. Camps may offer nutrition and sanitation services. Staging areas are locations where personnel and resources are stored awaiting activation.

THE PLANNING PROCESS

NIMS outlines the key steps in the planning process for incident management. The planning process may begin before the onset of an incident, such as in the case of a threat or impending disaster.[11] Each section is responsible for input into the planning process. While the incident commander ultimately develops objectives and approves resource orders, operations assigns and supervises resources. Planning will track resources, logistics orders resources, and finance/administration procures resources and manages costs.[6] Planning requires an accurate assessment of the situation, which resources are available, and what future events are likely to occur. It involves predicting the course of the incident and developing appropriate strategies to manage the event. An incident action plan for the following operational period should be written.

Five primary phases occur in the planning process (**Box 74-2**). The first is to understand the situation. Understanding the situation refers to both the size and type of emergency as well as what resources will be needed and are available. It is viewing the large picture of what is occurring at an incident. The next phase is to establish incident objectives and strategies. Objectives should entail overall incident goals, and the strategies are the means to obtain them. Strategies need to be reasonable and logistically sound. Developing the plan is the third phase of planning. This involves developing the actual tactics, assigning resources and equipment to specific tasks. Preparing and disseminating the plan is the fourth phase of the planning process. The actual plan will vary depending on the type of incident. Outline form is usually appropriate for an oral briefing, but a longer written plan should also be developed for complex incidents. Lastly, execute, evaluate, and revise the plan. This phase refers to putting the plan into action. After tasks are initiated, they should each be evaluated in order to create the next steps toward that goal. Revision of the plan contributes to the development of the plan for the next operational period. Actual progress needs to be taken into account and strategies may need to be reconsidered.

THE PLANNING P

The planning P is the diagrammatic representation of the planning process (**Figure 74-2**). The circular portion of the P is repeated in each planning operational period, whereas the linear portion is undertaken at the beginning of the incident only. The operational period is a variable length of time in which the tactical objectives are to be accomplished and the need to reevaluate the objectives emerges. This time period depends on factors specific to the incident, including the specific type and size of the event and the number and condition or available resources.[2] It is the task of the incident commander to determine the length of the operational period. The linear portion of the P is the initial response period. Five events comprise the initial response period: the incident or event, notifications, initial response and assessment, incident briefing using ICS form 201, and initial incident command or unified command meeting.

The incident command/unified command (IC/UC) objectives meeting marks the start of the cyclic portion of the planning P. At the onset of the incident, command identifies and outlines the overall objectives for the entire incident management. These objectives may be overwhelming, and the purpose of the division into operational periods is to break

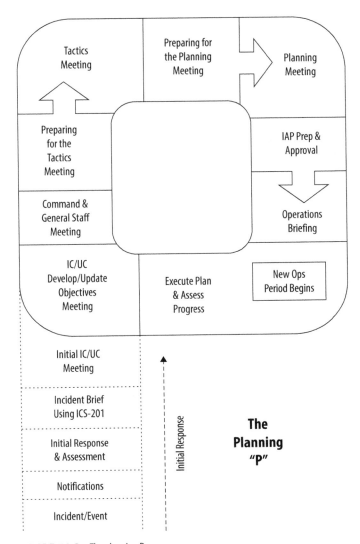

FIGURE 74-2. The planning P.

the larger objectives into manageable pieces. During the IC/UC objectives meeting, the specific goals for that period are determined. Any changes in strategy or tactics are taken into account. Next the command and general staff meeting occurs. During this meeting, communication and direction that need to be immediate are undertaken. Next, preparing for the tactics meeting and the tactics meeting ensue. The operations section chief leads the tactics meeting, whose aim is to devise and tweak tactical operations and to assign resources to accomplish particular tasks. Remember, objectives state what will be accomplished, strategies establish the general plan for accomplishing objectives, and tactics specify how each strategy will be accomplished.[2]

ICS form 215 records the operational planning from the tactics meeting. Following the tactics meeting is preparing for the planning meeting and the planning meeting. Preparing for the planning meeting includes analyzing ICS 215, writing a safety analysis (ICS 215A), and assessing resource efficiency and effectiveness of operations.[2] The planning meeting reviews the operational plan and is led by the planning section chief. The resource unit and the logistics section work together to delegate appropriate resources. During the planning meeting, safety concerns, policy issues, support requirements, and the incident action plan may all be discussed. After the planning meeting, the incident action plan preparation and approval occurs. Again, the planning section collates and prepares the IAP based on the information provided by the various sections. Ultimately the incident commander will review and approve

---

Box 74-2

Five Phases of Planning

1. Understand the situation.
2. Establish incident objectives and strategies.
3. Develop the plan.
4. Prepare and disseminate the plan.
5. Execute, evaluate, and revise.

the plan. ICS 202-206 are utilized in the development of the IAP. ICS 206, the incident medical plan, is a key component which may be prepared by the EMS physician. The operations briefing ensues, during which the IAP is presented to supervisors. This briefing marks the beginning of each operational period. Lastly, the plan is executed and assessed. Incident supervisors educate their staff on individual tasks and portions of the plan, while the operations section chief continues to assess the IAP implementation. Ultimately, the circular portion of the planning P begins again, with the IC/UC updating objectives for the event. In this manner, the goals of the incident continue to advance, while continuous assessment and revision of objectives, strategies, and tactics occur. The planning P provides an organized structure in which to perform these actions.

The ICS forms are a crucial element in the planning process (**Table 74-1**). While all forms may not be used at all types of incidents, they do provide a structured, uniform manner in which to compile and communicate important information. It is helpful to keep ICS forms organized in a binder or a laptop computer. Laminate copies provide the opportunity to write and rewrite the critical information through multiple operational periods.

SUMMARY

The ICS and NIMS systems have developed over the past years in response to issues and problems with managing incidents. The management structure of ICS is applicable to incidents of all type and size. NIMS is a national approach to managing emergency responses, utilizing the structure of ICS as a component. The EMS physician must be familiar with all aspects of these systems in order to function in the emergency environment. He or she must be capable of integrating into a variety of potential positions within the ICS structure, including command, operations, and technical specialists. The Federal Government offers a multitude of courses which can assist the EMS physician in building knowledge and confidence in different aspects of incident management (**Table 74-2**).

TABLE 74-2 Incident Command Courses

100.b: Introduction to the Incident Command System
200.b: ICS for Single Resources and Initial Action Incidents
300: Intermediate ICS for Expanding Incidents
400: Advanced ICS Command and General Staff—Complex Incidents
700.a: National Incident Management System (NIMS) An Introduction
800.b: National Response Framework (NRF) An Introduction

KEY POINTS

- The EMS physician should be familiar with the key elements of a functional and effective mass casualty incident response: interoperable communications; patient tracking; maintaining "usual procedures" as often as feasible instead of deploying disaster-specific procedures; utilizing NIMS by all disciplines and resources.
- MCI response begins with emergency preparedness planning.
- Planning should involve collaboration with all disciplines and resources that would respond and should be coordinated.
- The EMS physician may have many potential roles during an MCI. Role priorities should be addressed during the planning process.
- Disaster response practices that are significantly dependent on exchange of information between medical personnel are more prone to problems than processes that are not dependent on an exchange of information.
- Disaster response practices that differ from day-to-day health care practices, or do not encompass day-to-day health care practices, are more likely to give rise to problems than processes that remain essentially similar to day-to-day health care practices.
- The existence of a plan or a protocol does not prevent problems. Flexibility and adaptability must be reinforced during the planning and response processes.

REFERENCES

1. Buck DA, Trainor JE, Aguirre BE. A critical evaluation of the incident management system and NIMS. *JHSEM*. 2006;3(3):1-27.
2. U.S. Department of Homeland Security. ICS-300: Intermediate ICS for expanding incidents. 2008. http://training.fema.gov/emiweb/is/icsresource/trainingmaterials.htm.
3. Lindell MK, Perry RW, Prater CS. Organizing response to disasters with the incident command system/incident management system. International Workshop on Emergency Response and Rescue. Presentation, Oct 31, 2005, Taipei, Taiwan.
4. Stumpf J. Incident command system: the history and need. *Internet J Rescue Disaster Med*. 2001;2:1.
5. Hannestad SE. Incident command system: A developing national standard of incident management in the U.S. *Proceedings of the Second International ISCRAM Conference*, Brussels, Belgium; 2005.
6. Georgia Department of Community Health. *Incident Command System (ICS)*. Quick Series Publishing, Dollard-des-Ormeaux, QC, Canada, December 2010.
7. Reid WM, Brown LM, Landis DC. Leadership, collaboration, and effective principles and practices from a decade of training by a center for public health preparedness. *J Emerg Manag*. January-February 2014;12(1):31-44.
8. Klima DA, Seiler SH, Peterson JB, et al. Full-scale regional exercises: closing the gaps in disaster preparedness. *J Trauma Acute Care Surg*. September 2012;73(3):592-597.
9. Bigley GA, Roberts KH. The incident command system: high-reliability organizing for complex and volatile task environments. *Acad Manage J*. 2001;44(6):1281-1299.
10. Moynihan DP. The network governance of crisis response: case studies of incident command systems. *J Public Admin Res Theory*. 2009;19:895-915.
11. Perry RW. Incident management systems in disaster management. *Disaster Prev Manag*. 2003;12(5):405-412.

CHAPTER 75

Mass Casualty Management

Michael A. Redlener

Bradley Kaufman

INTRODUCTION

A mass casualty incident (MCI) is an event that produces or has the potential to produce multiple casualties requiring medical care. The goal of prehospital care is to provide the optimal level of care to save the most lives and minimize the morbidity of this type of event. For the purposes of this chapter, we will further define the term *mass casualty* as an event that challenges the everyday response capacity of a local response system requiring a change in mode of operation. This chapter will attempt to distill the essential elements of prehospital mass casualty management and planning.

OBJECTIVES

- Describe essential elements in planning for response to mass casualty.
- Describe on-scene responsibilities of EMS assets during a mass casualty response.
- Discuss the importance of patient tracking.
- Detail the role of EMS medical director during mass casualty management.
- Discuss some challenges of a multiagency response.
- Discuss prearranged roles of area hospitals and health care facilities during a mass casualty.
- List community and volunteer organizations that can expand the ability to care for patients during a mass casualty disaster.

SYSTEM EMERGENCY PREPAREDNESS AND PLANNING

Plans are nothing; planning is everything.

— Dwight D. Eisenhower

PLANNING

The planning phase of disaster preparedness is essential to mass casualty resource management. The development of response protocols for EMS, identification of emergency response capabilities, activation of the disaster response system, and regional/local interagency planning will create the framework for an effective response.[1-3] Prehospital medical care requires cooperation and coordination with many partners including government, hospital, and community resources.[4] Many communities perform hazard analysis to identify common and catastrophic scenarios that must be prepared for. Understanding the roles, responsibilities, and capabilities of each community, state and federal partner will promote a more efficient response.

EMS MASS CASUALTY MANAGEMENT TRAINING

EMS providers should be trained in the implementation of mass casualty scene management and incident command.[5] In fact, it is a requirement that first response agencies that receive federal funding are trained in Incident Command Systems (ICS) and National Incident Management Systems (NIMS). ICS, NIMS, and the federal response to disaster are all discussed in details in other chapters; however, it is important to mention here that the ability to have an interoperable, scalable response will allow the rapid incorporation of additional resources into a response effort that traverses local jurisdictions or requires a state or federal involvement.

DRILLS AND EXERCISES

Exercises are an essential step in the planning process. All components of a plan should be exercised, and then the interface for those individual components should be assessed in tabletop and full-scale exercises. Such exercises not only promote familiarization with the plans for all involved, but also identify deficiencies or areas for improvement. Subsequently the plans must undergo revisions and be reexercised. Therefore, the planning process may require less effort after initially developed, but remains a continuous cycle of evaluation and modification.[6]

Municipalities and states deal regularly with minor mass casualties, most of which do not impact the daily operations of EMS agencies. However, the principles of MCI management apply and these events can prove to be excellent trials for larger events. After-action reports should detail lessons learned and action plans to improve response.

ASPECTS OF MASS CASUALTY MANAGEMENT

MCI RECOGNITION AND ALERT

Plans must first take into account the process for notification of an incident and subsequent dispatch of resources including the process at the public safety answering center (PSAC). After an MCI, multiple calls to 9-1-1 may occur simultaneously.[7] Similarly, information and notifications often occur from other first response agencies (eg, police, fire) via radio communication or computer messages. Ideally, there should be an organized process for filtering and managing this information. An agency must identify the process for escalation of EMS response and declaration of an MCI. Should this occur prior to event confirmation by on-scene resources? Can this be determined by the first-line call-taker or must the PSAC supervisory personnel be required to make the determination? It is easy to imagine the implications on a system if the determination of an MCI is delayed, thereby delaying a sufficient EMS response. Similarly, unnecessary overresponse can also have detrimental effects—when units are removed from 9-1-1 response duties, there are less resources to respond to non-MCI emergencies. Furthermore, these decisions must often be made rather quickly. Establishing clear guidelines for such situations is critical.

From a medical and EMS standpoint, the Emergency Medical Dispatch (EMD) will generally take responsibility for dispatching prehospital EMS resources to the scene of an event. Ongoing communication between EMD and the field responders should continue as the situation develops. Only with constant, effective communication can incident commanders and medical leadership make good operational and medical decisions.

ON-SCENE MANAGEMENT

In the initial stages of an MCI, chaos should be expected as an event unfolds. Chemical or radiologic threats, an active shooter, building collapse or secondary devices can complicate an effective response.[7-9]

EMS agencies should have policies to establish a command structure immediately with the arrival of the first medical personnel that make clear considerations of scene safety.

Depending on the nature of the event, key response components should be established including an incident command post, triage/treatment areas, a casualty collection point and staging areas for resources.

As the scale and scope of the event becomes clear, the onsite incident command should be established per local protocol. The incident commander (IC) is responsible for operational and tactical decisions on the ground, resource allocation, and overall scene management. The medical branch director must work with the IC to establish the most appropriate patient care for any given situation. In general, EMS, if not the lead agency, will, per protocol, designate an individual to act as a medical branch director (**Box 75-1**).

The essential role of the Medical Branch director in an MCI is to balance the triage, treatment, and transport of patients to minimize the morbidity and mortality of any given event. The medical branch director must direct available resources based on the resource availability of a region. Triage is discussed in depth in a separate chapter; however, it is

---

Box 75-1

Responsibilities of the Medical Branch

1. Establishing command and control of medical operations
2. Identifying appropriate triage and treatment location(s), casualty collection points, and staging areas for EMS resources
3. Initiating patient triage
4. Performing immediate lifesaving efforts
5. Making transportation decisions
6. Maintaining situational awareness and communicating via ICS
7. Keeping personnel safe

Box 75-2

Implications of Self-Transported Patients

1. Self-transport of patients can confuse an organized response but should be expected.
2. The closest medical facilities/hospitals will be overwhelmed by self-transported patients.
   a. Consider transport to further hospital for "delayed" or stable patients who are being considered for treatment.
   b. Encourage hospitals to adopt surge plans that divert "minor" patients to nonambulance entrances.
3. Patients who are considered "contaminated" should be decontaminated on scene if stable.

---

worthwhile to mention that the scale of an event will skew the strategy (ie, if there is widespread facility or infrastructure destruction a greater proportion of care may occur in the prehospital setting).[10] If the number of critical patients are greater than the number of transport resources or if there is widespread distribution, then the role of on-scene medical direction, treatment, and disposition becomes more important. On the other hand, if there are an adequate number of EMS resources, triage will be essential to quickly transport critical patients to definitive care.

ESTABLISHING COMMAND AND CONTROL

The EMS providers at a mass casualty event take on the primary role for patient care and transport. The plans must first identify the person who will be directing the EMS actions. In general, the first EMS providers on the scene assume the command role until higher level EMS providers or officers arrive and assume control. This may be counterintuitive to providers who want to rush to an individual patient's rescue; however, first performing a rapid scene assessment and determination of need will better serve the MCI operation.

As higher level providers and leadership arrive to the scene, the command and control role typically transfers to those with higher authority. EMS providers are then assigned positions in the ICS format, which allows a clear line of reporting. There should be no confusion with regard to roles, responsibilities, and reporting.

TRIAGE, TREATMENT, CASUALTY COLLECTION, AND STAGING AREAS

The physical space where a mass casualty occurs will shape the operational context and thus the layout of how patients are cared for, where they are taken for safe immediate care and transport from the scene. Considerations should be made for CBRNE and provider safety (cold, warm, and hot zones) and issues related to ingress and egress of EMS vehicles.

Triage and Treatment Areas   Ideally, all mass casualty victims be transported from the scene immediately. However, in an MCI, usually, this is not possible. Therefore, it is necessary to 1) establish triage and treatment areas to separate critical from non-critical patients, perform life-saving treatments and develop a transport priority list; 2) Deploy treatment resources to dedicated areas, not an entire MCI scene and 3) Monitor multiple patients simultaneously.

Casualty Collection Point   The Casualty Collection point is a space designated by the medical branch director or IC to arrange for on-scene providers to meet transport resources.

Staging Area   The Staging Area is the site selected for resources to wait prior to arriving on the scene of an MCI. Selecting the staging area is key to ensuring that there is appropriate ingress and egress of emergency vehicles. Failure of appropriate staging or control of vehicles can contribute to delayed response and time to definitive care.[10]

EMS AND SELF-TRANSPORT OF MCI PATIENTS

The goal of EMS transport decision making is to transport the sickest patients who will benefit from definitive lifesaving care first. Rational triage and transportation decisions based on this goal are ideal. However, there will be many patients who will self-transport from the scene. Analyses of major MCIs demonstrate that this wave of patients arrive first to area emergency departments, causing operational strain to hospitals prior to the arrival of critical patients.[1,10] Some may believe they have not been physically affected, others will believe it is better to seek care independently; more often than not, they will be considered "minor" patients. Other people, not directly impacted by the incident will be concerned for themselves and/or their families and seek medical care. There are many accounts in the medical literature that demonstrate this phenomenon.[7] The closest hospital to an MCI will become quickly overwhelmed with less seriously injured patients and the "worried well." In Japan, after the Sarin subway attacks, out of 498 patients presenting to the closest hospital from the attack, only 19.9% arrived by Tokyo Metropolitan Fire Department vehicle, the remainder walked, arrived by taxi, or got a ride from a passerby[9] (**Box 75-2**).

COMMUNICATION

The tenants of effective radio and telephone communication are generally taught to EMS providers and used frequently without adverse consequence. However, it has been shown that the stress and chaos of an MCI can affect the quality of communication in general. Attention to the transfer of information will impact the overall ability of the system to respond.

First responders utilize several systems of communication. During an MCI, particularly an event that causes public health and infrastructure breakdown, effective communication strategy will underlie an effective response. In many complex emergencies, breakdown in communications have led to key failures in response.

PROVIDER SAFETY

As with any prehospital care, it is essential for medical personnel to understand the scene safety profile at an MCI. Any event that has produced a significant number of casualties must be thoroughly analyzed prior to the initiation of patient care for a hazardous environment (**Box 75-3**).

SPECIALTY RESOURCESS

EMS providers may have additional training that allows them to manage patients in unique circumstances. For instance, tactical EMTs and paramedics may join with a police department SWAT team to provide patient care in an unsecured environment. Similarly, EMS providers may have additional training for HAZMAT and rescue operations (eg, swift water, high angle, etc) and thereby be inserted into those unique environments.

Box 75-3

Key Operational Problem at the March 1995 Tokyo Subway Sarin Attack

Disregard for provider safety and patient decontamination:

Ten percent of EMTs from the Tokyo Metropolitan Fire Department (TMFD), the key prehospital medical provider, suffered from acute organophosphate poisoning due to secondary exposure from sarin gas vaporized from transported patients.

EMS Physician Role

Provision of subject matter expertise

Implementation of altered standards of care

Class orders

On-scene disposition of patients

The medical care provided may be limited by the environment, for instance, the ability to intubate or perform certain procedures in HAZMAT personal protective equipment. On the other hand, the MCI environment may actually require increased amount or level of prehospital medical care than what is normally provided. For instance, a patient entrapped in a confined space might benefit from additional medications for the treatment of crush syndrome or might require extremity amputation for extrication. Such scenarios should be considered in advance, and additional medical protocols might be prepared. Alternatively, an EMS physician might be required to manage such cases directly or via discretionary orders to the on-scene EMS providers.

EMS PHYSICIAN ROLE

The role of a medical director of an EMS agency changes based on the experience and history of each agency/locality. Advanced understanding of prehospital care and triage may benefit the providers on the ground. As first responders, EMS medical directors may improve the ability of prehospital providers to address the ongoing needs of the patients affected by mass casualty. The following list reflects responsibilities of the EMS physician that are key to prehospital care provision and will likely impact the overall system response effectiveness (**Box 75-4**).

Provision of subject matter expertise: Physicians can act as on-scene medical subject matter and clinical experts for IC with specific medical knowledge related to injury types (eg, blast, crush, burns), toxicological and biological exposures, radioactive contamination, and other advanced medical knowledge. This allows them to advise on the most appropriate patient care and triage strategies in complex or unusual scenarios.

Implementation of altered standards of care: This concept has been discussed by the Institute of Medicine in depth and it goes beyond standard triage—when patients of equally severe injury/disease require advanced care that is limited or unavailable.[12,13] In conjunction with operational leadership, EMS medical directors will be required to make justifiable and ethical decisions for who will get the care available. Physician leadership will be key to creating and implementing these standards.

Class orders: The use of antidote for a weapon of mass destruction or the activation of class orders may be necessary for situations that involve the use of chemical, biologic, or radiologic weapons. Caches of antidote may be mobilized with this order. EMT and first responders will be tasked with distribution and treatment with specialized care.

On-scene disposition of patients: The treatment and disposition of walking wounded and worried well patients may provide relief of the system surge burden. As is mentioned in the earlier section, one of the more challenging aspects of prehospital transport is preventing the overburdening of the closest hospital by patients' self-transporting. If patients can be seen by a provider and dispatched to their home or nonmedical facility, this can ease this concern.[14]

PATIENT TRACKING IN MASS CASUALTY

Patient tracking is essential for effective mass casualty care. In order to appropriately respond and plan in an MCI, prehospital medical leadership must understand numbers of patients, triage categories, patient movement, and distribution to hospitals.

There are many reasons to accurately track patients. Firstly, medical and operational leadership needs to understand the distribution of patients, most notably, critical patients in order to continue to make informed decisions related to patient transport.

In some events (eg, explosions), patients will not necessarily be readily identifiable, so tracking that includes location found will assist in identification of patients. As families begin the search for family members that may have been involved, the more information available to them, the higher the likelihood they will be able to find their loved one. From an operational standpoint, when victim/patient identification is improved, there is less of a likelihood that patient friends and family will disrupt ongoing medical operations.

Technology offers opportunities for improving patient tracking. RFID technology, barcodes on triage tags, and electronic patient record sharing are all methods that have been recommended and/or tested.

MASS CASUALTY INCIDENT: A MULTIAGENCY RESPONSE

MCIs are generally recognized to transcend the medical first response community. Local incident management should be preestablished. First response agencies, including EMS, should have defined role and protocolized interaction in an MCI.[15,16] Joint training and drills should reinforce these key relationships so that during mass casualty management, there is less confusion among responders. As the size, scope, or nature of the MCI evolves, the response can escalate as needed. High-profile or complex events will trigger a multiagency response from all levels of government and response network. The overlapping goals and aims of these responder agencies can increase activity and chaos on scene.

The challenge for the medical response is to identify and treat all victims of an MCI in as safe and secure manner as circumstances allow. Life safety and patient treatment ranks high in the goals of response. However, each agency will have priorities based on the goal of their operation. For instance, the goal of the police response will be to gather evidence and provide security to the public. Operational needs must be clearly identified and communicated with other responding agencies. **Box 75-5** demonstrates a typical large-scale event response from New York City (NYC) agencies.

INTEGRATION OF EMS RESPONSE TO HEALTH CARE NETWORK

Variability exists among regions with regard to information sharing and emergency planning. In an ideal world, relationships between EMS and hospitals will have been established and strengthened by drills and training. Real-time information about emergency department, surgical, and ICU bed availability will affect the transport decisions that prehospital providers make.

Identification and classification of all medical facilities in a community is essential. Knowledge of hospital resources should be a common component of a prehospital system. EMS physicians and providers know the everyday capabilities of each hospital, that is, which hospital is a trauma center, a STEMI center, etc.

During a mass casualty incident, EMS providers and emergency managers need to understand the surge capacity of the system. Each mass casualty scenario will challenge one or more aspect of a health care system. What if there are a high volume of pediatric patients? Burn patients? How will the system adjust to each eventuality? EMS physicians need to understand the regional planning for surge patient care in order to distribute patients to the most appropriate facilities. Additionally, it is essential to know the alternatives to traditional emergency care facilities.

Soon after the recognition of an MCI, the area hospitals should be notified. This task may be assigned to the communications personnel or a separate operations center of such resource exists. The EMS and other on-scene personnel should not be responsible for making such contacts as they will be extremely busy and on-scene communications may be limited. During the notification, the hospitals should be queried as to

Agencies Responding to a Large-Scale Event in NYC

1. EMS
2. FDNY
3. HAZMAT
4. HazTac
5. NYC Police Department
6. Port Authority Police Department
7. Metropolitan Transportation Authority Police Department
8. Emergency Services Unity
9. NYC Office of Emergency Management
10. Port Authority Office of Emergency Management
11. NYC Department of Environmental Protection
12. US Department of Homeland Security
13. NYS Office of Homeland Security
14. FBI/DOJ
15. Mayor's Office
16. Joint Terrorism Task Force
17. NYPD counterterrorism
18. NY State Police
19. NYC Sanitation
20. Medical Examiner
21. FEMA
22. Military/Department of Defense
23. National Guard
24. American Red Cross
25. Salvation Army
26. Centers for Disease Control
27. US Public Health Service
28. Con Ed
29. NYC Dept of Buildings
30. Port Authority
31. Metropolitan Transportation Authority
32. NY State Emergency Management Office
33. NMDS
34. PD Auxiliary
35. Regional EMS Council
36. US Environmental Protection Agency
37. US Transportation Security Admin
38. US National Transportation Safety Board
39. NYC Dept of Education
40. US Coast Guard
41. NY Department of Health
42. NYC Department of Health and Mental Hygiene

the number of critical and noncritical patients that they can handle, as well as specialty referral patients (eg, burn, trauma). This information is then relayed to the IC or medical branch director either verbally via radio or phone, or via an electronic message, to allow for improved decision making for patient transports. Hospital personnel must understand that the availability reported is taken into consideration; however, large numbers of patients may require EMS transports that can overwhelm an emergency department, and hospitals are required to plan for such events via the Hospital Incident Command System (HICS). Hospitals contacted may initiate plans to receive patients from an event, and yet may not receive any. Therefore, hospitals should similarly be contacted when MCI operations conclude to prevent them from unnecessarily anticipating patients (eg, keeping trauma areas cleared).

EXPANDING THE RESPONSE CAPACITY OF THE REGION

■ COMMUNITY PARTNERS

Community health clinics, schools, or other large public spaces can be retasked to provide care to less seriously injured or affected patients. These resources can reduce the burden to hospitals and emergency departments who will need to care for the more critical patients in the short and long term. In mass casualty incidents that occur and develop over an extended period of time, this will be a fluid process that planners and providers will need to address over time. Identification of these potential resources should occur prior to a mass casualty event. Plans should be in place that prepare these partners to take on these roles should it be required.

EMS leadership needs to develop policy prior to a mass casualty incident that delineates transport decisions to nontraditional facilities.

Mobile health clinics have been utilized to reach people and populations affected by natural disaster without access to adequate transportation.[17]

Federal resources, as discussed in Chapter 75, such as DMAT field hospitals, will be common alternatives for localities that have had their health care facilities overwhelmed or determined not to be operational.

■ MUTUAL AID AGREEMENTS

Mutual aid agreements augment local and/or regional medical capacities in times of medical need. There are several ways in which mutual aid is organized. Local EMS agencies will sign agreements with adjacent communities if their communities have increased demand on services.

If a region has become overwhelmed by an event, state-based resources and federal resources through FEMA can be made available based on community requests, including EMS resources specifically or entire disaster medical assistance teams (DMAT) and Urban Search and Rescue (USAR) teams.

■ AMERICAN RED CROSS AND OTHER AID ORGANIZATIONS

Nongovernmental organizations (NGOs) are common in the disaster response field. There are direct care organizations and those that provide support functions to the medical response community, providing important resources for patients and providers, including blood product distribution, relief supplies, etc. Also, NGO groups often assist in running facilities/shelters.

■ CREDENTIALING AND VOLUNTEERS

Health care professionals often volunteer their services to a community in need. This altruistic response must be tempered by a system to ensure quality and qualifications of providers. On a national and sometimes local level, a number of disaster medical response systems have attempted to deal with this problem.

■ MEDICAL RESERVE CORPS (MRC) AND COMMUNITY EMERGENCY RESPONSE TEAMS (CERT)

This federally guided effort recruits physicians and other medical professionals to a prescreened network of potential responders. In times of high demand or disruption of the established medical network, these physicians can fill or backfill necessary specialties. CERTs typically comprise nonmedically-trained citizens who have training in areas of disaster response and recovery.

REGIONAL PLANNING

Federal Emergency Management Agency Regional health care planning occurs through multiple modalities. Emergency Service Function 8 (ESF 8) is the federally sanctioned regional tool utilized to coordinate health care resources in the event of a disaster or true mass casualty event. EMS should be a key player in this group. Communication of challenges and needs should be made through this group.

CONCLUSION

While all MCIs will have unique characteristics that will influence the type of response that is made, it is important to identify the common processes associated with emergency response in MCI situations (**Box 75-6**).

As this chapter delineates each step of a disaster response, these themes will recur in the discussion of each. The lessons of each event described in the literature contribute to the overall understanding of the medical response; however, a systematic approach will provide prehospital/EMS system medical directors with a comprehensive approach to mass casualty preparedness and response.

Box 75-6

Factors Contributing to Failure of Disaster Response

- Communication: Processes in which exchange of information among medical personal plays a major role are more likely to be affected by problems than processes in which this is less relevant.

- Processes in which disaster circumstances differ from day to day health care, or do not figure in day-to-day health care, are more likely to give rise to problems than processes that remain essentially similar.

- The existence of a protocol or disaster plan governing a process does not prevent problems.

KEY POINTS

- The incident commander (IC) is responsible for operational and tactical decisions on the ground, resource allocation, and overall scene management.

- The medical branch leader must work with the IC to establish the most appropriate patient care for any given situation

- Community health clinics, schools, or other large public spaces can be retasked to provide care to less seriously injured or affected patients.

- EMS providers should be trained in the implementation of mass casualty scene management and incident command. It is a requirement that members of first response agencies, that receive federal funding, receive training in Incident Command Systems (ICS) and National Incident Management Systems (NIMS).

REFERENCES

1. Waeckerle JF; Disaster Planning and Response, *N Engl J*, 1991;324 (14):815-821.
2. Dunlop AL, Logue KM, Isakov AP. The engagement of academic institutions in community disaster response: a comparative analysis. *Public Health Rep*. 2014;129(suppl 4):87-95.
3. Rubin J. In defense of emergency plans. *J Environ Health*. September 2014;77(2):30-31.
4. After Action Report for the Response to the 2013 Boston Marathon Bombings, 2014, Produced by the Massachusetts Emergency Management Agency, Massachusetts Department of Public Health, City of Boston, et al accessed at http://www.mass.gov/eopss/docs/mema/after-action-report-for-the-response-to-the-2013-boston-marathon-bombings.pdf, p 38-40.
5. Blumenthal DJ, Bader JL, Christensen D, et al. A sustainable training strategy for improving health care following a catastrophic radiological or nuclear incident. *Prehosp Disaster Med*. February 2014;29(1):80-86.
6. Homeland Security Exercise and Evaluation Program (HSEEP), April 2013, Federal Emergency Management Agency accessed at http://www.fema.gov/media-library-data/20130726-1914-25045-8890/hseep_apr13_.pdf.
7. Lockey DJ, MacKenzie R, Redhead J, et al; Major Incident Report – London bombings July 2005: The immediate pre-hospital medical response; Resuscitation 66 (2005) ix-xii.
8. Maningas P, Robinson M, Mallonee S; The EMS Response to the Oklahoma City Bombing, *Preh Dis Med*;1997;12(2):80-85.
9. Okumura T, Suzuki K, Fukudu A, et al. The Tokyo Subway Sarin Attacks: Disaster Management, Part 1: Community Emergency Response. *Acad Emerg Med*. 1998;5(6):613-617.
10. Carresi A, The 2004 Madrid train bombings: an analysis of pre-hospital management. *Disasters*. 2007:41-65.
11. Hogan DE, Waeckerle JF, Dire DJ, Lillibridge SR, Emergency Department Impact of the Oklahoma City Terrorist Bombing, *Ann Emer Med*. 1999;34:160-167.
12. Hanfling D, Altevogt BM, Viswanathan K, Gostin LO, Crisis Standards of Care: A Systems Framework for Catastrophic Disaster Response, Institute of Medicine, National Academies Press, Washington DC 2012.
13. Rios C, Redlener M, et al. Addressing the Need, Ethical Decision Making in Disasters, Who Comes First? *Journal Of U.S.-China Medical Science*.
14. Redhead J, Ward P, Batrick N; The London Attacks – Response, Prehospital and Hospital Care. *N Engl J Med*. 2005; 353;6: 546-547.
15. Sabra JP, Cabañas JG, Bedolla J, et al. Medical support at a large-scale motorsports mass-gathering event: the inaugural Formula One United States Grand Prix in Austin, Texas. *Prehosp Disaster Med*. August 2014;29(4):392-398.
16. Jacobs LM, Wade DS, McSwain NE, et al. The Hartford Consensus: THREAT, a medical disaster preparedness concept. *J Am Coll Surg*. November 2013;217(5):947-953.
17. Krol DM, Redlener M, Shapiro A, Wajnberg A, A Mobile Medical Care approach Targeting Underserved Populations in post-Hurricane Katrina Mississippi. *Health Care for the Poor and Underserved*. 2007;18(2):331-340.

Federal Response and Interoperability

Dario Gonzalez

INTRODUCTION

This chapter will discuss the issue of disaster response by local, state, regional, municipal, and tribal authorities. Additionally, the issue of federal participation and the factors associated with an integrated and interoperable response process will be reviewed and federal response activities outlined. The management and mitigation of disaster response activities are multifaceted with significant negative consequences if not managed correctly. The federal assets available for local response and mitigation are significant and available for those that are aware of the full depth of resources.[1-7] The federal assets are not only limited to logistical support but also include human resources that are significant in their expertise and organizational skills. Knowledge of the Federal Response Plan and associated legal statutes allow for informed emergency management planning and modifying the incident impact.

OBJECTIVES

- Discuss, and review issues associated with interoperability.
- Review the Federal Response Plan.
- Review the Department of Defense (DoD) assets in disaster mitigation.
- Discuss National Disaster Medical System (NDMS)/Disaster Medical Assistance Team (DMAT) medical operations and structure.

INTEROPERABILITY AND EMS SYSTEM DESIGN

Interoperability is the process by which information, communication, and data systems are designed to easily and consistently connect/interface with each other independent of the manufacturer, management system, or operating platform. This would apply to federal, municipal, state, tribal routine and/or disaster operations with respect to incident communication, mitigation, and response. One example of successful interoperability can be found in casual Internet computer access. This task is carried out countless of times per day independent of the computer manufacturer, platform, or even operating system, yet we accept the impossibility of this when it comes to medical information sharing.

Applied to disaster and EMS operations, interoperability is the ability of simultaneous responders and/or agencies to be able to freely communicate and/or share data on a real-time basis. Unfortunately, prehospital health information (clinical, demographic, incident data) is not routinely managed in an interoperable platform. In this case information sharing between different emergency response agencies and/or federal partners at a disaster scene is at best a cumbersome process (and we accept this as a given fact). In the ideal world, the ability to integrate differing systems and organizations to seamlessly interface and operate efficiently and effectively with one another should be the norm.[8] This would allow all (local, civilian, federal, NGOs [nongovernmental organization] and military) end users to effectively perform disaster activities and enable end users to perform disaster operations as an integrated coordinated operation. This would allow for greater situational awareness and avoid duplication of services (ie, building searches).

Presently there are no existing national (or even regional) interoperability standards or guidelines for EMS systems or federal resources but concepts are in various stages of development and have been repeatedly identified as an issue (seen in Katrina and 9/11). Interoperability is defined by the Oxford Dictionary of the US Military as "... the ability of systems, units, or forces to provide services to and accept services from other systems, units, or forces and to use the services so exchanged to enable them to operate effectively together; the condition achieved among communications-electronics systems or items of communications-electronics equipment when information or services can be exchanged directly and satisfactorily between them and/or their users."[9]

Department of Defense (DoD) Northern Command (NORTHCOM) while conducting rescue operations during Hurricane Katrina noted a lack of common standards among communications platforms which did not allow first responders to directly communicate with federal assets (or even sometimes between federal responders).[1] In one situation, Urban Search and Rescue (USAR) assets were actively involved in a rescue of military and civilian personnel, from an overturned military truck in flood waters with multiple occupants. A circling military helicopter overhead produced significant wash of water over the victims while hovering over the incident location. The on-scene USAR group attempted to signal and contact the helicopter but was unsuccessful. Communication from ground FEMA (Federal Emergency Management Agency) USAR personnel to helicopter crew followed this process: USAR field operations to USAR base of operations that required a face to face with military personnel at the Zephyr base helipad to have them contact the circling helicopter to pull back (even though they were just above the civilian/military group). The rescue could not be affected until this was accomplished.

At this point in time, written communication (though inefficient) is the only universal method of interoperable information (data storage, transmission, and common information [language]) sharing that exists between civilian and/or federal assets. Interoperability is not just a technical concept, but is a practical information, communication, and management process. Existing EMS and military development is focused on single system needs (ie, NYC 9-1-1) and local operational needs, creating islands of development with closed information silos. This does not optimize resource utilization, but rather limits the effectiveness of a unified disaster response and mitigation process. Interoperability is not an all or nothing concept, but may in the future be implemented in a stepwise manner. A need exists for standards that create accurate, complete, private, secure data sharing systems. Interoperable health information systems should ideally work together within and across organizational boundaries in order to advance the effective/efficient delivery of health care resources for individuals and communities. This applies to different first-responder groups (local, neighboring, and distant EMS systems, police and fire) as well as federal (USAR, NDMS, DoD, etc) and civilian (Red Cross, Salvation Army, etc) groups.

Communications interoperability is probably the most critical necessary component in disaster and day-to-day EMS, military, and local government response (and mitigation) operations. Disaster operations fail or succeed as communication is maintained and managed. Communication interoperability avoids duplication of efforts and resources but requires crossing traditional jurisdictional lines of authority and reporting relationships (how, to or thru who). Traditional methods impair the free flow of critical "real-time" information and therefore situational awareness: disciplines (police vs EMS vs fire), civil versus military, federal versus municipal, or other responding agencies' (NGOs') ground operations to communicate with air assets (helicopter to ambulance). The goal is to allow any emergency responder to operate and work seamlessly with other systems without any special effort. Allow police, firefighters, EMS, military responding assets to better coordinate disaster efforts, that is, wireless communications that allows the sharing of information via voice and/or data platforms, in real time. Communication interoperability increases rescue operation efficiency and decreases redundancy/duplication of efforts while decreasing event impact (ie, single common evacuation and operations channel).

Interoperability planning allows for Standard Operating Procedures (SOPs), incident contingencies (Earthquake [EQ]), with Tsunami, with nuclear reactor containment failure), emergency evacuation procedures, medevac operations, or event deterioration (second EQ), event termination. Coordinated interagency decision making is required to establish priorities, support local municipalities, establish common rescue protocols (i.e. victim location, house marking post search, rescue, procedures, and body management-location).

National Incident Management System (NIMS) interoperability and compatibility mandates public/private partnerships to develop a functional integrated (technology use, support, technical integration), effective, efficient disaster response operation (data acquisition, utilization, interpretation, including information sharing), and incident management operations. This includes complimentary and compatible emergency management response and common and adapted standards, http://www.safecomprogram.gov/SAFECOM/interoperability/default.htm (including terminology). *NIMS STEP (Supporting Technology Evaluation Program)* is an attempt to develop an independent, objective assessment of commercial and government hardware/software projects. Interoperability is a critical component of the emergency management process (local and national) in order to foster the incident implementation of NIMS operations. In *Citations from FEMA 501, National Incident Management System:* "Systems operating in an incident management environment must be able to work together (across disciplines and jurisdictions) and not interfere but rather complement one another. Interoperability and compatibility are achieved through the use of tools such as common communications and data standards (ie, audio and video), digital data formats, equipment, and design standards." RapidCom was initiated by President Bush in 2004; this program mandated a minimum level of emergency response interoperability that ultimately resulted in coordinated efforts in the cities of Boston, Chicago, Houston, Jersey City, Los Angeles, Miami, New York, Philadelphia, San Francisco, and Washington. This program was to assess city communications interoperability capabilities, identify deficiencies, propose and initiate solutions. When completed, incident commanders within the identified jurisdictions would have the capability of communicating between command centers (within 1 hour of an incident). Emergency Response Interoperability Center (ERIC) had the stated goal, to ensure national interoperability utilizing 700-MHz network. To establish interoperability regulations, license requirements, and technical standards. Project participating federal departments included Department of Homeland Security (DHS), National Institute of Standards and Technology (NIST), Department of Justice (DOJ), and Department of Commerce (DOC). *Civil-military interoperability:* Strategic *concept* for the defense and security of the members of NATO, to better coordinate the military civilian emergency response sector within the NATO group (multinational *civil-military interoperability*).[2]

Systems interoperability allows for the capacity to operate effectively, efficiently, and seamlessly. Compatible communication frequencies provide the ability to share (where appropriate) confidential medical information via common platforms and being capable to easily transfer data between systems. Interoperability system deficiency was identified during the attacks on 9-1-1 on the World Trade Center and the Pentagon and during Hurricane Katrina disaster response, yet to date this issue has not been fully resolved.

INTEGRATION AND INTEROPERABILITY DURING SMALL AND LARGE-SCALE RESPONSES

Department of Defense (DoD) is capable of the deployment of large assets in response to the need for the support of domestic disaster relief. DoD normally functions in a supporting role, but the Hurricane Katrina response left many unanswered questions as to the preparedness of the involved states and the need for federal support function.

US military role in Hurricane Katrina relief operations consisted of ~72,000 service members assisted by 346 helicopters, 76 fixed-wing aircraft, 21 ships, amphibious landing crafts, satellite imagery, construction support, and mortuary teams. Thousands of Gulf coast residents were rescued and evacuated by military assets. The military provided greater than 30 million meals ready-to-eat (MRE) and 10,000 truckloads of ice and water for the civilian population. Hurricane Katrina was a Category 5 (with subsequent levee failure) and was of such a magnitude that there was a questionable level and capabilities of the municipality and state with respect to "preparedness" and their ability to save lives and

property. It was clear that first responders at the local and state levels were overwhelmed and the need for federal response was critical. There were problems encountered between all levels of government and multiple involved federal agencies with respect to rescue operation integration, and lines of authority (who is in charge, establish search areas, house access, etc).

President Bush suggested the leadership role in disaster relief operations be entrusted to the Department of Defense. For example, the United States Navy (USN) has within its ranks significant assets that can be utilized for domestic disaster response but at the same time limited ability to communicate or integrate with existing local entities. USN response to domestic disasters is a nontraditional role, based on an independent unilateral Navy-centric operation, with minimal civil integration, resources. This was more often an accident of chance rather than the result of emergency management planning. The USN brings significant capabilities (aircraft carriers, amphibious vessels, and other vessels) and expertise (communications, logistics) to the table. As the Navy responded to Katrina the local power and communication systems (ie, 9-1-1) were inoperable, limiting the response capabilities of the state and municipality as they attempted to respond, limit and mitigate the disaster. The local authorities had insufficient awareness of military capabilities and/or limitations, to such a point that assets like the USS Bataan were underutilized (and simply stood off shore without a significant mission assignment). You had to know who had what and how to get it! Issues to resolve were the coordination and integration of communication systems, and the legal procedure to acquire and utilize these resources. Utilization of emergency resources (including the Louisiana's National Guard) and equipment in the region lacked situational awareness regarding the impact of levee failures; insufficient civilian/military resources integration city to assist in the evacuation of the stranded population after Katrina's landfall. The National Guard forces employed under State Active Duty or Title 32 status are under the command and control of the governor of their state and were not considered part of federal military response efforts. They performed exemplary via military command to rescue countless individuals from roof tops.

DoD developed a rapid and massive response that occurred through two major components, Northern Command (NORTHCOM) and the National Guard, but this was as an independent response system. At the same time, the Louisiana National Guard deployed the majority of the personnel from state activations during the initial response period as directed by the governor. NORTHCOM spearheaded federal efforts under its Joint Task Force Katrina (JTFK) with the following federal military units: Air Force, Navy, Marines, and Army. It deployed 77 aircraft, 18 vessels, >10,000 navy personnel to support JTF-Katrina's operations. USNORTHCOM supported Department of Homeland Security (DHS) and Federal Emergency Management Agency (FEMA) and other federal agencies in disaster relief efforts for the mitigation of Hurricane Katrina with > 21,400 Active Duty personnel and 45,700 Army and Air National Guard members supported the effort in the Gulf Coast.[16] The traditional US Navy operations utilize the organization of a Carrier Strike Group, helicopters, and aircraft carrier jets, supported by other vessels and personnel, but were not significantly modified for civilian disaster response. During Hurricane Katrina, many of the vessels (USS Bataan, USS Truman, USS Iwo Jima, USNS Comfort) normally utilized as support vessels assumed the leading role for disaster response. The subsequent push of military personnel, materials, and equipment did not have the immediate impact that many had envisioned. A postdisaster review from independent Congressional committees[a,b] cited the

---

[a] Statement by Paul McHale, Assistant Secretary of Defense for Homeland Defense; Before the 109th Congress; Select Bipartisan Committee to Investigate the Preparation for and Response to Hurricane Katrina; United States House of Representatives; October 27, 2005

[b] Civil–Military Relations in Hurricane Katrina: A Case Study on Crisis Management in Natural Disaster Response; Chapter 22; Jean-Loup Samaan and Laurent Verneuil

TABLE 76-1 US Navy Resources Utilized in the Katrina Hurricane Response

Vessel Name/Type	Event Operation/Function
Amphibious Assault Vehicles (USS Iwo Jima)	Smaller versions of aircraft carriers (but large-profile amphibious assault vessels); different capabilities: transport, rapidly deploy, direct large numbers of Marines, vehicles, and equipment to shore on smaller landing craft and helicopters; diverse usable disaster vehicles
USS Bataan	First vessel to respond during Hurricane Katrina
USS Iwo Jima	Center for relief operations upon arrival on September 5, 2005; flagship for senior officials, including presidential visits, provided facilities and equipment to enable staff coordination, information dissemination, public affairs briefings. Proxy air traffic control agency (in lieu of the Federal Aviation Agency)
	Only functioning dental clinic in New Orleans; ~3000 meals per day for first responders and National Guard; produced 120,000 ga of water, 6.2 MW of electrical power to support ongoing relief activities while working pier side in New Orleans
Amphibious Assault Vehicles	Air evacuation, sea-based logistics, medical support, command, and control functions; may be utilized to launch smaller vessels, helicopters; amphibious platforms to assist in a coastal disaster response
Hospital ships (USNS Comfort)	Converted San Clemente–class super tankers, built to provide transcontinental oil delivery; not fully manned or operated at all times and maintained in a "reduced operating status"
	Response to Hurricane Katrina, USNS Comfort mobilized and steamed around Florida to the Gulf Coast in less than 3 days; treated >1528 patients aboard ship in Mississippi; 7000 patients received treatment at clinics and hospitals staffed by naval medical corpsman and doctors who deployed from the USNS Comfort. Outpatient and advanced care to residents in land-based facilities. Hospital ships not likely to provide immediate response following a disaster can provide ongoing long-term nonemergent care
	USNS Mercy, USNS Comfort's sister ship, provided postdisaster relief for 40 days following the 2004 tsunami disaster in Banda Aceh, Indonesia. USNS Mercy provided relief following March 2005 earthquake that struck near Nias Island, Indonesia, and World Trade Center attacks in New York City in September 2001
	Limited adaptability of hospital ships, limited berthing and medical capabilities make these vessels of limited value in the response to domestic disasters
High Speed Vessels (HSV-2 Swift)	High-speed catamaran, relatively low profile, with helicopter platform. Sustain rapid speeds in excess of 60 knots/hour; able to complete transoceanic crossings without being refueled; extendable ramp enables large diesel trucks to drive directly onto vessel (decreasing) on/off-loading time; little capability to expand services, ie, medical facilities and command areas (minimal situational adaptability); during completed three round-trip logistic runs from Pensacola to the Gulf Coast; rapid delivery of over 800 tons of water, materials, and supplies; capable of people movement
Aircraft Carriers (USS Harry S. Truman)	Single most expensive asset in the US military's inventory, (>$4.5 billion per vessel), historically provided air combat support; activation notification (by Naval Command) after the New Orleans levees failed
	Mass loading of food and water from nearby warehouses as the vessel steamed around Florida to the Gulf Coast, numerous helicopters were received on the flight deck. Altered the traditional mix of aircraft onboard the vessel (traditionally set aside for fighter jets); served as a fuel station; directed and supported air Search and Rescue operations; provide logistical support over extended distances to other vessels in the Gulf Coast; able to operate when air asset use is limited
	Primary normal focus to manage, support, and direct long-range air operations, the capabilities aboard the vessel would have to be significantly modified to accommodate close-in disaster response; lack of ship-to-shore assets limits disaster support role
	Able to support the delivery of logistical supplies (ie, 1-MW generator)
Supplies, communication capacity, medical resources, command and control functions on USN ships allow for utilization and support for state and local leaders as command and control platform	

Vessel name (after a person or a state) provided to identify the vessel.

Type: category of vessel for which it was designed, that is, aircraft carrier for launching of aircraft while out at sea, with the hull (classification codes for ships) designation of CV (aircraft carrier).

Data from JTF-Karteina SITREPS/NORTHCOM; Katrina LA DCO SITREPS; August to September 2005JTF-

NORTHCOM Katrina Timeline; 19 August to 11 October; NC JOC-OMB/NORTHCOM OPS DAILY; 24 August to 30 September 2005.

lack of situational awareness, inadequate materials, and poor communication with other organizations as negatively impacting the responsiveness of DoD units and personnel. Naval forces' positive effects included >8500 evacuations, medical aid >10,000, 14,000 berths, >2.2 million lb of emergency food and water. The US Navy communication systems regained control of airspace and area logistics reopened and dredged sea lanes to improve accessibility and restore river traffic. Helicopter pilots, mechanics, and air traffic controllers coordinated air support from navy vessels. Delivering goods and services into the region while also providing the lift capabilities to conduct evacuations and move logistical supplies (see **Table 76-1**).

In summary the integration among federal assets responding to Katrina had variable degrees of success and failure.[c,17-20] Communication interoperability is the key issue to success or failure or limited resolution of critical time sensitive events. Intrafederal resolution improved rescue activities and coordination. Civilian interoperability issues need more

extensive procedures, protocols, and equipment standardization to optimize rescue and recovery operations.

FEDERAL AGENCIES AND DISASTER RESPONSE

DHS is responsible for the coordinated management of a terrorist attack, natural disaster, or other large-scale emergency with a comprehensive response and recovery effort. It has the primary responsibility for ensuring that emergency response is managed in a professional manner. It was developed in an attempt to create a home for coordination and integration of multiple federal agencies and programs into a single, managing agency by the use of 16 DHS subcomponents with specific responsibilities and areas of expertise. These range from assessment of threats to intelligence analysis.

▣ FEDERAL EMERGENCY MANAGEMENT AGENCY

Federal Emergency Management Agency (FEMA) is the lead federal agency (part of DHS as of 3/1/2003) for consequence management of a

---

[c] The Federal Response to Hurricane Katrina: Lessons Learned,; February 2006

Box 76-1

National Incident Management System (NIMS)

- Command and management
- Preparedness
- Resource management
- Communications and information
- Management
- Supporting technologies
- Ongoing management and maintenance
- Incident Command System (ICS)
- National Incident Management Resource Typing System
- Emergency disaster management

large-scale event response to a natural or man-made disaster. It functions to support general population and emergency responders at a disaster incident with statutory authority for most federal disaster response activities (**Box 76-1**). It partners with state, local emergency management agencies, federal agencies, civilian groups (ie, American Red Cross, Salvation Army, etc) to assist and support (not supplant) response, mitigation, recovery, and preparedness. FEMA is composed of >3700 full-time employees with 4000 standby disaster assistance employees who are able to deploy to disaster locations.

NATIONAL RESPONSE PLAN

National Response Plan (NRP) is the guiding document that integrates federal and domestic disaster activities into an all-hazards approach addressing prevention, preparedness, response, mitigation, recovery plans. The NRP allows the use and collaboration of multiple agencies (local, state, federal) such as Federal Bureau of Investigation (FBI), Department of Defense (DoD), Department of Justice (DOJ), all under jurisdiction of Secretary of Homeland Security. Department of Defense are the military assets such as local commanding officers who are authorized to activate their on-site resources (command and control, personnel, and/or equipment) to meet the request of a local authority, without (pre-) formal permission from their formal chain of command (ie, formal disaster declaration). They will act to preserve life, decrease impact or disaster potential on a local population, including property. It is clear that these local disasters may have national impact: Katrina, Oklahoma City (OKC) Murrow Building Bombing, 9/11 WTC/Pentagon; therefore, early support and participation is critical. DoD responsibilities include Search and Rescue (with DHS/FEMA, US Coast Guard, Department of the Interior), patient movement (with Department of Health and Human Services), augment public health and medical services, provide logistic support, distribution of commodities to quarantined and/or isolated persons, provide manpower and security support to points of (ie, antibiotics) distribution, provide subject matter experts, manpower, and technical assistance to augment mortuary support operations, provide transportation support, provide continuity of government, augment communications for local, state, tribal, and federal communications resources for interoperability, provide base and installation support to other local, state, and federal agencies, ensure protection of defense industrial base, critical infrastructure, and mission assurance, and provide military assistance to civil disturbance for restoration of civil order as it relates to quarantine and isolation enforcement.

US MARINE CORPS' CHEMICAL BIOLOGICAL INCIDENT RESPONSE FORCE

US Marine Corps' Chemical Biological Incident Response Force (CBIRF) respond to a threat of a CBRNE (**C**hemical **B**iological **R**adiological **N**uclear **E**xplosive) incident to assist local, state, tribal, federal agencies;

conduct consequence management operations; agent detection, identification; Search and Rescue; personnel decontamination; emergency medical care, casualty stabilization.

PUBLIC HEALTH SERVICE COMMISSIONED CORPS

Public Health Service (PHS) Commissioned Corps, uniformed service of public health professionals: rapid response to public health needs; essential public health and health care services, prevent and control injury and spread of disease, assess food supply, drinking water, drugs, environment, global health; public health and clinical expertise in response to large-scale local, regional, and national public health emergencies and disasters.

CENTERS FOR DISEASE CONTROL

Centers for Disease Control (CDC) is charged with the protection of the public health and functions with state health departments and other organizations; developing and applying disease prevention and control (infectious disease, food borne, etc), environmental and occupational health. The Strategic National Stockpile (SNS) is the CDC's supply of a large quantity of medicine and medical supplies to be used in the event of a public health emergency (bioterrorist, flu pandemic, hurricane) of significant magnitude to cause local supplies to be insufficient for the general public.

NATIONAL DISASTER MEDICAL SYSTEM

National Disaster Medical System (NDMS) is a federally supported system to augment national medical response capability. It primarily supports Emergency Support Function 8 (ESF 8) and provides support to the military and the Department of Veterans Affairs medical systems in caring for casualties repatriated to the US from overseas armed conflicts. The Department of Health and Human and Services (DHHS) is the lead agency with system operational control and administered through Office of Emergency Response (OER), US Public Health Service (USPHS). Additional federal response and support groups include National Institute for Occupational Safety and Health (NIOSH), DHHS, Environmental Protection Agency (EPA), Occupational Safety & Health Administration (OSHA), the American Red Cross, the International Federation of Red Cross and Red Crescent Societies (IFRC), NVRT (or VMAT, American Veterinary Association), Urban Search and Rescue (USAR), US Fish and Wildlife Service (FWS), US National Response Team (NRT), Radiation Emergency Medical Management (REMM), Federal Medical Stations (FMSs), USAID's Office of Foreign Disaster Assistance (OFDA), Disaster Assistance Response Team (DART), Community Emergency Response Teams, and Citizen Corps (see **Table 76-2**).

NATIONAL RESPONSE FRAMEWORK

Provides guidelines for national response to disasters and emergencies (document attached): preparation and implementation; placed in effect on March 22, 2008, to address natural or man-made (terrorists, industrial) responses for communities, tribes, states, the federal government, private sectors, and nongovernmental entities to operate together. The National Response Framework (NRF) tries to establish best practices in a flexible and scalable response system, utilizing coordinated and integrated response. The plan identifies the emergency support functions (15 total) and annexes as a method used to identify and coordinate federal, NGO, private sector agency resources too effectively and efficiently deliver (direct) resources to local, city, state, tribal entities. It expands from single agency coordination with resources from multiple agencies to a fully operational multiagency, multijurisdictional response. Listed are the emergency support functions and ESF coordinators[2]: ESF 1 Transportation; ESF 2 Communications; ESF 3 Public Works and Engineering; ESF 4 Firefighting; ESF 5 Emergency Management; ESF 6 Mass Care, Emergency Assistance, Housing, and Human Services; ESF 7 Logistics Management and Resource Support; ESF 8 Health and Medical Services; ESF 9 Search and Rescue; ESF 10 Oil and Hazardous Materials

TABLE 76-2   Federal and Civilian Disaster Response Resources

Federal Response and Support Groups	Tasks and/or Function
National Institute for Occupational Safety and Health (NIOSH)	Occupational safety and health for workers; prevent work-related illness, injury, disability, and death
Department of Health and Human Services (DHHS)	Cabinet department, goal of protecting the health of citizens and providing essential human services
Environmental Protection Agency (EPA)	Protect general public from risks to human health and the environment; reduce environmental risk; enforce federal environmental laws
Occupational Safety & Health Administration (OSHA)	Primary federal agency charged with enforcement of safety and health legislation
The American Red Cross	Emergency response organization that offers humanitarian care to the victims of war, and natural disasters
The International Federation of Red Cross and Red Crescent Societies (IFRC)	Humanitarian organization, providing assistance to any nationality, race, religious beliefs, class or political opinions; relief operations to assist victims of disasters
	Red crescent is used in place of the Red Cross in many Islamic countries
NVRT (or VMAT, American Veterinary Association)	Individuals within the NDMS system with expertise in veterinary medicine, and pet and service animal needs following major disasters
Part of National Disaster Medical System (NDMS), DHHS, Assistant Secretary for Preparedness and Response (ASPR), Office of Preparedness and Emergency Operations (OPEO); Component of Emergency Support Function #8 (ESF-8), Health and Medical Services	Pets Evacuation and Transportation Standards Act (PETS Act)
Urban Search and Rescue	Location, rescue (extrication), and initial medical stabilization of victims trapped in confined spaces (collapse environments, victims of natural or man-made disasters); national asset of 27 teams across the country
Function under FEMA ESF 8	
US Fish and Wildlife Service (FWS)	Fire management to conserve, protect, and enhance fish, wildlife, plants, their habitats, and surrounding communities; AKA National Wild Life and Fire
US National Response Team (NRT); 16 Federal agencies	Emergency response to pollution incidents (oil and HAZMAT). Interagency group cochaired by the EPA and the US Coast Guard. Does not respond directly to incidents, supports the Regional Response Teams
Radiation Emergency Medical Management (REMM)	DHHS; provides evidence-based data for health care professionals about radiation emergencies (diagnosis and management)
Federal Medical Stations (FMSs)	Support to state-run field hospitals, special needs shelters with equipment, supplies, and personnel
	Stand-alone facility, augment mobile medical facilities
	Scalable (in size), modular, and rapidly deployable health and medical care. FMS units as large as ~5500 have been deployed. Provided care for people suffering from exacerbation of chronic disease and/or behavioral health conditions. Staffed by multidisciplinary, rapidly deployable Public Health service team. Not an acute care hospital, nursing facility
Citizen Corps	Volunteer service programs, administered locally and coordinated nationally by DHS, mitigate disaster, and prepare the population for emergency response through public education, training, and outreach
Community Emergency Response Teams	Citizen Corps program focused on disaster preparedness and teaching basic disaster response skills
	Volunteer teams are utilized to provide emergency support when disaster overwhelms the local emergency response services
Disaster Assistance Response Team (DART)	DoD asset, United States Agency for International Development's (USAID) under the Office of United States Foreign Disaster Assistance. Rapidly deployable team in response to international disasters (ie, Japan, Chile). Specialists, trained in disaster relief skills, to assist US embassies and USAID missions with the management of US government response to disasters
USAID's Office of Foreign Disaster Assistance (OFDA)	Seven-person Disaster Assistance Response Team
	On-site assessment and the consequences to the affected population

Federal Response and Support Groups: Other civilian and federal agencies utilized by the federal government to respond and mitigate national/local disasters. Tasks and/or Function: operation activities identified to each agency, organization, or entity.

Response; ESF 11 Agriculture and Natural Resources; ESF 12 Energy; ESF 13 Public Safety and Security; ESF 14 Long-Term Community Recovery; ESF 15 External Affairs. Each function has an identified agency based on expertise (HAZMAT, medical infrastructure) capabilities and equipment (firefighting personnel and equipment). Not an all or nothing system and may be implemented pre- (impending hurricane) or postincident (post-bombing incident) as the need occurs. This process is consistent with resource typing identified in National Incident Management System. The ESF coordinator is the management structure for a particular ESF with ongoing responsibility for each cell for as long as ongoing operations continue: response, recovery, and preparedness. They operate within the event established ICS (unified incident command structure). The use of DOD assets requires approval of Secretary of Defense. They are also responsible for Defense Support of Civil Authorities (DSCA) during domestic incidents. DoD's main role is operational and to provide assistance from one or more groups to accomplish necessary assigned tasks. They have defined lines of communication and

responsibility. Intergraded with state, local, and federal agencies or identified incident partners, in order to optimize resources utilization and to operate efficiently. DoD is considered a support entity for all ESFs (see **Table 76-3**). The NRF is based on all hazards approach and not event or threat specific, independent of scope and magnitude of incident.

NRF preparedness strives to stress preincident planning, preparation, and use of historical event lessons learned (**Figure 76-1**). Response: "... immediate actions to save lives, protect property and the environment, and meet basic human needs..."[d] with respect to the federal government role, it identifies instances of primary responsibility in catastrophic events where state, city, tribal resources are overwhelmed and/or require substantive support in resolving or recovering from the incident. This includes large numbers of casualties and/or damage (physical, cyber), or

---

[d] National Response Framework (NRF); January 2008

TABLE 76-3	Emergency Support Functions and Emergency Support Function Coordinators
ESF #1—Transportation **ESF Coordinator: Department of Transportation**	• Aviation/airspace management and control • Civilian military transportation support and safety • Restoration and recovery of transportation infrastructure • Movement restrictions • Damage and impact assessment
ESF #2—Communications **ESF Coordinator: DHS (National Communications System)**	• Coordination and support with telecommunications and information technology industries • Restoration and repair of telecommunications infrastructure • Protection, restoration, and sustainment of national cyber and information technology resources • Oversight of communications within the federal incident management and response structures
ESF #3—Public Works and Engineering **ESF Coordinator: Department of Defense (US Army Corps of Engineers)**	• Infrastructure protection and emergency repair • Infrastructure restoration: essential public services (including facilities) • Engineering services and construction management • Emergency contracting support for lifesaving and life-sustaining services
ESF #4—Firefighting **ESF Coordinator: Department of Agriculture (US Forest Service)**	• Coordination of federal firefighting activities • Support, locate, and suppress wildland, rural, and urban fires • Firefighting operations at mobilization and logistic centers
ESF #5—Emergency Management **ESF Coordinator: DHS (FEMA)**	• Coordination of incident management and response efforts • Issuance of mission assignments • Resource and human capital • Incident action planning • Financial management
ESF #6—Mass Care, Emergency Assistance, Housing, and Human Services **ESF Coordinator: DHS (FEMA)**	• Mass care • Emergency assistance • Disaster housing • Human services • Collect, evaluate, and disseminate event (and related) information to ease response and recovery activities
ESF #7—Logistics Management and Resource Support **ESF Coordinator: General Services Administration and DHS (FEMA)**	• Comprehensive, national incident logistics planning, management, and sustainment capability • Resource support (facility space, office equipment and supplies, contracting services, etc) • Provide equipment and personnel to responding federal resources • Upon state request, coordinate supplemental federal law
ESF #8—Health and Medical Services **ESF Coordinator: Lead agency: US Public Health Service, Department of Health and Human Services**	• Provides assistance for public health and medical care needs
ESF #9—Search and Rescue **ESF Coordinator: DHS (FEMA)**	• Lifesaving assistance • Search and Rescue operations: locate, provide initial medical care for trapped victims in collapsed structures

TABLE 76-3	Emergency Support Functions and Emergency Support Function Coordinators *(continued)*
ESF #10—Oil and Hazardous Materials Response **ESF Coordinator: Environmental Protection Agency**	• Support federal response to actual or potential HAZMAT release • Oil and hazardous materials (chemical, biological, radiological, TIC, etc) response • Environmental short- and long-term cleanup
ESF #11—Agriculture and Natural Resources **ESF Coordinator: Department of Agriculture**	• Nutrition assistance: for affected population, including distribution • Animal and plant disease and pest response • Food safety and security • Natural and cultural resources and historic properties protection • Safety and well-being of household pets and service animals
ESF #12—Energy **ESF Coordinator: Department of Energy**	• Energy infrastructure assessment, repair, and restoration • Energy industry utilities coordination • Energy forecast
ESF #13—Public Safety and Security **ESF Coordinator: Department of Justice**	• Facility and resource security • Security planning and technical resource assistance • Public safety and security support • Support to access, traffic, and crowd control
ESF #14—Long-Term Community Recovery **ESF Coordinator: DHS (FEMA)**	• Social and economic community impact assessment • Long-term community recovery assistance to states, tribes, local governments, and the private sector • Analysis and review of mitigation program implementation
ESF #15—External Affairs **ESF Coordinator: DHS**	• Emergency public information and protective action guidance • Media and community relations • Congressional and international affairs • Tribal and insular affairs

Federally identified Support Division (Function) and its operational responsibilities in order to coordinate the response to an incident by various Federal agencies.

Data from the Oxford Essential Dictionary of the U.S. Military; Copyright © 2001, 2002 by Oxford University Press, Inc

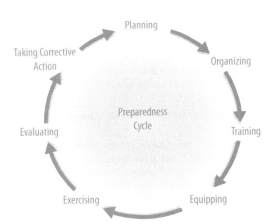

FIGURE 76-1. National Response Framework preparedness cycle. (Reprinted from FEMA. See https://www.fema.gov/national-preparedness-cycle.)

civil/federal/tribal governmental disruption affecting the general population, including infrastructure (daily operations), environment, or local, state, federal, tribal economy. It provides groundwork for first responders, local/state entities to support and/or participate as part of a unified national response. The NRP also addresses the use and partnership of DoD and its assets (**Table 76-4**).

TABLE 76-4	Department of Defense (DOD) US Northern Command in Domestic Disaster Response
Operational objectives	Coordinate defense support of civil authorities and provide domestic disaster relief: natural (hurricane) or man-made (WMD terrorist incidents)
	Participate in pandemic planning, response, and mitigation
	Utilized when civilian authorities are overwhelmed
Support under the National Response Plan	Should response forces be required, the governor has the authority to request federal support, directly from the president, who directs the Department of Homeland Security, as the primary federal agency, to respond accordingly
	Northern Command is ultimately the organization tasked to identify and deploy military assets in response
Operational Support	Assist local law enforcement's ability to interdict threats by using ground sensors, air surveillance radar, unmanned aerial systems, Stryker vehicles, and other detection platforms
	Detection of illegal drugs, including air reconnaissance to detect illegal drugs in public lands and forests
Intelligence Support	Intelligence collection, analysis, information sharing, imagery support
	Jointly participate in mission prioritization
	Law enforcement analysis training
Engineering Support	Defense Department engineers support law enforcement agencies by constructing roads, bridges, fences, vehicular barriers, and lights
General Support	Tunnel detection, transportation of law enforcement personnel and equipment using fixed-wing aircraft, mobile training teams (ie, special reaction team operations, desert survival, trauma management, chemical weapons detection, emergency response, patrolling, land navigation, and intelligence link analysis)
Emergency Support	Responding to emergencies or disasters immediate response and support for incidents under the National Response Plan provided under the Stafford Act
Immediate Response	Form of immediate action taken by a DOD component or military commander to aid civil authorities, the public, alleviate/prevent victim suffering, mitigate property damage
	Need civil authority assistance request
	May be initiated prior to disaster declaration in view of incident severity
	Local military commanders may provide immediate response for lifesaving measures or to mitigate and limit significant potential/actual property damage

Department of Defense (DOD) US Northern Command: aka NORTHCOM, responsibilities and description of activities.

Data from Hurricane Katrina: DOD Disaster Response; September 19, 2005; Steve Bowman, Specialist in National Defense Foreign Affairs, Defense, and Trade Division; Lawrence Kapp, Specialist in National Defense; Foreign Affairs, Defense, and Trade Division; Amy Belasco, Specialist in National Defense, Foreign Affairs, Defense, and Trade Division; Army Support During the Hurricane Katrina Disaster; James A. Wombwell; The Long War Series, Occasional Paper 29; US Army Combined Arms Center; Combat Studies Institute Press; Fort Leavenworth, Kansas;

Bowman, S., Kapp, L., Belasco, A: Hurricane Katrina: DOD Disaster Response; *Congressional Research Service ˜ The Library of Congress;* September 19, 2005.

Box 76-2

Statutory Authority

1. 10 U.S.C. § 375. Restriction on direct participation by military personnel.

2. American Recovery & Reinvestment Act (http://www.hhs.gov/recovery/)

3. Executive Order 12148, 44 Fed. Reg. 43239, designates DHS as the primary agency for coordination of federal disaster relief, emergency assistance, and emergency preparedness. Robert T. Stafford Disaster Relief and Emergency Assistance Act, PL 100-707, amended the Disaster Relief Act of 1974, PL 93-288, 88 Stat. 143; statutory authority for most federal disaster response activities especially as they pertain to FEMA and FEMA programs and processes for the federal government to provide disaster and emergency assistance.[10,11]

4. Homeland Security Act of 2002, Pub. Law 107-296, 116 Stat 2135 (2002), established the Department of Homeland Security with the mandate and legal authority to protect the American people from the continuing threat of terrorist.[11]

5. Homeland Security Presidential Directive-5: Management of Domestic Incidents, February 28, 2003, is intended to enhance the ability of the United States to manage domestic incidents by establishing a single, comprehensive National Incident Management System.

6. Military Cooperation with Civilian Law Enforcement Agencies Act

7. The Insurrection Act, 19 U.S.C 331-335 (2002). Authorize the President to direct armed forces to enforce the law to suppress insurrections and domestic violence. Military forces may be used to restore order, prevent looting, and engage in other law enforcement activities

8. The Posse Comitatus Act, United States federal law (18 U.S.C. § 1385), prohibits use of the Army or the Air Force for law enforcement purposes, except as otherwise authorized by the Constitution or statute.

9. Post Katrina Emergency Management Reform Act (PKEMRA)

10. Indian Tribe List Act of 1994, 25 U.S.C. 479a, Indian tribal governments as federally recognized entities.

The NRF uses National Incident Management System (NIMS) as basis and template for incident management (superseded "the National Response Plan" March 22, 2008). Sections of the NIMS include Command and Management, Preparedness, Resource Management, Communications and Information, Management, Supporting Technologies, Ongoing Management and Maintenance, Incident Command System (ICS), National Incident Management Resource Typing System, Emergency disaster management via an integrated/unified command structure and ICS (**Box 76-2**).

Note: Source location: NRF Resource Center (www.fema.gov/nrf). "The *NRF* is built on the following five principles[e]: Engaged partnerships, Tiered response, Scalable, Flexible, and Adaptable operational capabilities, Unity of effort through unified command, Readiness to act." National Response Framework document organization and content: Chapter I: Roles and Responsibilities, Emergency Management Actions at Local, Tribal, State, Federal, Private sector and NGOs, Chapter II: Response, National Response to an Incident, Chapter III: Response Organization, National Organization for Response Actions, Chapter IV: Planning Elements of National Planning Structures, Chapter V: Information for Online NRF Resource Center, and DHS/Federal Emergency Management Agency.

The overall goal of the development and implementation of the National Response Framework is to allow for directed and predictable response, stress need for realistic preparation and training, identify

---

[e]National Response Framework (NRF) – FACT SHEET

civilian and federal resource roles and responsibilities, and foster cooperative organized disaster response and incident command operations.

MOBILIZATION OF FEDERAL RESOURCES

The Federal Declaration Process[f] is based on the legal authority of the Robert T. The Stafford Disaster Relief and Emergency Assistance Act (*Stafford Act* (§401)[g] requires that for a declaration of disaster (and therefore aid) to be declared (by the president), a formal request for aid must be submitted by the governor of the affected state.[12]

The Federal Response Plan (FRP) initiates provisions of the Stafford Act (Public Law 93-288, as amended). It describes events that may be considered disasters, describes the basic mechanisms and structures through which federal aid and assistance may be provided, and outlines coordination of federal agencies to fulfill emergency support functions (ESF). This document specifies that when state capabilities are/may be exceeded, the governor may request federal assistance, including assistance under the Stafford Act. The response is initiated by a presidential declaration of a major disaster or emergency and incident results in significant damage to warrant federal disaster assistance to support and/or supplement local, state, tribal efforts. The affected governor will submit the request for declaration of disaster through the regional FEMA office (**Figure 76-2**).

State and federal officials will then conduct a preliminary damage assessment (PDA) to assess the potential impact and/or significance of the incident. This will determine impact on the affected population and infrastructure (as part of governors' request for aid). Subsequently the event should exceed the capability of the state to respond appropriately; governors' request shall include incident scope, nature, and impact; state's response to the incident (actual, proposed). As part of the request, governor must take appropriate action under state law and direct execution of the state's emergency plan and provide a dollar estimate of assistance required under the Stafford Act and commit to a cost sharing

process. This will then obtain a FEMA recommendation (based on the nature, scope, and governors' PDA) if forwarded to the president for action. The president may or may not declare that a disaster exists that requires federal assistance.

DMAT AND EMS/EMERGENCY MEDICINE PHYSICIANS

The Disaster Medical Assistance Team (DMAT) is a federally organized volunteer "rapid" response group to provide emergency medical services at disaster locations, where the medical infrastructure (hospitals, unburden medical staff) in the impact zone is compromised (**Figure 76-3**). It is intended to augment other federal response components as an organized group of medical professionals (to fill a vacuum as a freestanding medical resource). It is a component of the National Disaster Medical System and operates under the authority of Department of Health and Human Services (DHHS), while partnering with Department of Defense (DoD), Department of Veterans Affairs (VA), Federal Emergency Management Agency (FEMA), state and local governments, private businesses and civilian volunteers. This is a federally coordinated medical response activity designed to increase available postincident local medical capability and capacity. It also has the responsibility to assist Veterans Administration (VA) with movement of repatriated injured military personnel. NDMS is composed of multiple emergency response teams:

Disaster Medical Assistance Team (DMAT): provide medical care during disasters

National Medical Response Team (NMRT): mass decontamination and medical treatment secondary to a release of weapons of mass destruction, large-scale release of hazardous material

Disaster Mortuary Operations Response Team (MORT): fatality identification, management, and mortuary services

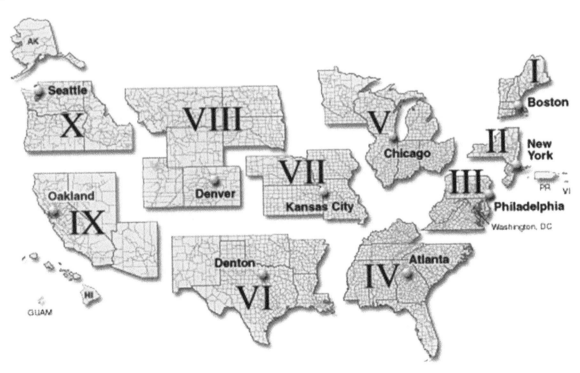

FIGURE 76-2. Regional FEMA offices. (Reprinted from FEMA. http://www.fema.gov/regional-operations.)

---

[f] The Declaration Process fema.gov website
[g] Robert T. Stafford Disaster Relief and Emergency Assistance Act, Public Law 93-288, Sections 5121-5206, et seq of Title 42 United States Code

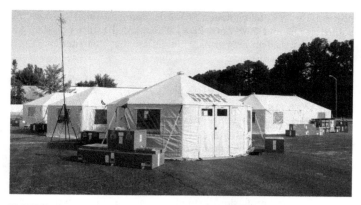

FIGURE 76-3. DMAT team encampment. (Reproduced with permission from Dr. John Lyng.)

National Veterinary Response Team (NVRT): veterinary care

National Pharmacy Response Team (NPRT): mass prophylaxis and/or vaccination

International Medical Surgical Response Team (IMSuRT): fully capable field surgical unit

National Nurse Response Team (NNRT): large number of nurses for prophylaxis and/or mass vaccination

The system is composed of 70 NDMS teams, 55 DMATs with 12 Type 1 DMATs. The Type 1 is described as self-sufficient, including medical and logistical support equipment, while the Type 2 is unable to be self-sufficient, it utilizes equipment left by other teams (capable of relieving a Type 1 team). The Type 3 DMAT is considered nondeployable and under development. Training, proficiency, experience establish team status (level).

The Deployment model is: self-sufficient for 72 hours, 14-day deployment, 35 selected staff members, provision of medical care: victims and/or responders, mass inoculations, medication dispensing, including victim reception (triage, treatment, and transport).

Team staffing structure consists of physicians, nurses, physician assistants, nurse practitioners, pharmacist, respiratory therapist, EMT/paramedic, and individuals with specific expertise and experience within a wide range of professions (medical and nonmedical); public health, emergency management, forensic sciences, etc. Each position has prerequisite training requirements including the maintenance of specific position certifications. Members of the NDMS (ie, DMAT) are federalized as temporary federal workers at the time of deployment and are therefore protected by federal health, life, and disability insurance (while deployed).

These teams may be utilized as a local, state, tribal resource. All teams function under the auspicious of a sponsoring organization, usually a medical center, nonprofit foundation, public health or safety agency, nonprofit, public, or private organization. The sponsoring agency is required to sign a Memorandum of Understanding (MOU) with the PHS, agreeing to administratively supports team, provide equipment, and logistical resources. Each team should have sufficient medical equipment (including medications), supplies, tents, generators, trucks, etc. Staff and equipment to be able to care for 200 victims per day, similar to urgent health care facility. The medical-administrative activities have tort protection during deployment. This is the same as the as National Guard, or Active Duty Military personnel. The Federal Tort Claims Act where the federal government becomes the defendant in the event of a malpractice claim. The members also have deployment job protection by the Uniformed Services Employment and Reemployment Act (USERRA) and are covered by federal health, life, and disability insurance while on deployment.

Refer to http://www.dmat.org/teamlinks.html for more information. The DMAT structure and function is defined by the National Response Framework (NRF). The emergency medicine physician role is a critical component and participant in the NDMS (DMAT) system. This is what allows it to operate in austere environments and to care for an unselected population (with chronic and acute medical concerns). Due to the nature of the unstructured incident and the unselected population there is limited role for selected subspecialists.

MILITARY RESOURCES RESPONDING TO A DOMESTIC DISASTER

Military assets have been utilized in domestic response to Hurricane Katrina (see **Table 76-5**) and internationally to the Japan 2011 Earthquake-Tsunami-Nuclear Reactor incident (see **Table 76-6**).[13,14,15] The operations fall the jurisdiction of the United States Northern Command aka USNORTHCOM aka NORTHCOM under Title 10; units provide support under the immediate response authority as directed by the Secretary of Defense to respond to the disaster situation. NORTHCOM civilian and federal support is limited by the Posse Comitatus Act. This prohibits Army, Air Force, Navy, Marine Corps, and National Guard from acting in a law enforcement capacity within the United States, except where expressly authorized the president, or Congress. It prohibits the use of federal military forces to "execute the laws," but military forces may provide civil support, but cannot become directly involved in law enforcement (ie, post-9/11 military patrols at airports). Coast Guard, under the Department of Homeland Security, is exempt from this act (enforces US laws, even as it operates as a service of the US Navy). Situations where act does not apply: National Guard operating under authority of state governor; Under *18 U.S.C. § 831*, Attorney General United States Attorney General may request the Secretary of Defense to provide emergency assistance if civilian law enforcement is unable to address threats involving nuclear materials, weapons, or release US Coast Guard, operating under the DHS.

SUMMARY

All disasters are local events, but many require assistance beyond the scope of the local, city, municipal, state, or tribal authorities. Disasters may result in significant injuries, loss of life, and property if appropriate resources are not brought to bear early in the incident (or preincident). An integrated (local, state, tribal, federal, NGO, and private sector) Disaster management response and operation is critical to minimizing or limiting the event consequences. The need for federal response is a component of local and national disaster response and mitigation. Potential environmental, economic consequences impacted/impaired health care response and/or delivery system can persist for an extended period of time. The impact on special needs populations, children, and impacted survivors require the municipality, state, Tribe to reestablish necessary services are a critical measure of the adequacy of disaster response. Large-scale evacuations with potential needs for evacuee sheltering and "temporary" housing are necessary planning components for any significant incident (ie, hurricane). There should be a plan for the reestablishment of first-responder services and law enforcement operations. Catastrophic events have the potential for not only a CONUS (Continental US) consequence but international (cross border) impact. Resolution will be based on a unified, organized, and rapid response. Communication has always been the Achilles' heel of disaster response. The lack of any national or regional communications, information sharing interoperability system or process will continue to hinder the safe and efficient management of any significant event. In the end, true interoperability is a function of the ability of individuals to operate in a cooperative, professional, and supportive manner.

TABLE 76-5	DoD Resources utilized during the Hurricane Katrina Response	
Asset	**Resources**	**Activities**
National Guard Task Force Eagle	72, 000 troops	Airborne, waterborne, ground Search and Rescue, medical assistance, repaired levees; cleared debris, security services, 15,436 rescues, delivered 217 tons of food and water, 248 tons of cargo and sandbags
	Note: 72,000 Total Active, Reserve, National Guard personnel involved in the Hurricane Katrina response	
	helicopters: 39 UH-60, 16 UH-1, 6 CH-47, 14 OH-58 including Blackhawks, 2 C-23 & 5 C-12 fixed-wing aircraft, 4000 military police	August 29-September 8: 6500 sorties, rescues >9600, transported 35,000, moved > 2100 tons of cargo
	Baptist Hospital	Transported 11 neonatal patients in incubators
	VA Hospital	Evacuated 11 ventilator patients, 60 in-patients
	Chalmette Hospital	Hemorrhaging pregnant woman, who was and expected to die without care, transported to Louisiana State University Medical Center in Baton Rouge
	St Bernard Parish jail	20 Patients removed from facility
528th Engineer Battalion	>200 Engineers	Ground Search and Rescue; removed > 120 million lb of trash and 36 million lb of rotting meat, installed 307 generators in affected area, repaired 310 structures
Army National Guard	Helicopters: 11 UH-60 Blackhawk, 4 CH-47 Chinook, and 1 C-23 fixed-wing aircraft	4000 Sorties, rescues > 17,875, moved > 12,315 to evacuation sites, delivered 600 tons of food and water, 634 tons of cargo, 1900 cases of MREs, 1800 cases of water, 3 million lb of sand into levee breaches, firefighting using buckets
		Initial problems air traffic control, but no aviation accidents occurred, Army helicopters rescued almost 3000 people
Texas National Guard	>1300 Guardsmen	Ground Search and Rescue, 2100 rescues, 300 military police, 120 engineers, water purification system, fuel tankers; medical unit: 5 doctors, 10 nurses, 30 physician's assistants, 30 medics
20th Special Forces Group		>3100 Rescues
1165th Area Support Medical Company (Puerto Rico)		Physicians, medical technicians, medical care: minor surgery, for soldiers and civilians
South Carolina National Guard		Two water purification detachments, engineers, helicopters, logistics support troops, military police, infantry, high-water vehicles
New Hampshire National Guard	500 Guardsmen	Ground Search and Rescue
Georgia/Louisiana National Guard		>50 High-water vehicles (HMMWVs: high mobility multipurpose wheeled vehicles) many for local police precincts
Colorado National Guard	700 Guardsmen	Ground Search and Rescue
Virginia National Guard	320 Guardsmen	Medical company, Forward Support Battalion, two transportation companies
Oregon National Guard	2000 Troops	Ground Search and Rescue
49th Movement Control Battalion	285 Trucks	Distributed 1.7 million gallons of water, 3.6 million meals, 11.5 million lb of ice
Company B helicopters	Dropped 1.7 million lb of sandbags into levee breaches, transported >1700 passengers, delivered >150,000 lb of cargo	
Logistics cell	Delivered 815,000 cases of MREs, 215,000 lb of ice, 837,000 bottles of water, 1.3 million gallons of fuel to the Active component	
13th Corps Support Command		Six reverse osmosis purification units, produced 600 gallons of potable water per hour, produced 142,000 gallons of water (for the troops)
JTF Katrina	Army, Navy, Marine, Air Force	1. Ground Search and Rescue
	USS Bataan, amphibious helicopter carrier: 3 MH-60 Seahawk, 2 MH-53E Sea Dragon helicopters	2. Levee repair: UH-60 helicopters picked up 3000-lb sandbags (3 million lb of sand) for levee repair
	Air Force: 5 HH-60 helicopters	3. 21,400 Active Duty personnel and 45,700 Army and Air National Guard members supported the effort in the Gulf Coast
	Army: 2 UH-60 Blackhawk helicopters	
	30 Additional helicopters; 143 fixed-wing aircraft	4. National Guard and Active Duty troops' response to Katrina became the largest domestic deployment of forces since the Civil War

DoD Resources: Department of Defense assets utilized by the federal government during disaster relief operation for Hurricane Katrina.

Data from JTF-Karteina SITREPS/NORTHCOM ; Katrina LA DCO SITREPS; August to September 2005;

NORTHCOM Katrina Timeline; 19 August to 11 October; NC JOC-OMB/NORTHCOM OPS DAILY; 24 August to 30 September 2005; THE US AIR FORCE RESPONSE TO HURRICANE KATRINA; Daniel L. Haulman; 17 November 2006.

TABLE 76-6   DoD Resources Utilized During the 2011 Japan Earthquake-Tsunami-Nuclear Reactor Incident Response

Service	Resource	Operation
US Navy	14 Ships (with associated aircraft), 17,000 sailors and Marines	Moving people and supplies, Search and Rescue, 129,000 gallons of water, 4200 lb of food; US personnel
	113 helicopter and 125 fixed-wing sorties, USS Essex (LHD 2), USS Harpers Ferry (LSD 49), USS Germantown (LSD 42), Marine Expeditionary Unit (2200)	low level radiation exposure; cleaned Sendai military airport; delivered two fire trucks; rescued victims from rooftops
	USS Ronald Reagan including H-60 helicopters: 3200 sailors and 2480 aviators and air wing personnel and 85 aircraft	Surveys at sea debris field; four drops of humanitarian supplies ashore;
		floating airport, refueling helicopters from the Japan Self Defense Force, Japan Coast Guard, fire and police units involved in rescue and recovery efforts ashore
	USS Tortuga (LSD 46), with heavy-lift helicopters	273 Japanese Ground Self-Defense Force troops, 93 vehicles and equipment moved
	USS Essex (LHD 2)	Humanitarian assistance and disaster relief (HADR) supplies:
	USS Blue Ridge (LCC 19)	> 45 pallets of surgical masks, water containers, water purifying tablets, health and comfort packs, blankets, insect repellant
	Ronald Reagan Carrier Strike Group: USS Chancellorsville (CG 62), USS Preble (DDG 88), USS Fitzgerald	33 Tons of humanitarian aid
	USNS Safeguard	Delivered high-pressure water pumps for Fukushima power plant
	Air Force C-17s and C-130s	Hauling supplies
	Sailors	Debris removal from beach from fishing village
	Navy P-3 Orion aircraft	Survey and assess the debris field at sea
	Four destroyers: USS Fitzgerald, USS John S. McCain, USS McCampbell, USS Curtis Wilbur with Japanese authorities, Search and rescue and recovery operations	
US Army	US Army Corps of Engineers	Disaster assessment team (debris removal), logistic and humanitarian missions
	50,000 Water bottles to disaster survivors	
	Ground operations	10 Person team of translators, communications experts, combat medics upon request of the Japanese Self-Defense Forces to assist with disaster assessment
	20,000 Troops, 140 aircraft, 20 ships	Support of Operation Tomodachi
	US military assistance to Japanese forces	>2 Million gallons of water, 189 tons of food, 11,960 gallons of fuel, 100 tons of relief supplies
	>1000 III Marine Expeditionary	Survivor recovery, personnel transport and relief supplies distribution
		>450 helicopter and aircraft missions survivor recovery, personnel transport and relief supplies distribution
		>129,000 lb of water, 4200 lb of food distributed; clear debris from airfields to allow logistic and humanitarian missions
US Marines	HMM-265	164 Support sorties carrying 130 passengers and transporting 94,230 lb of cargo supporting Operation Tomodachi; >42,000 lb of heating fuel to small villages in Japan's northern areas
	Transported from Okinawa on a WestPac Express High Speed Vessel	Forward Air Refueling Point (FARP), temporary refueling facility, facilitates continuous operation of aircraft
	Escorted by Japan Ground Self-Defense Force members III MEF (Fwd)	Establish Humanitarian Assistance Center; assets of: 67 tons, 11 Humvees, communication trucks, tactical vehicles, food, water, blankets
	Marine Expeditionary Force and Japan Self-Defense Force with CH-46E Sea Knight	Bottled food for Japanese population affected by the earthquake and tsunami
	Maine Corps	Clear debris from airfields to allow logistic and humanitarian missions
	Third Marine Expeditionary Force	Dispatched a small command and control team from Okinawa to mainland Japan and a Deployable Joint Command and Control System
	Eight CH-46E helicopters from Marine Medium Helicopter Squadron 265 Conduct relief operations	
US Air Force	Air Force C-17s and C-130s	Hauling supplies
	Unmanned Global Hawk aircraft	Aerial surveillance over the country including nuclear reactor; collect digital imagery of earthquake and tsunami damage (real-time imagery): Search and Rescue, mitigation and recovery
Japan	Japanese military CH-47 Chinook helicopters: dump seawater on damaged reactor of Unit 3 at the Fukushima complex	
Issues	Bandwidth shortages and network limitations	Inhibit communications, command and control: blocking access to a range of commercial Web sites (bandwidth to support mission-essential communications) using DoD Enterprise Level Protection System
	Conductivity	Intermittent Internet and communications issues: Pentagon shut down Internet to allow military use

DOD response to the DoD 2011 Japan Earthquake-Tsunami-Nuclear Reactor Incident. Military asset assignments and operational event activities. Part of the nuclear reactor "meltdown" mitigation project aka Operation Tomodachi; resource origin and function (assigned tasks).

Feickert, Andrew, Chanlett-Avery Emma; Japan 2011 Earthquake: U.S. Department of Defense (DOD) Response; Congressional Research Service, 7-5700, www.crs.gov, R41690; March 16, 2011.

- Identify areas where interoperability operations may be expanded or created.
- Establish and maintain an integrated operation.
- Clearly delineate responsible entities.
- Define reporting relationships and areas of responsibility.
- This process allows for multiple individual roles and responsibilities.
- Establish incident needs early in the event (including people and services).
- Allow for local, state, tribal control of the incident planning and management.
- Knowledge and use of incident management and the Federal Response Plans allow for common goals and operating procedures.
- Use of DoD assets allows for a shorter response, mitigation, and recovery phases.
- Event planning and management should be based on an all-hazards philosophy rather than an event (type) specific approach.
- Multiple serial and/or simultaneous or single events are possible.

REFERENCES

1. Bowman S, Kapp L, Belasco A. *Hurricane Katrina: DOD Disaster Response.* Congressional Research Service, The Library of Congress; Washington DC. September 19, 2005.
2. Tactics, techniques, and procedures. *Civil Support and the U.S. Army Newsletter.* December 2009;1-104.
3. Cronin RB, . U.S. Northern Command & defense support of civil authorities. *Civil Support and the U.S. Army Newsletter.* December 2009;25-32.
4. Feickert A, Chanlett-Avery E. Japan 2011 earthquake: U.S. Department of Defense (DOD) response. Congressional Research Service, 7-5700. March 16, 2011. www.crs.gov, R41690.
5. FEMA: ICS 700: Interoperability. http://emilms.fema.gov/IS700a NEW/NIMS01summary.htm.
6. Gay J E, Turso DL. *Integration and Interoperability: An Analysis to Identify the Attributes for System of Systems* [Thesis]. Monterey, CA: Postgraduate school; September 2008.
7. Homeland Security Presidential Directive-5 (HSPD-5). February 28, 2003. https://www.dhs.gov/sites/default/files/publications/Homeland%20Security%20Presidential%20Directive%205.pdf.
8. Jackson T. Power and domestic disaster response: exploring the role of naval vessels during Hurricane Katrina. *Liaison Online;* IV(1).
9. The Oxford Essential Dictionary of the U.S. Military; Copyright © 2001, 2002 by Oxford University Press, Inc.
10. The Posse Comitatus Act: a principle in need of renewal. Wash Univ Law Q; 75(2).
11. Public Law 107-296, the Homeland Security Act of 2002.
12. Robert T. Stafford Disaster Relief and Emergency Assistance Act, Public Law 93-288, Sections 5121-5206, et seq of Title 42 United States Codes.
13. Chen R, Sharman R, Chakravarti N, Rao HR, Upadhyaya SJ. Emergency response information system interoperability: development of chemical incident response data model. *J Assoc Inf Syste.* March 4, 2008.
14. Townsend FF. *The Federal Response to Hurricane Katrina: Lessons Learned.* February 2006. http://www.floods.org/PDF/Katrina_Lessons_Learned_0206.pdf.
15. Wombwell JA. *Army Support During the Hurricane Katrina Disaster: The Long War Series, Occasional Paper 29.* Fort Leavenworth, KS: Combat Studies Institute Press; 2005.
16. Rusiecki JA, Thomas DL, Chen L, Funk R, McKibben J, Dayton MR. Disaster-related exposures and health effects among US Coast Guard responders to Hurricanes Katrina and Rita: a cross-sectional study. *J Occup Environ Med.* August 2014;56(8):820-833.
17. Rutkow L. An analysis of state public health emergency declarations. *Am J Public Health.* September 2014;104(9):1601-1605.
18. Dillon RL, Tinsley CH, Burns WJ. Near-misses and future disaster preparedness. *Risk Anal.* 2014;34(10):1907-22.
19. Knox CC. Analyzing after-action reports from Hurricanes Andrew and Katrina: repeated, modified, and newly created recommendations. *J Emerg Manag.* March-April 2013;11(2):160-168.
20. Mintz A, Gonzalez W. National mass care strategy: a national integrated approach. *J Bus Contin Emer Plan.* Autumn 2013;7(1):33-43.

CHAPTER 77

Terrorism, Weapons of Mass Destruction, and Explosives

Anne Klimke
Michael Kowalski

INTRODUCTION

In the decade following the September 11, 2001, terrorist attacks, Americans have become more accustomed to the threat of terrorist attacks by weapons of mass destruction (WMD). Training for response to such events is now common for first responders and medical personnel. This chapter will present practical approaches to terrorist attacks involving WMD and explosives, an overview of specific types of explosives, and strategies for dealing with blast and burn injuries in the prehospital setting.

OBJECTIVES

- Define terrorism, domestic and international.
- Discuss specific threats to emergency responders to terrorist events.
- Discuss principles and strategies relating to the approach to a possible terrorist attack.
- Define the term *weapon of mass destruction*, and list examples.
- Discuss specific issues related to emergency response to various types of WMD events.
- Describe explosives and incendiaries and give examples.
- Discuss specific medical conditions associated to exposure to explosives and incineraries.
- Discuss signs of the possible presence of explosives on a scene (eg, pipe lengths, blasting caps, detonator cord, etc).

BACKGROUND

Terrorism is any violent act directed against people or property, which is intended to cause damage and/or death, instill fear, and disrupt normal activity among civilians while drawing attention to or furthering a specific nongovernmental group or cause.

Domestic terrorism in the United States refers to activities undertaken in the territorial jurisdiction of the United States which appear to be intended to intimidate or coerce a population or influence governmental policy by mass destruction, assassination, or kidnapping[1] [18 USC 2331(5)].

International terrorism refers to terrorist activities that would violate American criminal laws or the laws of any state and which occur outside the territorial jurisdiction of the United States or transcend national boundaries in terms of the means by which they are accomplished, the population they are meant to affect, or the locale in which the events occur or where the perpetrators seek asylum.[2]

Uses of chemical, biological, radiation, nuclear, and explosive (CBRNE) resources have been well described as possible terrorist scenarios. Explosives have long been weapons of choice for international attacks due to their relative ease of use, low cost, and high impact. In the Middle East, *improvised explosive devices* (IEDs) and suicide bombings occur with relative frequency. Although there have been fewer explosive attacks in the United States, notable examples from the past two decades include the use of stationary IEDs in the 1993 World Trade Center attack and the Centennial Park bombing during the 1996 Olympic Games in Atlanta, Georgia. *Vehicle-borne improvised explosive devices* (VBIED) were used in 1995 at the Oklahoma City Murrah Building bombing and the September 11, 2001, attacks on the World Trade Center and the Pentagon. There was also an unsuccessful VBIED attempt in Times Square in 2010. Internationally, explosives were second only to firearms as the most common method of attacks against civilians in 2010 and explosives were responsible for the highest number of civilian casualties.[3] Explosives, as a method of inflicting casualties, is now the leading method of murder chosen by terrorists around the world.[4]

All of these examples can be considered WMD attacks. The term *weapons of mass destruction*, however, has become an increasingly political term used to describe conventional and unconventional weaponry used to cause widespread damage or panic. Its connotation suggests terrorism, but it can be applied literally to many circumstances, including traditional warfare. In the immediate aftermath of an event, it may be difficult to determine if the event was intentional or accidental, and that determination may be of secondary importance. Many agencies are now using the more precise term *CBRNE* to describe chemical, biological, radiological, nuclear, or explosive events in an effort to devise a uniform response to such an event, regardless of its underlying nature. Accidental explosions may occur as a result of industrial accidents, compromised gas pipes, motor vehicle accidents, and many other etiologies. In many parts of the world, death or dismemberment from accidental landmine detonations are still common.[5]

Unfortunately, terroristic events in the United States are not a new phenomenon. Explosives have been utilized throughout the 20th century to inflict fear in civilian populations. In 1920, a horse-drawn wagon carrying 45 kg of dynamite and 230 kg of iron sash weights was parked in the financial district of New York City. At noon, on September 16, the explosive-laden wagon, detonated by a timing device, exploded along Wall Street, killing 23 people and injuring 400.

Bath Township, Michigan, was site to multiple bombings in May 1927. The attacks were responsible for the deaths of 45 people. A local farmer, devastated over financial matters, used stockpiled pyrotol and dynamite to blow up his farm, the Bath Consolidated School, and finally himself.

These historical examples involve soft targets. Potential targets for a terrorist event are generally categorized as soft or hard. *Soft targets* are generally undefended and easier to penetrate, like train stations and buses. An attack on these locations may inflict psychological distress and some civilian casualties; however, soft target attacks do not generally result in long-term disruption of daily activity. For example, the multiple London bombings on July 7, 2005, resulted in 52 deaths but the city largely returned to normal function by the next day.

Conversely, *hard targets* include essential, defended, or fortified infrastructure like military installations and airports which are considerably more protected. Increased security serves both as a deterrent and makes the sites more resistant to successful attacks.[6]

Nevertheless, a determined individual is all that is necessary to cause massive destruction and carnage. Would-be bombers are able to construct lethal explosives with minimal finances, resources, or expertise. Instructions to manufacture an explosive device are easily obtained via the Internet. If a bomber can obtain the necessary materials, remain inconspicuous, and transport the device, then he or she stands a good chance of deploying the device. For these reasons, it is imperative that civilian medical personnel begin to consider explosions as credible—or even likely—disasters.[7-10]

Twenty-four-hour news coverage now guarantees immediate media attention, and terrorists are acutely aware of how to manipulate propaganda through the media to advance their agendas. By striking highly populated or highly publicized locations, terrorists know they can inflict more casualties and garner more attention.

TYPES OF EXPLOSIVE DEVICES

Medical responders do not have to possess an exhaustive knowledge of explosives. Law enforcement organizations are more appropriate to pursue detailed forensic work regarding explosives. It is important,

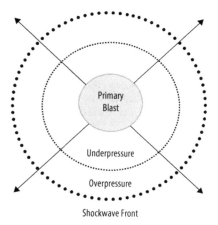

FIGURE 77-1. Primary blast with returning shockwave.

however, to understand the physics of an explosive device and the resulting aftermath. Knowledge of blast wave mechanics will allow a health care provider to search out blast-related injuries.

In general, explosive materials may be categorized into two types: low grade and high grade. A *low-grade explosive* is similar to gunpowder including fireworks and nitrostarch. These substances *deflagrate*, or undergo subsonic combustion, at less than 1000 m/s. This results in a subsonic reaction without a classic blast wave. Conversely, *high-energy explosives* detonate at about 4500 m/s and produce a supersonic shock wave.[11] Examples of high-grade explosives include trinitrotoluene (TNT), C-4, Semtex, nitroglycerin, dynamite, or ammonium nitrate fuel oil (ANFO).

Detonation of explosive material causes chemical bonds within the material to break down, rapidly converting solid or liquid material to gas.[5] The rapid breakdown of bonds creates an exothermic reaction, resulting in a superheated ball of gas. The gas expands outward in a radial pattern, causing a shockwave that propagates through the explosive material. The outwardly expanding wave displaces the surrounding medium, causing an increase in the surrounding atmospheric pressure (the *overpressure*). An uninterrupted blast wave continues moving outward but dissipates quickly in an open area. Immediately behind the area of increased atmospheric pressure is a zone of negative pressure. This underpressurized area subsequently creates a vacuum (see **Figure 77-1**). The resulting pressure phenomenon is best summarized by the Freidlander waveform (**Figure 77-2**). From an explosion, victims can sustain blunt trauma, penetrating trauma, thermal burns, and severe musculoskeletal trauma including amputation.[12]

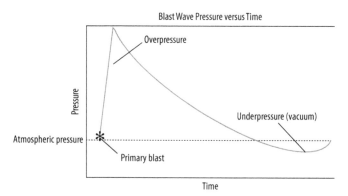

FIGURE 77-2. Waveform representing ideal open air blast as described by the modified Friedlander equation. (Dewey JM. The Shape of the Blast Wave: Studies of the Friedlander Equation. Presented at the 21st International Symposium on Military Aspects of Blast and Shock, Israel 2010)

IMPROVISED EXPLOSIVE DEVICES

Improvised explosive device (IED) is a general term that encompasses a wide range of devices. IEDs may vary in size, shape, and material. In their simplest form, IEDs are essentially any explosive material wired to a trigger device. The common characteristic of all devices is they have been adapted from their original intent.[13] A *vehicle-borne improvised explosive device (VBIED)* is an example of such a device. A VBIED is a vehicle packed with explosive material then detonated in a crowded location or driven to a target site. A home-borne IED is a house or building packed with explosives and detonated when targets approach or enter the structure.

IEDs may also consist of manipulated blast mines, explosive formed projectiles (EFP), and suicide/homicide bombs.[14] Typically, an IED is a nonstate sponsored explosive constructed out of available materials, most often military ordinance. These devices have recently gained worldwide notoriety as a favorite tool among insurgents in Iraq and Afghanistan.

The type of device a bomber constructs depends on the target and available resources. IEDs are popular because of the ease in which they can be built and concealed. The devices can be hidden along a road or thoroughfare.[15] Instead of a single device, IEDs may be strung together in a continuous "daisy chain" formation to increase damage and casualties.[13]

The explosive device may be activated remotely by the bomber or triggered by the victims themselves. An IED is triggered by tripwire, ignition fuse, mercury switch, or depressing a pressure plate. A bomb may also be detonated using a timer, radiofrequency, or cell phone, allowing the bomber to be in a location far from the explosion.

Terrorists may utilize shape charges, which add directionality to the blast. Other options include suicide/homicide bomb vest or other garment worn by the bomber, VBIEDs, and a variety of other devices to increase lethality.[16-18] Each weapon has qualities that a terrorist can take advantage of to accomplish his or her goal and escape detection.

INCENDIARY DEVICES

In addition to explosives, incendiary devices may be deployed to cause damage, inflict casualties, or incite panic. An *incendiary device* is designed to ignite and cause fire rather than explode. Explosions rarely cause fires because oxygen is depleted during the blast.[19] Explosives may cause burns because of thermal energy released during the rapid expansion phase of a blast. However, incendiary devices are specifically meant to ignite a fire and usually burn at high temperatures.

A classic example of an incendiary device is a Molotov cocktail (**Figure 77-3**), which consists of a bottle partially filled with a flammable substance. A rag, doused with a flammable liquid, is shoved into the bottle opening and the rag is lit. When the bottle is thrown, it shatters against a hard surface. The flame ignites the rest of the fluid and the ensuing flames are scattered over a larger area. The resulting fire can trigger an explosion if the open flame contacts other volatile substances.

CHEMICAL, BIOLOGIC, RADIATION, NUCLEAR DEVICES

Today, one of the largest security concerns for the nation is the combination of chemical, biologic, or radioactive substances with explosives. The addition of these agents would compound the fear resulting from an explosion alone. Intelligence agencies have found plans by terrorists to attempt just such an attack.[20] In most cases, an explosion utilizing chemical, biological, or radioactive agents would not result in many casualties; yet an attack involving CRBN would have exorbitant cleanup costs, incite panic, and cause logistical complications especially if it occurs in a highly populated area like New York City.[21]

A chemical substance, such as chlorine, could potentially be combined with an explosive. Chlorine, as with many chemicals, is transported by trains and trucks across the country. An explosive incident involving a chemical like chlorine could release a gas cloud into an unsuspecting populated area. In this case, because of a moving gas cloud, casualties would be located at the immediate scene, as well as downwind from the incident.

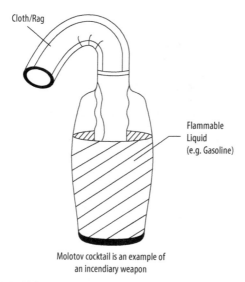

Cloth/Rag

Flammable
Liquid
(e.g. Gasoline)

Molotov cocktail is an example of
an incendiary weapon

FIGURE 77-3. Molotov cocktail.

This was the case in the Graniteville, SC, chlorine gas spill when a train collision released a gas cloud on January 6, 2005, killing nine people and leading to over 250 people seeking treatment for chlorine exposure.[22]

If a victim is within range of the blast, they will be exposed to typical blast-related injuries as discussed later in the chapter. If a victim is located outside the blast radius, he or she may be exposed to a substances dispersed by the blast. While the effects from exposure will vary by chemical or contaminant, the most likely result will be respiratory and mucosal irritation. Decontamination and removal from the source of exposure should be done as early as possible. Bronchodilators may be beneficial for respiratory distress from pulmonary irritation.

When an explosive device is combined with any radioactive substance, it becomes a *radiologic dispersal device* (RDD), also referred to as a "dirty bomb."[23] An RDD is postulated to be small enough to be portable so as to allow terrorists to remain inconspicuous. The detonation of such a device would not result in a traditional nuclear explosion but would cause panic and uncertainty as well as incur great financial cost to society because of the spread of radioactive contamination.

The effects of a blast following an RDD detonation would be confined to the immediate area and would account for most of the initial casualties. The radioactive substance, however, could be dispersed over a much larger area.[24-27] Because of their prevalence, the most likely radioactive substances to be incorporated into an RDD are Cs-137, Sr-90, Co-60, Am-241, and Pu-239.[23] Contamination occurring from the spread of radiation would hinder immediate rescue efforts and evacuation of survivors.

Victims may be grossly decontaminated through removal and disposal of their clothes and copious irrigation. Responders may minimize radiation exposure by following the International Commission on Radiological Protection recommendations including limiting time of exposure, increasing distance from primary contamination, and wearing proper protective and shielding equipment.[23,28] Victims without injuries but requiring decontamination should not be transported directly to hospitals; instead they should first be directed to a designated screening and decontamination area for proper assessment and decontamination as indicated.[29,30]

CONDITIONS THAT IMPACT CASUALTIES

Many conditions influence injury severity, morbidity, and mortality. These factors include the location in which the explosion occurs, the amount and type of explosive material utilized, the physical environment,

blast fragments, proximity of the victim to the blast, and how he or she is dressed.[31] Responders have no impact on any of these variables, but understanding the mitigating circumstances may help them assess the victims and the scene.

Explosive results can vary according to the properties of the materials incorporated to make the bomb. The duration of an explosion also depends on the amount of material that is utilized. As the amount of explosive material is increased, the size and strength of the resulting blast wave also increase.

Victims who are located nearest the primary blast fare worse than those who are further away. Because of the close proximity, death is often instantaneous or injuries so severe that survivability is greatly diminished. Responders must look for occult injuries in those who survive and were located near the explosion.

The pattern of injury and number of casualties depend on the environment in which the blast occurs. Arnold et al documented an immediate mortality rate of 25%, 0.8%, and 0.04% for structural collapse, enclosed blasts, and open area blasts, respectively. Structural collapse results in an increase in injury severity among casualties, as well as increased fatalities.[6,32]

There are three main types of mass casualty environments. These include enclosed area, open area explosion, and structural collapse.[31] Bus or train explosions may be considered as ultraconfined and result in higher mortality than other equivalent enclosed explosions. Bus explosions are considered, by some, as a separate environment since victims are packed closely together and tend to be more proximal to the epicenter of the blast.[33]

When explosions occur within an enclosure like a building or train, the damage is more severe and results in higher mortality.[34] Instead of dissipating in an exponential fashion, blast waves rebound and reverberate off surrounding walls and structures. The initial force of the wave becomes magnified when multiple reflected waves combine, resulting in an additive effect (**Figure 77-4**). Unlike open area blasts, increased distance from the primary explosion does not necessarily reduce injury severity. Cumulative wave forces may be two to nine times greater after reflecting off surrounding structures.[33] Survivors are more likely to sustain occult internal injuries, like blast lung.[34,35]

In an open-air explosion, a blast wave will dissipate more rapidly because there is nothing impeding the wave front. Barring structural interference, the force of the blast wave decreases by the cube of the distance from the site of primary explosion. In other words, victims located three times the distance from the primary site will experience a force 27 times less than those at the site of the blast.[36]

The medium in which the explosion occurs, impacts how efficiently a pressure wave is transmitted. An underwater explosion will cause a blast wave that propagates faster and maintains force for a longer duration than in air.[4] The propagation of a blast wave front is dependent on the amount of force that is transmitted from molecule to molecule within the medium. Due to water's increased density, the strength of a blast

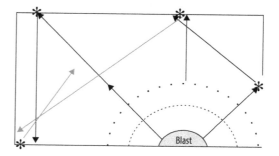

Blast

FIGURE 77-4. Combined wave forces in an enclosed space. Black arrows represent primary force of blast while red arrows represent subsequent increased force from combined blast waves.

wave is estimated to be three times greater in water than in open air.[36] Therefore, injuries and damage in water can be more severe at comparative distances.

When an explosion occurs, fragmented material from the bomb is hurled outward from the primary blast site. Shrapnel fragments consist of whatever material was used to construct the bomb and its casing. Bomb-makers also add additional materials to act as penetrating missiles. They may include bits of metal, screws, nails, bolts, and ball-bearings.[37] In the case of suicide bombers who wear their bombs, their bones, clothing, and accessories can also become projectiles. The force of a blast can transfer anything around the bomb into high-speed projectiles. The fragments are projected in all directions, causing additional penetrating injuries to victims. As a result, victims sustain both blunt injuries from the blast wave, and penetrating wounds from fragmentation and projectiles.[19]

APPROACHING THE INCIDENT

As with any disaster, the ability to respond to a CBRNE event begins in the planning and assessment phase with a hazards vulnerability assessment (HVA). This critical assessment includes identification of assets or potential targets, potential undesirable events, consequences and losses associated with each potential event, and risk stratification. The assessment should guide efforts at prevention, mitigation, and response. While the responsibility for implementing preventative measures usually lies primarily with law enforcement and security agencies, all first responders should be vigilant and able to function in prevention and mitigation capacities.

Should an event occur, responders in the operational setting need to be able to apply the general principles of scene safety, recognize the nature of the event, implement mass casualty management strategies, and call upon additional resources. Once an event has occurred, responders should approach the area as any hazardous materials event, keeping in mind that hazardous materials exposure and contamination could arise from an explosive dispersal device, be part of a secondary device, be released from the scene itself, or be transmitted via blood and bodily fluids originating from perpetrators or victims. The standard approach to HAZMAT scenes involves staging upwind, uphill, and upstream; accessing the scene from upwind to avoid vapor hazards; establishing hot, warm, and cold zones; ensuring safe ingress and egress routes; and decontaminating victims, responders, and equipment. Personal protective equipment should be chosen based on the responders' areas of operations, potential exposures, and detected or presumed threats. In the cold zone, level D protection in the form of uniforms, gloves, and simple respiratory masks may be sufficient. In other areas of operations, responders may require protection from multiple threats and may need to don more specialized, risk-specific PPE, such as level A or B HAZMAT suits, turnout gear, self-contained breathing apparatuses (SCBA), structural collapse gear, or tactical body armor, depending on the threat assessment. Only personnel trained to operate within the hot zone while wearing appropriate PPE should attempt to do so. In addition to being treated as HAZMAT scenes, all blast scenes should also be recognized as having the potential for continuing explosions, whether from unintentionally unexploded ordinance or from secondary devices intentionally placed to target first responders.

Oftentimes the first responders to a bombing will not have the specialized skills to detect all threats or recognize the full scope of the event, yet their initial survey can help guide the procurement of additional personnel and equipment. First responders' initial surveys can estimate the number of victims and detect additional threats such as building collapse, utility fires and explosions, and booby traps. Any indication of such threats should be passed along the chain of command to facilitate the timely deployment of medical personnel, heavy rescue equipment, search and rescue teams, structural engineers, HAZMAT and/or radiological teams, utility company personal, bomb squads or explosive ordnance disposal (EOD) teams, etc. After the initial assessment, medical first responders will transition into mass casualty incident (MCI) management and operations. The standardized MCI approach involves assigning a triage officer,

implementing triage operations, establishing treatment and transportation areas, organizing victim evacuation, and coordinating with local hospitals. Regardless of the triage method chosen, the goal of triage is the same: maximize the likelihood of survival in the greatest possible number of victims. At a blast scene, first responders can expect to see victims with severe burns, traumatic amputations, penetrating injuries from shrapnel, blast injuries, and smoke inhalation. Posttriage management should proceed in accordance with local operating protocols, and providers should keep in mind that triage is a dynamic process and patients' conditions may deteriorate rapidly. Those patients with more severe injuries should receive priority treatment, transportation, and evacuation. While this portion of MCI response is familiar to most first responders, bombing scenes require additional considerations. Blast scenes are dynamic scenes with the potential to become rapidly dangerous due to secondary blasts, fire, HAZMAT release, or structural collapse. With that in mind, responders may forego triaging in place in preference for a load-and-go approach within critical zones. When operating in hot or critical zones, medical personnel should be accompanied by security personnel who can observe for hazards and/or provide tactical cover. Responders should also be cognizant of the fact that perpetrators of the event may be among the injured. They or their security escorts should perform at least a cursory assessment for weapons or unexploded ordnance, since transporting these individuals to casualty collection points or health care facilities without clearing them of weapons could have devastating consequences.[38]

Accidental explosions may be caused by an electric arc or fire, but in the immediate moments after a disaster, both intentional and accidental scenes can be identical. Communities conduct extensive drills and education directed at the management of chemical, biological, radiological, and nuclear aspects of terrorism. Less investment has been made in training for pure explosion scenarios.

When a mass casualty event occurs, there are often conflicting accounts. The reports can be contradictory and confound the true details. In the moments after an explosion or fire, nonaccidental and accidental catastrophes can appear identical. When the London bombings occurred in 2005, conflicting reports included blown power transformers, underground fires, and numerous subway bombings after victims emerged from multiple train exits.[39]

Locations like buses and stadiums are more likely to be terrorism targets, whereas industrial sites may seem accidental. This logic may be deceiving if an industrial site has military connections or may be considered vital infrastructure. In these cases, terrorists may target sites for symbolic value rather than the number casualties. Furthermore, any location is subject to potential terrorism if someone has a personal vendetta, like a disgruntled employee.

Standard algorithms, like Advanced Trauma Life Support (ATLS), ensure that the same format is followed each time and details are not forgotten. This minimizes confusion in disturbing situations when emotions may impair a logical thought process.

First responders must be aware of possible malicious intent and maintain a high index of suspicion for further attacks due to the unknown etiology of a disaster. Regardless of whether the disaster was nonaccidental, or purposeful, the victims and providers are in continuous danger. Threats persist until all personnel are evacuated from the scene.

Further death or injury may occur due to secondary attacks, structural damage, building collapse, leaking gas lines, or chemical exposure. In the past, responders have been killed by falling debris.[40,41] When a building is destroyed, substances that cause topical or inhalation injury may be released, as was the case during the 2001 World Trade Center attacks. Long after the wreckage has been removed from Ground Zero, questions persist regarding inhalation injuries and exposures among responders.

In the past, terrorists have increased casualties by targeting responders and bystanders. Additional victims have been injured or killed by the detonation of secondary explosive devices at the scene or being fired upon by snipers. Spending extra time to safeguard the site by verifying remaining structures are stable, securing the proper equipment (PPE) and eliminating further threats can minimize further loss of life.[32]

TABLE 77-1 Summary of Indicated Mass-Casualty Prehospital Medical Care[40,46]

1. Victims who lack spontaneous respirations and palpable pulses, and those who have dilated pupils should be considered dead.
2. Perform airway management with C-spine control for unconscious victims and those with poor ventilation.
3. Perform needle thoracostomy and oxygen supplementation in the field or during transport.
4. Apply direct pressure and then tourniquets for extremity bleeding.
5. Intravenous fluid may be administered for patients who are hemodynamically unstable from blood loss if he or she can soon be stabilized in an operating facility.
6. Fracture reduction and splinting are indicated for patient stabilization during transport and to minimize blood loss.
7. Cover open wounds as soon as possible to minimize contamination.
8. On-scene CPR is not indicated.

First responders also play a preventative role by assisting in the detection of secondary explosive devices after intentional blasts. Responders should keep the blast area clear of unnecessary personnel until those with proper equipment clear the scene. The presence of a secondary explosive device can be easily overlooked among the carnage so rescuers should stay alert and aware of the environment.

Detection of further explosive devices is the responsibility of specially trained teams. They utilize equipment including robotic instruments with cameras, bomb-sniffing dogs, and sensors to detect specific chemicals.[42] Mammalian olfactory senses have been proven to be efficient detectors of explosive material and have been manipulated for such purposes.[43] It is well documented that the first wave of responders are secondary targets as well.[32] For this reason, the explosion site must be secured and any unexploded ordinances and bombs disarmed prior to evacuation and medical management of the victims.

Victims should be removed from the primary scene as quickly as possible. Any intervention necessary to stabilize the patient like a thoracostomy or intubation should be done to ensure safe transport. However, the majority of medical care should be carried out at a medical center. Rapid evacuation of responders and patients minimizes the risk of further injury to either group. Victims must be removed from the primary scene as quickly as possible without posing unnecessary risk to rescuers. Structural damage to surrounding infrastructure makes the environment dangerous for prolonged medical management on scene.[39]

Experience from the frequent bombings in Israel has provided a plethora of data regarding the most efficient management of victims at a scene. Einav et al recommend an algorithm of immediate on-scene triage with minimal medical intervention followed by immediate evacuation of critically injured victims to the nearest hospital and finally evacuation of the remaining survivors to surrounding hospitals.[40,44,45]

When triaging, or sorting, victims, there are four triage levels. The first requires immediate treatment and evacuation, the second group needs intervention but is presently stable, the third is described as "walking wounded" with minimal injuries and therefore requiring no immediate intervention, and the final group is likely to expire without the investment of considerable medical resources.[32] A summary of guidelines for mass-casualty medical field care as suggested by Stein et al is found in **Table 77-1**.[40,46]

As in the case of the 2005 London bombing, multiple locations may be attacked at once. The health care system is unable to prevent further mass casualty events. For this reason, as soon as a nonaccidental explosion is suspected, a central dispatch needs to be notified to prepare resources[39] A central Emergency medical services (EMS) dispatch is vital for proper resource utilization. Central coordination ensures patients are distributed appropriately among multiple healthcare facilities.[40]

INJURY PATTERNS

Victims of bombing incidents demonstrate unique injury patterns. Often, they will sustain serious injuries that involve at least three regions of his or her body.[19] Severe injuries to the head will likely result in a nonsurvivable condition. If the victim does survive, he or she may develop central nervous system disruption that presents later as a traumatic brain injury (TBI).

After an explosion, fatalities and injuries occur because of immense thermal energy, rapid expansion of gas, and a powerful shockwave that radiates outward.[5] Victims who are struck by a blast wave after an explosion will sustain variable injuries. The extent and severity of injuries depends on the factors previously discussed, for example, the victim's proximity to the blast, the type of blast, and location of the explosion.

In general, blast waves affect organ systems that consist of air-filled structures especially where there exists an air-tissue interface.[5] Such structures include the auditory, pulmonary, and gastrointestinal systems. Following an explosion, injuries may be classified as primary, secondary, tertiary, quaternary, and quinary.[47] A summary description of this classification system according to the Department of Defense (DOD) is summarized in **Table 77-2**.[48]

Critically injured blast victims have a different pattern of mortality than nonblast-related trauma victims. Historically, nonblast-related trauma victims experience a trimodal mortality pattern, whereas blast victims demonstrate a bimodal mortality pattern.[31]

Additionally, victims who were involved in structural collapse and crush-related incidents had increased rates of mortality both initially, and after 24 hours.[49]

Victims, who are involved in a structural collapse, experience higher rates of inhalational complications, crush injuries, and fractures. Victims from confined blasts sustain more pulmonary injuries, solid organ injury (SOI), burns, and TM rupture. Finally, open-air blast victims tend to receive more penetrating soft tissue wounds.[31] Wounds from penetrating injuries and foreign bodies can be hidden underneath clothing. Detection of every injury is difficulty without diagnostic equipment, so a high degree of suspicion for occult injuries is warranted even when victims appear well.[37]

TABLE 77-2 Blast Injuries

Blast Injury	Mechanism	Injury Pattern
I (Primary)	Direct tissue damage resulting from impact with blast wave front	Blunt trauma, blast lung, contusion, traumatic amputation of limbs, TM rupture, hollow organ rupture
II (Secondary)	Injuries resulting from impact with fragments and projectiles	Penetrating injuries, lacerations
III (Tertiary)	Injuries resulting from the displacement of victim's body	Acceleration/deceleration injuries, blunt injury, crush injuries
IV (Quaternary)	Additional injuries resulting from contact with explosive material and blast	Thermal burns, inhalation injury, toxic/chemical exposures
V (Quinary)	Injuries or symptoms as a result of contact with contaminants within explosive device	Bacterial exposure, biohazard exposure, radiation exposure

Adapted from Directive Department of Defense. Medical Research for Prevention, Mitigation, and Treatment of Blast Injuries. Number 6025.21E. 2006 [updated April 12, 2011; cited 2011 December 8]. http://dod-executiveagent.osd.mil/agentListView.aspx?ID=80.

Ocular injuries may consist of conjunctival abrasions, foreign bodies from penetrating fragments, or lens dislocation.[50] Victims can sustain burn injuries from chemical exposure or thermal heat from a blast. Blast burns occur more often on areas of exposed skin. Therefore, patterns of burn injury will be dependent on the type of clothing the victim is wearing. The most common sites that victims sustain burns are the hands and face.[51]

Blunt force trauma to the chest can affect the pulmonary and cardiac systems. Cardiac contusions following blunt force trauma to the chest can lead to dysrhythmias.[50] In the immediate seconds following the blast, victims may experience a period of apnea, which usually resolves without intervention (2). Blast lung is a potentially fatal injury in which hemorrhage and edema occurs at the air-tissue interface between the capillary bed and alveoli.[52] Additionally, victims may sustain pulmonary contusions, pneumothorax, pulmonary hemorrhage, or air embolism.[50]

Victims can suffer a wide variety of musculoskeletal injuries. Crush injuries with tissue destruction may occur from structural collapse of a building with subsequent entrapment. Compartment syndrome of the extremities is a concern following prolonged pressure on a body part. Fracture sites usually occur along the distal and proximal thirds of the upper and lower extremities.[5] Traumatic amputation most commonly occurs at the fracture sites of long bones.

The amount of pressure required to cause tympanic membrane (TM) damage is 2-5 PSI.[47] The absence of TM damage was once believed to be an indicator for the absence of severe occult injuries. However, Harrison et al demonstrated that the presence or absence of TM damage was not a sensitive indicator for injury severity.[53] Tinnitus and hearing loss may be temporary, but some survivors have reported permanent deafness.[5]

The gastrointestinal system appears to be injured more often in underwater blasts.[4] This may be from the abdominal exposure when victims are floating prone on the surface of the water. Victims can also sustain bowel contusions and less often, perforations.[5] He or she may also suffer solid organ injuries from primary or tertiary blast effects.[19]

A fetus may be protected from blast wave effects in utero. Most bodily damage occurs at an air-tissue interface.[5,47] Because the fetus is bathed in amniotic fluid, the risk of injury is reduced. However, the fetus may suffer injuries from a structural collapse, blunt trauma, and any systemic injuries that the mother may sustain.

In the process of triaging victims, one may commit errors such as over- or undertriaging. Great care should be taken to avoid these mistakes since incorrect designation may lead to misallocation of essential resources and contribute to increased mortality and morbidity.

While assessing injuries in order to triage victims after a mass casualty incident, it is important to recognize errors that might occur. Overtriage is the act of assigning noncritical patients to critical status.[35] Incorrect classification may result in the unnecessary expenditure of limited time and resources. Resources can be diverted from other, truly critical victims and detract from his or her care or even evacuation from a scene. This is acceptable during normal trauma but may contribute to increased mortality during a critical mass casualty incident.[54]

Blast victims may also be undertriaged. In contrast to overtriaging, blast injuries may be overlooked and the victims therefore do not receive the care they require in a timely manner.[34] Blast injuries can be deceiving and a critical injury may not be evident until the victim deteriorates.

The proper triage assignment of blast victims is difficult to balance. Designation of triage status often occurs in intense situations where responders are easily distracted and overwhelmed. Awareness of triaging errors will help minimize the above mistakes.

The Extended Focused Assessment with Sonography in Trauma (EFAST) exam with ultrasound equipment on scene may be helpful to assess for the presence of certain life-threatening injuries.[12] Conditions that may be detected early include pneumothorax, intra-abdominal fluid, or pericardial effusion.[37]

A few interventions should be considered before a victim is transported. Needle thoracostomy should be performed immediately if a pneumothorax is suspected. Endotracheal intubation on scene may be necessary for stabilization of victims with evidence of respiratory distress. Suspected pelvic fractures should undergo external stabilization before transport to minimize continued blood loss.

Long bone fractures should be splinted to avoid neurovascular damage, bleeding, and to minimize pain. Victims impaled by foreign bodies should have the objects removed only in the operating room. The object, itself, may act to tamponade a severe wound. However, it may be necessary to cut or shorten the object in order to safely transport.[49]

Burns should be covered to prevent further contamination, and intravenous fluid resuscitation can begin prior to transportation. With ocular exposures, early irrigation should continue for at least 60 minutes or until the pH of the eye is neutral.[49] These interventions should not delay mobilization of the victim but should begin as early as possible.

Advances in medical technology are significant in times of war. The impetus to decrease mortality and find effective treatments on the battlefield assists in tremendous gains in civilian medicine as well. The frequent bombings in Israel, as well as the wars in Iraq and Afghanistan over the past 10 years are no exception. Managing traumatic wounds sustained from blast injuries in IED explosions has allowed medical personnel to publish a great deal of literature on the subject. As a result of improved medical care and equipment, mortality from these wars is considerably lower than past conflicts.

KEY POINTS

- Every explosion incident should be considered intentional until proven otherwise.
- Explosives are responsible for the highest number of civilian casualties worldwide.
- Explosive materials may be categorized into two types: low grade and high grade.
- High-energy explosives detonate at about 4500 m/s and produce a supersonic shock wave.
- A blast causes an increase in the surrounding atmospheric pressure called the overpressure.
- Blast wave physics is best summarized by the Freidlander wave.
- IEDs have been adapted from their original intent and may include VBIED, HBIED, suicide vests, roadside bombs, or many other variations on the same concept.
- Explosions rarely cause fires because oxygen is depleted during a blast as opposed to an incendiary device, which is intended to cause fires.
- A chemical substance, such as chlorine, could potentially be combined with an explosive.
- An explosive device combined with any radioactive substance is referred to as a radiologic dispersal device (RDD).
- The most likely radioactive substances to be incorporated into an RDD are Cs-137, Sr-90, Co-60, Am-241, and Pu-239.
- The three types of mass casualty environments are enclosed, confined, and structural collapse.
- Blast fragments are mostly responsible for any fatalities and injuries.
- Additional victims have been injured or killed by the detonation of secondary explosive devices at the scene or being fired upon by snipers.
- The National Disaster Medical System (NDMS) was developed to assist in coordinating mass casualty operations.
- Blast injuries may be classified as primary, secondary, tertiary, quaternary, and quinary.
- The presence or absence of TM damage is not a sensitive indicator for injury severity.

REFERENCES

1. *18 U.S.C. § 2331(5)* United States Code, Title 18, Section 2331.

2. *18 U.S.C. § 2331(1)* United States Code, Title 18, Section 2331.

3. National Counterterrorism Center: Annex of Statistical Information. 2010 NCTC Report on Terrorism. The National Counterterrorism Center, Washington DC, April 30, 2011. http://www.dni.gov/files/documents/2010_report_on_terrorism.pdf.

4. Covey DC, Born CT. Blast injuries: mechanics and wounding patterns. *J Surg Orthop Adv*. Spring 2010;19(1):8-12.

5. Garner J, Brett SJ. Mechanisms of injury by explosive devices. *Anesthesiol Clin*. March 2007;25(1):147-160.

6. Barishansky RM, Jaskoll S. Are we ready for suicide bombings? *Emerg Med Serv*. February 2005;34(2):76-78, 84.

7. Thompson J, Rehn M, Lossius H, Lockey D. Risks to emergency medical responders at terrorist incidents: a narrative review of the medical literature. *Crit Care*. September 24, 2014;18(5):521.

8. Cole LA, Wagner K, Scott S, et al. Terror medicine as part of the medical school curriculum. *Front Public Health*. September 12, 2014;2:138.

9. Steering Committee on an All-of-Government Approach to Increase Resilience for International Chemical, Biological, Radiological, Nuclear, and Explosive (CBRNE) Events, Division on Earth and Life Studies, National Research Council. An All-of-Government Approach to Increase Resilience for International Chemical, Biological, Radiological, Nuclear, and Explosive (CBRNE) Events: A Workshop Summary. Washington, DC: National Academies Press (US); August 21, 2014.

10. Holstein B, Getts A, Jimenez J, Macgregor-Skinner G. Are American hospitals prepared to respond to a mass casualty chemical weapons attack? *J Healthc Prot Manage*. 2014;30(2):1-16.

11. Goh SH. Bomb blast mass casualty incidents: initial triage and management of injuries. *Singapore Med J*. January 2009;50(1):101-106.

12. Alfici R, Ashkenazi I, Kessel B. Management of victims in a mass casualty incident caused by a terrorist bombing: treatment algorithms for stable, unstable, and in extremis victims. *Mil Med*. December 2006;171(12):1155-1162.

13. GlobalSecurity.org. Improvised Explosive Devices (IEDs) / Booby Traps. http://www.globalsecurity.org/military/intro/ied.htm.

14. Ramasamy A, Hill AM, Clasper JC. Improvised explosive devices: pathophysiology, injury profiles and current medical management. *J R Army Med Corps*. December 2009;155(4):265-272.

15. Jones N, Thandi G, Fear NT, Wessely S, Greenberg N. The psychological effects of improvised explosive devices (IEDs) on UK military personnel in Afghanistan. *Occup Environ Med*. July 2014;71(7):466-471.

16. Heldenberg E, Givon A, Simon D, Bass A, Almogy G, Peleg K. Terror attacks increase the risk of vascular injuries. *Front Public Health*. May 30, 2014;2:47.

17. Singleton JA, Gibb IE, Bull AM, Mahoney PF, Clasper JC. Primary blast lung injury prevalence and fatal injuries from explosions: insights from postmortem computed tomographic analysis of 121 improvised explosive device fatalities. *J Trauma Acute Care Surg*. August 2013;75(2 suppl 2):S269-S274.

18. Edwards MJ, Lustik M, Eichelberger MR, Elster E, Azarow K, Coppola C. Blast injury in children: an analysis from Afghanistan and Iraq, 2002-2010. *J Trauma Acute Care Surg*. November 2012; 73(5):1278-1283.

19. Mayo A, Kluger Y. Terrorist bombing. *World J Emerg Surg*. 2006;1:33.

20. Bureau of Counterterrorism. Annual report on assistance related to international terrorism: fiscal year 2010. Office of the Coordinator for Counterterrorism. United States Department of State; April 19, 2011; Washington, DC.

21. Van Moore A Jr. Radiological and nuclear terrorism: are you prepared? *J Am Coll Radiol*. January 2004;1(1):54-58.

22. Dunning E, Oswalt JL. Train wreck and chlorine spill in Graniteville, South Carolina: transportation effects and lessons in small-town capacity for no-notice evacuation. *Transportation Research Record: Journal of the Transportation Research Board*. 2009;130-135.

23. Chin FK. Scenario of a dirty bomb in an urban environment and acute management of radiation poisoning and injuries. *Singapore Med J*. October 2007;48(10):950-957.

24. Katz SK, Parrillo SJ, Christensen D, Glassman ES, Gill KB. Public health aspects of nuclear and radiological incidents. *Am J Disaster Med*. Summer 2014;9(3):183-193.

25. Snyder E, Drake J, Cardarelli J, et al. Assessment of self-help methods to reduce potential exposure to radiological contamination after a large-scale radiological release. *Health Phys*. September 2014;107(3):231-241.

26. Urso L, Kaiser JC, Woda C, et al. A fast and simple approach for the estimation of a radiological source from localised measurements after the explosion of a radiological dispersal device. *Radiat Prot Dosimetry*. March 2014;158(4):453-460.

27. Reynolds SL, Crulcich MM, Sullivan G, Stewart MT. Developing a practical algorithm for a pediatric emergency department's response to radiological dispersal device events. *Pediatr Emerg Care*. July 2013;29(7):814-821.

28. Valentin J. Protecting people against radiation exposure in the event of a radiological attack. A report of the International Commission on Radiological Protection. *Ann ICRP*. 2005; 35(1):1-110, iii-iv.

29. Coleman CN, Lurie N. Emergency medical preparedness for radiological/nuclear incidents in the United States. *J Radiol Prot*. March 2012;32(1):N27-N32.

30. Hagby M, Goldberg A, Becker S, Schwartz D, Bar-Dayan Y. Health implications of radiological terrorism: Perspectives from Israel. *J Emerg Trauma Shock*. May 2009;2(2):117-123.

31. Arnold JL, Halpern P, Tsai MC, Smithline H. Mass casualty terrorist bombings: a comparison of outcomes by bombing type. *Ann Emerg Med*. February 2004;43(2):263-273.

32. Frykberg ER. Medical management of disasters and mass casualties from terrorist bombings: how can we cope? *J Trauma*. August 2002;53(2):201-212.

33. Kosashvili Y, Loebenberg MI, Lin G, et al. Medical consequences of suicide bombing mass casualty incidents: the impact of explosion setting on injury patterns. *Injury*. July 2009;40(7):698-702.

34. Leibovici D, Gofrit ON, Stein M, et al. Blast injuries: bus versus open-air bombings--a comparative study of injuries in survivors of open-air versus confined-space explosions. *J Trauma*. December 1996;41(6):1030-1035.

35. Born CT, Calfee R, Mead J. Blast injuries in civilian practice. *Med Health R I*. January 2007;90(1):21-24.

36. Ciraulo DL, Frykberg ER. The surgeon and acts of civilian terrorism: blast injuries. *J Am Coll Surg*. December 2006;203(6):942-950.

37. Aharonson-Daniel L, Klein Y, Peleg K. Suicide bombers form a new injury profile. *Ann Surg*. December 2006;244(6):1018-1023.

38. Texas A&M Engineering Extension Service. Participant Manual: Medical Preparedness and Response for Bombing Incidents. United States Department of Homeland Security. Federal Emergency Management Agency. Texas A&M Engineering Extension Service. College Station, TX, 2009.

39. Lockey D, Mackenzie R, Redhead J, et al. London bombings July 2005: The immediate pre-hospital medical response. *Resuscitation*. 2005;66(2):ix-xii.

40. Lucci EB. Civilian preparedness and counter-terrorism: conventional weapons. *Surg Clin North Am*. June 2006;86(3):579-600.

41. Hogan DE, Waeckerle JF, Dire DJ, Lillibridge SR. Emergency department impact of the Oklahoma City terrorist bombing. *Ann Emerg Med*. August 1999;34(2):160-167.

42. Singh S. Sensors—an effective approach for the detection of explosives. *J Hazard Mater*. June 1, 2007;144(1-2):15-28.

43. Corcelli A, Lobasso S, Lopalco P, et al. Detection of explosives by olfactory sensory neurons. *J Hazard Mater*. March 15, 2010; 175(1-3):1096-1100.

44. Cook CH, Muscarella P, Praba AC, Melvin WS, Martin LC. Reducing overtriage without compromising outcomes in trauma patients. *Arch Surg.* July 2001;136(7):752-756.

45. Einav S, Feigenberg Z, Weissman C, et al. Evacuation priorities in mass casualty terror-related events: implications for contingency planning. *Ann Surg.* March 2004;239(3):304-310.

46. Stein M, Hirshberg A. Medical consequences of terrorism. The conventional weapon threat. *Surg Clin North Am.* December 1999; 79(6):1537-1552.

47. Champion HR, Holcomb JB, Young LA. Injuries from explosions: physics, biophysics, pathology, and required research focus. *J Trauma.* May 2009;66(5):1468-1477; discussion 77.

48. Directive Department of Defense. Medical Research for Prevention, Mitigation, and Treatment of Blast Injuries. Number 6025.21E. 2006 [updated April 12, 2011; cited 2011 December 8]. http://dod-executiveagent.osd.mil/agentListView.aspx?ID=80.

49. DePalma RG, Burris DG, Champion HR, Hodgson MJ. Blast injuries. *N Engl J Med.* March 31, 2005;352(13):1335-1342.

50. Kluger Y, Kashuk J, Mayo A. Terror bombing-mechanisms, consequences and implications. *Scand J Surg.* 2004;93(1):11-14.

51. Wolf SJ, Bebarta VS, Bonnett CJ, Pons PT, Cantrill SV. Blast injuries. *Lancet.* August 1, 2009;374(9687):405-415.

52. Ritenour AE, Baskin TW. Primary blast injury: update on diagnosis and treatment. *Crit Care Med.* July 2008;36(7 suppl): S311-S317.

53. Harrison CD, Bebarta VS, Grant GA. Tympanic membrane perforation after combat blast exposure in Iraq: a poor biomarker of primary blast injury. *J Trauma.* July 2009;67(1):210-211.

54. Kluger Y. Bomb explosions in acts of terrorism—detonation, wound ballistics, triage and medical concerns. *Isr Med Assoc J.* April 2003;5(4):235-240.

Index

9 780071 775649